Diagnosis in
Chinese Medicine
A Comprehensive Guide

To the memory of my parents

For 16 years Giovanni Maciocia has been the one author in the field of oriental medicine whose books have become the essential study and practice texts for an entire generation in the West. With this long-awaited comprehensive book on diagnosis and differentiation of symptoms, he adds to this impressive body of work and no student nor practitioner will want to be without it.

Peter Deadman
Editor
Journal of Chinese Medicine
Author of 'A Manual of Acupuncture'

Maciocia has yet again made another very significant contribution to our field. His 'Diagnosis in Chinese Medicine' is incredibly comprehensive, clearly written with supporting examples from his vast clinical experience, and an important and very useful text for both students and seasoned practitioners.

Peter Valaskatgis
Chair of the Chinese Acupuncture Studies Dept.
New England School of Acupuncture

Maciocia draws on his many years of meticulous clinical observation and long and thorough study of the classics to provide a series of profound insights into human pathology and differential diagnosis that are invaluable to the modern practitioner of Chinese medicine.

Jeremy Ross Dr.Ac, BSc, MNIMH

Articulated and precise, the text by Giovanni Maciocia maps out for the inexperienced reader a safe path through clinical symptoms and signs; for those who are experts in the art, it is a most useful manual for consultation. This book is indispensable both for students and for practitioners of all levels.

Massimo Muccioli
Professor of Acupuncture and Diet Therapy, Director of Faculty of Chinese Herbal Medicine, Scuola Matteo Ricci, Bologna, Italy

Giovanni Maciocia has consistently provided the West with precise knowledge and profound clarity concerning Eastern medicine. This new work continues his unique scholar–practitioner tradition of teaching and writing that simultaneously supplies immediately practical information with direct clinical application with theoretical insight and wisdom that makes one consider and ponder and see the Eastern tradition from new perspectives. This is an invaluable addition to what can only be described as the ongoing 'Maciocia transmission'.

Ted Kaptchuk, OMD
Assistant Professor of Medicine
Harvard Medical School

Maciocia's new book on diagnosis brilliantly fills a gap in the existing literature. It appears encyclopedic yet is surprisingly useful in daily practice. While it is solidly based on Chinese medicine, this book guides the reader in applying the principles of traditional diagnosis to present-day Western patients. Physician acupuncturists will especially appreciate the book's easy access to discover the significance of symptoms and signs they encounter in their practices. It's a remarkably good book.

Joseph M. Helms, M.D.
President, Helms Medical Institute
Founding President, American Academy of Medical Acupuncture

Maciocia's 'Diagnosis in Chinese Medicine' is an indispensable tool for the interpretation of symptoms and signs. It is the first text that helps the practitioner to understand the significance of symptoms and signs making diagnosis and treatment strategies easier and more logical.

Dr Carlo Maria Giovanardi
President Italian Federation of Acupuncture Societies
Director Acupuncture College of Matteo Ricci Foundation, Bologna, Italy

For Churchill Livingstone:

Publishing Manager: Inta Ozols
Associate Editor: Karen Morley
Project Manager: Samantha Ross
Designer: Andy Chapman
Illustration Manager: Bruce Hogarth

Diagnosis in Chinese Medicine

A Comprehensive Guide

Giovanni Maciocia CAc (Nanjing)

Acupuncturist and Medical Herbalist, UK

Visiting Associate Professor at the Nanjing University of Traditional Chinese Medicine, Nanjing

Foreword by
Julian Scott, PhD, BAc, MBAcC
Private Practitioner, Bath, UK

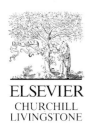

ELSEVIER
CHURCHILL
LIVINGSTONE

Edinburgh   London   New York   Oxford   Philadelphia   St Louis   Sydney   Toronto   2004

Churchill Livingstone
An imprint of Elsevier Limited

First published 2004
  Reprinted 2004, 2005

ISBN 0 443 06448 2

British Library Cataloguing in Publication Data
A catalogue record for this book is available from the British Library

Library of Congress Cataloging in Publication Data
A catalog record for this book is available from the Library of Congress

Notice
Medical knowledge is constantly changing. Standard safety precautions must be followed, but as new research and clinical experience broaden our knowledge, changes in treatment and drug therapy may become necessary as appropriate. Readers are advised to check the most current product information provided by the manufacturer of each drug to be administered to verify the recommended dose, the method and duration of administration, and contraindications. It is the responsibility of the practitioner, relying on experience and knowledge of the patient, to determine dosages and the best treatment for each individual patient. Neither the Publisher nor the author assumes any liability for any injury and/or damage to persons or property arising from this publication.

The Publisher

 your source for books, journals and multimedia in the health sciences
www.elsevierhealth.com

The
publisher's
policy is to use
**paper manufactured
from sustainable forests**

Printed in China

CONTENTS

Foreword *xxxv*
Preface *xxxvii*
Acknowledgements *xli*
Note on the translation of Chinese terms *xliii*
How to use this book *xlv*
Index of symptoms and signs *xlix*
List of abbreviations *liii*

PART 1
DIAGNOSIS BY OBSERVATION *1*
- INTRODUCTION *1*
- RELATIONSHIP BETWEEN THE FIVE SENSES, THE NINE ORIFICES AND THE INTERNAL ORGANS *2*
- RELATIONSHIP BETWEEN DIFFERENT AREAS OF THE FACE AND THE INTERNAL ORGANS *3*
- RELATIONSHIP BETWEEN THE FIVE TISSUES AND THE INTERNAL ORGANS *3*
- RELATIONSHIP BETWEEN THE FIVE SITES OF QI TRANSPORTATION AND THE YIN ORGANS *4*
- MANIFESTATIONS OF THE FIVE YIN ORGANS *4*
- THE 12 CUTANEOUS REGIONS *5*

SECTION 1
OBSERVATION OF THE BODY, MIND AND COMPLEXION *7*
INTRODUCTION *7*
- CORRESPONDENCE BETWEEN AN INDIVIDUAL PART AND THE WHOLE *7*
- OBSERVATION OF CONSTITUTIONAL TRAITS *9*

CHAPTER 1
OBSERVATION OF THE BODY SHAPE, PHYSIQUE AND DEMEANOUR *11*

INTRODUCTION *11*

CLASSIFICATION OF BODY SHAPE ACCORDING TO YIN AND YANG *12*
Body shape abundant in Yang *12*
Body shape abundant in Yin *13*
Body shape deficient in Yang *14*
Body shape deficient in Yin *14*
Body shape with Yin and Yang in balance *15*

CLASSIFICATION OF BODY SHAPE ACCORDING TO THE FIVE ELEMENTS *15*
Wood type *15*
Fire type *16*
Earth type *17*
Metal type *19*
Water type *19*
Clinical application of the Five Element types *21*

CLASSIFICATION OF BODY SHAPE ACCORDING TO PRENATAL AND POSTNATAL INFLUENCES *21*
Body shape with strong prenatal constitution *21*
Body shape with weak prenatal constitution *23*
Body shape with strong postnatal Qi *23*
Body shape with weak postnatal Qi *24*

CLASSIFICATION ACCORDING TO BODY BUILD *25*
Robust type *25*
Compact type *25*
Muscular type *26*
Thin type *26*
Overweight type *27*

CLASSIFICATION OF BODY SHAPE ACCORDING TO PAIN AND DRUG TOLERANCE *27*
Body shape indicating high pain and drug tolerance *27*
Body shape indicating low pain and drug tolerance *28*

CHAPTER 2
OBSERVATION OF THE MIND, SPIRIT AND EMOTIONS *31*

INTRODUCTION *31*

THE THREE ASPECTS OF THE SPIRIT *32*
The embodiment of the Spirit *32*
The vitality of the Spirit *32*
The lustre of the Spirit *33*

THE THREE CONDITIONS OF THE SPIRIT *33*
Strong Spirit *33*
Weak Spirit *34*
False Spirit *34*

THE SPIRIT AND CONSTITUTION *34*
Strong Spirit and strong constitution *35*
Weak Spirit and weak constitution *35*

Weak Spirit and strong constitution *35*
Strong spirit and weak constitution *36*

THE SPIRIT AND THE EMOTIONS *36*
Eyes *36*
Complexion *36*
Tongue *36*

CHAPTER 3
OBSERVATION OF THE COMPLEXION COLOUR *39*

INTRODUCTION *39*

DOMINANT AND GUEST COLOURS *40*
Dominant colours *40*
Guest colours *41*
Clinical significance *41*

OBSERVATION OF DIFFERENT ASPECTS OF COMPLEXION COLOUR *42*
Superficial or deep colour *42*
Distinct or obscure colour *42*
Scattered or concentrated colour *43*
Thin or thick colour *43*
Lustrous or lustreless colour *44*
Conforming or opposing colours *44*
Prognosis according to complexion colour *47*
Changes in complexion colour during a disease *49*
Complexion colours and emotions *49*

COMPLEXION COLOURS *50*
Normal complexion colour *50*
White complexion colour *51*
Sallow complexion colour *52*
Yellow complexion colour *52*
Red complexion colour *54*
Bluish/Greenish complexion colour *55*
Dark complexion colour *56*
Purple complexion colour *56*

CHAPTER 4
OBSERVATION OF BODY MOVEMENTS *59*

HEAD *59*
Tremor of the head *59*
Rigidity of the neck *59*

FACE *60*
Deviation of eye and mouth *60*
Facial paralysis (Bell's palsy) *60*
Facial tic *61*

LIMBS AND BODY *61*
Paralysis *61*
Tremor or spasticity of the limbs *62*
Twitching of the muscles *63*
Opisthotonos *63*
Contraction of the limbs *63*
Hemiplegia *64*
Tremor of the hands *64*
Tremor of the feet *64*
Contraction of the fingers *65*

SECTION 2
OBSERVATION OF PARTS OF THE BODY *67*
INTRODUCTION *67*

CHAPTER 5
OBSERVATION OF HEAD, FACE AND HAIR *69*

HEAD *69*
Dry scalp *69*
Redness and pain of the scalp *69*
Tremor of the head *70*
Swelling of the whole head *70*
Boils on the scalp *70*
Ulcers on the scalp *70*
Ulcers in the mastoid region *70*
Erosion of the scalp *70*
Head leaning to one side *70*
Head tilted backwards *70*
Late closure of the fontanelles *70*

FACE *70*
Acne *71*
Papular/macular eruptions *71*
Oedema of the face *71*
Swelling and redness of the face *71*
Swelling, redness and pain of the cheeks *71*
Ulcers below the zygomatic arch *71*
Lines on the face *71*
Deviation of eye and mouth *71*

HAIR *71*
Hair falling out *72*
Alopecia *72*
Dry and brittle hair *72*
Greasy hair *73*
Premature greying of the hair *73*
Dandruff *73*

CHAPTER 6
OBSERVATION OF THE EYES *75*

INTRODUCTION *75*

CHANNELS INFLUENCING THE EYES *76*

RELATIONSHIP BETWEEN THE INTERNAL ORGANS AND THE EYES *76*
The eyes and the Liver *76*
The eyes and the Kidneys *77*
The eyes and the Heart *77*
The eyes and the Stomach and Spleen *77*
The eyes and the Gall-Bladder *77*
The eyes and the Bladder *78*
The eyes and the Small Intestine *78*
The Five Wheels *78*
The Eight Ramparts *79*
The Eye System *79*

ASPECTS OF OBSERVATION OF THE EYES *80*
The lustre of the eyes *80*
The control of the eyes *80*

The normal eye *81*

OBSERVATION OF PATHOLOGICAL SIGNS OF THE EYE *81*
Abnormal colour *81*
Other features *82*

CHAPTER 7
OBSERVATION OF THE NOSE *87*

INTRODUCTION *87*

CHANNELS INFLUENCING THE NOSE *87*

RELATIONSHIPS BETWEEN THE NOSE AND THE INTERNAL
ORGANS *88*

ABNORMAL COLOUR *89*
Pale *89*
Yellow *89*
Red *89*
Bluish-greenish *89*
Reddish-purple *89*
Dark *90*

SWOLLEN NOSE *90*

FLAPPING ALAE NASI (THE OUTSIDE OF THE NOSTRILS) *90*

DRY NOSTRILS *90*

NOSEBLEED *90*

POLYPS *90*

ULCERS ON THE NOSE *90*

PAPULES ON THE NOSE *90*

CHAPTER 8
**OBSERVATION OF LIPS, MOUTH, PALATE, TEETH, GUMS
AND PHILTRUM** *93*

CHANNELS INFLUENCING THE MOUTH AND LIPS *93*

LIPS *94*
Abnormal colour *94*
Dry or cracked lips *96*
Peeled lips *96*
Swollen lips *96*
Trembling lips *96*
Inverted lips *96*
Drooping lips *96*

MOUTH *96*
Cold sores *97*
Cracked corners of the mouth *97*
Mouth ulcers *97*
Mouth open *97*
Deviation of mouth *97*
Dribbling from the corners of the mouth *98*

PALATE *98*
Abnormal colour *98*

TEETH AND GUMS *99*
Teeth *99*
Gums *100*

PHILTRUM *101*
Flat philtrum *102*
Stiff-looking philtrum *102*
Abnormal colour *102*

CHAPTER 9
OBSERVATION OF THE EARS *105*

INTRODUCTION *105*

CHANNELS INFLUENCING THE EARS *105*

EAR SIZE *106*
Large ears *106*
Small ears *106*
Swollen ears *107*
Contracted ears *107*

DRY AND CONTRACTED HELIX *107*

SORES ON THE EAR *107*

WARTS ON THE EAR *107*

ABNORMAL COLOUR *107*
Yellow helix *107*
Pale helix *107*
Bluish-greenish (*qing*) helix *107*
Dark helix *107*
Red helix *107*
Red back of the ear *108*
Swelling and redness of the concha *108*

DISTENDED BLOOD VESSELS ON THE EAR *108*

EXCESSIVE WAX PRODUCTION *108*

DISCHARGE FROM THE EARS *108*

CHAPTER 10
OBSERVATION OF THE THROAT AND NECK *109*

CHANNELS INFLUENCING THE THROAT AND NECK *109*

THROAT *110*
Redness on the throat *110*
Goitre *110*
Pulsation of the carotid artery *110*
Observation of the pharynx *110*
Swollen tonsils *111*
Abnormal tonsils colour *111*

NECK *112*
Neck length *112*
Rigidity of the neck *112*
Soft neck *113*
Deviated neck *113*
Neck width *113*
Swollen neck glands *114*

CHAPTER 11
OBSERVATION OF THE BACK *115*

CHANNELS INFLUENCING THE BACK *115*

ATROPHY OF THE MUSCLES ALONG THE SPINE *116*

RIGIDITY OF THE LOWER BACK *116*

SPINAL CURVE ABNORMALITIES *116*
Spine bent forward *116*
Scoliosis *117*
Lordosis *117*
Kyphosis *117*
Flattening of lumbar spine *118*
List of spine *118*

SKIN SIGNS *118*
Spots on the back *118*
Vesicles on the lower back *119*
Dryness and redness of the skin of the lower back *119*
Yellow colour of the lower back *119*
Skin marks on the lower back *119*
Boils on BL-23 Shenshu *119*
Papules or pustules on the buttocks *119*

CHAPTER 12
OBSERVATION OF WOMEN'S BREASTS *121*

INTRODUCTION *121*

CHANNELS INFLUENCING THE BREASTS *121*

BREAST SIZE *122*
Small breasts *122*
Breast distension *122*
Swollen breasts *122*
Redness and swelling of the breasts *122*

BREAST LUMPS *122*

NIPPLE ABNORMALITIES *124*
Milky nipple discharge *124*
Sticky yellow nipple discharge *124*
Bloody discharge from the nipple *124*
Inverted nipples *125*
Cracked nipples *125*

PEAU D'ORANGE SKIN *125*

CHAPTER 13
OBSERVATION OF THE HEARTBEAT *127*

INTRODUCTION *127*

HEARTBEAT DISPLACED DOWNWARDS *128*

HEARTBEAT DISPLACED UPWARDS *128*

HEARTBEAT DISPLACED TO THE LEFT *128*

HEARTBEAT DISPLACED TO THE RIGHT *128*

HEARTBEAT BELOW THE XYPHOID PROCESS *128*

CHAPTER 14
OBSERVATION OF THE HANDS *129*

INTRODUCTION *129*

ABNORMAL COLOUR *129*
Pale hands *129*
Red dorsum of the hands *129*
Red palms *129*

VENULES ON THE THENAR EMINENCE *130*

ATROPHY OF THE THENAR EMINENCE *130*

ATROPHY OF THE MUSCLES OF THE DORSUM OF THE HANDS *130*

TREMOR OF THE HANDS *130*

TINEA (RINGWORM) *130*

THE FINGERS *130*
Contraction of the fingers *130*
Spoon-shaped fingers *131*
Thin, pointed fingers *131*
Swollen fingers *131*
Cracked fingers *132*
Thickened fingers like cocoons *132*
Shrivelled and wrinkled fingers *132*

DEFORMED KNUCKLES *132*

THE PALMS *132*
Dry, cracked, peeling palms *132*
Sweaty palms *133*
Hand lines *133*

CHAPTER 15
OBSERVATION OF THE NAILS *137*

INTRODUCTION *137*

SURFACE ABNORMALITIES *137*
Ridged nails *137*
Indented nails *137*
Thin and brittle nails *138*
Thickening of the nails *138*
Coarse and thick nails *138*
Withered and brittle nails *138*
Withered and thickened nails *138*
Cracked nails *138*
Flaking nails *138*

TWISTED NAILS *139*

CURLING NAILS *139*

NAILS FALLING OFF *139*

ABNORMAL COLOUR *139*
  Nails with white spots *139*
  Pale-white nails *139*
  Dull-white nails *139*
  Red nails *139*
  Yellow nails *139*
  Bluish-greenish nails *139*
  Dark nails *139*
  Purple nails *139*

LUNULAE *140*

CORRESPONDENCE OF NAILS TO ORGAN SYSTEMS *140*
  Thumb *140*
  Index finger *140*
  Middle finger *141*
  Ring finger *141*
  Little finger *142*

CHAPTER 16
OBSERVATION OF THE CHEST AND ABDOMEN *143*

CHEST *143*
  Protruding chest *144*
  Sunken chest *144*
  Protruding sternum *144*
  Chest sunken on one side *144*
  Chest protruding on one side *145*
  Gynaecomastia *145*

ABDOMEN *145*
  Abdominal size *146*
  Abdominal masses *146*
  Umbilicus signs *147*
  Skin signs *147*

CHAPTER 17
OBSERVATION OF THE GENITALIA *149*

CHANNELS INFLUENCING THE GENITALIA *149*

PUBIC HAIR *150*
  Loss of pubic hair *150*
  Excessive pubic hair *150*

PENIS *150*
  Redness and swelling of the glans penis *150*
  Ulcers on the penis *150*
  Peyronie's disease *150*
  Priapism *150*
  Soft and withered penis *150*
  Long penis in children *150*

SCROTUM *150*
  Contracted scrotum *150*
  Loose scrotum *151*
  Scrotum drooping on one side *151*
  Swollen scrotum *151*
  Swollen and oozing scrotum *151*
  Abnormal colour *151*

VULVA AND VAGINA *151*
  Vulvar sores *151*
  Leukoplakia *151*
  Swelling of the vulva *151*
  Prolapse of the vagina *151*

CHAPTER 18
OBSERVATION OF THE FOUR LIMBS *153*

INTRODUCTION *153*

ATROPHY OF THE FOUR LIMBS *153*

FLACCIDITY OF THE FOUR LIMBS *154*

RIGIDITY OF THE FOUR LIMBS *154*

PARALYSIS OF THE FOUR LIMBS *154*

LIMB MOVEMENTS *155*
  Contraction of the four limbs *155*
  Convulsions of the four limbs *155*
  Tremor or spasticity of the four limbs *156*

OEDEMA OF THE FOUR LIMBS *156*

SWELLING OF THE JOINTS OF THE FOUR LIMBS *157*

CHAPTER 19
OBSERVATION OF THE LEGS *159*

LEGS SIGNS *159*
  Oedema *159*
  Atrophy *160*
  Paralysis *160*
  Arched legs *160*

GAIT *161*
  Festination *161*
  Unstable gait *161*
  Staggering gait *161*
  Stepping gait *161*
  Shuffling gait *161*

CHAPTER 20
OBSERVATION OF EXCRETIONS *163*

INTRODUCTION *163*

SPUTUM *163*

NASAL DISCHARGE *164*

SWEAT *164*

STOOLS *164*
  Colour *164*
  Consistency *165*
  Shape *165*

URINE *165*

MENSTRUAL BLOOD *166*
Colour *166*
Consistency *166*

VAGINAL DISCHARGE *166*
Colour *166*
Consistency *166*
Lochia *166*

CHAPTER 21
OBSERVATION OF THE SKIN *169*

INTRODUCTION *169*
Skin layers *169*
Types of skin lesion *170*

THE SKIN AND THE INTERNAL ORGANS *170*
The skin and the Lungs *170*
The skin and the Stomach and Spleen *172*
The skin and the Kidneys *172*
The skin and the Liver *173*
The skin and the Heart *173*
The skin and the Connecting channels *174*

SKIN SIGNS *174*
Skin colour *174*
Skin texture *175*
Skin of the forearm (inner aspect) *176*
The space between skin and muscles (*Cou Li*) *176*
Body hair *176*
Macules, papules, vesicles and pustules *176*
Dry skin *178*
Greasy skin *179*
Swelling of the skin *179*
Scales *179*
Erosion of the skin *179*
Rashes *180*
Fissures *180*
Skin ulcers *180*
Dermographism *181*

SKIN DISEASES *181*
Eczema *181*
Acne *182*
Psoriasis *183*
Urticaria *185*
Naevi *185*
Malignant melanoma *186*
Tinea *186*
Candida *187*
Herpes simplex *188*
Herpes zoster *188*
Warts *189*
Rosacea *189*

CHAPTER 22
OBSERVATION IN CHILDREN *191*

INTRODUCTION *191*

COMPLEXION *191*
Red *191*

Yellow *191*
Pale *192*
Bluish-greenish *192*

ORIFICES *192*
Eyes *192*
Ears *192*
Nose *192*
Mouth *193*
Urethra and anus *193*

BODY MOVEMENT *194*

SPINAL MUSCLES *194*

INDEX FINGER *194*
Veins on the index finger *194*
Creases on the index finger *195*

ROOT OF THE NOSE *199*

SECTION 3
TONGUE DIAGNOSIS *201*
INTRODUCTION *201*

CHAPTER 23
TONGUE DIAGNOSIS *203*

CONDITIONS FOR EXAMINING THE TONGUE *203*
Lighting *203*
Techniques of observation of the tongue *203*
External factors affecting the colour of the tongue *204*

AREAS OF THE TONGUE *204*

CLINICAL SIGNIFICANCE OF THE TONGUE *206*
Tongue-body colour *206*
Tongue-body shape *206*
Tongue coating *206*
Tongue spirit *207*

CHAPTER 24
TONGUE-BODY COLOUR *209*

TONGUE SPIRIT *209*

TONGUE-BODY COLOURS *210*
Pale *210*
Red *210*
Purple *212*

SUBLINGUAL VEINS *213*

CHAPTER 25
TONGUE-BODY SHAPE *215*

INTRODUCTION *215*

THIN *215*

SWOLLEN *216*

PARTIALLY SWOLLEN *216*

STIFF *216*

FLACCID *217*

LONG *217*

SHORT *217*

CRACKED *217*

DEVIATED *218*

MOVING *218*

QUIVERING *219*

TOOTHMARKED *219*

CHAPTER 26
TONGUE COATING *221*

PHYSIOLOGY OF TONGUE COATING *221*

CLINICAL SIGNIFICANCE OF TONGUE COATING *221*

PRESENCE OR ABSENCE OF COATING *222*

COATING WITH OR WITHOUT ROOT *222*

COATING THICKNESS *223*

COATING DISTRIBUTION *223*

COATING MOISTURE *223*

COATING TEXTURE *224*
  Sticky coating *224*
  Slippery coating *224*
  Mouldy coating *224*

TONGUE COATING IN EXTERNAL DISEASES *224*

CHAPTER 27
TONGUE IMAGES AND PATTERNS *227*

QI-DEFICIENCY TONGUES *227*

YANG-DEFICIENCY TONGUES *227*

BLOOD-DEFICIENCY TONGUES *228*

YIN-DEFICIENCY TONGUES *228*

THE TONGUE IN PHLEGM AND DAMPNESS *230*

THE TONGUE IN HEAT *230*

THE TONGUE IN COLD *230*

THE TONGUE IN QI AND BLOOD STAGNATION *231*

THE TONGUE IN INTERNAL WIND *231*

THE TONGUE IN EXTERNAL INVASIONS OF WIND *231*

PART 2
DIAGNOSIS BY INTERROGATION *233*
INTRODUCTION *233*

CHAPTER 28
INTRODUCTION *235*

NATURE OF DIAGNOSIS BY INTERROGATION *235*

NATURE OF 'SYMPTOMS' IN CHINESE MEDICINE *236*
  Tongue and pulse *237*

THE ART OF INTERROGATION: ASKING THE RIGHT QUESTIONS *237*

TERMINOLOGY PROBLEMS IN INTERROGATION *238*

PATIENTS' EXPRESSIONS *239*

PITFALLS TO AVOID IN INTERROGATION *239*

PROCEDURE FOR INTERROGATION *240*

TIME SCALE OF SYMPTOMS *241*

INTEGRATION OF INTERROGATION WITH OBSERVATION *242*

IDENTIFICATION OF PATTERNS AND INTERROGATION *242*

TONGUE AND PULSE DIAGNOSIS: INTEGRATION WITH INTERROGATION *243*

THE 10 TRADITIONAL QUESTIONS *249*
  Limitations of the 10 traditional questions *249*
  Questions on emotional state *250*
  Questions about sexual life *250*
  Questions on energy levels *250*

THE 16 QUESTIONS *250*

CHAPTER 29
PAIN *253*

INTRODUCTION *253*

AREA OF PAIN *255*

NATURE OF PAIN *255*
  Soreness *255*
  Pain with a sensation of heaviness *255*
  Distending pain *255*
  Pain with a feeling of fullness *256*
  Pain with a feeling of emptiness *256*
  Pain with a feeling of cold *256*
  Burning pain *256*
  Colicky pain *256*
  Spastic pain *256*
  Pain with a distressing feeling *256*
  Pain with a sensation of stuffiness *257*
  Pushing pain *257*
  Pulling pain *257*

Cutting pain *257*
Throbbing pain *257*
Boring pain *257*
Lurking pain *257*

TIME OF PAIN *257*

FACTORS AFFECTING PAIN *258*
Pressure *258*
Temperature *258*
Food and drink *258*
Bowel movement *258*
Movement and rest *258*

ORGAN VERSUS CHANNEL PAIN *259*

CHAPTER 30
FOOD AND TASTE *261*

INTRODUCTION *261*

MAIN PATTERNS OF DIGESTIVE SYMPTOMS *262*
Qi deficiency *262*
Qi stagnation *262*
Qi rebellious *262*
Blood stasis *262*
Dampness *262*
Phlegm *262*
Retention of food *262*

FOOD *264*

APPETITE *264*
Excessive hunger *264*
Aversion to food *264*
Hunger but no desire to eat *265*

TASTE *265*

NAUSEA AND VOMITING *266*

BELCHING *266*

SOUR REGURGITATION *267*

CHAPTER 31
STOOLS AND URINE *269*

INTRODUCTION *269*

STOOLS *270*
Frequency *270*
Consistency of stools *271*
Shape *272*
Colour *272*
Odour and sounds *273*
Abdominal pain related to evacuation *273*

URINE *274*
Frequency *274*
Colour *274*
Amount *275*

Difficulty in micturition *275*
Cloudiness *275*
Incontinence *275*
Urination at night *275*
Pain *275*
Smell *275*

CHAPTER 32
THIRST AND DRINK *277*

INTRODUCTION *277*

THIRST *278*

DRY MOUTH *279*

PREFERENCE FOR HOT OR COLD DRINKS *279*

ABSENCE OF THIRST *279*

CHAPTER 33
ENERGY LEVELS *281*

INTRODUCTION *281*

HISTORICAL BACKGROUND *282*

PATTERNS CAUSING TIREDNESS *282*

CHAPTER 34
HEAD *287*

INTRODUCTION *287*

HEADACHE *288*
Onset *288*
Time *288*
Location *288*
Character of pain *288*
Ameliorating or aggravating factors *289*
Internal and external origin *289*

DIZZINESS *295*

FAINTING *296*

FEELING OF DISTENSION OF THE HEAD *297*

FEELING OF HEAVINESS OF THE HEAD *297*

FEELING OF MUZZINESS (FUZZINESS) OF THE HEAD *297*

BRAIN NOISE *298*

FEELING OF COLD OF THE HEAD *298*

FEELING OF HEAT OF THE HEAD *299*

NUMBNESS/TINGLING OF THE SKIN OF THE HEAD *299*

ITCHY SCALP *299*

CHAPTER 35
FACE *301*

INTRODUCTION *301*

FACE *302*
Feeling of heat of the face *302*
Facial pain *302*
Feeling of numbness/tingling of the face *303*

NOSE *303*
Blocked nose *304*
Itchy nose *304*
Sneezing *304*
Runny nose *305*
Nose ache *305*
Nose pain *305*
Dry nostrils *306*
Loss of sense of smell *306*

TEETH AND GUMS *306*
Toothache *306*
Inflamed gums *307*
Bleeding gums *307*
Receding gums *307*

MOUTH AND LIPS *308*
Mouth ulcers *308*
Cold sores *309*

TONGUE *309*
Itchy tongue *309*
Numbness of the tongue *309*
Tongue pain *309*

CHAPTER 36
THROAT AND NECK *311*

INTRODUCTION *311*

CHANNELS INFLUENCING THE THROAT AND NECK *312*

THROAT *312*
Sore throat *312*
Dry throat *313*
Itchy throat *313*
Hoarse voice *313*
Feeling of obstruction in the throat *314*
Swollen and red tonsils *314*

NECK *315*
Goitre *315*
Painful or stiff neck *316*

CHAPTER 37
BODY *317*

INTRODUCTION *317*

ACHES IN THE WHOLE BODY *317*

PAIN IN THE JOINTS *318*

LOWER BACKACHE *318*

NUMBNESS/TINGLING *319*

ITCHING *319*

LOSS OF WEIGHT *319*

OBESITY *319*

CHAPTER 38
CHEST AND ABDOMEN *321*

CHEST *321*
Cough *322*
Chest pain *323*
Pain in the ribs *324*
Feeling of oppression of the chest *324*
Feeling of heat in the chest *325*
Palpitations *325*

ABDOMEN *326*
Sensations *326*
Areas of abdominal pain *327*

CHAPTER 39
LIMBS *337*

INTRODUCTION *337*

WEAKNESS OF THE LIMBS *338*

DIFFICULTY IN WALKING (ATROPHY/FLACCIDITY OF LIMBS) *338*

FEELING OF DISTENSION OF THE LIMBS *338*

FEELING OF HEAVINESS OF THE LIMBS *339*

MUSCLE ACHE IN THE LIMBS *339*

NUMBNESS/TINGLING OF THE LIMBS *339*

GENERALIZED JOINT PAIN *339*

TREMOR OF LIMBS *340*

UPPER LIMBS *341*
Pain and inability to raise the shoulder *341*
Pain in the elbow *342*
Pain in the hands *342*
Cold hands *342*
Hot hands *343*
Itchy hands *343*
Numbness/tingling of the hands *343*
Oedema of the hands *343*

LOWER LIMBS *343*
Pain in the hip *343*
Pain in the thigh *344*
Pain in the knees *344*
Weak knees *344*
Cramps in the calves *344*

Cold feet *344*
Pain in the feet *344*
Oedema of the feet *345*
Pain in the soles *345*
Burning sensation in the soles *345*

CHAPTER 40

SLEEP *347*

INTRODUCTION *347*

INSOMNIA *348*

EXCESSIVE DREAMING *349*

SOMNOLENCE *349*

CHAPTER 41

SWEATING *351*

INTRODUCTION *351*

CLINICAL SIGNIFICANCE OF SWEATING *352*
Exterior patterns *352*
Interior patterns *352*

PATHOLOGY OF SWEATING *352*

CLASSIFICATION OF SWEATING *353*
Area of body *353*
Time of day *353*
Condition of illness *353*
Quality of sweat *353*

ABSENCE OF SWEATING *353*

CHAPTER 42

EARS AND EYES *355*

EARS *355*
Tinnitus *356*
Deafness *357*
Earache *357*
Itchy ears *357*

EYES *357*
Eye pain *358*
Itchy eyes *359*
Feeling of distension of the eyes *360*
Streaming eyes *360*
Dry eyes *360*
Blurred vision *360*

CHAPTER 43

FEELING OF COLD, FEELING OF HEAT AND FEVER *361*

INTRODUCTION *361*

FEELING OF COLD *362*
Feeling of cold in interior conditions *363*
Feeling of cold in exterior conditions *365*
How to distinguish between external and internal causes
of feeling of cold *366*

SIMULTANEOUS FEELING OF COLD AND FEVER IN
EXTERIOR CONDITIONS *367*
Wind-Cold and Wind-Heat *369*
Summer-Heat *370*
Damp-Heat *370*
Dry-Heat *370*

ALTERNATING FEELING OF COLD AND FEELING OF
HEAT *370*

FEELING OF HEAT FROM INTERNAL CAUSES *371*

INTERIOR FEVER *372*
Acute fever *372*
Chronic fever *374*

FIVE-PALM HEAT *376*

CONTRADICTORY FEELINGS OF COLD AND HEAT IN
INTERNAL CONDITIONS *376*
Simultaneous deficiency of Kidney-Yin and
Kidney-Yang *376*
Blood deficiency with Empty-Heat *376*
Disharmony of the Penetrating Vessel *376*
Yin Fire *376*

CHAPTER 44

MENTAL–EMOTIONAL SYMPTOMS *379*

INTRODUCTION *379*

DEPRESSION *380*
Definition of depression *380*
Diagnosis of depression *381*
Depression in Chinese medicine *381*
Patterns in depression *382*

FEAR/ANXIETY *384*

IRRITABILITY/ANGER *385*

WORRY/OVERTHINKING *386*

SADNESS/GRIEF *387*

EXCESS JOY *388*

MENTAL RESTLESSNESS *388*

CHAPTER 45

SEXUAL SYMPTOMS *391*

INTRODUCTION *391*

MEN *392*
Impotence *392*
Lack of libido *392*
Premature ejaculation *393*
Nocturnal emissions *393*
Tiredness and dizziness after ejaculation *393*

WOMEN *393*
  Lack of libido *393*
  Headache soon after orgasm *394*

CHAPTER 46
WOMEN'S SYMPTOMS *395*

INTRODUCTION *395*

THE GYNAECOLOGICAL HISTORY *396*

BREAST SYMPTOMS *397*
  Breast lumps *397*
  Premenstrual breast distension *398*

MENSTRUATION *398*
  Amount of bleeding *399*
  Colour *400*
  Consistency *400*
  Cycle *400*
  Menarche *401*
  Menopause *401*
  Pain *401*
  Premenstrual symptoms *404*
  Other symptoms occurring around menstruation *405*

PREGNANCY AND CHILDBIRTH *406*
  Fertility *406*
  Miscarriage and abortion *408*
  Childbirth *408*
  Lactation *408*

VAGINAL DISCHARGE *409*

CHAPTER 47
CHILDREN'S SYMPTOMS *411*

INTRODUCTION *411*

MOTHER'S PREGNANCY *411*

CHILDBIRTH *412*

POSTPARTUM PROBLEMS *412*

CHILDHOOD DISEASES *412*

DIGESTIVE SYMPTOMS *412*

IMMUNIZATIONS *412*

RESPIRATORY SYMPTOMS AND EARACHE *412*
  Coughs and wheezing *413*
  Earache *413*
  Chronic catarrh *413*

SLEEP *413*

SLOW DEVELOPMENT *413*

CHAPTER 48
DIAGNOSING THE CAUSES OF DISEASE *415*

INTRODUCTION *415*

INTERACTIONS BETWEEN CAUSES OF DISEASE *416*
  Interaction of trauma with climate *416*
  Interaction of hereditary weak constitution with diet *416*
  Interaction of emotional problems at puberty with overwork *416*
  Interaction of weak Heart constitution and emotional problems *417*

THE FIVE STAGES OF LIFE *417*
  Childhood *417*
  Adolescence *417*
  Young adulthood *417*
  Middle age *418*
  Old age *418*

THE CAUSES OF DISEASE *418*
  Heredity *418*
  Emotions *420*
  Overwork *427*
  Diet *427*
  Climate *428*
  Trauma *428*
  Drugs including immunizations *429*
  Excessive sexual activity *430*

PART 3
DIAGNOSIS BY PALPATION *431*
INTRODUCTION *431*

CHAPTER 49
PULSE DIAGNOSIS *433*

INTRODUCTION *433*

THE 'NINE REGIONS' OF THE PULSE FROM THE 'YELLOW EMPEROR'S CLASSIC OF INTERNAL MEDICINE' *434*

THE PULSE IN THE 'CLASSIC OF DIFFICULTIES' *435*

THE THREE SECTIONS OF THE PULSE *436*

ASSIGNMENT OF PULSE POSITIONS TO ORGANS *438*
  Organ positions on the pulse *438*
  Reconciling different pulse arrangements *443*

THE THREE LEVELS *445*

METHOD OF PULSE TAKING *446*
  Time *446*
  Levelling the arm *446*
  Equalizing the breathing *447*
  Placing the fingers *447*

FACTORS AFFECTING THE PULSE *449*
  Season *449*
  Gender *450*

Age 450
Body build 450
Menstruation 451
Pregnancy 451
Fan Guan Mai and Xie Fei Mai 451

ATTRIBUTES OF THE NORMAL PULSE 451
Spirit 451
Stomach-Qi 451
Root 452

GUIDELINES FOR INTERPRETING THE PULSE 454
Feeling the pulse as a whole with three fingers 454
Feeling the spirit, Stomach-Qi and root 454
Feeling the three positions together first and then
individually 454
Feeling the three levels 455
Feeling the overall quality of the pulse, if there is
one 456
Feeling the pulse quality, strength and level of each
individual position by rolling and pushing the fingers 456
Counting the pulse rate 457

CLINICAL APPLICATION OF PULSE DIAGNOSIS 457
The pulse is often crucial in clinching a diagnosis 457
The pulse is essential to distinguish Deficiency from
Excess 457
The pulse is essential to determine the treatment
principle 458
The pulse in emotional problems 458
The pulse as an indicator of an organ problem 459
The pulse as an indicator of a heart problem 459
The pulse does not necessarily reflect all the aspects of a
disharmony 461
The pulse indicates disharmonies beyond the presenting
patterns 461
The pulse can indicate an underlying Deficiency in the
absence of symptoms 461
The pulse in cancer 462

INTEGRATION OF PULSE AND TONGUE DIAGNOSIS 463
Qi and Blood 463
Time factor 463
When the pulse is Rapid and the tongue is not Red 463
When the pulse is Slow and the tongue is Red 463
Pulse diagnosis adds detail to tongue diagnosis 463

LIMITATIONS OF PULSE DIAGNOSIS 464
It is subjective 464
It is subject to short-term influences 464

CHAPTER 50
PULSE QUALITIES 465

INTRODUCTION 465

FEELING AND IDENTIFYING THE PULSE QUALITY 466

THE EIGHT BASIC PULSE QUALITIES 467
Floating 467
Deep 469
Slow 470

Rapid 472
Empty 474
Full 475
Slippery 476
Choppy 477

EMPTY-TYPE PULSES 479
Weak 479
Fine 480
Minute 480
Soggy (Weak-Floating) 481
Short 481
Hollow 482
Leather 482
Hidden 483
Scattered 484

FULL-TYPE PULSES 485
Wiry 485
Tight 486
Overflowing 487
Big 488
Firm 489
Long 490
Moving 490

PULSES WITH IRREGULARITIES OF RATE OR RHYTHM 491
Knotted 491
Hasty 492
Hurried 492
Intermittent 493
Slowed-Down 494

THREE NON-TRADITIONAL PULSE QUALITIES 494
Irregular 494
Stagnant 495
Sad 495

CLASSIFICATION OF PULSE QUALITIES 496
The eight basic groups of pulse qualities 496
The different aspects for the classification of pulse
qualities 497
Classification of pulse qualities according to Qi, Blood
and Body Fluids patterns 497
Classification of pulse qualities according to the Eight
Principles 497
Classification of pulse qualities according to the Six Stages
patterns 498
Classification of pulse qualities according to the Four Levels
patterns 498
Classification of pulse qualities according to the Triple Burner
patterns 498

TERMINOLOGY 498

THE PULSE POSITIONS IN DETAIL 499
Left Front position (Heart) 500
Left Middle position (Liver) 501
Left Rear position (Kidney) 502
Right Front position (Lungs) 503
Right Middle position (Stomach and Spleen) 504
Right Rear position (Small Intestine and Kidney) 506

PULSE QUALITIES INDICATING DANGEROUS
CONDITIONS *506*

THE INFLUENCE OF DRUGS ON THE PULSE *507*

CHAPTER 51
PALPATION OF PARTS OF THE BODY *509*

INTRODUCTION *509*

PALPATION OF THE CHEST AND ABDOMEN *510*
Palpation of the chest *512*
Palpation of the abdomen *513*

PALPATION OF THE SKIN *516*
Body skin *516*
Forearm diagnosis *517*
Palpation of temples in children *518*

PALPATION OF HANDS AND FEET *519*
Temperature *519*
Palpation and comparison of dorsum and palm *520*
Palpation of feet and hands in children *520*
Palpation of the nails *520*

PALPATION OF ACUPUNCTURE POINTS *520*
Front Collecting (*Mu*) points *521*
Back Transporting (*Bei Shu*) points *522*
Source (*Yuan*) points *522*

CHAPTER 52
PALPATION OF CHANNELS *525*

INTRODUCTION *525*

CONNECTING CHANNELS *525*

MUSCLE CHANNELS *527*

PALPATION OF THE CHANNELS IN PAINFUL OBSTRUCTION
SYNDROME (*BI*) *527*

PALPATION OF CHANNELS *528*
Lung channel *528*
Large Intestine channel *528*
Stomach channel *529*
Spleen channel *530*
Heart channel *531*
Small Intestine channel *532*
Bladder channel *533*
Kidney channel *533*
Pericardium channel *534*
Triple Burner channel *535*
Gall-Bladder channel *536*
Liver channel *536*

PART 4
DIAGNOSIS BY HEARING AND SMELLING *539*
INTRODUCTION *539*

CHAPTER 53
DIAGNOSIS BY HEARING *541*

INTRODUCTION *541*

VOICE *541*
Normal voice *542*
The voice and the Five Elements *542*
Strength and quality of the voice *543*

SPEECH *544*

CRYING IN BABIES *544*

BREATHING AND SIGHING *544*
Breathing *544*
Pathological breathing sounds *545*
Sighing *545*

COUGHING AND SNEEZING *545*
Coughing *545*
Sneezing *546*

HICCUP *546*

BELCHING *546*

VOMITING *547*

CHAPTER 54
DIAGNOSIS BY SMELLING *549*

INTRODUCTION *549*

BODY ODOUR *549*

ODOUR OF BODILY SECRETIONS *550*
Breath *550*
Sweat *550*
Sputum *550*
Urine and stools *550*
Vaginal discharge and lochia *551*
Intestinal gas *551*

PART 5
SYMPTOMS AND SIGNS *553*
INTRODUCTION *553*

SECTION 1
SYMPTOMS AND SIGNS OF PARTS OF THE BODY *557*
INTRODUCTION *557*

CHAPTER 55
HEAD, HAIR AND FACE *559*

HEAD *559*
Dizziness *559*
Fainting *560*
Feeling of heaviness of the head *561*
Headache *561*
Feeling of distension of the head *562*
Feeling of muzziness (fuzziness) of the head *563*
Feeling of cold of the head *563*
Feeling of heat of the head *563*

Numbness of the head 563
Drooping head 563
Leaning of the head to one side 564
Tremor of the head 564
Brain noise 564
Swelling of the whole head 564
Ulcers in the mastoid region 564
Head tilted backwards 565

HAIR AND SCALP 565
Premature greying of the hair 565
Hair falling out 565
Alopecia 566
Dry and brittle hair 566
Greasy hair 566
Dandruff 567
Itchy scalp 567
Dry scalp 568
Redness and pain of the scalp 568
Boils on the scalp 568
Erosion of the scalp 568
Ulcers on the scalp 568

FACE 569
Acne 569
Feeling of heat of the face 569
Facial pain 571
Numbness of the face 572
Oedema of the face 572
Tic 572
Deviation of eye and mouth 573
Facial paralysis 573
Papular/macular eruptions 573
Swelling and redness of the face 573
Swelling, redness and pain of the cheeks 573
Ulcers below the zygomatic arch 574
Lines on the face 574

CHAPTER 56
FACE COLOUR 575

WHITE/PALE 575

YELLOW 576

RED 577

BLUISH/GREENISH 577

PURPLE 578

DARK 578

SALLOW 578

BLUSHING 579

CHAPTER 57
EARS 581

TINNITUS/DEAFNESS 581

ITCHY EARS 582

EARACHE 582

BLEEDING FROM THE EARS 583

DISCHARGE FROM THE EARS 583

EXCESSIVE WAX PRODUCTION 583

ABNORMAL SIZE 584
Swollen ears 584
Contracted ears 584

DRY AND CONTRACTED HELIX 584

SORES ON THE EAR 584

WARTS ON THE EAR 585

ABNORMAL HELIX COLOUR 585
Yellow 585
Pale 585
Bluish-greenish (Qing) 585
Dark 585
Red 586

RED BACK OF THE EAR 586

DISTENDED BLOOD VESSELS ON THE EAR 586

SWELLING AND REDNESS OF THE CONCHA 586

CHAPTER 58
NOSE 589

ABNORMAL COLOUR 589
Pale 589
Yellow 589
Red 590
Bluish-greenish 590
Reddish-purple 591
Dark 591

SNEEZING 591

BLOCKED NOSE 591

RUNNY NOSE 592

ITCHY NOSE 593

DRY NOSTRILS 593

NOSEBLEED 594

NOSE ACHE 595

NOSE PAIN 595

SWOLLEN NOSE 596

BAD SMELL *597*

LOSS OF SENSE OF SMELL *597*

POLYPS *598*

FLAPPING ALAE NASI (THE OUTSIDE OF THE NOSTRILS) *598*

ULCERS ON THE NOSE *598*

PAPULES ON THE NOSE *598*

CHAPTER 59

THROAT *601*

SORE THROAT *601*

REDNESS OF THE PHARYNX *602*

REDNESS AND SWELLING OF THE PHARYNX *602*

REDNESS AND EROSION OF THE PHARYNX *602*

SWOLLEN TONSILS *603*

PHLEGM IN THE THROAT *603*

GOITRE (SWELLING OF THE SIDES OF THE NECK) *604*

ITCHY THROAT *605*

DRY THROAT *605*

HOARSE VOICE OR LOSS OF VOICE *606*

WHITE PURULENT SPOTS IN THE THROAT *606*

FEELING OF OBSTRUCTION OF THE THROAT *607*

REDNESS ON THE THROAT *607*

CHAPTER 60

MOUTH, TONGUE, TEETH, GUMS, LIPS, PALATE AND PHILTRUM *609*

MOUTH *609*
Mouth ulcers *609*
Cold sores *610*
Cracked corners of the mouth *611*
Itching around the mouth *611*
Dribbling from the corners of the mouth *612*
Trembling mouth *612*
Mouth open *612*
Deviation of the mouth *613*

TONGUE *613*
Itchy tongue *613*
Painful tongue *613*
Numbness of the tongue *614*
Tongue ulcers *614*

TEETH *615*
Toothache *615*
Tooth cavities *616*

Loose teeth *616*
Grinding teeth *616*
Plaque *617*
Dry and white teeth *617*
Dry and dull teeth *617*
Yellow and dry teeth *618*
Grey teeth *618*
Upper teeth moist and lower teeth dry *618*

GUMS *618*
Inflamed gums *618*
Bleeding gums *619*
Receding gums *619*
Gums oozing pus *620*
Pale gums *620*
Red gums *620*
Purple gums *620*

LIPS *621*
Pale lips *621*
Red lips *621*
Purple lips *621*
Bluish-greenish lips *622*
Yellow lips *622*
Dry or cracked lips *622*
Trembling lips *623*
Peeled lips *623*
Swollen lips *623*
Inverted lips *624*
Drooping lips *624*
Abnormal lip colour in pregnancy *624*

PALATE *624*
Pale palate *624*
Dull-pale palate *624*
Yellow palate *625*
Red palate *625*
Purple palate *625*

PHILTRUM *625*
Flat philtrum *625*
Stiff-looking philtrum *625*
Pale philtrum *625*
Red philtrum *626*
Bluish-greenish philtrum *626*
Dark philtrum *626*

CHAPTER 61

EYES *627*

VISION *628*
Blurred vision and floaters *628*
Strabismus *628*
Myopia *629*
Hyperopia *629*
Decreased night vision *630*
Decreased visual acuity *630*
Sudden blindness *630*

ITCHY EYES *631*

DRY EYES *631*

HOT AND PAINFUL EYES 632

STREAMING EYES 633

DISCHARGE FROM THE EYES 634

EYE COLOUR 634
Yellow (sclera) 634
Red (sclera) 635
Bluish-greenish (sclera) 635
Dark (sclera) 636
Pale corners 636
Red corners 636

EYELIDS 637
Stye 637
Red eyelids 637
Dark eyelids 638
Green eyelids 638
Pale eyelids 638
Swollen eyelids 638
Boil on the eyelid 639
Pain of the eyelids 639
Flapping eyelids 639
Drooping eyelids 640
Loss of control of the eyelids 640
Nodules within the eyelids 640
Small red grains inside the eyelids 641
Redness inside the lower lids 641

GLAUCOMA 641

FEELING OF DISTENSION OF THE EYES 641

EYEBALL 642
Protruding eyeball 642
Sunken eyeball 643
Scaly eyeballs 643
Quivering eyeball 644
Eyeball turning up 644

ECCHYMOSIS UNDER CONJUNCTIVA 644

RED VEINS/MEMBRANE 645
Red veins in the eyes 645
Drooping red membrane 645
Red membrane in the corner of the eye 646

CORNEA 646
Corneal opacity 646
Scarring after corneal opacity 647

WHITE SPECKS 647

PUPILS 647
Red ring around the pupil 647
White membrane on the pupil in children 648
Yellow fluid between pupil and iris 648
Bleeding between pupil and iris 649
Dilated pupils 649
Contracted pupils 649

STARING, FIXED EYES 650

CLOSED EYES 650

OPEN EYES 650

INVERTED EYELASHES 650

CATARACT 651

CHAPTER 62
NECK, SHOULDERS AND UPPER BACK 653

NECK AND SHOULDERS 653
Stiff neck 653
Rigidity of the neck 654
Neck pain 654
Soft neck 654
Deviated neck 654
Wide neck 655
Thin neck 655
Swollen neck glands 655
Pulsation of the carotid artery 655
Shoulder ache 656
Frozen shoulder 656

UPPER BACK 656
Upper backache 656
Cold upper back 656
Hot upper back 656
Stiffness of the back as if wearing a tight belt 657

CHAPTER 63
CHEST 659

COUGH 659
Acute cough 659
Chronic cough 660
Coughing blood 660

BREATHLESSNESS 661

WHEEZING 662

PAIN 663
Chest pain 663
Pain in the ribs 664

FEELINGS IN THE CHEST AND HEART 664
Feeling of oppression of the chest 664
Feeling of distension of the chest 664
Feeling of heat of the chest 665
Heart feeling vexed 665
Feeling of stuffiness under the heart 666

PALPITATIONS 666
Palpitations under the heart 666

DISPLACED HEARTBEAT 667
Heartbeat displaced downwards 667
Heartbeat displaced upwards 667
Heartbeat displaced to the left 668

Heartbeat displaced to the right *668*
Heartbeat below the xyphoid process *668*

ABNORMAL CHEST SHAPE *668*
Protruding chest *668*
Sunken chest *668*
Protruding sternum *669*
Chest sunken on one side *669*
Chest protruding on one side *669*

GYNAECOMASTIA *669*

YAWNING *670*

SIGHING *670*

CHAPTER 64
LIMBS *671*

MUSCLE ACHE IN THE LIMBS *671*

PAIN IN THE LIMBS *672*

HANDS AND FEET *672*
Cold hands and feet *672*
Hot hands and feet *672*

ABNORMAL FEELINGS IN THE LIMBS *673*
Numbness/tingling of the limbs *673*
Feeling of heaviness of the limbs *673*
Feeling of distension of the limbs *674*

WEAKNESS AND ATROPHY *674*
Weakness of the limbs *674*
Atrophy of the limbs *674*
Flaccidity of the limbs *675*

LIMB SWELLING *675*
Oedema of limbs *675*
Swelling of the joints of the limbs *676*

LIMB MOVEMENT *676*
Rigidity of the limbs *676*
Paralysis of the limbs *676*
Contraction of the limbs *677*
Tremor or spasticity of the limbs *678*
Convulsions of the limbs *678*

CHAPTER 65
ARMS *679*

PAIN IN THE ELBOW *679*

HANDS *680*
Cold hands *680*
Hot hands *680*
Pale hands *681*
Red dorsum of the hands *681*
Red palms *681*
Sweaty palms *681*
Pain in the hands *682*
Itchy hands *683*

Numbness/tingling of the hands *683*
Tremor of the hands *684*
Oedema of the hands *684*
Deformed knuckles *684*
Tinea (ringworm) *684*
Dry, cracked and peeling palms *684*
Venules on the thenar eminence *685*
Atrophy of the thenar eminence *685*
Atrophy of the muscles of the dorsum of the hands *685*

FINGERS *686*
Swollen fingers *686*
Contraction of the fingers *686*
Spoon-shaped fingers *687*
Thin, pointed fingers *687*
Cracked fingers *687*
Thickened fingers *688*
Shrivelled and wrinkled fingers *688*

NAILS *688*
Ridged nails *688*
Thickening of the nails *688*
Coarse and thick nails *688*
Cracked nails *688*
Nails falling off *689*
Indented nails *689*
Thin and brittle nails *689*
Withered and brittle nails *689*
Withered and thickened nails *690*
Curling nails *690*
Flaking nails *690*
Twisted nails *691*
Nails with white spots *691*
Pale-white nails *691*
Dull-white nails *691*
Red nails *691*
Yellow nails *691*
Bluish-greenish nails *691*
Dark nails *692*
Purple nails *692*
Small or absent lunulae *692*
Large lunulae *692*

CHAPTER 66
LEGS *693*

FEET *693*
Oedema *693*
Cold feet *694*

ATROPHY OF THE LEGS *694*

PARALYSIS OF THE LEGS *695*

GAIT *695*
Festination *695*
Unstable gait *695*
Staggering gait *696*
Stepping gait *696*
Shuffling gait *696*

ARCHED LEGS *696*

PAIN *696*
  Pain in the thigh *696*
  Pain in the hip *697*
  Pain in the knee *697*
  Pain in the foot *697*
  Pain in the groin *698*
  Pain in the soles *698*

KNEES *698*
  Weak knees *698*
  Stiff knees *699*

WEAKNESS OF THE LEGS *699*

A FEELING OF HEAVINESS OF THE LEGS *699*

RESTLESS LEGS *700*

TREMOR OF THE LEGS *700*

CRAMPS IN THE CALVES *700*

LOWER LEG ULCERS *701*

TOE ULCERS *701*

BURNING SENSATION IN THE SOLES *701*

CHAPTER 67
LOWER BACK *703*

LOWER BACKACHE *703*

SCIATICA *704*

FEELING OF COLD AND HEAVINESS OF THE LOWER BACK *704*

WEAKNESS OF THE LOWER BACK AND KNEES *704*

STIFFNESS OF THE LOWER BACK *705*

COCCYX PAIN *705*

ATROPHY OF THE MUSCLES ALONG THE SPINE *705*

RIGIDITY OF THE LOWER BACK *705*

SKIN SIGNS *706*
  Spots on the back *706*
  Vesicles on the lower back *706*
  Dryness and redness of the skin of the lower back *706*
  Yellow colour of the lower back *706*
  Skin marks on the lower back *706*
  Boils on BL-23 Shenshu *706*
  Ulcers on the buttocks *706*
  Papules or pustules on the buttocks *707*

SPINAL CURVATURE *707*
  Scoliosis *707*
  Lordosis *707*
  Spine bent forward *707*
  Kyphosis *708*

Flattening of lumbar spine *708*
List of spine *708*

CHAPTER 68
BODY *709*

BODY ACHES *709*

PAIN IN THE JOINTS *710*

LOSS OF FEELING *710*
  Paralysis *710*
  Hemiplegia *711*
  Numbness/tingling *712*
  Numbness of half the body *712*

ITCHING *713*

OEDEMA *713*

WEIGHT CHANGE *713*
  Obesity *713*
  Loss of weight *714*

JAUNDICE *714*

TWITCHING OF MUSCLES *714*

OPISTHOTONOS *715*

CHAPTER 69
DIGESTIVE SYSTEM AND TASTE *717*

BELCHING *717*

REGURGITATION *718*
  Sour regurgitation *718*
  Regurgitation of food *718*

HICCUP *719*

HUNGER AND EATING *719*
  Poor appetite *719*
  Excessive hunger *720*
  Aversion to food *721*
  Hunger with no desire to eat *721*
  Gnawing hunger *721*
  Craving for sweets/constant picking *722*

SLEEPINESS AFTER EATING *722*

NAUSEA, RETCHING AND VOMITING *723*
  Nausea *723*
  Vomiting *724*
  Retching *725*
  Vomiting of blood *725*

DIFFICULTY IN SWALLOWING (DIAPHRAGM CHOKING) *726*

TASTE *726*
  Bitter taste *726*
  Sweet taste *727*

Salty taste *727*
Sour taste *727*
Sticky taste *728*
Loss of taste *728*
Foul breath *729*

CHAPTER 70
THIRST AND DRINK *731*

THIRST *731*

DRY MOUTH *732*

ABSENCE OF THIRST *733*

INCREASED SALIVATION *733*

CHAPTER 71
ABDOMEN *735*

INTRODUCTION *735*

PAIN *736*
Area below the xyphoid process *736*
Epigastric pain *737*
Hypochondrial pain *738*
Umbilical pain *738*
Central-lower abdominal pain *739*
Lateral-lower abdominal pain *740*

DISTENSION AND FULLNESS *740*
Abdominal distension *740*
Abdominal fullness *741*

ABNORMAL FEELINGS IN THE ABDOMEN *741*
Feeling of cold in the abdomen *741*
Feeling of pulsation under the umbilicus *742*
Feeling of energy rising in the abdomen *742*

BORBORYGMI *742*

FLATULENCE *743*

SKIN SIGNS *743*
Distended abdominal veins *743*
Lines *743*
Maculae *743*

ABDOMINAL MASSES *744*
Small, hypochondrial lumps *744*
Lumps in the epigastrium *744*

OEDEMA OF THE ABDOMEN *745*

ABNORMAL SIZE *745*
Thin abdomen *745*
Large abdomen *745*

SAGGING LOWER ABDOMEN *745*

UMBILICUS *745*
Protruding umbilicus *745*
Sunken umbilicus *745*

CHAPTER 72
DEFECATION *747*

DIARRHOEA OR LOOSE STOOLS *747*

DIARRHOEA WITH VOMITING *748*

CONSTIPATION *748*

ALTERNATION OF CONSTIPATION AND LOOSE
STOOLS *749*

INCONTINENCE OF FAECES *750*

BLOOD AND MUCUS IN THE STOOLS *750*

MUCUS IN THE STOOLS *751*

BLOOD IN THE STOOLS *751*

DIFFICULTY IN DEFECATION *751*

STRAINING IN DEFECATION *752*

CHAPTER 73
URINATION *753*

DARK URINE *753*

PALE AND ABUNDANT URINE *754*

TURBID URINE *754*

PAINFUL URINATION *754*

SCANTY AND DIFFICULT URINATION *755*

DIFFICULT URINATION *755*

FREQUENT URINATION *756*

DRIBBLING OF URINE *756*

INCONTINENCE OF URINE *757*

NOCTURNAL ENURESIS *757*

URINATION AT NIGHT *758*

BLOOD IN THE URINE *758*

SPERM IN THE URINE *759*

CHAPTER 74
ANUS *761*

ITCHING OF THE ANUS *761*

HAEMORRHOIDS *761*

ANAL PROLAPSE *762*

ANAL FISSURE *762*

ANAL FISTULA *762*

ANAL ULCERS *763*

CHAPTER 75
MEN'S SEXUAL AND GENITAL SYMPTOMS *765*

IMPOTENCE *765*

LACK OF LIBIDO *766*

EJACULATION *766*
  Premature ejaculation *766*
  Nocturnal emissions *767*
  Inability to ejaculate *767*
  Blood in the sperm *768*
  Cold-watery sperm *768*
  Tiredness and dizziness after ejaculation *768*

PRIAPISM *768*

COLD GENITALS *769*

SCROTUM *769*
  Contraction of the scrotum *769*
  Loose scrotum *769*
  Scrotum drooping to one side *769*
  Swollen scrotum *770*
  Swollen and oozing scrotum *770*
  Pale scrotum *770*
  Red scrotum *770*
  Purple scrotum *770*
  Dark scrotum *771*
  Itchy scrotum *771*

PENIS *771*
  Pain and itching of the penis *771*
  Soft and withered penis *771*
  Redness and swelling of the glans penis *772*
  Peyronie's disease *772*
  Ulcers *772*

SWELLING AND PAIN OF THE TESTICLES *773*

PUBIC HAIR *773*
  Loss of pubic hair *773*
  Excessive pubic hair *773*

CHAPTER 76
SWEATING *775*

SPONTANEOUS SWEATING *775*

NIGHT SWEATING *776*

SWEATING FROM COLLAPSE *776*

YELLOW SWEAT *777*

LOCALIZED SWEATING *777*
  Unilateral sweating *777*
  Sweating on the head *778*

Sweating on the chest *778*
Sweating of hands and feet *778*
Sweating of the palms *779*
Sweating in the axillae *779*

ABSENCE OF SWEATING *780*

CHAPTER 77
SKIN SIGNS *781*

GREASY SKIN *781*

DRY SKIN *782*

ERUPTIONS *782*
  Eczema *782*
  Psoriasis *783*
  Acne *783*
  Urticaria *784*
  Rosacea *785*
  Rash in the axillae *785*
  Red, itchy and swollen fingers *785*

INFECTIONS *785*
  Herpes simplex *785*
  Herpes zoster *786*
  Tinea *786*
  Candida *787*

GROWTHS AND MASSES *787*
  Warts *787*
  Naevi (moles) *787*
  Malignant melanoma *788*
  Furuncle (boil) on the head *788*
  Carbuncles on the neck *788*
  Carbuncles on the upper back *788*
  Nodules under the skin *788*

NECK ULCERS *789*

CHAPTER 78
EMOTIONAL SYMPTOMS *791*

PROPENSITY TO ANGER *791*

PROPENSITY TO WORRY *791*

SADNESS *792*

FEAR/ANXIETY *792*

TENDENCY TO BE EASILY STARTLED *793*

EXCESS JOY *794*

MENTAL RESTLESSNESS *794*

SEVERE TIMIDITY *795*

INAPPROPRIATE LAUGHTER *795*

CHAPTER 79
MENTAL AND EMOTIONAL SYMPTOMS *797*

DEPRESSION *797*

DEPRESSION AND MANIC BEHAVIOUR *798*
  Depressive phase *798*
  Manic phase *799*

ANXIETY *799*

IRRITABILITY *800*

SCHIZOPHRENIA *802*

CHAPTER 80
MENTAL DIFFICULTIES *803*

POOR MEMORY *803*

DIFFICULTY IN CONCENTRATION *804*

LEARNING DIFFICULTY IN CHILDREN *804*

HYPERACTIVITY *804*

CHAPTER 81
SLEEP PROBLEMS *807*

INSOMNIA *807*

EXCESSIVE DREAMING *808*

SOMNOLENCE *810*

SLEEP TALKING *810*

SLEEP WALKING *810*

SNORING *811*

CHAPTER 82
FEELING OF COLD, FEELING OF HEAT, FEVER *813*

FEELING OF COLD, SHIVERING *813*
  Exterior *813*
  Interior *814*

FEVER *814*
  Acute fever *814*
  Chronic fever *815*
  Tidal fever *816*
  Fever in cancer *816*
  Fever after chemotherapy *817*

FIVE-PALM HEAT *817*

CONTRADICTORY FEELINGS OF COLD AND HEAT *817*

CHAPTER 83
VOICE, SPEECH AND SOUNDS *819*

LOUD VOICE *819*

WEAK VOICE *820*

MUFFLED VOICE *820*

HOARSE VOICE *820*

NASAL VOICE *820*

SNORING *821*

SLURRED SPEECH *821*

INCOHERENT, INCESSANT SPEECH *821*

MUTTERING TO ONESELF *821*

DELIRIOUS SPEECH *822*

DIFFICULTY IN FINDING WORDS *822*

STUTTERING *822*

GROANING *822*

CRYING OUT *822*

SECTION 2
GYNAECOLOGICAL SYMPTOMS AND SIGNS *823*
INTRODUCTION *823*

CHAPTER 84
MENSTRUAL SYMPTOMS *825*

MENSTRUAL BLOOD *825*
  Pale menstrual blood *825*
  Purple menstrual blood *825*
  Menstrual clots *826*
  Sticky menstrual blood *826*
  Watery menstrual blood *826*

PERIODS *827*
  Early periods (short cycle) *827*
  Late periods (long cycle) *827*
  Irregular periods *827*
  Heavy periods *827*
  Scanty periods *828*
  Painful periods *828*
  Absence of periods *829*
  Mid-cycle bleeding *829*
  Periods that stop and start *830*
  Periods that return after the menopause *830*

CHAPTER 85
PROBLEMS AT PERIOD TIME *831*

PREMENSTRUAL TENSION *831*

HEADACHE *832*

BREAST DISTENSION *832*

FEVER *833*

BODY ACHES *833*

OEDEMA *833*

DIARRHOEA *833*

CONSTIPATION *834*

NOSEBLEED *834*

MOUTH ULCERS *834*

SKIN ERUPTIONS *834*

DIZZINESS *835*

VOMITING *835*

INSOMNIA *835*

EYE PAIN *835*

CHAPTER 86
PROBLEMS DURING PREGNANCY *837*

MORNING SICKNESS *837*

VAGINAL BLEEDING *838*

ABDOMINAL PAIN *838*

OEDEMA *838*

URINATION PROBLEMS *839*
Painful urination *839*
Retention of urine *839*
Blood in the urine *839*

CONSTIPATION *839*

ANXIETY *840*

DIZZINESS *840*

COUGH *840*

LOSS OF VOICE *840*

FEELING OF SUFFOCATION *841*

CONVULSIONS (ECLAMPSIA) *841*

PROBLEMS WITH THE FETUS *841*
Threatened miscarriage *841*
Fetus not growing *842*
Breech presentation *842*
Habitual miscarriage *842*

CHAPTER 87
PROBLEMS AFTER CHILDBIRTH *843*

RETENTION OF PLACENTA *843*

LOCHIA *843*

Persistent lochial discharge *843*
Retention of lochia *844*

PAIN *844*
Abdominal pain *844*
Join pain *844*
Hypochondrial pain *844*

VAGINAL BLEEDING *845*
Vaginal bleeding after childbirth *845*
Amenorrhoea after miscarriage *845*

URINARY DIFFICULTY *845*

CONSTIPATION *845*

SWEATING *846*

DIZZINESS *846*

OEDEMA *846*

FEVER *846*

BREAST MILK *847*
Breast milk not flowing *847*
Spontaneous flow of milk after childbirth *847*

POSTNATAL DEPRESSION/PSYCHOSIS *847*

COLLAPSE *847*

CONVULSIONS *848*

CHAPTER 88
BREAST SIGNS *849*

BREAST DISTENSION AND SWELLING *849*
Breast distension *849*
Swollen breasts *850*
Redness and swelling of the breasts *850*

BREAST PAIN *850*

BREAST LUMPS *850*

NIPPLES *851*
Milky nipple discharge *851*
Sticky yellow nipple discharge *851*
Bloody discharge from the nipple *851*
Cracked nipples *852*
Inverted nipples *852*

PEAU D'ORANGE SKIN *852*

SMALL BREASTS *852*

CHAPTER 89
MISCELLAENOUS GYNAECOLOGICAL SYMPTOMS *855*

INFERTILITY *855*

MENOPAUSAL SYNDROME *856*

ABDOMINAL MASSES *856*

VAGINAL DISCHARGE *857*
White *857*
Yellow *857*
Red-white *857*
Five-colour *857*

INFLAMMATION AND SWELLING *858*
Vaginal itching *858*
Genital eczema *858*
Vulvar sores *858*
Swelling of the vulva *858*

PROLAPSE *859*
Prolapse of uterus *859*
Prolapse of vagina *859*

LEUKOPLAKIA *859*

DYSPAREUNIA *859*

BLEEDING ON INTERCOURSE *859*

LACK OF LIBIDO *860*

PUBIC HAIR *860*
Loss of pubic hair *860*
Excessive pubic hair *860*

SECTION 3
PAEDIATRIC SYMPTOMS AND SIGNS *861*
INTRODUCTION *861*

CHAPTER 90
CHILDREN'S PROBLEMS *863*

FEVER *863*
Low-grade fever *864*

VOMITING *864*

DIARRHOEA *865*

RESPIRATORY PROBLEMS *865*
Cough *865*
Wheezing *865*

EAR PROBLEMS *865*
Earache *865*
Glue ear *866*

HOT PALMS AND SOLES *866*

CONSTITUTIONAL WEAKNESS *866*

CONSTIPATION IN INFANCY *867*

URINATION PROBLEMS *867*
Retention of urine in infancy *867*
Nocturnal enuresis *867*

CRYING *868*
Crying at night in babies *868*

DISTURBED SLEEP *868*

ACCUMULATION DISORDER *868*

WORMS *869*
Pinworms *869*
Roundworms *869*

FIVE FLACCIDITIES *869*

FIVE RETARDATIONS *869*

INFLAMMATION *869*
Acute skin rash *869*
Erysipelas *870*

JAUNDICE *870*

INFECTIONS *870*
Chickenpox *870*
Mumps *870*

FLAPPING OF NOSTRILS *870*

CONVULSIONS *870*
Acute *870*
Chronic *871*

FETUS TOXIN *871*

FONTANELLES *871*
Sunken fontanelles *871*
Raised fontanelles *871*
Late closure of fontanelles *872*

WHITE SPOTS ON THE PALATE AND TONGUE *872*

LONG PENIS *872*

PART 6
IDENTIFICATION OF PATTERNS *873*
INTRODUCTION *873*

SECTION 1
IDENTIFICATION OF PATTERNS ACCORDING TO THE
INTERNAL ORGANS *877*
INTRODUCTION *877*

CHAPTER 91
HEART *879*

HEART-QI DEFICIENCY *879*

HEART-YANG DEFICIENCY PATTERNS *879*
Heart-Yang deficiency *879*
Heart-Yang deficiency with Phlegm *880*

HEART-YANG COLLAPSE *880*

HEART-BLOOD DEFICIENCY *880*

HEART-QI AND HEART-BLOOD DEFICIENCY *880*

HEART-YIN DEFICIENCY PATTERNS *880*
  Heart-Yin deficiency *880*
  Heart-Yin deficiency with Empty-Heat *881*

HEART-QI AND HEART-YIN DEFICIENCY *881*

DEFICIENCY OF BOTH HEART-YANG AND HEART-YIN *881*

HEART-QI STAGNATION *881*

HEART-FIRE BLAZING *881*

PHLEGM PATTERNS *882*
  Phlegm-Fire harassing the Heart *882*
  Phlegm misting the Mind *882*

HEART-BLOOD STASIS *882*

HEART VESSEL OBSTRUCTION *882*

WATER OVERFLOWING TO THE HEART *883*

TURBID DAMPNESS SURROUNDING THE HEART *883*

COMBINED PATTERNS *883*

CHAPTER 92

SPLEEN *885*

SPLEEN-QI DEFICIENCY PATTERNS *885*
  Spleen-Qi deficiency *885*
  Spleen-Qi deficiency with Dampness *885*
  Spleen-Qi deficiency with Phlegm *886*

SPLEEN-YANG DEFICIENCY *886*

SPLEEN-BLOOD DEFICIENCY *886*

SPLEEN-QI SINKING *886*

SPLEEN NOT CONTROLLING BLOOD *886*

SPLEEN-YIN DEFICIENCY PATTERNS *887*
  Spleen-Yin deficiency *887*
  Spleen-Yin deficiency with Empty-Heat *887*

COLD-DAMPNESS IN THE SPLEEN *887*

DAMP-HEAT IN THE SPLEEN *887*

SPLEEN-HEAT *888*

PHLEGM OBSTRUCTING THE MIDDLE BURNER *888*

YIN FIRE FROM DEFICIENCY OF THE STOMACH AND
SPLEEN AND ORIGINAL-QI *888*

COMBINED PATTERNS *888*
  Spleen- and Stomach- Qi deficiency *888*
  Spleen- and Heart-Blood deficiency *888*
  Spleen- and Lung-Qi deficiency *889*
  Spleen- and Liver-Blood deficiency *889*

Obstruction of the Spleen by Dampness with stagnation
of Liver-Qi *889*

CHAPTER 93

LIVER *891*

LIVER-QI STAGNATION PATTERNS *891*
  Stagnation of Liver-Qi *891*
  Stagnant Liver-Qi turning into Heat *891*
  Liver-Qi stagnation with Phlegm *892*

REBELLIOUS LIVER-QI *892*

LIVER-YANG RISING *892*

LIVER-BLOOD STASIS *892*

LIVER-FIRE BLAZING UPWARDS *893*

DAMP-HEAT *893*
  Damp-Heat in the Liver *893*
  Damp-Heat in the Liver and Gall-Bladder *893*

LIVER-WIND *893*
  Extreme Heat generating Wind *893*
  Liver-Yang rising generating Wind *894*
  Liver-Fire generating Wind *894*
  Liver-Blood deficiency giving rise to Wind *894*
  Liver-Wind harbouring Phlegm *895*

LIVER-BLOOD DEFICIENCY PATTERNS *895*
  Liver-Blood deficiency *895*
  Liver-Blood deficiency with phlegm *895*

STAGNATION OF COLD IN THE LIVER CHANNEL *895*

LIVER-YIN DEFICIENCY PATTERNS *895*
  Liver-Yin deficiency *895*
  Liver-Yin deficiency with Empty Heat *896*

LIVER-QI DEFICIENCY *896*

LIVER PHLEGM-FIRE *896*

LIVER-YANG DEFICIENCY *896*

COMBINED PATTERNS *897*
  Rebellious Liver-Qi invading the Spleen *897*
  Rebellious Liver-Qi invading the Stomach *897*
  Liver-Fire insulting the Lungs *897*
  Liver- and Heart-Blood deficiency *898*

CHAPTER 94

LUNGS *899*

LUNG-QI DEFICIENCY PATTERNS *899*
  Lung-Qi deficiency *899*
  Lung-Qi deficiency with Phlegm *899*

LUNG-YANG DEFICIENCY *900*

LUNG-YIN DEFICIENCY PATTERNS *900*
  Lung-Yin deficiency *900*

Lung-Yin deficiency with Empty-Heat *900*
Lung-Yin deficiency with Phlegm *900*

LUNG-QI AND LUNG-YIN DEFICIENCY *900*

LUNG-DRYNESS *901*

INVASION OF LUNGS BY WIND *901*
Invasion of Lungs by Wind-Cold *901*
Invasion of Lungs by Wind-Heat *901*
Invasion of Lungs by Wind-Dryness *901*
Invasion of Lungs by Wind-Water *901*

LUNG-HEAT *902*

PHLEGM PATTERNS *902*
Damp-Phlegm in the Lungs *902*
Cold-Phlegm in the Lungs *902*
Phlegm-Heat in the Lungs *902*
Phlegm-Dryness in the Lungs *902*
Phlegm-Fluids in the Lungs *903*

LUNG-QI STAGNATION *903*

LUNG-QI COLLAPSE *903*

COMBINED PATTERNS *903*
Lung- and Heart-Qi deficiency *903*

CHAPTER 95
KIDNEYS *905*

KIDNEY-QI DEFICIENCY *905*

KIDNEY-YANG DEFICIENCY PATTERNS *905*
Kidney-Yang deficiency *905*
Kidney-Yang deficiency, Water overflowing *906*

KIDNEY-YIN DEFICIENCY PATTERNS *906*
Kidney-Yin deficiency *906*
Kidney-Yin deficiency with Empty-Heat *906*
Kidney-Yin deficiency, Empty-Heat blazing *906*
Kidney-Yin deficiency with Phlegm *907*

KIDNEY-YANG AND KIDNEY-YIN DEFICIENCY
PATTERNS *907*
Kidney-Yang and Kidney-Yin deficiency – predominance of
Kidney-Yin deficiency *907*
Kidney-Yang and Kidney-Yin deficiency – predominance of
Kidney-Yang deficiency *907*

KIDNEY-QI NOT FIRM *907*

KIDNEYS FAILING TO RECEIVE QI *908*

KIDNEY-ESSENCE DEFICIENCY *908*

COMBINED PATTERNS *908*
Kidney- and Liver-Yin deficiency *908*
Kidney- and Liver-Yin deficiency with Empty-Heat *909*
Kidney and Heart not harmonized (Kidney and Heart-Yin
deficiency with Heart Empty-Heat) *909*

Kidney- and Lung-Yin deficiency *909*
Kidney- and Lung-Yin deficiency with Empty-Heat *909*
Kidney- and Spleen-Yang deficiency *910*

CHAPTER 96
SMALL INTESTINE *911*

FULL-HEAT IN THE SMALL INTESTINE *911*

SMALL INTESTINE QI PAIN *911*

SMALL INTESTINE QI TIED *912*

SMALL INTESTINE DEFICIENT AND COLD *912*

INFESTATION OF WORMS IN THE SMALL INTESTINE *912*

CHAPTER 97
STOMACH *913*

STOMACH-QI DEFICIENCY *913*

STOMACH DEFICIENT AND COLD (STOMACH-YANG
DEFICIENCY) *913*

STOMACH-YIN DEFICIENCY PATTERNS *914*
Stomach-Yin deficiency *914*
Stomach-Yin deficiency with Empty-Heat *914*

DEFICIENCY OF STOMACH-YIN AND
STOMACH-YANG *914*

STOMACH-QI STAGNATION *914*

BLOOD STASIS IN THE STOMACH *915*

STOMACH-HEAT *915*

STOMACH-FIRE *915*

STOMACH PHLEGM-FIRE *915*

STOMACH DAMP-HEAT *916*

COLD INVADING THE STOMACH *916*

STOMACH-QI REBELLING UPWARDS *916*

RETENTION OF FOOD IN THE STOMACH *916*

CHAPTER 98
GALL-BLADDER *917*

DAMP-HEAT PATTERNS *917*
Damp-Heat in the Gall-Bladder and Liver *917*
Damp-Heat in the Gall-Bladder *917*

DAMP-COLD IN THE GALL-BLADDER *918*

GALL-BLADDER HEAT *918*

GALL-BLADDER DEFICIENT *918*

STAGNATION OF THE GALL-BLADDER WITH
PHLEGM-HEAT *918*

CHAPTER 99
LARGE INTESTINE *921*

DAMP-HEAT IN THE LARGE INTESTINE *921*

HEAT PATTERNS *921*
  Heat in the Large Intestine *921*
  Heat obstructing the Large Intestine *922*

COLD PATTERNS *922*
  Cold invading the Large Intestine *922*
  Large Intestine Cold *922*

LARGE INTESTINE DRYNESS *922*

DAMPNESS IN THE LARGE INTESTINE *922*

LARGE INTESTINE DEFICIENT AND COLD *923*

LARGE INTESTINE DEFICIENT AND DAMP *923*

COLLAPSE OF LARGE INTESTINE *923*

CHAPTER 100
BLADDER *925*

DAMP-HEAT IN THE BLADDER *925*

DAMP-COLD IN THE BLADDER *925*

BLADDER DEFICIENT AND COLD *926*

SECTION 2
IDENTIFICATION OF PATTERNS ACCORDING TO QI, BLOOD
AND BODY FLUIDS *927*

INTRODUCTION *927*

CHAPTER 101
**IDENTIFICATION OF PATTERNS ACCORDING TO QI,
BLOOD, YANG AND YIN** *929*

QI *929*
  Qi deficiency *929*
  Qi sinking *929*
  Collapse of Qi *929*
  Qi stagnation *929*
  Rebellious Qi *930*
  Qi obstructed *930*

BLOOD *930*
  Blood deficiency *930*
  Blood stasis *930*
  Blood-Heat *931*
  Blood-Dryness *931*
  Blood-Cold *931*

Loss of Blood *931*
Collapse of Blood *931*

YANG *932*
  Yang deficiency *932*
  Collapse of Yang *932*
  Clear Yang not ascending *932*

YIN *932*
  Yin deficiency *932*
  Yin deficiency with Empty-Heat *932*
  Collapse of Yin *932*
  Turbid Yin not descending *932*

COMBINED QI, BLOOD, YIN AND YANG *932*
  Yin and Yang both deficient *932*
  Qi and Blood both deficient *932*
  Qi and Yin both deficient *933*

CHAPTER 102
**IDENTIFICATION OF PATTERNS ACCORDING TO BODY
FLUIDS** *935*

DEFICIENCY OF BODY FLUIDS *935*

OEDEMA *935*

PHLEGM *936*
  Wind-Phlegm *936*
  Phlegm-Heat *936*
  Cold-Phlegm *936*
  Damp-Phlegm *936*
  Dry-Phlegm *936*
  Qi-Phlegm *936*
  Food-Phlegm *936*
  Phlegm with Blood stasis *937*
  Phlegm-Fluids *937*
  Phlegm under the skin *937*
  Phlegm in the channels *937*
  Phlegm misting the Heart *937*
  Phlegm in the joints *937*
  Phlegm in the Gall-Bladder *937*
  Phlegm in the Kidneys *937*
  Shock-Phlegm *937*
  Wine-Phlegm *938*

SECTION 3
IDENTIFICATION OF PATTERNS ACCORDING TO
PATHOGENIC FACTORS, FOUR LEVELS, SIX STAGES
AND THREE BURNERS *939*

INTRODUCTION *939*

CHAPTER 103
**IDENTIFICATION OF PATTERNS ACCORDING TO
PATHOGENIC FACTORS** *943*

INTRODUCTION *943*

WIND *943*
 Exterior Wind *944*
 Interior Wind *945*

COLD *946*
 Exterior Cold *946*
 Interior Cold *947*

SUMMER-HEAT *948*

DAMPNESS *948*
 External Dampness *949*
 Internal Dampness *950*

DRYNESS *950*
 External Dryness *951*
 Internal Dryness *951*

FIRE *951*

CHAPTER 104
IDENTIFICATION OF PATTERNS ACCORDING TO THE FOUR LEVELS *953*

INTRODUCTION *953*

DEFENSIVE-QI LEVEL *954*
 Wind-Heat *954*
 Summer-Heat *954*
 Damp-Heat *954*
 Dry-Heat *955*

QI LEVEL *955*
 Lung-Heat (Heat in chest and diaphragm) *955*
 Stomach-Heat *955*
 Intestines Dry-Heat (Fire) *955*
 Gall-Bladder Heat *955*
 Damp-Heat in Stomach and Spleen *956*

NUTRITIVE-QI LEVEL *956*
 Heat in Nutritive-Qi level *956*
 Heat in the Pericardium *956*

BLOOD LEVEL *957*
 Heat victorious agitates Blood *957*
 Heat victorious stirring Wind *957*
 Empty-Wind agitating in the Interior *957*
 Collapse of Yin *957*
 Collapse of Yang *957*

THE FOUR LEVELS IN A NUTSHELL *957*

LATENT HEAT *958*
 Lesser-Yang type *961*
 Bright-Yang type *961*
 Lesser-Yin type *962*

RELATIONS BETWEEN THE FOUR LEVELS, SIX STAGES AND THREE BURNERS *962*

CHAPTER 105
IDENTIFICATION OF PATTERNS ACCORDING TO THE SIX STAGES *965*

GREATER-YANG STAGE *965*
 Channel patterns *965*
 Organ patterns *966*

BRIGHT-YANG STAGE *967*
 Bright-Yang channel pattern *967*
 Bright-Yang organ pattern *967*

LESSER-YANG STAGE *967*

GREATER-YIN STAGE *967*

LESSER-YIN STAGE *968*
 Cold Transformation *968*
 Heat Transformation *968*

TERMINAL-YIN STAGE *968*

CHAPTER 106
IDENTIFICATION OF PATTERNS ACCORDING TO THE THREE BURNERS *969*

UPPER BURNER *969*
 Wind-Heat in the Lung Defensive-Qi portion *969*
 Heat in the Lungs (Qi Level) *969*
 Heat in the Pericardium (Nutritive-Qi level) *970*

MIDDLE BURNER *970*
 Heat in Bright-Yang *970*
 Damp-Heat in the Spleen *970*

LOWER BURNER *970*
 Heat in the Kidneys *970*
 Liver-Heat stirs Wind *970*
 Liver Empty-Wind *970*

CHAPTER 107
RESIDUAL PATHOGENIC FACTOR *973*

INTRODUCTION *973*

FORMATION OF RESIDUAL PATHOGENIC FACTOR *973*

DIAGNOSIS AND TREATMENT OF RESIDUAL PATHOGENIC FACTOR *975*
 How is it diagnosed? *975*
 Types of residual pathogenic factor *975*
 Effects of residual pathogenic factor *975*
 Treatment of residual pathogenic factor *975*

PHLEGM *976*
 Damp-Phlegm in the Lungs *976*
 Phlegm-Heat in the Lungs *976*

DAMPNESS *977*
  Dampness in the Stomach and Spleen *977*
  Damp-Heat in the Stomach and Spleen *977*
  Damp-Heat in the Gall-Bladder *977*
  Damp-Heat in the ears *977*
  Damp-Heat in the head *977*

HEAT *978*
  Heat in the Lungs *978*
  Heat in the Lungs with Dryness *978*
  Heat in the Stomach *978*
  Toxic Heat in the tonsils *979*

LESSER-YANG PATTERN *979*
  Lesser-Yang pattern (Six Stages) *979*
  Heat in the Gall-Bladder (Four Levels) *979*

SECTION 4
IDENTIFICATION OF PATTERNS ACCORDING
TO THE EIGHT PRINCIPLES, 12 CHANNELS,
EIGHT EXTRAORDINARY VESSELS AND
FIVE ELEMENTS *981*

INTRODUCTION *981*

CHAPTER 108
**IDENTIFICATION OF PATTERNS ACCORDING TO THE
EIGHT PRINCIPLES** *983*

INTRODUCTION *983*

INTERIOR–EXTERIOR *984*
  Exterior conditions *984*
  Interior conditions *985*

HOT–COLD *985*
  Hot conditions *985*
  Cold conditions *986*
  Combined Hot and Cold conditions *987*

FULL–EMPTY *988*
  Full conditions *990*
  Empty conditions *990*
  Combined Full–Empty conditions *990*

YIN–YANG *991*

CHAPTER 109
**IDENTIFICATION OF PATTERNS ACCORDING TO THE
12 CHANNELS** *993*

LUNGS *993*

LARGE INTESTINE *993*

STOMACH *994*

SPLEEN *994*

HEART *994*

SMALL INTESTINE *994*

BLADDER *995*

KIDNEYS *995*

PERICARDIUM *995*

TRIPLE BURNER *995*

GALL-BLADDER *996*

LIVER *996*

CHAPTER 110
**IDENTIFICATION OF PATTERNS ACCORDING TO THE
EIGHT EXTRAORDINARY VESSELS** *997*

INTRODUCTION *997*

GOVERNING VESSEL (DU MAI) *997*

DIRECTING VESSEL (REN MAI) *998*

PENETRATING VESSEL (CHONG MAI) *998*

COMBINED DIRECTING AND PENETRATING VESSEL
PATTERNS *999*
  Directing and Penetrating Vessels Empty *999*
  Directing and Penetrating Vessels unstable *999*
  Directing and Penetrating Vessels deficient and cold *999*
  Blood stasis in the Directing and Penetrating Vessels *1000*
  Blood stasis and Dampness in the Directing and Penetrating
  Vessels *1000*
  Full-Heat in the Directing and Penetrating Vessels *1000*
  Empty-Heat in the Directing and Penetrating Vessels *1001*
  Damp-Heat in the Directing and Penetrating Vessels *1001*
  Stagnant Heat in the Directing and Penetrating Vessels *1001*
  Full-Cold in the Directing and Penetrating Vessels *1001*
  Uterus deficient and cold *1002*
  Dampness and Phlegm in the Uterus *1002*
  Stagnant Cold in the Uterus *1002*
  Fetus Heat *1003*
  Fetus Cold *1003*
  Blood rebelling upwards after childbirth *1003*

GIRDLE VESSEL (DAI MAI) *1003*

YIN HEEL VESSEL (YIN QIAO MAI) *1004*

YANG HEEL VESSEL (YANG QIAO MAI) *1004*

YIN LINKING VESSEL (YIN WEI MAI) *1005*

YANG LINKING VESSEL (YANG WEI MAI) *1005*

CHAPTER 111
**IDENTIFICATION OF PATTERNS ACCORDING TO THE
FIVE ELEMENTS** *1007*

INTRODUCTION *1007*

GENERATING SEQUENCE PATTERNS *1007*
  Wood not generating Fire *1007*
  Fire not generating Earth *1008*

Earth not generating Metal *1008*
Metal not generating Water *1008*
Water not generating Wood *1008*

OVERACTING SEQUENCE PATTERNS *1008*
Wood overacting on Earth *1008*
Earth overacting on Water *1008*
Water overacting on Fire *1008*
Fire overacting on Metal *1008*
Metal overacting on Wood *1008*

INSULTING SEQUENCE PATTERNS *1009*
Wood insulting Metal *1009*
Metal insulting Fire *1009*
Fire insulting Water *1009*
Water insulting Earth *1009*
Earth insulting Wood *1009*

APPENDICES *1011*

Appendix 1 Case histories *1013*

Appendix 2 Prescriptions *1025*

Appendix 3 History of diagnosis in Chinese
Medicine *1051*

GLOSSARY OF CHINESE TERMS *1061*

BIBLIOGRAPHY *1067*

CHINESE CHRONOLOGY *1069*

INDEX *1071*

Colour plates can be found at the end of the book (pages P1–P25)

Foreword

It gives me great pleasure to write a foreword to this book, the latest in the series on the fundamentals of Chinese medicine. It follows the same high standard that we have come to expect. Here we see the principles of diagnosis presented clearly in relation to the differentiation of syndromes, one of the great theories of Chinese medicine.

Mr Maciocia was the first to attempt any book in the English language on diagnosis, with his excellent book on tongue diagnosis. That still remains the best textbook on the subject. Now he has succeeded in writing a more complete book on the whole subject. Presented for the first time are all the little details observable in clinic, which, when put together, form a complete whole. Some of this information comes from his tireless translation of Chinese texts, which are inaccessible to most Western practitioners; and part comes from his clinical experience with patients in the West. This makes the book all the more valuable, as the lifestyle in the West is so different from the Chinese lifestyle, that many of the clinical signs point in a different direction.

The practice of medicine is about relieving suffering. Human nature is complex and so the diseases and ailments which cause this suffering are also complex. When trying to unravel complexities of this nature, one needs a frame of reference on which to base understanding. The basis for understanding them is a philosophy which helps to understand life, and how people come to suffer in the first place. One of the glories of Chinese medicine is its foundation in a rich and holistic philosophy which incorporates all of human experience. Above all, it is a philosophy that recognizes the vast complexity of human nature. At its heart is the Yin–Yang theory, together with the theory of Five Transformations. But this is only the foundation. There are a multitude of other theories built on this – the theory of penetration by Cold, the theory of Warm Diseases, the theory of tonifying the Earth, to name but a few. At times some of these theories seem mutually incompatible.

In Chinese science and medicine, it is rare for a new theory to lead to the total abandonment of an old one. There is the feeling that if the ancestors said something, and took the trouble to write it down, then it must contain truths worthy of study. Out of respect for the ancestors, any new theory is grafted onto the old one. It is understood that there is no theory that is sufficiently complete to explain all of human behaviour. The human mind is too small, and the complexity of life is too great. When there are two theories that do not seem to fit with each other, this is not seen as a problem. There will be one theory that explains one situation, while there is another that explains a different one. This is a problem for the beginner in Chinese medicine, particularly one like myself who was brought up in the Western scientific tradition. At times, when learning Chinese medicine, it seemed as though one had to heed the advice of the Red Queen, to 'believe three impossible things before breakfast.' When one learns more, it slowly becomes clear that all theories have their application, and it is the context that is all-important.

Apparent inconsistencies of this nature are rare in Western science. The reason is that there is an unstated assumption that modern theories are good, and an improvement on old theories. Therefore the old theories are abandoned, and with it any danger of inconsistency. In medicine, the modern theories, based on microscopic observations of bacteria, viruses and genes, have superseded the old humoral theories, and relegated them to history. Unfortunately this process means that a lot that is valuable is thrown out at the same time. Although the theories of Hot and Cold permeate all other medical systems, and give a valuable indication of what medicine to prescribe, based on what the patient actually experiences, these phenomenological theories have been totally abandoned in favour of objective material tests. Subjective feelings, like the patient's will to live, have little place in modern Western medicine.

By contrast, in Chinese medicine, the role of the mind and consciousness is considered of great importance. In the very first term, the student of TCM learns that 'the Heart houses the Shen'. From the outset it is stated that there is a consciousness which is related to the body. It is implicit that the consciousness influences

the body, and vice versa. Right from the very start there is this recognition that human beings are more than mere walking lumps of flesh. All of life – movement, feelings, behaviour and physical body – are governed by the laws of Yin and Yang. They are in constant motion, constantly varying.

It is quite natural that one should have feelings of anger, compassion and anguish. Illness occurs when these get out of balance. Likewise, hot and cold, dry and damp are constantly varying. Thus the art of diagnosis in TCM is much more subtle. Not only does it involve assessing the state of the physical body, but it also involves assessing the emotional state, and the whole state of a person's life.

Diagnosis is based on the idea that there must be a fundamental imbalance in Yin and Yang for illness to occur, and that this imbalance will manifest in all areas of human experience. For example, the patient will show an imbalance in colour, movement, texture of skin, food preferences, music, clothes, sports, or styles of painting. On the body, the channels, the Elements, the Blood, and the whole way that Qi flows will be influenced by the imbalance.

This difference in the philosophical basis is evident when it comes to diagnosis. The philosophical basis for Western medicine is strongly biased towards the material basis of life, and diagnosis leans heavily in this direction. A diagnosis now depends more on tests than on the observation skills of the physician. The bacteria which are causing disease, or the part of the body that is dysfunctional, are considered to be the cause of the disease. For most physicians the emotional life of the patient is of negligible importance. Even less important would be their favourite colours. In Chinese medicine, the material components of the body are important, but so also is the emotional state of patients. Just as important is the spirit of patients and their Qi. The will to live is every bit as important as the microscopic components of the illness. When treating a stomach ulcer due to Liver invading the Stomach, the emotions have to be taken into account. The degree of inflexibility of a patient's anger is every bit as important as the size of the ulcer in assessing treatment and outcome.

'Western medicine is difficult to learn, but easy to practise. Chinese medicine is easy to learn, but difficult to practise.' These are the words of our late teacher, Dr J. F. Shen. At first sight, Chinese medicine seems very easy. There is not all that much to learn (by comparison with orthodox medicine). Although the present book is large, it contains almost all that can be said about diagnosis. The equivalent book in orthodox medicine might fill a whole shelf. However, one should not judge the richness of the medicine by a word count, for each word is part of a 'pith instruction', a sentence that contains a wealth of meaning, and needs to be interpreted by one who is experienced in the art. The instructions on diagnosis are short sentences to point the way, rather than give a detailed instruction.

Diagnosis, which means knowing, or understanding, a patient, is the heart of medicine. Once knowledge about the patient and his illness has been gathered and understood, then the nature of the illness and its likely course are known. The principles of treatment become clear and the progress of the illness predictable. But without a clear understanding of the patient and the condition being treated, the practitioner is fumbling in the dark. Treatment is haphazard and cure uncertain. Chinese medicine, although difficult to practise, comes to a more certain and more complete diagnosis, one which incorporates all aspects of a patient's life, and so comes to a more reliable treatment than Western medicine.

We are now living in a time of rapid change. The world of the 21st century is very different from the world that the author was born into. But human nature remains the same. People still have likes and dislikes, loves and hates, pleasures and pain. They still have to experience the constant fluctuations of Yin and Yang. They still have to witness their greatest pleasure turning into the source of their greatest pain. And all of this is built into the fabric of Chinese medicine. So, although society and lifestyle appears to change, Chinese medicine is still as relevant today as it has ever been. It still provides the basic framework for understanding people and their illness. Thus the art of diagnosis in Chinese medicine becomes richer and richer the more it is practised. The pith instructions in this book seem to become richer and more meaningful the longer they are used and the wider their field of application.

It is said in the Nei Jing that the superior doctor can predict disease before it occurs, the average doctor can diagnose disease when it is present, while the inferior doctor cannot even diagnose accurately when it has occurred. With this book, it will now be possible for more TCM practitioners to become superior.

2004   Julian Scott

Preface

This book on diagnosis in Chinese medicine complements my previous books: on the basic theory of Chinese medicine 'Foundations of Chinese Medicine', the application of this theory to the treatment of diseases 'Practice of Chinese Medicine', tongue diagnosis 'Tongue Diagnosis in Chinese Medicine' and gynaecology 'Obstetrics and Gynaecology in Chinese Medicine'.

The longer I practise, the more I appreciate the importance of diagnosis to Chinese medicine in particular and to medicine in general. Indeed, one could say that the value of Chinese medicine lies not in its theories of Yin–Yang, Five Elements, Eight Principles, etc., but in diagnosis itself. Chinese medicine diagnosis is so valuable because it starts firmly from the careful *examination* of the patient: this forms the basis of diagnosis in any type of medicine from any cultural background, including modern Western medicine.

Although it is not often appreciated, modern Western medicine used to be based on the careful examination of the patient, before technology and modern diagnostic aids took precedence over it. Technological tests have replaced a proper examination of the patient; this is the weakest link of Western medicine and it is also the reason why Chinese medicine, with its careful examination of the patient, appeals to many thousands of medical doctors all over the world.

An example from my practice is particularly apt to illustrate this point. A patient came to me for a one-off consultation (she lived in the USA) about persistent hip and back pain. She was 78 and for 4 years had been suffering from severe pain in the lower back irradiating towards the right hip. She went to see one of the top neurosurgeons in the USA who ordered a scan; purely on the basis of this and without a proper examination, he diagnosed a problem with the intervertebral spaces in the lumbar spine. He did not recommend an operation and the patient went on to suffer for another 2 years. She had been very active in her mid-seventies, playing tennis three times a week, but she could now hardly walk.

When I examined her, the first thing I noticed was that she walked with a limp, her body oscillating sideways. I have no osteopathic skills but I have observed over the years that people with a chronic back problem tend to walk leaning slightly forward; her walk was quite different and, in my experience, was related to a hip problem rather than a back problem. I took a detailed history and then asked her to lie down on the couch. I did the straight-leg lifting test (i.e. lifting her right leg with a straight knee); this elicited no pain in the back. I then abducted her right leg and this produced an intense pain in the hip. Everything pointed to a hip rather than a lower back problem. I was still very hesitant to question the diagnosis of an eminent neurosurgeon. I therefore rang a colleague in Italy who is an extremely skilled and knowledgeable osteopath and, while on the phone, he asked me to make the patient perform three other movements for diagnostic purposes. To my astonishment, he confirmed that the patient definitely suffered from a hip rather than a lower back pathology. I asked her to have an X-ray of the hip (which had not been ordered by her neurosurgeon) as soon as she went back to the USA. This she did and the X-ray showed that her right hip was completely and totally invaded by very severe osteoarthritis. She had a hip replacement, her pain has completely disappeared and she is back on the tennis court. She is now 80.

I report this case history as a glaring illustration of how the proper examination of the patient including a careful taking of the case history has been forgotten in Western medicine in favour of technological tests. Of course such tests are important, but they must follow and be guided by a proper examination of the patient.

Another example of the power of diagnosis in Chinese medicine springs to mind with a patient I saw a few months ago. She was a 29-year-old woman who had a severe pain in the back, lethargy and sickness, which had been diagnosed by her general practitioner (GP) as a kidney infection. She had been taking antibiotics for a week, which had made no apparent difference to the symptoms. After questioning the patient, it transpired that the pain, which was indeed in the area of the left kidney, was related to movement and was worse on breathing in. She had no fever (in fact she felt quite cold) and no urinary symptoms. Her pulse and tongue were unremarkable, other than the fact that the Liver and Gall-Bladder positions were Wiry and slightly Tight. The Kidney and Bladder pulse felt quite healthy and there was no sticky yellow coating on most of the tongue.

On the basis of the above, I felt that the GP's diagnosis of a kidney infection was unlikely to be correct and that the pain was more likely to come from a problem with the ribs (which is why the Liver and Gall-Bladder position on the pulse was affected): the aggravation of the pain on breathing strongly pointed to a rib problem as backache from a urinary infection would not be affected by breathing. I treated her accordingly and the pain immediately improved. An osteopath later confirmed that, in fact, the twelfth rib was displaced and that it was this that had been causing the pain.

This case history in another illustration of the importance of a proper *examination* of the patient (which the above-mentioned GP had omitted to do): this is the real strength of Chinese diagnosis and Chinese medicine in general. The strength of Chinese medicine diagnosis is precisely in the incredibly detailed examination of the patient approached from the four viewpoints of observation, interrogation, palpation and hearing/smelling.

Chinese medicine diagnosis is also strong in its holistic view of the body and mind. Probably no other form of diagnosis can make such a comprehensive, holistic and detailed assessment of a patient in a relatively short time, pulling all the different strands of diagnosis together. For example, as soon as a patient comes in, the practitioner of Chinese medicine exerts all his or her senses to their sharpest, observing the way the patient walks, the level of vitality, the strength of voice, the lustre of the eyes and complexion, the shape of the face, the complexion colour, the smell of the body, the hair, the tongue and, finally, the pulse.

Another motivation for writing a book on diagnosis is that I feel this is an area that has been neglected in modern China. In their eagerness to 'modernize' Chinese medicine and make it more acceptable to the biomedical establishment in China and in the West, modern Chinese doctors and teachers have tended to overlook the more subtle aspects of Chinese diagnosis, especially tongue and pulse diagnosis. Too often, in Chinese clinics, the clinical teacher will describe a pulse quality in a perfunctory way to *make* it agree with the clinical manifestations: if a patient has all the symptoms of Liver-Qi stagnation, the pulse *is* Wiry. This ignores the possibility that the pulse might be Choppy instead (indicating that the stagnation of Liver-Qi is secondary to a Liver-Blood deficiency). It is my wish that the more subtle aspects of Chinese diagnosis be preserved.

The book is divided into the traditional four major parts of Chinese diagnosis, that is, diagnosis by observation ('to look'), interrogation ('to ask'), palpation ('to touch') and auscultation ('to hear and to smell'). In addition to these four major parts, Part 5 covers symptoms and signs: whereas Part 1 Observation deals with signs and Part 2 Interrogation deals with symptoms, Part 5 Symptoms and Signs lists hundreds of different clinical manifestations, irrespective of which category they fall into, and arranges them according to the part of the body they affect.

The separation between observation and interrogation is made purely for didactic purposes and does not correspond to clinical reality where what is seen on observation and what is elicited on interrogation occurs simultaneously and may be integrated automatically. For example, the separation between dry skin (a sign in observation) and itchy skin (a symptom in interrogation) is artificial and unrealistic. Another good example is that of oedema of the ankles: the observation of this sign is immediately integrated with palpation of the area and interrogation of the patient.

Moreover, the combination of both symptoms and signs for each area corresponds also to how we normally proceed with the patient. For example, when a patient comes in and the clinical manifestations are mainly concentrated in one area of the body, we would naturally investigate that area first by asking about symptoms and observing any outward sign without distinction between interrogation and observation. Supposing a patient complains about blurred vision, we would immediately and automatically observe the eyes to see whether they are dry or bloodshot.

Part 6 lists the patterns of Chinese medicine from various points of view – that is, the Internal Organs, the pathogenic factors, Qi, Blood and Body Fluids, the Eight Principles, 12 channels, Four Levels, Six Stages, Three Burners and Five Elements. It should be noted that the patterns listed in Part 5 on Symptoms and Signs have been adapted to each particular symptom and will not necessarily correspond to the patterns in Part 6. For example, the pattern of Liver-Blood deficiency under a particular eye symptom will contain symptoms and signs slightly different from those given in the general pattern of Liver-Blood deficiency in Part 6. Part 6 lists treatment with acupuncture and herbal medicine whenever appropriate.

At the beginning of the book there is an index of all symptoms and signs contained in Part 5 with cross-references to Part 1 (Observation), Part 2 (Interrogation), Part 3 (Palpation) and Part 4 (Hearing and Smelling).

Appendix 1 contains case histories with a particular diagnostic significance, which are used to illustrate important principles of Chinese medicine theory. Appendix 2 lists all the herbal formulae mentioned in Part 6 on Patterns. Appendix 3 is a brief history of Chinese diagnosis.

Amersham, 2004   *Giovanni Maciocia*

Acknowledgements

Many teachers have inspired my interest in diagnosis. I am indebted to the late Dr J. H. F. Shen for imparting to me some of his knowledge and skill in pulse diagnosis which I have been trying to convey in this book.

Dr J. D. Van Buren was the first teacher who taught me the art of diagnosis by observation and I am grateful to him for inspiring me at the very beginning of my professional career.

I express my gratitude to all the teachers and staff of the Nanjing University of Traditional Chinese Medicine: studying and spending clinical periods there have been crucial to my professional development.

Rebecca Avern contributed greatly to the book with her suggestions and comments; she also saw the book through from the very beginning in all its stages and assisted me with editing: for this I am deeply grateful.

I am indebted to Dr Andreas Hoell for reading the manuscript and giving me many helpful suggestions and comments and to Isobel Cosgrove and Tim Davis for reading the manuscript and making many helpful suggestions derived from their clinical experience. Alan Papier read the manuscript and made many useful suggestions, for which I am grateful.

I wish to express my appreciation to Dr Jin Hui De and Ms Fu Zhi Wen for their invaluable help in the translation of Chinese texts.

I would also like to thank the staff at Churchill Livingstone, especially Inta Ozols, Dinah Thom, Samantha Ross and Karen Morley, for their professionalism, helpfulness and kindness.

Note on the translation of Chinese terms

The terminology used in this book generally follows that used in 'Foundations of Chinese Medicine', 'Practice of Chinese Medicine' and 'Obstetrics and Gynaecology in Chinese Medicine'. As in those books, I have opted for translating all Chinese medical terms with the exception of Yin, Yang, Qi and *cun* (unit of measurement).

I have also continued using initial capitals for the terms which are specific to Chinese medicine. For example, 'Blood' indicates one of the vital substances of Chinese medicine, whereas 'blood' denotes the liquid flowing in the blood vessels, for example 'In Blood deficiency the menstrual blood may be pale'. I use initial capitals also for all pulse qualities and for pathological colours and shapes of the tongue body. This system may not be ideal but it has served readers of my previous books well. As most teachers (including myself) use Chinese terms when lecturing (e.g. Yuan Qi rather than Original Qi), I have given each term in pinyin and Chinese characters whenever it is introduced for the first time.

I made the choice of translating all Chinese terms (with the exceptions indicated above) mostly for reasons of style: I believe that a well-written English text reads better than one peppered with Chinese terms in pinyin. Leaving Chinese terms in pinyin is probably the easiest option but this is not ideal because a single pinyin word can often have more than one meaning; for example, *jing* can mean 'channels', 'periods', 'Essence' or 'shock', while *shen* can mean 'Kidneys' or 'Mind/Spirit'.

I am conscious of the fact that there is no such thing as a 'right' translation of a Chinese medicine term and my terminology is not proposed in this spirit; in fact, Chinese medicine terms are essentially impossible to translate. The greatest difficulty in translating Chinese terms is probably that a term has many facets and different meanings in different contexts; thus it would be impossible for one translation to be 'right' in every situation. For example, the term *jue* (厥) has many different meanings; a translation can illustrate only one aspect of a multifaceted term. In fact, *jue* can mean a state of collapse with unconsciousness, coldness of hands and feet, or a critical situation of retention of urine. In other contexts it has other meanings: for example, *jue qi* (厥气) is a condition of chaotic Qi, *jue xin tong* (厥心痛) a condition of violent chest pain with cold hands, and *jue yin zheng* (厥阴证) the Terminal-Yin pattern within the Six-Stage identification of patterns characterized by Heat above and Cold below.

Although a diversity of translation of Chinese terms may present its problems, these are easily overcome if an author explains the translation in a glossary. Moreover, the problem arises only in the written form as, in my experience, most lecturers in colleges throughout the Western world normally prefer using pinyin terms rather than their counterparts in English (or any other Western languages). Thus, a lecturer will refer to Kidney-*jing* rather than 'Essence'. A diversity of translation of Chinese terms may even have a positive aspect as each author may highlight a particular facet of a Chinese term so that diversity actually enriches our understanding of Chinese medicine. If someone translates *zong qi* (宗气) as 'Initial Qi', for example, we learn something about that author's view and understanding of *zong qi*; the translation cannot be branded as *wrong* (I translate this term as 'Gathering Qi'). Another example: if someone translates *yang qiao mai* as 'Yang Motility Vessel', the translation captures one aspect of this vessel's nature; again, this could not be defined as wrong (I translate the name of this vessel as 'Yang Heel Vessel'). Trying to impose a standard, *right* translation of Chinese medicine terms may lead to suppression of healthy debate. I therefore hope that readers will continue to benefit from the diversity of translation of Chinese medical terms and draw inspiration from the rich heritage of Chinese medicine that it represents.

A glossary with Chinese characters, pinyin terms and English translation appears on page 1061.

How to use this book

The book is articulated into six parts and three appendices as follows:

Part 1 Observation
Part 2 Interrogation
Part 3 Palpation
Part 4 Hearing and Smelling
Part 5 Symptoms and Signs
Part 6 Patterns
Appendix 1 Case histories
Appendix 2 Prescriptions
Appendix 3 History of Chinese diagnosis

Part 1 on observation discusses the diagnostic significance of *signs* by body area (e.g. head, face, eyes, ears, limbs, etc.). Part 2 on interrogation describes the techniques used in asking questions about various parts of the body; this process of asking questions should elicit an account of *symptoms* from the patient. Part 3 on palpation includes pulse diagnosis and diagnosis from palpation of the abdomen and channels. Part 4 describes the diagnostic significance of sounds and smells. Thus, *signs* are described in Part 1 on observation and *symptoms* in Part 2 on interrogation.

Part 5 on symptoms and signs lists without discussion many symptoms and signs with their related patterns. I would like to stress that this part discusses the differentiation of patterns of *symptoms* and *signs*, and *not* diseases. For example, the reader will find the differentiation of patterns for the symptoms of dizziness and nausea, but not that for Meniere's disease (which manifests with dizziness and nausea). This is because it is the role of a book on diagnosis to discuss symptoms and signs, and that of a book on internal medicine to discuss diseases. This Part is linked to Parts 1 and 2 in so far as it lists clinical manifestations irrespective of whether they are symptoms or signs (Fig. F.1).

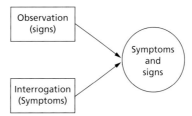

Fig. F.1 Link between observation, interrogation and symptoms and signs

Please note that all the symptoms and signs described in Parts 1 and 2 are covered in Part 5 on Symptoms and Signs, but not vice versa; that is, this Part may contain some less common symptoms and signs that are not in Parts 1 and 2.

All Parts of the book contain highlighted cross-references which link one Part to another. For example, under the heading of 'Red eyes' in Chapter 6 (Observation) there is a cross-reference linking this sign to Chapter 61 (Symptoms and Signs); vice versa, in Chapter 61 (Symptoms and Signs) under the sign of 'red eyes' there is a cross-reference linking this sign to Chapter 6 (Observation). This should facilitate navigation between the different parts of the book for each particular symptom or sign (Fig. F.2).

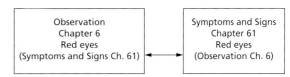

Fig. F.2 Link between Parts for each symptom or sign

There are three main ways to use this book, as follows:

1. The reader can read a particular chapter to gain an understanding of the diagnostic significance of

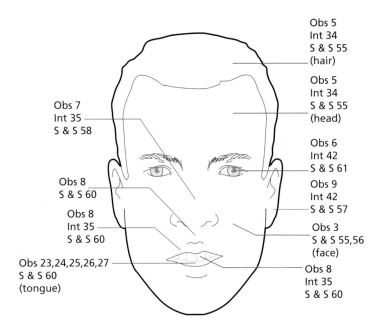

Obs 5
Int 34
S & S 55
(hair)

Obs 5
Int 34
S & S 55
(head)

Obs 7
Int 35
S & S 58

Obs 6
Int 42
S & S 61

Obs 8
S & S 60

Obs 9
Int 42
S & S 57

Obs 8
Int 35
S & S 60

Obs 3
S & S 55,56
(face)

Obs 23,24,25,26,27
S & S 60
(tongue)

Obs 8
Int 35
S & S 60

Fig. F.3 Map of face areas

a specific part of the body. For example, Chapter 3 contains a detailed discussion of the diagnostic significance of the complexion colour, which is an extremely important aspect of diagnosis. Likewise Chapter 49 in Part 3 contains a detailed discussion of the general principles of pulse diagnosis.

2. A second way to use the book is to 'dip' into it. If the reader is faced with a patient with symptoms and signs that clearly revolve around a particular area of the body, he or she may dip into the sections dealing with that particular part of the body. For example, if a patient presents with blurred vision, dry eyes and eye ache, these symptoms and signs can be looked up in Chapter 6 in Observation and Chapter 42 in Interrogation. Figure F.3 illustrates the main face areas with the relevant chapter numbers from Part 1 on observation, Part 2 on interrogation and Part 5 on symptoms and signs; Figure F.4 does the same for body areas.

3. A third way to use the book is for the reader to look up a particular symptom or sign encountered in the clinic, especially if this is an uncommon one such as sweating on one side of the body. The

symptom or sign should be read about in all parts of the book in which it appears (e.g. Parts 2 and 5, or Parts 1, 3 and 5). Each part may give slightly different information, or at least information from a different perspective, about that symptom or sign.

HOW TO MOVE BETWEEN DIFFERENT PARTS OF THE BOOK

To facilitate the link between the different parts of the book (Observation, Interrogation, Palpation and Hearing/Smelling), there is a symptoms index on page xlix. This lists each symptom that is in Part 5 Symptoms and Signs and links it to Parts 1 to 4 on observation, interrogation, palpation and hearing and smelling. For example, on looking up 'dry nostrils' (in Chapter 58 of Symptoms and Signs), the reader will find that this symptom is also discussed in Chapter 7 of Observation and 35 of Interrogation. In addition, there is a cross-reference under 'dry nostrils' in Symptoms and Signs which will also direct the reader to these other chapters.

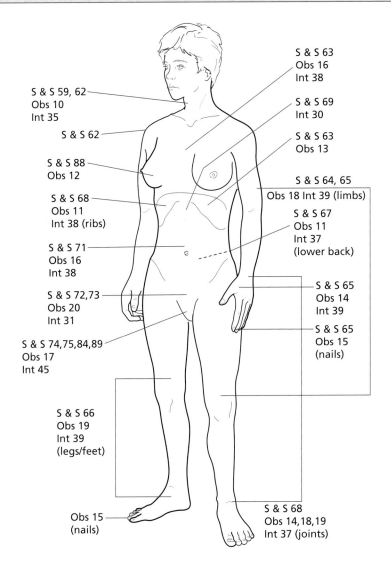

S & S 63
Obs 16
Int 38

S & S 59, 62
Obs 10
Int 35

S & S 69
Int 30

S & S 62

S & S 63
Obs 13

S & S 88
Obs 12

S & S 64, 65
Obs 18 Int 39 (limbs)

S & S 68
Obs 11
Int 38 (ribs)

S & S 67
Obs 11
Int 37
(lower back)

S & S 71
Obs 16
Int 38

S & S 72,73
Obs 20
Int 31

S & S 65
Obs 14
Int 39

S & S 65
Obs 15
(nails)

S & S 74,75,84,89
Obs 17
Int 45

S & S 66
Obs 19
Int 39
(legs/feet)

Obs 15
(nails)

S & S 68
Obs 14,18,19
Int 37 (joints)

Fig. F.4 Map of body areas

Index of symptoms and signs

Part number	5	1	2	3
HEAD AND FACE				
Head				
Brain noise	55		34	
Dizziness	55		34	
Drooping head	55			
Fainting	55		34	
Feeling of cold of the head	55		34	
Feeling of distension of the head	55		34	
Feeling of heat of the head	55		34	
Feeling of heaviness of the head	55		34	
Feeling of muzziness of the head	55		34	
Head leaning to one side	55	5		
Head tilted backwards	55	5		
Headache	55		34	
Numbness of the skin of the head	55		34	
Redness and pain of the scalp	55	5		
Swelling of the whole head	55	5		
Tremor of the head	55	4, 5		
Ulcers in the mastoid region	55	5		
Hair and scalp				
Alopecia	55	5		
Boils on the scalp	55	5		
Dandruff	55	5		
Dry and brittle hair	55	5		
Dry scalp	55	5		
Erosion of the scalp	55	5		
Greasy hair	55	5		
Hair falling out	55	5		
Itchy scalp	55		34	
Premature greying of the hair	55	5		
Redness and pain of the scalp	55	5		
Ulcers on the scalp	55	5		
Face				
Acne	55, 77	5		
Bluish/greenish complexion colour	56	3		
Dark complexion colour	56	3		
Deviation of eye and mouth	55	4, 5		
Facial pain	55			35
Facial paralysis	55	4		
Facial tic	55	4		
Feeling of heat of the face	55			35
Lines on the face	55	5		
Numbness/tingling of the face	55			35
Oedema of the face	55	5		
Papular/macular eruptions	55	5		

Part number	5	1	2	3
Purple complexion colour	56	3		
Red complexion colour	56	3		
Sallow complexion colour	56	3		
Swelling and redness of the face	55	5		
Swelling, redness and pain of the cheeks	55	5		
Ulcers below the zygomatic arch	55	5		
White/pale complexion colour	56	3		
Yellow complexion colour	56	3		
Ears				
Bleeding from the ears	57			
Bluish-greenish helix	57	9		
Contracted ears	57	9		
Dark helix	57	9		
Discharge from the ears	57	9		
Distended blood vessels on the ear	57	9		
Dry and contracted helix	57	9		
Earache	57		42	
Excessive wax production	57	9		
Itchy ears	57		42	
Pale helix	57	9		
Red back of the ear	57	9		
Red helix	57	9		
Sores on the ears	57	9		
Swelling and redness of the concha	57	9		
Swollen ears	57	9		
Tinnitus/deafness	57		42	
Warts on the ears	57	9		
Yellow helix	57	9		
Nose				
Bad smell	58			
Blocked nose	58		35	
Bluish-greenish nose	58	7		
Dark nose	58	7		
Dry nostrils	58	7	35	
Flapping alae nasi	58	7		
Itchy nose	58		35	
Loss of sense of smell	58		35	
Nose ache	58		35	
Nosebleed	58	7		
Nose pain	58		35	
Pale nose	58	7		
Papules on the nose	58	7		
Polyps	58			
Red nose	58	7		
Reddish-purple nose	58	7		
Runny nose	58	20	35	
Sneezing	58		35	

Part number	5	1	2	3
Swollen nose	58	7		
Ulcers on the nose	58	7		
Yellow nose	58	7		
Throat				
Dry throat	59		36	
Feeling of obstruction of throat	59		36	
Hoarseness/loss of voice	59		36	53
Itchy throat	59		36	
Phlegm in throat	59			
Redness of pharynx	59	10		
Redness/erosion of pharynx	59	10		
Redness and swelling of pharynx	59	10		
Redness on throat	59	10		
Sore throat	59		36	
Swelling of sides of neck (goitre)	59	10	36	
Swollen tonsils	59	10	36	
White purulent spots on the throat	59			
Mouth				
Cold sores	60	8	35	
Cracked corners of the mouth	60	8		
Deviation of the mouth	60	8		
Dribbling from corners of the mouth	60	8		
Itching around the mouth	60			
Mouth ulcers	60	8	35	
Mouth wide open	60	8		
Trembling mouth	60			
Tongue				
Itchy tongue	60		35	
Numbness of the tongue	60		35	
Painful tongue	60		35	
Tongue ulcers	60			
Teeth				
Dry and dull teeth	60	8		
Grey teeth	60	8		
Grinding teeth	60			
Loose teeth	60	8		
Plaque	60	8		
Tooth cavities	60	8		
Toothache	60		35	
Upper teeth moist/lower teeth grey	60	8		
White and dry teeth	60	8		
Yellow and dry teeth	60	8		
Gums				
Bleeding gums	60	8	35	

Part number	5	1	2	3
Gums oozing pus	60	8		
Inflamed gums	60	8	35	
Pale gums	60	8		
Purple gums	60	8		
Receding gums	60	8	35	
Red gums	60	8		
Lips				
Abnormal lip colour in pregnancy	60	8		
Bluish-greenish lips	60	8		
Drooping lips	60	8		
Dry or cracked lips	60	8		
Inverted lips	60	8		
Pale lips	60	8		
Peeled lips	60	8		
Purple lips	60	8		
Red lips	60	8		
Swollen lips	60	8		
Trembling lips	60	8		
Yellow lips	60	8		
Palate				
Dull-pale palate	60	8		
Pale palate	60	8		
Purple palate	60	8		
Red palate	60	8		
Yellow palate	60	8		
Philtrum				
Bluish-greenish philtrum	60	8		
Dark philtrum	60	8		
Flat philtrum	60	8		
Pale philtrum	60	8		
Red philtrum	60	8		
Stiff-looking philtrum	60	8		
Eyes				
Bleeding between pupil and iris	61			
Bluish-greenish eyes (sclera)	61	6		
Blurred vision and floaters	61		42	
Boil on the eyelid	61			
Cataracts	61			
Closed eyes	61			
Contracted pupils	61			
Corneal opacity	61			
Dark eyelids	61			
Dark eyes (sclera)	61	6		
Decreased night vision	61			
Decreased visual acuity	61			
Dilated pupils	61			
Discharge from the eyes	61	6		
Drooping eyelids	61			
Drooping red membrane	61			
Dry eyes	61		42	
Ecchymosis under conjunctiva	61			
Eyeball turning up	61			
Feeling of distension of the eyes	61		42	
Flapping eyelids	61			
Glaucoma	61			
Green eyelids	61			
Hot and painful eyes	61		42	
Hyperopia in children	61			
Inverted eyelashes	61			
Itchy eyes	61		42	
Loss of control of the eyelids	61			
Myopia	61			
Nodules within the eyelids	61			
Open eyes	61			
Pain of the eyelids	61			
Pale corners of the eyes	61	6		
Pale eyelids	61			
Protruding eyeball	61	6		
Quivering eyeball	61			

Part number	5	1	2	3
Red and hot eyelids	61	6		
Red corners of the eyes	61	6		
Red eyelids	61			
Red eyes (sclera)	61	6		
Red membrane in the corner of eye	61	6		
Red ring around the pupil	61			
Red veins in the eyes	61			
Redness inside the lower lids	61			
Scaly eyeballs	61			
Scarring after corneal opacity	61			
Small red grains inside the eyelids	61			
Staring, fixed eyes	61	6		
Strabismus	61	6		
Streaming eyes	61	6	42	
Stye	61			
Sudden blindness	61			
Sunken eyeball	61	6		
Swollen eyelids	61	6		
White membrane on pupil	61			
White specks	61	6		
Yellow eyes (sclera)	61	6		
Yellow fluid between pupils and iris	61			
TRUNK AND LIMBS				
Neck and shoulders				
Deviated neck	62	10		
Frozen shoulder	62			
Neck pain	62		36	
Pulsation of the carotid artery	62	10		
Rigidity of the neck	62	10		
Shoulder ache	62			
Soft neck	62	10		
Stiff neck	62		36	
Swollen neck glands	62	10		
Thin neck	62	10		
Wide neck	62	10		
Upper back				
Cold upper back	62		37	
Hot upper back	62			
Stiffness of the back as if wearing a tight belt	62			
Upper backache	62		37	
Chest				
Acute cough	63	20		53
Breathlessness	63			53
Chest pain	63		38	
Chest protruding on one side	63	16		
Chest sunken on one side	63	16		
Chronic cough	63			53
Coughing blood	63			
Feeling of distension of the chest	63			
Feeling of heat in the chest	63		38	
Feeling of oppression of the chest	63		38	
Feeling of stuffiness under the heart	63			
Gyaecomastia	63	16		
Heart feeling vexed	63			
Heartbeat displaced downwards	63	13		
Heartbeat displaced upwards	63	13		
Heartbeat displaced to the left	63	13		
Heartbeat displaced to the right	63	13		
Heartbeat below the xyphoid process	63	13		
Pain in the ribs	63		38	
Palpitations	63		38	
Palpitations under the heart	63			
Protruding chest	63	16		

Part number	5	1	2	3
Protruding sternum	63	16		
Sunken chest	63	16		
Wheezing	63			53
Four limbs				
Atrophy of the limbs	64	18	39	
Cold hands and feet	64			
Contraction of limbs	64	18		
Convulsions of the limbs	64	4,18		
Feeling of distension of the limbs	64		39	
Feeling of heaviness of the limbs	64		39	
Flaccidity of the limbs	64	18	39	
Hot hands and feet	64			
Muscle ache in the limbs	64		39	
Numbness of the limbs	64		39	
Oedema of the limbs	64, 65, 66, 68	18	39	
Pain in the limbs	64		39	
Paralysis of the limbs	64	18		
Rigidity of the limbs	64	18		
Swelling of the joints of the limbs	64	18		
Tremor or spasticity of the limbs	64, 66	4,18	39	
Weakness of the limbs	64		39	
Arms				
Atrophy of the muscles of the dorsum of the hand	65	14		
Atrophy of the thenar eminence	65	14		
Bluish-greenish nails	65	15		
Coarse and thick nails	65	15		
Cold hands	65		39	
Contraction of fingers	65	4,14		
Cracked fingers	65	14		
Cracked nails	65	15		
Curling nails	65	15		
Dark nails	65	15		
Deformed knuckles	65	14		
Dry, cracked and peeling palms	65	14		
Dull-white nails	65	15		
Flaking nails	65	15		
Hot hands	65		39	
Indented nails	65	15		
Itchy hands	65		39	
Large lunulae	65	15		
Nails falling off	65	15		
Nails with white spots	65	15		
Numbness/tingling of the hands	65		39	
Oedema of the hands	65, 64, 68	18	39	
Pain in the elbow	65		39	
Pain in the hands	65		39	
Pale hands	65	14		
Pale-white nails	65	15		
Purple nails	65	15		
Red dorsum of the hands	65	14		
Red nails	65	15		
Red palms	65	14		
Ridged nails	65	15		
Shrivelled and wrinkled fingers	65	14		
Small or absent lunulae	65	15		
Spoon-shaped fingers	65	14		
Sweaty palms	65	14		
Swollen fingers	65	14		
Thickened fingers	65	14		
Thickening of the nails	65	15		
Thin and brittle nails	65	15		

Part number	5	1	2	3
Thin, pointed fingers	65	14		
Tinea (ringworm)	65, 77	14		
Tremor of the hands	65	4,14		
Twisted nails	65	15		
Venules on the thenar eminence	65	14		
Withered and brittle nails	65	15		
Withered and thickened nails	65	15		
Yellow nails	65	15		
Legs				
Arched legs	66	19		
Atrophy of the legs	66	19		
Burning sensation in the soles	66		39	
Cold feet	66		39	
Cramps in the calves	66		39	
Festination	66	19		
Heaviness of the legs	66, 64		39	
Lower leg ulcers	66	21		
Oedema of the feet	66, 64, 68	18,19	39	
Pain in the foot	66		39	
Pain in the groin	66			
Pain in the hip	66		39	
Pain in the knee	66		39	
Pain in the soles	66		39	
Pain in the thigh	66		39	
Paralysis of the legs	66	19		
Restless legs	66			
Shuffling gait	66	19		
Staggering gait	66	19		
Stepping gait	66	19		
Stiff knees	66			
Toe ulcers	66	21		
Tremor of the legs	66, 64	4,18		
Unstable gait	66	19		
Weak knees	66		39	
Weakness of the legs	66			
Lower back				
Atrophy of the muscles along the spine	67	11		
Boils on BL-23 Shenshu	67	11		
Coccyx pain	67			
Dryness and redness of the skin of the lower back	67	11		
Feeling of cold and heaviness of the lower back	67			
Flattening of spine	67	11		
Kyphosis	67	11		
List of the spine	67	11		
Lordosis	67	11		
Lower backache	67		37	
Papules or pustules on the buttocks	67	11		
Rigidity of the lower back	67	11		
Sciatica	67			
Scoliosis	67	11		
Skin marks on the lower back	67	11		
Spine bent forward	67	11		
Spots on the back	67	11		
Stiffness of the lower back	67			
Ulcers on the buttocks	67	11		
Vesicles on the lower back	67	11		
Weakness of the lower back and knees	67			
Yellow colour of the lower back	67	11		
Body				
Body aches	68		37	
Hemiplegia	68	4		

Part number	5	1	2	3
Itching	68		37	
Obesity	68		37	
Oedema	68, 64, 65, 66	18,19	39	
Opisthotonos	68	4		
Pain in the joints	68		37	
Paralysis	68	4		
Twitching of muscles	68	4		
DIGESTIVE/URINARY SYSTEM				
Aversion to food	69		30	
Belching	69		30	53
Bitter taste	69		30	
Constant picking, Craving for sweets	69			
Difficulty in swallowing (diaphragm choking)	69			
Excessive hunger	69		30	
Gnawing hunger	69			
Hiccup	69			53
Hunger with no desire to eat	69		30	
Loss of sense of taste	69		30	
Nausea	69		30	
Poor appetite	69		30	
Pungent taste	69		30	
Regurgitation of food	69			
Retching	69			
Salty taste	69		30	
Sleepy after eating	69			
Sour regurgitation	69		30	53
Sour taste	69		30	
Sticky taste	69		30	
Sweet taste	69		30	
Vomiting	69		30	53
Vomiting of blood	69			
Thirst and drink				
Absence of thirst	70		32	
Dry mouth	70		32	
Increased salivation	70			
Thirst	70		32	
Abdomen				
Abdominal distension	71	16	38	
Abdominal fullness	71		38	
Abdominal masses	71	16		
Borborygmi	71			
Central-lower abdominal pain	71		38	
Distended abdominal veins	71	16		
Epigastric pain	71		38	
Feeling of cold in the abdomen	71		38	
Feeling of energy rising in the abdomen	71			
Feeling of pulsation under the umbilicus	71			
Flatulence	71			
Hypochondrial pain	71		38	
Large abdomen	71	16		
Lateral-lower abdominal pain	71		38	
Lines on the abdomen	71	16		
Lumps in the epigastrium	71	16		
Maculae on the abdomen	71	16		
Oedema of the abdomen	71	16		
Pain below the xyphoid process	71		38	
Protruding umbilicus	71	16		
Sagging lower abdomen	71	16		
Small hypochondrial lumps	71	16		
Sunken umbilicus	71	16		
Thin abdomen	71	16		
Umbilical pain	71		38	

Part number	5	1	2	3
Defecation				
Alternation of constipation and loose stools	72		31	
Blood and mucus in the stools	72	20	31	
Blood in the stools	72	20	31	
Constipation	72		31	
Diarrhoea or loose stools	72	20	31	
Diarrhoea with vomiting	72			
Difficulty in defecation	72		31	
Incontinence of faeces	72			
Mucus in the stools	72	20	31	
Straining in defecation	72		31	
Urination				
Blood in the urine	73	20	31	
Dark urine	73	20	31	
Difficult urination	73		31	
Dribbling of urine	73		31	
Frequent urination	73		31	
Incontinence of urine	73		31	
Nocturnal enuresis	73		31	
Painful urination	73		31	
Pale and abundant urine	73	20	31	
Scanty and difficult urination	73	20	31	
Sperm in the urine	73			
Turbid urine	73	20	31	
Urination at night	73		31	
Anus				
Anal fissure	74			
Anal fistula	74			
Anal prolapse	74			
Anal ulcers	74			
Haemorrhoids	74			
Itching of the anus	74			
MEN'S SEXUAL AND GENITAL SYMPTOMS				
Blood in the sperm	75			
Cold genitals	75			
Cold watery sperm	75			
Contraction of the scrotum	75	17		
Dark scrotum	75	17		
Excessive pubic hair	75	17		
Impotence	75			45
Inability to ejaculate	75			
Itchy scrotum	75			
Lack of libido	75			45
Loose scrotum	75	17		
Loss of pubic hair	75	17		
Nocturnal emissions	75			45
Pain and itching of the penis	75			
Pale scrotum	75	17		
Penis ulcers	75	17		
Peyronie's disease	75	17		
Premature ejaculation	75			45
Priapism	75	17		
Purple scrotum	75	17		
Red scrotum	75	17		
Redness and swelling of glans penis	75	17		
Scrotum drooping on one side	75	17		
Soft and withered penis	75	17		
Swelling and pain of the testicles	75			
Swollen/oozing scrotum	75	17		
Tiredness and dizziness after ejaculation	75			45
SWEATING				
Absence of sweating	76		41	
Night sweating	76		41	
Spontaneous sweating	76		41	
Sweating in the axillae	76			
Sweating on the chest	76	20	41	
Sweating from collapse	76		41	

Part number	5	1	2	3
Sweating of hands and feet	76	20	41	
Sweating on the head	76	20	41	
Sweating of the palms	76	20	41	
Unilateral sweating	76			
Yellow sweat	76	20	41	

SKIN

Part number	5	1	2	3
Acne	77, 55	21		
Candida	77	21		
Carbuncles on the upper back	77			
Dry skin	77	21		
Eczema	77	21		
Furuncle (boil) on the head	77			
Greasy skin	77	21		
Herpes simplex	77	21		
Herpes zoster	77	21		
Malignant melanoma	77	21		
Naevi	77	21		
Neck carbuncle	77			
Nodules under the skin	77			
Psoriasis	77	21		
Red, itchy and swollen fingers	77			
Rosacea	77	21		
Tinea	77	21		
Urticaria	77	21		
Warts	77	21		

MENTAL AND EMOTIONAL SYMPTOMS

Emotional symptoms

Part number	5	1	2	3
Easily startled	78			
Excess joy	78		44	
Fear/anxiety	78		44	
Inappropriate laughter	78			
Mental restlessness	78		44	
Propensity to anger	78		44	
Propensity to worry	78		44	
Sadness	78		44	
Severe timidity	78			

Mental and emotional symptoms

Part number	5	1	2	3
Anxiety	79		44	
Depression	79		44	
Depression and manic behaviour	79		44	
Irritability	79		44	
Schizophrenia	79			

Mental difficulties

Part number	5	1	2	3
Difficulty in concentration	80			
Hyperactivity	80			
Learning difficulty in children	80			
Poor memory	80			

Sleep

Part number	5	1	2	3
Excessive dreaming	81		40	
Insomnia	81		40	
Sleep talking	81			
Sleep walking	81			
Snoring	81, 83			53
Somnolence	81		40	

FEELING OF COLD, FEELING OF HEAT, FEVER

Part number	5	1	2	3
Contradictory feelings of cold and heat	82		43	
Feeling of cold, shivering	82		43	
Fever	82		43	
Five-palm heat	82		43	

VOICE AND SPEECH

Part number	5	1	2	3
Crying out	83			53
Delirious speech	83			
Difficulty in finding words	83			
Groaning	83			53
Hoarse voice	83			
Incoherent, incessant speech	83			
Loud voice	83			53
Muffled voice	83			
Muttering to oneself	83			
Nasal voice	83			
Slurred speech	83			
Snoring	83, 81			53
Stuttering	83			53
Weak voice	83			53

GYNAECOLOGICAL PROBLEMS

Menstrual symptoms

Part number	5	1	2	3
Absence of periods	84		46	
Early periods (short cycle)	84		46	
Heavy periods	84		46	
Irregular periods	84		46	
Late periods (long cycle)	84		46	
Menopausal syndrome	89		46	
Menstrual clots	84	20	46	
Mid-cycle bleeding	84	20		
Painful periods	84		46	
Pale menstrual blood	84	20	46	
Periods returning after the menopause	84			
Periods stopping and starting	84		46	
Purple menstrual blood	84	20	46	
Scanty periods	84		46	
Sticky menstrual blood	84	20	46	
Watery menstrual blood	84	20	46	

Problems at period time

Part number	5	1	2	3
Body aches	85			
Breast distension	85		46	
Constipation	85		46	
Diarrhoea	85		46	
Dizziness	85			
Eye pain	85			
Fever	85			
Headache	85		46	
Insomnia	85			
Mouth ulcers	85			
Nosebleed	85			
Oedema	85		46	
Premenstrual tension	85		46	
Skin eruptions	85			
Vomiting	85		46	

Problems of pregnancy

Part number	5	1	2	3
Abdominal pain	86			
Anxiety during pregnancy	86			
Blood in the urine during pregnancy	86			
Breech presentation	86			
Constipation during pregnancy	86			
Convulsions during pregnancy	86			
Cough during pregnancy	86			
Dizziness during pregnancy	86			
Feeling of suffocation during pregnancy	86			
Fetus not growing	86			
Habitual miscarriage	86		46	
Loss of voice during pregnancy	86			
Morning sickness	86		46	
Oedema during pregnancy	86		46	
Painful urination during pregnancy	86			

Part number	5	1	2	3
Retention of urine during pregnancy	86			
Threatened miscarriage	86		46	
Vaginal bleeding	86			

Problems after childbirth

Part number	5	1	2	3
Abdominal pain after childbirth	87			
Amenorrhoea after miscarriage	87			
Breast milk not flowing	87		46	
Collapse after childbirth	87			
Constipation after childbirth	87			
Convulsions after childbirth	87			
Dizziness after childbirth	87			
Fever after childbirth	87		46	
Hypochondrial pain after childbirth	87			
Joint pain after childbirth	87			
Oedema after childbirth	87			
Persistent lochial discharge	87	20		
Postnatal depression/psychosis	87		46	
Retention of lochia	87	20		
Retention of placenta	87			
Spontaneous flow of milk	87		46	
Sweating after childbirth	87		46	
Urinary difficulty after childbirth	87			
Vaginal bleeding after childbirth	87			

Breast signs

Part number	5	1	2	3
Bloody discharge from the nipple	88	12		
Breast distension	88	12	46	
Breast lumps	88	12	46	51
Breast pain	88			
Cracked nipples	88	12		
Inverted nipples	88	12		
Milky nipple discharge	88	12		
Peau d'orange	88	12		
Redness and swelling of the breast	88	12		
Small breasts	88	12		
Sticky yellow nipple discharge	88	12		
Swollen breasts	88	12		

Miscellaneous gynaecological symptoms

Part number	5	1	2	3
Abdominal masses	89, 71	16		
Bleeding on intercourse	89			
Dyspareunia	89			
Excessive pubic hair	89			
Genital eczema	89, 77	21		
Infertility	89		46	
Lack of libido	89		45	
Leukoplakia	89	17		
Loss of pubic hair	89			
Menopausal syndrome	89			
Prolapse of uterus	89			
Prolapse of vagina	89	17		
Swelling of the vulva	89	17		
Vaginal discharge	89	20	46	54
Vulvar sores	89	17		

CHILDREN'S PROBLEMS

Part number	5	1	2	3
Accumulation disorder	90		47	
Acute convulsions	90			
Acute skin rash	90			
Chickenpox	90			
Chronic convulsions	90			
Constipation in infancy	90			
Constitutional weakness	90			
Cough	90		47	

Part number	5	1	2	3
Crying	90			
Crying at night	90			
Diarrhoea	90			
Earache	90		47	
Erysipelas	90			
Fetus toxin	90			
Fever	90			
Five Flaccidities	90			
Five Retardations	90			

Part number	5	1	2	3
Flapping nostrils	90			
Glue ear	90			
Hot palms and soles	90			
Jaundice	90			
Late closure of fontanelles	90	5		
Long penis	90	17		
Low-grade fever	90			
Mumps	90			
Nocturnal enuresis	90			

Part number	5	1	2	3
Pinworms	90			
Raised fontanelles	90			
Retention of urine in infancy	90			
Roundworms	90			
Sunken fontanelles	90			
Vomiting	90			
Wheezing	90		47	
White spots on the palate and tongue	90			

LIST OF ABBREVIATIONS

CFIDS   chronic fatigue immune deficiency syndrome
CT   computerized tomography
HPV   human papilloma virus
lg   immunoglobulin
LGL   Lown-Ganong-Levine (syndrome)
MAOI   monoamine oxidase inhibitor
ME   myalgic encephalitis
MRI   magnetic resonance imaging
PET   positron emission tomography
SSRI   selective serotonin reuptake inhibitor
TB   tuberculosis
WPW   Wolff-Parkinson-White (syndrome)

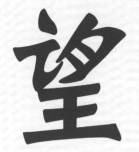

PART 1

DIAGNOSIS BY OBSERVATION

Part contents

SECTION 1
OBSERVATION OF THE BODY, MIND AND COMPLEXION
1 Observation of the body shape, physique and demeanour   11
2 Observation of the Mind, Spirit and emotions   31
3 Observation of the complexion colour   39
4 Observation of body movements   59

SECTION 2
OBSERVATION OF PARTS OF THE BODY
5 Observation of head, face and hair   69
6 Observation of the eyes   75
7 Observation of the nose   87
8 Observation of lips, mouth, palate, teeth, gums and philtrum   93
9 Observation of the ears   105
10 Observation of the throat and neck   109
11 Observation of the back   115
12 Observation of women's breasts   121
13 Observation of the heartbeat   127
14 Observation of the hands   129
15 Observation of the nails   137
16 Observation of the chest and abdomen   143
17 Observation of the genitalia   149
18 Observation of the four limbs   153
19 Observation of the legs   159
20 Observation of excretions   163
21 Observation of the skin   169
22 Observation in children   191

SECTION 3
TONGUE DIAGNOSIS
23 Tongue diagnosis   203
24 Tongue-body colour   209
25 Tongue-body shape   215
26 Tongue coating   221
27 Tongue images and patterns   227

INTRODUCTION

Diagnosis by observation is one of the most important aspects of Chinese diagnosis: in ancient times, it was considered the highest diagnostic art and the mark of a superior doctor who could diagnose simply by looking at a patient without any need to ask questions or to palpate. Observation of the patient is also the first diagnostic technique used as a patient comes in and a great deal of information can be obtained simply by observation, for example the patient's constitution, body type, Five-Element type and deviations from it, constitutional state of Yin and Yang, state of the Mind and Spirit, etc.

Diagnosis by observation in Chinese medicine is based on the principle that the Internal Organs and their disharmonies manifest themselves externally with what the ancient Chinese called 'images' (xiang). In disease, every aspect of the complex of clinical manifestations is an 'image' of an internal disharmony, for example a pulse image, a complexion image, a pattern image, a tongue image, etc. Chapter 10 of the 'Simple Questions' discusses the concept of 'images': *'The images of the five Yin organs can be deduced and categorized; the five Yin organs correspond to the five sounds which can be detected; the five colours can be observed. The combination of the pulse [image] with the colours can give us the whole picture.'*[1] The concept of correspondence between the Internal Organs and their external image manifestations can be found throughout the 'Simple Questions' and the 'Spiritual Axis'. For example, Chapter 37 of the 'Spiritual Axis' says: *'The five colours manifest on the face and through them we can observe the Qi of the five Yin organs.'*[2] Chapter 71 of the same book says: 'By observing the five colours, we can know the state of the 5 Yin organs; by feeling the pulse and

observing the colours, we can diagnose conditions of Heat or Cold and Painful Obstruction Syndrome.'[3]

> **!**
>
> **Remember:** in observation, avoid the two pitfalls: either missing important details though seeing the picture as a whole, or missing the whole picture while paying excessive attention to details.

When observing a patient, it is important to look at the whole picture, integrating the various aspects of observation, but also to pay attention to details. Therefore, there are two pitfalls we should avoid: either considering the whole picture but missing some important details in it, or paying excessive attention to small details but missing the whole picture.

Before discussing the various aspects of diagnosis by observation, it is useful to review the various correspondences between the Internal Organs and parts of the body, forming a 'map' of the body. These relationships are six:

- relationship between the five senses, the nine orifices and the Internal Organs
- relationship between areas of the face and the Internal Organs
- relationship between the five tissues and the Internal Organs
- relationship between the five sites of Qi transportation and the Yin organs
- manifestations of the five Yin organs
- the 12 cutaneous regions.

Relationship between the five senses, the nine orifices and the Internal Organs

The nine orifices are the two eyes, the two nostrils, the two ears, the mouth, the urethra and the anus. The orifices according to Chapter 37 of the 'Classic of Difficulties' are different:

The Five Yin Organs communicate internally with the seven upper orifices. Lung-Qi communicates with the nose: when the nose is in harmony we can detect smells. Liver-Qi communicates with the eyes: if the eyes are in harmony we can distinguish black from white [i.e. see]. Spleen-Qi communicates with the mouth: when the mouth is in harmony we can taste food. Heart-Qi communicates with the tongue: *when the tongue is in harmony we can taste the five flavours. Kidney-Qi communicates with the ears: when the ears are in harmony we can hear the five sounds. When the Five Yin Organs are not in harmony the seven orifices are blocked.*[4]

Thus, the 'Classic of Difficulties' mentions only the seven upper orifices but these differ from the list given above: they make up seven only if we count the eyes and ears as two but the nose as one. If we do this, the seven orifices are the two eyes, the two ears, the nose, the mouth and the tongue. This is the most common way of counting the upper orifices because it assigns them neatly to the five Yin organs. The two lower orifices, being the urethra and anus, are under the influence of the Kidneys.

Therefore the relationship between the nine orifices, the five senses and the Internal Organs is as shown in Table P1.1.

Table P1.1 Relationship between the nine orifices, the five senses and the Internal Organs

Orifice	Sense	Yin organ
Eyes (2)	Sight	Liver
Ears (2)	Hearing	Kidneys
Nose (1)	Smell	Lungs
Mouth (1)	Taste	Spleen
Tongue (1)	Taste	Heart
Urethra (1)		Kidneys
Anus (1)		Kidneys

As can be seen, the sense of touch is not included and the sense of taste is related both to the Spleen and the Heart. According to the above passage from the 'Classic of Difficulties', the Spleen is responsible for the sense of taste in general while the Heart is responsible for distinguishing the five flavours (sweet, sour, bitter, pungent and salty).

Chapter 59 of the 'Spiritual Axis' also describes the five sense organs as places where the energy of the Five Yin organs manifests when there are changes in colour:

When the area between the eyebrows [top of nose] is thin and moist, the disease is in the skin [i.e. Lungs]; when the lips are greenish, yellow, red, white or black, the disease is in the muscles [i.e. Spleen]; when the Nutritive Qi is moist, the disease is in Blood [i.e. Heart]; when the eyes are greenish, yellow, red, white or black, the disease is in the sinews [i.e. Liver]; when the ear is dry and full of dirt [ear wax?], the disease is in the bones [i.e. Kidneys].[5]

Relationship between different areas of the face and the Internal Organs

Each area of the face reflects the state of an Internal Organ. The 'Simple Questions' (Chapter 32) and the 'Spiritual Axis' (Chapter 49) give two different views of these relationships. Chapter 32 of the 'Simple Questions' mentions the correspondence of areas of the face to the five Yin organs in the context of Heat diseases: 'In Heat disease of the Liver, the left cheek becomes red; in Heat disease of the Heart, the forehead becomes red, in Heat disease of the Spleen, the nose becomes red; in Heat disease of the Lungs, the right cheek becomes red; in Heat disease of the Kidneys, the chin becomes red.'[6] Figure P1.1 shows the correspondence of face areas to Internal Organs according to the 'Simple Questions' and Figure P1.2 that according to the 'Spiritual Axis'.

The significance of the correspondence between areas of the face and the Internal Organs in diagnosis will be explored in greater detail later.

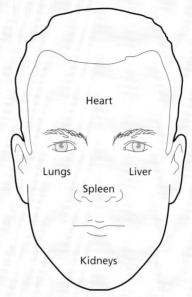

Fig. P1.1 Correspondence of facial areas to the Internal Organs according to the 'Simple Questions'

Relationship between the five tissues and the Internal Organs

Chapter 4 of the 'Simple Questions' establishes the correspondence between the five tissues and the five Yin organs. This is as follows:

Lungs	skin
Spleen	muscles
Liver	sinews
Heart	blood vessels
Kidneys	bones

The Lungs influence the skin in so far as they diffuse the Defensive Qi in the skin and the space between the skin and muscles (cou li); the Lungs also control the opening and closing of the pores and therefore sweating. The relationship between the Lungs and skin is very clear in atopic patients who suffer from both asthma and eczema.

The Spleen influences the muscles causing muscular weakness when it is deficient. The Liver influence the sinews which include tendons and cartilages: Liver-Blood, in particular, nourishes the sinews in the joints and ensures that they are properly fed and lubricated. The 'sinews' and their relationship with the Liver, however, have a broader meaning in Chinese medicine. For example, the nails are considered an extension of

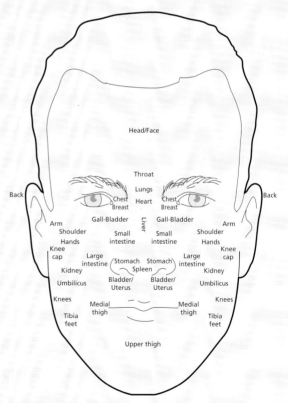

Fig. P1.2 Correspondence of facial areas to the Internal Organs according to the 'Spiritual Axis'

the sinews and tremors or convulsions in a patient suffering from internal Wind are said to be due to 'shaking of the sinews'.

The Heart governs Blood and influences the state of the blood vessels. The Kidneys influence the bones and bone marrow: in particular, it is the Kidney-Essence that nourishes the bones and bone marrow.

The five tissues readily show pathological states of their related organs. When the Lungs are deficient, the space between the skin and muscles is 'open' and the person may suffer from spontaneous sweating and will be prone to invasions of external Wind.

When the Spleen is deficient, the person will experience muscular weakness and general tiredness. If the Liver (and in particular Liver-Blood) is deficient, the sinews become vulnerable to invasion of Cold, Dampness or Wind; a deficiency of Liver-Blood may also cause a contraction of the sinews. Liver-Blood stasis or Liver-Qi stagnation may cause a stiffness of the sinews in the joints, while Liver-Wind may cause tremors of the sinews.

A deficiency of Heart-Blood may cause a weakness of the blood vessels while Heart-Blood stasis may cause a hardening of the blood vessels. A deficiency of the Kidney-Essence may cause brittle bones (osteoporosis).

Box P1.1 summarizes the five Yin organs and the five tissues.

> **BOX P1.1 THE FIVE YIN ORGANS AND THE FIVE TISSUES**
>
> Lungs: skin (pores open)
> Spleen: muscles (weak muscles)
> Liver: sinews (vulnerable to external invasions, stiffness)
> Heart: blood vessels (weakness or hardening)
> Kidneys: bones (brittle bones)

Relationship between the five sites of Qi transportation and the Yin organs

Chapter 4 of the 'Simple Questions' says,

The East wind comes in Spring and the Liver is often diseased affecting the neck ... The South wind comes in Summer and the Heart is often diseased affecting the chest and hypochondrial region. The West wind comes in Autumn and the Lungs are often diseased affecting the upper back and shoulders. The North wind comes in Winter and the Kidneys are often diseased affecting the thighs and the lower back. The Centre corresponds to Earth and the Spleen is often diseased affecting the spine.[7]

> **BOX P1.2 THE FIVE SITES OF QI TRANSPORTATION**
>
> * Neck: Liver
> * Chest: Heart
> * Upper back and shoulders: Lungs
> * Thighs and lower back: Kidneys
> * Spine: Spleen

Thus the 'Five sites of Qi transportation' (Box P1.2) where the Qi of the five Yin organs accumulates are the neck, the chest, the upper back and shoulders, the thighs and lower back and the spine for the Liver, Heart, Lungs, Kidneys and Spleen respectively.

Most of these correspondences are confirmed in practice and have some clinical relevance. For example, the neck is frequently affected by Liver disharmonies such as Liver-Qi stagnation or Liver-Yang rising causing a stiff neck; the relationship between the Heart and the chest is well known; the upper back is frequently affected by Lung disharmonies such as Lung-Heat, which may cause a pain in this area; the thighs may become weak when the energy of the Kidneys declines; the Spleen has an influence on the spine and the point SP-3 Taibai may be used to straighten the spine.

Manifestations of the five Yin organs

Chapter 9 of the 'Simple Questions' says:

The Heart ... manifests in the face, and nourishes the blood vessels; the Lung ... manifests in the body hair and nourishes the skin; the Kidneys ... manifest in the hair and nourish the bones; the Liver ... manifests in the nails and nourishes the sinews; the flourishing of the Spleen, Stomach, Large Intestine, Small Intestine, Triple Burner and Bladder ... manifests in the white skin around the lips, and nourishes the muscles.[8]

The manifestation sites of the five Yin organs (Box P1.3) are well known and widely used in practice. For example, the facial complexion as a whole reflects the state of the Heart; the body hair may become withered when the Lungs are weak; the hair becomes dull and brittle when the Kidneys are deficient and grey when the Kidney-Essence declines; the nails become brittle when Liver-Blood is deficient; the lips may become dry when Spleen-Yin is deficient or red when the Spleen has Heat.

The 12 cutaneous regions

Chapter 56 of the 'Simple Questions' says, 'The twelve cutaneous regions follow the course of the twelve main channels.'[9] The area on the skin overlying each main channel constitutes its cutaneous region (Fig. P1.3). This correspondence between wide skin sections and the channels and Internal Organs is of course crucial to many aspects of diagnosis by observation. The cutaneous region of a particular channel reflects its pathologies and those of the relevant organ. A pathology of the relevant channel may manifest on the corresponding cutaneous region with pain, discoloration, skin rashes, veins, venules, contraction of muscles, etc. Thus the cutaneous regions are very immediate and important diagnostic signs.

The most important implication of the cutaneous regions is that the influence of each channel is not restricted to its line of trajectory but spreads over a broad area around the channel, so that every part of the body is covered by a given channel.

The above discussion highlighted the various relationships between the Internal Organs and external manifestations: it is these relationships that make diagnosis by observation possible.[10]

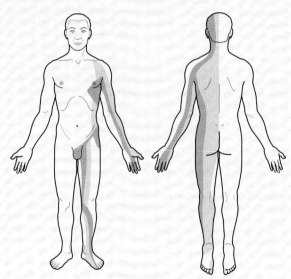

Fig. P1.3 The 12 cutaneous regions

NOTES

1. 1979 The Yellow Emperor's Classic of Internal Medicine – Simple Questions (Huang Di Nei Jing Su Wen 黄帝内经素问), People's Health Publishing House, Beijing, p. 75. First published c. 100BC.
2. 1981 Spiritual Axis (Ling Shu Jing 灵枢经), People's Health Publishing House, Beijing, p. 77. First published c. 100BC.
3. Ibid., p. 126.
4. Nanjing College of Traditional Chinese Medicine 1979 A Revised Explanation of the Classic of Difficulties (Nan Jing Jiao Shi 难经校释), People's Health Publishing House, Beijing, p. 91. First published c. AD100.
5. Spiritual Axis, p. 108.
6. Simple Questions, p. 189.
7. Ibid., p. 23.
8. Ibid., p. 67.
9. Ibid., p. 290.
10. The main Chinese source for the discussion of observation in Chinese diagnosis was Zhang Shu Sheng 1995 Great Treatise of Diagnosis by Observation in Chinese Medicine (Zhong Hua Yi Xue Wang Zhen Da Quan 中华医学望诊大全), Shanxi Science Publishing House, Taiyuan.

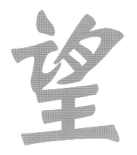

SECTION 1

OBSERVATION OF THE BODY, MIND AND COMPLEXION

Section contents

1 Observation of the body shape, physique and demeanour *11*
2 Observation of the Mind, Spirit and emotions *31*
3 Observation of the complexion colour *39*
4 Observation of body movements *59*

INTRODUCTION

Observation of the body includes observation of the body's shape, physique, demeanour and movements. The first things we observe as a patient comes in is probably the body shape, way of walking, general appearance, demeanour and personality. One can formulate a very good first impression of the patient's constitutional type in the first few minutes of the consultation simply by observing the above features. There are various ways of classifying body types and these are listed below bearing in mind that 'observation of the body' includes observation of the body's shape, physique, demeanour and personality.

Before describing and discussing the various body shapes and their clinical significance, we should first highlight two important principles of diagnosis by observation, i.e. the principle of correspondence between individual parts of the body and the whole, and the importance of observing and assessing constitutional traits. The latter is important because all the various body types reflect not a patient's actual, present disharmonies but his or her constitutional traits.

Correspondence between an individual part and the whole

One of the principles on which diagnosis by observation in Chinese medicine is based is that each single, small part of the body reflects the whole.

The face as a microsystem

The face is a very important example of this principle, as it is a reflection both of the Internal Organs and of various parts of the body. Chapter 32 of the 'Simple Questions' lists the correspondence of various parts of the face with Internal Organs, as follows: '*In Heat disease of the Liver, the left cheek becomes red; in Heat disease of the Heart, the forehead becomes red; in Heat disease of the Spleen, the nose becomes red; in Heat disease of the Lungs, the right cheek becomes red; in Heat disease of the Kidneys, the chin becomes red.*'[1] (See Fig. P1.1, p. 3.)

Chapter 49 of the 'Spiritual Axis' gives a more detailed map of the correspondence between Internal Organs and parts of the body and various areas of the face.[2] (See Fig. P1.2, p. 3.)

A careful observation of these face areas and their colours is an extremely important part of diagnosis by observation which should be always carried out. The correspondence between face areas and Internal Organs reveals three possible conditions:

- an actual disharmony, for example red cheeks may indicate Heat in the Lungs
- a constitutional trait, for example short earlobes may indicate weak Kidneys and short life
- an aetiological factor, for example a bluish colour on the forehead (related to the Heart according to the 'Simple Questions' correspondences) in a child may indicate prenatal shock.

The correspondence between face areas and Internal Organs should be integrated with the colour of the complexion in those areas and interpreted in the light of the Five Elements. For example, a greenish colour in the face area corresponding to the Spleen (i.e. the tip of the nose) indicates that the Liver is invading

the Spleen and that that particular Spleen disharmony is secondary to a Liver disharmony.

The ear as a microsystem

Ear acupuncture is a well-known application of the principle that a single, small part of the body reflects the whole: according to this theory, the ear resembles an upside-down fetus and there is a point in the ear pavilion that reflects a part or an organ of the body.

Microsystems over the whole body

According to recent theories, each part of the body is a miniature replica of the whole and can therefore reflect pathological changes of the whole body.

The following microsystems reflect this general hypothesis: ear acupuncture, facial colour diagnosis, iris diagnosis, tongue diagnosis, nose acupuncture, face acupuncture, foot acupuncture, etc. According to modern Chinese research, a certain part of the body can reflect the whole body: this principle can be used both in diagnosis and in treatment. Diseases of different parts of the body can be treated using points on a specific area of the body, such as the ear, hand or nose. Chinese researchers have identified 102 microsystems in the body as follows:

- metacarpal bone system: 5 on each side, 10 in total
- hand phalangeal bone system: 14 on each side, 28 in total
- radius system: 1 on each side, 2 in total
- ulna system: 1 on each side, 2 in total
- humerus system: 1 on each side, 2 in total
- femur system: 1 on each side, 2 in total
- tibia system: 1 on each side, 2 in total
- fibula system: 1 on each side, 2 in total
- metatarsal bone system: 5 on each side, 10 in total
- foot phalangeal bone system: 14 on each side, 28 in total
- ear system: 1 on each side, 2 in total
- face system: 1
- nose system: 1
- tongue system: 1
- body trunk system: 1
- neck system: 1
- scalp system: 1 in the middle, 1 on each side, 3 in total
- eye system: 1 on each eye, 2 in total
- foot system: 1 on each foot, 2 in total.[3]

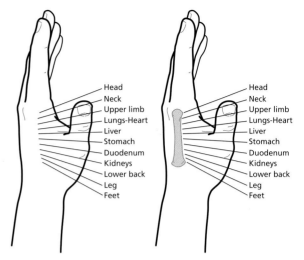

Fig. P1S1.1 Microsystems of diagnosis

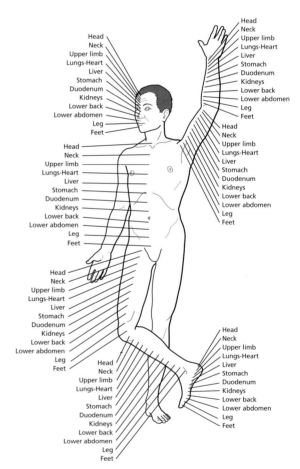

Fig. P1S1.2 Microsystems of the body according to Dr Zhang Ying Qing

This theory was first proposed by Zhang Ying Qing in 1973. In diagnosing and needling the side of the second metacarpal bone, he discovered that the points on this bone formed a pattern and constituted a miniature of the whole body (Fig. P1S1.1).

After repeated research, he discovered other microsystems all over the body (Fig. P1S1.2).

Observation of constitutional traits

The art of observation in Chinese medicine is based on two broad areas: observation of constitutional traits and observation of actual disharmony signs. For example, a tall, thin, sinewy body indicates a constitutional Wood type but it does not necessarily indicate any actual disharmony in the Liver or Gall-Bladder. Conversely, a person may belong constitutionally to a Fire type but have a pale-greenish complexion, brittle nails and dry hair indicating an actual Wood disharmony (in this example Liver-Blood deficiency).

Why is it necessary to observe constitutional traits if we need to treat the presenting disharmony? In the above example of a patient with a pale-greenish complexion, brittle nails and dry hair, we obviously need to nourish the Liver-Blood, whatever the observation of constitutional characteristics might indicate.

However, observation of constitutional traits is important for various reasons, described below.

1. A constitutional type indicates the *tendency* to certain disharmonies and it therefore allows us to forecast, and accordingly to prevent, a possible pathological development. For example, if a person with constitutional Yang excess suffers an invasion of Wind-Heat and a febrile illness, we can expect that person to have a strong tendency to develop an intense Heat pattern. In terms of the Four Levels, we can foretell that that person might enter the Qi level more quickly and with more Heat than another person: this means that we should be prepared for this and administer strong cooling herbs.

2. Observation of a constitutional type and tendency allows us to put the presenting disharmony into perspective, helping us to gauge its severity. For example, if a person with constitutional Yang excess develops a Heat pattern, that is a less severe situation than a Heat pattern in a person with constitutional Yin excess or constitutional Yang deficiency.

3. Observation of constitutional traits and the deviation or conformity of a person to his or her constitutional type gives us an idea of the severity of a problem and therefore prognosis. For example, it is better for a Wood type to have a Wood rather than a Fire disharmony. So, if a Wood type suffers from a Fire disharmony, this indicates a worse prognosis than that of a Fire type suffering from a Fire disharmony or a Wood type suffering from a Wood disharmony.

4. Observation of constitutional types is important to give patients an underlying treatment, irrespective of the presenting disharmony. It is always important to bear in mind the constitutional type and treat it accordingly. In the above example, if a person of a Wood type suffers from a Fire disharmony, it is obviously necessary to treat the presenting disharmony, but, perhaps afterwards, it would be good to treat also the Element type, that is Wood. The treatment of the underlying Element type is an important aspect of the preventive potential of Chinese medicine and it should always be applied.

5. Treatment of the constitutional Element type is particularly useful in the case of mental–emotional problems. For example, a Wood type might display some typical emotional traits such as indecision and inability to plan one's life: treatment of the Wood Element would help the person on a mental–emotional level, whatever other disharmony that person might suffer from.

6. Observation of the constitutional type and tendency of a patient allows us to forecast the type of disharmony that such a patient might be subject to in the future: this means that the preventive potential of Chinese medicine can be exploited to the full. For example, if people in their 40s display signs of constitutional Yang excess and also pertain to the Wood type, we know that such people may have a strong tendency to develop Liver-Yang rising with signs such as hypertension. This allows us to actively subdue Yang and pacify Wood even in the absence of any clinical manifestations.

7. Observation of the Element type is useful when a person displays all the traits of a certain Element type except for one detail; that is a bad sign even if that person may not suffer any disharmony yet. For example, if a person displays all the

BOX P1S1.1 THE IMPORTANCE OF OBSERVING CONSTITUTIONAL TRAITS

- A constitutional type indicates a *tendency* to certain disharmonies and therefore allows us to forecast and prevent a possible pathological development during the course of an illness.
- It allows us to put the presenting disharmony into perspective and helps us to gauge its severity.
- Deviation or conformity of a person to his or her constitutional type is a good measure of prognosis.
- It helps us to give patients a treatment appropriate to the underlying constitution, irrespective of the presenting disharmony.
- It is particularly useful in the treatment of mental–emotional problems.
- It allows us to forecast the type of disharmony that a patient might be subject to in the future and therefore to treat the patient preventatively.
- Deviation from an Elemental type in one detail may be a warning sign.

characteristics of the Fire type but walks slowly, this small detail tells us that something is amiss and that that person may develop a serious disharmony. This discrepancy might be particularly relevant in the case of the Fire type as we know that a Fire type may have a tendency to develop a serious pathology very suddenly.

Box P1S1.1 summarizes the important reasons for observing constitutional traits.

NOTES

1. 1979 The Yellow Emperor's Classic of Internal Medicine – Simple Questions (*Huang Di Nei Jing Su Wen* 黄帝内经素问), People's Health Publishing House, Beijing, p. 189. First published c. 100BC.
2. 1981 Spiritual Axis (*Ling Shu Jing* 灵枢经), People's Health Publishing House, Beijing, p. 97. First published c. 100BC.
3. Zhang Shu Sheng 1995 Great Treatise of Diagnosis by Observation in Chinese Medicine (*Zhong Hua Yi Xue Wang Zhen Da Quan* 中华医学望诊大全), Shanxi Science Publishing House, Taiyuan, p. 38.

Chapter **1**

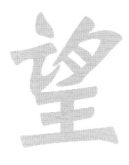

OBSERVATION OF THE BODY SHAPE, PHYSIQUE AND DEMEANOUR

Chapter contents

INTRODUCTION   *11*

CLASSIFICATION OF BODY SHAPE ACCORDING TO YIN AND YANG   *12*
   Body shape abundant in Yang   *12*
   Body shape abundant in Yin   *13*
   Body shape deficient in Yang   *14*
   Body shape deficient in Yin   *14*
   Body shape with Yin and Yang in balance   *15*

CLASSIFICATION OF BODY SHAPE ACCORDING TO THE FIVE ELEMENTS   *15*
   Wood type   *15*
   Fire type   *16*
   Earth type   *17*
   Metal type   *19*
   Water type   *19*
   Clinical application of the Five Element types   *21*

CLASSIFICATION OF BODY SHAPE ACCORDING TO PRENATAL AND POSTNATAL INFLUENCES   *21*
   Body shape with strong prenatal constitution   *21*
   Body shape with weak prenatal constitution   *23*
   Body shape with strong Postnatal Qi   *23*
   Body shape with weak Postnatal Qi   *24*

CLASSIFICATION ACCORDING TO BODY BUILD   *25*
   Robust type   *25*
   Compact type   *25*
   Muscular type   *26*
   Thin type   *26*
   Overweight type   *27*

CLASSIFICATION OF BODY SHAPE ACCORDING TO PAIN AND DRUG TOLERANCE   *27*
   Body shape indicating high pain and drug tolerance   *27*
   Body shape indicating low pain and drug tolerance   *28*

INTRODUCTION

The body shape of a person is determined by the prenatal constitution and subsequent postnatal nourishment: for this reason, the body shape of a person can give us an indication both of the constitutional *tendency* to a certain pathology and of an actual pathology resulting from postnatal influences. Observation of the body (including size, height, tone of skin and muscles, length of bones, etc.), as well as of demeanour and personality, is important to assess the constitution of a patient. Chapter 21 of the 'Simple Questions' says, '*In diagnosing diseases one should observe whether the patient is extrovert or timid and observe the state of the bones, muscles and skin in order to understand the condition so that we can diagnose and treat.*'[1] There are five different ways of classifying the body shape in Chinese medicine, which are described below:

1. According to Yin and Yang:
   —body shape abundant in Yang
   —body shape abundant in Yin
   —body shape deficient in Yang
   —body shape deficient in Yin
   —body shape with Yin and Yang in balance
2. According to the Five Elements:
   —Wood type
   —Fire type
   —Earth type
   —Metal type
   —Water type
3. According to prenatal and postnatal influences:
   —body shape with strong prenatal constitution
   —body shape with weak prenatal constitution
   —body shape with strong Postnatal Qi
   —body shape with weak Postnatal Qi

4. According to body build:
    —robust type
    —compact type
    —muscular type
    —thin type
    —overweight type
5. According to drug and pain tolerance:
    —body shape indicating high drug and pain tolerance
    —body shape indicating low drug and pain tolerance.

CLASSIFICATION OF BODY SHAPE ACCORDING TO YIN AND YANG

The possible body shapes according to Yin and Yang are:

> • body shape abundant in Yang
> • body shape abundant in Yin
> • body shape deficient in Yang
> • body shape deficient in Yin
> • body shape with Yin and Yang in balance.

Chapter 31 of Volume 4 of the 'Classic of Categories' (*Lei Jing*, 1624) summarizes the characteristics of people with a constitutional excess of Yin, people with a constitutional excess of Yang and people with a balance of Yin and Yang:

People gifted with pure Yin are known as the Greater-Yin type; those with a mixture of Yin and Yang but more Yin than Yang are known as the Lesser-Yin type; those with pure Yang are known as the Greater-Yang type; those with a mixture of Yin and Yang but more Yang than Yin are known as the Lesser-Yang type. Together with the type of people with equal Yang and Yin, these constitute the five different types of people. Therefore, for people with abundant-Yang constitution, it is advisable to use cooling methods of treatment. For people with abundant-Yin constitution, it is advisable to use warming methods of treatment.[2]

Body shape abundant in Yang
Observation

The body shape, demeanour and personality of a person with abundant Yang are as follows: strong body build, tendency to a red face, preference for cold, intol-

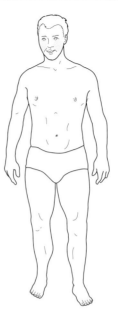

Fig. 1.1 Body shape abundant in Yang

erance of heat, preference for light clothes, lively character, active and talkative nature, loud voice, tendency to laugh, tendency to being a high achiever, decisiveness, assertiveness, walking with the chest and stomach projecting forward (Fig. 1.1).

Clinical significance

The above-mentioned features indicate abundant Yang (which could be of the Greater-Yang or Lesser-Yang type, as described in the quotations below). It is important to stress that such a body shape indicates only a constitutional *tendency* to excess of Yang and not necessarily an actual pattern of Yang excess. In pathological conditions, a person with an abundant-Yang constitution will have a tendency to excess of Yang, that is, Heat or Fire. In treatment, emphasis should be put on reducing Yang and nourishing Yin.

Quotations from the classics

The 'Spiritual Axis' in Chapter 72 says:

A Greater-Yang type of person looks arrogant with the chest and stomach projected forward as if the body was bending backwards. This is the picture of a Greater-Yang type of person. A Lesser-Yang type of person holds the head high while standing, and shakes the body while walking. The two hands are often held behind the body with the arms and elbows exposed on the side of the body. This is the picture of a Lesser-Yang type of person.[3]

. . .

A Greater-Yang type of person has excess of Yang and deficiency of Yin and it is necessary to examine them with great care and treat them so that the Yin is not reduced to the point of collapse. The Yang must be reduced but not excessively to the point of collapse, lest the patient develops madness.[4]

Chapter 67 of the same book says:

A person with abundant Yang is emotional and as warm as fire; he talks fast and is swollen with arrogance. It is because the Heart- and Lung-Qi of such a person are abundant; Yang-Qi is therefore plentiful and flows freely and vigorously. For this reason, it is easy to stimulate his spirit, and the Qi arrives quickly when acupuncture is given.[5]

The 'Golden Mirror of Medicine' (*Yi Zong Jin Jian*, 1742) points out in the chapter 'Keys to the Four Diagnostic Methods':

People with abundant Yang hold their head high while standing because it is in the nature of Yang to rise. They shake their body while walking because it is in the nature of Yang to move. They often hold their hands behind the body with the arms and elbows by the sides of the body as it is in the nature of Yang to be exposed. This is the picture of the personality of the Lesser-Yang type of people.[6]

The same book says:

The six external pathogenic factors attack people in the same way but diseases caused by them will have different manifestations in different people. Why? The reason is that a person's body can be either strong or weak, Qi can be full or deficient, and the internal organs can be of cold or hot. After the external pathogenic factors invade the body, they will transform according to the condition of the internal organs. Therefore, the syndromes vary. They can transform into deficient or excessive conditions, and into cold or hot conditions.[7]

This last quotation highlights an important principle of Chinese medicine: pathogenic factors tend to develop in their pathology according to the pre-existing constitution of the person. For example, if a person who is constitutionally abundant in Yang suffers an invasion of external Wind, this will develop into Wind-Heat, while if a person who is constitutionally abundant in Yin suffers the same invasion, the external Wind will manifest as Wind-Cold.

Body shape abundant in Yin
Observation

The typical characteristics of a person of the abundant-Yin type are: a tendency to obesity, relatively dark

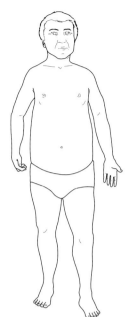

Fig. 1.2 Body shape abundant in Yin

complexion, loose muscles with thick skin, quiet, reticent and introverted nature, soft voice, a preference for heat and a desire to wrap up warm (Fig. 1.2).

Clinical significance

The above-mentioned features indicate an abundant-Yin constitution. It is important to stress that such a body shape indicates only a constitutional *tendency* to excess of Yin and not necessarily an actual pattern of Yin excess. In pathological conditions, a person with an abundant-Yin constitution will have a tendency to excess of Yin, that is, Cold, Dampness or Phlegm. Common patterns appearing in people with an abundant-Yin constitution include Cold, Dampness, Damp-Phlegm, Cold-Phlegm, Phlegm-Fluids, Qi stagnation, Blood stasis, etc. In treatment, emphasis should be put on reducing Yin, expelling Cold, resolving Dampness and Phlegm and tonifying Yang. At the same time, attention should be paid to regulating Qi and invigorating Blood.

Quotations from the classics

Chapter 72 of the 'Spiritual Axis' says:

Persons of the Greater-Yin type have a sombre countenance and pretend to be humble. They have the body build of a grown-up, but make themselves smaller by bending their back and knees slightly. This is the picture of a Greater-Yin type of person . . . They are restless while standing, and

walk as if to hide themselves. This is the picture of a Lesser-Yin type of person.[8]

...

Persons of the Greater-Yin type are constitutionally excessive in Yin and deficient in Yang. Their Yin and Blood are thick and turbid. Their Defensive Qi does not flow freely. Yin and Yang are not in a harmonious state, which leads to loose sinews and thick skin. When needling patients with an abundant-Yin constitution, only through reducing the Yin quickly and immediately can an improvement be expected.[9]

...

The Yellow Emperor asks: 'How is it that sometimes the body will react only after several acupuncture treatments?' Qi Bo answers, 'Such a person is excessive in Yin and deficient in Yang. The movement of Qi is restrained and therefore it is difficult for Qi to arrive when the patient is needled. This is the reason why the body will react to the acupuncture only after several treatments.[10]

The last passage clearly relates the ease or difficulty with which a patient reacts to acupuncture to the relative balance of Yin and Yang: patients with a constitutional abundance of Yin will react to acupuncture more slowly.

Body shape deficient in Yang
Observation
The typical characteristics of a person with the deficient-Yang type of body shape are as follows: overweight/swollen body, pale or pale-bluish complexion, listlessness, low spirits, slow movement, weak, loose muscles, a preference for warmth, aversion to cold, cold limbs and a desire to wrap up (Fig. 1.3).

Clinical significance
The above-mentioned body appearance indicates that the patient is constitutionally deficient in Yang. It is important to stress that such body shape indicates only a constitutional *tendency* to Yang deficiency: it does not necessarily follow that every person with such a body shape actually suffers from Yang deficiency.

When such a constitutional tendency does manifest with an actual Yang deficiency, these people will suffer symptoms of Cold, Cold-Dampness, Cold Phlegm, Damp-Phlegm and Phlegm-Fluids.

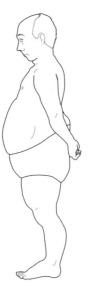

Fig. 1.3 Body shape deficient in Yang

Body shape deficient in Yin
Observation
The typical characteristics of a person with a deficient-Yin type of body shape are as follows: thin body build, sometimes red cheeks and lips, an excited look, a restless expression in eyes, a propensity to be excited, a feeling of heat and quick movements. People of Yin-deficient body shape are often deficient in Yin and excessive in Yang. The body is thin and tall with a long-

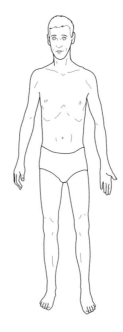

Fig. 1.4 Body shape deficient in Yin

shaped head, thin long neck, narrow shoulders and a narrow, long, flat chest. These people often bend forward when they walk or stand (Fig. 1.4).

Clinical significance

The above-mentioned features indicate a deficient-Yin constitution. It is important to stress that such a body shape indicates only a constitutional *tendency* to deficiency of Yin and not necessarily an actual pattern of Yin deficiency. In pathology, these patients will tend to Yin or Essence deficiency and hyperactivity of Yang. When they fall ill, they will easily develop Empty-Heat or Dryness.

Body shape with Yin and Yang in balance

Observation

The body shape with harmony of Yin and Yang is of medium build, not too tall or short, neither too stout nor thin. The movements are balanced and the personality is stable. People with such a constitution are better able to adapt themselves to changes caused by the stresses of life (Fig. 1.5).

Clinical significance

The above-mentioned features indicate a harmony of Yin and Yang. These people are less easily attacked by

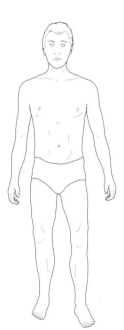

Fig. 1.5 Body shape with harmony of Yin and Yang

external pathogenic factors. When they do fall ill, the pathogenic factors are often not strong, the location of the disease is superficial and the disease itself is mild.

Quotations from the classics

Chapter 72 of the 'Spiritual Axis' says: *'People with the body shape with harmony of Yin and Yang look elegant and graceful.'*[11]

CLASSIFICATION OF BODY SHAPE ACCORDING TO THE FIVE ELEMENTS

The body shapes according to the Five Elements are:

- Wood type
- Fire type
- Earth type
- Metal type
- Water type.

Wood type

Observation

People of the Wood type have a subtle shade of green in their complexion, a relatively small head and long-shaped face, broad shoulders, straight back, tall, sinewy body and elegant hands and feet. In terms of personality, they have developed intelligence but their physical strength is poor. Hard workers, they think things over and tend to worry (Fig. 1.6, see also Plates 1.1 and 1.2 on p. P1).

Clinical significance

People of the Wood type often suffer from diseases caused by pathogenic factors in autumn and winter. They are in relatively good health in spring and summer.

Quotations from the classics

Chapter 64 of the 'Spiritual Axis' says:

The Wood type of people correspond to Shang Jiao of the note Jiao, which is one of the five notes and is related to the element of Wood. Their complexion colour is similar to that of the Green Emperor, who is one of the five heavenly emperors, and represents the East. Their complexion has a subtle green colour, they have a small head, long-shaped face, broad back and shoulders, straight body trunk and small hands and feet. They are intelligent, and keep their mind working hard. They are not strong physically. They

(a)

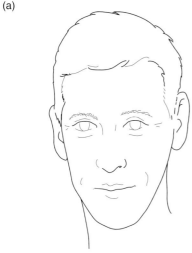

(b)

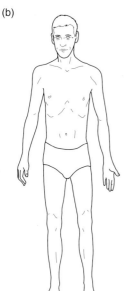

Fig. 1.6 Wood type: (a) face; (b) body

are often worried. They like Spring and Summer and dislike Autumn and Winter.[12]

...

People of the Wood type can tolerate Spring and Summer but not Autumn or Winter. In Autumn or Winter, they suffer from diseases caused by invasion of pathogenic factors.[13]

The chapter 'Key to the Four Diagnostic Methods' in the 'Golden Mirror of Medicine' (*Yi Zong Jin Jian*, 1742) says:

People of the Wood type respond to the colour green, which is at its best when, like green wood, there is moisture in it. People of the Wood type have a straight body just like the trunk of a tree. They have the so-called five kinds of Smallness, i.e. a small head, small hands and small feet, just like the twigs of a tree. They have the so-called five kinds of Thinness and Length, implying a long, thin body trunk and limbs, like the branches of a tree. Just as wood has various uses and can be cut in different ways as wanted, people of the Wood type are versatile, and are apt to intellectual work. Just as wood is seldom quiet [i.e. always swaying in wind and breeze], people of the Wood type tend to worry, and are often exhausted by what they do. If wood is not straight but is short and soft, it is not good timber for use.[14]

Box 1.1 summarizes the characteristics of the Wood type.

BOX 1.1 WOOD TYPE

- Greenish complexion
- Small head
- Long face
- Broad shoulders
- Straight back
- Sinewy body
- Tall
- Small hands and feet

Fire type

Observation

People of the Fire type have a red, florid complexion, wide teeth, a pointed, small head, possibly with a pointed chin, hair that is either curly or scanty, well-developed muscles of the shoulders, back, hips and head and relatively small hands and feet. In terms of personality, they are keen thinkers. The Fire type is quick, energetic and active. They are short-tempered. They walk firmly and shake their body while walking. They tend to think too much and often worry. They have a good spirit of observation and they analyse things deeply (Fig. 1.7, see also Plate 1.3 on p. P1).

Clinical significance

People of the Fire type are healthy in spring and summer but sick in autumn and winter from invasion of pathogenic factors. When compared with other Elemental types, people of the Fire type may tend to suffer a sudden death.

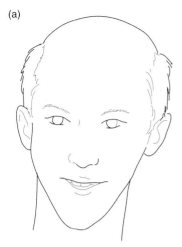

(a)

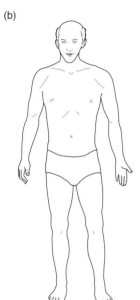

(b)

Fig. 1.7 Fire type: (a) face; (b) body

Quotations from the classics

Chapter 64 of the 'Spiritual Axis' says:

People of the Fire type correspond to Shang Zhi of the note Zhi, which is one of the five notes, and is related to the element of Fire. The colour of their complexion is similar to that of the Red Emperor, who was one of the five heavenly emperors, and represents the South. They have a red complexion, wide teeth, a thin small face, small head, well-developed and nice-looking shoulders, back, thighs and abdomen. They have small hands and feet. They walk with quick steps but tread the ground softly and soundlessly, and their body shakes as they walk. They are short-tempered. They act boldly and make light of money, but they are not

trustworthy. They worry too much. They have a good sense of judgment. The colour of their complexion is attractive, but they are short-tempered. They like Spring and Summer and dislike Autumn and Winter.[15]

. . .

People of the Fire type have a short life often ending with a sudden death. They can tolerate Spring and Summer but not Autumn or Winter. In Autumn or Winter they will suffer from diseases caused by invasion of pathogenic factors.[16]

The chapter 'Keys to the Four Diagnostic Methods' of the 'Golden Mirror of Medicine' says:

People of the Fire type have a red complexion which is best when it is also bright [i.e. with shen]. They have the so-called Five Pointed Structures, i.e. a pointed head, forehead, nose, face and mouth: they are similar to the pointed shape of a flame when it flares up . . . People of the Fire type are bold and daring because Fire is Yang in nature and rich in Qi. They make light of money, which is similar to the scattering nature of Fire. They are not trustworthy for just like a fire they are constantly changing. They tend to worry, mirroring the flickering of a flame. They move constantly just like a fire which is always moving. They are short-tempered, sharing fire's quickness and suddenness. If these people have symptoms of mental confusion and abnormality of Qi and colour, it means that their body is in disharmony.[17]

Box 1.2 summarizes the characteristics of the Fire type.

BOX 1.2 FIRE TYPE

- Red complexion
- Wide teeth
- Pointed, small head
- Well-developed shoulder muscles
- Curly hair or not much hair
- Small hands and feet
- Walking briskly

Earth type

Observation

People of the Earth type have a yellowish complexion, round-shaped face, relatively big head, wide jaws, well-developed and nice-looking shoulders and back, large abdomen, strong thigh and calf muscles, relatively small hands and feet, and well-built muscles of the whole body. They walk with firm steps without lifting

(a)

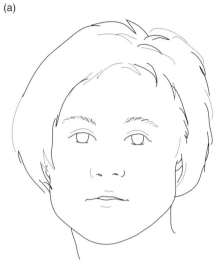

(b)

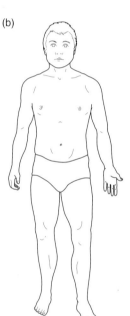

Fig. 1.8 Earth type: (a) face; (b) body

their feet very high. The Earth type is calm and generous, has a steady character, likes to help people and is not overambitious. It is easy to get on with (Fig. 1.8, see also Plate 1.4 on p. P1).

Clinical significance

People of the Earth type are in relatively good health in autumn and winter. They fall prey easily to invasions of pathogenic factors in spring and summer.

Quotations from the classics

Chapter 64 of the 'Spiritual Axis' says:

The Earth type of people correspond to Shang Gong of the note Gong which is one of the five notes, and is related to the element of Earth. Their complexion is similar in colour to that of the Yellow Emperor, who is one of the five heavenly emperors and represents the Centre. They have a yellow complexion, round-shaped face, large head and well-developed and nice-looking shoulders and back. The abdomen is large and their thighs and legs strong and well-built. They have small hands and feet, but well-developed muscles. Every part of their body, from the upper to the lower, is well proportioned. They walk steadily, and are trustworthy. They are calm and like to help people. They are not interested in pursuing power or position. They like to establish good relations with other people. They like Autumn and Winter and dislike Spring and Summer.[18]

The chapter 'Key to the Four Diagnostic Methods' of the 'Golden Mirror of Medicine' says:

People of the Earth type respond to the yellow colour, which is best when it is also shiny. They have the so-called Five Kinds of Roundness similar to the round shape of the Earth. They have the so-called Five Kinds of Solidity and Thickness which in nature resemble the solid Earth. They have the so-called Five Kinds of Shortness which is similar to the appearance of the Earth being solid and short. Although people with the Earth type of body have the characteristics of roundness, solidity, thickness and shortness, each person will have a particular, individual shape. The round face, the big head, the large abdomen and the well-built shoulders and legs all resemble the dense and solid appearance of the Earth. People of the Earth type are sincere and trustworthy. They take their time in doing things. They are calm at heart. All these characteristics mirror the nature of Earth in being honest and reliable.[19]

Box 1.3 summarizes the characteristics of the Earth type.

BOX 1.3 EARTH TYPE

- Yellowish complexion
- Round face
- Wide jaws
- Large head
- Well-developed shoulders and back
- Large abdomen
- Large thighs and calf muscles
- Well-built muscles

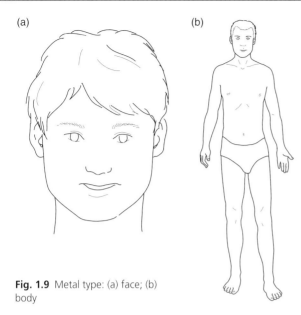

Fig. 1.9 Metal type: (a) face; (b) body

Metal type
Observation

People of the Metal type have a relatively pale complexion, a square-shaped face, a relatively small head, small shoulders and upper back, a relatively flat abdomen, and small hands and feet. They have a strong voice, move swiftly and have keen powers of thought. They are honest and upright. They are generally quiet and calm in a solid way, but also capable of decisive action when necessary. They have a natural aptitude for leadership and management (Fig. 1.9, see also Plate 1.5 on p. P2).

Clinical significance

People of the Metal type are in relatively good health in autumn and winter, but may suffer ill health in spring and summer.

Quotations from the classics

Chapter 64 of the 'Spiritual Axis' says:

People of the Metal type correspond to Shang [a musical note] while keeping still, but are intrepid and fierce when active. They have a natural aptitude for leadership and management . . . People of the Metal type correspond to Shang, which is one of the five notes and is related to the element of Metal. Their complexion is similar to that of the White Emperor, who is one of the five heavenly emperors and represents the West. They have a relatively pale complexion, a
small head, small shoulders and upper back, a flat abdomen, and small hands and feet. They have strong heels as if the bones grew outside rather than in. They are quick and swift in movement, and are honest and upright in personality. They are short-tempered. They appear quiet and calm when keeping still, but fierce and bold once they make a move. They have the talent to be officials. They like Autumn and Winter and dislike Spring and Sunmer.[20]

. . .

People of the Metal type can tolerate Autumn and Winter but not Spring or Summer when they may suffer diseases from invasion of external pathogenic factors.[21]

The chapter 'Keys to the Four Diagnostic Methods' of the 'Golden Mirror of Medicine' says:

People of the Metal type correspond to the colour white and their complexion is best when it is pure. They have the so-called Five Kinds of Squareness similar to the square structure of metal. They have the so-called Five Kinds of Moisture similar to the quality of metal under water. Individuals who deviate from the typical characteristic of Metal may not display square and regular features. If the muscles become thinner, their bones will show. These are all signs of exhaustion. People of the Metal type are quiet and calm when keeping still but fierce once in action. This mirrors the nature of metal which is silent and resilient. People of this kind are honest and upright as metal is pure and strong in quality. As officials, people of the Metal type are awesome and dignified just as metal is solemn.[22]

Box 1.4 summarizes the characteristics of the Metal type.

BOX 1.4 METAL TYPE

- Pale complexion
- Square face
- Small head
- Small shoulders and upper back
- Flat abdomen
- Strong voice

Water type
Observation

People of the Water type have a relatively dark complexion, wrinkles, a relatively big head, a round face and body, broad cheeks, narrow and small shoulders and a large abdomen. They keep their body in motion while walking and find it difficult to keep still. They

(a)
(b)

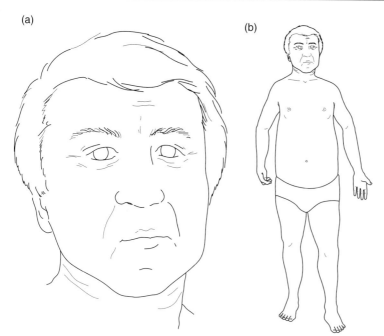

Fig. 1.10 Water type: (a) face; (b) body

have a long spine. The Water type is sympathetic and slightly laid-back. They are good negotiators and loyal to their work colleagues. They are aware and sensitive (Fig. 1.10, see also Plates 1.6 and 1.7 on p. P2).

Clinical significance

People of the Water type are often in relatively good health in autumn and winter but not in spring or summer when they may suffer diseases from invasion of external pathogenic factors.

Quotations from the classics

Chapter 64 of the 'Spiritual Axis' says:

People of the Water type correspond to Shang Yu of the note Yu, which is one of the five notes and is related to the Water element. Their complexion is similar in colour to that of the Black Emperor, who was one of the heavenly emperors and represents North. They have a relatively dark complexion, wrinkled face, a big head, broad cheeks, small shoulders and a large abdomen. Their hands and feet are seldom at rest, and their body quivers while walking. They have a long spine. They like Autumn and Winter and dislike Spring and Summer.[23]

The chapter 'Keys to the Four Diagnostic Methods' in the 'Golden Mirror of Medicine' says:

People of the Water type correspond to the colour purple, and their complexion is best when it possesses lustre. Their face is fat and uneven just as the sea's surface is vast and rolling with waves. They have the so-called Five Kinds of Fatness just as water is wide. They have the so-called Five Kinds of Tenderness mirroring the moistness of water. They have the so-called Five Kinds of Smoothness resembling the clear nature of water. With a fat body build, people of the Water type tend to have a mobile body when they walk, mirroring the flowing movement of water. This kind of people have no respect for anybody nor do they fear; like water, they always run to a lower place. They pretend to be humble but actually tend to be deceivers; water, too, feels empty and lacking a solid structure.[24]

Box 1.5 summarizes the characteristics of the Water type.

BOX 1.5 WATER TYPE
• Dark complexion   • Wrinkly skin   • Large head   • Broad cheeks   • Narrow shoulders   • Large abdomen   • Long spine

Clinical application of the Five Element types

The first thing to note is that very few people will display all the characteristics of a 'pure' Element type as there will always be deviations from the ideal type caused by life influences. For example, the Wood type should have a tall and slender body; however, if they overeat they may develop a large abdomen. It is important, therefore, when evaluating an Element type, to take into account all physical and behavioural characteristics of the patient. In the above example, if we drew a conclusion only from observation of the large abdomen, we might wrongly conclude that that person is an Earth type. Vice versa, an Earth type should have a relatively large abdomen and large thighs; however, if they lose weight due to a serious disease such as cancer, they may not have a large abdomen and thighs and we should pay attention to all the other physical characteristics.

Secondly, each Element type should have a strong point (Box 1.6) and a weakness in that area indicates a poor prognosis. For example, people of the Wood type should have strong sinews; if they do not, it indicates a possible illness. People of the Fire type should walk fast and their strong point should be the Heart and blood vessels; for the Fire type to walk slowly indicates a potential problem. People of the Earth type should have strong muscles; if they do not it indicates a weakness in the Stomach and Spleen and the tendency to rheumatism. People of the Metal type should walk slowly and deliberately and their voice should be strong; if they walk fast and their voice is weak it indicates a potential problem. People of the Water type should have strong Kidneys and may easily suffer from overindulgence in sexual activity.

BOX 1.6 STRONG POINTS OF ELEMENT TYPES

- Wood: strong sinews
- Fire: strong heart and blood vessels
- Earth: strong muscles
- Metal: strong voice
- Water: strong Kidneys

Thirdly, patients should be observed carefully and their Element type assessed so that deviations from the type can be noted. If a person has a certain trait which is unrelated to the person's particular type, the prognosis is worse than if the trait represents an exaggeration of a trait that is normal for that type. For example, people of the Fire type should walk fast; if they walk too fast it is not so bad as a Metal type walking fast (as the Metal type should walk slowly and deliberately). Another example: if a Metal type has too loud a voice, it is not so bad as another type having a loud voice.

Finally, the prognosis is better if a person of a certain Element type suffers from a disharmony in the same Element rather than in another Element. For example, it is better for a Wood type to suffer from a disharmony in this (for example Liver-Qi stagnation) than in another Element (for example Lung-Qi deficiency, Heart-Fire, Spleen-Yang deficiency or Kidney-Yin deficiency).

CLASSIFICATION OF BODY SHAPE ACCORDING TO PRENATAL AND POSTNATAL INFLUENCES

The body shapes according to prenatal and postnatal influences are as follows:

- body shape with strong prenatal constitution
- body shape with weak prenatal constitution
- body shape with strong Postnatal Qi
- body shape with weak Postnatal Qi.

Body shape with strong prenatal constitution

Observation

People with a strong prenatal constitution have a full and broad forehead and glabella (the frontal bone between the eyebrows). Their nose is long and wide. The area from the cheek to the front of the ear is wide with well-developed muscles. The lower jaw is high, thick and protruding. The ear is long, wide and regular-shaped with long ear-lobes. The eyes, nose, ears and mouth are well spaced and in the right proportion to each other. The philtrum (the vertical depression between the nose and mouth) is long. The complexion is normal in colour and lustrous. Breathing is even and smooth. The bones, muscles and skin are strong. The whole body is full of life.

Clinical significance

The above features indicate a good prenatal constitution: when this person is ill, the disease is easy to treat.

People with a strong prenatal constitution generally have a long life and they are able to survive even serious illnesses. A strong prenatal constitution often explains why one person can survive a serious disease such as cancer, where another person does not. A person with a strong constitution may also 'get away with' living in an unhealthy way and still live a long life. Of course, it is also possible to ruin a good prenatal constitution through unhealthy living. A good prenatal constitution is very often the crucial determining factor in prognosis.

To summarize, the main features indicating a good prenatal constitution are as follows (Fig. 1.11):

- broad forehead and glabella
- long and wide nose
- full cheeks
- strong lower jaw
- long ears with long ear-lobes
- well-proportioned eyes, nose, ears and mouth
- long philtrum
- normal complexion with lustre
- even and smooth breathing
- firm muscles and skin.

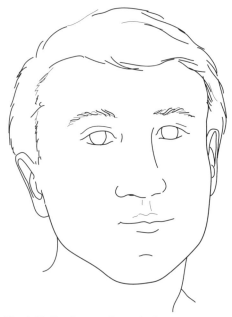

Fig. 1.11 Good prenatal constitution

Quotations from the classics

Chapter 37 of the 'Spiritual Axis' says:

A life as long as 100 years can be expected if the forehead and glabella are full and broad; the cheek and the area from the cheek to the front of the ear have well-developed muscles and protrude from the face, connecting a strong lower jaw and long ear lobes together; the eyes, nose, ears and mouth are well spaced and well proportioned; the face colour is normal. These people have abundant Qi and Blood. Their skin and muscles are strong. They respond well to acupuncture treatment.[25]

Chapter 54 of the same book says:

A person will have a long life if the five Yin organs are strong, blood circulates normally without obstruction, the skin is firm, the circulation of Nutritive and Defensive Qi is normal, breathing is regular, Qi circulates smoothly, and the six Yang organs transform and transport the food essences and body fluids smoothly to all parts of the body, maintaining its normal physiological functions . . . People with long life expectancy have long and deep nostrils. The muscles of the cheek and of the area from the cheek to the front of the ear are thick and high and well formed. The circulation of Nutritive and Defensive Qi is smooth. The upper, middle and lower parts of the face are in the right proportion, with well-developed and distinct muscles and prominent bones. People of this type can live out their normal life expectancy, or even up to the age of 100.[26]

Chapter 6 says:

People with a strong body build and relaxed skin, in whom Qi flows smoothly, will live a long life; while those with a strong body build but tense skin, in whom Qi stagnates, will die young. A strong build, a big pulse and a firm Exterior and Interior are signs of longevity; a strong build but a weak, empty pulse, a deficient Interior and a strong Exterior, with empty Qi, indicate a short life. A strong build but hollow, small zygomatic bones indicate weak bones and a short life expectancy; a strong build with well-developed muscles indicates long life; a strong build but with weak and underdeveloped muscles indicates a short life. These are all signs of pre-natal constitution which give an indication of life expectancy. As medical practitioners, we must understand the connection between body build and body shape so that we may have an idea of the patient's life expectancy.[27]

The chapter 'Keys to the Four Diagnostic Methods' in the 'Golden Mirror of Medicine' says: *'If the forehead is high, the glabella is full, the nose is high and straight, the*

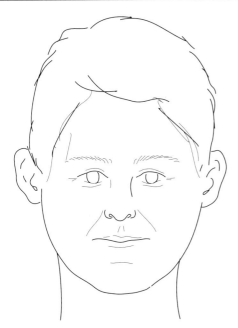

Fig. 1.12 Weak prenatal constitution

cheeks are full and the skeleton is well built, the person will have a long life expectancy.'[28]

Body shape with weak prenatal constitution

Observation

The physical features of people with a weak prenatal constitution are as follows: the eyes, nose, ears and mouth are close together; the forehead is narrow and the space between the eyebrows small; the nose is narrow with nostrils turned up and exposed; the philtrum is short; the cheek and the area between the cheek and the front of the ears are narrow; the ears are short, small and turning outwards; the lower jaw is flat, sunken, low and narrow; breathing is coarse and the skin is loose (Fig. 1.12).

Clinical significance

When the above-mentioned physical features are observed, they indicate that the person has a poor prenatal constitution. These people will have a tendency to suffer from a deficiency of Qi, Blood, Yin or Yang. Compared with people with a strong prenatal constitution, these people are more easily invaded by external pathogenic factors and, when this occurs, the treatment will be relatively more difficult.

Quotations from the classics

Chapter 37 of the 'Spiritual Axis' says:

When the five senses are not sharp, the forehead and glabella are narrow, the nose is small, the area between the cheek and the front of the ears is narrow, the lower jaw is flat and the ears turn outwards, the pre-natal constitution is poor even though the complexion and colour may be normal. These people are intrinsically unhealthy, even more so when they are ill.[29]

Chapter 54 of the same book says:

When the five Yin organs are weak, the nostrils are small and splay outwards, breathing is shallow, the cheek muscles are sunken, the pulse is thin and weak and the muscles are loose, the person is easily invaded by Wind-Cold. As a result, Qi and Blood become more deficient, and the circulation in the vessels is impaired, which will predispose the person to further invasions of pathogenic factors.[30]

Body shape with strong Postnatal Qi

Observation

Physical features indicating strong Postnatal Qi are as follows: ruddy complexion with lustre, strong body build with solid muscles and firm, elastic skin, shiny

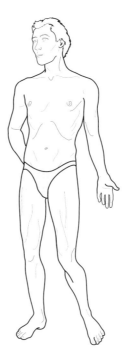

Fig. 1.13 Strong Postnatal Qi

hair with moisture, vigour and swift movements (Fig. 1.13).

Note that the features indicating strong Prenatal Qi relate more to the actual structure of the face, ears, nose, eyes and mouth and to the body build (i.e. inherited features), while the features indicating strong Postnatal Qi relate to lustre, hair, muscles (i.e. features subject to the state of Qi and Blood).

Clinical significance

The above features indicate a good Postnatal Qi. The Spleen and Stomach are strong, and they function properly. Qi, Blood, Yin and Yang are abundant and the body will not be easily attacked by external pathogenic factors. If there is any disease, it will be easy to treat.

Quotations from the classics

The chapter 'On the Pre-natal and Post-natal' of the 'Complete Works of Jing Yue' (*Jing Yue Quan Shu*, 1624) says:

If the pre-natal constitution is good, life will be long; if the pre-natal constitution is weak, life may be short. If people with a good pre-natal constitution take care of their post-natal Qi [with a good lifestyle and diet], they may live even longer; if people with a poor pre-natal constitution do not take care of their post-natal Qi [instead following a poor lifestyle and diet], their life may be even shorter. The build of the skeleton depends on the pre-natal constitution, while the build of the muscles depends on the post-natal Qi. The spirit [Shen] reflects the pre-natal constitution, while the complexion reflects the post-natal Qi. A deep colour of the complexion indicates long life, while a tender, light colour may indicate a short life. A strong, loud voice may indicate a long life, while a feeble voice may indicate a short one. A strong body build may indicate a long life while a weak body build may indicate a short one. One should also differentiate the mental state, paying attention to whether it is calm or restless: a calm mental state may indicate long life while a restless mental state may indicate a short one. As for the development of the body in youth, if a person appears weak when young, but grows stronger as he or she grows up, it is a good sign.[31]

Body shape with weak Postnatal Qi
Observation

The physical features of people with weak Postnatal Qi are as follows: poor energy, haggard, sallow complex-

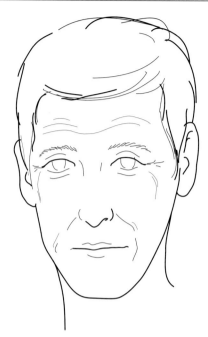

Fig. 1.14 Weak Postnatal Qi

ion, dry, withered hair, a thin, small build and loose skin without elasticity (Fig. 1.14).

Note that the features indicating weak Prenatal Qi relate more to the actual structure of the face, ears, nose, eyes and mouth and to the body build (i.e. inherited features), while the features indicating weak Postnatal Qi relate to lustre, hair, muscles (i.e. features subject to the state of Qi and Blood).

Clinical significance

When the above-mentioned physical features are observed, it indicates that the person has weak Postnatal Qi. The Spleen and Stomach are weak and Qi, Blood, Yin and Yang are deficient. The body will be easily invaded by pathogenic factors and any diseases will be of a deficient nature.

Quotations from the classics

The 'Complete Works of Jing Yue' says:

A person's life expectancy is determined by their pre-natal constitution. If the pre-natal constitution is good and the person receives good post-natal Qi, life expectancy may be long. If the pre-natal constitution is deficient, and the post-natal Qi is poor, life expectancy will be short. If people pay attention to this [i.e. influencing the pre-natal constitution through the post-natal nourishment], those with a short

life expectancy can increase it. If people neglect these factors [i.e. they ruin their pre-natal constitution through poor post-natal Qi], those with a high life expectancy can decrease it. What we are born with [i.e. our pre-natal constitution] can exceed what we can reach by our efforts [i.e. our post-natal Qi]; conversely, what can be reached by our efforts [i.e. our post-natal Qi] can exceed what we were born with [i.e. our pre-natal constitution]. The pre-natal constitution is largely determined by that of the parents while the post-natal Qi is determined by our own efforts.[32]

> **!**
>
> **Remember:** make an assessment of the constitution of the patient from the observation of the body shape. A strong or weak post- or prenatal constitution gives us an immediate idea of the patient's general health and prognosis.

CLASSIFICATION ACCORDING TO BODY BUILD

Chapters 38 and 59 of the 'Spiritual Axis' describe five types of body shape: robust, compact, muscular, thin and overweight. The physical characteristics of these five types generally coincide with those according to Yin and Yang mentioned above; for example, the robust type has a tendency to abundance of Yang, the thin type has a tendency to deficiency of Blood or Yin, the overweight type has a tendency to deficiency of Yang, etc.

The five body shapes described in these chapters of the 'Spiritual Axis' indicate inherited constitutional traits and not acquired ones; for example, the overweight type is constitutionally overweight from an early age and not someone who becomes overweight through overeating and lack of exercise.

The classification of the body type according to body build is as follows:

- robust type
- compact type
- muscular type
- thin type
- overweight type.

Robust type
Observation

People of the robust type have large, firm muscles, smooth moist skin, a large abdomen, intolerance to

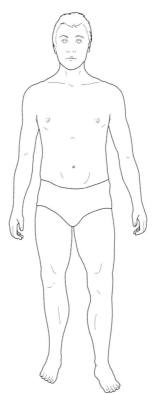

Fig. 1.15 Robust body type

heat and a preference for cold. Figure 1.15 shows a robust body type.

Clinical significance

The above-mentioned physical features indicate that the person has a constitutional abundance of Yang-Qi. Such a person has strong resistance to cold. These people will have a tendency to diseases of Hot nature.

Quotations from the classics

Chapter 59 of the 'Spiritual Axis' says: *'Robust people are rich in Qi, and abundant Qi will keep the body warm. Therefore, they have strong resistance to cold.'*[33]

Compact type
Observation

People of the compact type have the following physical features: a small skeleton, compact solid muscles, thick fat under the skin and a small but full body build. Figure 1.16 shows a compact body type.

Clinical significance

The above-mentioned physical features indicate that the person has a smooth circulation of Qi and Blood,

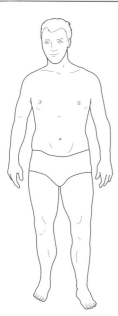

Fig. 1.16 Compact body type

but he or she may also have a tendency to Qi and Blood deficiency. The diseases these people suffer from are either Cold in nature due to deficiency of Qi, or are Hot in nature due to deficiency of Blood.

Quotations from the classics

Chapter 59 of the 'Spiritual Axis' says: *'The muscles of compact type of people are compact and solid, and their skin is full and tight . . . People with a compact body build have compact muscles but a small body . . . Although people with a compact body build have some fat, their body build is not big.'*[34]

Muscular type
Observation

The physical features of people of the muscular type are as follows: large skeleton, plump and solid body build with the skin and muscles compacted tightly together. Figure 1.17 shows a muscular body type.

Clinical significance

The above-mentioned physical features indicate that the person has abundant Blood and harmonious Qi. Such a person will not be easily invaded by pathogenic factors.

Quotations from the classics

Chapter 59 of the 'Spiritual Axis' says: *'People of the muscular type have skin and muscles tightly compacted*

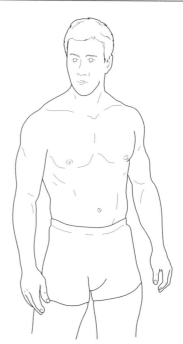

Fig. 1.17 Muscular body type

together . . . big, broad body size . . . and large limbs' and also: *'People of the muscular type have abundant Qi, their body build is full and strong and their Qi is harmonious.'*[35]

Thin type
Observation

People of the thin type have the following physical features: thin body build, thin muscles and lips and a feeble voice. Figure 1.18 shows a thin body type.

Clinical significance

The above-mentioned physical features indicate that the person's Qi and Blood circulate smoothly. Thin, pale people have a tendency to deficiency of Qi and Blood. In treatment, attention should be paid to tonifying and caution should be exercised when eliminating pathogenic factors. Thin people with a relatively dark complexion tend to suffer from Yin deficiency and possibly Empty-Heat. In herbal treatment, warm and drying herbs (which have a tendency to injure Yin) should be used with caution.

Quotations from the classics

Chapter 38 of the 'Spiritual Axis' says: *'Thin type of people have thin pale skin as well as thin muscles and lips.*

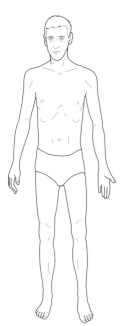

Fig. 1.18 Thin body type

They talk in a feeble voice. Their Blood is clear, and their Qi is smooth and slippery. Their Qi will dissipate easily, and their Blood will exhaust easily. Therefore, when needling these people, insertion should be superficial and the needles should be withdrawn quickly.'[36]

Overweight type
Observation

The overweight body type has loose skin and muscles, fat abdomen and thighs, moves slowly and often becomes breathless on walking.

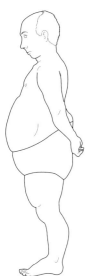

Fig. 1.19 Overweight body type

Clinical significance

The overweight body type indicates either an actual condition of Damp-Phlegm with Qi deficiency or a predisposition to it. Figure 1.19 shows an overweight type.

CLASSIFICATION OF BODY SHAPE ACCORDING TO PAIN AND DRUG TOLERANCE

The body shapes indicating high or low tolerance to drugs and pain may be either constitutional or the result of postnatal influences.

The body shape may be classified according to drug and pain tolerance as follows:

- body shape indicating high pain and drug tolerance
- body shape indicating low pain and drug tolerance.

Body shape indicating high pain and drug tolerance
Observation

People with a high drug (including herbs) and pain tolerance have certain physical features: the complexion is relatively dark, the body build is big and full with a strong skeleton, the tendons are soft, the muscles are loose and the skin firm.

Clinical significance

The above-mentioned physical features indicate that the person has strong drug and pain tolerance. When treating such a patient, the practitioner should be aware of the strong drug and pain tolerance and consider using medicines in relatively large doses.

Quotations from the classics

Chapter 53 of the 'Spiritual Axis' says:

The Yellow Emperor asks Shao Yu: 'People's tendons and bones can be strong or weak, the muscles can be solid or loose, the skin can be thick or thin, the space between skin and muscles can be firm or weak, how does this affect people's tolerance of pain caused by needling and the burning of the moxa? People's stomach and intestines can be strong or weak, how does this affect their tolerance of medicinal drugs? I hope that you will explain this to me in

detail.' Shao Yu answers: 'People with strong bones, soft tendons, relaxed muscles and thick skin, have a strong tolerance to pain. They can tolerate pain caused by needling as well as the burning of moxa.' The Yellow Emperor asks: 'How can you know that people can tolerate the burning pain of moxibustion?' Shao Yu answers: 'In the above-mentioned people who have strong bones, soft tendons, relaxed muscles and thick skin, if their complexion colour is relatively dark and their skeleton is well-built and strong, they can tolerate the burning pain of moxibustion. People with a thick stomach, dark complexion colour, solid skeleton and a large body build have sufficient Qi and Blood. They have a good tolerance to medicinal drugs.'[37]

Chapter 50 of the same book says:

The Yellow Emperor says: 'The tolerance of pain does not depend only on the courage of a person. A person who is brave but intolerant of pain, will act without fear in a difficult and dangerous situation, but he or she cannot stand pain. Vice versa, a person who is cowardly but tolerant of pain, will be panic-stricken in a difficult and dangerous situation, but he or she will tolerate pain. A person who is brave and also tolerant of pain is not afraid in a difficult and dangerous situation and can also tolerate pain. A person who is timid and intolerant of pain will be overwhelmed by difficulties, danger or pain: these people will be so afraid that their heads spin and their vision is blurred; they lose their voices and become pale; they cannot look people in the eye and their hearts beat violently. They are scared to death. I have encountered all these kinds of people, but I do not know what the causes are. I would like to know the reasons.' Shao Yu answers: 'Tolerance to pain depends on whether the skin is thin or thick and the muscles are solid or weak and loose or tense. It cannot be determined by the bravery or cowardice of a person.'[38]

Chapter 70 of the 'Simple Questions' says: 'For people who have strong drug tolerance, use medicines with strong flavours and medicinal action. For people who have weak drug tolerance, use medicines of mild flavour and medicinal action.'[39]

Body shape indicating low pain and drug tolerance
Observation
The body shape indicating a low tolerance of pain and drugs is as follows: a thin body, solid muscles and thin, tender, loose skin.

Clinical significance
The above physical features indicate that the person has a relatively lower tolerance to pain and medicinal drugs. Such a patient tends to complain more about the illness and does not tolerate Chinese herbal medicines well: we should therefore use lower doses when treating these patients.

Quotations from the classics
Chapter 53 of the 'Spiritual Axis' says: 'People with solid muscles and thin skin are intolerant of pain caused by needling and of the burning pain of moxibustion . . . People who are thin with a weak Stomach cannot tolerate the strong irritation of medicinal herbs.'[40]

NOTES

1. 1979 The Yellow Emperor's Classic of Internal Medicine – Simple Questions (Huang Di Nei Jing Su Wen 黄帝内经素问), People's Health Publishing House, Beijing, p. 138. First published c. 100BC.
2. Zhang Jie Bin 1982 Classic of Categories (Lei Jing 类经), People's Health Publishing House, Beijing, p. 99. First published in 1624.
3. 1981 Spiritual Axis (Ling Shu Jing 灵枢经), People's Health Publishing House, Beijing, p. 129. First published c. 100BC.
4. Ibid., p. 130.
5. Ibid., p. 123.
6. Wu Qian 1977 Golden Mirror of Medicine (Yi Zong Jin Jian 医宗金鉴), People's Health Publishing House, Beijing, vol. 2, p. 889. First published in 1742.
7. Cited in Zhang Shu Sheng 1995 Great Treatise of Diagnosis by Observation in Chinese Medicine (Zhong Hua Yi Xue Wang Zhen Da Quan 中华医学望诊大全), Shanxi Science Publishing House, Taiyuan, p. 44.
8. Spiritual Axis, p. 130.
9. Ibid., p. 130.
10. Ibid., p. 129.
11. Ibid., p. 130.
12. Ibid., p. 115.
13. Ibid., p. 115.
14. Golden Mirror of Medicine, vol. 2, p. 885.
15. Spiritual Axis, p. 115.
16. Ibid.
17. Golden Mirror of Medicine, p. 885.
18. Spiritual Axis, p. 115.
19. Golden Mirror of Medicine, vol. 2, p. 886.
20. Spiritual Axis, p. 116.
21. Ibid., p. 116.
22. Golden Mirror of Medicine, vol. 2, p. 886.
23. Spiritual Axis, p. 116.
24. Golden Mirror of Medicine, vol. 2, pp. 886–887.
25. Spiritual Axis, p. 78.
26. Ibid., p. 102.
27. Ibid., p. 19.
28. Golden Mirror of Medicine, vol. 2, p. 871.
29. Spiritual Axis, p. 78.
30. Ibid., p. 103.
31. Zhang Jing Yue 1986 The Complete Works of Jing Yue (Jing Yue Quan Shu 景岳全书), Shanghai Science and Technology Press, Shanghai, p. 19. First published in 1624.
32. Ibid., p. 19.

33. Spiritual Axis, p. 108.
34. Ibid., p. 108.
35. Ibid., p. 108.
36. Ibid., p. 79.

37. Ibid., p. 102.
38. Ibid., p. 99.
39. Simple Questions, p. 456.
40. Spiritual Axis, p. 102.

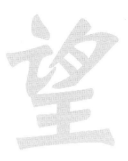

Chapter **2**

OBSERVATION OF THE MIND, SPIRIT AND EMOTIONS

Chapter contents

INTRODUCTION   31

THE THREE ASPECTS OF THE SPIRIT   32
  The embodiment of the Spirit   32
  The vitality of the Spirit   32
  The lustre of the Spirit   33

THE THREE CONDITIONS OF THE SPIRIT   33
  Strong Spirit   33
  Weak Spirit   34
  False Spirit   34

THE SPIRIT AND CONSTITUTION   34
  Strong Spirit and strong constitution   35
  Weak Spirit and weak constitution   35
  Weak Spirit and strong constitution   35
  Strong Spirit and weak constitution   36

THE SPIRIT AND THE EMOTIONS   36
  Eyes   36
  Complexion   36
  Tongue   36

INTRODUCTION

The Chinese character 'Shen' has many different meanings in Chinese medicine, the main ones being, of course, Mind and Spirit. It should be remembered here that I translate as 'Mind' the 'Shen' pertaining to and residing in the Heart, while I translate as 'Spirit' the total of the Five Spiritual Aspects, i.e. the Ethereal Soul (*Hun*) residing in the Liver, the Corporeal Soul (*Po*) residing in the Lungs, the Intellect (*Yi*) residing in the Spleen, the Will-Power (*Zhi*) residing in the Kidneys and the Mind (*Shen*) itself residing in the Heart.

> **!**
>
> **Remember**: I translate the *Shen* of the Heart as 'Mind' and the complex of *Hun, Po, Yi, Zhi* and *Shen* itself as 'Spirit'.

The Mind and Spirit are formed from the Prenatal Essences of the parents and are nourished by the Postnatal Essence of food and water taken in by the body. For example, Chapter 32 of the 'Spiritual Axis' says: *'The Mind and Spirit result from the transformation of the Essence of food and water.'*[1]

Chapter 9 of the 'Simple Questions' says:

Heaven provides human beings with the five Qi [air] and Earth provides human beings with the five flavours [food]. The air is absorbed through the nose, and is stored in the Lungs and Heart. It ascends to make the complexion bright and lustrous and the voice sonorous. The food is taken through the mouth, and is stored in the Stomach and Intestines. After the food is digested and absorbed, the food Essence is delivered to the five Yin organs and therefore nourishes the Qi of the five Yin organs. When the Qi of the five Yin organs is in a state of harmony, the body can trans-

form properly, body fluids are produced normally and the Mind and Spirit are formed.[2]

The Essence, Qi and Blood are the material foundation of the Mind and Spirit and, conversely, the Mind and Spirit are the external manifestation of Essence, Qi and Blood. Chapter 18 of the 'Spiritual Axis' says: *'The Stomach is in the Middle Burner, it opens into the Upper Burner, it receives Qi, excretes the dregs, evaporates the fluids, transforming them into a refined essence. This pours upwards towards the Lungs and is transformed into Blood ... Blood is the foundation of the Mind and Spirit.'*[3] All the above quotations highlight the relation between the Essence, Qi, Blood and the Mind/Spirit.

The 'Great Dictionary of Chinese Medicine' says: *'Human life originates from the Essence. It is maintained by Qi and manifested through the Mind and Spirit. Qi, Blood and Essence are the material foundation of the Mind and Spirit. Therefore, when Qi, Blood and Essence are sufficient, the Mind and Spirit are healthy. If there is deficiency of Qi, Blood and Essence, the Mind and Spirit suffer.'*[4]

Our physical features reflect the state of the Mind and Spirit and therefore the state of the Mind and Spirit can be gauged through the observation of the physical features.

As we know, Qi is a subtle life force which is manifested simultaneously in the body in all its physiological activities and in the Mind and Spirit in its emotional and thinking activities (Fig. 2.1). For example, the pathological condition of Liver-Qi stagnation manifests with physical signs such as abdominal distension and simultaneously with emotional signs such as depression or mood swings.

Therefore, the Mind, Spirit and emotions reflect the state of the internal organs and of Qi, Blood and Essence and, vice versa, the state of Qi, Blood and Essence influences the Mind, Spirit and emotions.

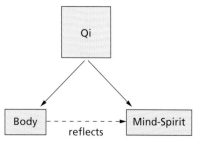

Fig. 2.1 Relationship between the body and the Mind and Spirit in Chinese medicine

Observation of physical features such as the lustre of the complexion and hair, the vitality of the eyes, the tone of voice, the body movement, the pulse, the tongue, etc., help us to assess the state of the Mind, the vitality of the Spirit and the emotional state.

THE THREE ASPECTS OF THE SPIRIT

When observing and assessing the Spirit of a person, we should examine three separate aspects:

- the embodiment of the Spirit
- the vitality of the Spirit
- the lustre of the Spirit.

The embodiment of the Spirit

Observation

The embodiment of the Spirit represents the outward physical manifestation of the Spirit in the body. If the embodiment of the Spirit is strong, a person will have good energy, a strong and solid body build, well-developed muscles, eyes with lustre and a lively expression, agile movements and keen reflexes. The whole body appears to be full of life. If the Spirit is weak, a person will have a weak or emaciated body, lack of energy, eyes without lustre, a dull complexion, slow movements, unsteady walk and slow reflexes. The whole body seems to lack vitality. In severe cases, there will also be mental confusion or lethargy, wasting muscles and a weak body with dull skin.

Clinical significance

The embodiment of the Spirit is the reflection of the Spirit in the body. If the embodiment of the Spirit is strong, it means that Yin, Yang, Qi and Blood are still abundant, pathogenic factors are not so strong, and there is no severe impairment of the internal organs yet. If the embodiment of the Spirit is weak, it shows that pathogenic factors are strong, Upright Qi is exhausted and the internal organs are depleted.

The vitality of the Spirit

Observation

The vitality of the Spirit is its manifestation in the general vitality of a person: the 'energy' radiated by people which reflects their Spirit. Observation of the

vitality of the Spirit is an integral part of the observation of the Spirit. If the vitality of the Spirit is vibrant, then a person will have a clear mind, high energy, a strong voice, regular breathing, clear thinking and quick reflexes. If the vitality of the Spirit is dull, a person will have low energy, a weak voice, dull expression, lethargy, apathy and, in severe cases, mental confusion.

Clinical significance

The vitality of the Spirit reflects the state of the Mind and Spirit and the relative strength of Qi and Blood of the internal organs and that of pathogenic factors. If the vitality of the Spirit of a person is vibrant, Qi and Blood are abundant, the internal organs are strong, pathogenic factors are weak and the disease is mild. If the vitality of the Spirit is dull, it indicates that Qi and Blood are deficient, the internal organs weak, pathogenic factors strong and the disease severe.

The chapter 'Key to the Four Diagnostic Methods' of 'The Golden Mirror of Medicine' says: *'In the beginning of a disease, the state of the Spirit is important. The reason is that if the Spirit is strong at the beginning of a disease, it means that pathogenic factors cannot defeat the Upright Qi, as it is still strong. If the Spirit is dull, it shows that the Upright Qi cannot resist pathogenic factors as it is deficient.'*[5]

The lustre of the Spirit

Observation

The lustre of the Spirit refers to the lustre of the complexion, hair and eyes; the Spirit is reflected in their lustre and observation of them is an essential part of the observation of the Spirit. If the lustre of the Spirit is bright, a person will have a normal, glowing complexion, clear sparkling eyes, shining hair, a lively expression and lustrous, supple skin. If the lustre of the Spirit is dull, a person will have a haggard complexion, withered, lifeless hair, dull eyes and a listless expression and dry, withered skin.

The chapter 'On compulsory observation of the Spirit while observing a disease' in the book 'Origin of Medicine' (*Yi Yuan*, 1861) says:

No matter what the colour is, there should be lustre (shen). In lustre, one can differentiate light and body. 'Light' refers to a bright appearance on the surface, while 'body' refers to the moisture below the surface of the skin. Light has no form and reflects Yang and Qi. Body has a form and reflects

Yin and Blood. If there is no abnormality of Qi and Blood, and Yin and Yang are in harmony, the lustre will have normal light and body.[6]

Clinical significance

The lustre of the Spirit reflects the state of the Internal Organs and the strength of Qi and Blood. If the lustre of the Spirit is rich, it indicates that the Internal Organs are functioning normally and Qi and Blood are abundant. When diseases occur, they are mild and the prognosis is good. If the lustre of the Spirit is lacking, this denotes that Qi and Blood are deficient, the Internal Organs are weak, pathogenic factors are strong and the prognosis is poor.

Box 2.1 summarizes the three aspects of the Spirit.

BOX 2.1 THE THREE ASPECTS OF THE SPIRIT

- The '**embodiment**' of the Spirit is the outward manifestation of the Spirit in the body itself
- The '**vitality**' of the Spirit is the outward manifestation of the Spirit as it is reflected in the 'energy' of the person
- The '**lustre**' of the Spirit is the outward manifestation of the Spirit as it is reflected in the lustre of the eyes and complexion

---

THE THREE CONDITIONS OF THE SPIRIT

When examining the state of the Mind and Spirit, there are three basic conditions:

- strong Spirit
- weak Spirit
- false Spirit.

Strong Spirit

Observation

The signs of a strong Spirit are: sparkling, clear eyes, a lively expression, a lustrous complexion, a clear and alert mind, keen reflexes, good energy, enthusiasm, normal breathing, a clear, ringing voice and agile body movements. This person will have high spirits, a positive approach to life, a stable personality, strong willpower, a clear sense of direction in life and a keen intellect.

Clinical significance

The above signs indicate that the person has a strong and healthy Mind and Spirit and, whatever problem that person might develop, the prognosis is good. The presence of a strong Spirit also means that that person will not suffer from emotional problems or, if these occur, will not be overwhelmed by them.

Weak Spirit

Observation

The signs of a weak Spirit are listlessness, lack of enthusiasm, dull eyes without sparkle, complexion without lustre, shallow breathing, a weak voice, slow body movements, confused thinking, tongue without 'spirit' (*Shen*), and possibly with a Heart crack, and a pulse without a wave. Such people will suffer from apathy, depression, lack of will-power, confusion about their path in life and a slow intellect.

Chapter 17 of the 'Simple Questions' describes the manifestation of a weak Spirit by observation of the head and eyes: *'The five Yin organs house the Spirit; they are essential for the body to be strong. The head is the residence of the Spirit: if the head droops and the eyes are deep-socketed and dull, it means that the Spirit is exhausted.'*[7]

The chapter 'Keys to the Four Diagnostic Methods' of 'The Golden Mirror of Medicine' also discusses the manifestations of lack of Spirit by observing the eyes, speech and mental condition of the patient and it says:

The Spirit is housed in the Heart. It is not substantial or visible but it manifests in the eyes. If the eyes look dull, it means that the Spirit is exhausted: it indicates a poor prognosis. If the eyes are bright and clear, it denotes that the Spirit is vital and the body is free of disease . . . If there is delirium and incoherent speech, it indicates that the Spirit is gone.[8]

Clinical significance

When the Spirit is weak all the organs are affected, the Essence and Qi suffer and, whatever disease the person might have, the prognosis is less good than in a person with a strong Spirit. A weak Spirit also means that that person is more prone to emotional problems or will be more easily overwhelmed by them.

False Spirit

The condition of 'False Spirit' usually appears only during the course of a severe, chronic disease. This occurs when a severely ill patient suddenly appears revitalized and in high spirits: this is called 'False Spirit' and it is usually a poor prognostic sign. The key factor in determining that this is a false appearance of the Spirit is the suddenness of the improvement; however, if the Spirit of a chronically ill patient improves slowly and gradually over several days, that is a good sign.

Observation

The typical manifestations of the False Spirit appear in the course of a severe chronic disease and they are as follows: the patient suddenly seems to be vigorous with a clear look in the eyes, talks incessantly and wants to meet family members, the appetite improves suddenly and the complexion suddenly becomes bright red almost as if the patient were wearing make-up. There is a precise description of the False Spirit in the book 'Chinese Medicine Diagnosis':

The False Spirit indicates the momentary improvement in energy of a patient during a severe, chronic disease: it is not a good sign but an omen of death. The manifestations of the False Spirit are as follows: in a patient suffering from a severe, chronic disease and previously suffering from a weak Spirit, suddenly the energy seems better, the eyes become bright, the patient suddenly talks a lot and wants to meet family members, the voice, previously feeble, suddenly becomes clear and loud, the complexion, previously dark, suddenly becomes bright red and the appetite suddenly comes back. These manifestations are due to the extreme exhaustion of the Essence and Qi. In such a circumstance, Yin fails to restrain Yang so that Yang floats outwards and upwards, causing the false appearance of an improvement. In ancient times, people compared it to the last flicker of a fading oil lamp or the last radiance of the setting sun. It is a dangerous sign indicating the separation of Yin and Yang.[9]

Clinical significance

If the manifestations of the False Spirit appear, it means that the Upright Qi is collapsing, and Yin and Yang are about to separate. Such patients often die within a short time.

THE SPIRIT AND CONSTITUTION

When observing the mental and emotional state of a person, it is important first of all to assess the relative strength of the Spirit compared with that of the consti-

tution, both the prenatal and postnatal as described above. The Spirit and the constitution are both reflections of the Essence and Qi of the body, the former in the mental–spiritual sphere and the latter in the physical sphere. Because of the close connection between the Spirit and the constitution of a person, generally a strong pre- and postnatal constitution is accompanied by a strong Spirit; conversely, a weak pre- and postnatal constitution is generally accompanied by a weak Spirit. However, there may be cases when there is a divergence between these two aspects, that is, the person has a strong pre- and postnatal constitution but a weak Spirit, or vice versa.

An assessment of the relative strength of the two is helpful in forming a prognosis, which will be discussed below. There are four possible situations:

- strong Spirit and strong constitution
- weak Spirit and weak constitution
- weak Spirit and strong constitution
- strong Spirit and weak constitution.

Strong Spirit and strong constitution
Observation

A person with a strong Spirit and strong constitution will have solid muscles, a lustrous normal complexion, a vigorous expression in shining eyes, a strong body, lustrous hair, agile movement and keen reflexes; on a mental–spiritual level, this person will have high spirits, a positive approach to life, a stable personality, strong will-power, a clear sense of direction in their life and a keen intellect.

Clinical significance

The above physical and mental characteristics indicate both a good constitution and a strong Spirit; the internal organs of such a person are strong and function normally, Qi and Blood are abundant and the Mind and Spirit are healthy. The body will not be easily invaded by pathogenic factors. Even if diseases occur, they can be easily cured. Chapter 19 of the 'Simple Questions' says: *'If the Upright Qi and the body build of a patient are both strong, any disease will be easy to treat. If the complexion is lustrous and bright, the patient will recover soon.'*[10] Chapter 20 of the same book says: *'If the body build and the Upright Qi are both strong, the patient will survive.'*[11]

Weak Spirit and weak constitution
Observation

A person with a weak Spirit and a weak constitution will be listless with an emaciated body build, a haggard complexion, dull eyes, withered hair and a feeble voice; from a mental–emotional point of view, such people will suffer from apathy, depression, lack of will-power, a confusion about their path in life and a slow intellect.

Clinical significance

The above characteristics indicate that the patient has both a weak Spirit and a weak constitution and there will be a deficiency of Yin, Yang, Qi or Blood. Any illness that such a person suffers from will tend to be long lasting and chronic and the body will be easily invaded by external pathogenic factors. The weak Spirit will also hamper an improvement in the physical condition. A simultaneous weakness of both the Spirit and the constitution generally indicates a poor prognosis.

Weak Spirit and strong constitution
Observation

A person with a weak Spirit and a strong constitution will have solid muscles, a strong body, lustrous hair, agile movement and keen reflexes, large bones, a brisk walk, but dull eyes without sparkle, a haggard complexion without lustre and a weak voice. From a mental–emotional point of view, such people will tend to suffer from apathy, depression, lack of will-power, a confusion about their path in life and a slow intellect.

Clinical significance

The combination of a weak Spirit and a strong constitution is usually seen in patients who are born with a strong prenatal constitution but whose Mind and Spirit are affected by life events. Although the treatment of such patients is more difficult than it would be if they had a strong Spirit, their strong constitution means that the prognosis is still relatively good and that the Mind and Spirit can recover their balance.

Chapter 19 of the 'Simple Questions' says: *'If the body build is strong and the Upright Qi and Mind weak, the disease is difficult to treat. If the complexion is dark without lustre, the disease is difficult to cure.'*[12]

Strong Spirit and weak constitution

Observation

A person with a strong Spirit and a weak constitution will suffer from chronic diseases and will have an emaciated body build, listlessness, a haggard complexion, dull eyes, withered hair, a feeble voice, coarse breath but a clear, loud voice and eyes with lustre; from the mental–emotional point of view, such patients will have high spirits, a positive approach to life, a stable personality, strong will-power, a clear sense of direction in their life and a keen intellect.

Clinical significance

The combination of a weak constitution and a strong Spirit may seem contrary to the fundamental tenet of Chinese medicine that sees the body and the Mind as an integrated whole; in fact, in general, a weak pre- and postnatal constitution will be accompanied by a weak Spirit. However, there are exceptions to this as some people seem to be able to maintain a strong Spirit despite a poor constitution.

The prognosis in this case is better than in the previous case because the strong Spirit, helped by treatment, is able to harness the healing powers of the body.

THE SPIRIT AND THE EMOTIONS

The emotional state of the patient is gauged primarily from observation of the eyes, the complexion and the tongue. The observation of these features must of course be closely integrated with the interrogation, listening to the voice and palpation of the pulse.

Eyes

Observation of the eyes to gauge the emotional state of the patient is based primarily on observation of the lustre and control of the eyes.

Lustre of the eyes refers to the brilliance, sparkle, glitter and vitality of the normal eye. Eyes with lustre indicate a normal state of the Mind and Spirit and, generally speaking, the absence of serious emotional problems. Eyes without lustre are dull, lack vitality and sparkle and look as if they were covered by a mist; this always indicates emotional problems of some nature. The extent to which the eyes lack lustre is directly related to the duration and intensity of the emotional problems: the duller the eyes, the deeper and more long standing are the emotional problems.

Control of the eyes refers to the gaze and movement of the eyes. If a person is able to fix the gaze and the eyes do not move but neither are they too fixed, the eyes have 'control'. If a person has a shifty gaze, if the eyes move too much or if they are fixed in a stare, they are 'uncontrolled'. Eyes without control indicate a relatively serious disturbance of the Mind and Spirit.

Complexion

A complexion with lustre is bright, moist and shining, while a lustreless complexion is dark, dull and somewhat dry. It is important to note that the lustre of the complexion is a diagnostic feature separate from the colour of the complexion; e.g. an abnormal yellow complexion could be with or without lustre.

A complexion with lustre indicates that the Mind and Spirit are relatively unaffected by emotional problems whereas a complexion without lustre indicates the presence of emotional problems. Similarly as for the eyes, the lack of lustre of a complexion is directly related to the intensity and duration of emotional problems: the duller the complexion, the deeper and more long standing the emotional problems.

Tongue

One of the main features to look for in the tongue to determine whether the patient is affected by emotional problems or not, is the presence of absence of a Heart crack (see Fig. 25.8, p. 217).

A Heart crack on the tongue is relatively narrow and it extends throughout the whole length of the tongue to the border of the tip. Such a crack indicates the tendency to emotional problems; the deeper the crack, the more intense the emotional problems.

A second pathological sign to look for on the tongue in emotional problems is a Red tip. Emotional stress generally leads to Qi stagnation and with time this leads to some Heat. As all emotions affect the Heart, emotional stress frequently manifests with a Red tip of the tongue, which reflects a certain degree of Heart-Heat. The redder the tip the more intense are the emotional problems, and a swelling and red points on the tip indicate an even more severe emotional problem.

The observation of these three features, eyes, complexion and tongue, should be closely integrated and each sign should be checked against the other two to give us

an idea of the intensity and duration of the emotional problems.

In terms of time scale, when a person is subject to emotional stress, the lustre of the eyes will be the first of these three to change, the complexion the second and the tongue the last (although this is just a general rule and there may be variations in practice). Therefore, for example, if the eyes lack lustre but the complexion has lustre and the tip of the tongue is not Red, this indicates that the emotional problems are of a relatively short duration; if, on the contrary, the eyes and complexion lack lustre and the tongue has a Red tip and a deep Heart crack, this indicates that the emotional problems suffered by the patient are very deep and long standing.

As indicated above, when diagnosing the emotional state of the patient, interrogation and observation must also be integrated with palpation of the pulse. In terms of time scale, the pulse will actually be the first to change. To summarize, therefore, the time scale of the changes observed in emotional problems is as follows:

- pulse
- eyes
- complexion
- tongue.

The observation of the lustre of the eyes is discussed also in Chapter 6, while that of the complexion is discussed in Chapter 3.

NOTES

1. 1981 Spiritual Axis (*Ling Shu Jing* 灵枢经), People's Health Publishing House, Beijing, p. 72. First published c. 100BC.
2. 1979 The Yellow Emperor's Classic of Internal Medicine – Simple Questions (*Huang Di Nei Jing Su Wen* 黄帝内经素问), People's Health Publishing House, Beijing, p. 67. First published c. 100BC.
3. Spiritual Axis, p. 52.
4. Cited in Zhang Shu Sheng 1995 Great Treatise of Diagnosis by Observation in Chinese Medicine (中华医学望诊大全), Shanxi Science Publishing House, Taiyuan, p. 65.
5. Ibid., p. 69.
6. Ibid., p. 69.
7. Simple Questions, p. 100.
8. Cited in Great Treatise of Diagnosis by Observation in Chinese Medicine, p. 71.
9. Ibid., p. 72.
10. Simple Questions, p. 128.
11. Ibid., p. 136.
12. Ibid., p. 128.

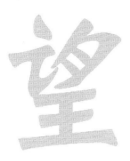

Chapter **3**

OBSERVATION OF THE COMPLEXION COLOUR

Chapter contents

INTRODUCTION   39

DOMINANT AND GUEST COLOURS   40
Dominant colours   40
Guest colours   41
Clinical significance   41

OBSERVATION OF DIFFERENT ASPECTS OF COMPLEXION
COLOUR   42
Superficial or deep colour   42
Distinct or obscure colour   42
Scattered or concentrated colour   43
Thin or thick colour   43
Lustrous or lustreless colour   44
Conforming or opposing colours   44
Prognosis according to complexion colour   47
Changes in complexion colour during a disease   49
Complexion colours and emotions   49

COMPLEXION COLOURS   50
Normal complexion colour   50
White complexion colour   51
Sallow complexion colour   52
Yellow complexion colour   52
Red complexion colour   54
Bluish/greenish complexion colour   55
Dark complexion colour   56
Purple complexion colour   56

INTRODUCTION

The colour and lustre of the complexion are the outward manifestations of the internal organs and of Yin, Yang, Qi and Blood. If the internal organs function normally and if Yin, Yang, Qi and Blood are abundant and balanced, the complexion will have normal colour and proper lustre; conversely, when Qi, Blood, Yin and Yang are weakened and the internal organs affected, the complexion acquires an abnormal colour.

The chapter 'On observation of the colour' in 'Principle and Prohibition for the Medical Profession' (*Yi Men Fa Lu*) says: '*When the five Yin organs are exhausted, the complexion colour becomes dark and lustreless . . . So the complexion colour is like a flag of the Spirit, and the Yin organs are the residences of the Spirit. When the Spirit is gone, the Yin organs are worn out, and the complexion colour becomes dark and lustreless.*'[1] As the above passage indicates clearly, observation of complexion colour is a very important diagnostic tool to assess the condition not only of Qi, Blood, Yin and Yang and of the internal organs, but also of the Mind and Spirit. Indeed from a Five-Element perspective, the facial complexion as a whole is a manifestation of the Heart and therefore the Mind and Spirit; this should never be forgotten in practice. Thus, if a woman has a very dull, sallow complexion it does indicate a Spleen-Qi deficiency and Dampness and possibly also Blood deficiency, but, at the same time, it also indicates that the Mind and Spirit are affected and suffering.

Yu Chang in 'Principles of Medical Practice' (1658) calls the complexion the 'banner of the Mind and Spirit' and he says: '*When the Mind and Spirit are flourishing, the complexion is glowing; when the Mind and Spirit are declining, the complexion withers. When the Mind is stable the complexion is florid . . .*'.[2]

The normal complexion should have 'lustre' and 'moisture'. 'Lustre' means that the complexion colour should be bright, glowing and with a shine to it; 'moisture' means that the complexion should look moist and the skin firm, indicating that there is moisture underneath it. There is a correspondence between these two aspects of the complexion and two of the attributes of the normal pulse: the lustre of the complexion corresponds to the spirit of the pulse, whereas the moisture of the complexion corresponds to Stomach-Qi of the pulse. Thus, we can say that if the complexion has lustre there is spirit; if it has moisture there is Stomach-Qi.

Observation of the complexion must be closely linked to the feeling of the pulse. The pulse shows the state of Qi, the complexion the state of the Mind and Spirit. If the pulse shows changes but the complexion is normal, this indicates that the problem is recent. If both the pulse and the complexion show pathological changes, this indicates that the problem is long standing.

The lustre of the complexion should also be checked against the lustre of the eyes. A change in the complexion always indicates a deeper or more long-standing problem. For example, a sustained period of overwork and inadequate sleep may cause the eyes to lack lustre (and the pulse to be Weak); if the complexion has not changed, this is not too serious and the person can recover easily by resting. If, however, the eyes lack lustre and the complexion is dull, without lustre, or dark, it indicates that the problem is not transient but deeper rooted.

Thus, in terms of time scale, the pulse changes first, the eyes second and the complexion last. Accordingly, if the pulse is affected but the eyes and the complexion are not, the problem is very recent; if pulse and eyes are affected (lacking in lustre), the problem is older (some months); if the pulse, eyes and complexion are all affected, the problem is even older (over 1 year).

DOMINANT AND GUEST COLOURS

Dominant colours

The normal complexion colour varies, of course, according to racial group but also according to Elemental types as described in Chapter 1. Wood types have a subtle greenish hue to their complexion, Earth types a subtle yellowish hue, Fire types a red hue, Metal types a white hue, and Water types a dark hue.

Therefore, the normal complexion colour is determined by race and prenatal influences and, in health,

remains the same throughout life. In disease, the complexion colour becomes pathological and will vary, obviously according to the racial group, but also according to Element type; for example, a pathological yellow colour in someone of the Wood type will be subtly different from that in someone of the Fire type. Such differences in pathological colours are, of course, even more evident in different racial groups; for example, the paleness of a Caucasian patient will differ from that of an Asian patient.

The basic inherited complexion colours, determined by race and Elemental type, are called 'dominant colours'. The chapter 'Keys to the Four Diagnostic Methods' in the 'Golden Mirror of Medicine' (*Yi Zong Jin Jian*) says: '*The colours of the five Yin organs manifest in people according to their body shape based on the Five Elements. Such colours never change throughout life. They are known as dominant colours.*'[3]

In addition, there are other factors related to environment and season which influence the complexion colour. Environmental conditions and lifestyle have an important influence on complexion colour so that what is a normal complexion colour for one person may not be so for another, even within the same racial group and Element type; this should be taken into account when diagnosing patients. For example, the normal complexion of a farmer who spends most of his life outdoors will obviously be different from that of an office worker: inevitably, the farmer's 'normal' complexion will be redder than the office worker's.

Chapter 12 of the 'Simple Questions' discusses environmental influences on the complexion:

The East is where Qi of all kinds of life in nature starts. It is an area close to seas and water and abounds in fish and salt. People who live in the East eat a lot of fish, and like salty food. Therefore they often have a relatively dark complexion and loose structures between the complexion and muscles. The South is where all kinds of life in nature grow vigorously, and where Yang flourishes. It is lower terrain, and has poor water and soil. There is often fog. People who live in the South like sour-flavoured and fermented food. Therefore, they often have a relatively red complexion and dense structures between the complexion and muscles.[4]

Obviously, the geographical references in the above passage refer to China and the dietary references refer to ancient China: however, the principle that the environment influences the complexion colour is still valid.

Box 3.1 summarizes the dominant colour.

Guest colours

'Guest' colours are those appearing on the Connecting channels of the face and limbs. The colours of the Yin Connecting channels follow those of the Main channels; that is, if the Main channels manifest with red colour, the Yin Connecting channel will also manifest with a red colour. The Yang Connecting channels are on the Yang surfaces and, being more superficial, they are more readily influenced by seasonal factors. Thus, the complexion may assume a certain colour owing to the seasonal and climatic influence on the Yang Connecting channels and such colour may contradict what one might expect from the Element type or pathological condition. For example, a patient with a pathological condition of the Heart (such as Heat) should have a reddish complexion; if the seasonal and climatic influence (e.g. spring) on the Yang Connecting channels predominates then the complexion may instead be greenish. This is called 'guest' colour and we should be able to recognize it in order to explain the anomaly.

Chapter 57 of the 'Simple Questions' says:

The Yellow Emperor asks: 'The Connecting channels are exposed to the exterior and manifest with five different colours which are green, yellow, red, white and black. What is the reason?' Qi Bo answers, 'The main channels have their regular colours, but the colours of the Connecting channels change according to the four seasons.' The Yellow Emperor asks, 'What are the normal colours of the main channels?' Qi Bo answers, 'Red for the Heart, white for the Lungs, green for the Liver, yellow for the Spleen and black for the Kidneys.' The Yellow Emperor asks, 'Do the colours of the Yin and Yang Connecting channels correspond to the regular colours of the related main channels?' Qi Bo answers, 'The colours of the Yin Connecting channels correspond to the regular colours of their related main channels, while those of the Yang connecting channels change in accordance with the four seasons. In cold weather, the circulation of Qi and Blood slows down and there is often a green or black colour. In warm and hot weather, Qi and Blood circulation is free and smooth, and there is usually a yellow or red colour. All these are normal phenomena, indicating the body is in a normal condition.'[5]

When the above passage talks about the 'normal colours of the main channels', it refers to the five main pathological colours of the face which are produced by the influence of the main Yin channels. For example, a pathological condition of the main channel of the Heart may produce a reddish complexion (of course this is seen strictly from a Five-Element point of view as, for example, Heart-Blood deficiency would manifest with a pale rather than red complexion). The passage then explains that, while the colour of the Yin Connecting channels accords with the predominant face colour, that of the Yang Connecting channels is influenced by the seasons and climate. Bearing in mind that the limbs are richly supplied by the Yang Connecting channels, one needs to observe the colour of the limbs as well as the face to gauge the seasonal influence of these channels. Such colours, compared with those deriving from racial group and Elemental type, are temporary and reversible and are known as the 'guest colours', which are not pathological.

It is important to differentiate between 'guest colours' due to environmental and climatic influences and actual abnormal colours due to pathological conditions.

Clinical significance

Observation of the complexion colour and lustre helps us to determine the pathology, location, nature and prognosis of a disease. When observing the complexion colour, attention should be paid to distinguishing the dominant colours, the guest colours and the abnormal colours. It is, of course, necessary to refer to the pulse, tongue and symptoms and also to take into account the patient's Element type.

For example, if someone of the Wood type has a slightly greenish complexion, this is in keeping with that type; if this person's complexion develops a reddish tinge (perhaps a superficial redness over the underlying greenish colour) during the summer, this is a 'guest' colour and is also normal. However, if the same person's complexion is very red and 'deep' (see below), it indicates not a 'guest' colour but a pathological condition of Heat.

Box 3.2 summarizes guest colours.

OBSERVATION OF DIFFERENT ASPECTS OF COMPLEXION COLOUR

The main aspects of complexion colour to observe are:

- superficial or deep colour
- distinct or obscure colour
- scattered or concentrated colour
- thin or thick colour
- lustrous or lustreless colour
- conforming or opposing colour
- prognosis according to complexion colour
- changes in complexion colour during a disease
- complexion colours and emotions.

Superficial or deep colour
Observation

The differentiation between superficial and deep colour is based on the 'depth' of the complexion's colour. A colour is defined as 'superficial' (see Plate 3.1 on p. P2) when it is seen clearly on the surface of the complexion, while it is defined as 'deep' when it appears to be on a level below the surface (see Plate 3.2 on p. P3).

Chapter 49 of the 'Spiritual Axis' says: '*The five colours are present in certain areas of the face. Recognizing whether the colours are superficial or deep helps us to understand the shallow or deep location of the pathogenic factors.*'[6] The chapter 'Keys to the Four Diagnostic Methods' in the 'Golden Mirror of Medicine' (*Yi Zong Jin Jian*) says:

The deep colour is relatively dark. It indicates that diseases are deep in the Interior. If it is also obscure and lustreless, it indicates that diseases are chronic and severe. The superficial colour is relatively light. It indicates that diseases are on the Exterior. If it is also bright and lustrous, it indicates that diseases are mild and newly-occurring.'[7]

The chapter 'Outline of the Ten Methods for Recognizing Qi' of '*Wang Zhen Zun Jing*' says:

'*The superficial colour is shown on the complexion, while the deep colour is hidden underneath the complexion. The superficial colour indicates Exterior diseases, and the deep colour indicates Interior diseases. If the colour is first superficial and later becomes deep, it reveals the movement of a disease from the Exterior to the Interior. If the colour is first deep and later becomes superficial, it reflects the movement of the disease from the Interior to the Exterior.*'[8]

Clinical significance

If the abnormal complexion colour is superficial and light, it indicates that the disease is mild and is located in the Exterior or in the Yang organs. It can be easily treated, and the prognosis is good. If the abnormal complexion colour is dark and deep, it means that the disease is severe and is located deep in the Interior or in the Yin organs. The treatment is relatively difficult, and the disease cannot be cured within a short time.

Chapter 15 of the 'Simple Questions' says:

If there are changes of the colours in the upper, lower, left and right regions of the face, efforts should be made to understand the location and prognosis of the diseases indicated by the respective colours. If the abnormal colour is light, it implies that the diseases are mild. Such patients can be treated with soups to nourish the body. They will recover in 10 days. If the abnormal colour is deep, it indicates that the disease is severe. Such patients should be treated with a herbal decoction. They will recover in 21 days. If the abnormal colour is even deeper, it means that the disease is much more severe. They must be treated with a herbal tincture to regulate the circulation in the channels. They will recover in 100 days. If the colour of the complexion is dark, haggard, vigourless and emaciated, it shows that the Spirit is gone, the disease cannot be treated and such patients will die in 100 days.[9]

BOX 3.3 SUPERFICIAL OR DEEP COLOUR

- Superficial colour: condition mild, Exterior, Yang
- Deep colour: condition severe, Interior, Yin

Box 3.3 summarizes superficial and deep colour.

Distinct or obscure colour
Observation

The differentiation between a 'distinct' or 'obscure' colour refers to the quality of the complexion colour: a distinct colour is bright and clear and manifests itself readily while an obscure colour is darkish, dull and lifeless as if 'trapped' inside the complexion. It is important to note that the differentiation between the distinct colour and the obscure colour of the complexion applies to any shade of pathological colour and both the distinct and obscure colours are abnormal; for example, a pathological, dull, yellow complexion may be either 'distinct' or 'obscure' (see Plates 3.3 and 3.4 on p. P3).

The chapter 'Outline of Ten Methods for Recognizing Qi' of '*Wang Zhen Zun Jing*' says:

The distinct, bright colour looks unfolded and the dark, obscure colour looks gloomy. The distinct colour indicates that the disease is of the Yang type; the obscure colour indicates that the disease is of the Yin type. If the distinct colour becomes obscure, it means that the disease has changed from the Yang to the Yin type. If the obscure colour becomes distinct, it means that the disease has changed from the Yin to the Yang type.[10]

Clinical significance

If an abnormal complexion looks distinct and bright, it indicates that the disease is of the Yang type, the location of the disease is superficial and the Upright Qi is not exhausted yet. If an abnormal complexion colour looks dark and obscure, it indicates that the disease is of the Yin type, the location of the disease is deep in the Interior, the Upright Qi is deficient and the disease is severe.

If in the course of a disease the complexion colour changes from distinct to obscure, it indicates that the disease is progressing from the Yang to the Yin organs, which is a poor sign. If it changes from obscure to distinct, it indicates that the disease is progressing from the Yin to the Yang organs, which is a good sign.

In treatment, for patients with an abnormal but distinct complexion colour, the emphasis of the treatment should be on eliminating pathogenic factors. For patients with an abnormal but obscure complexion colour, equal emphasis should be put on eliminating pathogenic factors and strengthening the Upright Qi.

BOX 3.4 DISTINCT OR OBSCURE COLOUR

- Distinct colour: Yang type of disease, superficial, Upright Qi not exhausted
- Obscure colour: Yin type of disease, deep, Upright Qi weakened

---

Box 3.4 summarizes distinct and obscure colours.

Scattered or concentrated colour
Observation

When considering abnormal complexion colours, another differentiation is that between 'scattered' and 'concentrated'. The scattered colour is thinly distributed and sparse, while the concentrated colour is densely distributed and aggregated (see Plates 3.5 and 3.6 on p. P3).

Chapter 49 of the 'Spiritual Axis' says: '*The observation whether the colour is scattered or concentrated tells us whether the disease is a long way off or imminent.*'[11]

The chapter 'Outline of ten methods for recognizing Qi' in '*Wang Zhen Zun Jing*' gives a different interpretation of the clinical significance of the scattered or concentrated colours:

The scattered colour is thinly distributed and 'open'; the concentrated colour is densely distributed and 'closed'. The scattered colour indicates that the disease has had a short duration, and is about to be alleviated. The concentrated colour indicates that the disease has had a long duration and will gradually become severe. If the abnormal colour is concentrated at first but changes later to being scattered, it indicates that the disease is about to be alleviated even though it has had a long duration. If the abnormal colour is scattered at first but changes later to being concentrated, it indicates that the disease is becoming severe even though it has had a short duration.'[12]

Clinical significance

When an abnormal complexion colour is scattered, this indicates that the disease is of short duration and mild nature, it will be treated relatively easily and the prognosis is good. When an abnormal complexion colour is concentrated, this indicates that the disease is of long duration and severe, pathogenic factors are strong, the treatment is relatively difficult and the prognosis is less good than in the case of a scattered colour.

BOX 3.5 SCATTERED OR CONCENTRATED COLOUR

- Scattered colour: mild disease, short duration, pathogenic factors not strong, prognosis good
- Concentrated colour: severe disease, long duration, pathogenic factors strong, prognosis not good

---

Box 3.5 summarizes scattered and concentrated colour.

Thin or thick colour
Observation

The differentiation between a thin colour and a thick colour is based on the 'thickness' of the colour. To understand this distinction one could think of paint:

the thin colour corresponds to a single skimpy coat of paint while the thick colour corresponds to several heavy coats of paint (see Plates 3.7 and 3.8 on pp. P3 and P4).

Clinical significance

A thin colour indicates a Deficiency while a thick colour indicates an Excess, that is, the presence of pathogenic factors. If the colour changes from thin to thick, it indicates that the condition is changing from one of Deficiency to one of Excess; if it changes from thick to thin, it indicates that the condition is changing from one of Excess to one of Deficiency.

BOX 3.6 THIN OR THICK COLOUR

- Thin colour: Deficiency
- Thick colour: Excess

Box 3.6 summarizes thin and thick colours.

Lustrous or lustreless colour
Observation

A lustrous complexion is bright, moist, vigorous and shining, while a lustreless complexion is dark, dull, gloomy and 'withered'. It is important to note that, in the context of pathology, an abnormal colour may be lustreless or lustrous. The presence of lustre in the complexion indicates a good prognosis, even if the colour is abnormal. The brightness of the complexion is a manifestation of the Spirit, while the lustre derives from the nourishment of Essence and Blood.

Clinical significance

If an abnormal complexion colour is lustrous, it denotes that the Spirit is not affected, pathogenic factors are not too strong, the condition is mild, the treatment relatively easy and the prognosis good. If an abnormal complexion colour is lustreless, it indicates that the Spirit has been affected, pathogenic factors are relatively strong, the Upright Qi is very deficient, the condition is severe, the treatment relatively difficult and the prognosis poor.

Chapter 49 of the 'Spiritual Axis' says: '*Observation of the lustre or lack of lustre of the complexion colour allows us to judge whether the prognosis is good or bad.*'[13]

If an abnormal colour of complexion acquires lustre, this indicates that the condition is improving, Upright Qi is returning, the Spirit is recovering and the prognosis is good; vice versa, if an abnormal lustrous colour of the complexion loses its lustre, this indicates that the Spirit is affected, the condition is worsening, Upright Qi is weakening and the prognosis is poor.

BOX 3.7 LUSTROUS OR LUSTRELESS COLOUR

- Lustrous colour: Spirit good, pathogenic factors not strong, condition mild, prognosis good
- Lustreless colour: Spirit weakened, pathogenic factors strong, condition severe, prognosis not good

---

Box 3.7 summarizes lustrous and lustreless colour.

Conforming or opposing colour
Observation

The differentiation between a 'conforming' colour and an 'opposing' colour is based on two distinct aspects: the first is whether the complexion colour accords with the prevailing disharmony; the second is whether the complexion colour accords with the prevailing disharmony according to the Five Elements and specifically according to the Generating and Overacting cycles.

Conforming or opposing colour according to pattern

According to the first aspect, a 'conforming' colour is in accordance with the condition of the patient; for example the patient has a Heat pattern and the complexion is red. An 'opposing' colour contradicts the patient's prevailing pattern; for example the patient has a clear Heat pattern but the complexion is pale. There can be several different explanations of a contradiction between the prevailing disharmony and the complexion colour, as follows:

- The complexion colour may contradict the main disharmony simply because the patient suffers from several different patterns and the complexion reflects one of them. For example, it would not be unusual for a person to suffer from chronic Spleen-Qi deficiency and therefore have a dull, pale-yellowish complexion but also to suffer from Heart-Fire.
- The complexion colour is influenced by seasonal influences; thus, a person may have a reddish complexion in the summer but suffer from chronic Spleen-Qi deficiency.

- The complexion colour strongly reflects the state of the Mind and Spirit and it may occasionally contradict the prevailing pattern. For example, a person may suffer from Liver-Fire but if this developed from the accumulated stagnant Qi deriving from deep emotional problems such as shock and guilt, the complexion may not be red but pale-bluish or greenish. In such cases, the complexion usually shows the deep, underlying emotional cause of the disharmony.
- In rare cases, there may be a 'false' complexion colour when there is a total separation of Yin and Yang and the patient suffers from 'false Yang' (red face, very cold limbs and slow pulse) or from 'false Yin' (very pale face, feeling of heat and red tongue).

Conforming or opposing colour according to the Five Elements

According to the second aspect, the conforming or opposing complexion colour is also decided on the basis of the Five Elements and one can distinguish four different situations when the complexion does not accord with the prevailing Element pattern. A practical example is the best way of describing these four possible situations. If a patient suffers from a Liver pattern but the complexion reflects the colour of the Mother Element (i.e. Water), this is called 'conforming colour'; if the complexion reflects the colour of the Child Element (i.e. Fire) this is called the 'slightly opposing colour' (Chinese books refer to it as 'opposition within conformity'); if the complexion reflects the

colour of the Element overacted upon (i.e. Earth) this is called 'opposing colour' (Chinese books refer to it as 'conformity within opposition'); if the complexion reflects the colour of the Element overacting on that of the prevailing pattern (i.e. Metal) this is called 'strongly opposing colour' (Table 3.1). The last scenario (i.e. when the complexion colour belongs to the Element that overacts on the Element of the prevailing pattern) is the most serious one. For example, if a patient suffers from a severe Spleen-Qi deficiency (Earth) but the complexion is green (Wood), this is a bad sign and it means that the condition will be more difficult to treat.

The conforming and opposing colours for diseases of the Five Elements are illustrated in Figures 3.1–3.5.

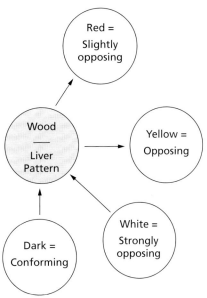

Fig. 3.1 Conforming and opposing colours in Liver patterns

Table 3.1 **Conforming and opposing complexion colours according to the Five Elements**					
Diseased Element	**Complexion**				
	Green	**Red**	**Yellow**	**White**	**Dark**
Wood		Slightly opposing	Opposing	**Strongly opposing**	Conforming
Fire	Conforming		Slightly opposing	Opposing	**Strongly opposing**
Earth	**Strongly opposing**	Conforming		Slightly opposing	Opposing
Metal	Opposing	**Strongly opposing**	Conforming		Slightly opposing
Water	Slightly opposing	Opposing	**Strongly opposing**	Conforming	

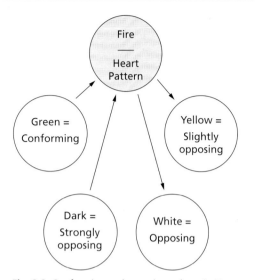

Fig. 3.2 Conforming and opposing colours in Heart patterns

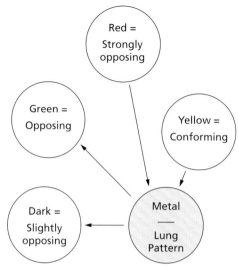

Fig. 3.4 Conforming and opposing colours in Lung patterns

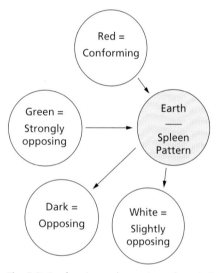

Fig. 3.3 Conforming and opposing colours in Spleen patterns

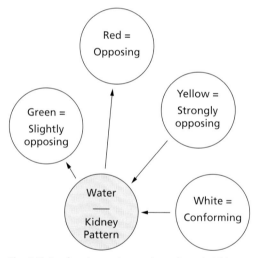

Fig. 3.5 Conforming and opposing colours in Kidney patterns

Clinical significance

The differentiation between a conforming or an opposing colour, whether according to pattern or the Five Elements, helps us to gauge the severity of the disease, the relative strength of pathogenic factors and Upright Qi and therefore the prognosis. If the complexion colour conforms with the disease condition, it indicates that the disease is mild, pathogenic factors are not strong, Upright Qi is still relatively intact, the treatment will be relatively easy and the prognosis is good. If the complexion colour opposes the disease condition, it indicates that the disease is severe, pathogenic factors are strong, Upright Qi is weak, the treatment will be relatively difficult and the prognosis is bad.

Of course, the conformity or opposition of the complexion colour according to the Five Elements is only one of the aspects to be considered in colour diagnosis. All other factors should be taken into account and, with regard to complexion in particular, the presence or absence of lustre overrides the others. In other words, if the complexion is dark, dull and without lustre, this indicates a poor prognosis even if the colour is conforming. Conversely, if the complexion has lustre the prognosis is good even if the colour is opposing.

Prognosis according to complexion colour

Observation

Complexion colour is used to determine prognosis in four ways: first by determining the presence or absence of lustre, secondly by paying attention to the 'thickness' of the colour, thirdly, by analysing the 'conforming' or 'rebellious' nature of the colour according to its movement between areas of the face, and fourthly by analysing the complexion colour in its conformity to or deviation from the seasonal influence. Thus, four aspects will be discussed:

> 1. Presence or absence of lustre
> 2. Thick or thin colour
> 3. Conforming or rebellious colour according to area of the face
> 4. Conformity or deviation of colour according to season.

1. Presence or absence of lustre

If a pathological complexion colour is bright, lustrous and contained, this is a sign of good prognosis; if it is dark, lustreless and fully revealed, it indicates poor prognosis. Shi Pa Nan in the 'Origin of Medicine' (1861) says: '*The shen of the complexion consists in lustre and body. Lustre means that the complexion appears clear and bright from the outside; body means that it is moist and with lustre in the inside.*'[14] If a complexion has such attributes, even if the colour is pathological, this indicates that the Mind and Spirit are stable and unaffected and therefore the prognosis is good.

Chapter 10 of the 'Simple Questions' differentiates between a good prognosis and a poor prognosis by observation of the five main pathological colours, comparing them with various objects that were in common daily use in ancient China (some of which

Table 3.2 Descriptions of pathological complexion colours in the 'Simple Questions'

Pathological colour	Good prognosis	Poor prognosis
Green	feather of a kingfisher	dead grass
Red	rooster comb	stagnant blood
Yellow	abdomen of a crab	bitter orange
White	pig's fat	dead bone
Dark	crow's feathers	coal ash

Table 3.3 Descriptions of healthy complexion colours in the 'Simple Questions'

Organ	Healthy complexion colour
Liver	thin piece of white silk covering a dark purple one
Heart	thin piece of white silk covering cinnabar
Spleen	thin piece of white silk covering snakegourd (*Gua Lou*) fruit
Lungs	thin piece of white silk covering a pink one
Kidneys	thin piece of white silk covering a purple one

will be unfamiliar to Westerners). The colours are given in Table 3.2.[15]

The same chapter also describes the five main healthy complexion colours, again comparing them with various objects (Table 3.3).[16]

It is interesting to note that the normal, healthy colours are described as being covered by a thin piece of white silk, which means that they should be rather subdued and subtle; it is also interesting that pathological colours are latent and manifest themselves when the 'thin piece of white silk' is removed.

Chapter 17 of the 'Simple Questions' describes the look of pathological colours with or without lustre in a slightly different way:

A red complexion should look like vermilion covered with white, not like ochre. A white complexion should look like feathers of a goose, not like salt. A blue complexion should look like moistened greyish jade, not like indigo. A yellow complexion should look like realgar covered with gauze, not like loess [the soil in North China along the Yellow River basin]. A black complexion should look like dark varnish, not like greyish charcoal.[17]

Dr Chen Shi Duo in 'Secret Records of the Stone Room' (1687) goes as far as saying: '*If the complexion is dark but with shen, the person will live even if the disease is serious. If the complexion is bright but without shen, the person will die even if there is no disease.*'[18]

If the complexion colour is bright, lustrous and contained, it indicates that, even though there is a pathological state, the Internal Organs are not weakened, pathogenic factors are not too strong, Stomach-Qi is still relatively intact, the disease is mild and the prognosis is good. If the complexion colour is dark, lustreless and fully revealed, it shows that the Internal Organs are weakened, pathogenic factors are strong, Stomach-Qi is exhausted, the disease is severe and the prognosis is poor.

2. Thin or thick colour

The 'thickness' of the facial complexion colour is directly related to the intensity of the pathological condition: a thin and superficial colour indicates either an exterior disease or a light pathogenic factor, while a thick and deep colour indicates an interior disease and a strong pathogenic factor. Therefore a change from a thick to a thin facial colour indicates that the pathogenic factors are getting weaker and the disease is retreating; by contrast, a change from a thin to a thick facial colour indicates that the pathogenic factors are getting stronger and the disease is advancing.

3. Conforming or rebellious colour according to area of the face

The conformity or rebellious nature of a colour must also be related to any movement of the colour from one area of the face to another.

A movement of a pathological facial colour from the top to the bottom part of the face indicates an improvement of the condition and is called 'conforming' movement; by contrast, a movement of a pathological colour from the bottom to the top part of the face indicates a worsening of the condition and is called 'rebellious' movement.

The 'Simple Questions' in Chapter 15 relates the conforming or rebellious movement of a facial colour (and therefore the prognosis) also to the left or right side of the face, making a distinction according to sex: 'In women, [a colour] on the right side indicates a rebellious [colour], while on the left side it is conforming. In men, [a colour] on the left side indicates a rebellious [colour], while on the right side it is conforming.'[19] This passage correlates the prognosis to the location of a pathological colour on the right or left side of the face in men and women: for example, in a woman, an excessively red colour is always pathological whether it is on the right or left but it is worse if it is on the right cheek; the reverse applies to a man.

4. Conformity or deviation of colour according to season

The complexion colour should be assessed carefully in the light of seasonal influences: if the influence of climatic factors of the seasons exceeds that of the pathology of the five Yin organs, it is a sign of a good prognosis; if the influence of the pathology of the five Yin organs exceeds that of the climatic factors of the seasons (the 'Guest Qi'), it is a sign of a bad prognosis.

The chapter 'Keys to the Four Diagnostic Methods' in the 'Golden Mirror of Medicine' (*Yi Zong Jin Jian*) says:

The Qi of the five Yin organs manifests with the five different [physiological] colours in accordance with the five different types of body shapes. Such colours will never change and are called Dominant Colours. The colours influenced by the climatic factors of the four seasons will change accordingly and are not the same all the time: they are called the Guest Colours. The climate in Spring corresponds to the Liver, and the complexion colour is relatively green. The climate in Summer corresponds to the Heart, and the complexion colour is relatively red. The climate in Autumn corresponds to the Lungs, and the complexion colour is relatively white. The climate in Winter corresponds to the Kidneys, and the complexion colour is relatively dark. The climate in Late Summer corresponds to the Spleen, and the complexion colour is relatively yellow. These colours are seen when the climatic changes in the seasons are normal. The Dominant Colours are a [physiological] manifestation of the five Yin organs, while the Guest Colours are produced by the climatic changes of the seasons. Therefore, [when observing] the complexion colour, if the influence of the climatic factors of the seasons exceeds that of the five Yin organs, it indicates a good prognosis. That is why it is said that the Guest colour replacing the Dominant colours is a sign of good prognosis. If the influence of the five Yin organs exceeds that of the climatic factors of the seasons, it is a sign of poor prognosis. That is why it is said that the Dominant Colours overtaking the Guest Colours is a sign of poor prognosis. The so-called replacing of the colours is found in the following situations: the complexion colour should be green [in Spring] but is white instead; the complexion colour should be red [in Summer] but is black instead; the complexion colour should be white [in Autumn] but is red instead; the complexion colour should be black [in Winter] but is yellow instead; and the complexion colour should be yellow [in Late Summer] but is green instead.[20]

Reading the above quotation, it should be noted that a poor prognosis is indicated when the dominant colour becomes pathological, when it manifests in the 'wrong' season and, specifically, when it belongs to the Element that overacts, along the Overacting cycle, on the Element of that particular season. For example, having a yellow (instead of greenish) complexion in springtime indicates a poor prognosis but the prognosis would be even worse if the complexion were white (because Metal overacts on Wood).

Box 3.8 summarizes the factors that affect prognosis.

Changes in complexion colour during a disease

Observation

When observing complexion colour, in addition to the above-mentioned aspects (i.e. whether the abnormal colour is superficial or deep, distinct or obscure, lustrous or lustreless, scattered or concentrated, conforming or opposing), attention should be paid also to observing any changes in the complexion in the course of a chronic disease.

Chapter 49 of the 'Spiritual Axis' says:

If the complexion colour looks contained and slightly bright, it indicates that the disease is mild. If the complexion colour is dark and lustreless, it means that the disease is severe. If the abnormal colour moves upwards [in the face], it is a sign of aggravation of the disease. If the abnormal colour moves downwards [in the face], like black clouds dissipating, it is a sign of the gradual alleviation of the disease.[21]

Clinical significance

The changes occurring in the complexion colour in the course of a disease reflect the changes in the relative strength of pathogenic factors and Upright Qi. Changes in the complexion colour indicating a worsening of the condition are as follows: from conforming to opposing, from thin to thick, from superficial to deep, from distinct to obscure, from scattered to concentrated, and from lustrous to lustreless. All these indicate that the disease is moving from the Exterior to the Interior, pathogenic factors are growing stronger, Upright Qi is getting weaker, the disease is becoming more severe and the treatment given is not effective. Changes in the complexion colour indicating an improvement in the condition are as follows: from opposing to conforming, from thick to thin, from deep to superficial, from obscure to distinct, from concentrated to scattered, and from lustreless to lustrous. All these signs indicate that the disease is moving from the Interior to the Exterior, pathogenic factors are subsiding, the Upright Qi is becoming stronger, the disease is getting better and the treatment received is effective.

Complexion colours and emotions

Specific signs in the complexion may indicate various emotions.

Anger usually manifests with a greenish tinge on the cheeks or under the eyes. If there is such a tinge on the forehead, it means that Liver-Qi has invaded the Stomach; if on the tip of the nose, that Liver-Qi has invaded the Spleen. Being prone to anger may also be manifested by eyebrows that meet in the centre. In some cases, if the anger is bottled up inside as resentment leading to long-standing depression, the complexion may be pale. This is due to the depressing effect of stagnant Liver-Qi on Spleen- or Lung-Qi. In such cases, the Wiry quality of the pulse will betray the existence of anger rather than sadness or grief (indicated by the pale complexion) as a cause of disease.

Excess joy may manifest with a red colour on the cheekbones.

Worry causes a greyish complexion and a skin without lustre because it knots Lung-Qi and affects the Corporeal Soul, which manifests on the skin.

Pensiveness may manifest with a sallow complexion because it depletes Spleen-Qi.

Fear shows with a bright-white complexion on the cheeks and forehead. If chronic fear causes deficiency of Kidney-Yin and the rising of Empty-Heat of the Heart, there will be a malar flush, with the underlying colour being bright-white.

Shock also causes a bright-white complexion. Shock early in childhood may manifest with a bluish tinge on the forehead. Such a bluish tinge there or around the mouth indicates a prenatal shock (while in the uterus).

Hatred often shows with a greenish complexion on the cheeks.

Craving shows with a reddish colour on the cheeks.

Guilt shows with a dark-ruddy complexion.

Box 3.9 summarizes the complexion colours associated with the emotions.

BOX 3.9 EMOTIONS AND COMPLEXION COLOURS

- Anger: greenish on cheeks or under eyes
- Excess joy: red on cheekbones
- Worry: greyish without lustre
- Pensiveness: sallow-yellow
- Fear: bright white on cheeks and forehead
- Shock: bright white or bluish
- Hatred: dull greenish without lustre
- Craving: reddish on cheeks
- Guilt: dark ruddy

COMPLEXION COLOURS

The complexion colours are:

- normal
- white
- sallow
- yellow
- red
- bluish/greenish
- dark
- purple.

Normal complexion colour

Observation

As 'normality' obviously varies from race to race, it is impossible to define a universal normal colour. We can, however, identify and define four essential characteristics of a normal complexion:

- lustre
- a subtle, slightly reddish hue
- 'contained', 'veiled' colour
- moisture.

The presence of lustre is an essential part of a normal complexion. Such a complexion is slightly shiny, vibrant in colour, lively, relatively bright and glowing. The presence of lustre in the complexion indicates that the Upright Qi is intact (even though there may be a pathology) and that the Mind and Spirit are healthy. The lustre of the complexion is equivalent to the spirit of the pulse (one of the attributes of the normal pulse) or of the eyes; they all indicate a good state of the Mind and Spirit.

The normal complexion should have a subtle, slightly reddish hue because the facial colour as a whole reflects the state of the Heart and a reddish hue indicates a good supply of Heart-Blood (and by implication, a good state of the Mind).

The colour of the facial complexion should be 'contained' as if there was a very thin, white silk veil over it. The book 'Wang Zhen Zun Jing' describes the normal complexion colour as being bright and lustrous and says: *'The complexion is bright because of the embodiment of the Spirit. It is lustrous because of the nourishment of the Essence and Blood.'*[22]

The normal complexion should be moist and look firm (because of the fluids underneath); a dry complexion is always a poor prognostic sign. The moisture of the complexion is equivalent to the Stomach-Qi of the pulse (one of the attributes of the normal pulse); they therefore both indicate that the patient's Stomach-Qi is intact (even though there may be pathogenic factors).

Apart from these four basic aspects of a normal complexion, the actual colour of course varies enormously according to race and even within the same racial group. The normal complexion colour for Caucasian people is a mixed white and slightly reddish colour which is lustrous, bright and contained. Within the Caucasian race, however, there can be considerable variations in normal complexion: for example, the normal complexion of a Norwegian person will be quite different from that of a Spaniard as the Mediterranean complexion is naturally slightly darker and of a more earthy colour than that of the northern European. The complexion of Chinese people is described in Chinese books as a mixed red and yellow colour, shown slightly, which is bright, lustrous and reserved.

The same wide variations may be observed in Asian, African and Afro-American people. For example, the complexion of people in north India is much lighter than that of Indians from the south.

Apart from racial differences, there can be wide variations in normal complexion in people of the same race due to other factors such as the influence of prenatal constitution, the profession, the area people come from and their working or living environment. However, complexion colour changes caused by the above-mentioned factors are not regarded as abnormal. For example, the normal complexion of a farmer will be rosier and redder than that of an office worker (see Plate 3.9 on p. P4).

Clinical significance

A bright, lustrous, white-reddish and 'contained' complexion colour in Caucasian people indicates strong Stomach-Qi, normal Internal Organs, ample Blood and good Spirit. This is regarded as a normal complexion colour. If such a complexion colour is observed in the process of a disease, it means that the duration of the disease is short, the pathogenic factors are weak, the Upright Qi is still strong, the treatment will be easy and the prognosis is good. Chapter 17 of the 'Simple Questions' says:

In the course of a disease, if the pulse is small and the complexion colour is normal, it is a disease with a short duration. If the pulse is normal but the complexion colour is abnormal, it is a disease with a long duration. If both the pulse and the complexion colour are abnormal, it is a disease with a long duration. If both the pulse and the complexion colour are normal, it is a disease with a short duration.'[23]

This highlights the connection between complexion colour and the duration of a disease.

BOX 3.10 ATTRIBUTES OF A NORMAL COMPLEXION

- Lustre: Spirit strong
- Subtle reddish hue: Heart-Blood abundant
- 'Contained', 'veiled' colour: no pathogenic factors
- Moisture: good state of fluids

Box 3.10 summarizes the attributes of a normal complexion.

White complexion colour

Symptoms and Signs, Chapter 56

There are several shades of white complexion:

- bright white
- dull white
- pale white
- sallow white
- bluish white.

Bright white
Observation

The bright-white complexion is of a brilliant and obvious white colour (see Plate 3.10 on p. P4).

Clinical significance

The bright-white complexion usually indicates Yang deficiency, which may affect especially the Spleen, Stomach, Lungs, Heart and Kidneys.

Dull white
Observation

The dull-white complexion has no lustre and is somewhat greyish (see Plate 3.11 on p. P4).

Clinical significance

The dull-white complexion also indicates Yang deficiency but of a more severe degree than that indicated by the bright-white complexion.

A dull-white complexion that looks like dry bones indicates Lung-Yang deficiency.

Pale white
Observation

The pale-white complexion is also somewhat bright like the bright-white complexion but to a lesser degree (see Plate 3.12 on p. P4).

Clinical significance

The pale-white complexion indicates Qi deficiency.

Sallow white
Observation

The sallow-white complexion is dull, without lustre and with a slight hint of yellow (see Plates 3.13 and Plate 3.14 on pp. P4 and P5).

Clinical significance

The sallow-white complexion indicates Blood deficiency. A further differentiation can be made according to subtle variations of the sallow-white colour. For example, a sallow-white complexion which is also very slightly bluish indicates severe Blood deficiency; a sallow-white complexion which is also slightly yellow indicates Qi deficiency not holding Blood with resulting bleeding; a sallow-white tip of the nose indicates Blood deficiency deriving from Spleen deficiency; a sallow-white complexion without lustre indicates Qi and Blood deficiency with Dryness, while a sallow-white and slightly yellow complexion in women after childbirth indicates exhaustion of Blood.

Bluish-white
Observation

The bluish-white complexion is bright-white with a subtle bluish hue.

Clinical significance

The bluish-white complexion indicates Cold that derives from Yang deficiency. The bright-white complexion described above may also indicate Cold but the emphasis is on Yang deficiency, whereas with the bluish-white complexion the emphasis is on Cold.

BOX 3.11 WHITE COMPLEXION COLOUR

- Bright white: Yang deficiency (Spleen, Stomach, Lungs, Heart, Kidneys)
- Dull white: severe Yang deficiency
- Pale white: Qi deficiency
- Sallow white: Blood deficiency
- Bluish-white: Cold

Box 3.11 summarizes the types of white complexion colour.

Sallow complexion colour

Symptoms and Signs, Chapter 56

Observation

The sallow complexion is pale, yellowish, dull and without lustre.

Clinical significance

The sallow complexion usually indicates Spleen-Qi deficiency with Dampness. In some cases it may indicate chronic Kidney-Yang deficiency; if it is greyish, it may indicate Blood stasis.

BOX 3.12 SALLOW COMPLEXION COLOUR

- Spleen-Qi deficiency with Dampness
- Kidney-Yang deficiency
- Blood stasis: sallow greyish

Box 3.12 summarizes sallow complexion colour.

Yellow complexion colour

Symptoms and Signs, Chapters 56 and 68

There are several types of yellow complexion:

- dull yellow
- greyish-yellow
- bluish-yellow
- floating, reddish-yellow
- floating yellow
- dry yellow
- ash-like yellow
- rich yellow
- bright yellow (jaundice).

Dull yellow
Observation

The dull-yellow complexion is relatively pale yellow, wan, sallow and without lustre (see Plate 3.15 on p. P5).

Clinical significance

The dull-yellow complexion always indicates a deficient, chronic condition and usually a deficiency of Blood. The dull-yellow complexion may also indicate a chronic deficiency of Spleen-Qi.

Greyish-yellow
Observation

The greyish-yellow complexion is dull, ashen and without lustre (see Plate 3.16 on p. P5).

Clinical significance

The greyish-yellow complexion is frequently seen in disharmonies of the Spleen and Liver characterized by Spleen-Qi deficiency and stagnation of Liver-Qi and/or Liver-Blood. This condition is frequently caused by deep emotional problems and symptoms may include severe abdominal distension, depression, irritability and poor digestion.

Bluish-yellow
Observation

A bluish-yellow complexion is primarily dark yellow with a slight bluish tinge; it is usually seen only in the elderly.

Clinical significance

A bluish-yellow complexion indicates Blood stasis with Damp-Heat.

Floating, reddish-yellow

Observation

A floating, reddish-yellow complexion is bright yellow with a slight red tinge and it gives the appearance of being on the surface of the skin.

Clinical significance

A floating, reddish-yellow complexion indicates an invasion of Wind-Heat.

Floating yellow

Observation

The floating yellow complexion is bright yellow and gives the impression of being on the surface of the skin (see Plate 3.17 on p. P5).

Clinical significance

A floating yellow complexion indicates an invasion of external Wind-Dampness.

Dry yellow

Observation

The dry-yellow complexion is dull and without lustre and the skin is dry, withered and without elasticity (see Plate 3.18 on p. P5).

Clinical significance

The dry-yellow complexion always indicates a disharmony of the Stomach and Spleen, usually due to Heat, which may be Full or Empty.

A thin, dry, yellow colour indicates Stomach Empty-Heat.

Ash-like yellow

Observation

The ash-like yellow complexion is dull, darkish and 'smoky'. It is darker than the greyish-yellow complexion (see Plate 3.19 on p. P5).

Clinical significance

The ash-like yellow complexion always indicates Dampness, often with Heat. It may indicate external Dampness, in which case the patient often suffers from body aches, or internal Dampness, in which case the complexion is slightly dryer and there are no body aches. The ash-like yellow complexion is also seen when Dampness is associated with Qi stagnation.

Rich yellow

Observation

The rich-yellow complexion is relatively bright and the colour is thick (see Plate 3.20 on p. P6).

Clinical significance

A rich-yellow complexion indicates Qi and Blood deficiency with Dampness.

Bright yellow (jaundice)

Observation

Patients with jaundice have yellow conjunctiva and a yellow complexion colour, which may be either bright yellow, orangey yellow or dark yellow as if smoked, yellow scanty urine, general weakness, listlessness and a greasy tongue coating.

Chapter 18 of the 'Simple Questions' says: '*Symptoms such as deep yellow urine and lethargy indicate jaundice. . . yellow conjunctiva indicates jaundice.*'[24] Chapter 74 of the 'Spiritual Axis' says: '*If the face is slightly yellow, the teeth filthy yellow, the nails yellow, this indicates jaundice. (If there are also symptoms and signs such as lethargy, deep yellow urine, poor appetite and a Small-Choppy pulse, it then indicates that it is the disease of the Spleen.)*'[25]

Clinical significance

The aetiology of jaundice, manifesting with yellow conjunctiva and a yellow complexion colour, is often related to poor diet and invasion by pathogenic factors such as Damp, Heat and Toxic Heat. It is often located in the Liver, Gall-Bladder, Spleen and Stomach. The nature of the disease is often one of either Damp-Heat, Cold-Damp, Toxic Heat, or Qi and Blood deficiency. Signs and symptoms such as a bright-yellow colour like an orange (called 'Yang yellow'), a Red tongue with a thick coating, yellow urine and abdominal distension indicate that the disease is caused by the accumulation of Damp-Heat in the Liver, Gall-Bladder, Spleen and Stomach. Signs and symptoms such as a

---

BOX 3.13 YELLOW COMPLEXION COLOUR

- Pale yellow: Spleen-Qi deficiency, Blood deficiency
- Greyish-yellow: Spleen-Qi deficiency with stagnation of Liver-Qi or Liver-Blood
- Dry yellow: Full- or Empty-Heat in Stomach and Spleen
- Ash-like yellow: Dampness
- Rich yellow: Qi and Blood deficiency with Dampness
- Bright yellow: Jaundice

dark-yellow, smoky colour (called 'Yin yellow') and a light-Red tongue body with a thick white coating indicate that the disease is caused by Cold-Damp being retained in the Liver, Gall-Bladder, Spleen and Stomach.

Box 3.13 summarizes the types of yellow complexion colour.

Red complexion colour

Symptoms and Signs, Chapter 56

A red complexion always indicates Heat, which may be Full or Empty; it indicates Empty-Heat particularly when only the cheeks are red. Redness of the complexion also indicates Empty-Heat when it is somewhat 'thin' or 'superficial' as defined above.

The clinical significance of the red complexion depends also on the location of the redness. There are three main types of red complexion:

- red cheeks
- red cheekbones
- floating red.

Red cheeks
Observation

In this case, the facial complexion is too red and the redness is located all over the cheeks; in some cases one cheek may be redder than the other. Usually the right cheek reflects the condition of the Lungs whereas the left one reflects the condition of the Liver (see Plates 3.21 and 3.22 on p. P6).

Clinical significance

A red facial complexion usually indicates Full-Heat, which may pertain to various organs, especially the Heart, Lungs, Liver or Stomach. In cases of Full Heat, the whole cheeks are of a full red colour. In some cases, a red complexion may be seen in Empty-Heat, in which case the red colour looks 'thinner' and it may come and go.

Red cheekbones
Observation

In this case, only the cheekbones are red and the colour is usually 'thinner' than that of Full-Heat; the redness of the cheekbones may come and go and often it appears only in the afternoon or evening (see Plates 3.23 and 3.24 on p. P6).

Clinical significance

Red cheekbones always indicate Empty-Heat, which may affect various organs and especially the Lungs, Heart, Stomach and Kidneys. The clinical significance may be further differentiated according to the type of redness and to the time of day when it appears.

A relatively thin red colour that looks like make-up and appears in the afternoon indicates Blood deficiency; if both cheekbones are deep red this indicates Empty-Heat; if both cheekbones are fresh red like threads it indicates Yin deficiency; if both cheekbones are pale red it indicates 'steaming from the bones' due to chronic Yin deficiency.

> **!**
>
> **Note**: do not assume that red cheekbones always indicate Yin deficiency; they may also indicate Blood deficiency especially if obvious in the afternoon (common in women).

Floating red
Observation

The floating red colour is a 'thin', floating, pale red that looks like rouge and may move from place to place (see Plate 3.25 on p. P6).

Clinical significance

The floating red colour generally indicates Empty-Heat. It is seen also in the pattern characterized by false Heat and true Cold, which means that the patient suffers from severe internal Cold and the separation of Yin and Yang which makes Yang 'float' to the top giving the false appearance of Heat. In fact, apart from the redness of the face, all the other signs and symptoms point to internal Cold (cold limbs, a desire to curl up, weak breathing, Pale and Short tongue and Slow pulse). However, this situation is rather rare.

Plates 3.26–3.31 on p. P7 illustrate thin/thick, superficial/deep and distinct/obscure red complexion colours.

BOX 3.14 RED COMPLEXION COLOUR

- Red cheeks: Full-Heat (Heart, Lungs, Liver, Stomach)
- Red cheekbones: Empty-Heat (Lungs, Heart, Stomach, Kidneys) or Blood deficiency
- Floating red: Empty-Heat or False Heat–true Cold

Box 3.14 summarizes the types of red complexion colour.

Bluish/greenish complexion colour

Symptoms and Signs, Chapter 56

'Bluish/greenish' is a translation of the Chinese word *qing* which can mean both blue and green. In the context of the Five Elements, it is the colour associated with Wood and it therefore makes more sense to translate it as green. In the context of facial diagnosis, *qing* can mean either bluish or greenish; for example, the *qing* colour may indicate a Liver pattern, in which case it would be greenish, or interior Cold, in which case it would be bluish (see Plate 3.32 on p. P8).

There are various types of bluish/greenish colour:

- pale greenish under the eyes
- dark bluish under the eyes
- white-bluish
- dull bluish
- bluish
- greenish.

Pale greenish under the eyes
Observation

A pale-greenish colour under the eyes is usually thin and rather bright.

Clinical significance

A pale-greenish colour under the eyes generally indicates Liver-Qi stagnation.

Dark bluish under the eyes
Observation

A dark-bluish colour under the eyes usually lacks lustre and is dull.

Clinical significance

A dark-blue colour under the eyes indicates Cold in the Liver channel.

White-bluish
Observation

The white-bluish complexion is bright.

Clinical significance

The white-bluish complexion generally indicates internal Cold or chronic pain.

Dull bluish
Observation

The dull-bluish complexion is ash-like and without lustre.

Clinical significance

The dull-bluish complexion indicates severe Heart-Yang deficiency with Blood stasis or chronic pain, or both. The duller and darker this complexion, the more severe is the condition.

Bluish
Observation

The bluish complexion is bright blue and it is usually confined to the lower part of the forehead or the space between the eyebrows in children.

Clinical significance

A bright-bluish complexion in the space between the eyebrows in children indicates Liver-Wind and it is often seen in convulsions.

A bluish complexion in pregnant women indicates Blood stasis and Yang deficiency and it is always a poor sign.

Greenish
Observation

The greenish complexion is dull green, somewhat greyish and without lustre.

Clinical significance

The greenish complexion always indicates a Liver pattern, which may be Liver-Qi stagnation, Liver-Blood stasis, Cold in the Liver channel or Liver-Wind.

A green complexion with a red tinge is seen in the Lesser-Yang syndrome. A green complexion with red eyes indicates Liver-Fire. Yellowish green cheeks indicate Phlegm with Liver-Yang rising often causing headaches.

A green nose indicates stagnation of Qi often causing abdominal pain. A dark, reddish-green complexion indicates stagnant Liver-Qi turning into Heat. A pale-green colour under the eyes indicates Liver-Blood deficiency. A grass-green indicates collapse of Liver-Qi.

Box 3.15 summarizes bluish/greenish complexion colour.

> **BOX 3.15 BLUISH/GREENISH COMPLEXION COLOUR**
>
> - Pale greenish under the eyes: Liver-Qi stagnation
> - Dark bluish under the eyes: Cold in the Liver channel
> - White-bluish: Cold or chronic pain
> - Dull bluish: severe Heart-Yang deficiency with Blood stasis, chronic pain
> - Bluish (in children): Liver-Wind
> - Greenish: Liver-Qi stagnation, Liver-Blood stasis, Cold in the Liver channel, Liver-Wind
> - Green with a red tinge: Lesser-Yang syndrome
> - Green with red eyes: Liver-Fire
> - Yellowish-green cheeks: Phlegm with Liver-Yang rising
> - Green nose: stagnation of Qi with abdominal pain
> - Dark reddish-green: stagnant Liver-Qi turning into Heat
> - Pale green under the eyes: Liver-Blood deficiency
> - Grass-like green: collapse of Liver-Qi

Dark complexion colour

Symptoms and Signs, Chapter 56

There are several types of dark complexion:

> - dark and dry
> - dull dark
> - faint dark
> - very dark.

Dark and dry
Observation

The dark and dry complexion is blackish, the skin is dry and withered and the ear-lobes are dry.

Clinical significance

The dark and dry complexion indicates severe Kidney-Yin deficiency.

Dull dark
Observation

The dark and dull complexion is blackish but faint and dim and the eye sockets are dark.

Clinical significance

The dark and dull complexion indicates severe Kidney-Yang deficiency with Empty-Cold.

A dark colour around the eye sockets indicates Kidney deficiency with Phlegm-Fluids or Cold-Dampness in the Lower Burner.

A dull-dark complexion like soot indicates the collapse of Kidney-Qi.

Faint dark
Observation

The faint-dark complexion is slightly blackish with a light hue and with a blackish colour around the eye sockets; the face might be swollen.

Clinical significance

The faint-dark complexion indicates severe Damp-Cold or Phlegm-Fluids.

Very dark
Observation

The very dark complexion is almost black, dull and without lustre.

Clinical significance

The very dark complexion indicates severe Blood stasis.

> **BOX 3.16 DARK COMPLEXION COLOUR**
>
> - Dark and dry: Kidney-Yin deficiency
> - Dull dark: Kidney-Yang deficiency with internal Cold
> - Dark around the eye sockets: Kidney deficiency with Phlegm-Fluids or Cold-Dampness in the Lower Burner
> - Dull dark like soot: collapse of Kidney-Qi
> - Faint dark: Damp-Cold or Phlegm-Fluids
> - Very dark: Blood stasis

Box 3.16 summarizes the types of dark complexion colour.

Purple complexion colour

Symptoms and Signs, Chapter 56

There are two types of purple complexion colour:

> - reddish-purple
> - bluish-purple.

Reddish-purple
Observation

The reddish-purple complexion approximates to the colour of a beetroot and is very similar to the colour of a reddish-purple tongue.

Clinical significance

The reddish-purple complexion indicates severe Blood stasis.

Bluish-purple
Observation

The bluish-purple complexion approximates to the colour of a blueberry but with a lighter hue and is very similar to the colour of the bluish-purple tongue.

Clinical significance

The bluish-purple complexion indicates severe internal Cold leading to Blood stasis. The bluish-purple complexion is also seen in cases of poisoning from food, drugs or toxic herbs.

BOX 3.17 PURPLE COMPLEXION COLOUR

- Reddish-purple: Blood stasis
- Bluish-purple: internal Cold leading to Blood stasis, or poisoning

---

Box 3.17 summarizes the types of purple complexion colour.

NOTES

1. Cited in Zhang Shu Sheng 1995 Great Treatise of Diagnosis by Observation in Chinese Medicine (*Zhong Hua Yi Xue Wang Zhen Da Quan* 中华医学望诊大全), Shanxi Science Publishing House, Taiyuan, p. 82.

2. Principles of Medical Practice 1658, cited in Wang Ke Qin 1988 Theory of the Mind in Chinese Medicine (*Zhong Yi Shen Zhu Xue Shuo* 中医神主学说), Ancient Chinese Medical Texts Publishing House, p. 56.

3. Cited in Great Treatise of Diagnosis by Observation in Chinese Medicine, p. 82.

4. 1979 The Yellow Emperor's Classic of Internal Medicine – Simple Questions (*Huang Di Nei Jing Su Wen* 黄帝内经素问), People's Health Publishing House, Beijing, p. 80. First published c. 100BC.

5. Ibid., p. 291.

6. 1981 Spiritual Axis (*Ling Shu Jing* 灵枢经), People's Health Publishing House, Beijing, p. 96. First published c. 100BC.

7. Wu Qian 1977 Golden Mirror of Medicine (*Yi Zong Jin Jian* 医宗金鉴), People's Health Publishing House, Beijing, vol. 2, p. 872. First published in 1742.

8. Cited in Great Treatise of Diagnosis by Observation in Chinese Medicine, p. 85.

9. Simple Questions, p. 89.

10. Cited in Great Treatise of Diagnosis by Observation in Chinese Medicine, p. 85.

11. Spiritual Axis, p. 98.

12. Cited in Great Treatise of Diagnosis by Observation in Chinese Medicine, p. 86.

13. Spiritual Axis, p. 98.

14. Shi Pa Nan 1861 Origin of Medicine (*Yi Yuan* 医元), cited in Wang Ke Qin 1988 Theory of the Mind in Chinese Medicine, p. 55.

15. Simple Questions, pp. 71–2.

16. Ibid., p. 72.

17. Ibid., p. 99.

18. Chen Shi Duo 1687 Secret Records of the Stone Room (*Shi Shi Mi Lu* 石室秘录), cited in Wang Ke Qin 1988 Theory of the Mind in Chinese Medicine, p. 56.

19. Simple Questions, p. 90.

20. Golden Mirror of Medicine, vol. 2, pp. 866–867.

21. Spiritual Axis, p. 97.

22. Cited in Zhang Shu Sheng 1995 Great Treatise of Diagnosis by Observation in Chinese Medicine, p. 89.

23. Simple Questions, p. 98.

24. Ibid. p. 114.

25. Spiritual Axis, p. 134.

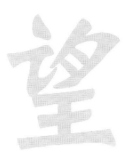

Chapter **4**

OBSERVATION OF BODY MOVEMENTS

Chapter contents

HEAD   *59*
  Tremor of the head   *59*
  Rigidity of the neck   *59*

FACE   *60*
  Deviation of eye and mouth   *60*
  Facial paralysis (Bell's palsy)   *60*
  Facial tic   *61*

LIMBS AND BODY   *61*
  Paralysis   *61*
  Tremor or spasticity of the limbs   *62*
  Twitching of the muscles   *63*
  Opisthotonos   *63*
  Contraction of the limbs   *63*
  Hemiplegia   *64*
  Tremor of the hands   *64*
  Tremor of the feet   *64*
  Contraction of the fingers   *65*

The discussion of 'body movements' includes both involuntary body movements and their opposite, that is, rigidity or paralysis.

HEAD

The signs discussed are:

- tremor of the head
- rigidity of the neck.

Tremor of the head

Observation, Chapter 5; Symptoms and Signs, Chapter 55

Observation

Tremor of the head consists of shaking of the head, with the head usually moving back and forth. The tremor ranges from the very slight with small amplitude to the very pronounced with large amplitude.

Clinical significance

A tremor of the head always indicates internal Wind, which itself stems from the Liver. Liver-Wind may be of the Full or Empty type: the Full type develops from Liver-Yang rising or Liver-Fire while the Empty type develops from Liver- and Kidney-Yin or Liver-Blood deficiency. The tremor of the head is pronounced in the Full type and slight in the Empty type. In a few cases, the cause may be exhaustion of Heart-Yin, in which case the tremor will usually be a fine one.

Rigidity of the neck
Observation

'Rigidity of the neck' indicates that the patient finds it difficult to bend the head forwards or backwards and to turn the head from side to side.

Clinical significance

In acute situations, rigidity of the neck may indicate an invasion of external Wind, in which case it will be accompanied by all the typical manifestations of an exterior invasion such as aversion to cold, fever, headache and a Floating pulse. Both Wind-Cold and Wind-Heat may cause rigidity of the neck but it is more likely to occur with an invasion of Wind-Cold (in fact, it is one of the chief symptoms of invasion of Wind-Cold as listed in the 'Discussion of Cold-induced Diseases' – see Bibliography, p. 1067). Another possible acute condition causing stiffness of the neck occurs when external Cold and Dampness invade the muscles of the neck, in which case there is also pronounced neck pain; this is a case of acute Painful Obstruction Syndrome and it is relatively common.

In chronic cases, stiffness of the neck is due either to a weakness of the Bladder channel in the neck occurring against a background of Kidney deficiency or to internal Wind, both of which are more common in the elderly.

Box 4.1 summarizes patterns underlying neck rigidity.

BOX 4.1 RIGIDITY OF THE NECK

- Rigidity with aversion to cold, Floating pulse: invasion of external Wind
- Rigidity and pain: invasion of external Cold and Dampness
- Slight rigidity and dizziness: Bladder and Kidney deficiency
- Slight rigidity and dizziness: Bladder and Kidney deficiency

---

FACE

The face signs discussed are:

- deviation of eye and mouth
- facial paralysis (Bell's palsy)
- facial tic.

Deviation of eye and mouth

Observation, Chapter 5; Symptoms and Signs, Chapter 55

Observation

Deviation of eyes and mouth consists in the mouth's being pulled towards the healthy side and an inability to close or open the eye completely; in addition, the patient finds it difficult to grimace, to bulge the cheeks, grin and whistle.

Clinical significance

Deviation of eye and mouth is a consequence of Wind-stroke and is usually seen in middle-aged or elderly people; it always indicates internal Wind affecting the muscles of the face.

When deviation of eyes and mouth follows a stroke, it is called central facial paralysis in Western medicine, as it arises from the central nervous system. In facial paralysis following Wind-stroke, the nerves above the eyes are not affected, that is, the movement of the eyebrows and furrowing of the forehead are normal. By contrast, in peripheral facial paralysis (Bell's palsy), the patient will be unable to raise the eyebrow or furrow the forehead on the paralysed side. Figure 4.1 shows the deviation of eye and mouth.

Facial paralysis (Bell's palsy)

Symptoms and signs, Chapter 55

Facial paralysis is due to an injury of peripheral nerves, whereas deviation of eyes and mouth following a stroke is due to the central nervous system. From a Chinese perspective, facial paralysis is due to an invasion of external Wind, whereas deviation of eyes and mouth following a stroke is due to internal Wind.

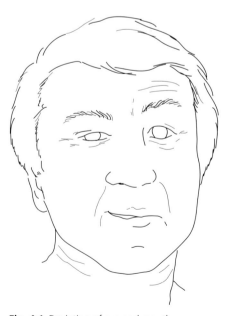

Fig. 4.1 Deviation of eye and mouth

Observation

Facial paralysis is characterized by deviation of the mouth, incomplete closure of one eye and inability to grimace, grin, bulge the cheeks, whistle, or raise the eyebrow and furrow the forehead on the affected side (see Plate 4.1 on p. P8).

Clinical significance

Facial paralysis is due to invasion of external Wind in the muscles of the face and primarily in the Bright-Yang channels.

Facial tic

Symptoms and Signs, Chapter 55

Observation

Tic consists in an involuntary twitching of the face muscles.

Clinical significance

In Chinese medicine a facial tic may be due to various patterns, among which are Liver-Qi stagnation, Liver-Blood deficiency, Liver-Wind, Liver-Wind with Phlegm and external Wind.

When due to Liver-Qi stagnation, facial tic will be accompanied by irritability, depression, tendency to crying, abdominal distension, headache and a Wiry pulse.

Liver-Blood deficiency causes facial paralysis by failing to nourish the muscles of the face and giving rise to Empty-Wind; other symptoms may include dizziness, blurred vision, dull-pale complexion and a Choppy pulse.

Liver-Wind may lead to facial tic because it is in the nature of internal Wind to cause involuntary movements. Facial tic caused by Liver-Wind is more common in the elderly and is accompanied by vertigo, headache, loss of balance and a Wiry pulse.

BOX 4.2 FACIAL TIC

- Tic and irritability, depression, Wiry pulse: Liver-Qi stagnation
- Tic and dizziness, blurred vision, Choppy pulse: Liver-Blood deficiency
- Tic and vertigo, Wiry pulse: Liver-Wind
- Tic and vertigo, nausea, Wiry-Slippery pulse: Liver-Wind with Phlegm
- Temporary tic: external Wind

In the elderly, Liver-Wind frequently combines with Phlegm, both of which may lead to facial tic. Other symptoms include vertigo, nausea, headache, a feeling of oppression of the chest, a tendency to being overweight, a Swollen tongue and a Wiry-Slippery pulse.

External Wind may cause a temporary facial tic.

Box 4.2 summarizes patterns underlying facial tic.

LIMBS AND BODY

The limb and body signs discussed are:

- paralysis
- tremor or spasticity of the limbs
- twitching of the muscles
- opisthotonos
- contraction of the limbs
- hemiplegia
- tremor of the hands
- tremor of the feet
- contraction of the fingers.

Paralysis

Observation, Chapters 18 and 19; Symptoms and Signs, Chapter 68

Paralysis is called *Tan Huan* in Chinese, which can be written with two different sets of characters, the second one of which means 'spread out' and 'relaxed' (see Glossary, p. 1061).

Observation

In paralysis, a weakness of the muscles of the four limbs impedes the proper function of the legs or arms, or both. Paralysis is seen only in chronic, protracted conditions and is usually, but not always, accompanied by flaccidity of the muscles, in which case, in Chinese medicine, it pertains to the disease category of Atrophy (*Wei* syndrome). In mild cases, paralysis consists in a weakness of arms or legs which creates a slowness of movement, whilst in severe cases movement of the arms or legs, or both, is severly impaired or completely impossible and the patient is confined to a wheelchair.

In Western medicine, this type of paralysis is frequently seen in spinal injuries or neurological diseases such as multiple sclerosis or motor-neurone disease.

Clinical significance

Paralysis may be due to many different patterns depending on the severity of the disease.

Generally speaking, in the beginning stages of paralysis there may be invasion of external Dampness occurring against a background of Deficiency.

In the later stages, paralysis is often due to a general deficiency of Qi and Blood, and in particular a deficiency of Stomach and Spleen, which become unable to transport Qi to the limbs.

In yet later stages, the main pattern emerging in paralysis is a deficiency of Liver and Kidneys, which may manifest with Yin or Yang deficiency. At such a stage, the condition is complicated by the possible development of pathogenic factors such as internal Wind (which may cause spasticity of the limbs), Blood stasis (which may cause pain in the limbs) or Phlegm (which may cause numbness of the limbs).

In acute febrile diseases which progress to the Blood level, Yin deficiency may develop leading to the severe malnourishment of the channels and therefore to paralysis; this is, for example, the pathology of the paralysis deriving from poliomyelitis.

Of course, paralysis deriving from a spinal injury is different as it is due to external trauma and does not fall under any of the above patterns. However, in a patient suffering from a paralysis from spinal injury, this condition itself will, in time, lead to a deficiency of Stomach and Spleen.

BOX 4.3 PARALYSIS

- Slight weakness of the limbs, feeling of heaviness: invasion of external Dampness
- Weakness of the limbs, difficulty in walking: deficiency of Qi and Blood (Stomach and Spleen)
- Severe difficulty in walking: deficiency of Liver and Kidneys

---

Box 4.3 summarizes patterns underlying paralysis.

Multiple sclerosis

Multiple sclerosis is an example of paralysis that is commonly seen in Western, industrialized countries and one can identify clearly the above patterns in its pathological development. There are four stages in the pathological progression of multiple sclerosis (Box 4.4). The very beginning stage is characterized by invasion of external Dampness and the symptoms are purely numbness and tingling. The second stage is characterized by deficiency of the Stomach and Spleen and at this stage the patient begins to experience difficulty in walking. The third stage is characterized by

---

BOX 4.4 MULTIPLE SCLEROSIS

1. Dampness: numbness and tingling
2. Stomach and Spleen deficiency: difficulty in walking
3. Deficiency of Liver and Kidneys: severe difficulty in walking and urinary incontinence
4. Internal Wind: spasticity of limbs
5. Blood stasis: pain in the limbs

---

deficiency of Liver and Kidneys, which fail to nourish the sinews and bones, and the patient experiences severe difficulty in walking and urinary incontinence deriving from the Kidney deficiency. The fourth stage is characterized by the development of pathogenic factors, which may be internal Wind, itself deriving from the Liver and Kidney deficiency and causing spasticity of the limbs, or Blood stasis causing pain in the limbs.

Tremor or spasticity of the limbs

Observation, Chapters 14 and 18; Interrogation, Chapter 39; Symptoms and Signs, Chapters 64 and 66

'Tremor or spasticity of the limbs' is a translation of the Chinese characters *zhi zhong*. *Zhi* means 'contraction or bending of the limbs' and *zhong* means 'relaxation or stretching of the limbs'; however, these two terms may indicate both spasticity and tremor of the limbs.

Observation

The patient may suffer from contraction, relaxation or tremor of the limbs.

Clinical significance

Spasticity or tremor of the limbs may be due to many different patterns. Liver-Wind is the most likely pattern to cause this condition in its three possible manifestations, that is, Full-Wind deriving from Liver-Yang rising or Liver-Fire, Empty-Wind deriving from Liver-Blood or Liver-Yin deficiency, or Wind combined with Phlegm. In cases of Full-Wind, the spasticity or tremor of the limbs is pronounced and the patient also suffers from pronounced vertigo. In cases of Empty-Wind, the spasticity or tremor is mild and the patient will display the symptoms of Liver-Blood or Liver-Yin deficiency. When Wind combines with Phlegm the patient will also suffer from numbness and heaviness of the limbs, the tongue is Swollen and the pulse is Wiry-Slippery. Epilepsy is an example of a disease usually characterized by internal Wind and Phlegm.

The same symptoms may be caused by a general deficiency of Qi and Blood failing to nourish the sinews and muscles, in which case they are mild.

Spasticity and tremor of the limbs may also appear at the Blood level (of the Four Levels) when the Heat generated by the febrile disease either leads to Liver-Wind or depletes the Yin to such an extent that Empty-Wind is generated.

Box 4.5 summarizes patterns underlying tremor or spacticity of the limbs.

BOX 4.5 TREMOR OR SPASTICITY OF THE LIMBS

- Severe spasticity or tremor with large amplitude, vertigo, Wiry pulse: Liver-Wind (Full type)
- Mild spasticity or tremor with small amplitude, dizziness, Fine-Wiry pulse: Liver-Wind (Empty type)
- Numbness and heaviness of the limbs, Swollen tongue, Wiry-Slippery pulse: Liver-Wind with Phlegm
- Mild spasticity or tremor of the limbs, tiredness, Pale tongue, Weak or Choppy pulse: Qi and Blood deficiency

---

Twitching of the muscles

Symptoms and Signs, Chapter 68

Observation

Twitching of the muscles consists in an involuntary quivering or vibration of the superficial muscles: in Western medicine this is called 'fasciculation'.

Clinical significance

Twitching of the muscles may be due to Yang deficiency, Water overflowing or Qi and Blood deficiency.

In Yang deficiency, twitching of the muscles is due to the Defensive Qi (which is Yang in nature) not nourishing the superficial muscles. Chapter 3 of the 'Simple Questions' says: *The refined part of Yang-Qi nourishes the Mind while the soft part nourishes the sinews.*[1]

Water overflowing indicates a condition of severe Yang deficiency leading to the accumulation of fluids, which may occur in the Heart, the Lungs or the muscles. The accumulation of Water in the muscles may cause them to twitch.

General Qi and Blood deficiency may also cause twitching of the muscles when Yang Qi fails to nourish the superficial muscles and Blood fails to nourish the muscles and sinews.

Box 4.6 summarizes patterns underlying twitching of the muscles.

BOX 4.6 TWITCHING OF THE MUSCLES

- Twitching with feeling of cold, tiredness, Deep-Slow pulse: Yang deficiency
- Twitching with oedema, coughing of profuse watery phlegm, Wet tongue: Water overflowing
- Twitching with tiredness, dizziness, Pale tongue, Weak or Choppy pulse: Qi and Blood deficiency

---

Opisthotonos

Symptoms and Signs, Chapter 68

Observation

Opisthotonos indicates a spasm in which the head and heel are bent backward and the body bent forward (Fig. 4.2).

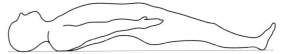

Fig. 4.2 Opisthotonos

Clinical significance

Opisthotonos is always due to Liver-Wind, which develops at the Blood level of a febrile disease. It may also occur after childbirth when the mother suffers from an infection but this is rarely seen in modern Western countries.

Contraction of the limbs

Observation, Chapter 18; Symptoms and Signs, Chapter 64

Observation

Contraction of the limbs consists in an involuntary clenching of the fists or contraction of the feet accompanied by rigidity of the affected limbs and the inability of the patient to stretch them. Contraction may affect any joint such as fingers, wrist, elbow, ankle and knees. Dupuytren's contracture, often involving the ring finger or the little finger, is an example of this condition.

Clinical significance

Contraction of the limbs may occur in various diseases such as arthritis, convulsions or Wind-stroke. The patterns causing it are usually general deficiency of Qi and Blood, internal Wind, Cold, Dampness, Phlegm or Blood stasis; in most cases the Liver and Kidney organs

are particularly involved because they nourish sinews and bones.

A general deficiency of Qi and Blood may cause a contraction of a particular joint due to Blood not nourishing the sinews. For example, a deficiency of Blood may affect the channels of the elbow and cause a contraction of that joint.

Internal Liver-Wind may cause contraction of any joint and this is frequently seen after an attack of Wind-stroke.

Cold by its very nature has a tendency to contract and may therefore cause a contraction of any joint; frequently seen in Painful Obstruction Syndrome, this often affects the elbow or knee and is accompanied by pain.

Dampness may cause contraction of a joint by obstructing the sinews and muscles; this is also seen in Painful Obstruction Syndrome and it affects particularly the wrist or fingers causing not only contraction but also swelling.

Phlegm may also cause contraction of a joint by obstructing the sinews, muscles and bones; this is seen in the late stages of Painful Obstruction Syndrome from Cold or Dampness complicated by Phlegm and it manifests not only with a contraction of the joint but also with bone deformities.

Blood stasis causes contraction and rigidity of joints because the Blood fails to nourish the sinews and bones and stagnates in the joints; this is seen also in the late stages of Painful Obstruction Syndrome from Dampness or Cold complicated by Blood stasis, which causes intense pain and rigidity.

Box 4.7 summarizes patterns underlying contraction of the limbs.

BOX 4.7 CONTRACTION OF LIMBS

- Mild contraction, tiredness, Pale tongue, Weak or Choppy pulse: Qi and Blood deficiency
- Pronounced contraction, vertigo, Wiry pulse: Liver-Wind
- Pronounced contraction and pain, feeling cold, ameliorated by heat: Cold
- Contraction of joints with swelling, feeling of heaviness: Dampness
- Contraction of joints with swelling and bone deformities: Phlegm
- Contraction and rigidity of joints with severe pain, Purple tongue: Blood stasis

---

Hemiplegia

Symptoms and Signs, Chapter 68

Observation

Hemiplegia consists in the unilateral paralysis of the arm or leg, or both.

Clinical significance

Hemiplegia is seen in the sequelae stage of Wind-stroke and the main patterns causing it are Liver-Wind and Phlegm. In protracted cases after a Wind-stroke, Blood stasis may also develop, which causes pronounced rigidity and pain of the limbs in addition to the paralysis.

Tremor of the hands

Observation, Chapter 14; Symptoms and Signs, Chapter 65

Observation

'Tremor of the hands' consists in an involuntary tremor of the hands or of the whole arm. The tremor may be very pronounced and with wide amplitude or very slight with a small amplitude. It may be unilateral or bilateral. The patient has difficulty holding a book, a spoon or a cup.

Clinical significance

Tremor of the hands always indicates internal Wind. Internal Wind may, in turn, develop from Liver-Yang rising, Liver-Fire, Liver-Blood deficiency or Liver- and Kidney-Yin deficiency. When it derives from Liver-Yang or Liver-Fire, the Wind is of a Full nature and the tremor is pronounced; when it derives from Deficiency, the Wind is of an Empty nature and the tremor is slight. In addition to the above patterns, in the elderly internal Wind is frequently complicated by Phlegm.

In alcoholics, a fine tremor of the hands is caused by Phlegm-Heat. In rare cases, retention of Dampness in the muscles and sinews of the hands may also cause a fine tremor.

Tremor of the feet

Symptoms and Signs, Chapter 66

Observation

'Tremor of the feet' consists in an involuntary tremor of the feet or of the whole leg, which may be unilateral

or bilateral. The patient has difficulty in walking and there may be atrophy of the lower limb.

Clinical significance

Tremor of the feet or legs is usually due to internal Wind of the Empty type, that is, deriving from Liver-Blood deficiency or Liver- and Kidney-Yin deficiency.

Contraction of the fingers

Observation, Chapter 14; Symptoms and Signs, Chapter 65

Observation

'Contraction of the fingers', which may be unilateral or bilateral, consists in an involuntary contracture of the fingers and permanent bending with inability to stretch the hand. The movement of the muscles and sinews above the wrist is normal.

Clinical significance

Contraction of the fingers is due either to deficiency of Blood or Yin, or both, or to invasion of Cold in the sinews and muscles, as in Painful Obstruction Syndrome. In the former case, the deficient Blood fails to nourish the sinews, which, in time, contract from lack of fluids; in the latter case, external Cold invades the sinews and muscles of the hands causing them to contract.

NOTES

1. 1979 The Yellow Emperor's Classic of Internal Medicine – Simple Questions (*Huang Di Nei Jing Su Wen* 黄帝内经素问), People's Health Publishing House, Beijing, p. 17. First published c. 100BC.

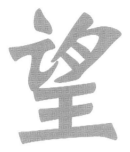

SECTION 2

OBSERVATION OF PARTS OF THE BODY

Section contents

 5 Observation of head, face and hair   69
 6 Observation of the eyes   75
 7 Observation of the nose   87
 8 Observation of lips, mouth, palate, teeth, gums and philtrum   93
 9 Observation of the ears   105
10 Observation of the throat and neck   109
11 Observation of the back   115
12 Observation of women's breasts   121
13 Observation of the heartbeat   127
14 Observation of the hands   129
15 Observation of the nails   137
16 Observation of the chest and abdomen   143
17 Observation of the genitalia   149
18 Observation of the four limbs   153
19 Observation of the legs   159
20 Observation of excretions   163
21 Observation of the skin   169
22 Observation in children   191

INTRODUCTION

This section discusses the observation of individual parts of the body. Section 1 dealt with the observation of the body shape, complexion and mental characteristics. These are the main things we would observe as the patient walks into our consulting room and they therefore give us the broad picture of that patient's constitution and potential disharmony.

After observing these general traits, we proceed to observing individual parts of the body, generally starting from the top and proceeding downwards. Some of these parts are observable as patients speak to us and some only when they undress and lie on the couch. Moreover, some of these parts are observed routinely (e.g. ears, hair, mouth, etc.) and some only if the patient asks us to (e.g. genitalia and women's breasts). Observation of the two excretions has been added here for completion although it is not carried out under normal clinical circumstances; this might be carried out if we see patients in their own home for an acute condition.

It is important to precede observation of individual parts of the body with the observation of the body shape and demeanour as a whole as described in the previous section. We should not give disproportionate importance to an individual part of the body (e.g. the ears) at the expense of observation of the body shape and demeanour as a whole. (Observation of the facial colours has been discussed in Chapter 3.)

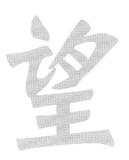

Chapter **5**

OBSERVATION OF HEAD, FACE AND HAIR

Chapter contents

HEAD   *69*
  Dry scalp   *69*
  Redness and pain of the scalp   *69*
  Tremor of the head   *70*
  Swelling of the whole head   *70*
  Boils on the scalp   *70*
  Ulcers on the scalp   *70*
  Ulcers in the mastoid region   *70*
  Erosion of the scalp   *70*
  Head leaning to one side   *70*
  Head tilted backwards   *70*
  Late closure of the fontanelles   *70*

FACE   *70*
  Acne   *71*
  Papular/macular eruption   *71*
  Oedema of the face   *71*
  Swelling and redness of the face   *71*
  Swelling, redness and pain of the cheeks   *71*
  Ulcers below the zygomatic arch   *71*
  Lines on the face   *71*
  Deviation of eye and mouth   *71*

HAIR   *71*
  Hair falling out   *72*
  Alopecia   *72*
  Dry and brittle hair   *72*
  Greasy hair   *73*
  Premature greying of the hair   *73*
  Dandruff   *73*

HEAD

In observation of the head, one should first of all make a general assessment of the patient's constitution based on the facial features. A person with a good constitution will generally have a head with smooth features, a broad forehead and long ears with thick ear-lobes. A person with a poor constitution will have a head that is too small or with uneven features and small ears with small ear-lobes.

The features discussed are as follows:

- dry scalp
- redness and pain of the scalp
- tremor of the head
- swelling of the whole head
- boils on the scalp
- ulcers on the scalp
- ulcers in the mastoid region
- erosion of the scalp
- head leaning to one side
- head tilted backwards
- late closure of the fontanelles.

Dry scalp

Symptoms and Signs, Chapter 55

A dry scalp indicates Liver- or Kidney-Yin deficiency, or both.

Redness and pain of the scalp

Redness and pain of the scalp indicate either an acute invasion of Wind-Heat or the flaring up of Liver-Fire.

Tremor of the head

Observation, Chapter 4; Symptoms and Signs, Chapter 55

Tremor of the head indicates internal Liver-Wind and is seen in Parkinson's disease in the elderly.

Swelling of the whole head

Symptoms and Signs, Chapter 55

A swelling of the face and the whole head with redness of the eyes is called 'Big Head Warm Disease', which is due to Wind-Heat with Toxic Heat invading the Upper Burner. It is often seen in parotitis.

Boils on the scalp

Symptoms and Signs, Chapter 55

Boils on the scalp are due to Liver-Fire, Damp-Heat in the Liver channel, or Toxic Heat.

Ulcers on the scalp

Symptoms and Signs, Chapter 55

Ulcers on the scalp are due to Liver-Fire, Damp-Heat in the Liver channel, or, if they are in the region of Du-20 Baihui, Heat in the Governing Vessel.

Ulcers in the mastoid region

Symptoms and Signs, Chapter 55

Ulcers in the mastoid region are due to Damp-Heat in the Gall-Bladder channel or to Liver-Fire.

Erosion of the scalp

Symptoms and Signs, Chapter 55

Erosion of the scalp (when the skin is broken) with itching and oozing of a fluid is due to Damp-Heat in the Liver channel.

Head leaning to one side

Symptoms and Signs, Chapter 55

If the head leans to one side and the patient is unable to keep it straight, this is due to either a deficiency and sinking of Spleen-Qi or a deficiency of the Sea of Marrow.

Head tilted backwards

Symptoms and Signs, Chapter 55

If the head is tilted backwards with eyes rolled up, this indicates internal Liver-Wind, which is frequently seen in acute febrile diseases in children.

Late closure of the fontanelles

Symptoms and Signs, Chapter 90

In babies, one should observe the fontanelles: late closure of the fontanelles indicates poor hereditary Kidney constitution. The posterior fontanelle usually closes about 2 months after birth, the sphenoid fontanelle closes at about 3 months, the mastoid fontanelle closes near the end of the first year, and the anterior fontanelle may not close completely until the middle or end of the second year.

BOX 5.1 HEAD SIGNS

- Dry scalp: Liver- /Kidney-Yin deficiency
- Red and painful scalp: Wind-Heat or Liver-Fire
- Tremor of head: Liver-Wind
- Swelling of head and face: Wind-Heat with Toxic Heat (parotitis)
- Boils on scalp: Liver-Fire, Damp-Heat or Toxic Heat
- Ulcers on scalp: Liver-Fire, Damp-Heat or Heat in the Governing Vessel
- Ulcers in the mastoid region: Damp-Heat in Gall-Bladder channel or Liver-Fire
- Erosion of skull with itching and oozing: Damp-Heat in the Liver channel
- Head leaning to one side: Spleen-Qi deficiency or deficiency of Sea of Marrow
- Head tilted backwards with eyes rolled up: Liver-Wind
- Late closure of fontanelles: poor hereditary Kidney constitution

---

Box 5.1 summarizes the head signs.

FACE

The most important aspect of observation of the face is the complexion colour, which has already been described in Chapter 3. Other diagnostic signs of the face include oedema, swelling, spots, ulcers and lines.

The following features are discussed:

- acne
- papular/macular eruptions
- oedema of the face
- swelling and redness of the face
- swelling, redness and pain of the cheeks
- ulcers below the zygomatic arch
- lines on the face
- deviation of eye and mouth.

Acne

Observation, Chapter 21; Symptoms and Signs, Chapters 55 and 77

Acne on the face is generally due to Damp-Heat, in chronic conditions occurring against a background of Qi deficiency. In severe cases when the pustules are very large and painful, it is due to Toxic Heat. If the pustules are of a dull-purplish colour, there is Blood stasis.

Papular/macular eruptions

Symptoms and Signs, Chapter 55

Papular eruptions on the face and nose indicate Lung-Heat while macular eruptions indicate Blood-Heat.

Oedema of the face

Symptoms and Signs, Chapter 55

Acute oedema of the face is due to invasion of the Lungs by Wind-Water; chronic oedema of the face is due to Spleen- and Lung-Yang deficiency.

Swelling and redness of the face

Symptoms and Signs, Chapter 55

Acute swelling and redness of the face indicate invasion of Wind-Heat with Toxic Heat such as is seen in infectious febrile diseases.

Swelling, redness and pain of the cheeks

Symptoms and Signs, Chapter 55

Swelling, redness and pain of the cheeks and below the mandible indicates invasion of Wind-Heat with Toxic Heat and it is usually seen in parotitis.

Ulcers below the zygomatic arch

Symptoms and Signs, Chapter 55

Ulcers below the zygomatic arch are due to Toxic Heat in the Stomach.

Lines on the face

Symptoms and Signs, Chapter 55

If there are lines on the face and the skin has a very uneven surface, this indicates Blood deficiency or Heat with Dryness, usually related to emotional stress.

Deviation of eye and mouth

Observation, Chapter 4; Symptoms and Signs, Chapter 55

A deviation of the eye and mouth that does not affect the eyebrows and forehead is due to internal Wind and is seen in patients suffering from Wind-stroke. A deviation of the eye and mouth with an inability to raise one eyebrow and furrowing of the forehead on one side indicates invasion of external Wind in the channels of the face and it is seen in Bell's palsy.

BOX 5.2 FACE SIGNS

- Acute oedema: invasion of Lungs by Wind-Water
- Chronic oedema: Lung- and Spleen-Yang deficiency
- Acute swelling and redness: Wind-Heat with Toxic Heat
- Acute swelling, redness and pain below mandible: Wind-Heat with Toxic Heat (parotitis)
- Ulcers below zygomatic arch: Toxic Heat in Stomach
- Papules on face and nose: Lung-Heat (Qi level)
- Macules on face and nose: Blood-Heat
- Lined face with uneven skin surface: Blood deficiency or Heat and Dryness
- Deviation of eye and mouth (not affecting eyebrows and forehead): facial paralysis from Wind-stroke
- Deviation of eye and mouth (affecting eyebrows and forehead): peripheral facial paralysis (Bell's palsy; external Wind invasion)

Box 5.2 summarizes the face signs.

HAIR

The development of the head and hair depends largely on the state of the Kidneys and Liver. The Kidneys influence the bones, which determine the structure of the head, and they govern the Marrow, which

determines the normal development of the brain. Both Kidneys and Liver influence the growth of hair and therefore its normal growth, colour and consistency depend on the Liver and Kidneys.

The patterns causing each of the hair signs discussed below are listed in greater detail in Chapter 55.

The following conditions are discussed:

- hair falling out
- alopecia
- dry and brittle hair
- greasy hair
- premature greying of the hair
- dandruff.

Hair falling out

Symptoms and Signs, Chapter 55

Observation

The term 'falling out' refers to a gradual loss of hair, or to its slow growth, or to excessively thin hair.

Clinical significance

The growth and the thickness of the hair depend largely on the state of the Liver and Kidneys and specifically on Liver-Blood and Kidney-Essence: therefore, a gradual loss of hair may be due to Liver-Blood deficiency or Kidney-Essence deficiency, or both. However, there are also Full causes of loss of hair and in particular Blood-Heat, which causes the hair to fall out by drying out the hair follicles; this Blood-Heat usually derives from Liver-Fire which rises up to the head causing the loss of hair.

Loss of hair frequently occurs after a serious disease that is either acute or chronic and lingering. Of course there may also be external causes of hair loss and an example of these is the loss occurring after a course of chemotherapy.

In some cases, baldness can occur in young people. If a young person shows no sign of Liver or Kidney

---

BOX 5.3 HAIR FALLING OUT

- Liver-Blood/Kidney-Essence deficiency
- Blood-Heat (from Liver-Fire)
- Serious, acute disease
- Chronic, protracted disease
- Chemotherapy

---

deficiency and has a strong body, this means that the baldness is a hereditary trait and has no clinical significance.

Box 5.3 summarizes the causes of falling-out hair.

Alopecia

Symptoms and Signs, Chapter 55

Observation

Alopecia refers to the sudden loss of hair, which usually falls out in clumps.

Clinical significance

Alopecia may be due to several factors: first, Blood-Heat (usually deriving from Liver-Fire) which dries out the hair follicles; or internal Wind rising to the head; or Blood stasis, when the stagnant Blood in the head prevents new Blood from nourishing the hair.

Box 5.4 summarizes the patterns underlying alopecia.

BOX 5.4 ALOPECIA

- Blood Heat: hair falling out in clumps, dry hair, feeling of heat, thirst, Red tongue, Rapid pulse
- Internal Wind: hair falling out in clumps, giddiness, Wiry pulse
- Blood stasis: hair falling out in clumps, dark complexion, Purple tongue

---

Dry and brittle hair

Symptoms and Signs, Chapter 55

Observation

The description refers to hair that is dry, brittle and excessively thin.

Clinical significance

The most common cause of dry and brittle hair is deficiency of Liver-Blood or Kidney-Yin, or both; as the Liver and Kidneys are the main organs that nourish the hair, this makes the hair dry, thin and brittle.

A general deficiency of Qi and Blood, usually involving Liver-Blood, may also cause the hair to become dry and brittle for the same reasons indicated above.

A deficiency of Stomach and Spleen may cause the hair to become excessively thin and brittle when it is

not nourished by the Food Essences produced by the Stomach. This condition is often caused by worry, pensiveness or excessive studying, which weakens the Spleen.

A chronic loss of blood, such as might happen in chronic menorrhagia, may also cause the hair to become dry and thin because there is not enough Blood to nourish it.

Box 5.5 summarizes the causes of dry and brittle hair.

BOX 5.5 DRY AND BRITTLE HAIR

- Liver-Blood/Kidney-Essence deficiency
- General Qi and Blood deficiency
- Stomach and Spleen deficiency
- Chronic loss of blood

Greasy hair

Symptoms and Signs, Chapter 55

Greasy hair is always a sign of Dampness (with or without Heat) or Phlegm.

Premature greying of the hair

Symptoms and Signs, Chapter 55

Observation

'Premature greying of the hair' refers to the hair becoming grey or white too early in a person's life; of course, whitening of the hair with age is normal and does not indicate a pathology.

Clinical significance

The most common cause of premature greying of the hair is deficiency of Liver-Blood or Kidney-Essence, or both, which fail to nourish the hair properly. Another cause is a general Qi and Blood deficiency. Hair turning white suddenly is usually due to Liver- and Heart-Fire caused by a shock or a very intense emotional upset such as anger.

Premature greying of the hair in a young person who has a strong body and is in good health is purely hereditary and has no clinical significance.

Hair turning yellow and dry usually indicates deficiency of Blood and Essence.

Box 5.6 summarizes the causes of premature greying of hair.

BOX 5.6 PREMATURE GREYING OF THE HAIR

- Liver-Blood/Kidney-Essence deficiency
- General Qi and Blood deficiency
- Liver- and Heart-Fire
- Hereditary

Dandruff

Symptoms and Signs, Chapter 55

Observation

Dandruff consists in small, white, dry scales which slough off the scalp.

Clinical significance

The most common cause of dandruff is Liver-Blood that is deficient and fails to nourish the scalp. If the production of dandruff is profuse and it comes in bouts, it is due to Liver-Wind usually stemming from Liver-Blood deficiency.

Dandruff may also be due to Heat conditions; in particular Liver-Fire, Damp-Heat in the Liver affecting the head, or Toxic Heat.

For a more detailed description of the patterns involved in dandruff see Part 5, Chapter 55.

Box 5.7 summarizes the causes of dandruff.

BOX 5.7 DANDRUFF

- Liver-Blood deficiency
- Liver-Wind
- Liver-Fire
- Damp-Heat in the Liver
- Toxic Heat

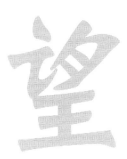

Chapter **6**

OBSERVATION OF THE EYES

Chapter contents

INTRODUCTION 75

CHANNELS INFLUENCING THE EYES 76

RELATIONSHIP BETWEEN THE INTERNAL ORGANS AND THE
EYES 76
  The eyes and the Liver 76
  The eyes and the Kidneys 77
  The eyes and the Heart 77
  The eyes and the Stomach and Spleen 77
  The eyes and the Gall-Bladder 77
  The eyes and the Bladder 78
  The eyes and the Small Intestine 78
  The Five Wheels 78
  The Eight Ramparts 79
  The Eye System 79

ASPECTS OF OBSERVATION OF THE EYES 80
  The lustre of the eyes 80
  The control of the eyes 80
  The normal eye 81

OBSERVATION OF PATHOLOGICAL SIGNS OF THE EYE 81
  Abnormal colour 81
  Other features 82

INTRODUCTION

From a Five-Element perspective, the eyes are the outlet of the Liver. Chapter 4 of the 'Simple Questions' says: *'The East direction corresponds to the colour green and the Liver which opens into the orifice of the eyes.'*[1] However, many other organs influence the eyes and, particularly from a diagnostic point of view, the eyes reflect the state of all the Internal Organs and therefore of the Mind and Spirit. In particular, the eyes reflect the state of the Mind and Spirit because of the close connection between the Eyes and the Heart. In fact, Chapter 81 of the 'Simple Questions' says: *'The Heart transports the Essence of the five Yin organs to the eyes; if the eyes are brilliant and with lustre, it shows that the person is happy and Qi is harmonious. If, on the contrary, the eyes lack lustre it indicates that the person is afflicted by worry and this is reflected in the brilliance of the eyes.'*[2] The same chapter says: *'The Spirit and the Essence of the Heart gather in the eyes.'*[3]

However, as mentioned above, many other organs also influence the eyes. Chapter 4 of the 'Spiritual Axis' says: *'Qi and Blood of the twelve channels and of the fifteen Connecting channels reach the orifices of the face so that the Yang-Qi brightens the eyes'.*[4] Chapter 71 of the same book says: *'By observing the five colours of the eyes, one can determine the state of the five Yin organs and therefore the prognosis.'*[5]

Therefore, as we can see, the essences and fluids of all the Internal Organs nourish and moisten the eyes: for this reason, the eyes can reflect the state of most Internal Organs and not just the Liver, to which they are related within the Five-Element scheme of correspondences. The 'Spiritual Axis' in Chapter 80 says:

The Essence of the five Yin and six Yang organs all reach the eyes which are the 'nest' of the Essence. The Essence of the

bones [and therefore of the Kidneys] manifests in the pupil; the Essence of the sinews [and therefore of the Liver] manifests in the iris; the Essence of Blood [and therefore of the Heart] manifests in the blood vessels and the canthus [of the eye]; the Essence of Qi [and therefore of the Lungs] manifests on the sclera; the Essence of the muscles [and therefore of the Spleen] manifests in the eyelids; therefore, the Essence of bones, sinews, blood and Qi together with the blood vessels form the Eye System which goes upwards entering the brain and backwards exiting at the nape of the neck.[6]

This statement from the 'Spiritual Axis' is important in two ways. First, it establishes a connection between the Internal Organs and the five parts of the eye that are called the Five Wheels. The Five Wheels are the pupil (corresponding to the Kidneys), the iris (corresponding to the Liver), the sclera (corresponding to the Lungs), the two corners of the sclera (corresponding to the Heart) and the eyelids (corresponding to the Spleen). Secondly, this chapter of the 'Spiritual Axis' describes an 'Eye System' composed of all the channels reaching the eye which enter the brain and exit at the nape of the neck.

The same chapter of the 'Spiritual Axis' also says:

The eyes manifest the Essence of the five Yin and six Yang organs, the Nutritive and Defensive Qi, and they are the place where the Qi of the Mind is generated... the eyes are the messengers of the Heart which houses the Mind. If the Mind and Essence are not co-ordinated and not transmitted one has visual hallucinations. The Mind, Ethereal Soul and Corporeal Soul are scattered so that one has bewildering perceptions.[7]

In conclusion, in diagnosis the eyes reflect the state of all the organs and of the Mind and Spirit.

> **!**
>
> **Remember**: the eyes reflect the state of *all* the organs, and of the Mind and Spirit.

The discussion of observation of the eyes will first of all look at the channels influencing the eyes and the various physiological relationships between the eyes and various organs. After discussing the physiological relationships between the Internal Organs and the eye, we shall discuss the particular aspects of the eyes that should be observed in clinical practice.

The various pathological colours of the sclera will be discussed and, finally, various other signs appearing in the eyes will be discussed. (Please note that many more signs related to the eyes are discussed in Part 5 Symptoms and Signs, Chapter 61.)

CHANNELS INFLUENCING THE EYES

The channels coursing through or around the eyes are illustrated in Figure 6.1. The pathways of the channels coursing through or around the eyes are as follows:

- The Stomach Main channel goes to the eye and connects with BL-1 Jingming.
- The Stomach Muscle channel connects with muscles around the orbit and with the Bladder Muscle channel.
- The Stomach Divergent channel goes to the forehead and down to enter the eye.
- The Heart Main, Connecting and Divergent channels all flow to the eye.
- The Bladder Main channel goes to the inner corner of the eye.
- The Bladder Muscle channel binds around the orbit.
- The Liver Main channel goes through the eye on its way to the vertex.
- The Gall-Bladder Main and Muscle channels go to the outer corner of the eye.
- The Directing and Penetrating Vessels go to the lower orbit of the eye (not shown in Fig. 6.1).
- The Yin and Yang Heel Vessels go to BL-1 Jingming (not shown in Fig. 6.1).

RELATIONSHIP BETWEEN THE INTERNAL ORGANS AND THE EYES

The eyes and the Liver

The relationship between the eyes and the Liver is, of course, very well known owing to the Five-Element correspondence. The Liver-Blood nourishes the eyes and produces normal vision. For example, the 'Spiritual Axis' in Chapter 17 says: '*Liver-Qi reaches the eyes, when the Liver is harmonized the eyes can distinguish the five colours.*'[8] It also says: '*The Liver stores Blood which allows us to see.*'[9] The 'Simple Questions' in Chapter 5 says: '*The Liver governs the eyes;*'[10] and in Chapter 4: '*The East corresponds to the green colour and the Liver which opens into the eyes.*'[11]

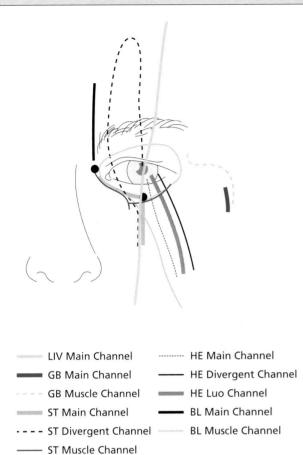

- LIV Main Channel
- GB Main Channel
- GB Muscle Channel
- ST Main Channel
- ST Divergent Channel
- ST Muscle Channel
- HE Main Channel
- HE Divergent Channel
- HE Luo Channel
- BL Main Channel
- BL Muscle Channel

Fig. 6.1 Channels coursing through the eyes

Liver-Yin also nourishes the eyes and, more specifically, it moistens them: in fact, dry eyes are often a symptom of Liver-Yin deficiency, while blurred vision is a symptom of Liver-Blood deficiency.

The eyes and the Kidneys

Like Liver-Blood, the Kidneys nourish the eyes; they also moisten the eyes and control the normal fluids that lubricate them. Many eye problems, especially in the elderly, are due to Kidney-Yin deficiency. The Kidneys also influence the intraocular pressure and glaucoma is often due to a Kidney deficiency.

The eyes and the Heart

The Heart Main channel reaches the eye internally, the Heart Connecting channel also reaches the eye, and the Heart Divergent channel connects with the Small Intestine channel at the inner canthus of the eyes.

The 'Spiritual Axis' in Chapter 10 says: '*The Heart channel connects with the Eye System.*'[12] In Chapter 11 it says: '*The Divergent channel of the Heart connects with the Eye System.*'[13] The same chapter also says: '*The Heart channel reaches the face and connects with the inner canthus of the eye.*'[14]

Therefore, Heart-Blood also nourishes the eye in a similar way to Liver-Blood, or, to put it differently, for Blood to reach the eye it needs the transporting action of Heart-Qi. The 'Simple Questions' also mentions the connection between the eye and the Heart in several places and Chapter 81 says: '*The Spirit and the Essence of the Heart gather in the eye.*'[15] It also says: '*The Heart is the focus of the Essence of the five Yin organs and its orifice is the eye.*'[16] The 'Spiritual Axis' in Chapter 80 says: '*The eye is the ambassador of the Heart.*'[17]

The significance of all the above statements is twofold. First, like the Liver, the Heart nourishes the eye and therefore many eye problems are related to a Heart pathology. Secondly, the Essence of the Heart, and therefore the Mind and Spirit, manifests in the eyes: this is an extremely important aspect of diagnosis as a careful observation of the eyes reveals the state of the Mind and Spirit.

The eyes and the Stomach and Spleen

The Stomach channel is closely connected to the eye as it starts just under the orbit of the eye. It transports the Food Essences to the eyes. The Spleen influences the eyelids and the muscles that control their opening and closing. Chapter 62 of the 'Spiritual Axis' says: '*Stomach-Qi flows upwards to the Lungs and on to the head via the throat and connects with the Eye System and from here enters the brain.*'[18] Chapter 31 of the 'Simple Questions' says: '*The Bright Yang controls the muscles and its channel flows to the nose and eyes.*'[19] Chapter 21 of the 'Spiritual Axis' says: '*The leg Bright Yang channel goes to the nose, the mouth and enters the Eye System.*'[20] Both the Divergent and the Muscle channels of the Stomach enter the eye. Chapter 13 of the 'Spiritual Axis' says: '*The Muscle channel of the Stomach . . . connects with the Greater Yang channel which controls the upper eyelid, while the Bright Yang channel controls the lower eyelid.*'[21] However, the prevalent view is that the Spleen controls both eyelids.

The eyes and the Gall-Bladder

The Gall-Bladder channel is closely connected to the eye as it starts at its outer corner. Chapter 10 of the

'Spiritual Axis' says: '*The Gall-Bladder channel starts from the lateral corner of the eye.*'[22] Chapter 11 of the same book says: '*The Gall-Bladder Divergent channel . . . scatters on the face, enters the Eye System and joins the Main channel at the external corner of the eye.*'[23] Chapter 13 says: '*The Muscle channel of the Gall-Bladder . . . binds around the external corner of the eye.*'[24] Thus, both the Divergent and the Muscle channel of the Gall-Bladder reach the eye.

The eyes and the Bladder

The Bladder channel starts at the inner corner of the eye. Its influence on the eye is a close one. Chapter 10 of the 'Spiritual Axis' says: '*The Bladder channel starts at the inner corner of the eye.*'[25] The Bladder Muscle channel is wrapped around the eye socket. Chapter 21 of the same book says: '*The leg Greater Yang channel penetrates the occiput, enters the brain, it connects with the eye and is called the Eye System.*'[26]

The eyes and the Small Intestine

Chapter 10 of the 'Spiritual Axis' says: '*A branch of the Small Intestine channel departing from the clavicle, goes to the neck and cheek to reach the lateral corner of the eye . . . another branch reaches the nose and arrives at the inner corner of the eye.*'[27] The Muscle channel of the Small Intestine also reaches the outer corner of the eye.

> **!**
>
> **Remember**: the Liver is *not* the only organ that influences the eyes.

BOX 6.1 THE EYES AND INTERNAL ORGANS

- Liver: Liver-Blood nourishes the eyes; Liver-Yin nourishes and moisturizes the eyes
- Kidneys: Kidney-Yin nourishes and moistens the eyes
- Heart: Heart-Blood nourishes the eyes; Heart-Qi transports Qi and Blood to the eyes
- Stomach and Spleen: Stomach transports food essences to the eyes: Stomach's Main, Muscle and Divergent channels reach the eyes; the Spleen controls the eyelids
- Gall-Bladder: the Gall-Bladder's Main, Divergent and Muscle channels reach the outer corner of the eyes; GB-1 connects with the Eye system
- Bladder: the Bladder's Main and Muscle channels reach the eyes; BL-1 connects with the Eye System
- Small Intestine: the Small Intestine's Main and Muscle channels reach the eyes

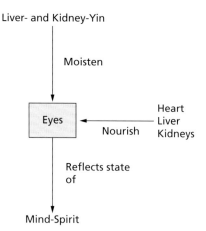

Fig. 6.2 Relationship of Internal Organs with the eyes

Box 6.1 and Figure 6.2 summarizes the relationships between the Internal Organs and the eyes.

The Five Wheels

The 'Five Wheels' is an ancient expression to indicate five areas of the eyes: the pupil, iris, corners of the sclera, the rest of the sclera and the eyelids. These Five Wheels are the Water Wheel, the Wind Wheel, the Blood Wheel, the Qi Wheel and the Muscle Wheel respectively. Figure 6.3 illustrates the Five Wheels.

The Five Wheels are as follows:

- The Wind Wheel is the iris; it is the essence of the sinews and pertains to the Liver.
- The Blood Wheel is the corners of the sclera of the eyes; it is the essence of the Blood and pertains to the Heart.
- The Qi Wheel is the rest of the sclera; it is the essence of Qi and pertains to the Lungs.
- The Muscle Wheel is the eyelids; it is the essence of the muscles and pertains to the Stomach and Spleen.
- The Water Wheel is the pupil, it is the essence of the bones and pertains to the Kidneys.

The significance of the Five Wheels is that it establishes a physiological relationship between those five parts of the eye and the Internal Organs. For example, the pupil pertains to the Kidneys and if it is excessively dilated it may indicate Kidney-Yang deficiency; the iris pertains to the Liver and its inflammation may indicate Liver-Heat; the sclera pertains to the Lungs and a

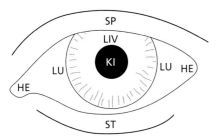

Fig. 6.3 The Five Wheels of the eye

change in its colour or texture may indicate a Lung pathology such as Lung-Heat; the corners of the eye pertain to the Heart and a redness there may indicate Heart-Fire; the eyelids pertain to the Stomach and Spleen and if, for example, they are drooping this may indicate sinking of Spleen-Qi, while if they are swollen and red they indicate Spleen-Heat. However, as always in the Chinese medicine system of correspondences, there are pathologies which escape such correspondences; for example, a redness of the sclera may be related to Heat in any organ and not just the Lungs.

The Eight Ramparts

The 'Eight Ramparts' are another way of classifying areas of the eye in relation to the Internal Organs. The classification according to the Eight Ramparts is broadly the same as that according to the Five Wheels, except that it is more detailed, especially in relation to the sclera, which is divided into three areas corresponding to the Lungs, Minister Fire and Triple Burner. (Fig. 6.4).

The Eight Ramparts are:

- Heaven Rampart corresponding to the sclera and pertaining to the Lungs and Large Intestine
- Earth Rampart corresponding to the eyelids and pertaining to the Stomach and Spleen
- Fire Rampart corresponding to the corners of the eye and pertaining to the Heart and Small Intestine
- Water Rampart corresponding to the pupil and pertaining to the Kidneys
- Wind Rampart corresponding to the iris and pertaining to the Liver and Gall-Bladder
- Thunder Rampart corresponding to the upper part of the outer sclera and pertaining to the Minister Fire
- Mountain Rampart corresponding to the outer corner and pertaining to the Pericardium
- Pool Rampart corresponding to the lower part of the inner sclera and pertaining to the Triple Burner.

The Eye System

Chapter 80 of the 'Spiritual Axis' mentions the Eye System (Fig. 6.5):

The Essences of the five Yin and six Yang organs all reach the eyes which are the 'nest' of the Essences. The Essence of the bones [and therefore of the Kidneys] manifests in the

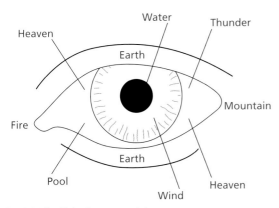

Fig. 6.4 The Eight Ramparts of the eye

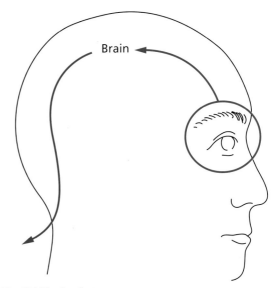

Fig. 6.5 The Eye System

pupil; the Essence of the sinews [and therefore of the Liver] manifests in the iris; the Essence of Blood [and therefore of the Heart] manifests in the blood vessels and the canthus [of the eye]; the Essence of Qi [and therefore of the Lungs] manifests on the sclera; the Essence of the muscles [and therefore of the Spleen] manifests in the eyelids; therefore, the Essences of bones, sinews, blood and Qi together with blood vessels [or channels] form the Eye System which goes upwards entering the brain and backwards exiting at the nape of the neck. Therefore, when pathogenic factors enter the occiput due to a deficiency condition of the body, they penetrate this pathway to the Eye System into the brain. This causes the brain to feel like 'turning' which causes a tightness of the Eye System; a tightness of the Eye System will cause the vision to be obfuscated and there is dizziness.[28]

The 'Eye System' is, therefore, the complex of channels, Connecting channels and blood vessels converging at the eyes and gathering the Qi and Essence of all organs, entering the brain and then exiting at the occiput. The Eye System essentially highlights the physiological relationship between the Internal Organs, together with their channels and blood vessels, the eyes and the brain. Modern Chinese texts often translate 'Eye System' as 'optic nerve'; this is, in my opinion, a reductionist view: although the Eye System is related to the optic nerve, it is not the same structure (in the same way that channels are related to, but are not the same as, the nerves running alongside them).

From an acupuncture perspective, many of the points around the eye socket have an influence on the brain and therefore the Mind.

> **!**
>
> **Remember**: many of the points around the eye socket have an influence on the brain and therefore the Mind through the Eye System.

ASPECTS OF OBSERVATION OF THE EYES

The lustre of the eyes

The lustre (*shen*) of the eyes refers to the brilliance, vitality, glitter and sparkle of the eyes, all of which reflect a normal state of the Mind and Spirit and therefore, in particular, of the Heart. However, as indicated

above, the Essence of the other Internal Organs also manifests in the eyes.

A good, normal lustre of the eyes indicates that, whatever the illness a person may be suffering from, the Mind and Spirit are still strong and that person's emotional and mental life is balanced and well integrated. This lustre is an extremely important sign and when present always points to a good prognosis. The normal lustre of the eyes is somewhat 'moist', that is, the eye looks well lubricated and not dry. However, the eye should not be too wet either.[29] As soon as a new patient sits down, I study first, and carefully, the lustre of the eyes.

When the Mind and Spirit are affected by long-standing emotional problems, the eyes may lose their lustre and become somewhat dull and lacking sparkle (see Plate 6.1 on p. P8). The degree of dullness of the eyes reflects the severity and duration of the emotional problems accurately: the duller the eyes, the more severe and long standing the emotional problems. In a few cases, however, the eyes can become dull and lose lustre from physical causes such as a serious disease or from a long course of chemotherapy. Barring the last cause of lack of eye lustre, I find this sign never to fail: even if a person tries hard to hide his or her emotional problems, lack of lustre of the eyes always tells the truth.

The 'Great Treatise of Ophthalmology' (*Yan Ke Da Quan*, 1644) relates the lustre of the eyes in particular to the Fire of the Gate of Life (*Ming Men*): '*The brightness of the Mind manifests with brilliance of the eyes. The brightness of the Mind has its origin in the Gate of Life (Ming Men) and it emerges to the Heart through the Gall-Bladder: therefore it is a manifestation of Fire.*'[30]

The control of the eyes

'Control' of the eyes refers to the movement or lack of movement of the eyeballs. Someone who has 'controlled' eyes is able to fix the gaze, the person will be able to look directly at other people and engage their gaze; the eyes do not move too much nor are they too fixed, they look stable and at ease. Uncontrolled eyes may manifest either with a fixed stare or with a shifty glance with excessive movement of the eyeballs; a person whose eyes are uncontrolled frequently looks down or away to avoid engaging another person's gaze.

The control of the eyes is quite separate from their lustre and one should not be surprised to see people

whose eyes appear to have lustre but lack control. Lack of control of the eyes indicates obstruction of the Mind's orifices and a troubled personality.

The normal eye

The normal eye is characterized by clear vision, a clear white sclera with a distinct border between sclera and iris, normal lustre, normal control, a bright appearance and normal moisture. The eyelids should not be swollen or red and should open and close normally; the inner corner should be pale red, moist and free from ulcers, sores or gum (sticky secretion collecting in the corner of the eye); the eye in general should be bright and have lustre and control indicating a good state of the Mind and Spirit; the eyeball should move normally, neither darting involuntarily nor staring fixedly; the sclera should have no spots, nebula or visible blood vessels.

The patterns causing each of the eye signs discussed below are listed in greater detail in Chapter 61.

OBSERVATION OF PATHOLOGICAL SIGNS OF THE EYE

Abnormal colour

The pathological colours of the eyes should be observed in the sclera. Chapter 72 of the 'Spiritual Axis' relates the five pathological colours of the sclera to the five Yin organs: *Red eyes indicate disease of the Heart, white of the Lungs, green of the Liver, yellow of the Spleen and black of the Kidneys.*[31]

Generally speaking, a yellow or red colour indicates Heat while a greenish or pale colour indicates Cold, and a bright colour indicates disease in the Yang while a turbid colour indicates disease in the Yin.

Yellow

Symptoms and Signs, Chapter 61

The most common cause of a yellow sclera is Damp-Heat. If Heat predominates, the sclera is a light and shiny yellow like tangerine peel; if Dampness predominates, the sclera is a dull yellow.

Cold-Dampness may also cause the sclera to become yellow, in which case it will be a dark and dull yellow.

Toxic Heat may cause the sclera to become deep yellow and bloodshot. Blood deficiency may also cause

the sclera to become yellow but in this case it would be a pale, light yellow.

Finally, Blood stasis may cause the sclera to be very dark yellow, almost brown.

Box 6.2 summarizes the patterns underlying a yellow sclera.

BOX 6.2 YELLOW SCLERA

- Damp-Heat: bright-yellow or dark-yellow sclera, feeling of heaviness, gum in the eyes, sticky-yellow tongue coating
- Cold-Dampness: dark, dull-yellow sclera, feeling of heaviness, cold limbs, abdominal pain
- Toxic Heat: deep-yellow and bloodshot sclera, gum in the eyes, Red tongue with red points
- Blood deficiency: pale-yellow sclera, dizziness, blurred vision, Choppy pulse
- Blood stasis: dark-yellow sclera, pain in the eye, Purple tongue

---

Red

Symptoms and Signs, Chapter 61

The red colour can be observed either in the sclera or at the corners of the eyes. A redness of the sclera indicates Heat, which may derive from any of the Internal Organs but the three most common ones are Heart-Fire, Liver-Fire and Lung-Heat.

Liver-Fire is probably the most common cause of a red sclera, in which case it may also be bloodshot and painful. Heart-Fire may also cause a red sclera, particularly in the two corners. Lung-Heat may cause a red sclera and this is especially seen in acute conditions of Lung-Heat or Phlegm-Heat in the Lungs occurring after an invasion of Wind. Heat in the Bladder may also sometimes cause a red sclera.

BOX 6.3 RED SCLERA

- Liver-Fire: bloodshot sclera, pain in the eye, bitter taste, Wiry-Rapid pulse
- Heart-Fire: red corners of the eyes, pain in the eye, palpitations, Red tip of the tongue
- Lung-Heat: cough, feeling of heat
- Phlegm-Heat in the Lungs: cough with expectoration of yellow sputum, feeling of oppression of the chest, Swollen tongue
- Heat in the Bladder: burning on urination, difficult urination
- Empty-Heat: pale-red sclera, thin, red blood vessels, night sweating, feeling of heat in the evening, Red tongue without coating

---

Apart from the conditions of Full-Heat listed above, Empty-Heat may also cause the sclera to become red in which case it would be pale red, or it might show thin, red blood vessels.

Box 6.3 summarizes the patterns underlying a red sclera.

Bluish-Greenish
Symptoms and Signs, Chapter 61

Liver-Wind may cause the sclera to become greenish, while internal Cold may cause it to become bluish. In some cases, severe, chronic deficiency of Kidney-Yin may cause the sclera to become dull greenish.

Box 6.4 summarizes the patterns underlying a bluish-greenish sclera.

BOX 6.4 BLUISH-GREENISH SCLERA

- Liver-Wind: greenish sclera, giddiness, tremor, Wiry pulse
- Internal Cold: bluish sclera, cold limbs, abdominal pain, Tight pulse
- Kidney-Yin deficiency: dull greenish sclera, dizziness, tinnitus, Floating-Empty pulse

---

Dark
Symptoms and Signs, Chapter 61

The most common cause of dark sclera is severe Full-Heat or Fire, which, as indicated above, may occur in many organs but especially Liver, Heart and Lungs. In such cases, the dark sclera can be considered as a further stage of red sclera.

Phlegm is also a common cause of dark sclera, in which case it is brownish and the eye sockets may also have a brown colour underneath the eyes. A chronic, severe deficiency of Liver- and Kidney-Yin may also cause the sclera to become dark.

A dull-dark appearance of the sclera may also be due to severe deficiency and dryness of Blood.

BOX 6.5 DARK SCLERA

- Liver-Fire: pain in the eye, bitter taste, headache, Red tongue with redder sides
- Heart-Fire: pain in the eye, palpitations, anxiety, Red tongue with redder tip
- Lung-Heat: cough, feeling of heat
- Phlegm: brownish-dark sclera, dull-white specks, dark sockets, Swollen tongue, Slippery pulse
- Liver- and Kidney-Yin deficiency: dizziness, tinnitus, night sweating, Floating-Empty pulse
- Deficiency and dryness of Blood: dull, dark sclera

Box 6.5 summarizes the patterns underlying a dark sclera.

Other features

White specks
Symptoms and Signs, Chapter 61

White specks may occur on the sclera or pupil. The most common cause of white specks is Phlegm, in which case they are often on the sclera and partially on the pupil. Severe, chronic Liver- and Kidney-Yin deficiency in the elderly may also cause dull-white specks on the sclera. Bright-white specks on the sclera are usually due to chronic Yang deficiency with internal Cold.

Box 6.6 summarizes the patterns underlying white spectra in the eye.

BOX 6.6 WHITE SPECKS

- Phlegm: white specks on sclera and pupil, blurred vision, sputum in the throat, feeling of oppression of the chest, Swollen tongue
- Liver- and Kidney-Yin deficiency: dull-white specks on sclera, dizziness, tinnitus, night sweating, Floating-Empty pulse
- Yang deficiency: bright-white specks, feeling of cold, loose stools, Deep-Weak pulse

---

Protruding eyeball
Symptoms and Signs, Chapter 61

One of the most common causes of protruding eyeball is in the Liver channel and this may manifest with many different Liver patterns such as Liver-Fire, Liver-Qi stagnation with Phlegm, Liver-Wind, Liver-Wind with Phlegm-Heat, Liver-Qi stagnation, Liver-Qi and Blood stagnation. Fire may also cause the eyeball to protrude and the two most common patterns causing this sign are Heart-Fire and Toxic Heat.

Deficiency may also cause the eyeball to protrude slightly, and especially a Kidney deficiency or a deficiency of Qi and Blood. Finally, the eyeball may protrude in chronic conditions of cough and asthma with rebellious Lung-Qi.

(For a detailed list and description of these patterns, see Chapter 61 in Part 5.)

Sunken eyeball
Symptoms and Signs, Chapter 61

Sunken eyeball is always due to Deficiency, which may be a chronic deficiency of Qi or a sudden deficiency of

Spleen-Qi induced by food poisoning. Another cause of sunken eyeball is collapse of Yin or Yang.

Box 6.7 summarizes the patterns underlying protruding eyeball.

BOX 6.7 PROTRUDING EYEBALL

- Liver-Fire: red, hot and painful eye, bitter taste, Red tongue with redder sides
- Heart-Fire: red and painful eye, anxiety, insomnia, palpitations, Red tongue with redder tip
- Liver-Qi stagnation with Phlegm: feeling of distension of the eye, irritability, feeling of oppression of the chest, Swollen tongue, Wiry pulse
- Liver-Wind: giddiness, tremor, Wiry pulse
- Liver-Wind with Phlegm-Heat: giddiness, tremor, feeling of oppression of the chest, phlegm in the throat, Swollen tongue, Wiry-Slippery pulse
- Liver-Qi stagnation: feeling of distension of the eye, streaming eyes, irritability, Wiry pulse
- Qi stagnation and Blood stasis: feeling of distension and pain of the eye, irritability, Purple tongue
- Toxic Heat: red sclera, gum in the eye, red and painful eye, fever, Red tongue with red points
- Deficiency of Kidney Yin and Yang: slightly protruding eyeball, dizziness, tinnitus, backache
- Qi and Blood deficiency: slightly protruding eyeball, tiredness, palpitations, poor appetite, loose stools
- Rebellious Lung-Qi: chronic cough or asthma
- Invasion of Wind-Heat: fever, aversion to cold, pain and itchiness in the eye, Floating-Rapid pulse

---

Strabismus
Symptoms and Signs, Chapter 61

The most common cause of strabismus in children is a deficiency of Kidney-Essence. In adults, the two most common patterns of strabismus are Liver-Wind or Liver-Yang rising. Other patterns which may cause strabismus include a chronic, severe deficiency of Qi and Blood of the Liver, internal Cold, Blood stasis, Toxic Heat and Phlegm. (For a detailed list and description of symptoms of these patterns, see Chapter 61.)

Box 6.8 summarizes the patterns underlying strabismus.

Staring, fixed eyes
Symptoms and Signs, Chapter 61

'Staring, fixed eyes' describes a condition in which the eyes are wide open and the pupils are staring and not moving.

Heart-Fire and Phlegm-Heat in the Heart are the two most common patterns causing staring and fixed eyes. In both cases, this symptom always indicates a disturbance of the Mind and Spirit with obfuscation of the Mind's orifices.

Abnormal colour of the eyelids
Symptoms and Signs, Chapter 61

Both eyelids reflect the state of the Spleen; the lower eyelid also reflects the state of the Stomach. Redness and swelling of the upper eyelid indicates Spleen-Heat, whereas redness and swelling of the lower eyelid indicates Stomach-Heat. If both eyelids are red, this usually indicates Damp-Heat in the Spleen. Redness of the eyelids with acute onset may be due to invasion of Wind-Heat. A redness inside the lower eyelid indicates Full-Heat; a thin, red line inside the lower eyelid indicates Empty-Heat. A redness of the eyelids like

---

BOX 6.8 STRABISMUS

- Kidney-Essence deficiency: strabismus from early childhood
- Liver-Wind: giddiness, tremor, Wiry pulse
- Liver-Yang rising: dizziness, tinnitus, headache, Wiry pulse
- Severe deficiency of Qi and Blood of the Liver: exhaustion, blurred vision, dizziness, Choppy pulse
- Internal Cold: feeling of cold, cold limbs, Tight-Slow pulse
- Blood stasis: headache, mental restlessness, Purple tongue
- Toxic Heat: fever, gum in the eyes, Red tongue with red points
- Phlegm: dizziness, nausea, muzziness of the head, blurred vision, Swollen tongue

---

BOX 6.9 ABNORMAL EYELID COLOURS

- Red and swollen upper lid: Spleen-Heat
- Red and swollen lower lid: Stomach-Heat
- Both lids red: Damp-Heat in Spleen
- Red lids with acute onset: Wind-Heat
- Redness inside lower lids: Full-Heat
- Thin, red line inside lower lids: Empty-Heat
- Red lids like cinnabar with small water blisters: Damp-Heat in Stomach and Spleen
- Red, itchy and hot lids with watery eyes: Wind, Heat, Dampness or Heart-Fire
- Dark lids: Kidney deficiency
- Greyish, dull, sooty lids: Cold-Phlegm
- Dark, red, swollen lids: Phlegm-Heat
- Dark lids with dull-yellow complexion: Wind-Phlegm
- Green lids: Stomach-Cold
- Pale colour inside lids: Blood or Yang deficiency
- Pale colour surrounded by yellow inside the lids: retention of food

---

cinnabar with small water blisters indicates Damp-Heat in the Stomach and Spleen. Red, itchy and hot eyelids with watery eyes are due to Wind, Heat, Dampness or Heart-Fire.

Dark eyelids indicate Kidney deficiency; greyish, dull, sooty eyelids indicate Cold-Phlegm; dark, red and swollen eyelids indicate Phlegm-Heat; dark eyelids with a dull-yellow complexion may indicate Wind-Phlegm; green eyelids indicate Stomach-Cold.

A pale colour inside the eyelids indicates either Blood or Yang deficiency, whereas a pale colour surrounded by yellow inside the eyelids indicates retention of food.

Box 6.9 summarizes the patterns underlying abnormal eyelid colour.

Swollen eyelids

Symptoms and Signs, Chapter 61

A swelling of the eyelids can derive either from Heat or from Cold. When it derives from Heat it could be due to invasion of external Wind-Heat or to Spleen Damp-Heat (as the Spleen controls the eyelids). A gradual swelling of the eyelids is usually due either to Water overflowing with oedema or to Cold-Dampness. A description of the patterns causing swelling of the eyelid can be found in Chapter 61.

Box 6.10 summarizes the patterns underlying swollen eyelids.

BOX 6.10 SWOLLEN EYELIDS

- Red and swollen lids: Damp-Heat in Spleen
- Pale and swollen lids: Cold-Dampness in Spleen
- Acute swelling of lids: Wind-Heat
- Gradual swelling of lids: Water overflowing or Cold-Phlegm

Streaming eyes

Interrogation, Chapter 42; Symptoms and Signs, Chapter 61

There are traditionally two types of streaming eyes: one is called '*liu lei*', which indicates runny and streaming eyes and is described here; the other is '*yan chi*', which indicates a thick discharge and is described under 'Discharge from the eyes'.

The most common cause of streaming eyes lies in the Liver channel: many different Liver patterns can cause this symptom, among them Liver-Blood deficiency, Liver-Heat, Liver-Fire and Liver-Yin deficiency. The Heart channel also reaches the eye and Heart-Fire may cause streaming eyes. The Kidneys control the fluids in the eyes and a deficiency of this

organ, whether of Yin or of Yang, may also cause streaming eyes. Finally, invasions of external Wind may cause streaming eyes with a sudden onset. (For a detailed description of the patterns causing streaming eyes, see Chapter 61.)

Box 6.11 summarizes the patterns underlying streaming eyes.

BOX 6.11 STREAMING EYES

- Liver-Blood deficiency: mildly streaming eyes when exposed to wind
- Liver-Heat (Fire): profusely streaming eyes
- Liver-Yin deficiency: mildly streaming eyes in the evening
- Heart-Fire: streaming eyes when upset
- Kidney deficiency: streaming eyes, worse when tired
- External Wind: streaming eyes with sudden onset

Discharge from the eyes

Symptoms and Signs, Chapter 61

'Discharge from the eyes' indicates a relatively thick, sticky discharge, different from that of streaming eyes, which is characterized by excessive tears. The most common cause of a discharge from the eyes is Heat (Fire), especially in the Liver or Heart, or Empty-Heat, especially of the Liver, Heart or Lungs. Invasion of external Wind-Heat may also cause a discharge from the eyes. (For a detailed description of patterns causing a discharge from the eyes, see Chapter 61.)

Box 6.12 summarizes the patterns underlying eye discharges.

BOX 6.12 DISCHARGE FROM THE EYES

- Liver-Fire: sticky yellow discharge
- Heart-Fire: sticky yellow discharge, worse when upset
- Liver-Yin deficiency with Empty-Heat: sticky discharge in the evening
- Heart-Yin deficiency with Empty-Heat: sticky discharge in the evening
- Lung-Yin deficiency with Empty-Heat: sticky discharge with cough
- Wind-Heat: sticky discharge with acute onset

Abnormal colours of the corners of the eyes

Symptoms and Signs, Chapter 61

The inner corners of the eyes are called 'large corners' in Chinese medicine, while the outer corners are called 'small corners'. Many different channels reach the corners of the eyes (Table 6.1).

Table 6.1 Relationship between channels and corners of the eyes

	Inner corner	Outer corner
Heart	Main channel	Main channel
Small Intestine	Main channel	Muscle channel
Gall-Bladder		Main and Muscle channel
Bladder	Main channel	
Triple Burner		Main and Muscle channel
Yin and Yang Heel Vessels	Yin and Yang Heel Vessels	

A redness of the corners of the eyes always indicates Heat, which may be external or internal and Full or Empty. Invasion of external Wind-Heat may cause a redness of the corners of the eyes. Full-Heat of various organs can cause a redness of the corners of the eyes: Lung-Heat usually causes a redness of the inner corner, Heart-Heat (Fire) a redness of the outer corner and Liver-Fire a redness of either corner.

Empty-Heat deriving from Yin deficiency may cause a redness and dryness of either corner of the eye; this may be due to Yin deficiency of various organs and especially Lungs, Heart, Liver and Kidneys.

Damp-Heat may also cause a redness of either corner, usually together with a sticky yellow discharge of the eye.

Redness starting from the inner corners of the eyes and extending towards the centre indicates a pathol-ogy of the Yin and Yang Heel vessels (Yin and Yang Qiao Mai). (For a description of the patterns causing red corners of the eyes, see Chapter 61.)

Pale corners of the eye is due to either Blood deficiency (of the Liver or Heart) or Yang deficiency (of the Spleen or Kidneys). (For a description of the patterns causing pale corners of the eyes, see Chapter 61.)

Box 6.13 summarizes the patterns underlying abnormal colours in the eye corners.

Abnormal colour of the eye sockets

Dark eye sockets usually indicate Phlegm; dark-purple eye sockets indicate severe Blood stasis. A bluish colour in the lower part of the eye socket usually indicates a Kidney deficiency; a swelling of the lower part of the eye socket extending down towards the cheek indicates a pathology of the Large Intestine. A pale-greenish colour under the eyes generally indicates Liver-Qi stagnation. A dark-blue colour under the eyes indicates Cold in the Liver channel.

Box 6.14 summarizes patterns underlying abnormal colours in the eye sockets.

BOX 6.14 ABNORMAL COLOUR OF EYE SOCKETS

- Dark: Phlegm
- Dark purple: Blood stasis
- Bluish: Kidney deficiency
- Swelling of lower part of socket extending towards cheek: Large Intestine pathology
- Pale greenish: Liver-Qi stagnation
- Dark blue: Cold in Liver channel

BOX 6.13 ABNORMAL COLOUR OF CORNERS OF THE EYES

- Redness of outer corner: Heart-Fire
- Redness of inner corner: Lung-Heat
- Redness of either corner: Liver-Fire, invasion of external Wind-Heat
- Redness of inner corner in the evening: Lung-Yin deficiency with Empty-Heat
- Redness of outer corner in the evening: Heart-Yin deficiency with Empty-Heat
- Redness of either corner in the evening: Liver-Yin deficiency with Empty-Heat, Kidney-Yin deficiency with Empty-Heat
- Redness of either corner with sticky-yellow discharge: Damp-Heat
- Redness starting from the inner corners extending towards the centre: Yin and Yang Heel Vessels pathology
- Pale corners of the eyes: Blood deficiency (of Liver or Heart); or Yang deficiency (of Spleen or Kidneys)

NOTES

1. 1979 The Yellow Emperor's Classic of Internal Medicine – Simple Questions (*Huang Di Nei Jing Su Wen* 黄帝内经素问), People's Health Publishing House, Beijing, p. 25. First published c. 100BC.
2. Ibid., p. 572.
3. Ibid., p. 573.
4. 1981 Spiritual Axis (*Ling Shu Jing* 灵枢经), People's Health Publishing House, Beijing, p. 129, para 11. First published c. 100BC.
5. Ibid., p. 128.
6. Ibid., p. 151.
7. Ibid., pp. 151–152.
8. Ibid., p. 50.
9. Ibid., p. 50.
10. Simple Questions, p. 36.
11. Ibid., p. 25.
12. Spiritual Axis, p. 32.
13. Ibid., p. 40.
14. Ibid., p. 40.
15. Simple Questions, p. 572.
16. Ibid., p. 572.

17. Spiritual Axis, p. 151.
18. Ibid., p. 112.
19. Simple Question, p. 184.
20. Spiritual Axis, p. 56.
21. Ibid., p. 44.
22. Ibid., p. 35.
23. Ibid., p. 40.
24. Ibid., p. 43.
25. Ibid., p. 33.
26. Ibid., p. 56.

27. Ibid., p. 33.
28. Ibid., p. 151.
29. Eyes that are too wet (though obviously not when crying or because of a condition such as allergic rhinitis) may indicate a strong sexual drive.
30. Great Treatise of Ophthalmology (*Yan Ke Da Quan* 眼科大全 1644) cited in Ma Zhong Xue 1989 Great Treatise of Chinese Diagnostic Methods (*Zhong Guo Yi Xue Zhen Fa Da Quan* 中国医学诊法大全), Shandong Science Publishing House, p. 23.
31. Spiritual Axis, pp. 133–134.

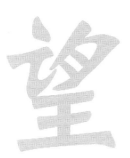

Chapter **7**

OBSERVATION OF THE NOSE

Chapter contents

INTRODUCTION 87

CHANNELS INFLUENCING THE NOSE 87

RELATIONSHIPS BETWEEN THE NOSE AND THE INTERNAL ORGANS 88

ABNORMAL COLOUR 89
  Pale 89
  Yellow 89
  Red 89
  Bluish-greenish 89
  Reddish-purple 89
  Dark 90

SWOLLEN NOSE 90

FLAPPING ALAE NASI (THE OUTSIDE OF THE NOSTRILS) 90

DRY NOSTRILS 90

NOSEBLEED 90

POLYPS 90

ULCERS ON THE NOSE 90

PAPULES ON THE NOSE 90

INTRODUCTION

The nose was called in ancient China the 'Bright Hall' (*ming tang*) of the face and it is a place where the clear Yang converges. The nose is the convergence of clear Yang for two reasons: first, because it takes in air, which is Yang in nature, and, secondly, because the Governing Vessel ('Governor' of all Yang energies) flows through the nose. In pathological conditions when clear Yang does not ascend to the nose, turbid Yin accumulates there causing conditions such as chronic sinusitis or rhinitis.

Another reason for the nose being called the Bright Hall in ancient times is related to Chinese face reading, according to which the nose represents the years from 41 to 49 in a person's life. Since these were considered to be the times when people established their career on a firm basis, the nose was compared to a hall – the most important room in a Chinese house in ancient times.

The patterns causing each of the nose signs discussed below are listed in greater detail in Part 5, Chapter 58.

CHANNELS INFLUENCING THE NOSE

The nose is influenced primarily by the Lung channel because the Lung 'opens' into the nose and controls the sense of smell. Chapter 37 of the 'Spiritual Axis' says: '*The nose is the sense organ of the Lungs*'[1] and Chapter 17 says: '*Lung-Qi penetrates the nose, when the nose is harmonized it can smell.*'[2] Chapter 4 of the 'Simple Questions' says: '*The West corresponds to the white colour and it is related to the Lungs which opens into the nose.*'[3] The Song dynasty doctor Chen Wu Ze said: '*The nose is the orifice of the Lungs through which we*

breathe and smell; in the nose Yang-Qi ascends and Yin-Qi descends so that it is the passage of Clear Qi.'[4] It is interesting to note that the Lung channel does not actually reach the nose and it therefore influences the nose through the Large Intestine channel.

The pathways of the channels flowing through or around the nose are as follows:

- both the Main and Muscle channels of the Large Intestine channel flow to the bottom of the nose (and influence the sense of smell)
- the Stomach channel connects with the nose
- the Bladder Muscle channel reaches the bridge of the nose
- the Governing Vessel flows downwards through the nose.

The channels flowing through or around the nose are illustrated in Figure 7.1.

Through their channels, the Large Intestine and Governing Vessel influence the sense of smell and cause symptoms such as sneezing in allergic rhinitis or nasal discharge in sinusitis.

Box 7.1 summarizes the channels influencing the nose.

BOX 7.1 CHANNELS INFLUENCING THE NOSE

- Lung Main channel (although it does not go to the nose)
- Governing Vessel
- Large Intestine Main and Muscle channels
- Stomach Main channel
- Bladder Muscle channel

RELATIONSHIPS BETWEEN THE NOSE AND THE INTERNAL ORGANS

Apart from the relationship between the nose and these channels, the shape and colour of the nose have particular diagnostic significance in facial diagnosis. In fact, pathological colours of the nose may reflect pathology of other organs such as the Liver and Spleen. Chapter 37 of the 'Spiritual Axis' says: *'The Bright Hall [nose] can have five [pathological] colours reflecting the Qi of the five Yin organs.'*[5] Different parts of the nose are related to different organs and these are illustrated in Figure 7.2. Chapter 19 of the 'Spiritual Axis' says: *'The bone of the Bright Hall [bridge of the*

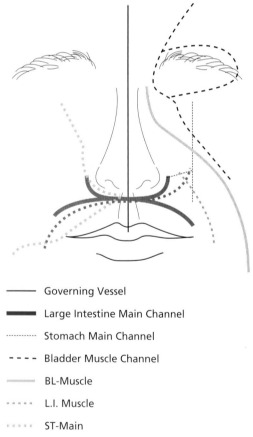

———— Governing Vessel

▬▬▬ Large Intestine Main Channel

············ Stomach Main Channel

- - - - Bladder Muscle Channel

———— BL-Muscle

· · · · · L.I. Muscle

· · · · · ST-Main

Fig. 7.1 Channels coursing through the nose

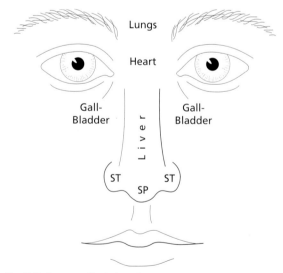

Fig. 7.2 Organs reflected on the nose

nose] should be high, even and straight; the state of the five Yin organs can be determined from the centre of the nose, while the state of the six Yang organs from the sides.'[6]

ABNORMAL COLOUR

Pale

Symptoms and Signs, Chapter 58

A pale nose may indicate Stomach- and Spleen-Qi deficiency with Empty-Cold; in such cases the pallor is primarily at the tip.

Blood deficiency (usually of the Liver) may cause the bridge of the nose to become pale. Among the Full conditions Phlegm-Fluids may cause the tip of the nose to become pale and swollen. A white and very dry nose indicates severe Lung-Qi deficiency.

Box 7.2 summarizes the patterns underlying a pale nose.

BOX 7.2 PALE NOSE

- Pale tip: Stomach- and Spleen-Qi deficiency with Empty-Cold
- Pale bridge: Liver-Blood deficiency
- Pale and swollen tip: Phlegm-Fluids
- Pale and dry: Lung-Qi deficiency

Yellow

Symptoms and Signs, Chapter 58

The yellowness ranges from a fresh, bright yellow to a dull yellow. If the yellowness is caused by Damp-Heat (usually in the Spleen), it will be bright if Heat predominates and dull if Dampness predominates.

A chronic Spleen-Qi deficiency with retention of Dampness is a common cause of a dull-yellow colour, usually at the tip of the nose. Spleen-Qi deficiency with Phlegm may cause the nose to become yellow and dry.

BOX 7.3 YELLOW NOSE

- Bright yellow: Damp-Heat in Spleen with predominance of Heat
- Dull yellow: Damp-Heat in Spleen with predominance of Dampness
- Yellow and dry: Phlegm with Spleen-Qi deficiency
- Dull, dark yellow: Liver-Blood stasis
- Bright yellow and dry tip: Spleen-Heat
- Yellow and swollen tip: Phlegm-Fluids

Liver-Blood stasis may cause a dull, dark yellow on the bridge of the nose. Spleen-Heat causes the tip of the nose to become bright yellow and dry. Finally, Phlegm-Fluids may cause the tip of the nose to become yellow and swollen.

Box 7.3 summarizes the patterns underlying a yellow nose.

Red

Symptoms and Signs, Chapter 58

Lung-Heat may cause a redness of the nose, especially on the upper part of the bridge. Liver-Fire is a common cause of redness of the central part of the bridge. Full- or Empty-Heat of the Spleen may cause a redness of the tip of the nose. Finally, the bridge of the nose may become red in invasions of Wind-Heat.

Box 7.4 summarizes the patterns underlying a red nose.

BOX 7.4 RED NOSE

- Red in upper part: Lung-Heat
- Red in central part: Liver-Fire
- Red tip: Spleen-Heat or Empty-Heat
- Red bridge with acute onset: Wind-Heat

Bluish-greenish

Symptoms and Signs, Chapter 58

Liver-Blood stasis may cause the nose bridge to become greenish, whereas Phlegm-Fluids may turn the nose tip bluish. Internal Cold may cause the bridge of the nose to become bluish.

Box 7.5 summarizes the patterns underlying a bluish-greenish nose.

BOX 7.5 BLUISH-GREENISH NOSE

- Greenish bridge: Liver-Blood stasis
- Bluish tip: Phlegm-Fluids
- Bluish bridge: internal Cold

Reddish-purple

Symptoms and Signs, Chapter 58

A reddish-purple nose always indicates Blood stasis occurring against a background of Heat. Blood stasis may occur in the Liver, in which case the bridge of the nose would be reddish-purple; in the Heart, in which case the area of the bridge between the eyes is reddish-

purple; or in the Stomach, in which case the alae nasi (the outside of the nostrils) become reddish purple.

Box 7.6 summarizes the patterns underlying a reddish-purple nose.

BOX 7.6 REDDISH-PURPLE NOSE

- Reddish-purple bridge: Liver-Blood stasis
- Reddish-purple in upper bridge between eyes: Heart-Blood stasis
- Reddish-purple nostrils: Blood stasis in Stomach

Dark

Symptoms and Signs, Chapter 58

A dark nose may be very dark, bluish-purple or may reach the point of being dull black. Dull blackness may indicate extreme Heat and a dark bluish-purple extreme deficiency, especially of the Kidneys. A dark and dry nose indicates Kidney-Yin deficiency, often deriving from excessive sexual activity. A dark-yellowish nose suggests Blood stasis. A dark nose appearing in a woman after childbirth may indicate a severe deficiency of Lungs and Stomach.

Box 7.7 summarizes the patterns underlying a dark nose.

BOX 7.7 DARK NOSE

- Dull black: extreme Heat (usually of Liver)
- Dark bluish-purple: extreme Deficiency
- Dark and dry: Kidney-Yin deficiency
- Dark yellowish: Blood stasis
- Dark nose in woman after childbirth: severe deficiency of Lungs and Stomach

---

SWOLLEN NOSE

Symptoms and Signs, Chapter 58

The nose can become swollen from Damp-Heat, Phlegm or Heat: the latter may derive from the Lungs, Heart or Liver. If the nose is swollen from Heat it will also be red, whereas if it is swollen from Phlegm it will be greasy. Empty Heat of the Heart or Kidneys may also cause the nose to swell.

FLAPPING ALAE NASI (THE OUTSIDE OF THE NOSTRILS)

Symptoms and Signs, Chapter 58

The most common cause of flapping alae nasi is Lung-Heat in acute conditions. It may also appear in Lung-Empty Heat and in external invasions of Wind-Heat.

DRY NOSTRILS

Interrogation, Chapter 35; Symptoms and Signs, Chapter 58

Dry nostrils can be caused either by Heat or Empty-Heat, usually affecting the Lung or Stomach channel. In acute febrile diseases, dry nostrils may be caused by Toxic Heat; in the beginning stages of respiratory infections they are caused by invasions of Wind-Heat.

NOSEBLEED

Symptoms and Signs, Chapter 58

The two main causes of nosebleed, as in other forms of bleeding, are Heat agitating the Blood or deficient Qi unable to hold Blood. In the case of nosebleed, the organs most frequently involved are Liver, Stomach and Lungs (with patterns of Heat) or the Spleen (deficient Spleen-Qi not holding Blood). Acute nosebleed may be caused by invasion of Wind-Heat.

POLYPS

Symptoms and Signs, Chapter 58

Polyps in the nose are caused either by Damp-Heat in the Stomach and Spleen or by Phlegm affecting the Lungs. Polyps caused by Damp-Heat are frequently seen in chronic sinusitis.

ULCERS ON THE NOSE

Symptoms and Signs, Chapter 58

Ulcers on the nose are usually due either to Lung-Heat or to Damp-Heat in the Stomach and Spleen.

PAPULES ON THE NOSE

Symptoms and Signs, Chapter 58

Red papules on the nose may indicate Stomach-Heat, Lung-Heat, or, if they are dark, Blood-Heat in the Lungs.

NOTES

1. 1981 The Yellow Emperor's Classic of Internal Medicine: Spiritual Axis (*Ling Shu Jing* 灵枢经), People's Health Publishing House, Beijing, p. 78. First published c. 100BC.
2. Ibid., p. 50.
3. 1979 The Yellow Emperor's Classic of Internal Medicine – Simple Questions (*Huang Di Nei Jing Su Wen* 黄帝内经素问), People's Health Publishing House, Beijing, p. 27. First published c. 100BC.

4. Cited in Ma Zhong Xue 1989, Great Treatise of Chinese Diagnostic Methods (*Zhong Guo Yi Xue Zhen Fa Da Quan* 中华医学望诊大全), Shandong Science Publishing House, Shandong, p. 56.

5. Spiritual Axis, p. 78.

6. Ibid., p. 96.

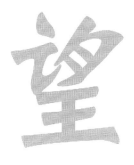

Chapter **8**

OBSERVATION OF LIPS MOUTH, PALATE, TEETH, GUMS AND PHILTRUM

Chapter contents

CHANNELS INFLUENCING THE MOUTH AND LIPS   *93*

LIPS   *94*
  Abnormal colour   *94*
  Dry or cracked lips   *96*
  Peeled lips   *96*
  Swollen lips   *96*
  Trembling lips   *96*
  Inverted lips   *96*
  Drooping lips   *96*

MOUTH   *96*
  Cold sores   *97*
  Cracked corners of the mouth   *97*
  Mouth ulcers   *97*
  Mouth open   *97*
  Deviation of mouth   *97*
  Dribbling from the corners of the mouth   *98*

PALATE   *98*
  Abnormal colour   *98*

TEETH AND GUMS   *99*
  Teeth   *99*
  Gums   *100*

PHILTRUM   *101*
  Flat philtrum   *102*
  Stiff-looking philtrum   *102*
  Abnormal colour   *102*

CHANNELS INFLUENCING THE MOUTH AND LIPS

From a Five-Element perspective, the mouth and lips are the orifice of the Spleen, but they are related to many other channels. The Spleen channel is closely related to both mouth and lips and Chapter 5 of the 'Simple Questions' says: *'The Spleen controls the mouth'*[1] and Chapter 4 of the same book says: *'The centre pertains to the yellow colour, it connects with the Spleen which opens into the mouth.'*[2] Chapter 17 of the 'Spiritual Axis' says: *'Spleen-Qi penetrates within the mouth, when the Spleen is harmonized, the mouth can taste the five flavours.'*[3] Chapter 37 of the same book says: *'The mouth and lips are the orifice of the Spleen.'*[4] and Chapter 47 says: *'When the lips are full, the Spleen is strong; when the lips are withered, the Spleen is weak; when the lips are hard, the Spleen has a Full condition; when the lips are large but soft, the Spleen is depleted. When both lips are in a good condition the Spleen is healthy; when the lips are deviated upwards, the Spleen is severely depleted.'*[5]

The Stomach channel is, of course, closely connected to the mouth because its Main and Muscle channels both flow around the mouth. Chapter 40 of the 'Spiritual Axis' says: *'The clear Qi of the Stomach ascends to the mouth.'*[6] The Large Intestine channel also flows to the lower part of the nose and its Muscle channels bind at the side of the nose.

The mouth and lips are therefore influenced primarily by the Spleen, Stomach and Large Intestine channels; however, the Liver channel also wraps around the lips and so do the Penetrating and Directing Vessels. Chapter 10 of the 'Spiritual Axis' says: *'The Liver channel flows around the inside of the lips.'*[7] The Governing Vessel penetrates through the upper lip and the upper gum. Internally, other channels flow to the

inside of the mouth and the tongue and, in particular, the Heart Connecting channel, the Kidney Main and Divergent channel.

As the Heart houses the Mind, it controls all the senses and therefore also the mouth and taste.

The saliva is mostly under the control of the Stomach, Spleen and Kidneys, and a normal level of moisture in the mouth indicates a normal state of the Body Fluids.

The channels flowing to or around the mouth are illustrated in Figure 8.1, and Box 8.1 summarizes them.

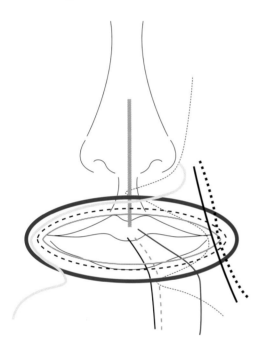

___ Large Intestine Main Channel

········· Stomach Main Channel

——— Heart Connecting Channel (to tongue)

- - - - Kidney Main Channel (to tongue)

——— Kidney Divergent Channel (to tongue)

▬▬▬ Governing Vessel

——— Liver Main Channel

- - - - Directing Vessel

▬▬▬ Penetrating Vessel

——— S T-Muscle

ı▪▪▪▪▪ S T-Main

Fig. 8.1 Channels flowing around the mouth

> **BOX 8.1 CHANNELS FLOWING TO OR AROUND THE MOUTH AND LIPS**
>
> - Stomach Main and Muscle channels
> - Large Intestine
> - Liver
> - Penetrating Vessel
> - Directing Vessel
> - Heart Connecting channel
> - Kidney Main and Divergent channels
> - Governing Vessel

LIPS

The following lip signs will be discussed:

> - abnormal colour (pale, red, purple, bluish-greenish and yellow lips, abnormal lip colour in pregnancy)
> - dry or cracked lips
> - peeled lips
> - swollen lips
> - trembling lips
> - inverted lips
> - drooping lips.

The colour of the lips primarily reflects the state of the Spleen, Heart and Liver. It also reflects conditions of Blood deficiency, Yang deficiency, Heat and Blood stasis. The normal lips, like the complexion, should be pale red and slightly moist, and not swollen, withered, contracted or quivering. The normal pale-red colour of the lips reflects the normal condition of Qi and Blood, their moistness reflects the normal condition of Body Fluids, and their normal movement reflects a normal condition of the Mind and Spirit.

The patterns causing each of the lip signs discussed below are listed in greater detail in Part 5, Chapter 60.

Abnormal colour
Pale lips
Symptoms and Signs, Chapter 60

When the lips are paler than the normal pale red, they indicate either Blood or Yang deficiency of the Spleen or Liver. In cases of Blood deficiency, especially of the Liver, they might also be slightly dry, while in cases of Yang deficiency they are usually moist. Pale-greyish

lips the colour of paper indicate severe Blood deficiency. For a more detailed description of the patterns involved, see Chapter 60.

Box 8.2 summarizes the patterns underlying pale lips.

> **BOX 8.2 PALE LIPS**
>
> * Pale and slightly dry: Blood deficiency of the Spleen or Liver
> * Pale and moist: Yang deficiency of the Spleen or Liver
> * Pale greyish: severe Blood deficiency

Red lips

Symptoms and Signs, Chapter 60

Red lips are always caused by Heat, which can be Full or Empty, and acute or chronic. Full-Heat of most organs, and especially the Lungs, Heart, Stomach, Liver, Kidneys and Spleen, may cause the lips to be red and swollen; Empty-Heat of the same organs may cause the lips to be red and dry. Acute invasions of Wind-Heat may also cause the lips to become bright red but this happens mostly in children; at the Qi level of acute febrile diseases, the lips also become bright red and they are also cracked and dry in cases of Fire. For a more detailed description of the patterns involved, see Chapter 60.

Box 8.3 summarizes the patterns underlying red lips.

> **BOX 8.3 RED LIPS**
>
> * Red and swollen: Full-Heat especially of the Lungs, Heart, Stomach, Liver, Kidneys and Spleen
> * Red and dry: Empty-Heat of the Lungs, Heart, Stomach, Liver, Kidneys and Spleen
> * Bright red (mostly in children): acute invasions of Wind-Heat, Qi level of acute febrile diseases
> * Bright red, cracked and dry: Fire

Purple lips

Symptoms and Signs, Chapter 60

Purple lips may reflect Blood stasis, in which case they tend to be reddish-purple, or Cold (which may be Full or Empty), in which case they tend to be bluish-purple. Bluish-purple and dark lips indicate extreme Cold. Long-standing retention of Phlegm in the Lungs often leads to Blood stasis and this may also cause the lips to be bluish-purple. Finally, the lips may become reddish-purple at the Nutritive-Qi or Blood levels in acute febrile diseases. For a more detailed description of the patterns involved, see Chapter 60.

Box 8.4 summarizes the patterns underlying purple lips.

> **BOX 8.4 PURPLE LIPS**
>
> * Reddish-purple: Blood stasis, Nutritive-Qi or Blood levels of acute febrile diseases
> * Bluish-purple: Full- or Empty-Cold, retention of Phlegm in the Lungs

Bluish-greenish lips

Symptoms and Signs, Chapter 60

'Bluish-green' is a translation of the Chinese word *qing*. The colour *qing* may be either bluish or greenish depending on the pattern involved. The lips may become bluish in case of Cold, which may be Full or Empty, and greenish in case of Blood stasis, which may affect Heart, Lungs, Stomach or Liver. For a more detailed description of the patterns involved, see Chapter 60.

Box 8.5 summarizes the patterns underlying bluish-greenish lips.

> **BOX 8.5 BLUISH-GREENISH LIPS**
>
> * Bluish: Full- or Empty-Cold
> * Greenish: Blood stasis of Heart, Lungs, Stomach or Liver

Yellow lips

Symptoms and Signs, Chapter 60

Yellow lips are usually caused by Dampness in the Stomach and Spleen, which may be associated with Heat or Cold; another possible cause of yellow lips is Full-Heat with Blood stasis. For a more detailed description of the patterns involved, see Chapter 60.

Box 8.6 summarizes the patterns underlying yellow lips.

> **BOX 8.6 YELLOW LIPS**
>
> * Dampness in the Stomach and Spleen with Heat or Cold
> * Full-Heat with Blood stasis

Abnormal lip colour in pregnancy

Symptoms and Signs, Chapter 60

Florid, red and full lips indicate a good state of the Penetrating Vessel and an easy childbirth. Pale lips in pregnancy indicate Blood deficiency and possibly a difficult childbirth. A white colour and dryness of the

corners of the mouth indicate severe Blood deficiency and also the possibility of a difficult birth. Bluish lips in pregnancy indicate Blood stasis from Cold and are always considered to be a dangerous sign. A bluish face and dark lips or a dark face and bluish lips in pregnancy also signal danger.

Box 8.7 summarizes patterns underlying abnormal lip colour in pregnancy.

BOX 8.7 ABNORMAL LIP COLOUR IN PREGNANCY

- Pale: Blood deficiency
- White and dryness of the corners of the mouth: severe Blood deficiency
- Bluish: Blood stasis from Cold

Dry or cracked lips

Symptoms and Signs, Chapter 60

The most common causes of dry lips are Stomach- and Spleen-Yin deficiency or Liver-Blood deficiency. Full-Heat or Empty-Heat may also cause the lips to become dry and cracked. Severe, long-standing Blood stasis may lead to the same effect because stagnant Blood prevents the proper generation and movement of Body Fluids. In acute cases, invasion of Wind-Heat can cause dry lips.

If the upper lip is dry, it indicates Lung-Heat or Heat in the Large Intestine. If the lower lip is dry, it indicates Heat in the Stomach. If the lips are dry but red, the condition is not severe and the prognosis is good. If they are dry but dark, the condition is more serious and the prognosis less good. For a more detailed description of the patterns involved, see Chapter 60.

Box 8.8 summarizes the patterns underlying dry, cracked lips.

BOX 8.8 DRY, CRACKED LIPS

- Dry and slightly red: Spleen-Yin deficiency
- Dry and pale: Liver-Blood deficiency
- Dry, cracked and red: Full-Heat (of Stomach and Spleen)
- Dry and slightly red: Empty-Heat (of Stomach and Spleen)
- Dry and purple: Blood stasis
- Dry with acute onset: Wind-Heat
- Dry upper lip: Heat in Lungs or Large Intestine
- Dry lower lip: Stomach-Heat
- Dry and red: prognosis good
- Dry and dark: prognosis not good

Peeled lips

Symptoms and Signs, Chapter 60

'Peeled lips' refers to lips that are peeled, fresh red, cracked and swollen. The causes of this are either Spleen-Heat or Spleen-Yin deficiency with Empty-Heat.

Swollen lips

Symptoms and Signs, Chapter 60

A swelling of the lips always indicates Heat, usually either Damp-Heat or Toxic Heat affecting the Stomach and Spleen. An acute swelling of the lips may also be due to an allergic reaction. For a more detailed description of the patterns causing swollen lips, refer to Chapter 60.

Trembling lips

Symptoms and Signs, Chapter 60

The most common cause of trembling lips is Spleen-Qi deficiency. It may also be caused by Blood deficiency with Empty-Wind or Stomach-Fire.

Inverted lips

Symptoms and Signs, Chapter 60

Inverted lips may be caused either by a severe Yang or a severe Yin deficiency. Contracted lips which do not cover the teeth, with a short philtrum, in the course of a serious disease indicate collapse of Spleen-Yin.

Drooping lips

Symptoms and Signs, Chapter 60

Drooping lips may be caused either by sinking of Spleen-Qi or deficiency of Spleen- and Kidney-Yang.

MOUTH

The patterns causing each of the mouth signs discussed below are listed in greater detail in Chapter 60.

The following mouth signs will be discussed:

- cold sores
- cracked corners of the mouth
- mouth ulcers
- mouth open
- deviation of mouth
- dribbling from the corners of the mouth.

Cold sores

Interrogation, Chapter 35; Symptoms and Signs, Chapter 60

A sudden attack of cold sores at the corner of the mouth or on the edge of the upper lip may be due to an external invasion of Wind-Heat. Chronic or recurrent cold sores at the corner of the mouth or on the edge of the lower lip may be caused by a Stomach pathology, either Damp-Heat, Heat or Yin deficiency with Empty-Heat. Heat or Damp-Heat in the Large Intestine may also cause cold sores, which in this case would be on the upper lip.

Box 8.9 summarizes the patterns underlying cold sores.

> **BOX 8.9 COLD SORES**
> - Sudden-onset cold sores at the corner of the mouth/edge of the upper lip: external invasion of Wind-Heat
> - Chronic or recurrent cold sores at the corner of the mouth/edge of the lower lip: Damp-Heat, Heat or Yin deficiency with Empty-Heat
> - Cold sores on the upper lip: Heat or Damp-Heat in the Large Intestine

Cracked corners of the mouth

Symptoms and Signs, Chapter 60

Cracked and dry corners of the mouth are due either to Stomach-Heat or to Stomach-Yin deficiency with or without Empty-Heat.

Box 8.10 summarizes the patterns underlying cracked corners of the mouth.

> **BOX 8.10 CRACKED CORNERS OF THE MOUTH**
> - Stomach-Heat
> - Stomach-Yin deficiency with or without Empty-Heat

Mouth ulcers

Interrogation, Chapter 35; Symptoms and Signs, Chapter 60

The most common causes of mouth ulcers are Stomach-Heat, when the ulcers have a red rim and will appear on the gums or inside the cheeks, and Heart-Fire, when the ulcers will be on the tip of the tongue. Mouth ulcers may also derive from a deficiency either of Yin (normally accompanied by some Empty-Heat) or of Stomach- and Spleen-Qi. A sudden attack of ulcers inside the cheeks may accompany an external invasion of Wind.

Box 8.11 summarizes the patterns underlying mouth ulcers.

> **BOX 8.11 MOUTH ULCERS**
> - Ulcers with red rim on gums/inside cheeks: Stomach-Heat
> - Ulcers on the tip of tongue: Heart-Fire
> - Deficiency of Yin, or Stomach- and Spleen-Qi
> - Sudden-onset ulcers inside the cheeks: external invasion of Wind

Mouth open

Symptoms and Signs, Chapter 60

'Mouth open' means that the person keeps the mouth open all the time. The most common cause of the mouth being wide open is deficiency of Lung-Qi with retention of Phlegm in the Lungs. Patients suffering from asthma often have their mouth open as they struggle to breathe and this itself usually indicates Lung-Qi deficiency and Phlegm in the Lungs.

The mouth could also be slightly open from Heart-Heat and, in this case, it usually reflects emotional problems.

Box 8.12 summarizes the patterns underlying 'mouth open'.

> **BOX 8.12 MOUTH OPEN**
> - Mouth wide open: deficiency of Lung-Qi with retention of Phlegm in the Lungs
> - Mouth open with struggling for breath: Lung-Qi deficiency and Phlegm in the Lungs
> - Mouth slightly open: Heart-Heat

Deviation of mouth

Symptoms and Signs, Chapter 60

There are two basic causes of deviation of the mouth: one is internal Liver-Wind, the other is invasion of external Wind in the channels of the face. From a Western perspective, the former usually corresponds to central paralysis (which is caused by a lesion of the central nervous system), while the latter is called peripheral paralysis and is caused by a lesion of the peripheral nerves (Fig. 8.2).

In some cases, deviation of the mouth may be caused by Liver-Qi stagnation, in which case it is not a permanent deviation but one that comes and goes according to the emotional state. A general deficiency of Qi and Blood may cause a slight deviation of the mouth. Finally, Toxic Heat affecting the Lesser-Yang

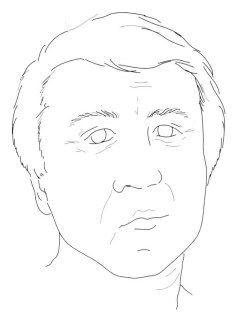

Fig. 8.2 Deviation of mouth

and Bright-Yang channels of the face may also cause deviation of the mouth.

Box 8.13 summarizes the patterns underlying deviation of the mouth.

BOX 8.13 DEVIATION OF MOUTH

- Internal Liver-Wind (central paralysis)
- Invasion of external Wind in face channels (peripheral paralysis)
- Toxic Heat affecting the Lesser-Yang and Bright-Yang channels of the face
- Deviation that comes and goes with the emotional state: Liver-Qi stagnation
- Slight deviation: general deficiency of Qi and Blood

Dribbling from the corners of the mouth

Symptoms and Signs, Chapter 60

Dribbling from the corners of the mouth may be caused by Qi deficiency of the Spleen or Lungs, or both, usually with Empty-Cold. Internal Wind, often combined with Phlegm, in the elderly is a common cause of dribbling from the corners of the mouth and this symptom is frequently seen after an attack of Wind-stroke. An invasion of external Wind in the channels of the face (the same pathology as in facial paralysis) may also cause dribbling from the corners of the mouth.

Heat in the Stomach and Spleen may also cause dribbling from the corners of the mouth.

Box 8.14 summarizes the patterns underlying dribbling.

BOX 8.14 DRIBBLING FROM THE CORNERS OF THE MOUTH

- Qi deficiency of the Spleen/Lungs, often with Empty-Cold
- Internal Wind, often combined with Phlegm, in the elderly
- Invasion of external Wind in the face channels
- Heat in the Stomach and Spleen

PALATE

The normal palate should be pale red, bright and moist. It can be divided into five areas, each corresponding to one of the Yin organs (Fig. 8.3).

Abnormal colour

The following palate signs will be discussed:

- pale palate
- dull-pale palate
- yellow palate
- red palate
- purple palate.

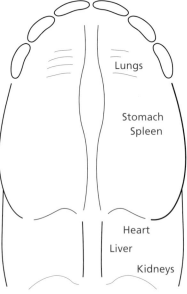

Fig. 8.3 Areas of the palate corresponding to the Yin organs

The patterns causing each of the palate signs discussed below are listed in greater detail in Chapter 60.

Pale palate

Symptoms and Signs, Chapter 60

This describes a palate that is too pale and looks like the skin of milk; it indicates deficiency of Stomach and Spleen.

Dull-pale palate

Symptoms and Signs, Chapter 60

A dull-pale palate indicates Blood deficiency or Qi and Blood deficiency.

Yellow palate

Symptoms and Signs, Chapter 60

A yellow palate indicates a pathology of the Stomach and Spleen, and in particular an Empty pathology if it is dull yellow and a Full pathology (such as Damp-Heat) if it is bright yellow.

Red palate

Symptoms and Signs, Chapter 60

A red palate indicates Full-Heat, which may derive from any organ, but in particular the Stomach, Lungs and Liver.

Purple palate

Symptoms and Signs, Chapter 60

A purple palate indicates Blood stasis.

Box 8.15 summarizes the patterns underlying abnormal palate colours.

BOX 8.15 ABNORMAL PALATE COLOURS

- Pale: deficiency of Stomach and Spleen
- Dull-pale: Blood/Qi deficiency
- Dull yellow: Empty pathology of Stomach and Spleen
- Bright yellow: Full pathology (such as Damp-Heat) of Stomach and Spleen
- Red: Full-Heat particularly of Stomach, Lungs and Liver
- Purple: Blood stasis

TEETH AND GUMS

The teeth and gums are closely related to the Stomach, Large Intestine and Kidneys. Chapter 63 of the 'Spiritual Axis' says: *'The teeth are at the end of the Stomach channel.'*[8] Chapter 10 of the same book says:

'The Stomach channel . . . enters the region of the upper teeth.'[9] The same chapter also says: *'The Large Intestine channel . . . enters the region of the lower teeth.'*[10] The Governing Vessel also influences the upper and lower gums in the midline of the body. The Kidney organ and channel specifically influence the teeth because the teeth are considered to be an extension of the bones.

Chapter 1 of the 'Simple Questions' describing the 7- and 8-year cycles of women and men clearly relates the development and decay of bones to the flourishing and decline of Kidney-Qi: *'When a girl is 7 years old, Kidney-Qi is flourishing and the teeth grow . . . when she is 21 Kidney-Qi is at its peak and the second teeth are fully grown . . . when a boy is 8 years old, Kidney-Qi is flourishing and the teeth grow . . . when he is 24 Kidney-Qi is at its peak and the second teeth are fully grown . . . when he is 64 the teeth fall out.'*[11] The gums are also influenced by the Kidneys.

Box 8.16 summarizes the channels influencing the teeth and gums.

BOX 8.16 CHANNELS INFLUENCING THE TEETH AND GUMS

- Stomach (gums)
- Large Intestine (gums)
- Kidneys (teeth and gums)
- Governing Vessel (teeth and gums)

The following teeth signs will be discussed:

- tooth cavities
- loose teeth
- plaque
- dry and white teeth
- dry and dull teeth
- yellow and dry teeth
- grey teeth
- upper teeth moist and lower teeth dry.

The patterns causing each of the teeth and gum signs discussed below are listed in greater detail in Chapter 60.

Teeth

Tooth cavities

Symptoms and Signs, Chapter 60

From the Chinese perspective, cavities may be caused by Damp-Heat in the Stomach channel, by Stomach- and Spleen-Qi deficiency and by a Kidney deficiency.

Loose teeth

Symptoms and Signs, Chapter 60

Again, from the Chinese perspective, teeth may become loose either from Heat or Empty-Heat of the Stomach or Large Intestine, or both, or from a Kidney deficiency (which may be of Yin or Yang). Stomach-Heat and Empty-Heat of the Spleen or Kidneys may all cause loose teeth.

Plaque

Symptoms and Signs, Chapter 60

The most common causes of plaque are Stomach-Heat or Heat in the Kidneys and Stomach. Another possible cause is Kidney-Yin deficiency.

Box 8.17 summarizes patterns underlying bad teeth.

BOX 8.17 BAD TEETH

- Cavities: Damp-Heat in the Stomach channel, Stomach- and Spleen-Qi or Kidney deficiency
- Loose teeth: Heat or Empty-Heat of the Stomach/Large Intestine/Spleen/Kidneys, Kidney-Yin or -Yang deficiency
- Plaque: Heat in the Kidneys/Stomach, Kidney-Yin deficiency

Dry and white teeth

Symptoms and Signs, Chapter 60

'White' here indicates teeth that are bright white and dry. The most common cause of white, dry teeth is either external Heat injuring the body fluids, or Stomach-Heat.

Dry and dull teeth

Symptoms and Signs, Chapter 60

'Dry and dull teeth' indicates teeth that are white but dull and very dry like old bones that have been exposed to the sun for a long time. The most common cause of dry and dull teeth is a Kidney-Yin deficiency with or without Empty-Heat; in the case of Empty-Heat, the teeth will be particularly dry. Another possible cause is Blood deficiency.

Yellow and dry teeth

Symptoms and Signs, Chapter 60

The most common cause of 'yellow and dry teeth' is Damp-Heat in the Stomach and Spleen, with a predominance of Heat. Another possible cause of yellow and dry teeth is a long-standing Kidney-Yin deficiency.

In a few cases, it may be due to long-standing accumulation of Cold. This happens when the accumulation of Cold in the abdomen impairs the circulation of Yang-Qi in the Greater-Yang and Bright-Yang channels, resulting in the accumulation of Yang energy in the top part of these channels and in the Governing Vessel over the teeth.

Grey teeth

Symptoms and Signs, Chapter 60

The most common cause of grey teeth is Kidney-Yin deficiency with Empty-Heat. Greyish teeth the colour of ash indicate Stomach- and Kidney-Yin deficiency with turbid Dampness.

Box 8.18 summarizes patterns underlying abnormal teeth colour.

BOX 8.18 ABNORMAL TEETH COLOUR

- Dry and white: external Heat injuring the body fluids, Stomach-Heat
- Dry and dull: Kidney-Yin deficiency with/without Empty-Heat, Blood deficiency
- Yellow and dry: Damp-Heat in the Stomach and Spleen, Kidney-Yin deficiency, accumulation of Cold
- Grey: Kidney-Yin deficiency with Empty-Heat
- Ash-like grey: Stomach- and Kidney-Yin deficiency with turbid Dampness

---

Upper teeth moist and lower teeth dry

Symptoms and Signs, Chapter 60

When the upper teeth are moist and the lower teeth dry, it indicates Kidney-Yin deficiency with Empty-Heat in the Heart.

Gums

The following gum signs will be discussed:

- inflamed gums
- bleeding gums
- receding gums
- gums oozing pus
- pale gums
- red gums
- purple gums.

The patterns causing each of the gum signs discussed below are listed in greater detail in Chapter 60.

Inflamed gums

Interrogation, Chapter 35; Symptoms and Signs, Chapter 60

The most common cause of inflamed gums is Heat or Empty-Heat in the Stomach or Large Intestine, or both. Yin Fire may also cause inflamed gums.

Bleeding gums

Interrogation, Chapter 35; Symptoms and Signs, Chapter 60

Deficient Spleen-Qi not holding blood is the most common cause of chronic bleeding gums. Stomach-Fire is also a common cause of bleeding gums, in which case the gums would be red and swollen and this symptom by itself allows us to differentiate Stomach-Fire from Stomach-Heat. Empty-Heat in the Stomach or Kidneys may also cause bleeding gums. Finally, Yin Fire may also cause bleeding gums.

Receding gums

Interrogation, Chapter 35; Symptoms and Signs, Chapter 60

The most common cause of receding gums is Qi and Blood deficiency. Receding gums may also be caused by Stomach-Fire or Kidney-Yin deficiency with Empty-Heat.

Gums oozing pus

Symptoms and Signs, Chapter 60

The most common cause of gums oozing pus is Stomach-Fire but in chronic conditions it may be caused by a severe deficiency of Qi and Blood.

Box 8.19 summarizes patterns underlying gum problems.

BOX 8.19 GUM PROBLEMS

- Inflamed: Heat or Empty-Heat in the Stomach/Large Intestine, Yin Fire
- Bleeding: Deficient Spleen-Qi not holding blood, Empty-Heat in Stomach/Kidneys, Yin Fire
- Bleeding, red and swollen: Stomach-Fire
- Receding: Qi and Blood deficiency, Stomach-Fire, Kidney-Yin deficiency with Empty-Heat
- Gums oozing pus: Stomach-Fire
- Gums oozing pus (chronic): severe deficiency of Qi and Blood

---

Pale gums

Symptoms and Signs, Chapter 60

Pale gums may reflect a Spleen-Qi deficiency, a Blood deficiency or a Spleen-Yang deficiency with Empty-Cold.

Red gums

Symptoms and Signs, Chapter 60

Red gums reflect Heat or Empty-Heat in the Stomach or Spleen. If they are also swollen and painful, this indicates Stomach-Fire. Slightly red gums, without swelling, and loose teeth that are painful in the afternoon indicate Kidney-Yin deficiency with Empty-Heat.

Purple gums

Symptoms and Signs, Chapter 60

The most common cause of purple gums is Blood stasis in the Stomach.

Box 8.20 summarizes patterns underlying abnormal gum colours.

BOX 8.20 ABNORMAL GUM COLOURS

- Pale: Spleen-Qi or Blood deficiency, Spleen-Yang deficiency with Empty-Cold
- Red: heat or Empty-Heat in the Stomach or Spleen
- Red, swollen and painful: Stomach-Fire
- Slightly red without swelling, with loose teeth painful in the afternoon: Kidney-Yin deficiency with Empty-Heat
- Purple: Blood stasis in the Stomach

PHILTRUM

The philtrum is the area between the bottom of the nose and the upper lip, defined by the two vertical ridges (Fig. 8.4).

The philtrum area is influenced by the Large Intestine channel and by the Governing Vessel. In

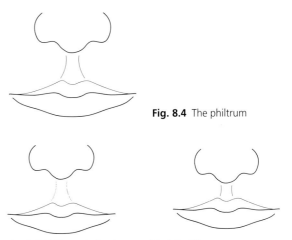

Fig. 8.4 The philtrum

Fig. 8.5 Philtrum indicating possible infertility

facial diagnosis, it reflects the state of the Bladder and Uterus. The philtrum should be well defined by the two vertical ridges and well proportioned, that is, not too long or too short. In face reading, the shape and appearance of the philtrum is related to fertility in women: a shallow philtrum with poorly defined vertical ridges or a very short philtrum indicates either infertility or difficulty in conceiving (Fig. 8.5).

In observing the philtrum, one should note its shape and its colour. In terms of shape, the philtrum may be too flat and undefined or too pronounced with stiff-looking ridges. The pathological colours of the philtrum include pale, red, bluish-greenish or dark.

The following philtrum signs will be discussed:

- flat philtrum
- stiff-looking philtrum
- abnormal colour (pale philtrum, red philtrum, bluish-greenish philtrum and dark philtrum).

The patterns causing each of the philtrum signs listed below are discussed in more detail in Chapter 60.

Flat philtrum

Symptoms and Signs, Chapter 60

The flat philtrum is poorly defined and the vertical ridges are not pronounced. The most common significance of a flat philtrum is a Kidney deficiency. It may also indicate Damp-Heat in the Stomach and Spleen (Fig. 8.6).

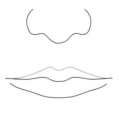

Fig. 8.6 Flat philtrum

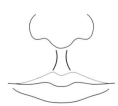

Fig. 8.7 Stiff-looking philtrum

Stiff-looking philtrum

Symptoms and Signs, Chapter 60

The stiff-looking philtrum is pronounced, its vertical ridges are overly defined and the upper lip curls up slightly (Fig. 8.7).

A stiff-looking philtrum generally indicates Blood stasis.

Abnormal colour
Pale philtrum

Symptoms and Signs, Chapter 60

A pale philtrum indicates either Qi deficiency or Cold, which may be of the Full or Empty type.

Red philtrum

Symptoms and Signs, Chapter 60

A red philtrum indicates either Blood-Heat, often in the Uterus, or, in acute cases, external invasion of Wind-Heat.

Bluish-greenish philtrum (qing)

Symptoms and Signs, Chapter 60

A bluish philtrum indicates internal Cold while a greenish philtrum indicates a Liver pattern, often stagnation of Liver-Qi.

Dark philtrum

Symptoms and Signs, Chapter 60

A dark philtrum indicates chronic Blood-Heat or Damp-Heat in the Lower Burner.

Box 8.21 summarizes philtrum signs.

BOX 8.21 PHILTRUM SIGNS

- Flat: Kidney deficiency, Damp-Heat in the Stomach and Spleen
- Stiff-looking: Blood stasis
- Pale: Qi deficiency, Full- or Empty-Cold
- Red: Blood-Heat, often in the Uterus, external invasion of Wind-Heat
- Bluish: internal Cold
- Greenish: Liver pattern, often stagnation of Liver-Qi
- Dark: chronic Blood-Heat, Damp-Heat in the Lower Burner

NOTES

1. 1979 The Yellow Emperor's Classic of Internal Medicine – Simple Questions (*Huang Di Nei Jing Su Wen* 黄帝内经素问), People's Health Publishing House, Beijing, p. 39. First published c. 100BC.

2. Ibid., p. 27.
3. 1981 Spiritual Axis (*Ling Shu Jing* 灵枢经), People's Health
   Publishing House, Beijing, p. 50. First published c. 100BC.
4. Ibid., p. 78.
5. Ibid, p. 91.
6. Ibid., p. 81.

7. Ibid., pp. 35–36.
8. Ibid., p. 114.
9. Ibid., p. 31.
10. Ibid., p. 31.
11. Simple Questions, pp. 5–6.

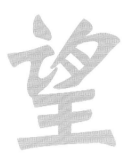

Chapter **9**

OBSERVATION OF THE EARS

Chapter contents

INTRODUCTION   *105*

CHANNELS INFLUENCING THE EARS   *105*

EAR SIZE   *106*
   Large ears   *106*
   Small ears   *106*
   Swollen ears   *107*
   Contracted ears   *107*

DRY AND CONTRACTED HELIX   *107*

SORES ON THE EAR   *107*

WARTS ON THE EAR   *107*

ABNORMAL COLOUR   *107*
   Yellow helix   *107*
   Pale helix   *107*
   Bluish-greenish (*qing*) helix   *107*
   Dark helix   *107*
   Red helix   *107*
   Red back of the ear   *108*
   Swelling and redness of the concha   *108*

DISTENDED BLOOD VESSELS ON THE EAR   *108*

EXCESSIVE WAX PRODUCTION   *108*

DISCHARGE FROM THE EARS   *108*

INTRODUCTION

The ears are related to the Kidneys. Chapter 17 of the 'Spiritual Axis' says: '*Kidney-Qi opens into the ears, when the Kidneys are harmonized the ears can detect the five sounds.*'[1] Chapter 5 of the 'Simple Questions' says: '*The Kidneys govern the ears.*'[2] Chapter 37 of the 'Spiritual Axis' says: '*The ears are the sense organ of the Kidneys.*'[3] Although the relationship between the ears and the Kidneys is very strong, other organs also influence the ears. For example, the Heart has an influence on the physiology and pathology of the ear. Chapter 4 of the 'Simple Questions' says: '*The South corresponds to the colour red and to the Heart which opens into the ear.*'[4]

CHANNELS INFLUENCING THE EARS

All the Yang channels reach or enter the ears. Both Lesser Yang channels, that is the Gall-Bladder and Triple Burner, have a strong influence on the ear also, the former circling around the ear and the latter entering the ear. These two channels are particularly involved in acute ear pathologies characterized by either Wind-Heat or Damp-Heat affecting the ears. The Small Intestine channel intersects with the Gall-Bladder channel in the region of the ear and enters the ear at SI-19 Tinggong. The Bladder channel also intersects with the Gall-Bladder channel in the region of the ear. The internal pathway of the Stomach channel also reaches the ear, while the Muscle channel of the Large Intestine travels to the front of the ear.

The pathways of the channels flowing to the ears are summarized in Box 9.1 and illustrated in Figure 9.1.

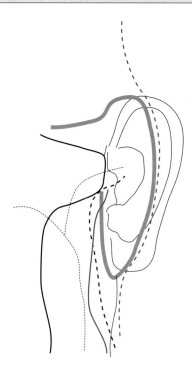

Gall-Bladder Main Channel

- - - - Triple Burner Main Channel

- - - - Bladder Main Channel

·············· Large Intestine Connecting Channel

———— Stomach Main Channel

———— Small Intestine Main Channel

Fig. 9.1 Channels flowing to the ears

BOX 9.1 CHANNELS INFLUENCING THE EAR

- Gall-Bladder
- Triple Burner
- Small Intestine
- Bladder
- Stomach
- Large Intestine Muscle channel

!

Remember: the ear is influenced not only by the Kidney channel.

The normal ear should be first of all proportionate in size to the head, it should be relatively moist, its flesh should be full but supple and the helix should be pale red and moist.

For a more detailed description of the patterns appearing in symptoms and signs related to the ears, see Chapter 57.

The following ear signs will be discussed:

- large ears
- small ears
- swollen ears
- contracted ears
- dry and contracted helix
- sores on the ear
- warts on the ear
- abnormal colour (yellow, pale, bluish-greenish, dark and red helix, red back of the ear, swelling and redness of the concha)
- distended blood vessels on the ear
- excessive wax production
- discharge from the ears.

Although the ear may present pathological signs like any other part of the face, the clinical significance of the observation of the ears is that they can give us an indication also of the constitution of the person; for example, large ears with long ear-lobes indicate a good constitution.

EAR SIZE

Large ears

The ears should be proportionate to the size of the head and therefore what is a 'large' ear for one person might be 'normal' for another. A large ear generally indicates a good hereditary constitution, a constitutional tendency to abundance of Qi and Blood and a propensity to Full conditions. However, it does so only if it is proportionate to the size of the head, well shaped and does not stick out, and if the lobe is long and well formed.

Small ears

Small ears generally indicate a poor hereditary constitution (especially if the lobe is very small), a constitutional tendency to deficiency of Qi and Blood and a propensity to Deficiency conditions.

Swollen ears

Symptoms and Signs, Chapter 57

Swollen ears are generally due to Heat or Damp-Heat, which may derive from various organs but particularly from the Gall-Bladder. (See Plate 9.1 on p. P8.) Another possible cause of swollen ears is invasion of Wind-Water in the Lungs.

Contracted ears

Symptoms and signs, Chapter 57

Contracted ears look somewhat 'crumpled' and 'squashed'. Contracted ears are generally due to deficiency of Body Fluids, which may derive either from Heat injuring the Body Fluids or from Yin deficiency. A less common cause of contracted ears is a severe stasis of Blood in the abdomen with abdominal masses: the severely stagnant Qi and Blood fail to nourish the muscles and flesh so that the person loses weight and the ears become contracted. This situation could, for example, occur with carcinomas of the abdomen.

DRY AND CONTRACTED HELIX

Symptoms and Signs, Chapter 57

The most common cause of a contracted, dry helix with a rough and scaly texture is Blood stasis, sometimes combined with Damp-Heat. A dry and dark helix may also be due to Kidney-Yin deficiency. A jagged helix indicates chronic Blood stasis.

SORES ON THE EAR

Symptoms and Signs, Chapter 57

Sores on the ear are always due to Heat. They may derive from various organs but are particularly related to the Liver and Gall-Bladder. Another cause of acute sores on the ear is invasion of Wind-Heat in the Lesser Yang channels.

WARTS ON THE EAR

Symptoms and Signs, Chapter 57

Warts on the ear are generally due to Heat in the Liver and Gall-Bladder but they may also be due to Heat in the Stomach channel (as the deep pathway of the Stomach channel goes to the ear).

ABNORMAL COLOUR

Yellow helix

Symptoms and Signs, Chapter 57

Damp-Heat is the most common cause of a yellow helix, in which case it would be bright yellow if Heat predominates and dull yellow if Dampness predominates. Another possible cause of a yellow helix is Blood stasis deriving from Heat, in which case the helix will be dull, dark yellow.

Pale helix

Symptoms and Signs, Chapter 57

A pale helix is due either to Yang deficiency (when it will be bright pale) or to Blood deficiency (when it will be dull pale). A less common cause of a pale helix is invasion of Wind-Water in the Lungs. A 'thick', deep, white colour indicates Qi deficiency with Phlegm.

Bluish-greenish (*qing*) helix

Symptoms and Signs, Chapter 57

Blood stasis is the main cause of a bluish-greenish helix. The helix is greenish if the Blood stasis derives from Heat and bluish if it derives from Cold. A particular case of bluish-greenish helix is that seen in children suffering from acute convulsions from internal Wind.

Dark helix

Symptoms and Signs, Chapter 57

The helix may become dark either from Blood stasis or from chronic Heat. A greenish-dark helix indicates Kidney-Yin deficiency.

Red helix

Symptoms and Signs, Chapter 57

A red helix generally indicates Heat, especially of the Heart or Lungs, or both; it may also indicate Heat in the Lesser-Yang channels or Damp-Heat in the Liver and Gall-Bladder. A floating, red colour of the helix is due to Kidney-Yin deficiency with Empty-Heat. (See Plate 9.2 on p. P8.)

Red back of the ear

Symptoms and Signs, Chapter 57

The usual cause of redness at the back of the ear is invasion of Wind-Heat. It is also seen in the beginning stages of measles.

Swelling and redness of the concha

Symptoms and Signs, Chapter 57

Damp-Heat in the Liver and Gall-Bladder is the most common cause of redness and swelling of the concha. In chronic conditions, Kidney-Yin deficiency with Empty-Heat may also cause a redness and swelling of the concha, while in acute conditions Toxic Heat may cause it.

DISTENDED BLOOD VESSELS ON THE EAR

Symptoms and Signs, Chapter 57

The two main causes of visible distended blood vessels in the ear are Lung-Qi deficiency with retention of Phlegm, and Blood stasis.

EXCESSIVE WAX PRODUCTION

Symptoms and Signs, Chapter 57

Excessive wax production is usually caused by Phlegm, which may affect various organs. Another common cause of excessive wax production is Damp-Heat in the Liver and Gall-Bladder. Deficiency conditions causing excessive wax production include Spleen- and Kidney-Yang deficiency and Kidney-Yin deficiency with Empty-Heat.

DISCHARGE FROM THE EARS

Symptoms and Signs, Chapter 57

In acute cases, discharge from the ear can be due to invasion of Wind-Heat affecting the Lesser-Yang channels or to Damp-Heat in the Liver and Gall-Bladder; the latter may also cause ear discharge in chronic conditions. Both Kidney-Yin deficiency with Empty-Heat and Spleen-Qi deficiency with Dampness may cause an intermittent, thin discharge from the ear.

Box 9.2 summarizes the patterns underlying ear discharge.

BOX 9.2 EAR DISCHARGE

- Acute: invasion of Wind-Heat affecting the Lesser-Yang channels, Damp-Heat in the Liver and Gall-Bladder
- Chronic: Damp-Heat in the Liver and Gall-Bladder
- Intermittent, thin discharge: Kidney-Yin deficiency with Empty-Heat, Spleen-Qi deficiency with Dampness

---

NOTES

1. 1981 The Yellow Emperor's Classic of Internal Medicine – Spiritual Axis (*Ling Shu Jing* 灵枢经), People's Health Publishing House, Beijing, p. 50. First published c. 100BC.
2. 1979 The Yellow Emperor's Classic of Internal Medicine – Simple Questions (*Huang Di Nei Jing Su Wen* 黄帝内经素问), People's Health Publishing House, Beijing, p. 41. First published c. 100BC.
3. Spiritual Axis, p. 78.
4. Simple Questions, p. 26.

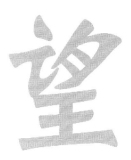

Chapter **10**

OBSERVATION OF THE THROAT AND NECK

Chapter contents

CHANNELS INFLUENCING THE THROAT AND NECK **109**

THROAT *110*
  Redness on the throat *110*
  Goitre *110*
  Pulsation of the carotid artery *110*
  Observation of the pharynx *110*
  Swollen tonsils *111*
  Abnormal tonsils colour *111*

NECK *112*
  Neck length *112*
  Rigidity of the neck *112*
  Soft neck *113*
  Deviated neck *113*
  Neck width *113*
  Swollen neck glands *114*

CHANNELS INFLUENCING THE THROAT AND NECK

Practically all channels, with the exception of the Bladder, flow through the throat but the most important channels involved in the various symptoms and signs of this area are the Directing Vessel for the front of the neck (throat area), the Stomach and Large Intestine for the sides of the throat, the Triple Burner and Gall-Bladder for the sides of the neck and the Governing Vessel and Bladder channel for the back of the neck.

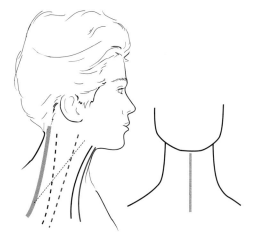

——— Large Intestine Channel (Main, Divergent, Muscle and Connecting)

——— Stomach Channel (Main, Divergent, Muscle and Connecting)

– – – Triple Burner Channel (Main, Divergent and Muscle)

·········· Small Intestine Channel (Main, Divergent and Muscle)

– – – Gall-Bladder Channel (Main, Divergent and Muscle)

▰▰▰ Bladder Channel (Main, Divergent and Muscle)

▭▭▭ Directing Vessel

Fig. 10.1 Channels flowing through the neck

BOX 10.1 CHANNELS INFLUENCING THE THROAT AND NECK

- Directing Vessel: front of the neck/throat area
- Stomach and Large Intestine: sides of throat
- Triple Burner and Gall-Bladder: sides of neck
- Governing Vessel and Bladder: back of neck

The pathways of the channels flowing through the neck are illustrated in Figure 10.1 and summarized in Box 10.1.

The symptoms and signs related to throat and neck are discussed in Chapters 59 and 62 respectively in Part 5.

THROAT

Redness on the throat

Symptoms and Signs, Chapter 59

By 'throat' here is meant not the inside of the throat (pharynx) but a redness on the skin outside.

A redness on the throat area (usually in the front and sides) always indicates Heat, which may be Full or Empty, and it often appears during the consultation when the patient is answering questions. This redness is usually due to Full- or Empty-Heat of the Heart or Lungs.

Goitre

Interrogation, Chapter 36; Symptoms and Signs, Chapter 59

The most common cause of goitre is Liver-Qi stagnation with Phlegm, usually occurring against a background of Spleen-Qi deficiency. It may also be caused by Phlegm and Blood stasis, Liver-Fire blazing with Phlegm or Heart- and Liver-Yin deficiency with Phlegm (Fig. 10.2).

Pulsation of the carotid artery

Symptoms and Signs, Chapter 62

Normally, carotid pulsations may be visible just medial to the sternocleidomastoid muscles, but 'pulsation of the carotid artery' signifies an excessive pulsation that is clearly visible. This may indicate either Water overflowing to the Heart or chronic Phlegm in the Lungs.

Observation of the pharynx

Symptoms and Signs, Chapter 59

To observe the pharynx, ask the patient to open the mouth; press the tongue down firmly with a disposable tongue blade, far enough back to get a good view of the pharynx but not so far as to cause gagging. Simultaneously ask the patient to say 'ah' or to yawn. Inspect the palate, the tonsils and the pharynx at this time (Fig. 10.3).

The pharynx should always be observed when a patient complains of acute or chronic 'sore throat': if the pharynx mucous membrane is red, it indicates Heat or Empty-Heat. In the many cases when patients complain of sore throat but there is no redness of the pharynx, the cause is often either stagnation of Qi (of the Liver or Lungs) or Yin deficiency (of the Lungs or Kidneys, or both).

If the pharynx is deep red on observation, it indicates Full-Heat, which may be exterior or interior. The inside of the throat may become red in acute invasions of Wind-Heat affecting the Lung channel and this is especially common in children. In interior conditions, a redness of the inside of the throat may be due to Full-

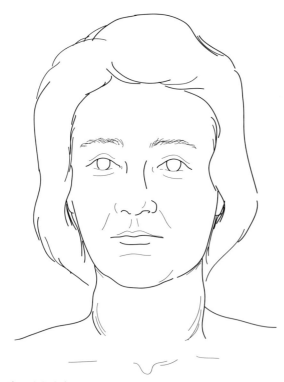

Fig. 10.2 Goitre

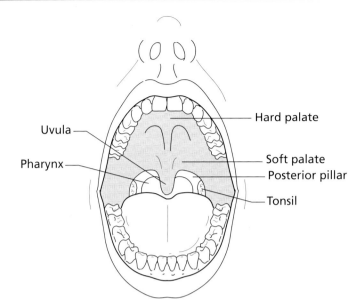

Uvula

Pharynx

Hard palate

Soft palate

Posterior pillar

Tonsil

Fig. 10.3 Pharynx

Heat in the Lungs or Stomach and Intestines, the latter being more common in children. If the inside of the throat is pale red, this indicates Empty Heat affecting the Lung or Kidney channel, or both.

Erosion, redness and swelling of the pharynx indicate Toxic Heat; this is seen more frequently in children suffering from acute upper respiratory infections.

Erosion, swelling and a yellowish-red colour of the pharynx, together with foul breath and a thick-yellow tongue coating, indicate Full Heat in the Stomach and Intestines, which, again, is more common in children.

A chronic erosion of the pharynx that comes and goes is usually due to Empty-Heat, which may affect Stomach, Lungs or Kidneys.

Chronic erosion and dryness of the pharynx that come and go with greyish ulcers, no swelling and a dry but not painful throat indicate chronic, severe Yin deficiency.

Chronic erosion of the pharynx with ulcers that have raised, hard edges indicates Blood stasis mixed with Phlegm-Heat.

Box 10.2 summarizes these pharynx signs.

Swollen tonsils

Symptoms and Signs, Chapter 59

Swollen tonsils of a normal colour indicate retention of Dampness or Phlegm occurring against a background of Qi deficiency. This is seen frequently in children with retention of a residual pathogenic factor (e.g. Dampness or Phlegm) after repeated acute upper respiratory infections. If both tonsils are affected, it generally indicates a greater severity than if only one is affected.

A chronic swelling of the tonsils in children is often accompanied by a chronic swelling of the adenoids, itself also a sign of retention of residual Dampness or Phlegm.

Abnormal tonsils colour

Red and swollen tonsils

Symptoms and Signs, Chapter 59

Red and swollen tonsils indicate Heat or Toxic Heat often in the Stomach or Large Intestine channel, or both. The tonsils should always be inspected in acute invasions of Wind-Heat, particularly in children. Red

---

BOX 10.2 PHARYNX SIGNS

- Deep red: Heat (interior or exterior)
- Pale red: Empty-Heat
- Erosion, redness and swelling: Toxic Heat
- Erosion, swelling, yellowish-red: Heat in Stomach
- Chronic erosion that comes and goes: Empty-Heat
- Chronic dryness and erosion with greyish ulcers: severe Yin deficiency
- Chronic erosion with ulcers that have raised, hard edges: Blood stasis with Phlegm-Heat

and swollen tonsils are frequently seen in children during acute upper respiratory infections. During acute invasions of Wind-Heat, a swelling and redness of the tonsils indicate a more severe degree of Wind-Heat and often the presence of Toxic Heat; they also point to an involvement of the Stomach or Large Intestine channel, or both, and tell us that the child has probably a pre-existing condition of Heat, often Stomach-Heat.

Chronic redness and swelling of the tonsils that come and go indicate either chronic Heat in the Stomach or Large Intestine channel, or both (more common in children and often due to a residual pathogenic factor), or Empty-Heat in the Lung channel. In both cases, the swelling and redness may be intermittent and less pronounced than in acute cases. Chronic redness and swelling of the tonsils used to be called 'milky moth' (*ru e*) when they resemble the wings of a moth and have a milky fluid on them.

If both tonsils are affected, it generally indicates a greater severity than if only one is affected.

Red and swollen tonsils with exudate

Symptoms and Signs, Chapter 59

Red and swollen tonsils with exudate, usually seen during acute upper respiratory infections and more common in children, definitely indicate an invasion of Wind-Heat (as opposed to Wind-Cold), and this may be complicated by Toxic Heat in the Stomach or Large Intestine channel, or both.

A swelling of the tonsils from Toxic Heat was called 'stone moth' (*shi e*) because the two tonsils look like the wings of a moth and have the hardness of a stone. If both tonsils are affected, it generally indicates a greater severity than if only one is affected.

Greyish tonsils

Greyish tonsils are often seen at the acute stage of glandular fever (mononucleosis).

BOX 10.3 TONSILS SIGNS

- Swollen, normal coloured: retention of Dampness or Phlegm with Qi deficiency
- Red and swollen: Heat or Toxic Heat in Stomach/Large Intestine channel
- Red and swollen during an invasion of Wind-Heat: severe Wind-Heat with toxic heat
- Chronic redness and swelling: chronic Heat in the Stomach/Large Intestine, Empty-Heat in the Lung channel
- Greyish: acute glandular fever

Box 10.3 summarizes patterns underlying tonsils signs.

NECK

Neck length

Long neck

A long neck is generally a sign of a good hereditary constitution (Fig. 10.4).

Short neck

A short neck may indicate a weak hereditary constitution of the Spleen and Kidneys (Fig. 10.5).

Rigidity of the neck

Symptoms and Signs, Chapter 62

This term refers not to the patient's subjective sensation but rather to a neck that looks rigid on observation and feels hard on palpation. Rigidity of the neck may be due to Cold in the channels as it occurs in

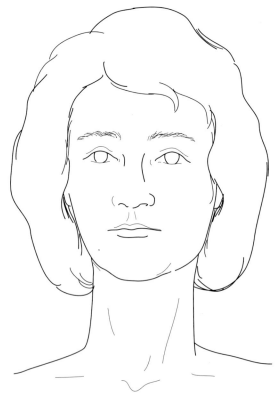

Fig. 10.4 Long neck

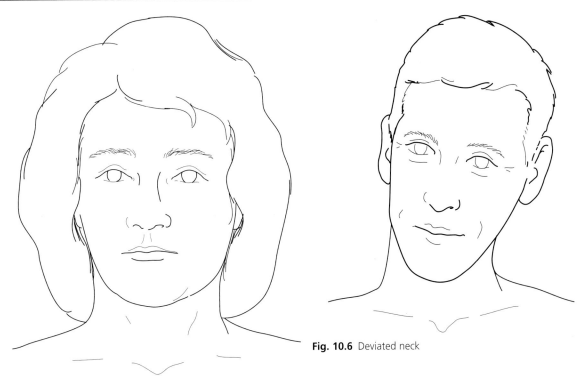

Fig. 10.5 Short neck

Fig. 10.6 Deviated neck

Painful Obstruction Syndrome. It may also be due to a Liver pattern and especially Liver-Qi stagnation, Liver-Yang rising or Liver-Wind.

Soft neck

Symptoms and Signs, Chapter 62

A neck with muscles that look soft and feel soft on palpation generally indicates severe deficiency of Qi and Blood or deficiency of Kidney-Yang.

Deviated neck

Symptoms and Signs, Chapter 62

A deviated neck (leaning to one side) is due either to a weak hereditary Kidney constitution or to severe stagnation of Liver-Qi (Fig. 10.6).

Neck width
Wide neck

Symptoms and Signs, Chapter 62

A wide neck may indicate Qi stagnation with Phlegm, Phlegm with Blood stasis, or Liver-Fire (Fig. 10.7).

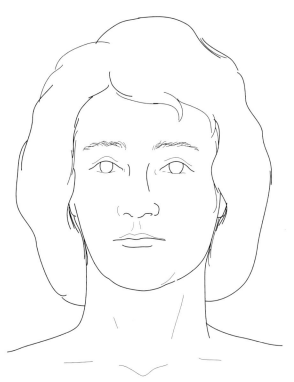

Fig. 10.7 Wide neck

Thin neck

Symptoms and Signs, Chapter 62

A thin neck may indicate a severe deficiency of Qi and Blood or chronic Yin deficiency (Fig. 10.8).

This is often seen when the patient, who is usually an elderly man, has the Chinese disease symptom of *ye ge* ('diaphragm choking'). The patient will be suffering weight loss, exhaustion, difficulty in swallowing, and will feel as if food is stuck between the throat and the diaphragm.

Swollen neck glands

Symptoms and Signs, Chapter 59

Figure 10.9 shows the location of the neck glands.

An acute swelling of the glands of the neck is usually due to an invasion of Wind-Heat with Toxic Heat; in other words a swelling of the neck glands during an invasion of Wind-Heat indicates that there is also Toxic Heat. This is common, for example, in the acute stage of glandular fever (mononucleosis). In chronic conditions, a swelling of the glands of the neck may also indicate Toxic Heat but one that generally

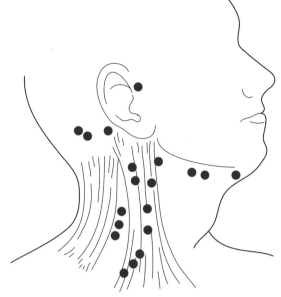

Fig. 10.9 Neck glands

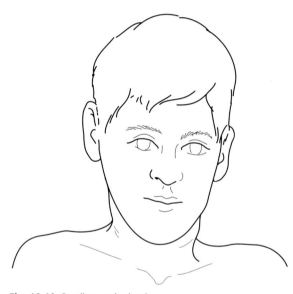

Fig. 10.10 Swollen neck glands

occurs against a background of Qi or Yin deficiency, or both.

In chronic cases, a swelling of the glands of the neck may be due to Toxic Heat with Blood stasis, or to Phlegm (Fig. 10.10).

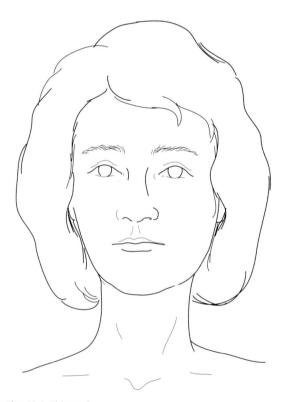

Fig. 10.8 Thin neck

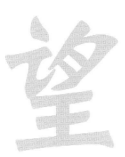

Chapter **11**

OBSERVATION OF THE BACK

Chapter contents

CHANNELS INFLUENCING THE BACK   *115*

ATROPHY OF THE MUSCLES ALONG THE SPINE   *116*

RIGIDITY OF THE LOWER BACK   *116*

SPINAL CURVE ABNORMALITIES   *116*
  Spine bent forward   *116*
  Scoliosis   *117*
  Lordosis   *117*
  Kyphosis   *117*
  Flattening of lumbar spine   *118*
  List of spine   *118*

SKIN SIGNS   *118*
  Spots on the back   *118*
  Vesicles on the lower back   *119*
  Dryness and redness of the skin of the lower
    back   *119*
  Yellow colour of the lower back   *119*
  Skin marks on the lower back   *119*
  Boils on BL-23 Shenshu   *119*
  Papules or pustules on the buttocks   *119*

CHANNELS INFLUENCING THE BACK

The upper back is influenced by the Governing Vessel and by the Bladder and Lung channel; the lower back is influenced by the Governing Vessel and the Bladder and Kidney channels. In more detail, the pathways of the channels flowing through the back are as follows (Fig. 11.1):

- The Bladder Main channel flows twice over the back.
- The Bladder Divergent channel ascends along the spine.
- The Bladder Muscle channel flows through the muscles alongside the spine.
- The Kidney Main channel enters the sacrum and flows through the lumbar spine.
- The Kidney Divergent channel ascends alongside the spine and connects with the Girdle Vessel at the level of BL-23 Shenshu.
- The Kidney Connecting channel spreads into the lumbar vertebrae.
- The Kidney Muscle channel ascends alongside the spine.
- The Governing Vessel ascends over the spine and a branch enters the sacrum and the lumbar vertebrae.
- The Governing Vessel Connecting channel connects with the Bladder channel and spreads through the spine.
- The Spleen Muscle channel adheres to the spine.

Box 11.1 summarizes the channels influencing the back.

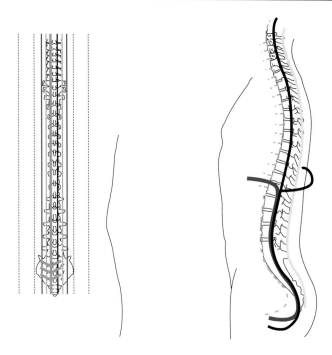

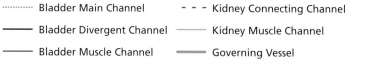

.... Bladder Main Channel   - - - Kidney Connecting Channel

———— Bladder Divergent Channel   ———— Kidney Muscle Channel

———— Bladder Muscle Channel   ▬▬▬▬ Governing Vessel

▬▬▬ Kidney Main Channel   - - - - - Governing Vessel Connecting Channel

▬▬▬ Kidney Divergent Channel   ———— Spleen Muscle Channel

Fig. 11.1 Channels flowing through the back

BOX 11.1 CHANNELS INFLUENCING THE BACK

- Governing Vessel
- Bladder
- Lung (upper back only, through the Large Intestine Divergent channel)
- Kidneys
- Spleen (Muscle channel)

ATROPHY OF THE MUSCLES ALONG THE SPINE

Symptoms and Signs, Chapter 67

Atrophy of the muscles along the spine indicates a Spleen deficiency because the Spleen nourishes all muscles but it also has a direct influence on the spine.

RIGIDITY OF THE LOWER BACK

Symptoms and Signs, Chapter 67

Rigidity of the lower back indicates either retention of Damp-Cold in the lower back or Blood stasis.

SPINAL CURVE ABNORMALITIES

Spine bent forward

Symptoms and Signs, Chapter 67

Bending forward of the spine indicates a hereditary Kidney-Essence deficiency, a deficiency of Marrow and a weakness of the Governing Vessel.

Scoliosis

Symptoms and Signs, Chapter 67

Scoliosis is an abnormal lateral curvature of the spine (Fig. 11.2). Congenital scoliosis is always due to a deficiency of Kidney-Essence. Acquired scoliosis is due either to a Kidney deficiency with Blood stasis or to retention of Wind-Dampness in the channels of the back.

Lordosis

Symptoms and Signs, Chapter 67

Lordosis is an accentuation of the normal lumbar curve (Fig. 11.3). Congenital lordosis is due to a deficiency of Kidney-Essence, while acquired lordosis may be due to a deficiency of the Stomach and Spleen, retention of Wind-Dampness in the channels of the back, or a deficiency of Yin of the Liver or Kidneys.

Kyphosis

Symptoms and Signs, Chapter 67

Kyphosis is a rounded convexity of the spine and upper back at the level of the thoracic vertebrae (Fig. 11.4). It is common in the elderly, more so in women. Kyphosis

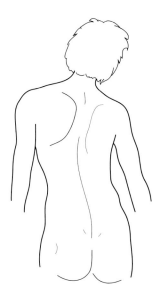

Fig. 11.2 Scoliosis

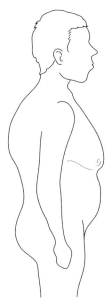

Fig. 11.4 Kyphosis

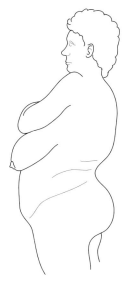

Fig. 11.3 Lordosis

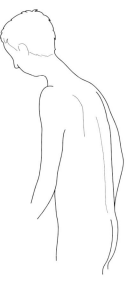

Fig. 11.5 Flattening of lumbar spine

indicates a decline of Kidney-Essence; in young people it indicates a congenital deficiency of Kidney-Essence.

Flattening of lumbar spine

Symptoms and Signs, Chapter 67

Flattening of the lumbar spine consists in a decreased lumbar curve (Fig. 11.5). It is often due to a pronounced spasm of the lumbar muscles and decreased spinal mobility; it may suggest the possibility of a herniated lumbar disc. The cause may be Liver-Qi stagnation, Liver-Blood stasis or Cold in the lower back.

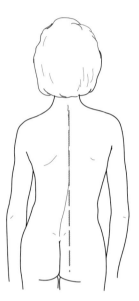

Fig. 11.6 List of spine

List of spine

Symptoms and signs, Chapter 67

A list is a lateral tilt of the spine (Fig. 11.6). When a plumb line dropped from T1 falls to one side of the gluteal cleft, a list is present. This may be due to a herniated disc or to spasm of the paravertebral muscles. It usually indicates Qi stagnation, Blood stasis or Damp-Cold in the lower back.

Box 11.2 summarizes patterns underlying spinal curve abnormalities.

SKIN SIGNS

Spots on the back

Symptoms and Signs, Chapter 67

Spots on the back consisting in red papules may indicate invasion of Wind-Heat with Toxic Heat in acute cases or, in chronic cases, Damp-Heat or Qi stagnation turning into Heat. The diagnostic significance of such spots depends also on the location: if they are located in the upper part of the back, in the area between T1 and T6, they reflect a pathology of the Lungs; if they are located in the central part of the back between T6 and T11, they reflect pathologies of the Heart and Liver; if they are located in the lower back, below T11, they reflect a pathology of the Kidneys.

Small, pinhead pustules, the size of millet grains, usually indicate either Damp-Heat or Phlegm-Heat and their significance also varies according to the location. If they are located in the upper back, they indicate a pathology of the Greater-Yang channels, often of external origin; if they are located in the mid back, they indicate Heat or Toxic Heat, often from emotional problems; if they are located in the lower back, they

---

BOX 11.2 SPINAL CURVE ABNORMALITIES

- Spine bent forward: hereditary Kidney-Essence deficiency, deficiency of Marrow, weakness of Governing Vessel
- Congenital scoliosis: Kidney-Essence deficiency
- Acquired scoliosis: Kidney deficiency with Blood stasis, retention of Wind-Dampness in back channels
- Congenital lordosis: Kidney-Essence deficiency
- Acquired lordosis: Stomach and Spleen or Liver/Kidney-Yin deficiency, retention of Wind-Dampness in back channels
- Kyphosis: decline of Kidney-Essence in elderly, congenital Kidney-Essence deficiency in young
- Flattening of lumbar spine: Liver-Qi stagnation, Liver-Blood stasis, Cold in lower back
- List of spine: Qi stagnation, Blood stasis, Damp-Cold in lower back

---

BOX 11.3 SPOTS AND PUSTULES ON THE BACK

Spots
- Between T1 and T6: Lungs pathology
- Between T6 and T11: Heart/Liver pathology
- Below T11: Kidney pathology

Pustules
- Small pinhead pustules: Damp-Heat or Phlegm-Heat
- Upper Back: Greater-Yang Channels
- Middle Back: Heat or Toxic Heat
- Lower Back: Kidney deficiency with Empty-Heat

usually indicate Empty-Heat from Kidney deficiency, often due to excessive sexual activity.

Box 11.3 summarizes pathologies underlying spots and pustules located in different positions on the back.

Vesicles on the lower back

Symptoms and Signs, Chapter 67

Vesicles filled with clear fluid on the lower back, which look like a string of pearls, indicate retention of Damp-Heat.

Dryness and redness of the skin of the lower back

Symptoms and Signs, Chapter 67

A red and dry macular rash on the skin of the lower back that is itchy and hot indicates Liver- and Heart-Fire.

Yellow colour of the lower back

Symptoms and Signs, Chapter 67

A yellow colour of the lower back with small vesicles indicates Damp-Heat in the Spleen and Kidneys.

Skin marks on the lower back

Symptoms and Signs, Chapter 67

A discoloration of the skin of the lower back that looks like long markings in the skin, often resembling a belt, and is neither itchy nor painful, indicates a pathology of the Girdle Vessel and a Kidney deficiency often due to excessive sexual activity.

Boils on BL-23 Shenshu

Symptoms and Signs, Chapter 67

A boil on BL-23 Shenshu indicates Phlegm occurring against a background of Kidney deficiency.

Papules or pustules on the buttocks

Symptoms and Signs, Chapter 67

Papules or pustules on the buttocks indicate Damp-Heat in the Bladder channel.

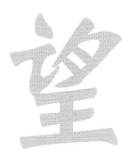

Chapter **12**

OBSERVATION OF WOMEN'S BREASTS

Chapter contents

INTRODUCTION   *121*

CHANNELS INFLUENCING THE BREASTS   *121*

BREAST SIZE   *122*
  Small breasts   *122*
  Breast distension   *122*
  Swollen breasts   *122*
  Redness and swelling of the breasts   *122*

BREAST LUMPS   *122*

NIPPLE ABNORMALITIES   *124*
  Milky nipple discharge   *124*
  Sticky yellow nipple discharge   *124*
  Bloody discharge from the nipple   *124*
  Inverted nipples   *125*
  Cracked nipples   *125*

PEAU D'ORANGE SKIN   *125*

INTRODUCTION

The routine observation in clinical practice does not normally include a woman's breasts, but is carried out when a patient reports specific breast problems such as tenderness, pain or lumps.

The symptoms and signs related to the breast are discussed in Part 5, Chapter 88.

CHANNELS INFLUENCING THE BREASTS

The channels coursing through the breasts are illustrated in Figure 12.1.

As we can see, the main channels influencing the breast are the Liver, Stomach and Penetrating Vessel: in addition, the Muscle channels of the Heart, Pericardium and Gall-Bladder also flow through the breast. In the internal anatomy of the breast, the

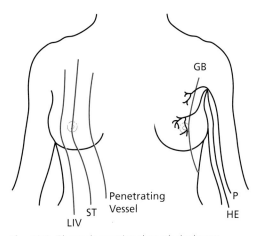

Fig. 12.1 Channels coursing through the breast

various structures are influenced by the following channels or tissues:

- glandular lobes: Stomach channel
- milk ducts: Stomach channel and Penetrating Vessel
- nipple: Liver channel
- areola: Penetrating Vessel
- adipose tissue in breast: fat tissue (*Gao*)
- connective tissue compartments: Membranes (*Huang*)
- blood vessels in the breast: Penetrating Vessel.

Box 12.1 summarizes the channels influencing the breasts.

BOX 12.1 CHANNELS INFLUENCING THE BREASTS

- Liver
- Stomach
- Penetrating Vessel
- Heart Muscle channel
- Pericardium Muscle channel
- Gall-Bladder Muscle channel

BREAST SIZE

Small breasts

Symptoms and Signs, Chapter 88

By 'small breasts' here is not meant breasts that are constitutionally small but that have become small. If the breasts become smaller, it indicates Qi and Blood deficiency or Yin deficiency. The sagging of the breasts may indicate Stomach deficiency or dryness of the Blood.

Breast distension

Interrogation, Chapter 46; Symptoms and Signs, Chapter 88

Breast distension is both a subjective sensation and an objective sign. The patient is uncomfortably aware of the distension of the breasts, and this distension is visible. It is very common in premenstrual syndrome. By far the most usual cause of this sign is Liver-Qi stagnation. It should be remembered that Qi stagnation can occur also in the Lungs and Lung-Qi stagnation may also cause breast distension. A slight breast dis-

tension may also occur with a Spleen and Kidney deficiency.

Swollen breasts

Symptoms and Signs, Chapter 88

A more severe stage of distension is the swelling of the breasts, which are noticeably larger than normal and often also painful. Swelling of the breasts is mostly due to Liver-Qi stagnation but with concurrent Phlegm. In a few cases, it may be due to Phlegm occurring against a background of Spleen- and Kidney-Yang deficiency.

Redness and swelling of the breasts

Symptoms and Signs, Chapter 88

Redness and swelling of the breasts usually indicate the presence of Heat, often Toxic Heat, combined with either Phlegm or Blood stasis. It is usually accompanied by breast pain and it may correspond to mastitis in Western medicine.

BREAST LUMPS

Interrogation, Chapter 46; Palpation, Chapter 51; Symptoms and Signs, Chapter 88

There are four broad categories of breast lumps in Western medicine: cysts, fibroadenomas, breast nodularity or carcinoma of the breast.

Cysts   Also called fibrocystic disease, these constitute the most common benign condition of the breast. They are usually bilateral and they feel soft and moveable on palpation. From the Chinese point of view, they are usually due to Phlegm. Cysts are most common between the ages of 30 and 50.

Fibroadenoma   This is the next most common benign breast disease, and occurs most often in young women. The adenoma is usually a single, unilateral lump and, on palpation, it feels harder than a cyst. From the Chinese point of view, it is due either to Blood stasis or to a combination of Blood stasis and Phlegm. Fibroadenomas are most common between the ages of 20 and 30.

Breast nodularity and tenderness   These occur in the breast before menstruation and usually decrease after the period. From the Chinese point of view, breast nodularity is due to a combination of Liver-Qi stagnation and Phlegm. It is most common between the ages of 30 and 50.

Carcinoma of the breast This usually presents with a single, painless, unilateral, immoveable, hard lump with indistinct margins. Its incidence is highest after the age of 50. It is nearly always due to a combination of Phlegm and Blood stasis occurring against a background of disharmony of the Penetrating and Directing Vessels. In carcinoma of the breast, there may be Toxic Heat in addition to Phlegm and Blood stasis. Phlegm is usually manifested by a Swollen tongue with sticky coating, and Blood stasis by a Purple colour on the breast areas of the tongue (Fig. 12.2) and Toxic Heat by a Red tongue with a thick, dry, dark-yellow coating and red points.

The three most common patterns leading to the formation of breast lumps (benign or malignant) are Qi stagnation, Blood stasis and Phlegm, but the first of these, Qi stagnation, usually accompanies the second and third as well. In Chinese medicine the Qi stagnation that leads to the formation of breast lumps is usually considered to be the result of emotional stress: this may be Liver-Qi stagnation, caused by such emotions as anger, resentment or repressed frustration, or Lung-Qi stagnation caused by sadness, worry or grief. Both conditions affect the breast and may lead to the formation of lumps.

> **!**
>
> **Remember**: Qi stagnation affecting the breast may derive not only from the Liver but also from the Lungs.

Case history 12.1 illustrates a pattern underlying a breast lump.

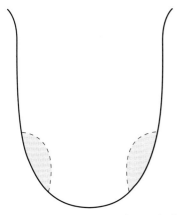

Fig. 12.2 Areas corresponding to the breast on the tongue

Case history 12.1

A 39-year-old woman had been suffering from a lump in the left breast (upper-left quadrant) for 5 years: the size of the lump had varied in relation to her menstrual cycle, increasing slightly before the period and decreasing afterwards. The lump was sometimes also painful. A biopsy, mammogram and MRI scan had confirmed the absence of any malignancy. The lump was neither a fibroadenoma nor a cyst and had been described simply as 'breast tenderness and nodularity'. On palpation, the lump was firm but not too hard, elongated and mobile. There was no lymph node involvement in the axilla.

Her periods were regular, not painful, not too heavy or scanty; she did suffer from premenstrual distension of the breasts and abdomen. She had no other symptoms, apart from a tendency to loose stools.

On observation, her complexion was dull and sallow and her eyes were slightly 'staring'; there was also a horizontal red vein starting from the outer corner of the left eye and reaching the edge of the pupil (Fig. 12.3; see also Plate 12.1 on p. P8). In addition, the white under the pupil was visible (this is not normally visible).

Her tongue was Red on the sides and tip, had a yellow coating and teeth marks in the left breast area (Fig. 12.4). Her pulse was Slippery on the whole, the left side was Slippery and Wiry, especially so on the Liver position, while the left-Front position was rela-

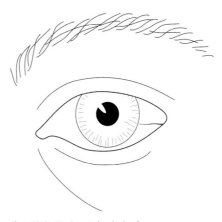

Fig. 12.3 Horizontal vein in the eye

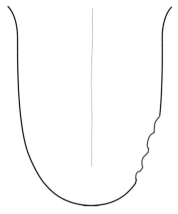

Fig. 12.4 Teeth marks in the left breast area

tively Overflowing; the pulse was also slightly Rapid (84).

Diagnosis: In breast lumps, the most common pathogenic factors are Liver-Qi stagnation, Liver-Blood stasis and Phlegm appearing in varying combinations. In this case, there are signs of all three patterns. There is Liver-Qi stagnation because of the premenstrual distension, the varying size of the lump in relation to the menstrual cycle and the Wiry pulse. There is Liver-Blood stasis because the lump is firm and slightly painful and the pulse is Wiry. There is Phlegm because the pulse is Slippery. Liver-Qi stagnation and Liver-Blood stasis are the predominant patterns compared with Phlegm. The chronic Liver-Qi stagnation has given rise to Liver-Heat and Heart-Heat, as evidenced by the Red sides and tip on the tongue: this is also confirmed by the rapidity of the pulse and the Overflowing quality on the Heart pulse.

The teeth marks in the left breast area on the tongue indicate that the breast pathology occurs against a background of Spleen-Qi deficiency, which is also confirmed by the tendency to loose stools. The slightly staring look of the eyes indicates that the Mind and Spirit are disturbed from emotional problems which, on interrogation, she confirmed having. The showing of the white under the pupil is generally a poor prognostic sign. The red vein in the left eye was in the Heart and Lung area and in the lower part of the sclera corresponding to the chest.[1]

BOX 12.2 FACTORS IN BREAST LUMPS

- Qi stagnation
- Blood stasis
- Phlegm

Box 12.2 summarizes the factors underlying breast lumps.

NIPPLE ABNORMALITIES

Milky nipple discharge

Symptoms and signs, Chapter 88

A milky nipple discharge is usually due to a deficiency condition: it may be a severe deficiency of Qi and Blood, or a deficiency of Spleen- and Kidney-Yang; in some cases, it may also be due to Liver-Qi stagnation.

Sticky yellow nipple discharge

Symptoms and signs, Chapter 88

A sticky-yellow nipple discharge is due either to Damp-Heat in the Liver channel or to Toxic Heat. In Western medicine, this may be caused by duct ectasia or epithelial hyperplasia.

Bloody discharge from the nipple

Symptoms and Signs, Chapter 88

As in all forms of bleeding, the two main causes are either Blood-Heat or Qi not holding Blood. In cases of a bloody discharge from the nipple, Toxic Heat is a common cause, especially in acute conditions. In chronic conditions, stagnant Liver-Qi turning into Heat may also cause an intermittent bloody nipple discharge. As for Deficiency conditions, a deficiency of the Liver and Kidneys and of the Penetrating Vessel may cause an intermittent bloody nipple discharge with pale blood.

BOX 12.3 NIPPLE DISCHARGES

- Milky: Qi and Blood deficiency, Spleen- and Kidney-Yang deficiency, Liver-Qi stagnation
- Sticky yellow: Damp-Heat or Toxic Heat in the Liver channel
- Bloody: Blood-Heat, Toxic Heat, Qi deficiency, stagnant Liver-Qi turning into Heat, deficiency of Liver and Kidneys

---

Box 12.3 summarizes patterns underlying nipple discharges.

Inverted nipples

Symptoms and Signs, Chapter 88

The inverting of a nipple is usually caused by complex pathologies; it may be due to Liver-Qi and Liver-Blood stagnation combined with Phlegm, or to Toxic Heat in the Blood combined with Blood stasis. From a Western medicine perspective, an inverted nipple may indicate an advanced stage of carcinoma of the breast.

Cracked nipples

Symptoms and Signs, Chapter 88

Cracked nipples may be caused either by stagnant Liver-Qi turning into Fire or by Liver-Yin deficiency with Blood-Heat.

PEAU D'ORANGE SKIN

Symptoms and Signs, Chapter 88

'Peau d'orange' refers to the appearance of an area of the breast that is covered with small dimples so that its texture resembles the rind of an orange. This may be due to Liver-Qi and Liver-Blood stagnation combined with Phlegm, or to Toxic Heat in the Blood combined with Blood stasis. From a Western medicine perspective, peau d'orange may indicate an advanced stage of carcinoma of the breast.

NOTES

1. See Maciocia G 1999 The Foundations of Chinese Medicine. Churchill Livingstone, Edinburgh. p. 147.

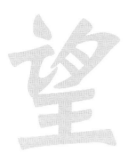

Chapter **13**

OBSERVATION OF THE HEARTBEAT

Chapter contents

INTRODUCTION   *127*

HEARTBEAT DISPLACED DOWNWARDS   *128*

HEARTBEAT DISPLACED UPWARDS   *128*

HEARTBEAT DISPLACED TO THE LEFT   *128*

HEARTBEAT DISPLACED TO THE RIGHT   *128*

HEARTBEAT BELOW THE XYPHOID PROCESS   *128*

INTRODUCTION

Observation of the heartbeat refers to observation of the pulsation of the left ventricle. In surface anatomy the left ventricle of the heart forms the organ's left border and produces the apical impulse, that is, the heart systolic beat, which can be felt in the fifth intercostal space, 7 to 9 centimetres from the midsternal line and either on the midclavicular line or just medial to it (Fig. 13.1). Although the pulsation of the left ventricle can always be felt on palpation, it cannot be observed under normal circumstances: it is only when there is a pathological state of the heart that the beat becomes visible on observation. Tangential lighting helps to detect an abnormal pulsation.

The pulsation of Xu Li

The heartbeat of the left ventricle, which can be felt in the fifth intercostal space, was called *Xu Li* in ancient Chinese medicine, which is another name for the Great Connecting channel of the Stomach. This channel cuts through the diaphragm and the lungs and exits below the left breast producing the heartbeat. It is also said to be the area where the Gathering Qi (*Zong Qi*) converges.

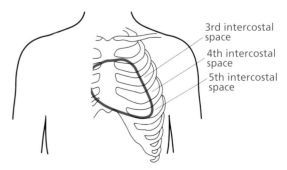

3rd intercostal space
4th intercostal space
5th intercostal space

Fig. 13.1 Location of the apical beat

The Gathering Qi itself is said to govern the heart and lung channels.

The *Xu Li* is described in Chapter 18 of the 'Simple Questions', which says: *'The Great Connecting channel of the Stomach is called Xu Li. It cuts through the diaphragm and connects with the lungs, it exits below the left breast and its beat is the beating of the Gathering Qi.'*[1] It is interesting therefore that, although the pulsation in the fifth intercostal space is obviously the pulsation of the left ventricle, in Chinese medicine it is also related to the Stomach and for this reason the Stomach channel has an important influence on the heart (both in a Chinese and a Western sense) and especially the heart rhythm. Besides the Stomach, the apical beat is also related to the Lungs, as it reflects the 'beating' of the Gathering Qi.

As mentioned above, if the heartbeat in the fifth intercostal space can be observed, it indicates an abnormal state of the heart by definition.

A more detailed description of the symptoms and signs related to each pattern will be given in Part 5, Chapter 63.

HEARTBEAT DISPLACED DOWNWARDS

Symptoms and Signs, Chapter 63

When displaced downwards, the heartbeat can be observed in the sixth intercostal space. From the Western medical point of view, this may be caused by hypertension, congenital heart disease, myocarditis or enlargement of the heart in heart failure.

From a Chinese perspective, the most likely patterns to appear in the above heart conditions are Qi deficiency with Blood stasis, Liver- and Kidney-Yin deficiency (especially in the elderly), Phlegm-Fluids obstructing the Heart or Toxic Heat invading the Heart.

HEARTBEAT DISPLACED UPWARDS

Symptoms and Signs, Chapter 63

When the heartbeat is displaced upwards, it can be observed in either the fourth or the third intercostal space. From the Western medical point of view this may be caused by hypertension, ascites, enlargement of the right heart or a tumour in the abdominal cavity.

From a Chinese medical perspective the most likely patterns to appear in the above conditions are Yang

deficiency with Water overflowing or Liver-Blood stasis with Water overflowing.

HEARTBEAT DISPLACED TO THE LEFT

Symptoms and Signs, Chapter 63

When the heartbeat is displaced to the left, it can be seen lateral to the midaxillary line. From a Western medical point of view, that may occur in pleuritis of the right side of the chest or in congestive cardiac failure.

From the Chinese medical point of view, the most likely patterns to appear in this condition are Phlegm-Fluids in the chest and hypochondrium, or Phlegm-Heat in the Lungs.

HEARTBEAT DISPLACED TO THE RIGHT

Symptoms and Signs, Chapter 63

When the heartbeat is displaced to the right, it can be observed medial to the midaxillary line. From a Western medical point of view, this may be due to a congenital heart condition or pleuritis of the left side of the chest.

From a Chinese medical point of view, the most likely patterns to appear in this condition are Qi deficiency with Blood stasis and Phlegm-Fluids in the chest and hypochondrium.

HEARTBEAT BELOW THE XYPHOID PROCESS

Symptoms and Signs, Chapter 63

From the Western medical point of view, a heartbeat below the xyphoid process may be observed in defects of the tricuspid valve, right heart disease, emphysema or enlargement of the right heart.

From the Chinese medical point of view, the most likely patterns to appear in these conditions are Heart-Blood stasis or Heart-Qi deficiency.

NOTES

1. 1979 The Yellow Emperor's Classic of Internal Medicine – Simple Questions (*Huang Di Nei Jing Su Wen* 黄帝内经素问), People's Health Publishing House, Beijing, p. 111. First published c. 100BC.

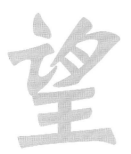

Chapter **14**

OBSERVATION OF THE HANDS

Chapter contents

INTRODUCTION   *129*

ABNORMAL COLOUR   *129*
  Pale hands   *129*
  Red dorsum of the hands   *129*
  Red palms   *129*

VENULES ON THE THENAR EMINENCE   *130*

ATROPHY OF THE THENAR EMINENCE   *130*

ATROPHY OF THE MUSCLES OF THE DORSUM OF THE
HANDS   *130*

TREMOR OF THE HANDS   **130**

TINEA (RINGWORM)   **130**

THE FINGERS   *130*
  Contraction of the fingers   *130*
  Spoon-shaped fingers   *131*
  Thin, pointed fingers   *131*
  Swollen fingers   *131*
  Cracked fingers   *132*
  Thickened fingers like cocoons   *132*
  Shrivelled and wrinkled fingers   *132*

DEFORMED KNUCKLES   *132*

THE PALMS   *132*
  Dry, cracked, peeling palms   *132*
  Sweaty palms   *133*
  Hand lines   *133*

INTRODUCTION

Observation of the hands has always formed a relatively important aspect of diagnosis and it is mentioned in several chapters of the 'Simple Questions' and 'Spiritual Axis' as well as in the 'Discussion of Origin of Symptoms in Diseases' (*Zhu Bing Yuan Huo Lun*, AD610 by Chao Yuan Fang).[1] The description of index finger diagnosis in children was discussed by the Tang dynasty doctor Wang Chao in the book 'Illustrated Formula of the Water Mirror' (*Shui Jing Tu Jue*).[2]

A more detailed description of the hand signs and symptoms described below can be found in Part 5, Chapter 65.

ABNORMAL COLOUR

Pale hands

Symptoms and Signs, Chapter 65

Pale hands are usually due to either Yang deficiency or Blood deficiency. Heart-Yang or Lung-Yang deficiency in particular may cause the hands to be pale. As for Blood deficiency, pale hands are usually caused by Heart-Blood or Liver-Blood deficiency.

Red dorsum of the hands

Symptoms and Signs, Chapter 65

Red dorsum of the hands is generally due to Full-Heat, in particular of the Heart, Lungs or Stomach.

Red palms

Symptoms and Signs, Chapter 65

Red palms are generally due to Empty-Heat, in particular of the Heart, Lungs or Stomach.

VENULES ON THE THENAR EMINENCE

Symptoms and Signs, Chapter 65

The thenar eminence shows the state of the Stomach. Chapter 10 of the 'Spiritual Axis' relates the colour of the thenar eminence to the state of the Stomach and says: *'When the Stomach has Cold, the thenar eminence is bluish; when the Stomach has Heat, the thenar eminence is reddish; if it is suddenly black, it indicates chronic Painful Obstruction Syndrome; if it is sometimes red, sometimes dark and sometimes bluish it indicates alternation of Heat and Cold; if it is bluish and short, it indicates deficiency of Qi.'*[3] Chapter 74 of the same book says: *'When the thenar eminence has bluish venules, it indicates Cold in the Stomach.'*[4]

Bluish or bluish-purple venules on the thenar eminence generally indicate Cold in the Stomach; if they are bluish but short they indicate deficiency of Qi or Empty-Cold from Stomach-Yang deficiency. Reddish venules indicate either Full-Heat or Empty-Heat (usually of the Stomach and/or Lungs), if they are reddish-purple they may indicate Blood stasis in the Stomach; and if yellowish-red, there is Damp-Heat in the Stomach.

ATROPHY OF THE THENAR EMINENCE

Symptoms and Signs, Chapter 65

The size and consistency of the thenar eminence are related to the state of the Stomach. When the thenar eminence is full, the state of the Stomach is good.

Atrophy of the thenar eminence may be due to deficiency of Yang of the Stomach, Spleen and Kidneys, or deficiency of Yin of the Stomach, Liver and Kidneys.

ATROPHY OF THE MUSCLES OF THE DORSUM OF THE HANDS

Symptoms and Signs, Chapter 65

Atrophy of the muscles of the dorsum may be due to deficiency of Liver-Blood, deficiency of Kidney-Yin or deficiency of Qi of the Stomach and Spleen.

TREMOR OF THE HANDS

Symptoms and Signs, Chapter 65

Tremor of the hands is a sign of internal Wind, which may be of the Full or Empty type. Internal Wind is always related to the Liver, and Liver-Wind or Wind-Phlegm in the Liver are the most frequent cause of tremor of the hands. Empty-Wind of the Liver causes a fine tremor of the hands; it may derive from Blood or Yin deficiency. Internal Wind, which may develop suddenly following a deep shock or a great fright, may also cause tremor of the hands.

In alcoholics, a fine tremor of the hands is caused by Phlegm-Heat. In rare cases, retention of Dampness in the muscles and sinews of the hands may also cause a fine tremor.

Box 14.1 summarizes patterns underlying hand tremor.

BOX 14.1 TREMOR OF THE HANDS

- Hand tremor: Full- or Empty-Wind, most commonly Liver-Wind or Wind-Phlegm in the Liver
- Fine tremor: Empty Liver-Wind from Blood or Yin deficiency, retention of Dampness in the muscles and sinews of the hands
- Tremor following shock or fright: internal Wind
- Fine tremor in alcoholics: Phlegm-Heat

TINEA (RINGWORM)

Observation, Chapter 21; Symptoms and Signs, Chapters 65 and 77

Tinea, a fungal infection of the skin, is characterized by disc-like skin lesions with sharply defined, raised borders which expand peripherally and clear centrally. There may be red scaling with itching as well as vesicles. Continuous scratching may result in lichenification (thickening and hardening of the skin). In Chinese medicine, tinea of the hands is due to an external invasion of Wind-Heat or Damp-Heat.

When tinea affects the nails, in Chinese medicine it is called Goose Claw Wind.

THE FINGERS

Contraction of the fingers

Symptoms and Signs, Chapter 65

Contraction of the fingers with normal movement of the wrist joint and all the joints above it is called Chicken Claw Wind. The most common cause of this contraction of the fingers is Liver-Blood or Liver-Yin deficiency; the Dupuytren contraction of the ring or little finger is a typical example of it (Fig. 14.1).

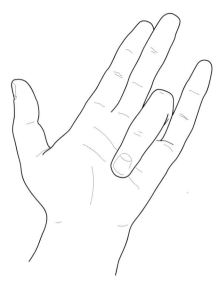

Fig. 14.1 Contraction of the ring finger

Two other causes of contraction of the fingers are Cold in the joints or stagnation of Qi from emotional problems; in the latter case the contraction of the fingers comes and goes according to the emotional state.

BOX 14.2 CONTRACTION OF THE FINGERS

- Liver-Blood or Liver-Yin deficiency (e.g. Dupuytren contraction)
- Cold in the joints
- Contraction that comes and goes according to the emotional state: stagnation of Qi from emotional problems

---

Box 14.2 summarizes patterns underlying contraction of the fingers.

Spoon-shaped fingers

Symptoms and Signs, Chapter 65

Spoon-shaped fingers (Fig. 14.2) usually indicate a Lung pathology, which may be Cold-Phlegm in the Lungs, Phlegm-Heat in the Lungs, or Lung and Kidney-Yin deficiency. They are usually seen only in patients suffering from chronic lung diseases such as emphysema, tuberculosis (TB) of the lungs, or chronic obstructive pulmonary disease. In some cases, spoon-shaped fingers may also indicate a Heart pathology.

Thin, pointed fingers

Symptoms and Signs, Chapter 65

Thin, pointed fingers are generally related to the state of the Stomach (Fig. 14.3) and may indicate Cold-Dampness in the Stomach, Damp-Heat in the Stomach or severe deficiency of Stomach- and Spleen-Qi.

Swollen fingers

Symptoms and Signs, Chapter 65

The most obvious and common cause of swelling of the fingers is Painful Obstruction Syndrome from Dampness, which may be Cold-Dampness, Wind-Dampness or Damp-Heat. Other causes of swelling of the fingers include Blood stasis (of the Heart or Liver)

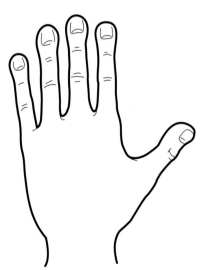

Fig. 14.2 Spoon-shaped fingers

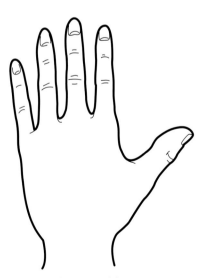

Fig. 14.3 Thin, pointed fingers

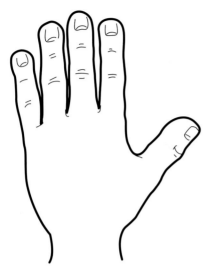

Fig. 14.4 Swollen fingers

or oedema, which, in the case of the hands, is due to deficiency of Yang of the Lungs and Spleen. In the elderly, swollen fingers may also be due to Liver- and Kidney-Yin deficiency with Blood-Heat (Fig. 14.4).

Box 14.3 summarizes patterns underlying swollen fingers.

BOX 14.3 SWOLLEN FINGERS

- Painful Obstruction Syndrome (Cold-Dampness, Wind-Dampness or Damp-Heat)
- Heart- or Liver-Blood stasis, oedema from Lung- and Spleen-Yang deficiency
- Blood stasis (of the Heart or Liver), oedema of the hands due to deficiency of Yang of the Lungs and Spleen in the elderly

---

Cracked fingers

Symptoms and Signs, Chapter 65

Cracked fingers are generally due to Blood deficiency or to Blood stasis. In some cases cracked fingers may also be due to Yang deficiency with Empty-Cold.

Thickened fingers like cocoons

Symptoms and Signs, Chapter 65

Thickening of the fingers so that they look like cocoons is due to general deficiency of Qi and Blood.

Shrivelled and wrinkled fingers

Symptoms and Signs, Chapter 65

Shrivelled and wrinkled fingers indicate a severe loss of fluids such as that which occurs after profuse sweating, vomiting, or diarrhoea.

DEFORMED KNUCKLES

Symptoms and Signs, Chapter 65

Deformed knuckles are seen in the late, chronic stages of Painful Obstruction Syndrome with Phlegm. In chronic Painful Obstruction Syndrome, there is a severe disruption of the transformation and movement of the fluids in the joints which, under the 'steaming' action of Heat, creates Phlegm in the joints. Thus, Phlegm is the central pathogenic factor causing deformed knuckles; it may be combined with other conditions such as Heat, Cold, Blood stasis or Qi or Yin deficiency, or both (Fig. 14.5).

THE PALMS

Dry, cracked, peeling palms

Symptoms and Signs, Chapter 65

Dry, cracked and peeling palms are generally due to Blood deficiency (of the Liver or Heart, or both); if the dryness is very pronounced and the hands are also itchy, it indicates Wind in the skin.

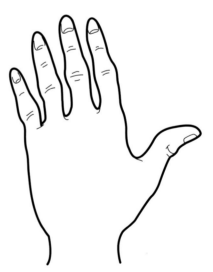

Fig. 14.5 Deformed knuckles

Sweaty palms

Symptoms and Signs, Chapter 65

Sweating of the palms is related primarily to the Heart and Lung channels and may be due to either deficiency of Qi or Yin or to Heat in one of these two organs.

Hand lines

Changes in the lines of the palms of the hands can indicate certain pathologies.

Description of the lines

The main hand lines to be observed are illustrated in Figure 14.6. The lines are the life line, the head line, the emotions line, the health line and the so-called Jade Pillar. Figure 14.7 illustrates the normal lengths of the emotions line and life line.

Description of abnormal signs on the lines

The abnormal signs appearing on the lines may be shaped like stars, crosses, triangles, ovals, squares, hashes, links of a chain or rope (Fig. 14.8).

Diseases indicated on the lines

The diseases indicated on the lines are as follows:

Diseases of the digestive system

In ulcerative colitis, there is a star-shaped sign on the distal or proximal end of the life line (Fig. 14.9).

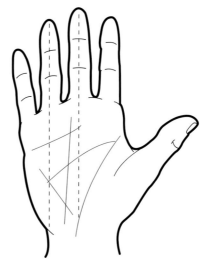

Fig. 14.7 Normal length of emotions and life lines

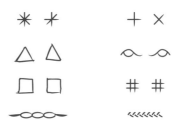

Fig. 14.8 Abnormal signs on the lines

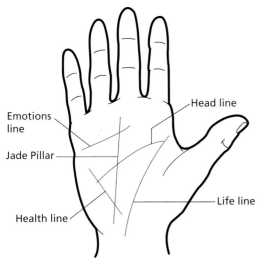

Fig. 14.6 Main hand lines

Emotions line
Jade Pillar
Health line
Head line
Life line

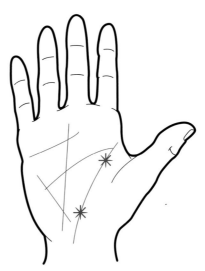

Fig. 14.9 Signs on the life line showing diseases of the digestive system

In gastritis, there is a star-shaped sign on the proximal end of the life line (Fig. 14.9).

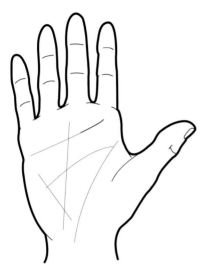

Fig. 14.10 Lines showing hypertension

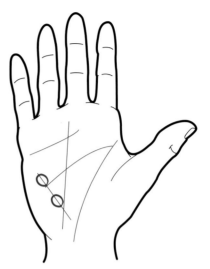

Fig. 14.12 Signs on the health line in asthma

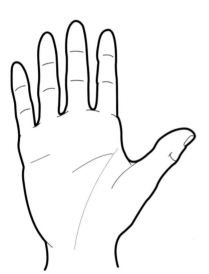

Fig. 14.11 Lines showing coronary heart disease

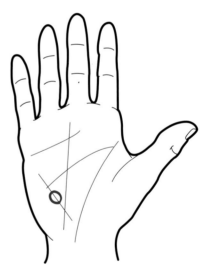

Fig. 14.13 Signs on the health line in TB of the lungs

Circulatory diseases

In hypertension, the emotions line extends radially beyond its natural boundary (Fig. 14.10).

In coronary heart disease; both the emotions line and the head line are shorter than normal (Fig. 14.11).

Respiratory diseases

In asthma, there are oval-shaped signs at either end of the health line (Fig. 14.12).

In TB of the lungs, there are oval-shaped signs in the middle of the health line (Fig. 14.13).

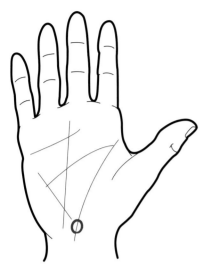

Fig. 14.14 Signs on the life line in urinary diseases

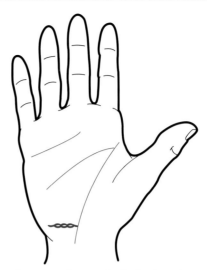

Fig. 14.16 Signs on the life line in male sexual dysfunctions

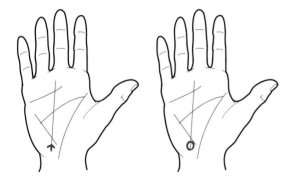

Fig. 14.15 Signs on the Jade Pillar line in gynaecological diseases

Diseases of the urinary system

In nephritis, urinary infections, prostatitis, or prostatic hypertrophy, there is an oval-shaped sign at the proximal end of the life line (Fig. 14.14).

Diseases of the reproductive system

In endometriosis, salpingitis, myomas, or ovarian cysts, there is an arrow-shaped or oval sign at the proximal end of the Jade Pillar (Fig. 14.15).

In erectile dysfunction or impotence, there are horizontal chain links near the proximal end of the life line (Fig. 14.16).

(a)

(b)

(c)

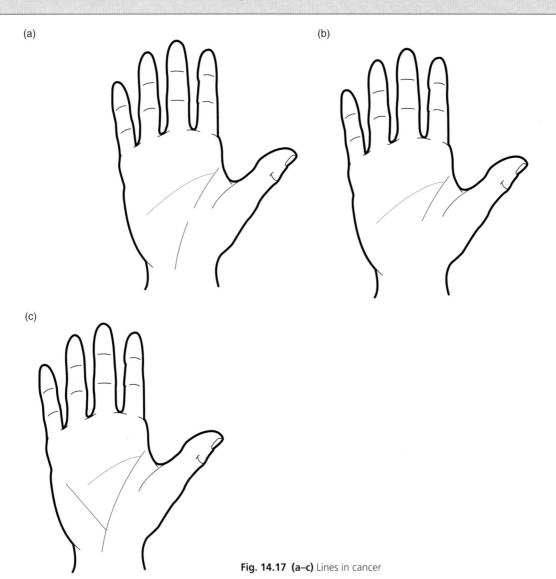

Fig. 14.17 (a–c) Lines in cancer

Cancer

Here the life line is broken, is short, or merges with the health line (Figs. 14.17a–c).

NOTES

1. Zhang Shu Sheng 1995 Great Treatise of Diagnosis by Observation in Chinese Medicine (*Zhong Hua Yi Xue Wang Zhen Da Quan* 中华医学望诊大全), Shanxi Science Publishing House, Taiyuan.
2. Ibid.
3. 1981 Spiritual Axis (*Ling Shu Jing* 灵枢经), People's Health Publishing House, Beijing, p. 129, para 37. First published c. 100BC.
4. Ibid., p. 133.

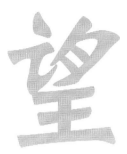

Chapter **15**

OBSERVATION OF THE NAILS

Chapter contents

INTRODUCTION   *137*

SURFACE ABNORMALITIES   *137*
  Ridged nails   *137*
  Indented nails   *137*
  Thin and brittle nails   *138*
  Thickening of the nails   *138*
  Coarse and thick nails   *138*
  Withered and brittle nails   *138*
  Withered and thickened nails   *138*
  Cracked nails   *138*
  Flaking nails   *138*

TWISTED NAILS   *139*

CURLING NAILS   *139*

NAILS FALLING OFF   *139*

ABNORMAL COLOUR   *139*
  Nails with white spots   *139*
  Pale-white nails   *139*
  Dull-white nails   *139*
  Red nails   *139*
  Yellow nails   *139*
  Bluish-greenish nails   *139*
  Dark nails   *139*
  Purple nails   *139*

LUNULAE   *140*

CORRESPONDENCE OF NAILS TO ORGAN SYSTEMS   *140*
  Thumb   *140*
  Index finger   *140*
  Middle finger   *141*
  Ring finger   *141*
  Little finger   *142*

INTRODUCTION

The nails are influenced by the Liver (particularly Liver-Blood) and they are considered to be the accumulation of the 'excess' of the sinews. Normal nails should be smooth, slightly bulging, slightly convex, relatively thick and bright. Such nails indicate a good state of the Liver and particularly Liver-Blood.

When observing nails, one should pay attention to their texture and colour. For example, brittle or ridged nails indicate a deficiency of Liver-Blood.

A more detailed description of the nail signs described below can be found in Part 5, Chapter 65.

SURFACE ABNORMALITIES

Ridged nails

Symptoms and Signs, Chapter 65

Longitudinal ridges in the nails are generally due to Liver-Blood deficiency or Liver-Yin deficiency.

Indented nails

Symptoms and Signs, Chapter 65

Nails take about 150–180 days to grow and horizontal indentations may appear in the course of a serious disease. From the location of a horizontal indentation, we can therefore gauge roughly the time of onset of the disease. Figure 15.1 illustrates two nails in section with two indentations corresponding to two different times of onset of a disease, one roughly 120 days, the other approximately 30 days.

Apart from indicating the onset of a disease, in general terms indentations of the nails may be due to deficiency and dryness of Liver-Blood, general deficiency of Qi and Blood, or Heat injuring fluids.

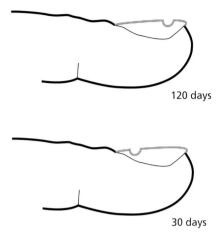

Fig. 15.1 Nail indentations showing disease onset at approximately 120 and 30 days

Moreover, small indentations of the nails are also seen in chronic skin diseases such as eczema and psoriasis, in which case the clinical significance is different, simply indicating chronic Liver-Blood deficiency.

Thin and brittle nails

Symptoms and Signs, Chapter 65

Thin and brittle nails generally indicate Qi and Blood deficiency, and particularly Liver-Blood deficiency. In severe cases, they may also indicate a deficiency of Kidney-Essence.

Thickening of the nails

Symptoms and Signs, Chapter 65

Thickening of the nails may be due to Liver-Fire, Liver-Blood stasis, or Phlegm.

Coarse and thick nails

Symptoms and Signs, Chapter 65

Coarse and thick nails generally indicate Qi and Blood deficiency with Blood-Dryness generating Wind, which often happens in chronic psoriasis. In some cases, coarse and thick nails may indicate accumulation of Dampness.

Withered and brittle nails

Symptoms and Signs, Chapter 65

Withered and brittle nails are generally due to a deficiency of Liver-Blood or Liver-Yin. In some cases, they may also be due to Liver-Blood stasis, in which case the withering of the nails is caused not by a lack of nourishment of Liver-Blood but by stagnant Liver-Blood being unable to reach the nails.

In some cases, Liver-Fire may cause the nails to become withered and brittle. If this occurs and the nails look scaly, it indicates a severe Kidney deficiency.

Withered and brittle nails in some cases may be due to Phlegm in the joints and this is seen in cases of chronic Painful Obstruction Syndrome with Phlegm, in patients suffering from rheumatoid arthritis. The withering of the nails observed in psoriasis is usually due to either deficiency and Dryness of Liver-Blood or stasis of Liver-Blood.

In acute cases, withered nails may appear in the aftermath of a febrile disease resulting in Blood- and Yin-deficiency with Blood-Dryness and Empty-Heat.

Withered and thickened nails

Symptoms and Signs, Chapter 65

Withered and thickened nails are dry, brittle, thicker than normal, irregular, greyish and lacking lustre. This type of nail is generally due to a severe deficiency of Stomach and Spleen, a deficiency and Dryness of Liver-Blood and Liver-Yin, or a combination of Damp-Heat with Toxic Heat.

Cracked nails

Symptoms and Signs, Chapter 65

Cracked nails indicate either a general deficiency of Qi and Blood or a deficiency and Dryness of Liver-Blood. In some cases, cracked nails may be caused by Full conditions and especially by Liver-Fire. In the elderly, cracked nails may also be due to Yin deficiency.

Flaking nails

Symptoms and Signs, Chapter 65

Scaly, flaky nails indicate a Kidney and Spleen deficiency with retention of Dampness.

Box 15.1 summarizes patterns underlying nail surface abnormalities.

BOX 15.1 NAIL SURFACE ABNORMALITIES

- Ridged nails: Liver-Blood or Liver-Yin deficiency
- Indented nails: Deficiency and Dryness of Liver-Blood, Qi and Blood deficiency, Heat injuring Body Fluids
- Thin and brittle nails: deficiency of Liver-Blood, Qi and Blood, or Kidney-Essence
- Thickening of the nails: Liver-Fire, Liver-Blood stasis, Phlegm
- Coarse and thick nails: Qi and Blood deficiency, Blood-Dryness generating Wind, Dampness
- Withered and brittle nails: deficiency of Liver-Blood or Liver-Yin, Liver-Blood stasis, Liver-Fire, Kidney deficiency, Phlegm, aftermath of febrile disease with Blood-Dryness and Empty-Heat
- Withered and thickened nails: Stomach and Spleen or Liver-Yin deficiency, Liver-Blood deficiency and Dryness, Damp-Heat with Toxic Heat
- Cracked nails: Liver-Blood deficiency and Dryness, Qi and Blood deficiency, Liver-Fire, Liver- and Kidney-Yin deficiency

TWISTED NAILS

Symptoms and Signs, Chapter 65

Twisted nails are due to a deficiency of Liver-Blood.

CURLING NAILS

Symptoms and Signs, Chapter 65

Nails may curl either down or up, like hooks, and the curling always indicates a chronic condition with Qi and Blood deficiency combined with Blood stasis.

NAILS FALLING OFF

Symptoms and Signs, Chapter 65

If the nails become swollen, hot and painful, then produce pus and later fall off, this indicates Toxic Heat, usually affecting the Liver.

ABNORMAL COLOUR

Nails with white spots

Symptoms and Signs, Chapter 65

Nails with white spots indicate Qi deficiency.

Pale-white nails

Symptoms and Signs, Chapter 65

Pale-white nails are generally due to Blood deficiency of the Liver and Spleen.

Dull-white nails

Symptoms and Signs, Chapter 65

Dull-white nails are generally due to Spleen- and Kidney-Yang deficiency, or to a sudden loss of Body Fluids such as happens in profuse vomiting, diarrhoea or sweating.

Red nails

Symptoms and Signs, Chapter 65

Red nails are simply due to Heat, and generally to Full-Heat, which may be related to any organ.

Yellow nails

Symptoms and Signs, Chapter 65

Yellow nails indicate Damp-Heat, which may be affecting the Stomach and Spleen or Liver and Gall-Bladder. If the colour is fresh yellow, it is a favourable sign: either the Damp-Heat is not serious or it is receding. If it is a dull and dark yellow, the Damp-Heat is serious or is advancing.

Bluish-greenish nails

Symptoms and Signs, Chapter 65

Bluish nails indicate Blood deficiency with internal Cold, while greenish nails (generally seen only in children's diseases) indicate severe Spleen-Qi deficiency with internal Wind. Bluish-greenish nails may also be due to Blood stasis.

Dark nails

Symptoms and Signs, Chapter 65

Dark nails generally indicate either a Kidney deficiency, which may be of Yin or Yang, or Blood stasis.

Purple nails

Symptoms and Signs, Chapter 65

Purple nails generally indicate Blood stasis of the Liver. If the nails are reddish-purple in febrile diseases this indicates Heat at the Blood level.

Box 15.2 summarizes patterns underlying abnormal nail colour.

BOX 15.2 NAIL COLOURS

- White spots: Qi deficiency
- Pale white: Blood deficiency of the Liver and Spleen
- Dull white: Spleen- and Kidney-Yang deficiency, sudden loss of Body Fluids
- Red: Heat, generally Full-Heat
- Yellow: Damp-Heat of Stomach and Spleen or Liver and Gall-Bladder
- Bluish: Blood deficiency with internal Cold
- Greenish: severe Spleen-Qi deficiency with internal Wind (generally only in children)
- Bluish-greenish: Blood stasis
- Dark: Kidney-Yin or -Yang deficiency, Blood stasis
- Purple: Liver-Blood stasis
- Reddish-purple in febrile disease: Heat at the Blood level

LUNULAE

Symptoms and Signs, Chapter 65

The lunulae are the white 'crescents' visible at the base of the nails. Generally speaking, their visible presence on the thumb and fingers indicates good health; according to some doctors, the little finger does not normally have a lunula.

Generally speaking, the nail bed (being red) reflects the state of Yang-Qi, while the lunula, being white, reflects the state of Yin and Essence. In men, the lunula of the thumb should be roughly 3 mm wide, decreasing proportionately on the index, middle and ring

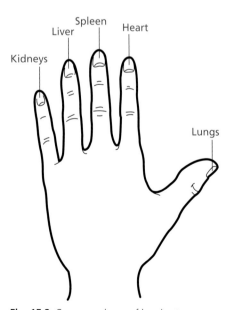

Fig. 15.2 Correspondence of lunulae to organs

fingers and usually not showing at all on the little finger. In women, the lunulae are generally smaller than in men.

The less the lunulae are visible, the poorer is the health of the individual. Conversely, excessively large lunulae indicate a tendency to excess of Yang and deficiency of Yin. If the lunulae dwindle and disappear from sight, this indicates internal Cold or Yang deficiency.

The lunula of the thumb corresponds to the Lungs, that of the index finger to the Heart, that of the middle finger to the Spleen, that of the ring finger to the Liver and that of the little finger to the Kidneys (if it shows at all) (Fig. 15.2). The lunula of a particular finger shows a Full condition of its relevant organ if it is too large or an Empty condition if it is too small.

CORRESPONDENCE OF NAILS TO ORGAN SYSTEMS

The nails of individual fingers correspond to the state of various organs, with a correspondence that is not always related to the channel of that particular finger.

Thumb

The thumbnail reflects diseases of the head, including brain, eyes, ears, nose, throat and mouth. Figure 15.3 shows the areas of the thumbnail that correspond to the above.

Index finger

The nail of the index finger reflects diseases of the Upper and Middle Burners, including oesophagus,

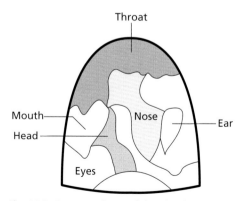

Fig. 15.3 Correspondence of thumbnail areas to organs

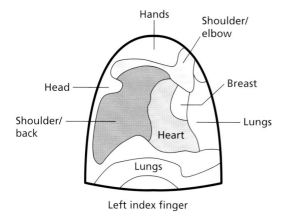

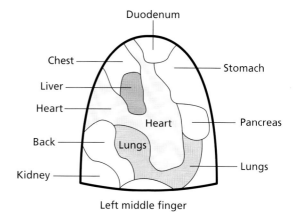

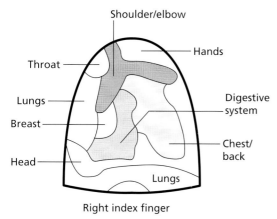

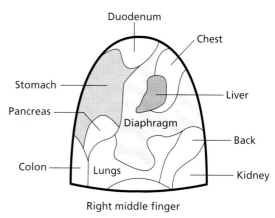

Fig. 15.4 Correspondence of the nail of the index finger to organs

Fig. 15.5 Correspondence of the nail of the middle finger to organs

chest, breast, lungs, heart, upper back, shoulder and throat, and also of the head, shoulder, back, elbow and hands. The areas vary between the right and left index finger and these are illustrated in Figure 15.4.

Middle finger

The nail of the middle finger reflects diseases of the Middle and Lower Burners. The nail of the right index finger reflects diseases of the stomach, duodenum, diaphragm, liver, pancreas, kidneys and colon, also the back and lungs. The nail of the left index finger reflects diseases of the same organs but also includes the heart (Fig. 15.5).

Ring finger

The nail of the ring finger also reflects diseases of the Middle and Lower Burners. That on the right hand reflects disease of the liver, gall-bladder, pancreas, kidneys, small intestine, large intestine, bladder and reproductive system, and also the knee. That on the left hand reflects diseases of the spleen, pancreas, uterus, urinary passages, fallopian tubes, external genitalia and anus, as well as the kidneys, liver, small intestine, large intestine, back and knee (Fig. 15.6).

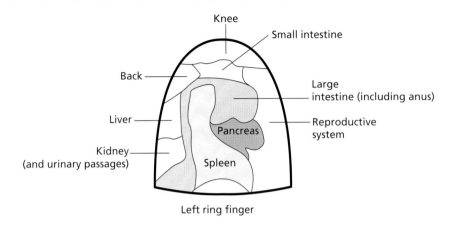

Left ring finger

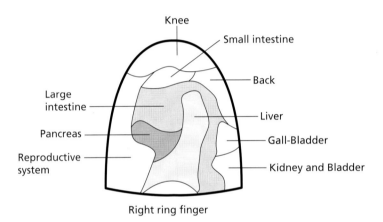

Right ring finger

Fig. 15.6 Correspondence of the nail of the ring finger to organs

Little finger

The nail of the little finger reflects diseases of the ankle, feet and metatarsal bones (Fig. 15.7).

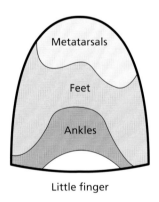

Little finger

Fig. 15.7 Correspondence of the nail of the little finger to the parts of the body

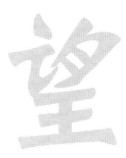

Chapter 16

OBSERVATION OF THE CHEST AND ABDOMEN

Chapter contents

CHEST   *143*
  Protruding chest   *144*
  Sunken chest   *144*
  Protruding sternum   *144*
  Chest sunken on one side   *144*
  Chest protruding on one side   *145*
  Gynaecomastia   *145*

ABDOMEN   *145*
  Abdominal size   *146*
  Abdominal masses   *146*
  Umbilicus signs   *147*
  Skin signs   *147*

CHEST

The front of the chest is influenced by the Lung and Heart channel and by the Directing and Penetrating Vessels; the sides of the chest are influenced by the Gall-Bladder and Liver channels (Fig. 16.1).

For a more detailed description of the patterns causing chest signs, see Part 5, Chapter 63.

Box 16.1 summarizes the channels influencing the chest.

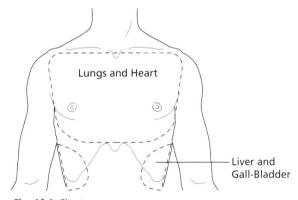

Lungs and Heart

Liver and Gall-Bladder

Fig. 16.1 Chest areas

BOX 16.1 CHANNELS INFLUENCING THE CHEST

- Lungs
- Heart
- Directing Vessel
- Penetrating Vessel
- Gall-Bladder (sides of chest)
- Liver (sides of chest)

Protruding chest

Symptoms and Signs, Chapter 63

The most common cause of a protruding chest (Fig. 16.2) is chronic retention of Phlegm in the Lungs. Other causes include severe, chronic Liver-Qi stagnation or Blood stasis in the chest.

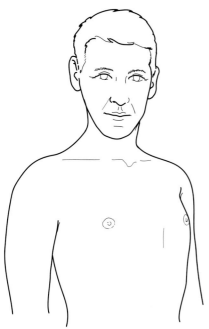

Fig. 16.2 Protruding chest

Sunken chest

Symptoms and Signs, Chapter 63

The most common cause of a sunken chest (Fig. 16.3) is a deficiency of Qi or Yin of the Lungs. A Kidney deficiency may also cause a sunken chest.

Protruding sternum

Symptoms and Signs, Chapter 63

The protruding sternum (Fig. 16.4) is either hereditary, in which case it is due to a constitutional deficiency of the Lungs and Kidneys, or it is caused by retention of Phlegm in the Lungs.

Chest sunken on one side

Symptoms and Signs, Chapter 63

The chest can become sunken on one side (Fig. 16.5) either because of a deficiency of the Lungs, specifically affecting one lung, or because of retention of Phlegm-Fluids, often with Blood stasis.

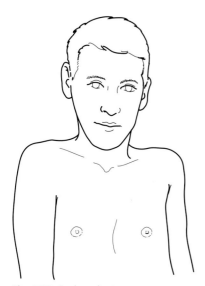

Fig. 16.3 Sunken chest

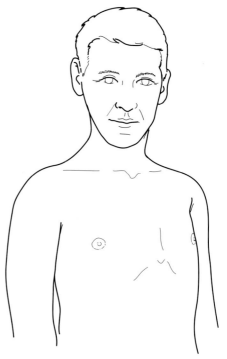

Fig. 16.4 Protruding sternum

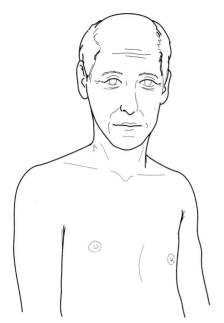

Fig. 16.5 Chest sunken on one side

Chest protruding on one side

Symptoms and Signs, Chapter 63

The chest can become protruding on one side (Fig. 16.6) from Phlegm-Fluids in the Lungs, severe Liver-Qi stagnation or Heart-Qi deficiency with Blood stasis.

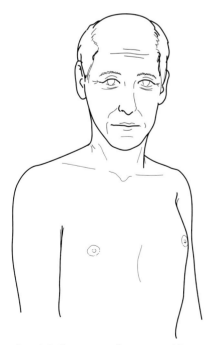

Fig. 16.6 Chest protruding on one side

Gynaecomastia

Symptoms and Signs, Chapter 63

Gynaecomastia indicates a swelling of the breast in males. It may be due to either Liver-Blood stasis or Damp-Heat in the Penetrating Vessel.

ABDOMEN

The regions of the abdomen in Chinese medicine are shown in Figure 16.7.

The area under the heart is the small area immediately below the xyphoid process extending approximately 2 inches (5 cm) and bordered by the ribs. It is influenced both by the Heart and the Stomach channels and by the Penetrating Vessel.

The epigastrium is the area between the xyphoid process and the umbilicus but excluding the hypochondrial area. It is related to the Stomach and Spleen channels.

The hypochondrium includes the two areas below the rib cage and its edges which are influenced by the Liver and Gall-Bladder channels.

The area around the umbilicus is influenced by the Spleen, Liver, Kidney and Small Intestine channels.

The central-lower abdominal area (*Xiao Fu*) is between the umbilicus and the symphysis pubis. This area is influenced by the Liver, Kidney, Bladder and Large Intestine channels and by the Directing Vessel; in women, it is also influenced by the Uterus.

The lateral-lower abdominal areas (*Shao Fu*) are influenced by the Liver and Large Intestine channels, and by the Penetrating Vessel.

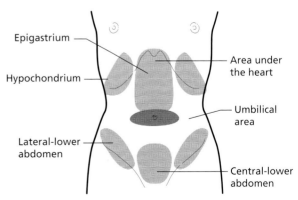

Fig. 16.7 Abdominal areas

Observation of the abdomen is an important part of observation in the clinic and one that should always be carried out in conjunction with palpation of the abdomen. In particular, observation of the abdomen is important because the epigastrium reflects the state of Stomach and Spleen (the Root of Postnatal Qi) and the lower abdomen that of the Kidneys (the Root of Prenatal Qi).

For a more detailed discussion of the patterns involved in abdominal signs, see Part 5 Symptoms and Signs, Chapter 71.

Abdominal size
Abdominal distension
Interrogation, Chapter 38; Symptoms and Signs, Chapter 71

Abdominal distension is both a symptom and a sign, that is, it is a subjective feeling of bloating but also an objective, distended feeling of the abdomen like a drum on palpation. The distended abdomen looks swollen and on palpation it is hard but relatively elastic, like an inflated balloon. In severe cases, the whole abdomen can be distended like a ball or a frog's belly. By far the most common cause of abdominal distension is Qi stagnation, which is usually related to the Liver, Spleen or the Intestines. Liver-Qi stagnation is the most common cause of abdominal distension, which may involve both the epigastrium and the lower abdomen. Stagnation of Qi in the Intestines will also cause abdominal distension and in this case there will be other symptoms such as loose stools or constipation. Spleen-Qi deficiency may cause slight abdominal distension.

In severe cases, when the whole abdomen may look like a ball or a frog's belly, this may be due to Damp-Phlegm in the Lower Burner or oedema of the abdomen.

Box 16.2 summarizes the patterns underlying abdominal distension.

BOX 16.2 ABDOMINAL DISTENSION

- Distension of epigastrium and the lower abdomen: Liver-Qi stagnation
- Distension with loose stools or constipation: Qi stagnation in Intestines
- Slight distension: Spleen-Qi deficiency
- Severe distension: Damp-Phlegm in the Lower Burner, oedema of the abdomen

---

Large abdomen
Symptoms and Signs, Chapter 71

A large, fat abdomen indicates Phlegm occurring against a background of Spleen deficiency. Again, allowance should be made for the Elemental type body structure: for example, a large abdomen is relatively normal in an Earth type but not in a Metal type.

Oedema of the abdomen
Symptoms and Signs, Chapter 71

Oedema of the abdomen is always due to a deficiency of Yang, which may be of the Spleen or of the Kidneys, in which case the ankles will be swollen as well.

Sagging lower abdomen
Symptoms and Signs, Chapter 71

The sagging abdomen is usually seen in obese people; it is swollen but soft and hangs down. If not due to obesity, the sagging abdomen is usually seen only in the elderly and it may be due to Damp-Phlegm in the lower abdomen or to a severe deficiency of Spleen- and Kidney-Yang associated with Damp-Phlegm. A sagging abdomen always involves a deficiency of the Directing and Penetrating Vessels and a slackening of the Membranes (*Huang*) and the Ancestral Muscles (*Zong Jin*), which are controlled by the Penetrating Vessel.

Thin abdomen
Symptoms and Signs, Chapter 71

A thin and emaciated abdomen may indicate a severe deficiency of Qi and Blood, which is often seen in serious diseases such as cancer; however, it may also simply indicate the condition of Yin deficiency. When observing the abdomen, allowance should be made for the Elemental type body structure; for example, a thin abdomen is relatively normal in a Metal type but not in an Earth type.

Abdominal masses
Symptoms and Signs, Chapters 71 and 89

Abdominal masses are called *Ji Ju*. *Ji* indicates actual abdominal masses which are fixed and immovable; if there is an associated pain, its location is fixed. These masses are due to stasis of Blood and I call them 'Blood masses'. *Ju* indicates abdominal masses which come and go, do not have a fixed location and are movable. If there is an associated pain, it too comes and goes and

changes location. Such masses are due to stagnation of Qi and I call them 'Qi masses'.

Actual abdominal lumps therefore pertain to the category of abdominal masses and specifically *Ji* masses, that is, Blood masses.

Another name for abdominal masses was *Zheng Jia*, *Zheng* being equivalent to *Ji*, that is, acute, fixed masses, and *Jia* being equivalent to *Ju*, that is, non-substantial masses from stagnation of Qi. The term *Zheng Jia* normally referred to abdominal masses occurring only in women; but although these masses are more frequent in women, they do occur in men as well.

Visible lumps in the lower abdomen are usually due to Qi stagnation, Blood stasis, Damp-Phlegm or Damp-Heat in the lower abdomen. As in the case of epigastric lumps, abdominal lumps visible on observation indicate an advanced stage which is usually seen in cancer of the uterus, large ovarian cysts or large myomas.

If due to Qi stagnation, abdominal lumps normally feel soft and come and go with emotional moods; if due to Blood stasis they feel hard on palpation and are usually associated with pain; if from Damp-Heat they may also be painful and, when palpated, very tender; if from Damp-Phlegm they feel softer than do lumps from Blood stasis or Damp-Heat. A typical example of an abdominal lump from Blood stasis is a myoma, while an example of that from Damp-Phlegm or Damp-Heat is an ovarian cyst.

Box 16.3 summarizes the two types of abdominal masses.

BOX 16.3 TYPES OF ABDOMINAL MASSES

- Qi (*Ju* or *Jia*): relatively soft masses that come and go
- Blood (*Ji* or *Zheng*): hard, fixed masses

Lumps in the epigastrium
Symptoms and Signs, Chapter 71

Visible epigastric lumps are usually due to Damp-Phlegm, Blood stasis or Phlegm and Blood stasis in the Middle Burner. Obviously, when a lump is visible on observation (rather than palpation), it is quite advanced and is seen in serious diseases such as stomach cancer, liver cancer, cancer of the oesophagus or enlargement of the liver or spleen.

Small hypochondrial lumps
Symptoms and Signs, Chapter 71

Small hypochondrial lumps resembling a string of pearls indicate Liver-Blood stasis.

Umbilicus signs
Protruding umbilicus
Symptoms and Signs, Chapter 71

A protruding umbilicus may be due to Empty-Cold with Qi stagnation, to Blood stasis with oedema in the abdomen, or to severe Spleen and Kidney deficiency. Empty-Cold with Qi stagnation is seen more frequently in children, whereas the pattern of Blood stasis with oedema is seen more frequently in the elderly.

Sunken umbilicus
Symptoms and Signs, Chapter 71

A sunken umbilicus may be due to Blood stasis with sinking of Qi, or to Damp-Heat in the abdomen.

Skin signs
Distended abdominal veins
Symptoms and Signs, Chapter 71

From a Chinese perspective, distended abdominal veins represent the Blood Connecting channels, which are a network of secondary Connecting channels where the blood pools. Thus, by definition, visible distended veins in the abdomen indicate a pathology of the Blood Connecting channels and, being in the abdomen, a pathology of the Penetrating Vessel. The Penetrating Vessel is the Sea of Blood and controls all the Blood Connecting channels, in particular those of the abdomen, and of the medial sides of the legs. If the distended veins are purple they indicate Blood stasis, if red Blood-Heat, and if bluish Cold.

Lines on the abdomen
Symptoms and Signs, Chapter 71

Lines on the abdomen are wide streaks which look like stretch marks (indeed, stretch marks are one type of such 'lines'). They may be blue or purple – blue indicating Blood stasis from Cold associated with Yang deficiency, and purple indicating Blood stasis with Blood-Heat associated with Yin deficiency. Such lines are frequently seen in patients who have been on oral corticosteroids for a long time.

Maculae on the abdomen
Symptoms and Signs, Chapter 71

Maculae on the abdomen always indicate a Blood pathology, which is Blood-Heat if they are red, Blood stasis if they are purple and Blood-Heat with Yin deficiency if they are scarlet red.

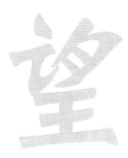

Chapter **17**

OBSERVATION OF THE GENITALIA

Chapter contents

CHANNELS INFLUENCING THE GENITALIA   *149*

PUBIC HAIR   *150*
  Loss of pubic hair   *150*
  Excessive pubic hair   *150*

PENIS   *150*
  Redness and swelling of the glans penis   *150*
  Ulcers on the penis   *150*
  Peyronie's disease   *150*
  Priapism   *150*
  Soft and withered penis   *150*
  Long penis in children   *150*

SCROTUM   *150*
  Contracted scrotum   *150*
  Loose scrotum   *151*
  Scrotum drooping on one side   *151*
  Swollen scrotum   *151*
  Swollen and oozing scrotum   *151*
  Abnormal colour   *151*

VULVA AND VAGINA   *151*
  Vulvar sores   *151*
  Leukoplakia   *151*
  Swelling of the vulva   *151*
  Prolapse of the vagina   *151*

CHANNELS INFLUENCING THE GENITALIA

The genitals are related primarily to the Liver and Kidney channels and to the Directing, Penetrating and Governing Vessels. The Liver Connecting channel, in particular, loops around the genitalia. Although the influence of the Directing Vessel on the genitalia is obvious, that of the Governing Vessel is often overlooked.

The 'Simple Questions' (Chapter 60) describes an anterior branch of the Governing Vessel that flows to the external genitalia both in men and women, and to the pubic bone and from here ascends up the

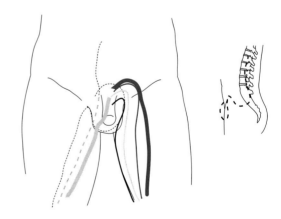

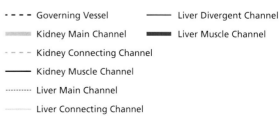

- - - - Governing Vessel   ———— Liver Divergent Channel

▒▒▒▒ Kidney Main Channel   ■■■■ Liver Muscle Channel

- - - - Kidney Connecting Channel

———— Kidney Muscle Channel

·········· Liver Main Channel

———— Liver Connecting Channel

Fig. 17.1 Pathways of channels influencing the genitalia

abdomen on the same trajectory as the Directing Vessel (Fig. 17.1 right).[1]

The pathways of the channels flowing through the genitalia are as follows (Fig. 17.1):

- A branch of the Governing Vessels flows down to the genitalia.
- The Kidney Main, Connecting and Muscle channels flow through the genitalia.
- The Liver Main, Connecting, Divergent and Muscle channels wrap around the genitalia.

(For a more detailed description of the patterns involved in the above genitalia signs, see Part 5, Chapters 75 and 89.)

PUBIC HAIR

Symptoms and Signs, Chapters 75 and 89

There are two items of observation regarding pubic hair:

- loss of pubic hair
- excessive pubic hair.

Loss of pubic hair

Loss of pubic hair may be due to a decline of Kidney-Essence. This decline is normal in the elderly; in younger people, it may result from a severe Spleen- and Kidney-Yang deficiency.

Excessive pubic hair

The term 'excessive' here indicates not so much the quantity as the extent of pubic hair and it refers to people whose pubic hair occupies a large area, extending down the legs and up towards the umbilicus. Excessive pubic hair, so defined, may be due to either Phlegm combined with Blood stasis or Kidney-Yin deficiency with Empty-Heat.

PENIS

Symptoms and Signs, Chapter 75 and 90

Redness and swelling of the glans penis

Redness and swelling of the glans penis may be due either to Toxic Heat or to Damp-Heat in the Liver channel.

Ulcers on the penis

This condition is characterized by redness, macular spots, erosion and oozing ulcers on the glans penis or the shaft, or both. This is usually accompanied by pain. The main causes of this condition are either Toxic Heat or Damp-Heat in the Liver channel.

Peyronie's disease

Peyronie's disease is an unnatural curvature of the penis, noticeable during an erection. It may prevent a complete erection, owing to plaque or scar tissue inside the penis, or it may render erection painful so that intercourse is impossible.

The most common causes of Peyronie's disease are:

- Blood stasis
- Dampness in the Liver channel
- Cold in the Liver channel.

Priapism

Priapism (abnormally prolonged erection) is due either to a deficiency of Kidney-Yin with Empty-Heat or to Damp-Heat in the Liver channel.

Soft and withered penis

A soft and withered penis in adults may be due to Liver-Qi deficiency, to Kidney deficiency (either Yin or Yang), or to Phlegm and Blood stasis in the Lower Burner.

Long penis in children

If a child's penis is abnormally long, almost the size of an adult's, this condition may be due to a hereditary Kidney-Yin deficiency, to sinking of Spleen-Qi, to Phlegm with Blood stasis in the Lower Burner, or to Damp-Heat in the Liver channel.

SCROTUM

Symptoms and Signs, Chapter 75

Contracted scrotum

The most common cause of contracted scrotum is stagnation of Cold in the Liver channel. It may also be seen in collapse of Yin or Yang.

Loose scrotum

A loose scrotum is due either to a deficiency of the Liver and Kidneys (usually Yang deficiency) or to sinking of Spleen-Qi.

Scrotum drooping on one side

A scrotum drooping on one side indicates a condition in which one side of the scrotum is swollen when the person is standing up but retracted when lying down; in Western medicine, this indicates inguinal hernia. From a Chinese perspective the patterns involved in this condition are Empty-Cold in the lower abdomen, Damp-Phlegm in the lower abdomen, Liver-Blood stasis or Damp-Heat in the Liver.

Swollen scrotum

A swollen scrotum may be due to Spleen- and Kidney-Yang deficiency, Damp-Heat in the Liver channel, sinking of Spleen-Qi, Heart-Yang deficiency or Liver-Blood deficiency generating Empty internal Wind.

Swollen and oozing scrotum

If the scrotum is swollen, red and oozing a sticky fluid, this condition is due either to Damp-Heat or to Toxic Heat in the Liver channel.

Abnormal colour

Pale scrotum

A pale scrotum is due to either Spleen- or Kidney-Yang deficiency.

Red scrotum

A red scrotum is due either to Damp-Heat or to Toxic Heat in the Liver channel.

Purple scrotum

A purple scrotum is due either to Liver-Blood stasis or to Damp-Heat with Blood stasis in the Liver channel.

Dark scrotum

A dark scrotum is due either to stagnation of Cold in the Liver channel or to Kidney-Yang deficiency.

VULVA AND VAGINA

Symptoms and Signs, Chapter 89

Vulvar sores

Vulvar sores may be due to Damp-Heat in the Liver channel or to Toxic Heat with Blood stasis in the Liver channel.

Leukoplakia

Leukoplakia may be due to Damp-Heat in the Liver channel or to long-standing Blood deficiency accompanied by Dampness.

Swelling of the vulva

Swelling of the vulva may be due to Toxic Heat with Blood stasis in the Liver channel, Damp-Phlegm in the Lower Burner, or Damp-Heat and Toxic Heat in the Liver channel.

Prolapse of the vagina

Prolapse of the vagina is always due to sinking of Qi, which may be that of the Spleen or Kidneys, or both.

NOTES

1. 1979 The Yellow Emperor's Classic of Internal Medicine – Simple Questions (*Huang Di Nei Jing Su Wen* 黄帝内经素问), People's Health Publishing House, Beijing, p. 320. First published c. 100BC.

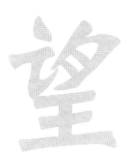

Chapter **18**

OBSERVATION OF THE FOUR LIMBS

Chapter contents

INTRODUCTION   *153*

ATROPHY OF THE FOUR LIMBS   *153*

FLACCIDITY OF THE FOUR LIMBS   *154*

RIGIDITY OF THE FOUR LIMBS   *154*

PARALYSIS OF THE FOUR LIMBS   *154*

LIMB MOVEMENTS   *155*
  Contraction of the four limbs   *155*
  Convulsions of the four limbs   *155*
  Tremor or spasticity of the four limbs   *156*

OEDEMA OF THE FOUR LIMBS   *156*

SWELLING OF THE JOINTS OF THE FOUR LIMBS   *157*

INTRODUCTION

Observation of the limbs includes observation of their skin, muscles, blood vessels and sinews. Therefore, although the overall condition of the limbs is related to the Stomach and Spleen, observation of the skin, muscles, sinews and blood vessels can reveal the state of the Lungs, Spleen, Liver and Heart respectively.

The symptoms and signs relative to the four limbs are in Chapters 64, 65 and 66 of Part 5.

ATROPHY OF THE FOUR LIMBS

Interrogation, Chapter 39; Symptoms and Signs, Chapter 64

Atrophy of the four limbs may range from a very slight thinning of the muscles to a complete wasting of the muscles such as is seen in the advanced stage of some neurological problems (e.g. motor neurone disease). The most common cause of atrophy of the limb muscles is a deficiency of the Stomach and Spleen, which results from the Stomach's not transporting the Food-Essences there. Another possible cause of atrophy of the four limbs, which usually involves the Heart, Spleen and Liver, is Qi and Blood deficiency. In more advanced stages, atrophy of the four limbs may be caused by Liver- and Kidney-Yin deficiency, or Spleen- and Kidney-Yang deficiency.

In children, atrophy of the four limbs is due either to a deficiency of Stomach and Spleen or to a congenital Kidney-Essence deficiency and it is one of the Five Flaccidities seen in children (see Ch. 90). The Chinese name for the condition that causes a child to have flaccid leg muscles and swollen knees is Crane Knee Wind, which is due to a deficiency of Yin of the three leg channels combined with invasion of Damp-Cold in the knees.

Box 18.1 summarizes the patterns underlying atrophy of the limbs.

BOX 18.1 ATROPHY OF THE FOUR LIMBS

- Stomach and Spleen deficiency
- Qi and Blood deficiency
- Liver- and Kidney-Yin deficiency
- Spleen- and Kidney-Yang deficiency
- Kidney-Essence deficiency (children)
- Spleen-, Liver- and Kidney-Yin deficiency with Damp-Cold in the knees (children)

FLACCIDITY OF THE FOUR LIMBS

Interrogation, Chapter 39; Symptoms and Signs, Chapter 64

The term 'flaccidity' indicates that the muscles are flaccid, soft and limp but not atrophied (as in atrophy of the muscles).

In acute cases, flaccidity of the four limbs may be due to invasion of Wind-Heat in the Lungs, later becoming interior Heat and injuring the Body Fluids of the Stomach and Spleen. In chronic cases, the flaccidity may result from Damp-Heat affecting the Stomach and Spleen in Full cases, or from a deficiency of the Stomach and Spleen in Empty conditions. In severe, chronic cases, flaccidity of the four limbs is often due to a deficiency of Kidney-Yin.

In children under 5 years, acute cases of flaccidity of the four limbs are due to an invasion of Wind-Heat that quickly progresses to the Interior, turns into interior Heat and damages the Body Fluids, which leads to malnourishment of the channels; this is the pathology of limb flaccidity caused by infectious diseases such as poliomyelitis. In interior conditions, flaccidity of the four limbs in children is due to retention of Damp-Heat or to Qi deficiency with Blood stasis occurring against a background either of poor hereditary constitution or of poor postnatal nutrition.

Box 18.2 summarizes the patterns underlying flaccidity of the limbs.

BOX 18.2 FLACCIDITY OF THE FOUR LIMBS

- Lung-Heat injuring body fluids (acute)
- Damp-Heat in the Stomach and Spleen (chronic)
- Stomach and Spleen deficiency (chronic)
- Kidney-Yin deficiency
- Invasion of Wind-Heat
- Qi deficiency with Blood stasis
- Retention of Damp-Heat

RIGIDITY OF THE FOUR LIMBS

Symptoms and Signs, Chapter 64

Rigidity of the four limbs means that the patient is unable to flex or extend the wrist, elbow, knee or ankle joints. It has many causes. In acute cases with sudden onset, it is due to invasion of Wind; such a rigidity is obviously of short duration and resolves itself once the Wind has been expelled.

In interior conditions, one common cause of rigidity of the four limbs is Liver-Yang rising or Liver-Wind in the elderly. Another is of course seen in Painful Obstruction (*Bi*) Syndrome, especially when caused by Dampness complicated by Phlegm in chronic cases, in which case the limb rigidity is accompanied by swelling and pain of the joints.

In the elderly, an inability to flex the joints is often due to retention of Phlegm in the channels together with internal Wind. A rigidity of the limbs accompanied by pain in the joints or muscles, or both, and worsening at night, is due to Blood stasis.

In Empty conditions, rigidity of the limbs may be due to a deficiency of Liver- and Kidney-Yin, or of Spleen- and Kidney-Yang, and this is more common in the elderly.

Box 18.3 summarizes patterns underlying limb rigidity.

BOX 18.3 RIGIDITY OF THE FOUR LIMBS

- Invasion of external Wind (acute)
- Liver-Yang rising
- Liver-Wind (elderly)
- Painful Obstruction Syndrome with Dampness
- Phlegm with internal Wind in the channels (elderly)
- Blood stasis
- Liver- and Kidney-Yin deficiency
- Spleen- and Kidney-Yang deficiency

PARALYSIS OF THE FOUR LIMBS

Symptoms and Signs, Chapter 64

Paralysis of the four limbs may range from a very slight limitation of movement, such as a tendency to drag a foot, to complete paralysis, as is seen in paraplegia following a fracture of the spine.

The main causes of paralysis of the four limbs are a Stomach and Spleen deficiency, a general deficiency of Qi and Blood and a deficiency of Yin of the Liver and

Kidneys. There are also Full causes of paralysis such as retention of Dampness in the muscles and Blood stasis.

The hemiplegia that occurs after a stroke is due to retention of Wind and Phlegm in the channels of the limbs on one side. The underlying pathology leading to a stroke is usually quite complex and includes Phlegm, internal Wind and Heat, usually occurring against a background of deficiency of Qi and Blood or of Yin.

Box 18.4 summarizes the patterns underlying limb paralysis.

BOX 18.4 PARALYSIS OF THE FOUR LIMBS

- Stomach and Spleen deficiency
- Qi and Blood deficiency
- Liver- and Kidney-Yin deficiency
- Dampness in the muscles
- Blood stasis
- Phlegm and internal Wind in the channels

LIMB MOVEMENTS

Contraction of the four limbs

Symptoms and Signs, Chapter 64

In acute cases with sudden onset, contraction of the four limbs may be caused by invasion of Wind and this is always of short duration and self resolving. In Full conditions, the contractions may be caused by Dampness obstructing the muscles, or by Heat injuring the Body Fluids of the limb channels.

In Empty conditions, the most common cause of contraction of the four limbs is Liver-Blood or Liver-Yin deficiency. In the elderly, a common example usually deriving from Liver-Blood or Liver-Yin deficiency is the Dupuytren contraction, which usually involves either the ring finger or the little finger (see Fig. 14.1 on p. 131).

Box 18.5 summarizes patterns underlying contraction of the four limbs.

BOX 18.5 CONTRACTION OF THE FOUR LIMBS

- Acute contraction with sudden onset: invasion of Wind
- Full conditions: Dampness obstructing the muscles, Heat injuring the Body Fluids of the limb channels
- Empty conditions: Liver-Blood or Liver-Yin deficiency
- Dupuytren contraction of ring/little finger: Liver-Blood or Liver-Yin deficiency (elderly)

Convulsions of the four limbs

Symptoms and Signs, Chapter 64

Convulsions of the four limbs always indicate internal Wind. In Chinese medicine, convulsions are considered to be due to the 'shaking' of the tendons and this is another reason why the Liver is always involved in this pathology.

In chronic, interior conditions, internal Wind is generated as the end result of a long pathological process, usually involving the Liver. In acute, febrile diseases, internal Wind is generated either directly from extreme Heat or from Yin deficiency, usually at the Blood level of the Four Levels. Whether the origin is internal or external, one can distinguish two types of internal Wind: one Full, characterized by strong convulsions with high amplitude; the other Empty, characterized by weak and infrequent convulsions with small amplitude, such as twitching.

In acute febrile diseases, internal Wind can develop quickly, even in a matter of days, when the Heat reaches the Blood level of the Four Levels. If Heat generates Wind, this causes strong convulsions of the four limbs. If Empty-Wind develops from Yin deficiency (itself caused by the Heat burning up the Body Fluids), the convulsions of the four limbs are less pronounced and may be infrequent.

In interior conditions, convulsions or twitchings of the four limbs are caused by internal Liver-Wind, which may derive either from Liver-Yang rising or from Liver-Blood deficiency.

If a newborn baby suffers from slight, intermittent convulsions but looks completely normal in between the attacks, its convulsions are due to invasion of external Wind combined with prenatal shock and poor hereditary constitution. The convulsions are more likely to occur in spring and autumn and they are due to a deficiency of the Spleen and Kidneys. Because the sinews lack nourishment, they are easily attacked by external Wind.

Convulsions in women after childbirth (now relatively rare) are due to Liver-Blood deficiency generating Liver-Wind.

Epilepsy is of course a type of convulsions of the four limbs due to internal Wind. Called *dian xian*, according to Chinese medicine it is caused both by internal Wind and by Phlegm obstructing the Mind's orifices, and the pathology involves Liver, Spleen and Kidneys.

Epileptic attacks during pregnancy or after childbirth are generally due to Liver- and Kidney-Yin

deficiency and Blood deficiency giving rise to Liver-Wind.

Box 18.6 summarizes patterns underlying convulsions of the limbs.

BOX 18.6 CONVULSIONS OF THE FOUR LIMBS

- Convulsions in acute febrile diseases: Full- or Empty-Wind
- Convulsions in chronic, internal diseases: Liver-Wind from Liver-Yang rising or Liver-Blood deficiency
- Small, intermittent convulsions in babies: external Wind with prenatal shock and poor constitution:
- Convulsions after childbirth: Liver-Wind from Liver-Blood deficiency
- Epileptic convulsions: Liver-Wind and Phlegm

Tremor or spasticity of the four limbs

Observation, Chapter 4; Interrogation, Chapter 39; Symptoms and Signs, Chapter 64

Tremor consists in a shaking, trembling or quivering either of the arms or the legs, or both. It ranges from a very pronounced shaking with wide amplitude to a quiver that is so fine and in amplitude so small that it is almost imperceptible. Tremor of the hands is more common than tremor of the legs. The cause is always Liver-Wind; as with convulsions, it may be either the Full or Empty type, the former being characterized by a pronounced shaking of the limbs and the latter by a fine tremor.

The most common cause of tremor of the four limbs, especially in the elderly, is a combination of Liver-Wind and Phlegm affecting the channels and sinews. Liver-Yang rising by itself may also give rise to internal Wind and tremors. Another common cause of tremors is Liver-Wind deriving from Liver-Blood deficiency; this is more common in women and will cause a fine tremor. Liver- and Kidney-Yin deficiency are also a common cause of tremors in the elderly.

In alcoholics, a fine tremor of the hands is caused by Damp-Heat. In rare cases, retention of Dampness in the muscles and sinews of the hands may cause a fine tremor of the hands.

A general deficiency of Qi and Blood failing to nourish the sinews and muscles may cause a mild, fine tremor of the limbs.

Spasticity and tremor of the limbs may also appear at the Blood level (of the Four Levels) when the Heat generated by the febrile disease either leads to Liver-Wind or depletes the Yin so that Empty-Wind is generated.

Box 18.7 summarizes the patterns underlying tremor of the limbs.

BOX 18.7 TREMOR OR SPASTICITY OF THE FOUR LIMBS

- Phlegm and internal Liver-Wind
- Liver-Yang rising generating Liver-Wind
- Liver-Blood deficiency giving rise to Liver-Wind
- Liver- and Kidney-Yin deficiency giving rise to Liver-Wind
- Damp-Heat (alcoholics)

OEDEMA OF THE FOUR LIMBS

Observation, Chapter 19; Interrogation, Chapter 39; Symptoms and Signs, Chapters 64, 65, 68

There are two types of oedema, one called 'water oedema' (*Shui Zhong*) and the other 'Qi oedema' (*Qi Zhong*). Water oedema is due to Yang deficiency and is always pitting oedema, that is, the skin pits and it changes colour on pressure. Qi oedema is due to either Qi stagnation or Dampness and the skin does not pit, nor does it change colour on pressure.

Another classification is that of Yang and Yin oedema: the former is of the Full type and is due to invasion of Wind, Dampness or Toxic Heat, whereas the latter is of the Empty type and is due to a deficiency of Spleen- or Kidney-Yang, or both. In Yin oedema there is marked pitting on pressure, whereas in Yang oedema there is little or no pitting. From a Western perspective, absence of pitting indicates oedema due to hypothyroidism.

When observing the limbs for oedema, we should always palpate the oedematous area and check whether or not the skin pits on palpation. If pressing the skin with the thumb leaves a dent that takes a long time to spring back, this indicates the so-called 'water' oedema, that is, oedema due to retention of fluids; if pressing the skin with the thumb forms no dent, this indicates 'Qi oedema' and it is due to Qi stagnation or Dampness.

True oedema is generally due to deficient Yang; the fluids which it is unable to transform, transport and excrete properly accumulate in the space between the skin and muscles (*Cou Li*).

Yang deficiency is the most common cause of oedema of the limbs: Lung-Yang deficiency affects primarily the hands, Kidney-Yang deficiency primarily the feet and Spleen-Yang deficiency both. Oedema of the four limbs may also derive from retention of

Dampness in the muscles, which may be associated either with Cold or with Heat.

Qi stagnation affecting the muscles may also cause oedema of the limbs, in which case it will be of the non-pitting type. In the elderly, oedema of the limbs may also derive from Qi deficiency and Blood stasis. Finally, acute oedema of the hands and face only may be due to invasion of the Lungs by Wind-Water, which is a type of Wind-Cold.

Box 18.8 summarizes the patterns underlying oedema of the limbs.

deriving from Dampness. In chronic conditions, Dampness develops into Phlegm, which obstructs the joints and causes further swelling and bone deformities. In adult patients, and especially women, it is very common for Painful Obstruction Syndrome and swelling of the joints of the four limbs to occur against a background of Blood deficiency. If, in addition to being swollen, the joints are also red and hot to the touch, this indicates retention of Damp-Heat.

Box 18.9 summarizes patterns underlying swelling of the joints.

BOX 18.8 OEDEMA OF THE LIMBS

- Oedema of the hands: Lung-Yang deficiency
- Oedema of the feet: Kidney-Yang deficiency
- Oedema of the four limbs: Spleen-Yang deficiency, Dampness
- Oedema of the four limbs (non-pitting): Qi stagnation
- Oedema of limbs in elderly: Qi deficiency and Blood stasis
- Acute oedema of the hands: invasion of the Lungs by Wind-Water

---

BOX 18.9 SWELLING OF THE JOINTS OF THE FOUR LIMBS

- Chronic swelling: Painful Obstruction (*Bi*) Syndrome, especially from Dampness
- Chronic swelling with bone deformities: Phlegm obstructing the joints
- Swelling in women: Blood deficiency
- Swollen, red joints hot to the touch: retention of Damp-Heat

---

SWELLING OF THE JOINTS OF THE FOUR LIMBS

Symptoms and Signs, Chapter 64

A swelling of the joints of the four limbs is always due to Painful Obstruction (*Bi*) Syndrome, especially that

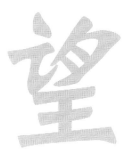

Chapter **19**

OBSERVATION OF THE LEGS

Chapter contents

LEG SIGNS   *159*
  Oedema   *159*
  Atrophy   *160*
  Paralysis   *160*
  Arched legs   *160*

GAIT   *161*
  Festination   *161*
  Unstable gait   *161*
  Staggering gait   *161*
  Stepping gait   *161*
  Shuffling gait   *161*

Observation of legs includes both observation of the legs themselves and also of the gait.

The symptoms and signs related to the legs are in Chapter 66 of Part 5.

LEG SIGNS

Oedema

Observation, Chapter 18; Interrogation, Chapter 39; Symptoms and Signs, Chapters 64, 66, 68

Oedema is generally caused by Yang deficiency of the Lung, Spleen or Kidneys or by retention of Dampness. When oedema affects the legs, it is due either to a Spleen-Yang deficiency, a Kidney-Yang deficiency or a combination of the two. In some cases, oedema may also be due to an accumulation of Dampness in the legs, which prevents the proper transformation of fluids; in this case, besides showing oedema, the legs will look generally puffy. Oedema caused by deficiency of Yang or Dampness shows pitting, that is, the skin pits on pressure. In a few cases, oedema may be due to stagnation of Qi and Blood in the legs, in which case it is non-pitting (Fig. 19.1).

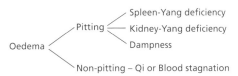

Fig. 19.1 Causes of oedema of the legs

Case history 19.1 illustrates a pattern of Spleen- and Kidney-Yang deficiency underlying leg oedema.

Case history 19.1

A 51-year-old man had been suffering from oedema of the legs and abdomen, breathlessness, night sweating and inability to lie down for 8 months. A Western diagnosis revealed that he suffered from congestive cardiac failure. He also experienced a feeling of heat in the head and a feeling of throbbing of the head; from a Western diagnostic point of view this was due to hypertension. On interrogation, it transpired that he also experienced a feeling of pressure in the right eye in the morning, tinnitus, thirst and a tendency to diarrhoea.

He was slightly overweight and his body shape was of the Fire type, having a relatively round body shape, round head and small hands and feet. However, the Fire type should walk briskly and talk fast, whereas this patient walked and talked rather slowly. His complexion was dull pale.

His tongue was very slightly Pale, very slightly Red on the sides with a deep Heart crack and a sticky-white tongue coating. His pulse was Weak on both Rear positions, but especially on the right, Weak on the right Front position and Slippery on the left Front position.

Diagnosis: First of all, the contradiction between the Fire body shape and his slow walk and talk indi- cates straight away a potential problem in the Fire Element and the Heart. This is confirmed by the pres- ence of the deep Heart crack on the tongue, which usually indicates either severe emotional problems (which was not the case in this patient) or a heart problem. The heart problem is also confirmed by the Slippery quality on the Heart position, which is all the more striking considering the Weak quality of most of the other pulses. When only the Heart pulse is Slippery, especially in its lateral or medial aspects, this often indicates the possibility of heart disease in a Western sense. Thus, in this patient, the contradiction between the body type and his walking and talking, the pulse and the tongue all clearly indicate the possi- bility of an actual heart disease, which was of course confirmed by the Western diagnosis.

In terms of patterns, there is a deficiency of Spleen- and Kidney-Yang manifested by the tinnitus, ten- dency to diarrhoea and Weak pulse on both Rear positions, with Water overflowing to the Heart, which is manifested by the oedema, breathlessness and inability to lie down. In addition to these two patterns there is also Liver-Yang rising (stemming from the Kidney deficiency) manifesting with a feeling of heat and throbbing of the head, thirst, pressure in the eye and Red sides of the tongue.

Atrophy

Symptoms and Signs, Chapter 66

The most common cause of atrophy of the legs is a chronic deficiency of the Stomach and Spleen. Another cause is a deficiency of Yin of the Liver and Kidneys (more common in the elderly).

Paralysis

Symptoms and Signs, Chapter 66

Paralysis of the legs may be due to chronic Stomach- and Spleen-Qi deficiency, to Liver- and Kidney-Yin deficiency or to Wind-Phlegm in the limbs. The first two patterns are seen in neurological conditions and the third is seen in the sequelae stage of Wind-stroke.

Arched legs

Symptoms and Signs, Chapter 66

Arched legs, which may be bowed outward or inward, in children are due to a congenital deficiency of the

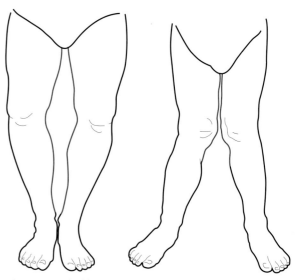

Fig. 19.2 Arched legs

Liver and Kidneys, or of the Stomach and Spleen (Fig. 19.2).

GAIT

Festination

Symptoms and Signs, Chapter 66

Festination refers to a walk characterized by leaning forwards almost to the point of falling, so that the patient needs to take quick and small steps. Once the patient starts walking it is difficult to stop. The causes of this way of walking are usually a severe, chronic deficiency of Liver- and Kidney-Yin or a severe deficiency of Qi and Blood, in both cases with internal Wind.

Unstable gait

Symptoms and Signs, Chapter 66

The unstable gait is characterized by the patient raising the leg very high and dropping it suddenly; the paces are wide, the walk is unstable and such patients will fall easily if they close their eyes. They lose balance also when they are standing. This gait is due to a chronic and severe Kidney- and Liver-Yin deficiency or a severe deficiency of Qi and Blood, in both cases with internal Wind.

Staggering gait

Symptoms and Signs, Chapter 66

The staggering gait consists in swaying from side to side when walking, as if in a state of drunkenness. This gait may be due to Phlegm and Blood stasis obstructing the legs, or to a severe deficiency of Kidney- and Liver-Yin.

Stepping gait

Symptoms and Signs, Chapter 66

The stepping gait consists in the patient raising the leg high and dropping the foot with the toes only touching the ground as if stepping over an obstacle. This type of gait is due to a severe Kidney- and Liver-Yin deficiency or Qi and Blood deficiency, in both cases with internal Wind.

Shuffling gait

Symptoms and Signs, Chapter 66

The shuffling gait consists in the patient not lifting the feet up when walking. It is due to a severe deficiency of Liver- and Kidney-Yin, often combined with Wind-Phlegm. This gait is commonly seen in people suffering from Parkinson's disease.

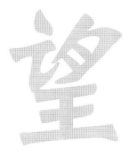

Chapter **20**

OBSERVATION OF EXCRETIONS

Chapter contents

INTRODUCTION   *163*

SPUTUM   *163*

NASAL DISCHARGE   *164*

SWEAT   *164*

STOOLS   *164*
   Colour   *164*
   Consistency   *165*
   Shape   *165*

URINE   *165*

MENSTRUAL BLOOD   *166*
   Colour   *166*
   Consistency   *166*

VAGINAL DISCHARGE   *166*
   Colour   *166*
   Consistency   *166*
   Lochia   *166*

INTRODUCTION

Generally, the term 'observation of the excretions' would include observation of urine, stools, vaginal discharge and menstrual blood, as well as of sputum, nasal discharge and sweat. As the doctor normally finds out about the first group of excretions through interrogation rather than observation, the reader should refer also to the Interrogation section, Part 2, Chapters 31 and 46.

SPUTUM

Interrogation, Chapter 38; Hearing and smelling, Chapter 54; Symptoms and Signs, Chapter 63

Sputum is always, by definition, a manifestation of Phlegm retained in the Lungs. The colour and consistency of the sputum give us an indication of the nature of the condition: Hot or Cold, or Deficient or Excess.

White and dilute sputum indicates Cold-Phlegm, which is usually associated with a Yang deficiency of the Spleen or Kidneys, or both.

White and sticky sputum indicates Damp-Phlegm in the Lungs, while yellow and sticky sputum indicates Phlegm-Heat in the Lungs. If yellow and sticky sputum is also purulent, this indicates Toxic Heat in the Lungs. Very dark sputum the colour of coffee grounds indicates Phlegm-Heat in the Lungs with a predominance of Heat injuring the blood vessels.

Blood-streaked sputum indicates either Phlegm-Heat in the Lungs or, if it is scanty, Lung-Yin deficiency with Empty-Heat.

Box 20.1 summarizes sputum signs.

BOX 20.1 SPUTUM

- White and dilute: Cold-Phlegm
- White and sticky: Damp-Phlegm
- Yellow and sticky: Phlegm-Heat
- Yellow, sticky and purulent: Toxic Heat
- Dark like coffee grounds: Phlegm-Heat at Blood level
- Blood streaked: Phlegm-Heat
- Scanty and blood streaked: Empty-Heat

NASAL DISCHARGE

Interrogation, Chapter 35; Symptoms and Signs, Chapter 58

Nasal discharge may indicate either Phlegm or Dampness: for example, a sticky-yellow nasal discharge in a person suffering from acute bronchitis indicates Phlegm-Heat, while the nasal discharge of a person suffering from sinusitis indicates Damp-Heat. In some cases, it may not fall into either category but is due simply to an impairment of the Lungs' diffusing and descending of fluids; examples of this are the chronic nasal discharge of allergic rhinitis or the acute nasal discharge seen in the common cold.

Generally, a white, watery and dilute nasal discharge indicates Cold Phlegm. Such a nasal discharge is frequently seen either in allergic rhinitis or in the common cold: in the former case it is due to deficient Lung-Qi failing in the diffusing and descending of the fluids; in the latter it is due to external Wind impairing the Lungs' diffusing and descending of fluids.

A white and sticky nasal discharge may indicate either an external invasion of Wind-Heat or chronic retention of Dampness in the nose and sinuses. A sticky-yellow nasal discharge indicates chronic retention of Damp-Heat in the nose and sinuses.

A blood-streaked nasal discharge may indicate either Phlegm-Heat in the Lungs or Damp-heat in the nose or sinuses.

Box 20.2 summarizes patterns underlying nasal discharges.

BOX 20.2 NASAL DISCHARGE

- White, watery, dilute: Cold-Phlegm; in rhinitis, Lung-Qi deficiency; in the common cold, external Wind.
- White, sticky: Dampness or Wind-Heat
- Yellow, sticky: Damp-Heat
- Blood-streaked: Phlegm-Heat or Damp-Heat

SWEAT

Interrogation, Chapter 41; Hearing and smelling, Chapter 54; Symptoms and Signs, Chapter 76

Sweating is generally due either to Heat or to a deficiency (of Qi, Yang or Yin).

Sweat that looks like drops of oil, especially on the forehead, indicates collapse of Yang. Yellow sweat indicates Damp-Heat in the Stomach and Spleen, while profuse, incessant sweating all over the body indicates either Stomach-Heat in acute conditions or severe deficiency of Yang in chronic conditions.

Sweating on the head indicates Heat or Damp-Heat in the Stomach or Empty-Heat deriving from Kidney-Yin deficiency. In children, sweating on the head is usually due to retention of food.

Sweating on the nose indicates Damp-Heat in the Lungs or Stomach, or both. Sweating on the hands indicates deficiency of Qi or Yin of the Lungs or Heart, or Heat in the Lungs or Heart. Sweating of the palms and soles indicates Kidney-Yin deficiency.

Box 20.3 summarizes patterns underlying sweating.

BOX 20.3 SWEAT

- Sweat like drops of oil on the forehead: collapse of Yang
- Yellow: Damp-Heat in Stomach and Spleen
- Profuse, incessant: Stomach-Heat or Yang deficiency
- Sweating on head: Heat or Damp-Heat in Stomach or Empty-Heat from Kidney-Yin deficiency
- Sweating on head in children: retention of food
- Sweating on the nose: Damp-Heat in the Lungs/Stomach
- Sweating on the hands: Qi or Yin deficiency of Lungs/Heart, or Heat in Lungs/Heart
- Sweating of palms and soles: Kidney-Yin deficiency

STOOLS

Interrogation, Chapter 31; Hearing and smelling, Chapter 54; Symptoms and Signs, Chapter 72

Colour

Normal stools are light brown in colour. Pale-yellow stools indicate Empty-Heat (of Spleen, Large Intestine or Kidneys). Dark-yellow stools indicate Full-Heat (of the Large Intestine). Dark stools may indicate the presence of occult blood and they generally indicate Heat (of the Large Intestine).

Pale, almost white stools indicate Cold in the Large Intestine. Green stools indicate Liver-Qi invading the Spleen. Red stools indicate the presence of fresh blood and this may be due either to Heat in the Large Intestine or to Spleen-Qi deficiency. Greenish-bluish stools indicate the penetration of external Cold into the Large Intestine (common in babies). Black or very dark stools indicate Blood stasis.

Consistency

The normal stool is well formed, not loose, not too dry and floating.

An excessively dry stool indicates either Heat in the Intestines, Blood deficiency (of the Liver) or Yin deficiency (which may affect the Large Intestine, Spleen, Liver or Kidneys).

Loose stools generally indicate a deficiency of the Spleen or Kidneys, or both. A deficiency of the Spleen is by far the most common cause of chronic diarrhoea or loose stools; a Kidney deficiency is a common cause of chronic diarrhoea in the elderly. If the diarrhoea is severe and very watery it usually indicates Yang deficiency (of the Spleen or Kidneys, or both), while loose stools usually indicate Spleen-Qi deficiency.

There are, however, also Full causes of diarrhoea, which are principally Dampness (which could be associated with Heat or Cold) and Cold in the Spleen and Intestines.

The presence of mucus in the stools indicates Dampness while the presence of blood indicates deficient Spleen-Qi not holding Blood, Damp-Heat or Blood stasis in the Intestines.

Undigested food in the stools indicates Spleen-Qi deficiency.

Sticky stools that necessitate brushing the toilet with a toilet brush every time indicate Dampness in the Intestines.

Shape

Stools like small pellets indicate Liver-Qi stagnation or Heat if they are also dry. Long and thin stools like pencils indicate Spleen-Qi deficiency (but bear in mind that they could also indicate carcinoma of the bowel). (See Figure 31.1 on p. 272.)

Box 20.4 summarizes the patterns underlying abnormal stools.

BOX 20.4 STOOLS

Colour
- Light brown: normal
- Pale yellow: Empty-Heat
- Dark yellow: Full-Heat
- Dark: Heat
- Pale: Cold
- Green: Liver-Qi invading Spleen
- Red: Large Intestine Heat or Spleen-Qi deficiency
- Greenish-bluish: Cold in Large Intestine
- Very dark, black: Blood stasis

Consistency
- Dry stools: Heat in Intestines, Blood or Yin deficiency
- Diarrhoea with mucus: Dampness in the Intestines
- Loose stools and diarrhoea: Spleen-Qi, Kidney or Yang deficiency or Dampness
- Diarrhoea with blood: Damp-Heat or Spleen-Qi deficiency
- Undigested food in the stools: Spleen-Qi deficiency
- Mucus in the stools: Dampness in the Intestines
- Blood in the stools: Spleen-Qi not holding Blood, Damp-Heat or Blood stasis
- Sticky stools: Dampness in the Intestine

Shape
- Bitty stools like pellets: Liver-Qi stagnation or Heat
- Long-thin stools like pencils: Spleen-Qi deficiency

URINE

Interrogation, Chapter 31; Hearing and smelling, Chapter 54; Symptoms and Signs, Chapter 73

The colour of the urine gives a good indication of the Hot and Cold condition of the patient. Normal urine is pale yellow. Pale urine indicates Cold in the Bladder or Kidney-Yang deficiency; dark urine indicates Heat in the Bladder or Kidney-Yin deficiency. It should be remembered that the colour of the urine is affected when the person drinks a lot of water (becoming paler than it would otherwise be) and also when the person takes Vitamin B, which makes the urine bright yellow.

Blood in the urine indicates either Qi deficiency (of the Spleen and Kidneys), Heat in the Bladder or Kidney-Yin deficiency.

Very dark urine, like soya sauce, indicates a kidney disease such as kidney failure or glomerulonephritis.

Turbid urine indicates Dampness in the urinary passages. Urine with small flakes of mucus indicates Damp-Heat in the Bladder.

Box 20.5 summarizes urine signs.

BOX 20.5 URINE

- Pale: Cold in the Bladder or Kidney-Yang deficiency
- Dark: Heat in the Bladder or Kidney-Yin deficiency
- Red (with blood): Qi deficiency, Heat in the Bladder or Kidney-Yin deficiency
- Turbid urine: Dampness in the urinary passages
- Mucus flakes: Damp-Heat in Bladder

MENSTRUAL BLOOD

Interrogation, Chapter 46; Hearing and smelling, Chapter 54;

Symptoms and Signs, Chapter 84

Colour

The colour of the menstrual blood varies slightly during the period. In general, it is usually dark red, being lighter at the beginning, deep red in the middle, and pinkish at the end of the period. The following are the main patterns with regard to colour:

- **Blood-Heat**: dark red or bright red
- **Blood deficiency**: pale
- **stasis of Blood**: blackish, very dark
- **Full-Cold**: purplish
- **Empty-Cold**: brownish like soya-bean sauce and dilute
- **Empty-Heat in Blood**: scarlet red.

Consistency

The normal flow does not coagulate and there are no clots; the blood is neither dilute nor thick. The following are the main patterns with regard to the consistency of menstrual blood:

- **stasis of Blood or Cold in the Uterus**: clotted, with dark, dull clots
- **Heat**: clotted, with dark but fresh-looking clots
- **stasis of Blood**: large clots
- **Cold in the Uterus**: small dark clots, but blood not dark
- **Blood or Yin deficiency**: watery
- **Dampness or Damp-Heat in the Uterus**: sticky.

Box 20.6 summarizes menstrual blood signs.

BOX 20.6 MENSTRUAL BLOOD

Colour
- Dark red: Blood-Heat
- Bright red: Blood-Heat
- Pale: Blood deficiency
- Dark: Blood stasis
- Purplish: Full-Cold
- Brownish and dilute: Empty-Cold
- Scarlet red: Blood Empty-Heat

Consistency
- Clotted with dark, dull clots: Blood stasis or Cold
- Clotted with dark, fresh-looking clots: Blood-Heat
- Large dark clots: Blood stasis
- Small dark clots in bright blood: Cold in the Uterus
- Watery blood: Blood or Yin deficiency
- Sticky blood: Dampness or Damp-Heat

VAGINAL DISCHARGE

Interrogation, Chapter 46; Hearing and smelling, Chapter 54;

Symptoms and Signs, Chapter 89

Colour

Vaginal discharges may vary in colour from white, through yellow or greenish to red.

White discharge is due to Cold. Cold can derive from Spleen- or Kidney-Yang deficiency, or from exterior Cold-Dampness.

Yellow discharge indicates Heat, usually Damp-Heat in the Lower Burner. A greenish discharge is a result of Damp-Heat in the Liver channel, and a red and white colour also indicates Damp-Heat.

Yellow or red discharge with white pus after menopause is due to Toxic Heat.

Consistency

A watery discharge may indicate Cold-Dampness, or a Deficiency condition, or both. A thick discharge shows Damp-Heat, or an Excess condition, or both.

Lochia

Hearing and smelling, Chapter 54; Symptoms and Signs, Chapter 87

Abundant and pale lochia generally indicate Qi deficiency; abundant and red lochia are due to Blood-Heat or Empty-Heat in the Blood; while abundant and dark lochia indicate Blood stasis or Qi deficiency with

Blood stasis. Scanty lochial discharge, if dark, usually indicates Blood stasis; if pale, it may also be due to a severe deficiency of Qi and Blood. A scanty lochial discharge may also be due to Cold obstructing the Uterus.

Box 20.7 summarizes patterns underlying vaginal discharges.

BOX 20.7 VAGINAL DISCHARGE

Colour
- White: Cold
- Yellow: Heat or Damp-Heat
- Greenish: Damp-Heat in Liver Channel
- Red and White: Damp-Heat
- Yellow-red with white pus after the menopause: Toxic Heat

Consistency
- Watery: Cold-Dampness/deficiency
- Thick: Damp-Heat

Chapter **21**

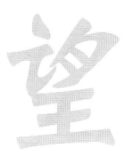

OBSERVATION OF THE SKIN

Chapter contents

INTRODUCTION   169
   Skin layers   169
   Types of skin lesion   170

THE SKIN AND THE INTERNAL ORGANS   170
   The skin and the Lungs   170
   The skin and the Stomach and Spleen   172
   The skin and the Kidneys   172
   The skin and the Liver   173
   The skin and the Heart   173
   The skin and the Connecting channels   174

SKIN SIGNS   174
   Skin colour   174
   Skin texture   175
   Skin of the forearm (inner aspect)   176
   The space between skin and muscles (Cou Li)   176
   Body hair   176
   Macules, papules, vesicles and pustules   176
   Dry skin   178
   Greasy skin   179
   Swelling of the skin   179
   Scales   179
   Erosion of the skin   179
   Rashes   180
   Fissures   180
   Skin ulcers   180
   Dermographism   181

SKIN DISEASES   181
   Eczema   181
   Acne   182
   Psoriasis   183
   Urticaria   185
   Naevi   185
   Malignant melanoma   186
   Tinea   186
   Candida   187
   Herpes simplex   188
   Herpes zoster   188
   Warts   189
   Rosacea   189

INTRODUCTION

Observation of the skin is an important aspect of observational diagnosis. It includes observing the skin colour, skin texture, skin pores and the body hair as well as, of course, any abnormal manifestations on the skin such as various skin diseases, moles, warts or naevi.

Skin layers

Ancient Chinese medicine had its own conception of the skin as made up of different layers and muscles. This conception was similar to that of modern Western medicine. The various layers and muscles in the structure of the skin are:

1. Superficial layer of skin (*Fu*)
2. Deep layer of skin (*Ge*)
3. Subcutaneous muscles (*Ji*)
4. Fat and muscles (*Fen Rou*)
5. Space between skin and muscles (*Cou Li*)
6. Skin pores, including sebaceous glands (*Xuan Fu*).

Fu indicates the superficial layer of skin (i.e. the epidermis), which is influenced mostly by the Lungs. *Ge* indicates the deep layer of skin (i.e. the dermis), which is influenced by the Lungs, Liver and Kidneys. *Ji*, a word that is sometimes translated as 'flesh', indicates the subcutaneous muscles and this structure is influenced by the Spleen and Liver. *Fen Rou* indicates two structures, i.e. fat (influenced by the Spleen, Kidneys and Directing Vessel) and muscles near the bones (influenced by the Spleen and Liver). *Cou Li* (therefore, the space between skin and muscles) is

influenced by the Lungs and Spleen.[1] *Xuan Fu* are the pores (including the sebaceous glands) through which the sweat comes out and they are influenced by the Lungs and Spleen.

Box 21.1 summarizes the organs influencing each layer of the skin.

BOX 21.1 ORGANS INFLUENCING LAYERS OF THE SKIN

- *Fu*: Lungs
- *Ge*: Lungs, Liver and Kidneys
- *Ji*: Spleen and Liver
- *Fen* (of *Fen Rou*): Spleen, Kidneys and Directing Vessel
- *Rou* (of *Fen Rou*): Spleen and Liver
- *Cou Li*: Lungs
- *Xuan Fu*: Lungs

Types of skin lesion

Figure 21.1 shows the various types of skin lesions.

THE SKIN AND THE INTERNAL ORGANS

The skin and the Lungs

As a whole, the skin is influenced by the Lungs. Chapter 10 of the 'Simple Questions' says: *'The Lungs are connected to the skin and control the state of the body hair.'*[2] The Lungs also control the opening and closing of the pores and this function is related to the Lung's diffusing of Defensive Qi to the skin. The pores were

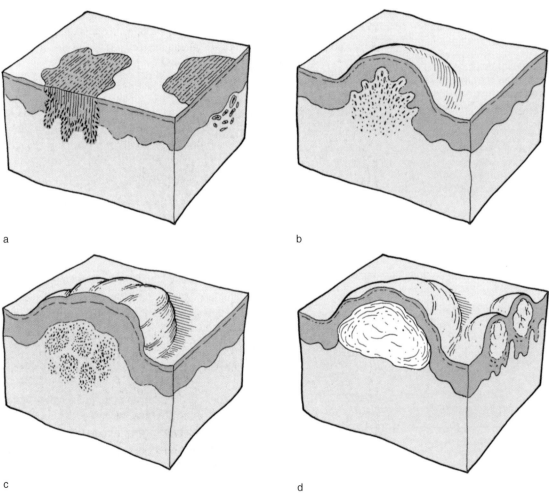

a

b

c

d

Fig. 21.1 Skin lesions. a, macule; b, papule; c, dermatofibroma; d, vesicles; e, pustule; f, epidermal cyst; g, wheal; h, psoriasis plaque; i, white and silvery scale; j, ulcer (From Gawkrodger 1992, An Illustrated Colour Text of Dermatology, pp. 12–13, with permission of Churchill Livingstone.)

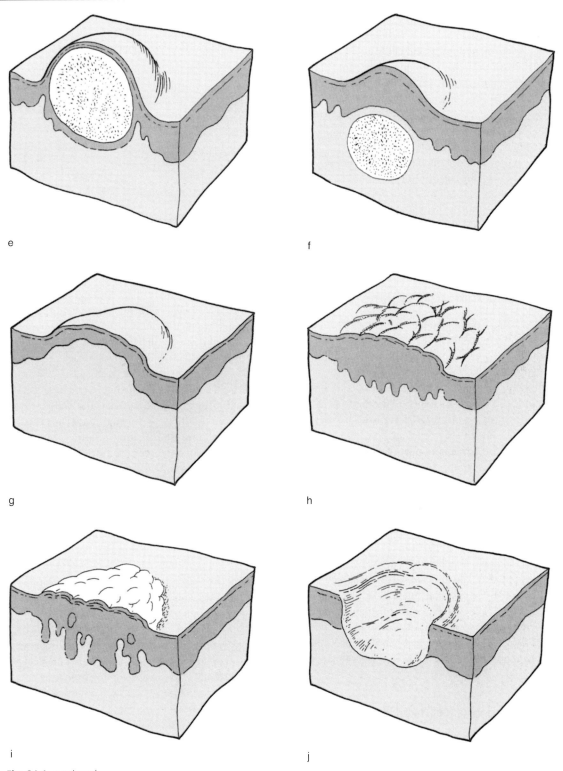

e

f

g

h

i

j

Fig. 21.1 *continued*

called 'sweat holes' (*Han Kong*) and their function is to discharge turbid Qi and sweat. The Defensive Qi and, therefore, the Lung's opening and closing of the pores, is a manifestation of the protective function of the Defensive Qi against the invasion of pathogenic factors. When the Defensive Qi is properly regulated, the pores are closed on exposure to a pathogenic factor and properly open during exercise or on exposure to hot weather. A weakness of Lung-Qi and of the Defensive Qi may lead to 'flaccidity' of the pores and result in their being too open: this facilitates the invasion of pathogenic factors. In pathology, a weakness of Lung-Qi, and therefore of the Defensive Qi in the space between the skin and muscles, causes acute skin diseases due to invasion of external Wind such as urticaria.

The skin and the Stomach and Spleen

The Stomach and Spleen produce Qi and Blood and the turbid part of Qi forms the Defensive Qi while the clear part forms Nutritive Qi. The Defensive Qi, through the diffusing of Lung-Qi, reaches the skin, warming it and regulating the opening and closing of the pores. On the other hand, the Stomach fluids also reach the skin through the diffusing of Lung-Qi, moistening it. The Stomach is also one of the origins of Body Fluids, part of which go to the Lungs and part of which go to the Kidneys. Kidney-Yang warms the Body Fluids deriving from the Stomach; the turbid part is excreted as urine and the pure part goes to the skin via the Triple Burner and the Bladder channel in the back.

The Spleen also controls the muscles immediately below the skin as well as the adipose tissue located there. In pathology, a deficiency of the Spleen may affect these structures and cause diseases such as scleroderma. Of course, Dampness resulting from a deficiency of the Spleen is the cause of many common skin diseases such as eczema, herpes, acne, etc. A failure of Spleen-Qi in holding blood in the vessels may cause bleeding under the skin and therefore red maculae.

The skin and the Kidneys

The Kidneys also influence the skin in other ways. First of all, although the Lungs diffuse Defensive Qi, and the Stomach and Spleen contribute to Defensive Qi's production, the Defensive Qi stems from the Lower Burner and from the Kidneys. Defensive Qi is Yang in nature

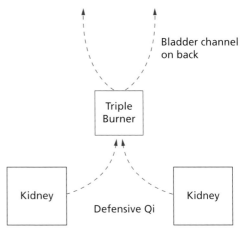

Fig. 21.2 Relationship between the Kidneys, Defensive Qi and skin

and it is therefore influenced by Kidney-Yang and the Fire of the Gate of Life. The Kidneys also play an important role in the distribution of Defensive Qi to all other channels and parts of the body with the aid of the Triple Burner and the Bladder channel. The Back Transporting points where the Defensive Qi infuses to the Internal Organs are situated in the back along the Bladder channel. This is because the Defensive Qi emerges from the Kidneys, through the Triple Burner, and flows up along the Bladder channel. Moreover, when the Defensive Qi emerges in the morning after flowing in the Yin organs at night, it starts from the Kidney channel (Chapter 76 of the 'Spiritual Axis')[3] (Fig. 21.2).

Therefore, when the Kidneys are deficient, the Defensive Qi may also be deficient. This deficiency in the skin gives rise to skin diseases. In particular, a deficiency of the Kidneys, with its consequent failure to irrigate the skin with Defensive Qi, is often at the root of complex, modern skin diseases such as lupus erythematosus or scleroderma.

Apart from a Kidney deficiency and impairment of the Defensive Qi circulation in the skin, these diseases are often associated with Yin Fire, that is, a pathological rise of the Minister Fire upwards stemming from a deficiency of the Original Qi (*Yuan Qi*). In such diseases, there are superficial manifestations on the skin but the root cause is a Kidney deficiency and a deficiency of the Original Qi; this also explains the often contradictory signs of a red rash on the skin of the face and a Pale tongue.

The Triple Burner also influences the skin and, in particular, the skin's moisture, because it plays such an important role in the metabolism of fluids. One import-

ant aspect of the Triple Burner, in fact, is the diffusion of fluids in the Upper Burner, the separation and transformation of fluids in the Middle Burner and the excretion of fluids in the Lower Burner. As heat is needed to transform and excrete fluids, the Triple Burner relies on that derived from the Fire of the Gate of Life in between the Kidneys. From this point of view, the Triple Burner's function of transporting and excreting fluids is inseparable from its location between the Kidneys where the Fire of the Gate of Life resides. For this reason, the Triple Burner is closely related to the Original Qi.

Chapter 66 of the 'Classic of Difficulties' states:

The Motive Force (Dong Qi) that resides between the Kidneys below the umbilicus is the source of life (ming) and the root of the twelve channels and that is why it is called Original [Qi]. The Triple Burner is the emissary of the Original Qi.[4] *It penetrates through the three Burners and spreads to the five Yin and the six Yang organs. Original Qi is the honorary name for the Triple Burner and that is why the places where [the Qi of the Triple Burner] stops in turn are called Origin [Source] points. Therefore diseases of the five Yin and the six Yang organs can be reflected on the Origin [Source] points.*[5]

As the Original Qi, which resides between the Kidneys, is the basis for the Triple Burner and transforms fluids that affect the skin, this is another way in which the Kidneys influence the skin (Fig. 21.3).

Chapter 47 of the 'Spiritual Axis' illustrates the connection between the skin and the Kidneys and Triple Burner: '*The Kidneys are connected with the Triple Burner and the Bladder which influence the pores and body hair.*'[6] Another passage from Chapter 64 of the 'Simple Questions' also illustrates the relationship between the Kidneys and the skin: '*When there is a pathogenic factor in the Kidneys, the skin is affected and there is a rash.*'[7]

Therefore, if the Kidneys are healthy, the skin is moistened and has lustre. If the Kidneys are deficient (in particular Kidney-Yin), the fluids are deficient and the skin loses moisture and becomes dry and lustreless. The thickening and hardening of the skin seen in scleroderma may be caused by a deficiency of Kidney-Yin in chronic cases. If Kidney-Yang is deficient, the fluids accumulate in the space between the skin and muscles and cause oedema.

The skin and the Liver

The Liver influences the skin through Liver-Blood. Like Kidney-Yin, Liver-Blood moistens and nourishes the skin and a deficiency of Liver-Blood is a common cause of dry skin, especially in women (of course, Liver-Yin deficiency may also bring this about). Liver-Fire, on the other hand, has a heating effect on the skin and is the underlying pattern in many skin diseases.

The skin and the Heart

The Heart influences the skin in a similar way to the Liver: Heart-Blood moistens and nourishes the skin just as Liver-Blood does. The influence of Heart-Blood in skin diseases, however, is seen especially on the face.

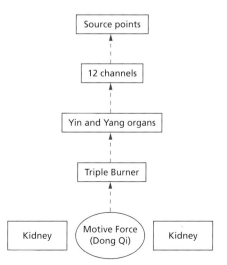

Fig. 21.3 Relationship between Kidneys, Triple Burner and skin

> **BOX 21.2 INFLUENCES OF THE INTERNAL ORGANS ON THE SKIN**
>
> - Lungs: pores, body hair and sweat
> - Stomach and Spleen: adipose tissue below the skin, vessels below the skin, moisture of the skin
> - Kidneys: moisture, Defensive Qi in the space between skin and muscles
> - Liver: moisture and lustre
> - Heart: moisture, blood vessels under the skin

Box 21.2 summarizes the influences of the Internal Organs on the skin.

Thus, from the diagnostic point of view, the skin reflects first of all the state of the Body Fluids, and therefore of the organs mentioned above, and also conditions of Heat or Cold, Fullness or Emptiness and of Yin or Yang.

The skin and the Connecting channels

The blood vessels (venules) visible on the surface of the skin are always a reflection of the Connecting channels. When they become visible, the blood vessels are an expression of the percolation of the Blood Connecting channels towards the surface of the skin (the Blood Connecting vessels at the deep level of the Connecting channels).

Chapter 17 of the 'Spiritual Axis' says: *'The Main channels are in the Interior, their branches are horizontal [or crosswise] forming the Luo channels: branching out from these are the Minute Luo. When these are Full with stagnant Blood they should be drained with bleeding with needle; when they are deficient, they should be tonified with herbs'.*[8] Chapter 10 of the same book says: *'The Main channels are deep and hidden between the muscles and cannot be seen; only the Spleen channel can be seen as it emerges from above the internal malleolus and it has no place to hide. The Luo channels are superficial and can be seen.'*[9] The same chapter also says: 'When the Luo channels are greenish-bluish it indicates Cold and pain; when they are red it indicates Heat.'[10]

Macules are a reflection of the Blood Connecting channels and red macules indicate Blood-Heat, while purple ones indicate Blood stasis. Bluish macules indicate pain and Blood stasis. **Papules** indicate Heat in the Connecting channels. **Vesicles** indicate Dampness in the space between skin and muscles and the Connecting channels. **Pustules** indicate Toxic Heat in the Connecting channels.

Apart from the blood vessels, the colour of the skin itself reflects the condition of the Connecting channels; red indicates Heat, green indicates pain, purple indicates Blood stasis, and bluish indicates Blood stasis and pain.

SKIN SIGNS

Skin colour

'Skin colour' refers to the colour of the body skin itself, as distinct from the complexion (discussed in Chapter 3). It does not refer to skin rashes, which will be discussed separately. The colours discussed are:

- pale
- red
- yellow
- bluish-greenish
- dark.

Of course, when observing body-skin colour one should take into account individual variations due to race and occupation. This has already been discussed in Chapter 3 dealing with observation of the complexion. For example, a body skin that might be described as 'pale' in a Mediterranean person would be normal in a Swedish person. Generally speaking, the colours described below apply to any racial group: for example, the body skin of an African-American or an Indian may be pale in colour, like a Caucasian's, although it will obviously look different.

The pathological colours described below may not necessarily appear all over the body, but may manifest in various localized places; the location of the pathological colour gives an indication of the organ and channel involved. If a large area is affected, this generally indicates that an organ is involved, whereas if the pathological colour appears along a definite line it indicates that the channel is involved. For example, if the epigastrium is generally very pale, it may indicate a condition of Yang deficiency of the Stomach, whereas if there is a redness appearing along the Lung channel it may indicate Heat in that particular channel rather than in the organ (although it would not exclude Heat in the organ as well).

Pale body skin

A pale body skin may indicate Qi, Yang or Blood deficiency. In Qi deficiency the body skin is slightly pale, in Yang deficiency it is pale and bright, while in Blood deficiency it is pale and dull.

Red body skin

A red body skin generally indicates Heat. If the redness appears suddenly and the colour is bright red, this indicates Full Heat; if the redness appears gradually and the colour is red but dull and dry, it indicates Empty Heat; if the colour is dark red and dull, it indicates Blood stasis. A 'floating' red colour (i.e. the red looks like 'rouge' applied to the surface of the skin) indicates Empty-Heat.

A redness of the body skin in acute cases is common in invasions of Wind-Heat; in such cases, besides the face, the neck and arms may also become red.

Yellow body skin

A dull-yellow body skin indicates Dampness or chronic Qi and Blood deficiency, while a bright-yellow skin indicates Damp-Heat. With an acute onset, this indicates the possibility of jaundice. One can distinguish five different yellow colours:

- dampness yellow
- dull yellow
- stagnant-Blood yellow
- jaundice yellow
- 'thick' yellow.

These colours are described in Table 21.1.

Bluish-greenish body skin

As usual, 'bluish-greenish' is a translation of the Chinese word '*qing*'. A bluish colour of the body skin generally indicates Cold; such a colour is common on the Bladder channel in the buttocks and legs and is frequently seen in patients suffering from sciatica.

A greenish colour of the body skin generally indicates Qi or Blood stagnation; such a colour is common on the face and abdomen.

In newborn babies, a greenish colour on the buttocks and back indicates a poor constitution and Accumulation Disorder.

Dark body skin

A dark body skin generally indicates severe Kidney deficiency. In Chinese medicine this particular colour was called 'dark jaundice' (*Hei Dan*) although it has nothing to do with jaundice. The Kidney deficiency manifesting with this colour was attributed to excessive sexual activity in old times; for this reason, this colour was also called 'women-fatigue jaundice' (*Nu Lao Dan*). In reality, this Kidney deficiency may be caused by other factors (such as overwork) besides excessive sexual activity.

A dark skin colour may also be caused by Blood stasis, in which case it will be dark without lustre and it will be associated with a purple colour of the lips and nails.

BOX 21.3 SKIN COLOURS

- Pale: Qi, Yang or Blood deficiency
- Red: Heat, Empty-Heat or Wind-Heat
- Yellow: Qi and Blood deficiency, Dampness, Damp-Heat, jaundice
- Bluish: Cold
- Greenish: Qi or Blood stagnation
- Dark: Kidney deficiency

Box 21.3 summarizes the patterns underlying different skin colours.

Skin texture

Apart from the colour, other aspects of the skin should be considered:

- lustre
- moisture
- texture
- growths on the skin.

Lustre

Lustre in relation to the skin has already been described in the chapter on Complexion (Chapter 3). A body skin with lustre indicates a good state of Body Fluids and of the Lungs, Stomach and Liver.

Table 21.1 Differentiation of five types of yellow

Type	Pathology	Main symptoms	Other symptoms	Differential signs
Dampness yellow	Dampness in the space between skin and muscles	Skin dull yellow with a 'smoky' appearance	Muscle ache or joint ache	Eyes not yellow
Dull yellow	Qi and Blood deficiency	Face and whole body dull yellow	Palpitations, tiredness, loose stools, blurred vision	Eyes not yellow
Stagnant-Blood yellow	Blood stasis	Dull, lustreless and dry yellow body skin	Abdominal pain	Eyes not yellow
Jaundice yellow	Dampness in Liver and Spleen, bile overflowing into skin	Body and eyes yellow	Dark urine, hypochrondrial distension, nausea	Eyes yellow
Thick yellow	Hookworms in intestines, Qi and Blood deficiency	Whole body yellow, some paleness within the yellow	Hunger, desire to eat strange objects	Eyes not yellow

Moisture

The moisture of the skin reflects the nourishment of the skin by Body Fluids and Blood; a normal moist state of the skin therefore reflects a healthy state of Body Fluids and Blood, and of the Liver and Kidneys primarily.

Texture

The skin should be firm but elastic and its surface should be smooth; this reflects a healthy state of the Lungs and Spleen. A rough texture may be due to Lung-Qi deficiency, while if the skin feels hardened it may indicate Dampness or Blood stasis.

Growths

Growths may take the form of vesicles, papules, pustules, moles, warts, etc. and they will be described below.

Skin of the forearm (inner aspect)

Besides palpation, the skin of the inner aspect of the forearm should be observed for slackness, tightness, moistness, dryness, protrusion and shrinking.

If the inner aspect of the forearm looks slack and loose, this indicates Heat; if it is tight, it indicates Cold. If the forearm is moist, this indicates Wind invasion; if it is dry it indicates Blood or Yin deficiency. If the forearm skin seems to be protruding and sticking out it indicates a Full condition; if it looks shrinking and withered, it indicates an Empty condition.

Palpation of the forearm is discussed in Chapter 51.

The space between skin and muscles (Cou Li)

The space between the skin and muscles, called *Cou Li*, is where the Defensive Qi flows and where sweat comes from.[11] The state of the space can be deduced by observing the state of the pores, sweat and skin texture. One should differentiate between a state of openness or closure and one of looseness or tightness.

The state of openness or closure of the space between the skin and the muscles can be judged by the sweating: the presence of sweating indicates that the space between the skin and muscles is open (either through Heat or Yang deficiency); its absence indicates that the space is closed.

A state of excessive openness of the space between skin and muscles facilitates the invasion of external pathogenic factors, while a state of excessive closure renders the person prone to fever and generally Heat.

If the skin is tight and thick, it indicates that the space between skin and muscles is tight, which is caused by a Full condition of the Triple Burner and Bladder; if the skin is loose and thin, it indicates that the space between the skin and muscles is loose, which is caused by an Empty condition of the Triple Burner and Bladder.

Body hair

The body hair indicates the state of the Lungs. One should examine its moistness, lustre and integrity.

If the body hair is lustrous, this indicates good Lung-Qi; if it is not, it indicates weak Lung-Qi. If the body hair is strong and long, this indicates good Qi and Blood; if it is short and weak, it indicates deficiency of Qi and Blood. If the body hair is brittle and breaks easily, this indicates weak Lung-Qi.

If the body hair stands on end, this indicates an invasion of Wind-Cold. If the body hair falls off, it indicates Lung-Heat or Lung-Qi deficiency.

Macules, papules, vesicles and pustules

Macules

A macule, called *ban* in Chinese, is a localized, flat area of colour change without elevation or infiltration of the skin: when a finger is passed over it, the macule does not stick out. A macule can be hypopigmented, as in vitiligo, pigmented, as in a freckle, or erythematous (red), as in a capillary haemangioma (the swollen and superficial capillaries seen frequently on the legs of the elderly).

Yang macules occur in diseases of external origin, have a sudden onset and appear first when the Heat reaches the Nutritive-Qi or Blood level. They generally appear on the chest first and are sparse and red in colour; then they gradually extend to the four limbs, becoming more dense and darker in colour as the patient grows feverish. A good prognosis is indicated by lightening of their colour, lessening of their concentration and receding from the limbs; a poor prognosis is indicated by darkening of their colour, increase in their density and spreading along the limbs.

Yin macules start gradually and are not associated with an external origin or a febrile disease: they are generally due either to chronic Blood-Heat or to Qi deficiency.

One should differentiate the shape, density and colour of the macules. The shape of a macule can be loose or tight: a loose macule looks like a wine stain and indicates a good prognosis; a 'tight' macule looks like the tip of a knitting needle and indicates that Toxic Heat and Blood-Heat are severe and that the prognosis is poor.

The density of the macules is also important: the more dense they are, the more intense is the Blood-Heat.

As for the colour, one should differentiate the following colours of macules:

- red
- purple
- black
- white.

Red macules

Red macules always indicate Heat. In the course of a febrile disease, haemorrhagic macules may appear at the Nutritive-Qi or Blood level and they should always be considered as a dangerous sign. Meningitis is an example of an acute febrile disease that manifests with haemorrhagic macules when it reaches the Nutritive-Qi or Blood level. Macules can be differentiated from papules (see below) by pressing them: if they disappear on pressure they are papules, if not, they are macules. A good method is to use a glass: if the spot disappears when the side of a glass is pressed against it, it is a papule; if not, it is a macule. In the course of acute, febrile diseases, especially in children, it is vital to distinguish papules from macules because the latter indicate the progression of a disease to the Blood level, which is always a dangerous sign. For example, if a child falls ill with meningitis the appearance of macules is a dangerous sign which should always be taken seriously.

The darker the macules, the more intense is the Blood-Heat.

> **!**
>
> **Remember**: in the course of an acute, febrile disease, especially in children, it is vital to distinguish between papules and macules. Papules disappear when the side of a glass is pressed against them, macules do not.

Purple macules

Purple macules indicate Blood-Heat with Blood stasis. (See Plates 21.1 and 21.2 on p. P9.)

Black macules

Black macules indicate very severe Blood-Heat and a dangerous condition. If they are black but bright and clear, the condition, although severe, can be treated. If they are black, dark and murky, this indicates that there is severe Blood-Heat and Toxic Heat and the condition is dangerous and the prognosis poor. If they are black, dull, unclear and edged with red it indicates that, although the illness is severe, the patient can be treated.

White macules

White macules may indicate Qi and Blood stagnation, Blood deficiency or Kidney-Yin deficiency.

Papules

A papule, in Chinese called *Qiu Zhen*, is a small, solid and usually well-demarcated elevation of the skin, generally defined as less than 5 mm in diameter. Papules may be flat-topped as in lichen planus or dome-shaped as in acne.

Red papules always indicate Heat. The Heat may be in any organ but the most frequent locations are the Lungs and Stomach. In terms of levels, the Heat manifested by papules may be at any level, that is, external Wind-Heat, Heat at the Qi level or Heat at the Blood level. Papules frequently reflect Heat combined with Dampness or Phlegm.

Dark-red or purple papules indicate Heat with Blood stasis. Chronic papular eruptions may be due to Spleen-Qi deficiency with Dampness. Papules with a crust indicate Blood or Yin deficiency.

A wheal, called *Feng Tuan* in Chinese, is a type of papule (although it may also be a plaque) characterized by a transitory, compressible elevation of skin with dermal oedema, red or white in colour. Urticaria is a typical example of skin eruptions with wheals. Pale wheals are caused by invasion of Wind-Cold or Yang deficiency; red wheals are caused by Heat or Empty-Heat; dark, purple wheals indicate Blood stasis. (See Plate 21.3 on p. P9).

A plaque, in Chinese called *Ban*, is a type of papule: it is a palpable, plateau-like elevation of skin, usually more than 2 cm in diameter. Certain psoriasis lesions are typical examples of plaques. The clinical

significance of plaques is the same as that of papules, that is, red plaques signify Heat while dark ones indicate Heat with Blood stasis. The fact that the Chinese name for plaques is the same as that for macule (*Ban*) should not induce us to infer that plaques indicate Blood-Heat (as do macules). (See Plate 21.4 on p. P9.)

Vesicles

A vesicle, in Chinese called *Shui Pao*, is a small blister (usually less than 5 mm in diameter) consisting of clear fluid accumulated within or below the epidermis. A vesicle larger than 5 mm is called a *bulla*. (See Plate 21.5 on p. P10.)

Vesicles are a classic sign of Dampness, large ones usually indicating Damp-Heat and small ones indicating Dampness with underlying Spleen deficiency.

Table 21.2 differentiates between macules, papules and vesicles.

Pustules

A pustule, in Chinese called *Nong Pao*, is a visible collection of free pus in a blister. Pustules may indicate infection (as in a furuncle or infected eczema) but not always, as the pustules seen in psoriasis, for example, are not infected.

Pustules usually indicate Toxic Heat or Damp-Heat mixed with Toxic Heat. The Heat is often related to the Lungs, Stomach or Spleen. (See Plate 21.6 on p. P10.)

Box 21.4 summarizes the patterns underlying these skin growths.

Dry skin

Symptoms and signs, Chapter 77

The most common cause of dry skin is Liver-Blood deficiency; this is especially common in women. Liver-Yin and Kidney-Yin deficiency are a common cause of

---

BOX 21.4 MACULES, PAPULES, VESICLES, PUSTULES

Macules
Red: Heat at Nutritive-Qi or Blood level
Purple: Blood-Heat with Blood stasis
Black: severe Blood-Heat, dangerous
White: Blood stasis, Blood deficiency, Kidney-Yin deficiency

Papules
- Red: Heat
- Dark red or purple: Heat with Blood stasis.
- Chronic, on–off: Spleen-Qi deficiency with Dampness
- Papules with crust: Blood or Yin deficiency
- Wheal: invasion of Wind-Cold if pale; Heat or Empty-Heat if red; Blood stasis if dark or purple
- Plaque: Blood-Heat if red; Blood stasis if dark

Vesicles
- Dampness

Pustules
- Toxic Heat
- Damp-Heat with Toxic Heat

---

dry skin in the elderly. In some cases, a dry skin may be due to Stomach-Yin deficiency.

A particular type of dry skin is that due to chronic Blood stasis; due to the interaction and mutual exchange between Blood and Body Fluids, stagnant Blood may impair the circulation of Body Fluids and this may cause the skin to become dry. Dry skin from Blood stasis occurs only in chronic cases when the Blood stasis is severe and it is more common in the elderly. It is fairly easy to distinguish between dry skin due to Blood stasis and that due to Yin or Blood deficiency because in the former the skin is also dark and lacks lustre and the nails are often dark or purple and dry and withered. Apart from that, there will be some general symptoms and signs of Blood stasis.

Box 21.5 summarizes the patterns underlying dry skin.

Table 21.2 Differentiation between macules, papules and vesicles

	Shape	Distribution	Aftermath
Macules	Large spots, level with skin, cannot be felt on touch, do not disappear on pressure	Chest, abdomen, back, face most of all. Seldom on limbs	Do not leave trace
Papules	Like small grains or beans, sticking out, can be felt on palpation, disappear on pressure	Same as above	Leave trace
Vesicles	Round, small spots, filled with fluid, usually white, shaped like grains of rice, or sometimes like pearls; can be felt on palpation	Chest, abdomen, axillae, neck. Seldom on limbs	Leave trace

BOX 21.5 DRY SKIN

- Dark: Kidney deficiency
- Liver- and Kidney-Yin deficiency
- Stomach-Yin deficiency
- Chronic Blood stasis

Greasy skin

Symptoms and Signs, Chapter 77

Greasy skin is always due either to Dampness or Phlegm. The greasy skin from Phlegm is usually accompanied also by a certain 'puffiness' of the skin.

Swelling of the skin

Observation, Chapter 18; Interrogation, Chapter 39; Symptoms and Signs, Chapter 64

Swelling of the skin may be due to accumulation of fluids under the skin as in oedema, stagnation of Qi or Dampness. Excluding the swelling due to Dampness, there are two main types of oedema: 'Water oedema' (*Shui Zhong*) and 'Qi Oedema' (*Qi Zhong*).

Water oedema is due to accumulation of fluids in the space between the skin and muscles usually from a dysfunction of the Lungs (not diffusing fluids), Spleen (not transforming fluids) and Kidneys (not transforming and excreting fluids). With Water oedema, there is pitting. Usually a distinction is made between Yang Water oedema, which has an acute onset, is of external origin and affects the top part of the body (usually with involvement of the Lungs), and Yin Water oedema, which has a slow onset, is of internal origin and affects the middle and lower parts of the body (usually with involvement of the Spleen and Kidneys).

Qi oedema is due to Qi stagnation in the space between the skin and muscles and there is no pitting on pressure. It may also be due to Dampness or Phlegm obstructing the space between the skin and muscles and impairing the Spleen's transformation and transportation of fluids, in which case there may be pitting.

There is a third, less common, type of skin swelling due to Blood stasis; this is called **Blood oedema**. In this case, the skin is swollen, dark, purple and without lustre. This swelling is often associated with joint pain.

BOX 21.6 OEDEMA

- Water oedema: Lung, Spleen and Kidney deficiency
- Qi oedema: Qi stagnation, Dampness or Phlegm
- Blood oedema: Blood stasis

Box 21.6 summarizes the patterns underlying skin oedema.

Scales

A scale, called *Lin Xiao* in Chinese, is an accumulation of thickened, horny-layer keratin in the form of readily detached fragments. Scales usually indicate an inflammatory change and thickening of the epidermis. They may be fine, as in pityriasis, white and silvery, as in psoriasis, or large and resembling fish scales, as in ichthyosis. (See Plate 21.7 on p. P10.)

In chronic skin diseases, dry scales are usually due to deficient and dry Blood giving rise to Wind; it should be noted here that 'Wind' in the context of skin diseases is different from external Wind or Internal Wind. In acute or subacute skin diseases, scales may be due to Heat and will therefore also appear in Damp-Heat. One should not assume that scales cannot appear when there is Dampness: eczema is a typical example of this situation. Oily scales are due to accumulation of Damp-Heat.

Erosion of the skin

Skin erosion is a superficial break in the epidermis, not extending into the dermis, which heals without scarring. Erosion is often seen after the appearance of vesicles or pustules.

Red erosion with oozing of a yellow fluid indicates Damp-Heat. Erosion with exudate of thick yellow fluid indicates Damp-Heat with Toxic Heat. Erosion with oozing of thin-watery fluids indicates Dampness with underlying Spleen deficiency.

BOX 21.7 SCALES AND EROSION

Scales
- Dry: deficiency and Dryness of Blood with Wind
- Red: Heat or Damp-Heat
- Oily: Damp-Heat

Erosion of skin
- Erosion with oozing of yellow fluid: Damp-Heat
- Erosion with exudate of thick yellow fluid: Damp-Heat with Toxic Heat
- Erosion with oozing of thin watery fluid: Dampness with Spleen-Qi deficiency

Box 21.7 summarizes the patterns underlying scales and erosion.

Rashes

A rash, called *Zhen* in Chinese, is a redness of the skin caused by vasodilatation. The Western medical name is erythema. The main rashes to be differentiated are measles, German measles, chickenpox and urticaria.

Measles (morbillus), called 'Hemp Rash' (*Ma Zhen*) in Chinese, once a common childhood infection, is now rare in developed countries but in developing countries is still common and still a major cause of child mortality.

German measles (rubella), called 'Wind Rash' (*Feng Zhen*) in Chinese, is a common childhood infection with a benign course.

Chickenpox (varicella), called 'Water Pox' (*Shui Dou*) in Chinese, is a common childhood infection characterized by Dampness.

The differentiation of the rash in these three diseases is made in Table 21.3.

Fissures

A fissure (or crack) is a linear split in the epidermis, often just extending into the dermis. From the Chinese point of view, fissures are due to a disharmony of Qi and Blood, Blood deficiency or Kidney-Yin deficiency.

Skin ulcers

Western pathology and diagnosis

An ulcer is a circumscribed area of skin loss extending through the epidermis into the dermis. Ulcers are usually the result of impairment of the vascular nutrient supply to the skin, often caused by peripheral arterial disease. Ulcer formation is preceded by itching, pain, erythema, oedema, breakage of the skin and oozing. When the ulcer is formed, there is loss of epidermis; as the ulcer progresses, the opening becomes wider and deeper. (See Plates 21.8 and 21.9 on pp. P10 and P11.)

Chinese pathology and diagnosis

In Chinese medicine two types of ulcers are differentiated: *Yang* ulcers have edges that protrude clearly, are clearly defined and are shaped like a basin; *Yin* ulcers do not have protruding edges, they are shallower, their edges are not clearly defined and there is more oozing. Yang ulcers are predominantly caused by a Full condition and have a better prognosis than Yin ulcers, which are characterized by a mixture of Deficiency and Excess.

The main patterns giving rise to ulcers are accumulation of Damp-Heat, Spleen-Qi deficiency with Dampness, Qi stagnation and Blood stasis and Liver- and Kidney-Yin deficiency.

Ulcers caused by Damp-Heat are characterized by hardened and rounded edges and oozing of a thick yellow fluid.

Ulcers caused by Spleen-Qi deficiency with Dampness are characterized by a greyish-white tissue inside the ulcer and oozing of a clear fluid.

Ulcers caused by Qi stagnation and Blood stasis are characterized by surrounding skin swelling with a purple colour, pain and varicosities.

Ulcers caused by Liver- and Kidney-Yin deficiency are characterized by deep-red surrounding skin and absence of pain.

Box 21.8 summarizes the patterns underlying ulcers.

Table 21.3 Differentiation of measles, German measles and chickenpox

	Measles	German measles	Chickenpox
General symptoms	High fever, cough, listlessness	Low fever, child not so ill, swelling of glands behind ears	Low fever, child not so ill
Onset of rash	Appears gradually, about 3 days after onset	Appears rather suddenly, complete in 24 hours	Appears after 1–2 days
Colour of rash	Dark red	Pale red	White, red around
Shape of papules	Protruding papules, large or small, first loosely distributed, then dense, no itching	Papules small, round, loosely and evenly distributed, itching	Round, ranging in size from rice grain to bean, filled with fluid
Distribution of rash	First behind ears and neck, then face, trunk and limbs. Also hands and feet. Rash densely distributed	First on face, then trunk, limbs, not on hands and feet. They can go quickly	On face, trunk, limbs, very few on hands and feet
Marks	Leaves mark	No mark	Leaves concavities

BOX 21.8 SKIN ULCERS

- Hardened with round edges and oozing of thick yellow fluids: Damp-Heat
- Greyish-white tissue and oozing of clear fluid: Spleen-Qi deficiency with Dampness
- Swelling of surrounding skin, purple colour, pain and varicosities: Qi stagnation or Blood stasis
- Deep-red surrounding skin, no pain: Liver- and Kidney-Yin deficiency

---

Dermographism

Dermographism (literally meaning 'writing on the skin') indicates the red wheals that may appear when the skin is stroked with a hard object such as the end of a pencil or a nail. From the Western point of view, this is due to the exaggerated release of histamine from the mast cells in the skin; this occurs in atopic individuals and is due to the presence of abnormal levels of immunoglobulin E (IgE) around the mast cells of the skin. (See Plate 21.10 on p. P11.)

From a Chinese perspective, dermographism indicates the presence of Wind in the skin, often Wind-Heat. If the patient suffers from atopic eczema, it indicates that Wind-Heat predominates; if the patient suffers from allergic asthma, it indicates that there is Wind and Heat in the Lungs.

SKIN DISEASES

Eczema

Symptoms and Signs, Chapters 77, 89

Western pathology and diagnosis

Eczema is the commonest skin disease seen in practice. In the UK, eczema and acne make up the highest proportion of skin diseases while, in general practice, eczema accounts for 30% of patients presenting with a skin problem. A complete discussion of the aetiology and pathology of eczema (both from a Western and a Chinese point of view) is beyond the scope of this book and I will concentrate on the diagnostic aspects, that is, how to recognize eczema and differentiate between it and other skin diseases. This is not a simple task since there are very many different types of eczema presenting in many different ways. In Western medicine, the term 'dermatitis' is generally now preferred to that of 'eczema'.

The most commonly seen eczema in practice is atopic eczema in children and babies. In babies, there is usually an exudative, vesicular rash on the face and hands. After 18 months, the pattern changes to the familiar involvement of the elbow and knee creases, neck, wrists and ankles. The face often shows erythema and infraorbital folds. Lichenification (from scratching), excoriation and dry skin are common and palmar markings are increased. Scratching and rubbing cause most of the clinical signs.

In adults, the commonest manifestation is hand dermatitis, exacerbated by irritants and with a past history of atopic eczema. A small number of adults have a chronic, severe form of generalized and lichenified atopic eczema. Exacerbations are often elicited by stress.

It should be remembered that many acute, sudden exacerbations are due to skin infection from *Staphylococcus aureus* rather than the eczema itself: skin infections in eczema are common as the skin is excoriated and therefore prone to invasion of bacteria. An acute infection is characterized by sudden aggravation of the eczema, papular or pustular rash and pronounced erythema. (See Plates 21.11–21.20 on pp. P11–P13.)

Chinese pathology and diagnosis

The modern Chinese name for eczema is 'Damp Rash' (*Shi Zhen*) clearly indicating the idea that Dampness is always present in eczema.

!

Remember: in eczema, there is *always* Dampness, even if the skin is not oozing.

Acute eczema is characterized by intense itching, vesicles, erythema (redness), swelling of the skin. Chronic eczema is characterized by itching, erythema, swelling of the skin, crusting, scaling, lichenification (thickening of the skin with increased skin markings), excoriation, and erosion. Chronic eczema may be weeping or dry: weeping eczema indicates the predominance of Dampness, whereas dry eczema indicates the predominance of Heat. However, it should be remembered that in eczema there is always some Dampness as there are always fluid-filled vesicles under the epidermis (which causes the swelling of the skin); when these vesicles come to the surface, the eczema weeps. Furthermore, in atopic dermatitis the superficial stratum corneum of the skin is damaged so that the

skin cannot hold moisture properly; this means that the skin becomes dry as a consequence rather than as a cause of the eczema.

The main pattern seen in atopic eczema is Damp-Heat with one or the other factor predominant (see above). In chronic eczema in adults, there is also Damp-Heat, but the the condition is characterized by Empty conditions as well and primarily a Spleen deficiency and a Blood deficiency and Dryness, with Blood failing to nourish the skin. Itching is caused by the Dampness or, in chronic cases, by the Wind generated by the Blood deficiency.

Wind also plays a role in chronic eczema in combination with Damp-Heat. Wind will manifest with the location of the rash on the upper part of the body and with intense itching. If the eczema is concentrated in the lower part of the body, this indicates the prevalance of Dampness. In chronic eczema in adults, Wind is also generated by the deficiency and Dryness of the Blood.

If the skin oozes a yellow fluid, it indicates the prevalence of Damp-Heat, while if it oozes a clear fluid, it indicates Dampness against a background of Spleen deficiency. If the skin oozes after scratching it also indicates Dampness, while if it bleeds after scratching, it indicates Blood-Heat. If the skin oozes a thick, sticky yellow fluid, it may indicate the possibility of a skin infection from *S. aureus*; this is a common complication of eczema.

Case history 21.1 illustrates a pattern underlying dry eczema.

Box 21.9 summarizes the patterns underlying eczema.

Acne

Observation, Chapter 5; Symptoms and Signs, Chapters 55 and 77

Western pathology and diagnosis

Acne is a chronic inflammation of the pilosebaceous units, producing comedones, then papules, pustules or cysts, and eventually possible scars. Acne has an equal sex incidence but tends to affect women earlier than men, although the peak age for clinical acne is 18 years in both sexes.

As for the clinical presentation, comedones are either open (blackheads, which are dilated pores with black plugs of melanin-containing keratin) or closed (whiteheads, which are small, cream-coloured, dome-shaped papules). They appear at about the age of 12 years and evolve into inflammatory papules, pustules or cysts. The sites of predilection (face, shoulders, back and upper chest) have many sebaceous glands. The severity of acne depends on its extent and the type of lesion, with cysts being the most destructive. Scars

Case history 21.1

A 29-year-old woman had been suffering from atopic eczema since she was a few months old. The manifestations were typical of atopic eczema manifesting with a dry red rash, scaliness, thickening of the skin and intense itching. The location of the eczema was confined to the top part of the body. The eczema became worse during a pregnancy and after childbirth. Her eczema was also aggravated with cyclical regularity every 7 years. Her tongue was slightly Red, with red points on the front part, a Stomach crack and not enough tongue coating. Her pulse was very Weak on the right Front position and Overflowing on the left at the middle level.

She was very thin and restless, tapping her fingers on the table as she talked.

Diagnosis: The immediate presenting pattern of the eczema is Empty-Heat in the Blood with Wind-Heat in the skin. The Empty-Heat in the Blood is manifested by the red, dry rash and the tongue being Red without enough coating; the Wind-Heat is manifested by the intense itching and the location of the eczema on the top part of the body. There is also a Yin deficiency of the Lungs and Stomach manifested by the Stomach crack and Weak pulse on the right Front position. The Yin deficiency is also manifested by the thin body and by her restless behaviour, tapping her fingers on the table as she talks.

Underlying this, there is also a deficiency of the Defensive-Qi systems of the Lungs and Kidneys and especially of the Lungs; this is manifested by the Weak pulse on the right Front position and by the aggravation of the eczema during pregnancy and after childbirth. An interesting feature of this case is the cyclical aggravation of the eczema every 7 years, which is in perfect accordance with the Chinese view on 7-year cycles in a woman's life as described in the first chapter of the 'Simple Questions'.

BOX 21.9 ECZEMA

- Weeping eczema: Damp-Heat with predominance of Dampness
- Dry eczema: Damp-Heat with predominance of Heat
- Chronic eczema in adults: Damp-Heat with Spleen-Qi deficiency and Blood deficiency
- Itchy eczema: Dampness or Wind generated by Blood deficiency
- Eczema in upper part of body: Damp-Heat with Wind
- Eczema in lower part of the body: Damp-Heat with prevalence of Dampness
- Skin oozing a clear fluid: Dampness with Spleen deficiency
- Oozing a yellow fluid: Damp-Heat
- Oozing a thick, sticky yellow fluid: possibly infection of skin
- Oozing a fluid after scratching: Dampness
- Bleeding after scratching: Blood-Heat

BOX 21.10 ACNE

- Whiteheads and blackheads on the forehead, nose, upper back and chest: Lung-Heat
- Whiteheads and blackheads around the mouth, on the chest and upper back: Stomach-Heat
- Red papules around the nose, mouth and eyebrows, worse before/during menstruation: Blood-Heat
- Painful pustules, inflamed cysts on upper back and chest: Toxic Heat
- Deep, painful, inflamed nodules, pus-filled cysts, pitting and scarring: Damp-Heat with Toxic Heat and Blood stasis
- Long-lasting papules which take a long time to resolve: Lung- and Spleen-Qi deficiency often combined with Dampness

---

Box 21.10 summarizes the patterns underlying acne.

may follow healing especially of cysts. (See Plates 21.21–21.24 on pp. P13 and P14.)

Psoriasis

Symptoms and Signs, Chapter 77

Chinese pathology and diagnosis

From the Chinese perspective, the main causes of acne are:

- **Lung-Heat**: this is characterized by papular whiteheads and blackheads usually on the forehead, around the nose and on the upper back and chest.
- **Stomach-Heat**: this is characterized by papular whiteheads and blackheads usually around the mouth and on the chest and upper back.
- **Blood-Heat**: this is characterized by red papules usually around the nose, mouth and eyebrows. This type of acne is often worse before and during menstruation.
- **Toxic Heat**: this is characterized by pustules which may be painful. It may also manifest with inflamed cysts. The most frequently affected sites are the upper back and chest.
- **Damp-Heat with Toxic Heat and Blood stasis**: this is characterized by deep, painful, inflamed nodules and pus-filled cysts. This type usually leaves pitting and scarring.
- **Lung- and Spleen-Qi deficiency**: this is often an underlying condition combined with Dampness and characterized by long-lasting papules which take a long time to resolve.

Western pathology and diagnosis

Psoriasis is a chronic, non-infectious, inflammatory dermatosis characterized by well-demarcated erythematous plaques topped by silvery scales. The peak onset of psoriasis is in the second and third decades. It is unusual in children under 8 years of age.

About 35% of patients show a family history of the disease. There is a 25% probability that if one of a child's parents has psoriasis the child will be similarly affected, but this increases to 60% if both parents have psoriasis.

Psoriasis's appearance ranges from the typical chronic plaques involving the elbows to the acute, generalized pustular form. There are many different types of psoriasis:

- **Plaque**: this consists in well-defined, disc-shaped plaques involving elbows, knees, scalp or hair margin.
- **Guttate**: this is an acute symmetrical eruption of 'drop-like' lesions usually on the trunk and limbs. This form usually affects adolescents or young adults and may follow a streptococcal throat infection.
- **Flexural**: this affects the flexures of the axillae, the areas under the breasts and groin. It is usually seen in the elderly.

- **Localized**: localized psoriasis may be seen on palms and soles, fingers and nails, scalp.
- **Generalized pustular**: this is a rare type of psoriasis characterized by pustules all over the body. Sheets of small, sterile, yellowish pustules develop on an erythematous background and may spread rapidly. The onset is often acute and the patient is unwell, with fever and malaise.
- **Nails**: thimble pitting is the commonest change in this type of psoriasis, followed by separation of the distal edge of the nail from the nail bed. There is subungual hyperkeratosis with a build-up of keratin beneath the distal edge of the nail, mostly affecting the toenails.
- **Psoriatic arthritis**: this is an autoimmune disease characterized by the simultaneous occurrence of psoriasis and arthritis which resembles rheumatoid arthritis.

Another diagnostic sign of psoriasis is the Auspitz's sign – that is, scraping of the superficial scales will typically reveal tiny bleeding points.

As there are many types of psoriasis, other skin diseases may easily be wrongly diagnosed as psoriasis. Table 21.4 illustrates the differential diagnosis of the most common types of psoriasis (i.e. for each type of psoriasis, the table lists other skin diseases which may look like psoriasis). Although Chinese medicine treats skin diseases primarily according to the presenting pattern and not according to the type of skin disease, in the particular case of psoriasis it is important to differentiate it from other diseases because of its prognosis; psoriasis is usually more difficult to treat. (See Plates 21.25–21.31 on pp. P14–P16.)

Table 21.4 Differential diagnosis of various types of psoriasis

Type of psoriasis	Differential diagnosis
Plaque psoriasis	Psoriasiform drug eruption
Palmoplantar psoriasis	Hyperkeratotic eczema, Reiter's disease
Scalp psoriasis	Seborrhoeic dermatitis
Guttate psoriasis	Pityriasis rosea
Flexural psoriasis	Candidiasis of the flexures
Nail psoriasis	Fungal infection of the nails

Chinese pathology and diagnosis

The patterns causing psoriasis are:

- **Blood-Heat**: this is characterized by red macules or papules that increase and proliferate rapidly. Red scales pile up and are easily shed when scratched.
- **Blood deficient and dry**: this is characterized by pale and very dry plaques which are covered by a thin layer of white scales. The course of the disease is slow with new lesions appearing sporadically.
- **Blood stasis**: this is characterized by dark-purple plaques covered by thick scales. In chronic psoriasis only, lichenification may appear.
- **Damp-Heat**: this is characterized by dark-red macules or papules covered by greasy or thick, crust-like scales. The skin weeps. There may also be pustules. The sites affected are usually the palms, soles and skin flexures.
- **Toxic Heat**: this is characterized by erythematous or pustular lesions which develop and spread rapidly, often piling up together. There are red scales that shed easily and there is itching, burning and pain.
- **Liver- and Kidney-Yin deficiency**: this is characterized by pale-red macules covered by a thin layer of greyish-white scales. A chronic condition, it is usually seen in the elderly.

BOX 21.11 PSORIASIS

- Red macules or papules with red scales that shed when scratched: Blood-Heat
- Pale, very dry plaques with a thin layer of white scales, new lesions appearing sporadically: Blood deficient and dry
- Dark-purple plaques with thick scales, lichenification in chronic psoriasis: Blood stasis
- Dark-red macules or papules with greasy or thick, crust-like scales, weeping skin, possibly pustules, on palms, soles and skin flexures: Damp-Heat
- Erythematous/pustular lesions spreading rapidly, with red scales that shed easily, itching, burning and pain: Toxic Heat
- Chronic pale-red macules with a thin layer of greyish-white scales (elderly): Liver- and Kidney-Yin deficiency

In addition to the above patterns, there is also nearly always Wind in psoriasis. Wind causes intense itching and also dryness: thus, it is important to remember that Dryness is not always a symptom of Blood deficiency.

Box 21.11 summarizes the patterns underlying psoriasis.

Urticaria

Symptoms and Signs, Chapter 77

Western pathology and diagnosis

Urticaria is a skin eruption characterized by transient, itchy wheals due to acute, dermal oedema. The cause is an allergic reaction. The lesions result when mast cells release histamine, which produces vasodilatation and the characteristic wheals.

Urticaria can be acute or chronic. Acute urticaria is typically due to an IgE-mediated type I reaction. The allergen is usually a food (e.g. shellfish or peanuts) or a drug. In some cases urticaria may also be due to insect stings or bites, desensitizing injections or inhalants such as pollen, moulds or animal dander. Some women develop urticaria during menstruation. Acute urticaria normally manifests with a sudden onset of red and very itchy wheals which rapidly spread all over the body. The lesions may be small or may enlarge to as much as 20 cm across. Chronic urticaria is characterized by pale-red or pink itchy wheals which typically last less than 24 hours and disappear without a trace. Often no allergen can be identified. Urticaria may also be caused by exposure to cold, heat or sun. (See Plates 21.32 and 21.33 on p. P16.)

Chinese pathology and diagnosis

In Chinese medicine, urticaria is called *Feng Yin Zhen*, which means 'Wind hidden rash'. In both acute and chronic urticaria, there is usually always an underlying pattern of Wind in the skin. A very common pattern, 'Wind' in the skin, manifests primarily with intense itching, either all over the body or moving from place to place, and in chronic cases, such as psoriasis, with Dryness of the skin; just as wind, in nature, dries up the soil, Wind in the skin may dry up the skin in chronic cases. Wind in the skin is neither an external type of Wind (because it does not cause exterior symptoms, such as aversion to cold, or fever) nor an internal type of Wind (because it does not cause tremors or paralysis).

In acute urticaria, Wind, especially Wind-Heat, predominates. It causes intense itching with sudden onset, and red wheals spreading rapidly; the more intense the itching, the stronger the Wind. In chronic urticaria, Wind may be combined with a Stomach and Spleen deficiency and Dampness, which usually makes the patient prone to food allergies. In this case, the wheals may exude a clear fluid, the itching is less intense and the wheals come and go with a chronic course. In chronic cases, Wind in the skin frequently occurs as a result of deficiency and Dryness of Blood; in such cases, the wheals may be pale red and the itching is less intense than in acute urticaria. This condition is more common in women and may be associated with menstruation or arise after childbirth.

Both acute and chronic urticaria may be accompanied by Blood-Heat, in which case the wheals are very large and bright red and, besides itching, the patient has an intense feeling of heat and the skin is very hot to the touch. Finally, chronic urticaria may be complicated by Blood stasis, in which case the wheals are purple and may last a long time.

Box 21.12 summarizes the patterns underlying urticaria.

BOX 21.12 URTICARIA

- Intense itching, sudden onset, red wheals which spread rapidly: Wind-Heat
- Wheals exuding a clear fluid, less intense itching, coming and going: Wind, Stomach- and Spleen-Qi deficiency, Dampness
- Pale red wheals, less intense itching: deficiency and Dryness of Blood
- Large, bright-red wheals, itching, feeling of heat, skin hot to touch: Blood-Heat
- Purple wheals which last a long time: Blood stasis

Naevi

Symptoms and Signs, Chapter 77

Western pathology and diagnosis

A naevus is a benign proliferation of one or more of the normal constituent cells of the skin. Naevi may be present at birth or may develop later. The most common naevi are those containing a benign collection of melanocytic naevus cells, commonly known as moles.

A differentiation between moles and other types of skin lesions is given in Table 21.5. (See Plate 21.34 on p. P17.)

Table 21.5 Differentiation of naevi

Lesion	Distinguishing features
Freckle	Tan-coloured macules on sun-exposed sites
Lentigo	Usually multiple with onset in later life
Seborrhoeic wart	Stuck-on appearance, warty lesions, easily confused with moles
Haemangioma	Vascular but may show pigmentation
Dermatofibroma	On legs, firm and pigmented
Pigmented, basal cell carcinoma	Often on face, pearly edge, increase in size, may ulcerate
Malignant melanoma	Variable colour and outline, increase in size, may be inflamed or itchy

Chinese pathology and diagnosis

Moles which are present from birth are an inherited trait without any clinical significance. Moles that develop later in life generally indicate Liver-Blood Heat, Damp-Heat or Blood stasis (if they are dark).

Box 21.13 summarizes the patterns causing moles.

BOX 21.13 CHINESE PATHOLOGY OF MOLES

- Blood-Heat (Liver)
- Damp-Heat
- Blood stasis

Malignant melanoma

Symptoms and Signs, Chapter 77

Western pathology and diagnosis

Malignant melanoma is a malignant tumour of melanocytes, usually arising in the epidermis. It is the most lethal of the main skin tumours and has increased in incidence over the last few years. It is particularly common in Australia, accounting for 40% of common dermatological disorders (compared with 7% in the UK).

There are four main variants of malignant melanoma.

- **Superficial, spreading, malignant melanoma**: this is characterized by macules, particularly on the legs and more commonly in females (50% of UK cases). (See Plates 21.35 and 21.39 on p. P17 and P18.)
- **Nodular, malignant melanoma**: this is characterized by pigmented nodules which may grow rapidly and ulcerate (25% of UK cases). (See Plate 21.36 on p. P17.)
- **Lentigo, malignant melanoma**: this is characterized by dark macules, especially on the face and particularly in the elderly (15% of UK cases). (See Plate 21.37 on p. P17.)
- **Acral, lentiginous, malignant melanoma**: this is characterized by plaques particularly on palms and soles (10% of UK cases). (See Plate 21.38 on p. P18.)

Chinese pathology and diagnosis

In Chinese medicine, malignant melanomas are usually due to Blood-Heat and Blood stasis: the darker their colour, the more Blood stasis there is. The differentiation is also made on the basis of the skin lesion. Macules always indicate Blood-Heat with Blood stasis, plaques indicate Blood-Heat with Damp-Heat and nodules indicate Blood stasis.

Box 21.14 summarizes the patterns underlying malignant melanoma.

BOX 21.14 MELANOMA

- Macules: Blood-Heat with Blood stasis
- Plaques: Blood-Heat with Damp-Heat
- Nodules: Blood stasis

Tinea

Symptoms and signs, Chapter 77

Western pathology and diagnosis

The most common fungal infection is tinea. Tinea presents with disc-like lesions consisting of a clearly defined round erythema expanding outwards and often clearing in the centre; there is itching and some scaling. There are many types of tinea, including the following:

- **Tinea corporis** (of the body): this is characterized by single or multiple plaques with scaling and erythema, especially at the edges. The lesions enlarge slowly with central clearing, leaving a ring pattern, hence the name ringworm. (See Plates 21.40 and 21.41 on p. P18.) It may also manifest with pustules or vesicles.
- **Tinea manuum** (of the hand): this is characterized by a unilateral, diffuse, powdery scaling of the palm. (See Plate 21.42 on p. P18.)
- **Tinea capitis** (of the head): this is characterized by an inflamed, pustular swelling of the scalp. (See Plate 21.43 on p. P19.)
- **Tinea pedis** (athlete's foot): this is characterized by an itchy, interdigital maceration with vesicles. (See Plate 21.44 on p. P19.)
- **Tinea cruris** (of the groin): this is characterized by scaling and erythema in the groin area spreading to the upper thigh. (See Plate 21.45 on p. P19.)
- **Tinea unguium** (of the nails): this is characterized by separation of the nail from the nail bed, thickening and brittleness of the nail, which becomes yellow, and subungual hyperkeratosis.

Chinese pathology and diagnosis

From the Chinese point of view, tinea of the head may be due to Wind-Heat, Damp-Heat or Toxic Heat, while tinea of the other parts of the body is mostly due to Damp-Heat or Toxic Heat. When due to Wind-Heat, tinea affects the head and may move from place to place. When due to Damp-Heat, it is characterized by a red and moist rash with vesicles usually with a fixed location but spreading slowly. When due to Toxic Heat, it is characterized by an intensely red rash with red papules that spreads quickly.

Box 21.15 summarizes the pathology of tinea.

BOX 21.15 TINEA

- Tinea of head: Wind-Heat
- Red rash with vesicles: Damp-Heat
- Intensely red rash with papules: Toxic Heat

Candida

Symptoms and Signs, Chapter 77

Western pathology and diagnosis

Candida albicans is a physiological fungus which is found in the mouth and gastrointestinal tract; when it multiplies too rapidly it can produce opportunistic infections.

Predisposing factors include:

- moist skin folds
- obesity
- diabetes mellitus
- pregnancy
- poor hygiene
- humid environment
- wet work occupation
- use of broad-spectrum antibiotics
- excessive consumption of sugar

Infections by *Candida albicans* may affect the following areas:

- **Genitals**: this is characterized by itchiness, soreness and redness of the vulva and vagina in women ('thrush'). White plaques adhere to inflamed mucous membranes and a white vaginal discharge may occur. Men develop similar changes on the penis. Thrush can be spread by sexual intercourse.
- **Flexures**: this is characterized by a moist, glazed and macerated appearance of the flexures under the breasts in women, axilla, groin or between the fingers or toes.
- **Oral**: this is characterized by white plaques adhering to an erythematous mouth mucosa. It is often caused by use of broad-spectrum antibiotics.
- **Systemic**: this is characterized by red nodules on the skin; it occurs in immunosuppressed patients such as those suffering from AIDS or those undergoing long-term corticosteroid therapy.

(See Plates 21.46 and 21.47 on p. P19.)

Chinese pathology and diagnosis

From the Chinese point of view, fungal infections are usually caused by Dampness, which may be combined

with either Cold or Heat but more frequently with Heat. Acute fungal infections are usually due to Damp-Heat, whereas chronic fungal infections are characterized by Dampness but they always occur against a background of chronic Spleen-Qi deficiency. Candida infections of the gastrointestinal system often manifest on the tongue with small, peeled patches with a white ring around them and a white-sticky coating in between.

Herpes simplex

Symptoms and Signs, Chapter 77

Herpes is a viral infection, of which there are two types: **herpes simplex**, which is due to infection from herpesvirex hominis, and **herpes zoster** (shingles), which is due to infection from varicella zoster.

Western pathology and diagnosis

Herpes simplex is a common, acute, vesicular eruption which is highly contagious. After the primary infection, the latent, non-replicating virus resides mainly within the dorsal root ganglia from where it can reactivate, invade the skin and cause recurrent lesions. There are two types of herpes simplex virus: type one is usually facial and type two usually genital. Type one infection manifests with vesicles on the lips and around the mouth; they quickly erode and are painful. The illness may be accompanied by fever, malaise and local lymphadenopathy. Type two infection usually occurs after sexual contact in young adults who develop acute vulvovaginitis, penile or perianal lesions.

Recurrent attacks are the hallmark of herpes simplex infection and they occur at a similar site each time, usually on the lips, face or genitals. (See Plates 21.48 and 21.49 on p. P20.) The outbreak of vesicles is often preceded by tingling or burning, crusts form within 48 hours and the infection fades after a week.

Chinese pathology and diagnosis

From the Chinese point of view, herpes simplex is nearly always characterized by Damp-Heat because vesicles by definition indicate Dampness. However, different types may be distinguished according to the manifestations and location of the lesions. Lesions occurring in the upper part of the body such as lips and mouth are due to a combination of Damp-Heat and Wind-Heat. Lesions which occur regularly and repeatedly around the mouth and on the lips may be

due to Damp-Heat in the Stomach and Spleen, while genital lesions are due to Damp-Heat mostly in the Liver channel. In the elderly, recurrent herpes simplex infections often occur against a background of Yin deficiency and Empty-Heat so that there is an underlying Empty-Heat, which predisposes the person to recurrent infection and Damp-Heat in the acute stages. If the eruptions become pustular or papular and are very painful, they indicate the presence of Toxic Heat as well as Damp-Heat.

BOX 21.16 HERPES SIMPLEX

- Lesions in upper body: Damp-Heat with Wind-Heat
- Lesions around mouth: Damp-Heat in Stomach and Spleen
- Genital lesions: Damp-Heat in Liver channel
- Recurrent infections (elderly): Damp-Heat with Yin deficiency and Empty-Heat
- Painful papular or pustular eruptions: Damp-Heat with Toxic Heat

---

Box 21.16 summarizes the patterns underlying herpes simplex.

Herpes zoster

Symptoms and Signs, Chapter 77

Western pathology and diagnosis

Herpes zoster is an acute vesicular eruption occurring in the dermatomal distribution caused by a recrudescence of the varicella zoster virus. It nearly always occurs in people who have had varicella (chickenpox). Pain, tenderness and tingling in the dermatome precedes the eruption by 3 to 5 days. Erythema and grouped vesicles follow, scattered within the dermatomal area. The vesicles become pustular and then form crusts, which separate in 2 to 3 weeks to leave scarring. Herpes zoster is normally unilateral and two-thirds of patients are over 50 years of age. (See Plate 21.50 on p. P20.)

Chinese pathology and diagnosis

From the Chinese point of view, herpes zoster is also always due to Damp-Heat because of its vesicular and erythematous eruption, but a further differentiation can be made according to the manifestations and location of the lesions. If the lesions are located in the thoracic or hypochondrial region, they are due to Damp-Heat in the Liver and Gall-Bladder channels.

Generally speaking, in lesions occurring in the neck and ophthalmic region (which is common in the elderly), in addition to Damp-Heat there is also Wind-Heat. Wind-Heat is also indicated if itching is very intense. If the lesions are pustular, they indicate the presence of Toxic Heat; if they are dark and very painful, they indicate Blood stasis, which also is common in the elderly.

Box 21.17 summarizes the pattern underlying herpes zoster.

BOX 21.17 HERPES ZOSTER

- Lesions in trunk: Damp-Heat in Liver and Gall-Bladder
- Lesions on neck and around eyes, itchy: Damp-Heat with Wind-Heat
- Papules or pustules: Toxic Heat
- Dark and painful papules: Blood stasis (in addition to Toxic Heat)

Warts

Symptoms and signs, Chapter 77

Western pathology and diagnosis

Warts are common and benign, cutaneous tumours due to infection of epidermal cells with human papilloma virus (HPV). The virus infects by direct inoculation and is caught by touch, sexual contact or in swimming pools.

Common warts present as dome-shaped papules or nodules, usually on the hands or feet. (See Plate 21.51 on p. P20.)

Plane warts are smooth, flat-topped papules often slightly brown in colour, commonest on the face and hands. (See Plate 21.52 on p. P21.)

Plantar warts are seen in children and adolescents on the soles of the feet.

Genital warts affect the penis in males and the vulva and vagina in women. (See Plate 21.53 on p. P21.) The warts present as small papules.

Chinese pathology and diagnosis

From the Chinese point of view, common, plane and plantar warts are usually due to a combination of Blood deficiency and Dryness, Blood-Heat and Blood stasis depending on whether the warts are pale and dry, red or dark brown. Genital warts are usually due to Damp-Heat in the Liver channel, which may be complicated also with Toxic Heat if the warts are pustular and painful.

Box 21.18 summarizes the pathology of warts.

BOX 21.18 WARTS

- Pale and dry: Blood deficient and dry
- Red: Blood-Heat
- Dark brown: Blood stasis
- Genital: Damp-Heat in Liver channel
- Painful, pustular: Toxic Heat

Rosacea

Symptoms and Signs, Chapter 77

Western pathology and diagnosis

Rosacea is a chronic, inflammatory, facial dermatosis characterized by erythema and pustules. The earliest symptom of rosacea is usually flushing of the cheeks which is followed by erythema, telangiectasia (dilated dermal blood vessel), papules and pustules. Rosacea lacks the comedones of acne and occurs in an older age group. (See Plates 21.54 and 21.55 on p. P21.)

Chinese pathology and diagnosis

From the Chinese point of view, rosacea may be due to the following patterns:

- **Heat in the Lungs and Stomach**: this is characterized by a red, papular rash of the cheeks.
- **Toxic Heat**: this is characterized by a red, pustular rash of the cheeks with swelling of the nose.
- **Blood-Heat**: this is characterized by a red, papular rash of the cheeks often aggravated before or during the menstrual cycle.
- **Blood stasis**: this is characterized by a dark-red or reddish-purple papular or pustular rash of the cheeks and nose.

Box 21.19 summarizes the pathology of rosacea.

BOX 21.19 ROSACEA

- Red, papular rash on cheeks: Lung- and Stomach-Heat
- Red, pustular rash of the cheeks with swelling of nose: Toxic Heat
- Red, papular rash on the cheeks aggravated during the period in women: Blood-Heat
- Dark-red or reddish-purple papular or pustular rash of the cheeks and nose: Blood stasis

NOTES

1. *Cou Li* (腠里 **)** is a difficult term to translate and one that is interpreted differently by modern Chinese doctors. *Cou* indicates 'spaces' or 'interstices' and it refers to all the spaces in the body, especially the small spaces (as opposed to large cavities such as the chest and abdomen) all over the body, including the space between skin and muscles, which is probably the most clinically relevant. *Li* means 'texture', 'grain' (as in the grain of wood) or 'pattern', and it indicates the texture of skin and the Internal Organs: it refers to the organized way in which the skin and organs are arranged, forming a 'texture' or 'pattern'. The 'Synopsis of Prescriptions from the Golden Cabinet' says: '*Cou is the place of the Triple Burner where the Original True [Essence] converges and Qi and Blood concentrate; Li is the texture of the skin and Internal Organs*' (He Ren 1981 A New Explanation of the Synopsis of Prescriptions from the Golden Cabinet *Jin Gui Yao Lue Xin Jie* 金匮要略新解), Zhejiang Science Publishing House, Beijing, p. 2). I translate *Cou Li* as 'space between skin and muscles'. Although this is not strictly accurate, because there are other spaces and because it ignores the *Li* part of it, it is the most clinically relevant. In the context of skin, therefore, *Cou Li* is the space between skin and muscles.
2. 1979 The Yellow Emperor's Classic of Internal Medicine – Simple Questions (*Huang Di Nei Jing Su Wen* 黄帝内经素问), People's Health Publishing House, Beijing, p. 70. First published c. 100BC.
3. 1981 Spiritual Axis (*Ling Shu Jing* 灵枢经), People's Health Publishing House, Beijing, p. 129. para 139. First published c. 100BC.
4. Clavey gives a different interpretation of the words *bie shi* (别使), which are usually translated as 'emissary' or 'special emissary'. According to him, the words should be translated as 'makes separate'. In other words, if this interpretation is correct, the Triple Burner separates the undifferentiated Original Qi and directs it into different channels and organs to perform its various functions. I personally feel that this interpretation is probably more correct. (Clavey, S. 1995 Fluid Physiology and Pathology in Traditional Chinese Medicine, Churchill Livingstone, Edinburgh, p. 21.)
5. Nanjing College of Traditional Chinese Medicine 1979 A Revised Explanation of the Classic of Difficulties (*Nan Jing Jiao Shi* 难经校释), People's Health Publishing House, Beijing, p. 144. First published c. AD100.
6. Spiritual Axis, p. 92.
7. Simple Questions, p. 353.
8. Spiritual Axis, p. 50.
9. Ibid., p. 37.
10. Ibid., p. 37.
11. The term *Cou Li* actually indicates more complex structures of the body and it includes all 'spaces' between organs and between channels: functionally, the *Cou Li* is connected to the Triple Burner. In this context, I will again translate it as 'space between skin and muscles' but the reader should bear in mind that this is only one of the *Cou Li* 'spaces'. Furthermore, while *cou* means 'spaces' or 'interstices', *li* means 'pattern' or 'texture' and it refers to the striae of the Internal Organs. I therefore translate *Cou Li* as 'space between skin and muscles' in the appropriate context, even though this is only one of the meanings of *Cou Li*. (See also Note 1 above.)

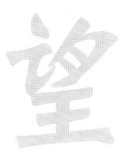

Chapter **22**

OBSERVATION IN CHILDREN

Chapter contents

INTRODUCTION   *191*

COMPLEXION   *191*
  Red   *191*
  Yellow   *191*
  Pale   *192*
  Bluish-greenish   *192*

ORIFICES   *192*
  Eyes   *192*
  Ears   *192*
  Nose   *192*
  Mouth   *193*
  Urethra and anus   *193*

BODY MOVEMENT   *194*

SPINAL MUSCLES   *194*

INDEX FINGER   *194*
  Veins on the index finger   *194*
  Creases on the index finger   *195*

ROOT OF THE NOSE   *199*

INTRODUCTION

Observation in children follows broadly the same rules as that of adults. There are, however, some items of observation which apply only to children. These are in particular:

- complexion
- orifices
- body movement
- spinal muscles
- index finger veins and creases
- root of the nose.

COMPLEXION

The characteristics of the normal complexion in children are the same as in adults, i.e. the complexion should be rosy and have proper depth, lustre and moisture.

Red

Children are prone to Heat conditions and a red complexion is fairly common. It always indicates Heat and may pertain to the Lungs, Stomach, Heart or Liver. In Lung-Heat the cheeks, in particular the right cheek, are red. Stomach-Heat is common in children and this may cause a redness on both cheeks, especially in the lower part.

Yellow

A yellow complexion always indicates a Stomach and Spleen disharmony, which may be a Stomach- and

Spleen-Qi deficiency (in which case the complexion would be pale yellow) or Dampness in the Stomach and Spleen (in which case the complexion would be bright yellow). A yellowish complexion in children may also indicate retention of food.

Pale

A pale complexion in children generally indicates Qi or Yang deficiency and usually of the Spleen or Lungs, or both.

Bluish-greenish

A bluish complexion indicates Cold or shock, while a greenish complexion indicates Wind or Pain. A greenish colour around the mouth usually indicates Liver-Wind (in children normally after a febrile disease), abdominal pain from Cold or Liver-Qi invading the Spleen. A bluish colour on the forehead pertains to the Heart and it indicates shock, while a bluish colour on both the forehead and chin in a baby may indicate pre-natal shock.

BOX 22.1 COMPLEXION COLOURS

- Red: Heat
- Right cheek red: Lung-Heat
- Both cheeks red: Stomach-Heat
- Pale yellow: Stomach- and Spleen-Qi deficiency
- Bright yellow: Dampness in Stomach and Spleen
- Dull yellow: retention of food
- Pale: Qi or Yang deficiency
- Bluish: cold or shock
- Greenish: Liver-Wind, abdominal pain from Cold, Liver-Qi invading the Spleen
- Bluish on the forehead: shock (heart)
- Bluish on the forehead and chin in a baby: prenatal shock

Box 22.1 summarizes the complexion colours.

ORIFICES

The orifices observed in children are the eyes, ears, nose, mouth, urethra and anus.

Eyes

A redness of the sclera indicates either external Wind-Heat or internal Heat. A yellowish colour of the sclera indicates Dampness, while a bluish-greenish colour of the sclera indicates Liver-Wind.

Streaming red eyes may indicate measles. Red and cracked corners of the eyes indicate Damp-Heat in the Intestines and retention of food.

'White membrane on the pupil in children' is called *Gan Yi* in Chinese, which means Childhood Nutritional Impairment Nebula; it consists of a white membrane covering the pupil, often starting with the symptom of decreased vision at night. As its name implies, it occurs in children suffering from nutritional impairment. A nebula is a translucent, greyish corneal haze, scarring or opacity. For a more detailed discussion of this sign, see Part 5, Chapter 61.

Box 22.2 summarizes the patterns underlying eye signs.

BOX 22.2 EYES

- Red eyes: Wind-Heat or internal Heat
- Yellowish eyes: Dampness
- Bluish-greenish eyes: Liver-Wind
- Streaming, red eyes: measles
- Red and cracked corners of the eyes: Damp-Heat in the Intestines
- White membrane on the pupil: Childhood Nutritional Impairment

---

Ears

Small and contracted ears indicate poor hereditary Kidney constitution. Redness at the back of the ears indicates Wind-Heat; if the body is also hot and the face red, it may indicate chickenpox. If the helix of the ear is bluish-greenish, it indicates either abdominal pain from Cold or Liver-Wind after a febrile disease.

Box 22.3 summarizes the patterns underlying ear signs.

BOX 22.3 EARS

- Small and contracted ears: poor hereditary Kidney constitution
- Redness at the back of the ears: Wind-Heat
- Body hot and face red: chickenpox
- Bluish-greenish helix: abdominal pain from Cold, Liver-Wind after febrile disease

---

Nose

A runny nose with white-watery discharge in acute cases indicates an invasion of Wind-Cold. If the discharge is yellowish, this indicates Wind-Heat. A white,

watery nasal discharge in a chronic condition indicates allergic rhinitis and it is due to Lung-Qi deficiency.

A blocked nose with difficulty in breathing generally indicates Dampness or Damp-Heat in the nose; this is very common in children and it is usually a residual pathogenic factor after repeated external invasions (especially when treated with antibiotics). A flapping of the nostrils in a child with fever indicates Phlegm-Heat in the Lungs and it is a relatively serious sign. Sweating on the nose in chronic conditions indicates Lung-Qi deficiency.

Box 22.4 summarizes the patterns underlying nose signs.

BOX 22.4 NOSE

- Runny nose with watery white discharge (acute): invasion of Wind-Cold
- Runny nose with yellowish discharge: Wind-Heat
- Runny nose with watery, white nasal discharge (chronic): allergic rhinitis due to Lung-Qi deficiency
- Blocked nose with breathing difficulty, especially in children: Dampness or Damp-Heat in the nose
- Flapping of the nostrils with fever (children): Phlegm-Heat in the Lungs
- Sweating on the nose (chronic): Lung-Qi deficiency

Mouth

Observation of the mouth includes observation of the lips, gums and throat.

The lips pertain to the Spleen and pale lips indicate Spleen-Qi deficiency whereas red lips indicate Heat in the Spleen and Heart. If the lips are dark and dry, this indicates a severe injury of Yin after a febrile disease.

Swollen and red gums indicate Stomach-Heat, retention of food or worms.

The throat should always be observed in children. In acute cases, a redness of the throat indicates Wind-Heat; in chronic cases, a redness of the throat is often due to Heat in the Stomach and Intestines.

Erosion, redness and swelling of the pharynx indicate Toxic Heat. This is seen more frequently in children suffering from acute upper respiratory infections.

Swollen tonsils of a normal colour indicate retention of Dampness or Phlegm occurring against a background of Qi deficiency. This is seen frequently in children with retention of a residual pathogenic factor (e.g. Dampness or Phlegm) after repeated acute upper respiratory infections.

A chronic swelling of the tonsils in children is often accompanied by a chronic swelling of the adenoids, itself also a sign of retention of residual Dampness or Phlegm.

Red and swollen tonsils indicate Heat or Toxic Heat often in the Stomach or Large Intestine channel, or both. The tonsils should always be inspected in acute invasions of Wind-Heat, particularly in children. Red and swollen tonsils are frequently seen in children during acute upper respiratory infections. During acute invasions of Wind-Heat, a swelling and redness of the tonsils indicates a more severe degree of Wind-Heat and often the presence of Toxic Heat; it also points to an involvement of the Stomach or Large Intestine channel, or both. It also tells us that the child probably has a pre-existing condition of Heat, often Stomach-Heat.

A chronic redness and swelling of the tonsils that comes and goes indicates either chronic Heat in the Stomach or Large Intestine channel, or both (more common in children and often due to a residual pathogenic factor), or Empty-Heat in the Lung channel. In Chinese medicine, a chronic redness and swelling of the tonsils was called 'milky moth' (*ru* 乳): the tonsils look like a moth's wings and have a milky fluid on them.

Red and swollen tonsils with exudate indicate Toxic Heat in the Stomach or Large Intestine channel, or both; they are usually seen during acute upper respiratory infections and are more common in children. Their presence definitely indicates an invasion of Wind-Heat (as opposed to Wind-Cold) and it indicates that it is complicated by Toxic Heat.

A swelling of the tonsils from Toxic Heat was called 'stone moth' (*shi e*): the two tonsils look like a moth's wings and have a stony hardness.

In any of the above pathologies of the tonsils, if both tonsils are affected, it generally indicates a greater severity than if only one is affected.

Box 22.5 summarizes patterns underlying signs in the mouth, lips, gums, throat and tonsils.

Urethra and anus

A yellowish and wet skin in the genital area indicates Damp-Heat. A persistent nappy (diaper) rash indicates Damp-Heat in the Liver channel. A sore and irritated anus may indicate worms, while itching in the anus at night may indicate pinworms.

> ## BOX 22.5 MOUTH, LIPS, GUMS, THROAT AND TONSILS
>
> - Pale lips: Spleen-Qi deficiency
> - Red lips: Spleen- and Heart-Heat
> - Dark and dry lips: severe injury of Yin
> - Swollen red gums: Stomach-Heat, Retention of food or worms
> - Red throat: Wind-Heat or Heat in Stomach and Intestines
> - Erosion, redness and swelling of the pharynx: Toxic Heat
> - Swollen tonsils: Dampness or Phlegm (background of Qi deficiency)
> - Red and swollen tonsils: Heat or Toxic Heat in the Stomach/Large Intestine
> - Red, swollen and purulent tonsils: Toxic Heat
> - On–off chronic redness and swelling of the tonsils: Heat in the Stomach/Large Intestine, Empty-Heat in the Lungs

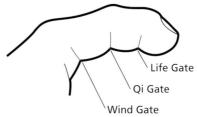

Fig. 22.1 Index finger Gates

BODY MOVEMENT

In general, the rules governing observation of children's body movements are the same as in adults. I will therefore highlight only the aspects that are peculiar to children.

The most important difference between adults and children is that it is normal for children to be much more active and to move around during a consultation. Apart from this, the same principles apply, that is, if the child is listless and excessively quiet it indicates Deficiency, while if the child moves around excessively and is hyperactive it indicates a Full condition. Full conditions which may cause excessive movement in children are Heat in the Stomach and Intestines, Heart-Fire or Liver-Fire.

When observing children's body movements, allowance should be made for any natural shyness of a child in the presence of a doctor: for example, a child may be shy and extremely quiet during the consultation but be a 'terror' at home!

SPINAL MUSCLES

Observation of the spinal muscles is carried out principally in babies. If the spinal muscles are very soft and flabby, this indicates a constitutional Spleen deficiency.

INDEX FINGER

Veins on the index finger

In children under 3 years, observation of the index finger is used for diagnosis of acute diseases. The three creases of the index finger are called Wind Gate, Qi Gate and Life Gate, starting from the proximal crease (Fig. 22.1). The left index finger is observed in boys and the right index finger in girls. Observation is carried out by rubbing the finger first and observing any veins appearing on the side of the finger.

Observation of the veins on the index finger in acute diseases in children under 3 years is carried out first of all to assess the seriousness of the condition. If any veins appearing on the finger extend just beyond the Wind Gate, this indicates that the pathogenic factor is in the Connecting channels only, it is relatively light and the condition is benign. If any veins appearing on the index finger extend just beyond the Qi Gate, the pathogenic factor is in the Main channels, it is deeper and the condition is more serious. If any veins on the finger extend just beyond the Life Gate, the pathogenic factor is in the Internal Organs, it is deep and the condition is life threatening.

The veins appearing on the index finger in young children should be differentiated according to the following criteria:

> - depth of colour
> - intensity of colour
> - actual colour
> - movement of veins
> - concentration of colour
> - length of veins
> - thickness.

Depth of colour

'Depth' of colour refers not to the shade but the visibility of the veins on the finger. If the veins are superficial and clearly visible on the surface, they indicate that the disease is on the Exterior and is of external origin; if they are deep and hidden, it indicates either that the disease is in the Interior and is of internal origin, or that an external pathogenic factor has become internal.

Intensity of colour

'Intensity' of colour refers to its 'thickness': if it is thin, the disease is benign; if it is 'thick', the disease is more severe. If the veins disappear easily on massaging the finger, this indicates Deficiency; if they do not disappear easily on massaging and look 'hidden', it indicates Excess.

Actual colour

The actual colour of the veins should be observed. Fresh-red veins indicate an external invasion of Wind-Cold or Wind-Heat, reddish-purple veins the presence of internal Heat, bluish-purple veins Wind-Heat, bluish veins a Liver-Wind condition, often with convulsions, light-red veins Empty-Cold, white veins Childhood Nutritional Impairment, yellow veins a Spleen condition, and dark-purple veins an obstruction of the Blood Connecting channels.

Movement of veins

The 'movement' of the veins refers to a vein that is relatively thick and pulsates strongly but not smoothly and looks congested. This may indicate a Full condition with strong pathogenic factors: stagnation of Qi and Blood, stagnation of Damp-Phlegm or retention of food.

Concentration of colour

Concentration of colour refers to the density of the colour of the veins: a concentrated colour is 'tightly packed' whereas a less concentrated one is more sparse.

The more concentrated the colour, the more severe the disease. The degree of concentration also indicates the character of the pattern – that is, a more concentrated colour indicates a Full condition and a sparse one an Empty condition.

Length of veins

The length of the veins should be observed: long veins indicate that the disease is progressing and short veins that the disease is retreating.

Thickness

The thickness of the veins should also be observed: thick veins indicate Heat and Full conditions, whereas thin veins indicate Cold and Empty conditions.

BOX 22.6 VEINS ON THE INDEX FINGER

Depth
- Superficial: Exterior disease
- Deep: Interior disease

Intensity
- Thin: benign disease
- Thick: severe disease
- Veins that disappear on massaging: Deficiency
- 'Hidden' veins that don't disappear: Excess

Colour
- Fresh-red: external Wind
- Reddish-purple: internal Heat
- Bluish-purple: Wind-Heat
- Bluish: Liver-Wind
- Light-red: Empty-Cold
- White: Childhood Nutritional Impairment
- Yellow: Spleen deficiency
- Dark-purple: Blood stasis

Movement
- Thick vein pulsating strongly: Full condition, strong pathogenic factors

Length
- Long: disease progressing
- Short: disease retreating

Thickness
- Thick: Heat, Full conditions
- Thin: Cold, Empty conditions

Box 22.6 summarizes patterns indicated by the index finger vein.

Creases on the index finger

The palmar surface of the index finger should be observed for creases. A round crease with a 'tail', called 'long pearl' in traditional Chinese medicine (Fig. 22.2), indicates Accumulation Disorder. A round crease without a tail, called 'flowing pearl', indicates internal Heat (Fig. 22.3).

A long crease which looks like a snake with its head on the distal end of the palmar surface of the index finger, called 'snake going away', indicates a digestive problem characterized by vomiting and diarrhoea (Fig. 22.4). A long crease which looks like a snake with

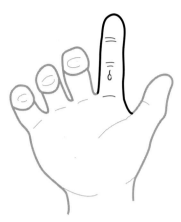

Fig. 22.2 'Long pearl' crease

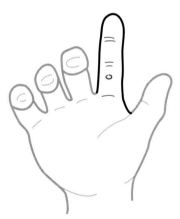

Fig. 22.3 'Flowing pearl' crease

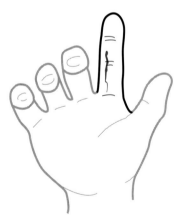

Fig. 22.4 'Snake going away' crease

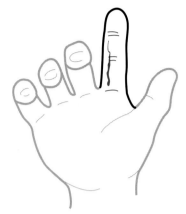

Fig. 22.5 'Snake returning' crease

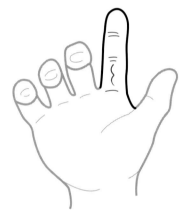

Fig. 22.6 'Bow facing inside' crease

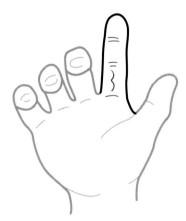

Fig. 22.7 'Bow facing outside' crease

its head on the proximal end of the palmar surface of the index finger, called 'snake returning', indicates Accumulation Disorder (Fig. 22.5).

A crease looking like a bow facing towards the middle finger, called 'bow facing inside', indicates an external invasion of Wind (Fig. 22.6). A crease

looking like a bow facing away from the middle finger, called 'bow facing outside', indicates Phlegm-Heat (Fig. 22.7).

A diagonal crease extending from the radial to the ulnar side with the upper part on the ulnar side indicates an external invasion of Wind-Cold (Fig. 22.8). A diagonal crease extending from the ulnar to the radial side with its upper part on the radial side indicates an external invasion of Cold (Fig. 22.9).

A straight crease which looks like a needle (Fig. 22.10) or, if longer, like a spear (Fig. 22.11), indicates Phlegm-Heat. A long, vertical crease extending through the whole index finger indicates an excess pattern of the Liver (often involving Liver-Wind) with severe Spleen deficiency (Fig. 22.12).

A curved crease indicates Liver-Wind (Fig. 22.13). A crease with its end shaped like a hook indicates deficiency of Yang of the Stomach and Spleen with internal Cold (Fig. 22.14). A curved crease with three bends that looks like a worm indicates Accumulation Disorder (Fig. 22.15). Three creases that resemble the

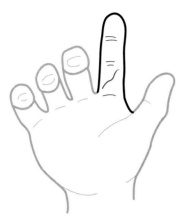

Fig. 22.8 Diagonal crease extending from the radial to the ulnar side

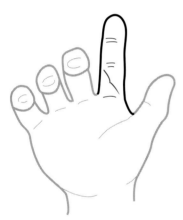

Fig. 22.9 Diagonal crease extending from the ulnar to the radial side

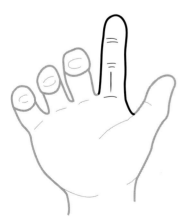

Fig. 22.10 'Needle' crease

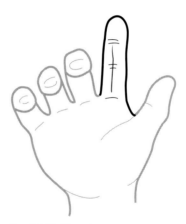

Fig. 22.11 'Spear' crease

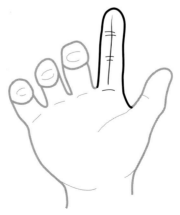

Fig. 22.12 Long, vertical crease

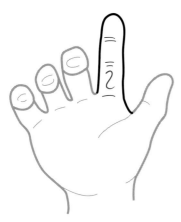

Fig. 22.13 Curved crease

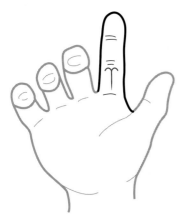

Fig. 22.14 Crease with end shaped like a hook

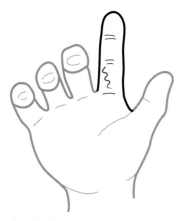

Fig. 22.15 'Worm' crease

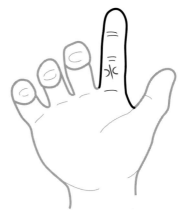

Fig. 22.16 Three creases

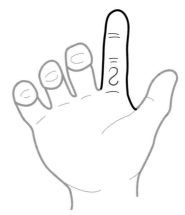

Fig. 22.17 S-shaped crease

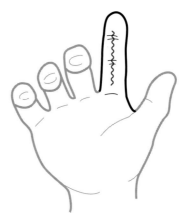

Fig. 22.18 'Fish-bone' crease

Chinese character for 'Water' (somewhat like two letters 'k' back to back) indicate chronic cough (Fig. 22.16). A curved crease which looks like an 's' indicates chronic vomiting and diarrhoea and Childhood Nutritional Impairment (Fig. 22.17).

A long crease that looks like a fish-bone indicates Liver-Wind and convulsions (Fig. 22.18). A crease

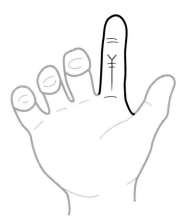

Fig. 22.19 Branching out crease

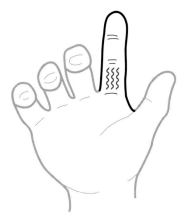

Fig. 22.20 Three irregular creases

dividing out into two small branches at its upper end also indicates Liver-Wind and convulsions (Fig. 22.19). Three squiggly creases indicate intestinal worms (Fig. 22.20).

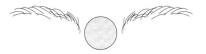

Fig. 22.21 The root of the nose area

ROOT OF THE NOSE

The root of the nose (the part of the nose between the eyes) can be used diagnostically in children under the age of 4 years. It reflects specifically the condition of the Stomach and Spleen (Fig. 22.21).

If the root of the nose is dark-greenish, it indicates retention of food or, in infants, problems with feeding and generally a Full condition.

If the root of the nose is light-greenish, it indicates digestive problems of an Empty nature. If there are bluish blood vessels on the root of the nose, it indicates abdominal pain due to retention of food or Cold.

Greenish maculae on the root of the nose indicate chronic diarrhoea from retention of food.

Box 22.7 summarizes patterns reflected by the root of the nose.

BOX 22.7 ROOT OF THE NOSE

- Dark greenish: retention of food
- Light greenish: Empty condition
- Bluish vessels: abdominal pain
- Greenish macules: chronic diarrhoea

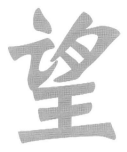

SECTION 3

TONGUE DIAGNOSIS

Section contents

23 Tongue diagnosis *203*
24 Tongue-body colour *209*
25 Tongue-body shape *215*
26 Tongue coating *221*
27 Tongue images and patterns *227*

INTRODUCTION

Tongue diagnosis is a very important part of diagnosis by observation. The strength of tongue diagnosis lies in its clarity and objectivity. Especially when compared with pulse diagnosis, tongue diagnosis is quite objective: when a tongue is too Red or too Pale, this can be observed objectively. Another important strength of tongue diagnosis is its capacity to shed light on complicated conditions. For example, a simultaneous deficiency of Kidney-Yin and Kidney-Yang is quite common in women over 40 and especially in menopausal women. This simultaneous deficiency can give rise to confusing hot and cold manifestations: the tongue will indicate quite clearly whether there is a predominance of Kidney-Yang or Kidney-Yin deficiency.

The principal aspects of tongue diagnosis are the tongue-body colour, the tongue-body shape and the coating. The tongue reflects the state of the Internal Organs and that of Qi and Blood. From the Eight-Principle point of view, it clearly reflects Heat–Cold, Full–Empty and Yin–Yang conditions.

For a more detailed discussion of tongue diagnosis see G Maciocia, 1995, 'Tongue Diagnosis in Chinese Medicine', Eastland Press, Seattle.

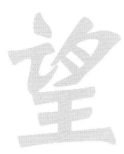

Chapter **23**

TONGUE DIAGNOSIS

Chapter contents

CONDITIONS FOR EXAMINING THE TONGUE   *203*
  Lighting   *203*
  Techniques of observation of the tongue   *203*
  External factors affecting the colour of the
    tongue   *204*

AREAS OF THE TONGUE   *204*

CLINICAL SIGNIFICANCE OF THE TONGUE   *206*
  Tongue-body colour   *206*
  Tongue-body shape   *206*
  Tongue coating   *206*
  Tongue spirit   *207*

CONDITIONS FOR EXAMINING THE TONGUE

Lighting

Proper lighting is absolutely essential for a correct examination of the tongue and the only good lighting is natural light on a sunny day. The room where the patient is examined should have an abundant source of natural light; for example, no proper natural light can ever be achieved in a basement. Even in daylight, the colour of the tongue can be interpreted properly indoors only if the day is sunny. On a cloudy day the colour of the tongue cannot be accurately observed indoors; if the patient is examined on such a day, it is advisable when observing the tongue to ask the patient to stand next to a window or even outdoors. Obviously, it is seldom possible to achieve ideal conditions. If it is necessary to observe the tongue on a cloudy day or in the afternoon or evening, I find that the best artificial light is that of a halogen bulb and the best way to observe the tongue is by means of a table lamp fitted with one of these bulbs.

Techniques of observation of the tongue

One should not ask the patient to hold the tongue out for longer than approximately 15 seconds because the longer the tongue is extended the darker it will tend to become. If we need longer than 15 seconds to observe the tongue, which we normally do, we should ask the patient to withdraw the tongue, close the mouth and extend the tongue again; this can be done several times without affecting its body colour.

It is very important to examine the tongue systematically following always the same order, which should be as follows:

- tongue-body colour
- tongue-body shape
- coating
- tongue spirit.

I would strongly recommend following this systematic order of observation of the tongue because the above order reflects the relative clinical importance of each item. For example, the tongue-body colour reflects conditions of Heat or Cold and deficiency of Yin or Yang in various organs, and especially the Yin organs; it should therefore be always the first aspect to be observed. The tongue-body shape often simply adds information to that gleaned from observation of the tongue-body colour; for example, if the tongue is Pale from Yang deficiency, its swelling will simply indicate that the Yang deficiency is particularly pronounced. The tongue coating reflects more the condition of the Yang organs and it is easily influenced by short-term factors, which makes it relatively less important than observation of the tongue-body colour in chronic conditions.

External factors affecting the colour of the tongue

The most obvious external factors affecting the colour of the tongue are highly coloured foods, sweets, drinks or pastilles. If a patient's tongue has a very obvious, unusual, bright colour, always ask what he or she has been eating.

Spicy foods such as cayenne pepper and curry may tend to make the tongue slightly redder soon after consumption. Tobacco smoking usually colours the coating yellow, and in regular smokers this is permanent. However, this cannot be written off as no more than a false appearance due to an external factor; in fact, tobacco, which has a hot energy, will tend to create Heat.

Medicines

Some medicines affect the appearance of the tongue and the most common ones are antibiotics. These tend to make the tongue partially peeled, that is, the loss of small patches of coating. Therefore, when I see such a tongue, the first thing I ask is whether the patient is on antibiotics or has taken them recently (Fig. 23.1). In my experience, the effect of the antibiotics on the tongue lasts for about 2 weeks after stopping the

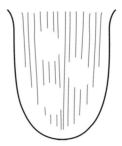

Fig. 23.1 Partially peeled tongue from antibiotics

course. Judging from the effects of antibiotics on the tongue, we can deduce that they injure Stomach-Yin.

Oral corticosteroids tend to make the tongue Red and Swollen, while inhaled bronchodilators (such as salbutamol) may cause the tip of the tongue to become Red, but only after many years of use.

Anti-inflammatory drugs such as phenylbutazone paradoxically cause the tongue to develop red points.

Most cytotoxic drugs used for cancer tend to create a very thick, dark-yellow or brown coating and also to make the tongue-body Red.

AREAS OF THE TONGUE

In men and women alike, the tongue-body can be divided into three areas: the rear corresponding to the Lower Burner, the middle to the Middle Burner and the front to the Upper Burner (Fig. 23.2).

Therefore, according to this division, the front third of the tongue reflects the state of the Heart and Lungs, the middle third that of the Stomach, Spleen, Liver and Gall-Bladder and the rear third that of the Kidneys, Bladder and Intestines. Figure 23.3 illustrates the areas corresponding to the Internal Organs in detail.

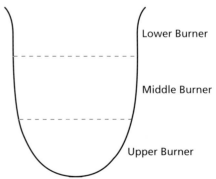

Fig. 23.2 Divisions of the tongue according to the Three Burners

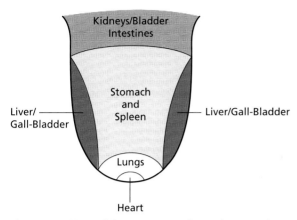

Fig. 23.3 Divisions of the tongue according to the Internal Organs

The relative position of the Heart and Lung areas on the tongue should be explained in relation to redness, swelling, cracks or Purple colour.

When there is Lung-Heat, this will make the whole front of the tongue Red *including* the Heart area (even though the Heat is only in the Lungs and not in the Heart) (Fig. 23.4); when there is Heart-Heat only the tip of the tongue becomes Red (Fig. 23.5).

As far as swelling is concerned, a swelling of the tip itself indicates a Heart pathology, usually Heart-Heat. (Fig. 23.6). A Lung-related swelling usually appears

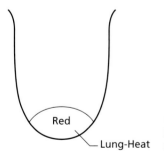

Fig. 23.4 Tongue indicating Lung-Heat (Red in the front third)

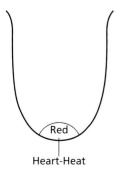

Fig. 23.5 Tongue indicating Heart-Heat (Red tip)

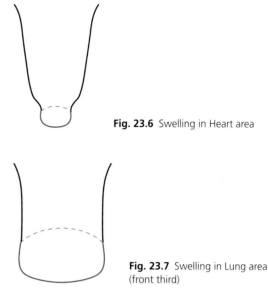

Fig. 23.6 Swelling in Heart area

Fig. 23.7 Swelling in Lung area (front third)

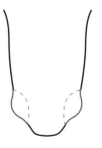

Fig. 23.8 Swelling in Lung area (sides)

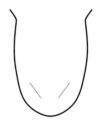

Fig. 23.9 Lung cracks

either in the whole front third (Fig. 23.7) or on the sides between the Heart area and the Stomach and Spleen area (Fig. 23.8).

As far as cracks are concerned, Lung cracks are usually located in the area between the tip and the centre (Fig. 23.9).

A Purple colour on the sides of the tongue between the tip and centre may be related to the Lungs or Heart. It indicates Blood stasis and, in lung disease, it is seen in chronic asthma or emphysema, while in heart disease it is seen in coronary heart disease or angina. The Purple patch may be unilateral or bilateral

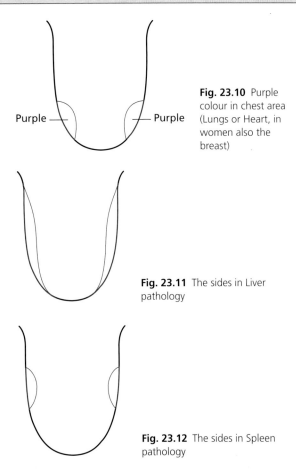

Fig. 23.10 Purple colour in chest area (Lungs or Heart, in women also the breast)

Fig. 23.11 The sides in Liver pathology

Fig. 23.12 The sides in Spleen pathology

(Fig. 23.10). In women, in addition, a Purple colour in that area may also indicate a breast pathology.

Although the sides of the tongue correspond to Liver and Gall-Bladder, they may also, under certain circumstances, reflect conditions of the Spleen. A pathology of the Liver, such as Heat, is reflected along the whole side of the tongue, while one of the Spleen is also reflected on the sides but only in the central section. This applies to both redness and swelling, and Figures 23.11 and 23.12 illustrate this difference.

CLINICAL SIGNIFICANCE OF THE TONGUE

The importance of tongue diagnosis lies mostly in the fact that it nearly always shows the true condition of the patient; this is, of course, most useful in complicated conditions when there may be contradictory signs of Heat and Cold or of Yin and Yang deficiency. For example, in menopausal conditions, when there is

often a simultaneous deficiency of Kidney-Yin and Kidney-Yang and contradictory symptoms of Heat and Cold, the tongue clearly shows whether there is a predominance of Yin or Yang deficiency as it will be Red in the former case and Pale in the latter.

The clinical significance of the tongue must be related to its various aspects as follows.

Tongue-body colour

The tongue-body colour reflects primarily the state of the Yin organs and Blood and it shows conditions of Heat or Cold and of Yin or Yang deficiency.

The tongue body's own colour is visible through the tongue coating and it is important not to confuse the two. Generally speaking, the tongue coating does not extend right to the edge of the tongue and therefore the sides of the tongue can show us the tongue-body colour if the coating is very thick. Observation of the tongue-body colour includes that of red points, which usually, but not always, occur on a Red tongue.

Examination of the body colour should also always include an examination of the veins under the tongue.

The normal Stomach fluids tend to make the tongue Pale whereas Heart-Blood tends to redden it; the influence of these two organs therefore causes the normal tongue to be Pale Red indicating a good state of Stomach fluids and Heart-Blood.

Tongue-body shape

The tongue-body shape reflects primarily conditions of Deficiency or Excess and observation of it adds more information to that gleaned from the tongue-body colour.

Observation of the tongue-body shape includes consideration of the shape itself: its thickness (Thin, Swollen, etc.), its suppleness (Stiff, Flabby, etc.), its surface (cracks, etc.), and its involuntary movements (Quivering, Moving, etc.).

The normal tongue-body shape is supple, not Swollen, not Thin and without cracks.

Tongue coating

The tongue coating reflects primarily the state of the Yang organs and especially of the Stomach. It also reflects conditions of Deficiency or Excess and of Heat or Cold.

The tongue coating is formed when some of the fluids generated in the process of the Stomach's digestion of food flow up and create its coating. A thin, white tongue coating, therefore, indicates a good state of Stomach-Qi while a rootless or an absent tongue coating indicates weakening of Stomach-Qi.

The tongue coating should be thin enough for the tongue-body colour to be seen through it.

Tongue spirit

The tongue 'spirit' refers to the general appearance of the tongue: this is called *shen* in Chinese and it is much the same as the *shen* of the complexion and eyes, (i.e. referring to the qualities of brightness, sheen and vitality). One can therefore distinguish two types of tongue: one with spirit, the other without spirit.

A tongue with spirit denotes certain qualities of liveliness, suppleness, vitality and brightness of the tongue-body; a tongue without spirit looks lifeless, rather stiff, rather dark and dull.

A tongue without spirit denotes a poor prognosis or that the condition is more difficult to treat.

For a detailed discussion of tongue diagnosis see 'Tongue Diagnosis in Chinese Medicine'.[1]

NOTES

1. G Maciocia 1995 Tongue Diagnosis in Chinese Medicine, Eastland Press, Seattle.

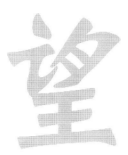

Chapter **24**

TONGUE-BODY COLOUR

Chapter contents

TONGUE SPIRIT   *209*

TONGUE-BODY COLOURS   *210*
　Pale   *210*
　Red   *210*
　Purple   *212*

SUBLINGUAL VEINS   *213*

TONGUE SPIRIT

The tongue 'spirit' refers to the general appearance of the tongue: this is called *shen* in Chinese and it is much the same as the *shen* of the complexion and eyes, that is, referring to the qualities of brightness, sheen and vitality. One can therefore distinguish two types of tongue: one with spirit, the other without spirit.

A tongue with spirit denotes certain qualities of liveliness, suppleness, vitality and brightness of the tongue body; a tongue without spirit looks lifeless, rather stiff, rather dark and dull. One can use the analogy of a piece of meat in a butcher's shop: the tongue with spirit looks like a fresh piece of meat, while the tongue without spirit looks like an old piece of meat which has become dark, greyish and lifeless.

The spirit should be observed in particular on the root of the tongue because the root reflects the state of the Kidneys and the spirit of this area reflects the condition of the Kidney-Essence. The Kidney-Essence is the foundation of life and the absence of spirit on the root of the tongue indicates a severe deficiency of the Kidneys and therefore the tendency to ill health. The tongue spirit is basically a prognostic sign as a tongue with spirit indicates that the patient may recover relatively easily whereas a tongue without spirit indicates that, whatever the patient may suffer from, the treatment may be prolonged.

It is important to remember that the tongue spirit has nothing to do with other pathological signs on the tongue; in other words, the patient may have a tongue that is pathological in many respects (e.g. Red with a thick coating), but if it has spirit this indicates that the Kidney-Essence is still strong and that the body can fight off pathogenic factors.

TONGUE-BODY COLOURS

The tongue-body colour reflects primarily the state of the Yin organs and Blood and it shows conditions of Heat or Cold and of Yin or Yang deficiency. The normal body colour is pale red. Traditionally five pathological colours are described, that is, Pale, Red, Dark-Red, Purple and Blue. However, the clinical significance of the Dark-Red tongue is essentially the same as that of the Red tongue and the clinical significance of the Blue tongue is essentially the same as that of the Bluish-Purple tongue: therefore, the pathological colours may be narrowed down to three: Pale, Red and Purple.

Pale

The Pale tongue is paler than normal. The pallor ranges from a very slight paleness to a paleness so extreme that the tongue is almost white. (See Plate 24.1 on p. P22.)

The Pale tongue indicates either Yang deficiency or Blood deficiency; in Yang deficiency it will tend to be slightly wet, whereas in Blood deficiency it will tend to be slightly dry. The latter is much more common in women. If it is only slightly Pale this may also indicate Qi deficiency.

The tongue is often Pale only on the sides. If the pallor is all along the sides this indicates Liver-Blood deficiency; if it is only in the central section it indicates Spleen-Blood deficiency. In severe cases of Liver-Blood deficiency the sides may also become orangey.

The Pale tongue normally has a coating, and a Pale tongue without coating indicates severe Blood deficiency; this is relatively rare and it is usually seen only in women.

Box 24.1 summarizes the patterns underlying a Pale tongue.

BOX 24.1 PALE TONGUE

- Pale and slightly wet: Yang deficiency
- Pale and slightly dry: Blood deficiency
- Slightly pale; Qi deficiency
- Pale on the sides all along edges: Liver-Blood deficiency
- Pale on the sides in central section: Spleen-Blood deficiency
- Pale-orangey or pale without coating: severe Liver-Blood deficiency

---

Red

The Red tongue is redder than the normal colour. Although traditionally two shades are described (i.e. Red or Dark-Red), the clinical significance of these two is essentially the same. (See Plate 24.2 on p. P22.)

A Red tongue always indicates Heat, which may be Full or Empty. Therefore, when we observe a Red tongue the first thing we should ask ourselves is whether it has a coating or not. If the tongue is Red with a coating with root (whatever its colour) this indicates Full-Heat; if the tongue is Red without a coating, or coated only partially, or with a rootless coating (whatever its colour), it indicates Empty-Heat.

It should be stressed that a Red tongue without coating indicates specifically Empty-Heat rather than Yin deficiency, although obviously it arises from the latter. In other words, it is the lack of coating that indicates the Yin deficiency and the redness (without coating) that indicates Empty-Heat. The implication of this is, of course, that there are many tongue types that indicate Yin deficiency while the tongue-body is not Red.

Box 24.2 summarizes the patterns underlying Red tongue and tongue coating.

BOX 24.2 RED TONGUE AND TONGUE COATING

- Red tongue with coating: Full-Heat
- Red tongue without coating: Empty-Heat
- Normal tongue without coating: Yin deficiency

The tongue-body may be Red in specific areas, especially the tip, the front third, the centre or the sides. A Red tip of the tongue (Fig. 24.1) indicates Heart-Heat (Full or Empty); if the tip only is Red, this indicates that the condition of Heart-Heat is slight, whereas if the whole tongue is Red and the tip redder it indicates that

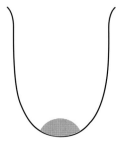

Fig. 24.1 Red tip

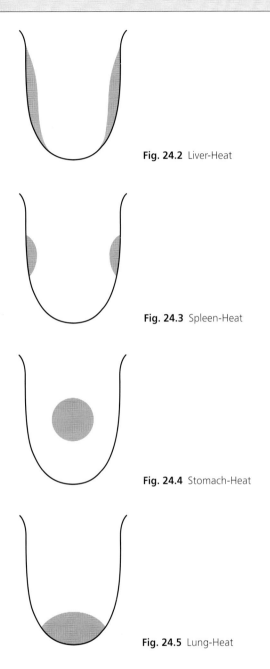

Fig. 24.2 Liver-Heat

Fig. 24.3 Spleen-Heat

Fig. 24.4 Stomach-Heat

Fig. 24.5 Lung-Heat

Red points

Before defining red points, we should define the red 'grains'. Ancient Chinese books on tongue diagnosis say that the physiological Minister Fire ascending to communicate with the Heart forms red grains on the surface of the tongue (bearing in mind that the tongue is the offshoot of the Heart). These red grains are normal and indicate that the physiological Minister Fire is in a healthy state, that is, it is neither excessive nor deficient. When the Minister Fire becomes pathological from various life influences, it flares upwards causing the red grains to become redder and to protrude from the surface of the tongue so that they become more visible: when this happens they are called red 'points'. Therefore red points are always pathological and they indicate a pathological state of the Minister Fire flaring upwards. Red points always indicate Heat to a degree greater than when the tongue is just Red. The intensity of their colour and their distribution clearly correlate with the intensity of the Heat: the more intense the colour and the more dense the distribution, the stronger is the Heat. (See Plate 24.5 on p. P22.)

Red 'spots' look the same as red points except that they are larger and they are usually seen only on the root of the tongue. Like red points, red spots also indicate Heat but with the additional component of some Blood stasis.

Red points are frequently seen on the tip, sides, centre or root of the tongue. Red points on the tip are relatively common and they indicate Heart-Fire, usually deriving from emotional stress. Red points on the sides in the Liver area indicate Liver-Heat (Liver-Fire), whereas red points in the centre indicate Stomach-Heat (Fig. 24.6). However, Stomach-Heat may also be reflected in red points on the sides but only in the middle section of the tongue and along a broader strip.

there is generalized Heat and severe Heart-Heat. (See Plate 24.3 on p. P22.)

Red sides all along the edge indicate Liver-Heat (Fig. 24.2, see also Plate 24.4 on p. P22), while a redness on the sides only in the central section indicates either Stomach-Heat or Spleen-Heat (Fig. 24.3).

If the tongue is Red in the centre it indicates Stomach-Heat (Fig. 24.4); if it is Red in the front third (including the tip) it indicates Lung-Heat (Fig. 24.5).

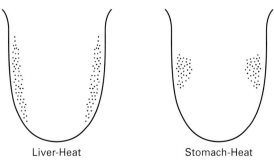

Liver-Heat   Stomach-Heat

Fig. 24.6 Red points indicating Liver-Heat or Stomach-Heat

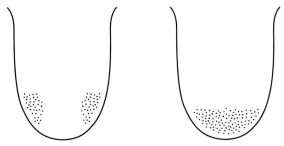

Fig. 24.7 Red points indicating Lung-Heat

With Lung-Heat, red points may appear either in the chest area or in the whole front third of the tongue, as opposed to the very tip as in the case of Heart-Heat (Fig. 24.7).

Red points on the root indicate Heat, usually Damp-Heat, in the Bladder or Intestines.

Red points in external diseases

The significance of red points in external diseases is different from that in internal diseases. First of all, red points in acute external diseases definitely indicate an invasion of Wind-Heat as opposed to Wind-Cold.

In external diseases the density of the red points reflects not only the intensity of the pathogenic factor but also its progression towards the Interior; thus if, in the course of an acute external disease, the red points become denser this indicates not only that the pathogenic factor has become stronger but that it is beginning to penetrate into the Interior.

The distribution of the red points also reflects the stages of penetration of an external pathogenic factor. In the very beginning stages of an invasion of external Wind, the red points may be more concentrated on the front third or on the sides. In this context, these two

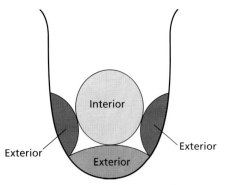

Fig. 24.8 Areas corresponding to Interior and Exterior in acute, external diseases

areas correspond to the Exterior of the body while the centre of the tongue corresponds to the Interior (Fig. 24.8).

Thus if after a few days, the red points from these two areas extend towards the centre of the tongue, it indicates that a pathogenic factor is penetrating into the Interior.

BOX 24.3 RED POINTS

- Red points: Heat
- Red spots: Heat with some Blood stasis
- Red points on the tip: Heart-Fire
- Red points on the sides: Liver-Heat
- Red points in the centre: Stomach-Heat
- Red points on the sides in central section: Stomach-Heat
- Red points on the sides in chest area: Lung-Heat
- Red spots on the root: Damp-Heat in the Lower Burner
- Red points in external diseases: Wind-Heat

Box 24.3 summarizes the patterns underlying red points on the tongue.

Purple

A Purple tongue always indicates Blood stasis, which itself may derive from Cold or from Heat. (See Plates 24.6, 24.7 and 25.3 on pp. P22, P23 and P24.) Internal Cold contracts and obstructs the circulation of Blood, leading to Blood stasis; Heat leads to Blood stasis by condensing the Body Fluids and Blood. When Blood stasis derives from Cold, the tongue is Bluish-Purple while when it derives from Heat, it is Reddish-Purple. Therefore the Bluish-Purple tongue indicating Cold derives from a Pale tongue while the Reddish-Purple tongue derives from a Red tongue (Fig. 24.9).

A tongue becomes Purple only after a prolonged time, usually years: therefore it always indicates a chronic condition and for this reason it is far more common in the elderly. The Purple colour of the tongue indicates potentially serious conditions and in the presence of such tongue-body colour we should always invigorate Blood and eliminate stasis (as well as expelling internal Cold in the case of Blood stasis deriving from Cold and clearing Heat in the case of Blood stasis deriving from Heat), even in the absence of any symptom of Blood stasis. Serious conditions relating to Blood stasis in Chinese medicine include cancer, coronary heart disease, stroke and hypertension.

The tongue can be only partially Purple and the most common areas are the sides (Liver or chest area)

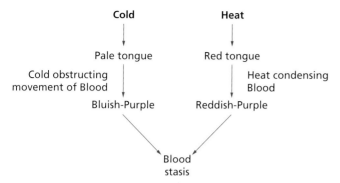

Fig. 24.9 Development of Bluish-Purple or Reddish-Purple tongue

of the tongue, the centre and the front third; the most frequent occurrence is on the sides in the Liver area. Strangely, the tongue is never Purple on the tip only and Blood stasis in the Heart usually manifests in the chest/breast area instead (see below).

A Purple colour on the sides in the Liver area (Fig. 24.10) indicates Blood stasis in the Liver, which may occur in any of the areas influenced by the Liver channel, for example Liver-Blood stasis in the hypochondrium, epigastrium, lower abdomen and Uterus. (See Plate 24.8 on p. P23.) It is interesting to note that, although the Uterus is in the Lower Burner, whose state is reflected in the back third of the tongue, Blood stasis in the Uterus is manifested with a Purple colour not on the root of the tongue but on the sides in the Liver area.

A Purple colour on the sides in the chest area (Fig. 24.11) indicates Blood stasis in the chest (which may include Heart or Lungs) or, in women only, the breasts. In lung diseases, a Purple colour in the chest area is seen in chronic obstructive pulmonary disease such as chronic asthma, bronchitis or emphysema. In heart diseases, a Purple colour in the chest area is seen in coronary heart disease. In addition, in women a Purple colour in the chest/breast area may indicate a breast pathology such as breast lumps, whether benign or malignant. Observation of the breast area in women suffering from carcinoma of the breast is an important prognostic factor because if this area is clearly Purple the prognosis is poor, whereas if it is not the prognosis is good. A Purple colour in the breast area is also sometimes seen in women without any breast pathology; this may indicate the predisposition to breast lumps and one should therefore invigorate Blood and eliminate stasis in the breasts even in the absence of symptoms and signs. (See Plate 24.9 on p. P23.)

A Purple colour in the centre of the tongue indicates Blood stasis in the Stomach, whereas a Purple colour in the front third indicates Blood stasis in the Lungs.

Box 24.4 summarizes patterns underlying Purple tongue areas.

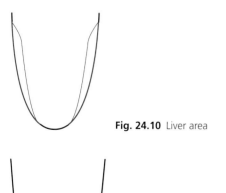

Fig. 24.10 Liver area

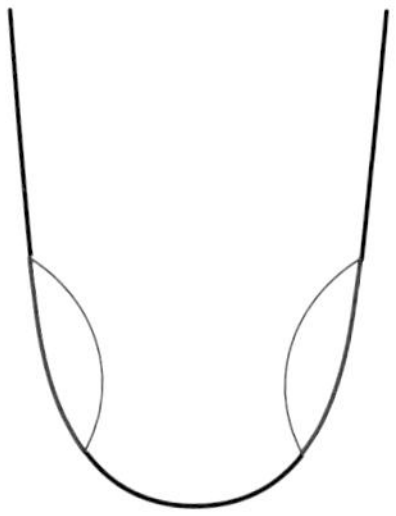

Fig. 24.11 Breast/chest areas

BOX 24.4 PURPLE AREAS ON THE TONGUE

- Liver areas: Liver-Blood stasis or Blood stasis in the Uterus
- Breast/chest areas: Blood stasis in the Heart or breast
- Centre: Blood stasis in the Stomach

SUBLINGUAL VEINS

The sublingual veins should always form part of a routine examination of the tongue body. Under normal conditions, the two veins under the tongue are barely visible and they have a very faint, pale-red colour.

When they become clearly visible, they are by definition pathological. (See Plate 24.10 on p. P23.) One should observe the size and the colour of the sublingual veins.

If the veins are distended but not dark, this indicates Qi deficiency, if they are too thin in relation to the sides of the tongue and the patient's body itself, this indicates Yin deficiency.

The most important sign with regard to sublingual veins is their Purple colour. If they are distended and dark Purple, this indicates Blood stasis, usually in the Upper Burner (Lungs or Heart) but it may also refer to the Liver. Distended and dark sublingual veins are more common in the elderly and they give an early indication of Blood stasis before the rest of the tongue body becomes Purple. Observation of the sublingual veins therefore has an important preventative value. Dark and dry sublingual veins indicate severe Yin deficiency with Empty-Heat. Dark, swollen and wet veins indicate Lung, Spleen and Kidney deficiency with accumulation of fluids.

Such observation is important also in chronic Painful Obstruction Syndrome. If the sublingual veins are reddish and shiny, they indicate Damp-Heat; if they are yellowish, Dampness, while if they are white and slippery, Cold-Dampness, and if they are swollen, white and sticky, Dampness and Blood stasis.

In modern China, some doctors consider the appearance of sublingual veins as a useful prodromal sign of certain diseases.[1] The main signs are as follows:

- dark-purple: hardening of the brain arteries
- distended, dark and crooked: hardening of arteries, hypertension (if the veins protrude a lot and look like earthworms, the disease is severe)
- small nodules like rice or wheat grains: hardening of arteries and heart disease.

Boxes 24.5 and 24.6 summarize the conditions underlying sublingual veins in Chinese and Western medicine.

BOX 24.5 SUBLINGUAL VEINS

- Distended (not dark): Qi deficiency
- Thin: Yin deficiency
- Distended and dark: Blood stasis in the Upper Burner
- Dark and dry: severe Yin deficiency with Empty-Heat
- Dark, swollen and wet: Lung, Spleen and Kidney deficiency with accumulation of fluids
- Reddish and shiny: Damp-Heat
- Yellowish: Dampness
- White and slippery: Cold-Dampness
- Swollen, white and sticky: Dampness and Blood stasis

BOX 24.6 SUBLINGUAL VEINS IN WESTERN MEDICINE

- Dark purple: hardening of the brain arteries
- Distended, dark and crooked: hardening of arteries, hypertension (if the veins protrude a lot and look like earthworms, the disease is severe)
- Small nodules like rice or wheat grains: hardening of arteries and heart disease

---

NOTES

1. Zhang Shu Min, The Diagnostic Significance of Sub-lingual Veins in Arteriosclerosis (*She Xia Mai Luo Zai Zhen Duan Dong Mai Ying Hua Zhong de Yi Yi* 舌下脉络在诊断动脉硬化中的意义), in Journal of Chinese Medicine (*Zhong Yi Za Zhi* 中医杂志), no. 12, 2000, p. 759.

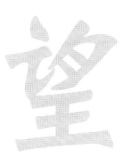

Chapter **25**

TONGUE-BODY SHAPE

Chapter contents

INTRODUCTION *215*

THIN *215*

SWOLLEN *216*

PARTIALLY SWOLLEN *216*

STIFF *216*

FLACCID *217*

LONG *217*

SHORT *217*

CRACKED *217*

DEVIATED *218*

MOVING *218*

QUIVERING *219*

TOOTHMARKED *219*

INTRODUCTION

Observation of the tongue-body shape reveals primarily conditions of Deficiency or Excess and it adds more information to that gleaned from observation of the tongue-body colour. For example, a Pale tongue may indicate Yang deficiency, but if, in addition to being Pale, it is also very Swollen this indicates that the Yang deficiency is severe and that it has led to the accumulation of Dampness or Phlegm. In this example, the tongue-body shape reflects the Full condition generated by Dampness or Phlegm.

To give another example, if a tongue lacks coating, this indicates Yin deficiency, but if in addition it is also very thin it indicates that the Yin deficiency is quite severe. In this example, the tongue-body shape reflects the severity of a deficiency condition. To give yet another example, if the tip of the tongue is Red this indicates Heart-Heat or Heart-Fire usually deriving from emotional problems, but if the tip is also swollen it indicates that a condition of Heart-Heat or Heart-Fire is more severe.

THIN

'Thin' refers to the thickness, not the width, of the tongue. The 'body' of the tongue is formed by fluids and Blood and a Thin tongue therefore always indicates a deficiency either of Blood or of Yin fluids. In the former case, it will also be Pale while in the latter case it will be Red.

A Thin tongue is actually not common, probably because Dampness and Phlegm, which make the tongue Swollen, are such common and predominant pathogenic factors. As they tend to make the tongue Swollen, even if the patient has a concurrent severe

Blood deficiency, this would not manifest on the tongue-body shape. In my practice, for example, out of 2378 patients, less than 2% have a Thin tongue while nearly 37% have a Swollen tongue.

SWOLLEN

The size of the tongue body has to be related to the size of the head of the person: what might be 'Swollen' for someone may be normal for another. (See Plate 25.1 on p. P23.) As the thickness of the tongue body depends on the supply of fluids and Blood, a Swollen tongue body indicates an accumulation of fluids, which may be Dampness, Phlegm or oedema. Thus a swelling of the tongue always indicates a Full condition and particularly one characterized by Dampness or Phlegm. Although Dampness and Phlegm usually arise from a Qi or a Yang deficiency, the swelling of the tongue body reflects the Full condition created by these two pathogenic factors.

PARTIALLY SWOLLEN

While a total swelling of the tongue always indicates Dampness or Phlegm, a partial swelling may indicate other pathologies such as Qi deficiency, Qi stagnation or Heat. The areas where a partial swelling is most commonly seen are the sides in the Liver or chest area, the tip and the front third.

A swelling on the sides in the Liver area (Fig. 25.1) is very common and it usually indicates Liver-Heat; it is nearly always associated with a Red colour in the same area.

A swelling on the sides in the chest/breast area (Fig. 25.2) generally indicates either retention of Phlegm in the chest or breast or Lung-Qi deficiency.

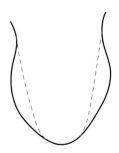

Fig. 25.1 Swelling in the Liver area

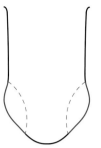

Fig. 25.2 Swelling in the chest/breast area

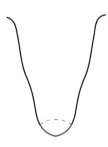

Fig. 25.3 Swelling of the tip of the tongue

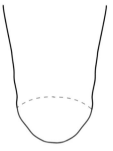

Fig. 25.4 Swelling of the front third of the tongue

A swelling of the tip of the tongue (Fig. 25.3), usually associated with a Red colour, is very common and it indicates Heart-Heat or Heart-Fire deriving from severe emotional problems.

A swelling of the front third of the tongue (Fig. 25.4) indicates retention of Phlegm in the Lungs. (See Plate 25.2 on p. P23.)

STIFF

A Stiff tongue lacks the normal suppleness and flexibility. It looks hard and stiff. It indicates internal Wind, Blood stasis or severe Yin deficiency. (See Plate 25.3 on p. P24.)

FLACCID

A flaccid tongue is flabby and, in severe cases, it has a crumpled look. It always indicates lack of Body Fluids or Blood.

LONG

A Long tongue is rather narrow and, when extended, protrudes further than normal. Not commonly seen, it always indicates Heat.

SHORT

A Short tongue appears to be contracted and the patient is unable to extend it out of the mouth cavity. The significance of the Short tongue depends on the body colour because it can indicate two opposite conditions: if it is Pale it indicates severe internal Cold and Yang deficiency; while if it is Red and without coating it indicates severe Yin deficiency. In the first instance, the patient cannot extend the tongue enough because internal Cold contracts the muscles, while in the latter instance this happens because there are not enough fluids in the tongue.

CRACKED

Generally, cracks on the surface of the tongue indicate Yin deficiency or the tendency to it but, though this is the most common cause, there are others such as Dampness or deficiency of the Original Qi. Horizontal cracks (Fig. 25.5) indicate Yin deficiency, usually of the Stomach or Kidneys, or both, and they are more commonly seen in the elderly.

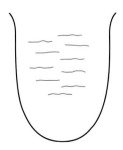

Fig. 25.5 Horizontal cracks

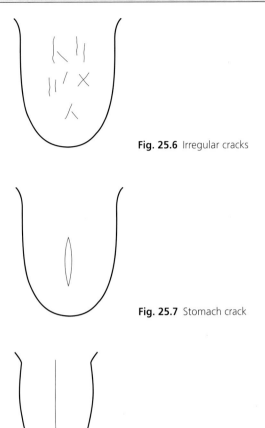

Fig. 25.6 Irregular cracks

Fig. 25.7 Stomach crack

Fig. 25.8 Heart crack

Irregular cracks (Fig. 25.6) usually indicate Stomach-Yin deficiency or the tendency to it. (See Plate 25.4 on p. P24.)

A central short crack in the midline of the tongue (Fig. 25.7) is very common and it indicates Stomach-Yin deficiency, or the tendency to it. (See Plate 25.5 on p. P24.)

A central long crack in the midline of the tongue (Fig. 25.8) is also common and its clinical significance depends on its depth and on the colour of the tongue body, especially the tip. (See Plates 25.6 and 25.7 on p. P24.)

If the Heart crack is shallow and the body colour normal, this simply indicates a constitutional tendency to Heart patterns and it does not have a specific clinical significance. However, if a person has such a crack, any emotional stress from which he or she might suffer will have deeper repercussions than for someone without a Heart crack. According to Dr J. H. F. Shen, a shallow Heart crack on a normal body colour may also

indicate heart disease in the parents or even grand-parents.

If the Heart crack is deep, it indicates that the person may suffer from a Heart pattern due to emotional stress, all the more so if the tip is also Red. One could describe different situations of emotional stress in order of increasing severity as manifested on the tongue as follows:

- shallow Heart crack, normal body colour
- no Heart crack, Red tip
- deep Heart crack, normal body colour
- shallow Heart crack, Red tip
- deep Heart crack, Red tip
- deep Heart crack, Red tip with red points
- deep Heart crack, Red tongue with redder tip and red points
- deep Heart crack, Red tongue with redder and swollen tip and red points.

Short, transverse cracks on the sides (Fig. 25.9) are a clear sign of Spleen-Yin deficiency. This is not common and is not a common condition often described among the Spleen patterns; such cracks are the easiest way of identifying such a pattern (see Plate 25.5 on p. P24.)

Short, transverse cracks behind the tip in the Lung area (Fig. 25.10) usually indicate a past Lung pathology such as pneumonia, whooping cough or repeated

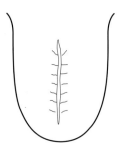

Fig. 25.11 Deep midline cracks with small cracks

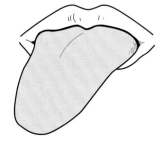

Fig. 25.12 Deviated tongue

lung infections during childhood. As such cracks reflect past pathologies, they do not have a major clinical significance.

An extremely deep midline crack with other small cracks branching out from it (Fig. 25.11) is usually seen in a Red tongue without coating. It indicates a severe Kidney-Yin deficiency with Empty-Heat in the Kidneys and Heart.

DEVIATED

The Deviated tongue deviates to one side when extended (Fig. 25.12).

The most common clinical significance of a Deviated tongue is internal Wind and this type of tongue is most commonly seen in the elderly. In a young person it may be related to a Heart deficiency.

MOVING

The Moving tongue moves *slowly* from side to side with large-amplitude movements when it is extended and the patient cannot control its movement. It always indicates internal Wind and is usually seen in the elderly.

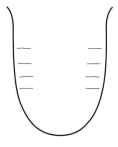

Fig. 25.9 Transverse Spleen cracks

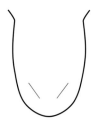

Fig. 25.10 Lung cracks

QUIVERING

The Quivering tongue trembles *rapidly* and with small-amplitude movements as it is extended. The most common clinical significance of a Quivering tongue in chronic conditions is Spleen-Qi or Spleen-Yang deficiency.

TOOTHMARKED

The tongue with teethmarks (Fig. 25.13) indicates chronic Spleen-Qi deficiency, but since a tongue with a normal body shape can have teethmarks, do not assume that the presence of teethmarks necessarily means it is Swollen. (See Plate 25.8 on p. P24.)

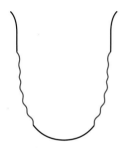

Fig. 25.13 Tongue with teethmarks

Box 25.1 summarizes the patterns underlying different tongue-body shapes.

BOX 25.1 TONGUE-BODY SHAPE

- Thin: Blood deficiency (if Pale); Yin deficiency (if without coating)
- Swollen: Phlegm or Dampness
  —Swollen sides all along edge (and Red): Liver-Heat
  —Swollen sides in central section (and Pale): chronic Spleen-Qi deficiency
  —Swollen on the sides in chest–breast area: Phlegm in chest or breast
  —Swollen tip (and Red): Heart-Fire
  —Swelling of front third: Phlegm in Lungs
- Stiff: internal Wind, Blood stasis, severe Yin deficiency
- Flaccid: lack of Body Fluids, Blood deficiency
- Long: Heat
- Short: severe Yang deficiency (if wet); severe Yin deficiency (if peeled and Red)
- Cracked: Yin deficiency
  —central long, thin midline crack: constitutional Heart deficiency with tendency to emotional problems
  —central, short, wide crack in the centre: constitutional Stomach deficiency
  —short, transverse cracks on the sides: Spleen-Yin deficiency
  —short, diagonal crack in Lung area: past Lung disease
  —very deep, midline crack with other cracks stemming from it: Kidney-Yin deficiency
- Deviated: Liver-Wind, or Heart deficiency (in young person)
- Moving: Liver-Wind
- Quivering: Spleen-Qi deficiency
- Teethmarks: Spleen-Qi deficiency

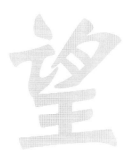

Chapter **26**

TONGUE COATING

Chapter contents

PHYSIOLOGY OF TONGUE COATING *221*

CLINICAL SIGNIFICANCE OF TONGUE COATING *221*

PRESENCE OR ABSENCE OF COATING *222*

COATING WITH OR WITHOUT ROOT *222*

COATING THICKNESS *223*

COATING DISTRIBUTION *223*

COATING MOISTURE *223*

COATING TEXTURE *224*
  Sticky coating *224*
  Slippery coating *224*
  Mouldy coating *224*

TONGUE COATING IN EXTERNAL DISEASES *224*

PHYSIOLOGY OF TONGUE COATING

The Stomach rots and ripens food, and during the process of digestion a small amount of what the ancient Chinese books called 'turbidity' or 'turbid fluids' escapes upwards to reach the tongue: this forms a coating. Therefore the presence of a coating indicates the normal functioning of Stomach-Qi. A normal coating should be white and thin enough to see the body colour through it. Although the tongue coating reflects primarily the physiological activity of the Stomach, the Spleen and the Kidneys also play a role in its formation; for this reason, if a tongue lacks a coating this may indicate Stomach-Yin or Kidney-Yin deficiency, or both.

It should be noted that the tongue coating is naturally thicker at the root of the tongue and thinnest towards the tip, and that the coating does not extend to the very edges of the tongue.

CLINICAL SIGNIFICANCE OF TONGUE COATING

The tongue coating reflects primarily the state of the Yang organs and especially of the Stomach. It also reflects conditions of Deficiency or Excess and of Heat or Cold (Box 26.1).

Observation of the tongue coating needs to be based on a careful analysis of the history of the patient because the tongue coating changes very rapidly in acute conditions and can reflect short-term variations. For example, a yellow tongue coating in the centre indicates Stomach-Heat and this could equally be a chronic condition of Stomach-Heat or simply an acute stomach upset. We therefore need to enquire carefully to exclude the possibility that the yellow coating

merely reflects an acute but passing condition. Apart from the history, the brightness of the coating can give us an indication of its duration: the duller the coating, the more chronic is the condition.

As the coating reflects primarily the condition of the Yang organs, its thickness and particularly its distribution give a clear indication of a pathology affecting one of the Yang organs. For example, the sides of the tongue reflect the condition of the Liver and Gall-Bladder and we can differentiate between these two by referring to the body colour or coating, that is, if the body colour is affected it indicates a Liver pathology, whereas if the coating is affected it indicates a Gall-Bladder pathology. Similarly for the root of the tongue: if the root of the tongue is Red without coating this indicates Kidney-Yin deficiency with Empty-Heat, whereas if it has a thick coating it indicates a pathology of one of the Yang organs of the Lower Burner (Bladder or Intestines).

The tongue coating also gives us a good indication of Deficiency and Excess conditions because a thick coating with root always reflects a Full condition while a coating without root or the complete absence of coating always reflects a Deficiency condition. This will be described in more detail below.

The tongue coating gives also a very clear indication of the Hot or Cold nature of a condition but, as indicated above, it may merely reflect a passing, acute condition.

Box 26.1 summarizes the significance of a tongue coating.

BOX 26.1 CLINICAL SIGNIFICANCE OF TONGUE COATING

- Yang organs
- Deficiency–Excess
- Heat–Cold

PRESENCE OR ABSENCE OF COATING

The presence or absence of coating tells us primarily about the state of the Stomach-Qi. If the tongue has a coating with root, it indicates that the Stomach-Qi is still intact even if the excessive thickness or colour of the coating is pathological. Excluding the case of a normal, thin white coating, the tongue with coating usually indicates a Full condition precisely because the Stomach-Qi is intact. A tongue without coating indi-

cates that the Stomach-Qi is severely weakened and therefore a Deficiency condition. Therefore, it is better to have a thick, pathological coating with root than not to have a coating.

How does the coating disappear from the tongue surface? In chronic conditions, the tongue coating disappears gradually over a long time (usually years); in acute conditions, and especially acute, febrile diseases in children, the coating may disappear very quickly in a matter of days.

In chronic conditions characterized by the absence of coating, with treatment the coating should return gradually and quite slowly; this is a positive sign. If the coating appears suddenly on a tongue that previously lacked it, this is a bad sign; for example, in a patient with cancer the sudden return of coating to a particular area of the tongue may indicate a metastasis of the corresponding organ.

Conversely, if a tongue has a very thick, pathological coating, its sudden total or partial disappearance in the course of a disease is a poor prognostic sign because it indicates the sudden depletion of Stomach-Qi. However, the clinical significance is different if a thick tongue coating becomes normal as a result of treatment; as indicated above, the tongue coating can change much more quickly than the tongue-body colour.

COATING WITH OR WITHOUT ROOT

We can compare the tongue coating to grass: it should 'grow' out of the tongue body just as grass grows out of the soil and it should have 'roots' just as grass stems have roots in the earth. A coating with root reflects the normal functioning of Stomach-Qi even if the coating may be pathological (e.g. too thick and dark yellow). A coating without root resembles mown grass scattered on barren ground: it looks as if it has been 'added' on top of the tongue rather than growing out of it. (See Plates 26.1a and b on p. P25.) In severe conditions, the rootless coating may look like salt or snow sprinkled on top of the tongue. A rootless coating indicates the beginning of the weakening of Stomach-Qi in the course of a chronic disease. Therefore, it is better to have a thick, pathological coating with root than to have a thin coating without root.

It should be emphasized that the coating with root is not necessarily thin, although that is the most common situation. The coating without root can also

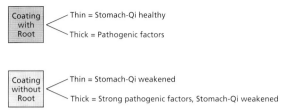

Fig. 26.1 Clinical significance of coating with or without root according to thickness

be thick and often sticky: this represents the worst scenario because it indicates that, on the one hand, Stomach-Qi is weakened and, on the other, that there is a significant pathogenic factor (against which the body is unable to fight due to the Stomach-Qi deficiency) (Fig. 26.1). For this reason it is obviously better to have a thin rather than a thick coating without root. (See Plate 26.1c on p. P25.)

Box 26.2 summarizes the four different situations seen in coating with and without root.

> ## BOX 26.2 COATING WITH OR WITHOUT ROOT
>
> - Thin coating with root: healthy Stomach-Qi
> - Thick coating with root: strong pathogenic factor, Stomach-Qi still intact
> - Thin coating without root: beginning of weakening of Stomach-Qi
> - Thick coating without root: strong pathogenic factor, Stomach-Qi weakened

COATING THICKNESS

The normal coating is thin and it should be possible to see the tongue body through it. If the tongue body cannot be seen, the tongue coating is too thick. The thickness of the tongue coating reflects the strength of the pathogenic factor clearly and accurately: the thicker the coating the stronger the pathogenic factor. If a thin coating becomes thick, this indicates that the pathogenic factors are getting stronger or that they are penetrating deeper into the Interior. The latter situation applies to conditions of acute, external diseases, which will be explained in greater detail below. Therefore, if we are treating a patient with a thick tongue coating, we should expect it to become gradually thinner. In some cases, a thick tongue coating can revert back to normal even after a very short time.

As mentioned above, a thick coating may be with or without root but the clinical significance of its thickness is the same – that is, it reflects the strength of a pathogenic factor.

COATING DISTRIBUTION

Generally speaking, the same areas that reflect changes in the tongue-body colour also reflect changes in the tongue coating, but there are some differences. For example, the tongue coating never extends to the very tip or the very edges of the tongue.

The most common locations where a thick coating is observed are in the centre and on the root of the tongue. A thick coating in the centre reflects the presence of a pathogenic factor in the Stomach, which may be Cold, Heat, Dampness or Phlegm depending on the colour and consistency of the coating, whereas a thick coating on the root reflects the presence of a pathogenic factor in the Bladder or Intestines.

A pathogenic factor in the Gall-Bladder (Fig. 26.2) may be manifested in a variety of ways; the most common one is a bilateral or unilateral coating that comes forward in one or two strips on the edges. (See Plate 26.2 on p. P25.)

COATING MOISTURE

The normal coating should be relatively moist, indicating a good supply and movement of Body Fluids. If the coating is too dry, it indicates either Heat or Yin deficiency. If the coating is too wet, it indicates severe Yang deficiency.

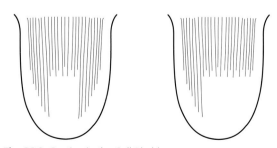

Fig. 26.2 Coating in the Gall-Bladder area

COATING TEXTURE

The normal coating texture should be like the hairs of a very fine brush, in Western medicine corresponding to the filiform papillae. The individual 'hairs' (filiform papillae) should be clearly seen and they should not be too dry or too wet. Pathological textures of the coating make it sticky, slippery or mouldy.

Sticky coating

The sticky (also called greasy) coating has an oily but coarse appearance and the individual papillae can still be seen. (See Plate 26.3 on p. P25.) To visualize a sticky coating, one can use the analogy of a toothbrush of very fine, natural hair spread with butter or lard: the toothbrush will appear very greasy but the individual hairs can still be seen. Thus, although the sticky coating is greasy and oily, it may also be, in addition, dry. This may seem a contradiction but it is not. To use the same analogy, we can think of a toothbrush with very fine hairs which has been spread with butter and left for several days; after that time, it will still have a greasy appearance but it will be dry. Thus, we should not identify 'stickiness' of the tongue coating with wetness.

The sticky coating indicates either Dampness or Phlegm and especially the latter. The sticky coating is extremely common: in my practice out of a database of 2378 patients nearly 30% have such a coating.

Slippery coating

The slippery coating has a greasy look. It is characterized by the fact that the individual papillae cannot be easily distinguished as they seem to be covered by an oily fluid. To compare the slippery with the sticky coating, the former is oilier and the individual papillae cannot be distinguished, whereas the latter is coarser and the individual papillae can be distinguished. The slippery coating, like the sticky coating, also indicates Dampness or Phlegm but predominantly Dampness.

Mouldy coating

The mouldy coating looks thick, patchy and crumbly. Chinese books describe it as 'tofu'; to use a Western analogy, it could be described as 'cottage cheese'. The mouldy coating also looks greasy and is by definition without root.

The mouldy coating indicates also Dampness or Phlegm but against a background of Stomach-Yin deficiency with Empty-Heat. Empty-Heat plays a role in the formation of the Phlegm indicated by the mouldy coating in evaporating the fluids. The mouldy coating is seen only in the elderly.

BOX 26.3 COATING TEXTURE

- Sticky coating: Dampness or Phlegm (especially latter)
- Slippery coating: Dampness or Phlegm (especially the former)
- Mouldy coating: Dampness or Phlegm with Stomach-Yin deficiency

---

Box 26.3 summarizes the patterns underlying different coating textures.

TONGUE COATING IN EXTERNAL DISEASES

In external diseases from invasion of Wind, the interpretation of the tongue coating is quite different from that of internal diseases.

In external diseases the thickness of the coating reflects, not only the intensity of the pathogenic factor, but also its progression towards the Interior: thus, if in the course of an acute external disease, the coating becomes thicker it indicates that not only has the pathogenic factor become stronger but that it is beginning to penetrate into the Interior.

The coating in external diseases reflects Hot and Cold influences in the same way as in internal diseases, but there are differences. The most important difference is that the coating tends to be white in the very beginning stages of an invasion of Wind even if it is Wind-Heat. If during an acute external disease the coating turns from white to yellow, this means there is not only a change from Cold to Heat (although a white coating may appear also in Wind-Heat), but also a penetration of the pathogenic factor into the Interior.

The distribution of the coating also reflects the stages of penetration of an external pathogenic factor. In the very beginning stages of an invasion of external Wind, the coating may be more concentrated

on the front third or on the sides. In this context, these two areas correspond to the Exterior of the body while the centre of the tongue corresponds to the Interior. (See Fig. 24.8 on p. 212.)

Thus, if after a few days the coating from these two areas extends towards the centre of the tongue, it indicates that a pathogenic factor is penetrating into the Interior.

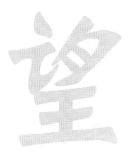

Chapter **27**

TONGUE IMAGES AND PATTERNS

Chapter contents

QI-DEFICIENCY TONGUES   *227*

YANG-DEFICIENCY TONGUES   *227*

BLOOD-DEFICIENCY TONGUES   *228*

YIN-DEFICIENCY TONGUES   *228*

THE TONGUE IN PHLEGM AND DAMPNESS   *230*

THE TONGUE IN HEAT   *230*

THE TONGUE IN COLD   *230*

THE TONGUE IN QI AND BLOOD STAGNATION   *231*

THE TONGUE IN INTERNAL WIND   *231*

THE TONGUE IN EXTERNAL INVASIONS OF WIND   *231*

QI-DEFICIENCY TONGUES

The tongue-body colour reflects primarily the condition of Blood rather than Qi and therefore a mild deficiency of Qi may not manifest on the tongue at all. In long-standing cases of Qi deficiency the tongue may become slightly Pale.

Severe Spleen-Qi deficiency may manifest with a swelling on the sides of the tongue in the central section (Fig. 27.1). (See also Plate 27.1 on p. P25.) This swelling differs from a Liver swelling in that it is much wider and it is more in the central section of the tongue (Middle Burner).

Stomach-Qi deficiency manifests with a rootless coating or with lack of coating in the centre (with the tongue-body colour still normal).

YANG-DEFICIENCY TONGUES

In Yang deficiency the tongue is definitely Pale and it tends also to be slightly wet. In severe Yang deficiency, the tongue may also become Swollen but the swelling itself is due to the presence of Dampness or Phlegm rather than the Yang deficiency itself.

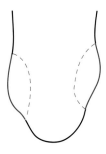

Fig. 27.1 Swelling on the sides from Spleen-Qi deficiency

> **!**
> A Swollen tongue does not indicate Yang deficiency but rather Dampness or Phlegm.

When the tongue is Pale, one cannot generally identify which is the main organ involved. For example, the tongue's Paleness may be due to Spleen-Yang deficiency, Kidney-Yang deficiency, or both, and we cannot deduce from the tongue alone which is the case. The only guideline one can follow is that the more Pale and Swollen the tongue is, the more likely it is that the cause is Kidney-Yang deficiency.

BLOOD-DEFICIENCY TONGUES

In Blood deficiency the tongue is also Pale but tending to be slightly dry. In severe cases of Blood deficiency, the tongue should be Thin as well as Pale but, for the reasons explained above, this is seldom the case.

Liver-Blood deficiency is frequently indicated by a Pale colour on the sides in the Liver area. Although the tip corresponds to the Heart, the tip is never Pale on its own in Heart-Blood deficiency; in this condition, however, the tongue may become Pale in the chest area (see Fig. 23.8 p. 205).

YIN-DEFICIENCY TONGUES

The tongue coating is formed during the process of the Stomach's digestion of food and, as we have seen above, the normal tongue should have a thin, white coating, which indicates a good state of Stomach-Qi. The normal coating is formed by the 'turbid fluids' produced by the Stomach's process of digestion and is therefore an expression of the normal state of Stomach fluids and therefore Qi and Yin.

If Stomach-Qi is weakened, the very first sign of this on the tongue will be a rootless coating in the centre; if Stomach-Qi gets weaker the coating will be rootless all over the tongue and if Stomach-Qi deficiency progresses to Stomach-Yin deficiency the tongue will lack a coating entirely. As the Stomach is the origin of fluids, a tongue without coating always indicates a deficiency of Stomach-Yin. Of course, a tongue without coating is also seen in deficiency of Yin of other organs but, whichever other organ is involved, it always indicates Stomach-Yin deficiency. For example, the tongue may lack a coating in the front indicating Lung-Yin deficiency but, because the coating is a reflection of Stomach-Qi and Stomach-Yin, we can say that in this case there is a deficiency of Yin of both the Lungs and Stomach. In terms of treatment this means that, whenever we see a tongue without coating, Stomach-Yin should always be nourished whatever other organ is involved.

It is most important to stress that Yin deficiency on the tongue is manifested by the lack of coating and *not* by the redness of the tongue body. Thus, if a tongue has a normal body colour and lacks coating we can say that it indicates Yin deficiency, whereas if it is Red and lacks a coating it indicates Yin deficiency with Empty-Heat. Therefore, the lack of coating by itself indicates Yin deficiency, whereas the lack of coating associated with the redness of the tongue body indicates Yin deficiency with Empty-Heat. In other words, although Empty-Heat arises from Yin deficiency, eventually, especially in the beginning stages, Yin deficiency may and does occur frequently without Empty-Heat, in which case the tongue lacks a coating but is not Red.

> **!**
> **Remember**: Yin deficiency is manifested by the lack of coating, not by the redness of the tongue, i.e.:
> • lack of coating: Yin deficiency
> • lack of coating and redness: Yin deficiency and Empty-Heat.

We can look upon Stomach-Yin deficiency as the beginning of a Yin deficiency that will eventually affect other organs. However, this does not mean that a Yin deficiency is always indicated by Stomach-Yin deficiency. For example, it is quite possible for someone to suffer from Lung-Yin deficiency without Stomach-Yin deficiency manifesting on the tongue coating. However, if the Yin deficiency manifests with a lack of coating, we can say that there is some underlying Stomach-Yin deficiency.

We can identify several stages of Yin deficiency according to the tongue coating and the body colour. As far as the Stomach is concerned, Stomach-Qi deficiency usually precedes Stomach-Yin deficiency and the very first and lightest sign of Stomach-Qi deficiency would be a rootless coating in the centre. At the other end of the scale, the most severe type of Yin deficiency (by this time with Empty-Heat) would be a

tongue that is Red, completely without coating and possibly with cracks indicating both Stomach-Yin and Kidney-Yin deficiency. We can therefore say that the tongue coating or the absence of it reflects a progression from Qi deficiency to Yin deficiency usually starting with the Stomach and gradually affecting other organs.

The most common stages of this process that we can identify are as follows:

- **Normal tongue with thin-white coating with root**: indicates good Stomach-Qi.
- **Rootless coating in the centre, normal body colour**: indicates the beginning of Stomach-Qi deficiency (Fig. 27.2).
- **Rootless coating all over, normal body colour**: indicates Stomach-Qi deficiency (Fig. 27.3 and Plates 26.1.a b on p. P25).
- **Rootless coating all over but missing in the centre, normal body colour**: indicates the beginning of Stomach-Yin deficiency (Fig. 27.4). A variation of this tongue would be that the centre is Red, which indicates Stomach-Yin deficiency with Empty-Heat (not affecting other organs) (Fig. 27.5).
- **Coating missing all over, normal body colour**: indicates advanced Stomach-Yin deficiency. A variation of this tongue would be that the centre is Red, which indicates advanced Stomach-Yin deficiency with Empty-Heat (not affecting other organs).
- **Coating missing all over, Red body colour**: indicates advanced Yin deficiency with Empty-Heat of the Stomach and other organs, notably the Kidneys. A variation of this tongue would be that, in addition to the above signs, the tongue also has a deep, midline Stomach crack and other scattered cracks, which simply indicate a more severe condition of Yin deficiency of the Stomach and Kidneys (Fig. 27.6).

Any of the first five tongues indicated above could also have a central Stomach crack or scattered Stomach cracks (Figs 27.2–27.5), which would simply indicate a pre-existing tendency to Stomach-Yin deficiency.

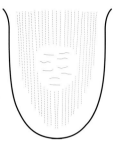

Fig. 27.2 Tongue with rootless coating in the centre

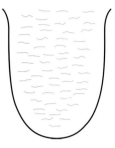

Fig. 27.3 Tongue with rootless coating all over

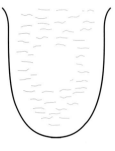

Fig. 27.4 Tongue with rootless coating all over but missing in the centre

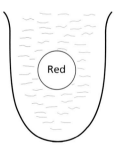

Red

Fig. 27.5 Tongue with rootless coating all over, missing in the centre and Red in the centre

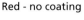

Red - no coating

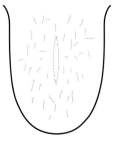

Fig. 27.6 Tongue with no coating, Red body colour, deep, midline Stomach crack and other scattered Stomach cracks

---

BOX 27.1 DEFICIENCY PATTERNS

Qi deficiency
- General Qi deficiency: slightly Pale
- Spleen-Qi deficiency: teethmarks or swollen on sides in central section
- Stomach-Qi deficiency: rootless coating
- Yang deficiency: Pale and slightly wet

Blood deficiency
- General Blood deficiency: Pale and slightly dry
- Liver-Blood deficiency: Pale on the sides

Yin deficiency
- General Yin deficiency: lack of coating
- Stomach-Yin deficiency: lack of coating in the centre
- Lung-Yin deficiency: lack of coating in the front third
- Kidney-Yin deficiency: lack of coating all over, Red body

THE TONGUE IN PHLEGM AND DAMPNESS

Both Phlegm and Dampness may manifest with a Swollen tongue and a sticky coating. However, in the case of Phlegm the swelling of the tongue is predominant, whereas in the case of Dampness the coating is predominant. Although both Phlegm and Dampness may derive from Qi deficiency, Qi deficiency on its own does *not* cause the tongue to be Swollen; therefore a Swollen tongue indicates not Qi deficiency but rather the presence of a pathogenic factor, that is, Phlegm or Dampness.

The tongue coating will differ slightly depending on whether there is Dampness or Phlegm present. Dampness causes the coating to appear more slippery and smooth, whereas a coating indicating Phlegm tends to be slightly rough and sticky.

THE TONGUE IN HEAT

Heat always manifests with a Red body colour and when examining a Red tongue the first question I ask myself is whether the tongue has a coating or not: a Red tongue with a coating with root (whatever its colour) indicates Full-Heat whereas a Red tongue without coating (or with a rootless coating) indicates Empty-Heat.

!

- **Full-Heat**: Red tongue with coating
- **Empty-Heat**: Red tongue without coating

When observing a Red tongue indicating Heat, we should identify the level of the Heat in accordance with the identification of patterns according to the Four Levels. Although the theory of the Four Levels was developed to explain the symptoms and signs of acute febrile diseases, it can be applied to conditions of chronic Heat. Indeed, much of the knowledge regarding Red tongues and red points derives from the theory of the Four Levels.

At the Defensive-Qi level, the tongue may be Red or slightly Red on the front or sides, or both, in the areas corresponding to the Exterior in the context of invasions of external Wind. (See Fig. 23.4 on p. 205.)

At the Qi level, the tongue is Red with a yellow, dark yellow, brown or even black coating. However, within the Qi level one can distinguish the two conditions of Heat or Fire. Heat is more superficial than Fire and can be cleared with pungent-cold herbs. Fire is deeper than Heat and needs to be drained with bitter-cold herbs. Within the theory of the Six Stages, the Bright-Yang channel pattern corresponds to Heat (of the Stomach) and the Bright-Yang organ pattern corresponds to Fire. Within the theory of the Four Levels the pattern of Stomach-Heat corresponds to Heat, whereas that of Dry Heat in the Stomach and Intestines corresponds to Fire. The tongue corresponding to Heat is Red with a yellow coating, whereas that corresponding to Fire is darker Red and with a dry, dark-yellow, brown or even black coating.

At the Nutritive-Qi and Blood levels, the tongue is Red and dry without a coating because at these levels the Fire has injured Yin.

Box 27.2 summarizes the tongue signs according to the Four Levels.

BOX 27.2 THE FOUR LEVELS AND THE TONGUE

- Slightly Red on the sides/front: Defensive-Qi level
- Red with dark-yellow coating: Qi level
- Red without coating: Nutritive-Qi level
- Dark Red without coating, dry: Blood level

THE TONGUE IN COLD

Cold affecting a Yin organ will manifest primarily on the tongue-body colour, which becomes Pale. For example, Spleen-Yang deficiency commonly manifests with a Pale tongue. Cold affecting a Yang organ will

manifest primarily on the tongue coating. For example, Cold in the Stomach manifests with a white coating in the centre.

When assessing the tongue in Cold patterns, we must distinguish Full- from Empty-Cold. Full-Cold manifests primarily on the coating, which becomes thick and white, while Empty-Cold manifests primarily on the colour and moisture of the tongue body, which becomes Pale and slightly wet.

THE TONGUE IN QI AND BLOOD STAGNATION

The tongue-body colour reflects the condition of Blood more than that of Qi. Therefore, in conditions of Qi stagnation the tongue-body colour may be unchanged, whereas in Blood stasis the tongue-body colour will become Purple. Chinese books frequently state that Liver-Qi stagnation manifests with a Purple tongue but I disagree with this as, in my opinion, a Purple colour on the sides always indicates Blood stasis.

In severe and long-standing conditions of Liver-Qi stagnation, the sides in the Liver area may become Red. However, in this case too, we can say that the tongue-body colour may reflect the condition of Blood primarily because the redness of the sides of the tongue indicates that long-standing Qi stagnation has given rise to Heat. Thus, the redness on the sides reflects the Heat rather than the Qi stagnation.

Blood stasis may manifest also with a Purple and dark colour of the sublingual veins. As mentioned above, this normally reflects the early stages of Blood stasis, particularly when it occurs in the Middle and Upper Burners.

THE TONGUE IN INTERNAL WIND

In internal Wind, the tongue may be Stiff, Moving or Deviated. Stiff is probably the most common way in which internal Wind manifests; the Moving tongue is not frequently seen, while the Deviated tongue indicating internal Wind is usually seen only in patients suffering from Wind-stroke.

THE TONGUE IN EXTERNAL INVASIONS OF WIND

As far as the body colour is concerned, in external invasions of Wind-Cold the tongue-body colour does not change. In invasions of Wind-Heat the tongue-body colour may become Red in the front or sides, or both, and, especially in children, it may also have red points in these areas. As far as the coating is concerned, this reflects invasions of external Wind only when the pathogenic factor is particularly strong, in which case the coating becomes thick. In the very beginning stages of invasion of Wind, the coating is white even with Wind-Heat; in other words, in the context of external invasions of Wind, a white colour of the coating indicates the early stage of invasion whereas a yellow colour indicates a later stage.

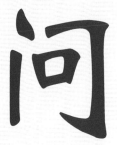

PART 2

DIAGNOSIS BY INTERROGATION

Part contents

28 Introduction *235*
29 Pain *253*
30 Food and taste *261*
31 Stools and urine *269*
32 Thirst and drink *277*
33 Energy levels *281*
34 Head *287*
35 Face *301*
36 Throat and neck *311*
37 Body *317*
38 Chest and abdomen *321*
39 Limbs *337*
40 Sleep *347*
41 Sweating *351*
42 Ears and eyes *355*
43 Feeling of cold, feeling of heat and fever *361*
44 Mental–emotional symptoms *379*
45 Sexual symptoms *391*
46 Women's symptoms *395*
47 Children's symptoms *411*
48 Diagnosing the causes of disease *415*

INTRODUCTION

This part deals with the diagnostic method based on asking. This is the central art of diagnosis not only because we need to elicit information from the patient but also because the way the patient talks during the interrogation is in itself a very important diagnostic sign reflecting the underlying physical, emotional and mental condition of the patient. Moreover, it is through the interrogation process that we interact with the patient; therefore, the skill, tact and compassion with which we conduct the interrogation has a profound influence on the therapeutic results themselves. Thus, the process of 'interrogation' of the patient is far more than a set of rules about which questions to ask and how to ask them: it is the heart of the therapeutic encounter between the practitioner and the patient; it is the crucible in which the healing takes place.

Diagnosis by interrogation is one of the four pillars of the Chinese diagnostic methods and one that should always be carried out. If the patient is unconscious or is a baby or a small child, the questions should be put to a close relative.

The discussion of the interrogation procedure will be articulated under the following headings (Chapter 28):

- nature of diagnosis by interrogation
- nature of 'symptoms' in Chinese medicine
- the art of interrogation: asking the right questions
- terminology problems in interrogation
- patients' expressions
- pitfalls to avoid in interrogation

- procedure for interrogation
- time scale of symptoms
- integration of interrogation with observation
- identification of patterns and interrogation
- tongue and pulse diagnosis: integration with interrogation
- the 10 traditional questions
- the 16 questions.

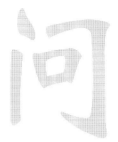

Chapter **28**

INTRODUCTION

Chapter contents

NATURE OF DIAGNOSIS BY INTERROGATION   235

NATURE OF 'SYMPTOMS' IN CHINESE MEDICINE   236
  Tongue and pulse   237

THE ART OF INTERROGATION: ASKING THE RIGHT QUESTIONS   237

TERMINOLOGY PROBLEMS IN INTERROGATION   238

PATIENTS' EXPRESSIONS   239

PITFALLS TO AVOID IN INTERROGATION   239

PROCEDURE FOR INTERROGATION   240

TIME SCALE OF SYMPTOMS   241

INTEGRATION OF INTERROGATION WITH OBSERVATION   242

IDENTIFICATION OF PATTERNS AND INTERROGATION   242

TONGUE AND PULSE DIAGNOSIS: INTEGRATION WITH INTERROGATION   243

THE 10 TRADITIONAL QUESTIONS   249
  Limitations of the 10 traditional questions   249
  Questions on emotional state   250
  Questions about sexual life   250
  Questions on energy levels   250

THE 16 QUESTIONS   250

NATURE OF DIAGNOSIS BY INTERROGATION

We can distinguish two aspects to the interrogation: a general one and a specific one.

In a ***general*** sense, the interrogation is the talk between doctor and patient to find out how the presenting problem arose, the living and working conditions of the patient and the emotional and family environment. The aim of an investigation of these aspects of the patient's life is ultimately to find the cause or causes of the disease rather than to identify the pattern; finding the causes of the disease is important in order for the patient and doctor to work together to try to eliminate or minimize such causes (Fig. 28. 1). How to find the cause of disease is discussed in Chapter 48.

In a ***specific*** sense, the interrogation aims at identifying the prevailing pattern of disharmony in the light of whatever method of pattern identification is applicable, for example according to the Internal Organs, according to the channels, according to the Four Levels, etc.

Box 28.1 summarizes these aspects of interrogation.

It is important not to blur the distinction between these two aspects of interrogation; enquiring about the

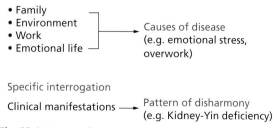

General interrogation

- Family
- Environment
- Work
- Emotional life

→ Causes of disease (e.g. emotional stress, overwork)

Specific interrogation

Clinical manifestations → Pattern of disharmony (e.g. Kidney-Yin deficiency)

Fig. 28.1 Interrogation

BOX 28.1 THE TWO ASPECTS OF INTERROGATION

- **General**: asking about lifestyle, work, emotions, diet, etc. to determine the cause of disease
- **Specific**: asking about clinical manifestations to determine the patterns of disharmony

patient's family situation, environment, work and relationships gives us an idea of the *cause*, not the *pattern* of the disharmony. Knowing that a patient is a business man with a heavy work burden, an antagonistic relationship with his employers or marital problems does not tell us which might be the prevailing *pattern* of disharmony but simply that stress and emotional tension are likely to be the *cause* of the disharmony; this knowledge is essential when working with the patient to try to eliminate or minimize the causes of disease.

During the course of the interrogation, we ask about many symptoms that may be apparently unrelated to the presenting problem; we do this in order to find the pattern (or patterns) of disharmony that underlie the presenting problem. For example, a patient may present with chronic backache which we suspect may be due to a Kidney-Yang deficiency with Dampness. By asking about bowels and urination, for example, we may find that there are other symptoms of Dampness in one of these two systems and this would confirm the original diagnosis of Dampness as the cause of the backache.

Not all symptoms and signs add up to one pattern of disharmony: indeed, most patients will suffer from at least two *related* patterns of disharmony. To use the above example again, in this case enquiring about urination and defecation may confirm to us that this patient does indeed suffer from Kidney-Yang deficiency with Dampness. These two patterns are related because deficient Kidney-Yang fails to warm, move, transform and excrete fluids properly, which may accumulate in the form of Dampness. Moreover, an enquiry about other areas of questioning beyond the lower back and urination is always important because it may reveal other patterns of disharmony, which may be *unrelated* to the patterns of disharmony causing a patient's presenting symptoms. To continue the above example, it may be that an enquiry about bowels, urination and other systems reveals a condition of Qi stagnation, which may be unrelated to the presenting problem.

Diagnosis by interrogation is intimately related to pattern identification: one cannot be carried out without a thorough knowledge of the other. Without a knowledge of pattern identification, interrogation would be a meaningless and aimless process of asking questions without a clear idea of what to make of the answers and how to use these to arrive at a diagnosis. On the other hand, a knowledge of pattern identification without a thorough understanding of diagnostic methods would be useless as we would lack the skills and tools to arrive at a pattern identification. Thus, a knowledge of pattern identification is the essential prerequisite to form a diagnosis, but skill in the diagnostic art is the means by which a diagnosis is made.

> **!**
>
> **Remember**: the questions asked during the interrogation must always be guided by our attempt to confirm or exclude a pattern of disharmony.

NATURE OF 'SYMPTOMS' IN CHINESE MEDICINE

Diagnosis by interrogation is based on the fundamental principle that symptoms and signs reflect the condition of the Internal Organs and channels. The concept of symptoms and signs in Chinese medicine is broader than in Western medicine. Whilst Western medicine mostly takes into account symptoms and signs as subjective and objective manifestations of a disease, Chinese medicine takes into account many different manifestations as parts of a whole picture, many of them not related to an actual disease process. Chinese medicine uses not only 'symptoms and signs' as such but many other manifestations to form a picture of the disharmony present in a particular person. Thus, the interrogation extends well beyond the 'symptoms and signs' pertaining to the presenting complaint. For example, if a patient presents with epigastric pain as the chief complaint, a Western doctor would enquire about the symptoms strictly relevant to that complaint (e.g. Is the pain better or worse after eating? Does the pain come immediately after eating or two hours later? Is there regurgitation of food? etc.). A Chinese doctor would ask similar questions but many others too, such as 'Are you thirsty?', 'Do you have a bitter taste in your

mouth?', 'Do you feel tired?', etc. Many of the so-called symptoms and signs of Chinese medicine would not be considered as such in Western medicine. For example, absence of thirst (which confirms a Cold condition), inability to make decisions (which points to a deficiency of the Gall-Bladder), dislike of speaking (which indicates a deficiency of the Lungs), propensity to outbursts of anger (which confirms the rising of Liver-Yang or Liver-Fire), desire to lie down (which indicates a weakness of the Spleen), dull appearance of the eyes (which points to a disturbance of the Mind and emotional problems), deep midline crack on the tongue (which is a sign of propensity to deep emotional problems), and so on. Whenever I refer to 'symptoms and signs' (which I shall also call 'clinical manifestations'), it will be in the above context.

Tongue and pulse

It is important to stress that the tongue and the pulse are signs that may determine a diagnosis, even in the complete absence of symptoms. In other words, a Slippery pulse is as much a sign of Phlegm as expectoration of sputum, and a persistently Weak pulse on the Kidney position is as much as sign of Kidney deficiency as other symptoms.

For example, a young woman may have a persistently Weak Kidney pulse without any symptoms of Kidney deficiency: the Weak Kidney pulse is as much a symptom of Kidney deficiency as backache, dizziness and tinnitus and we can therefore safely assume that this patient suffers from a Kidney deficiency. However, a particular pulse position may become Weak only temporarily through various lifestyle influences and we can reach a diagnostic conclusion only when the pulse has a particular quality consistently over a period of a few weeks or more.

The same applies to tongue signs which may appear in the absence of symptoms. For example, a Swollen tongue with a sticky coating indicates Phlegm even in the absence of other symptoms of Phlegm. In other words, such a tongue is as much a sign of Phlegm as expectoration of sputum.

> **!**
>
> **Remember**: the tongue or pulse *alone* are enough to confirm the presence of a pattern of disharmony.

THE ART OF INTERROGATION: ASKING THE RIGHT QUESTIONS

Diagnosis by interrogation is of course extremely important as, in the process of identifying a pattern, not all the information is given by the patient. Indeed, even if it were, it would still need to be organized in order to identify the pattern or patterns. Sometimes the absence of a certain symptom or sign is diagnostically determinant and patients, of course, would not report symptoms they do not experience. For example, in distinguishing between a Heat and a Cold pattern, it is necessary to establish whether a person is thirsty or not, and the absence of thirst would point to a Cold pattern. The patient would obviously not volunteer the information of 'not being thirsty'.

The art of diagnosis by interrogation consists in asking relevant questions in relation to a specific patient and a specific condition. A certain pattern may be diagnosed only when the 'right' questions are asked; if we are not aware of a specific pattern and do not ask relevant questions, we will never arrive at a correct diagnosis. For example, if we do not know the existence of the pattern of 'rebellious Qi of the Penetrating Vessel,' we will obviously not ask the questions which might lead us to diagnose such a pattern (see below).

The interrogation should not consist of blindly following the traditional list of questions; it should be conducted following a 'lead' with our asking a series of questions to confirm or exclude a pattern, or patterns, of disharmony that comes to our mind during the exchange of question and response. Therefore, when we ask the patient a question we should always ask ourselves *why* we are asking that question. During an interrogation, we should be constantly shifting or reviewing our hypotheses about the possible patterns of disharmony, trying to confirm or exclude certain patterns by asking the right questions.

For example, a patient may present with chronic headaches and, even at this very early stage, we are already making a hypothesis about the possible pattern of disharmony on the basis of our experience and our knowledge, that is, we are thinking of Liver-Yang rising because we know it is by far the most common cause of chronic headaches. We therefore ask questions about the character and location of the pain: if the patient says that the pain is throbbing and is located on the temples, even these few details would

almost certainly confirm the diagnosis of Liver-Yang rising. However, we should never stop there and reach premature conclusions. Instead we should ask further questions to confirm or exclude the existence of other patterns which also cause headaches. For example, Phlegm is another common cause of chronic headaches and we therefore ask this patient first about other characteristics of the headaches which may confirm Phlegm, and also about possible symptoms of Phlegm in other parts of the body: 'Does the patient experience a feeling of muzziness in the head?' 'Is the headache sometimes dull and accompanied by a feeling of heaviness?' If the answer to these questions is affirmative, we conclude that Phlegm might be a further cause of the headaches. We then ask other questions related to Phlegm in other parts of the body; in this particular case, we might ask whether the patient occasionally expectorates sputum or sometimes experiences a feeling of oppression in the chest. (Fig. 28.2).

Another example of the importance of asking the right questions to confirm or exclude our hypothesis about the pattern or patterns of disharmony is rebellious Qi of the Penetrating Vessel. Rebellious Qi in the Penetrating Vessel may cause a wide range of symptoms affecting the whole torso. These may include: lower abdominal fullness and pain, painful periods, umbilical fullness and pain, epigastric fullness and pain, a feeling of energy rising in the abdomen, a feeling of tightness of the chest, slight breathlessness, palpitations, a feeling of lump in the throat, a feeling of heat in the face, and anxiety (of course not all these symptoms need to be present). It may well be that the patient reports only the symptoms of painful periods and a feeling of lump in the throat: if we are not familiar with the pattern of rebellious Qi in the Penetrating

Vessel we may not ask the right questions to uncover other related symptoms and we may therefore attribute painful periods to Cold in the Uterus (for example) and the feeling of a lump in the throat to stagnation of Liver-Qi. Even should we uncover other symptoms mentioned above, if we are not familiar with the pattern of rebellious Qi in the Penetrating Vessel we may wrongly attribute the above symptoms to a confusing number of patterns involving many organs instead of seeing that they are connected with the pattern of rebellious Qi of the Penetrating Vessel.

TERMINOLOGY PROBLEMS IN INTERROGATION

A potential problem for practitioners in the West is that the interrogation and the various expressions used to express symptoms are derived from Chinese experiences and culture and a Western patient would not necessarily use the same expressions. This is a problem, however, that can be overcome with experience. After some years of practice, we can learn to translate the Chinese way of expressing symptoms and find correlations more common to Western patients. For example, whereas a Chinese man might spontaneously say that he has a 'distending pain', an English-speaking Western patient might say that he feels 'bloated' or 'bursting'. The words are different, but the symptom they describe is the same. With practice and acute observation we gradually build up a 'vocabulary' of symptoms as described by Western patients. For example, I have come to interpret the peculiar English expression 'a feeling of butterflies in the stomach' as a symptom of rebellious Qi in the Penetrating Vessel.

The translation from Chinese of the terms related to certain symptoms may also present some problems. The traditional terms are rich with meaning and sometimes very poetic and are more or less impossible to translate properly because Western language cannot convey all the nuances intrinsic in a Chinese character. For example, I translate the word *Men* as a 'feeling of oppression'; an analysis of the Chinese character, however, which portrays a heart squashed by a door, conveys the feeling of oppression in a rich, metaphorical way. What cannot be adequately translated is the cultural use of this term in China often to imply that the person is rather 'depressed' (as we intend this term in the West) from emotional problems. As Chinese

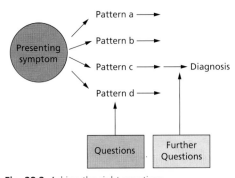

Fig. 28.2 Asking the right questions

patients seldom admit openly to being 'depressed', they will often say they experience a feeling of *Men* in the chest.

Another example is the term *Xin Fan*, which I translate as 'mental restlessness': the Chinese characters contain the radical for 'heart', indicating an emotional cause of this feeling, and the radical for 'fire', indicating the heating effect of emotional stress on the Internal Organ; the translation cannot possibly do justice to the Chinese term and convey its rich inner meaning.

Yet another interesting example is the use of the word *Ku* to describe certain symptoms: *Ku* means 'bitter' and is sometimes used to indicate a pain's severity. However, the word *Ku* in China has also a definite emotional connotation implying that the person has had a 'bitter' life and bitter life experiences.

We should not, however, overemphasize the terminology problems due to cultural differences between China and the West. Quite frequently, Western patients report symptoms exactly as they are in Chinese books. For example, a patient recently told me quite spontaneously 'I am often thirsty but I do not feel like drinking'.

PATIENTS' EXPRESSIONS

It is only after the patient has finished relating the main problems that we can start asking questions systematically on the basis of the '10 questions' (see below), but always following the lead given by what the patient has told us. Often patients have a good insight as to the main problem in their life; often this is the first 'problem' they report. For example, when asked about what the main problem was, a 48-year-old man said that he was *at a cross-roads in his life*, that he *felt dissatisfied with his work* and that he *was searching for something more meaningful in his life*. This is a good example of how a patient spontaneously volunteers information about existential doubts which are obviously at the root of the physical problems. Of course, it is not always like this: very many patients cannot see or do not want to see the existential and spiritual problems in their life and present with a long list of physical symptoms which hide the true root of their existential *dis-ease*.

At the beginning of the interrogation, it is important to let patients speak freely and to make a note of the actual expressions they use; these are usually quite suggestive and indicative of the patient's problem and sometimes also of the aetiology. For example, if a patient describes feeling 'impotent' about a certain situation, it conveys the idea that the patient feels frustrated (and, in the case of a man, it may also indicate sexual impotence). It is particularly important to make a note of the actual expression used by a patient especially when this is repeated in the course of the interrogation. For example, a patient may use the expression 'trapped' two or three times, clearly indicating that emotional frustration may be at the root of the problem.

In some cases patients refer to a particular part of the body several times in the course of the interrogation and this gives a strong indication of the possible pattern involved. For example, a patient suffering from chronic mental–emotional problems may refer to the 'throat' three or four times during the course of the interrogation, saying things such as, 'I feel a lump in the throat when I'm upset', 'My throat often feels dry', or 'I feel my heart in my throat': this may suggest a condition of Qi stagnation in the Liver or Lungs.

The practice of Chinese medicine in the West presents us with new challenges which Chinese practitioners do not have in China. Western patients often seek treatment in search of an existential and spiritual balance, which is not the case in China. We therefore need to adapt our diagnosis and treatment to the needs of Western patients. For example, a woman said that she sought treatment because she wanted 'more integration, rhythm and earthedness in her life'. We therefore need to develop a new knowledge of patterns and diagnosis which allows us to interpret the needs of our patients as they report them. In this particular example, I interpreted this patient's lack of 'earthedness' as being due to a severe Kidney deficiency which made her feel 'without root' (it would have been a mistake to interpret her word 'earthedness' in a literal sense as necessarily pointing to a deficiency in the Earth element).

PITFALLS TO AVOID IN INTERROGATION

The specific interrogation (as defined above), based on questions that concern the patient's clinical manifestations, is aimed at finding the *pattern* of disharmony; the

general interrogation (about the patient's lifestyle, family situation, emotional environment, living conditions, etc.) is aimed at finding the cause of disease. It would be wrong to confuse the two and to deduce the pattern of disharmony from the enquiry about the patient's lifestyle, work and family life. I have noticed this occurring in practice many times when a student or practitioner brings a patient to me for a second opinion: I frequently hear comments such as 'Andrew is under a lot of stress at work and he **therefore** suffers from Liver-Qi stagnation'. This is an example of how a practitioner may confuse the general enquiry about the patient's life to find the *cause* of the disease with the specific enquiry about clinical manifestations to find the *pattern* of disharmony. In other words, to go back to the above example, it would be totally wrong to *assume* that Andrew suffers from Liver-Qi stagnation on the basis of an enquiry about his lifestyle, work, etc.: such a diagnosis can be made only on the basis of a specific enquiry about his clinical manifestations. Patients might well have a lot of stress in their life, but this does not necessarily cause Liver-Qi stagnation as emotional strain may cause many other patterns.

Another possible pitfall is to make a diagnosis of a pattern of disharmony on the basis of vague and woolly concepts deduced from observation of the patient's lifestyle – for example, 'Betty seems to be a very "woody" person, so I thought there was Liver-Qi stagnation'. Of course, a diagnosis of a person's prevailing Element on the basis of the body shape, mannerism, gait and voice is important (see Chapter 1), but this does not always coincide with the prevailing pattern; in other words, a Wood-type person will not necessarily suffer from a Liver pattern of disharmony.

A word of caution about the conducting of the interrogation is called for. As mentioned above, the interrogation is conducted with close reference to pattern identification and the questions are aimed at confirming or excluding the existence of a certain pattern of disharmony in the patient. The diagnostic process starts with observation skills as soon as a patient walks in; for example, if a woman patient looks pale, talks with a low voice, and complains of tiredness and poor appetite, we immediately think of Spleen-Qi deficiency as a possible pattern, and thus further questions aim to confirm or disprove the existence of this pattern. In Chinese medicine, however, it is easy to conduct the interrogation in a way that might influence the patient and elicit the symptoms that will force the clinical manifestations into a preconceived

pattern; this is a real danger of Chinese diagnosis. The only way to eliminate this danger is to keep an open mind; this is extremely important. Going back to the above example, we must at all times be prepared to contemplate the real possibility that this patient might *not* suffer from Spleen-Qi deficiency, or that Spleen-Qi deficiency might not be the only or even the main pattern or problem.

Box 28.2 summarizes pitfalls in interrogation.

> ### BOX 28.2 PITFALLS IN INTERROGATION
>
> - Do not use information about the patient's lifestyle to deduce the *pattern* of disharmony (you may deduce the *cause* of disease from it).
> - Do not rely exclusively on a patient's Elemental type to diagnose a pattern of disharmony.
> - Remember to keep an open mind when diagnosing the patterns of disharmony.

PROCEDURE FOR INTERROGATION

The interrogation generally follows on from the observation of the patient's facial colour, body shape and body movement and hearing the patient's voice and other sounds: thus observation precedes interrogation. As soon as the patient comes in, the diagnostic process has already started: we observe the movement of the patient (whether slow or quick, for example), the complexion, the body shape, to assess it in terms of Five Elements, the sound of the voice and any smell emanating from the patient.

I usually start the interrogation by asking the patient about the main problems that bring him or her to me: I let the patient speak freely first without interrupting. I always make a note of any peculiar expressions the patient might use. As indicated above, Western patients will obviously use different expressions from those used by Chinese patients. I never discount a patient's turn of phrase as it can usually be interpreted in terms of Chinese diagnosis.

Examples of peculiar descriptions of symptoms from my practice with English patients might include 'a feeling of butterflies in the stomach', a 'feeling as if the stomach is having an argument with itself', etc. As the patient is describing the main problem or problems, I am already thinking of various patterns of disharmony that might be causing it or them, and I therefore start asking questions to confirm or exclude the particular pattern of disharmony I had in mind.

After patients have finished reporting the main problems for which they are seeking help, and after I have broadly decided on the patterns of disharmony involved, I then proceed to ask more questions, generally following either the traditional 10 questions or the 16 questions that are indicated later in this chapter. This is done for two reasons: first, because the answers to these further questions may confirm the patterns of disharmony diagnosed and, second, because they may bring up other problems which the patient has overlooked.

I generally look at the tongue and feel the pulse towards the end of the interrogation, again to confirm further the patterns of disharmony. However, it is important to note that the tongue and pulse are not simply used to confirm the diagnosis of a pattern of disharmony: very often they clearly show the existence of other patterns which were not evident from the symptoms and signs. In this case, we should never discount the findings of the tongue and pulse but we should always ask further questions to confirm the patterns of disharmony shown by the tongue and pulse. Even if there are no further symptoms, we can still rely on the tongue and pulse signs as the basis to diagnose a certain pattern of disharmony. For example, a patient may come to us complaining of dizziness and, on the basis of symptoms and signs, we diagnose that the prevailing pattern causing the dizziness is that of Phlegm. When we then observe the tongue, we find that the tongue, besides being Swollen (indicating Phlegm) is also clearly Purple; this is a definite sign of Blood stasis even if the patient has no symptoms of it.

In a few cases, the tongue and pulse may show conditions that are actually opposite to that indicated by the patterns of disharmony. For example, a person may suffer from a very clear Yang deficiency and the pulse is Rapid or, vice versa, the person has clear symptoms and signs of Heat but the pulse is Slow. We should never discount these contradictory signs and we should always try to find their cause.

TIME SCALE OF SYMPTOMS

After this step, I would continue asking other questions, broadly following the 16 questions discussed below to find out whether there are other symptoms and signs that the patient might have forgotten about. This is always followed by asking about past history of any other diseases or operations.

When asking about various problems the patient has or has had, it is important to establish the exact time of onset. It is my experience that patients nearly always underestimate the length of time that they have suffered from a particular problem. Therefore if, when asked how long the particular problem has existed, a patient says 'I cannot remember exactly, probably 5–7 years', we can be almost certain that the onset was at the higher point of the range offered by the patient, that is, 7 years or more.

Establishing the time of onset of a problem accurately is important in many cases because it may establish a causality that neither the patient nor the doctor or consultant has observed, and this happens frequently in practice. Examples of events (besides the traditional causes of disease, e.g. emotional problems, diet, etc.) that may be the unrecognized trigger of a particular problem are:

- an operation
- an accident
- an immunization
- the menarche
- the menopause
- childbirth.

For example, a patient may develop abdominal pain after an abdominal operation from adhesions; someone may develop backache and neck ache after an accident which had been forgotten; postviral fatigue syndrome (myeloencephalitis, ME) may develop after a series of immunizations prior to travel abroad; young girls suffering from migraine may have forgotten that the onset coincided with the menarche (this has important repercussions on the diagnosis and treatment); a change in the emotional state may be related to the onset of the menopause; asthma or migraine may start after childbirth.

Box 28.3 summarizes the main 'trigger events' in patients' lives.

BOX 28.3 TRIGGER EVENTS IN PATIENTS' LIVES

- An operation
- An accident
- An immunization
- The menarche
- The menopause
- Childbirth

INTEGRATION OF INTERROGATION WITH OBSERVATION

The interrogation should be integrated seamlessly with observation. All the time while the patient is talking we should observe the facial complexion, the eyes and other features; this is important not only for the observation itself but also to observe any changes that take place during the interrogation. For example, frequently women develop a light, red rash on the neck as they relate their symptoms; I interpret this as a sign of Liver-Heat and one that often reflects the emotional origin of a problem.

Another possible change that should be observed during the interrogation is a change in the tone and pitch of voice. If the voice becomes weaker and sounds sad, this indicates that sadness or grief are at the root of the problem, in particular of the specific problem being related. For example, if a woman's voice becomes weak and sad as she reports that her periods have stopped, it may indicate that sadness or grief affecting the Lungs and Heart are the root of this particular problem. Conversely, if the voice becomes stronger and assumes a higher pitch as the patient relates a particular problem, it may indicate that that problem is due to anger or repressed anger. Often a patient may try to hide a particular emotion; for example by laughing inappropriately during the interrogation; the hidden emotion is often sadness or grief, especially in societies where expression of one's feelings is somewhat discouraged.

IDENTIFICATION OF PATTERNS AND INTERROGATION

After the patient has finished describing the main problem or problems, we start asking questions to organize the presenting symptoms and signs into patterns. While we ask questions, we still observe the complexion, eyes, shape of facial features, sound of voice, smells, etc., to be integrated with the findings from the interrogation. Once we are reasonably confident in having identified the pattern or patterns involved, we must continue the interrogation often to *exclude* or confirm the presence of other patterns that may stem from the existing ones. For example, if there is Liver-

Blood deficiency, I would always check whether this has given rise to Heart-Blood deficiency (especially if the observation leads me to believe this) and would therefore ask questions to exclude (or confirm) the presence of this pattern. If there is a Liver deficiency, in women especially (for example, if a woman suffers from amenorrhoea), even though the pattern of Liver-Blood deficiency may be very clear, I would always check whether there is a Kidney deficiency. If there is Liver-Qi stagnation, I would check whether this has given rise to some Heat; if there is a Spleen deficiency, I would check whether there is also a Stomach deficiency, etc.

It is important to remember, therefore, that the interrogation is aimed not only at finding out the main pattern or patterns of disharmony but often also at excluding certain patterns of disharmony. Table 28.1 shows the main patterns that I usually exclude or confirm in the presence of a presenting pattern.

Table 28.1 Patterns to exclude or confirm in the presence of presenting patterns

Presenting pattern	Pattern to exclude or confirm
Liver-Qi stagnation	Liver-Blood deficiency
Liver-Qi stagnation	Stagnant Liver-Qi turning into Heat
Liver-Qi stagnation	Liver-Blood stasis
Liver-Blood deficiency	Heart-Blood deficiency (and vice versa)
Liver-Blood deficiency	Liver-Yin deficiency
Liver-Blood deficiency	Kidney deficiency
Liver-Yang rising	Liver-Yin deficiency
Liver-Yang rising	Kidney deficiency
Liver-Yang rising	Liver-Blood deficiency
Liver-Yang rising	Liver-Fire
Liver-Fire	Heart-Fire
Heart-Blood deficiency	Liver-Blood deficiency
Heart-Fire	Liver-Fire
Heart-Yin deficiency	Kidney-Yin deficiency
Spleen-Qi deficiency	Spleen-Yang deficiency
Spleen-Qi deficiency	Stomach-Qi deficiency
Spleen-Qi deficiency	Dampness (and vice versa)
Spleen-Yang deficiency	Kidney-Yang deficiency
Lung-Qi deficiency	Spleen-Qi deficiency
Lung-Yin deficiency	Kidney-Yin deficiency
Kidney-Yang deficiency	Spleen-Yang deficiency
Kidney-Yin deficiency	Liver-, Heart- or Lung-Yin deficiency
Invasion of Wind	Check for symptoms of interior transmission

TONGUE AND PULSE DIAGNOSIS: INTEGRATION WITH INTERROGATION

Finally, I look at the tongue and feel the pulse: this is done not only to *confirm* the pattern or patterns identified from the interrogation but also to see whether the tongue and pulse indicate the presence of patterns not evident from the clinical manifestations. This occurs frequently in practice and is the real value of tongue and pulse diagnosis; if tongue and pulse diagnosis were used simply to confirm a diagnosis, there would be no point in carrying out this step.

Very often the tongue and pulse add valuable information to the findings from interrogation and should never be discounted. For example, a patient may complain of various symptoms and we diagnose Liver-Qi stagnation; if the tongue has a deep Heart crack, this tells us that the patient has a constitutional tendency to Heart patterns and a constitu-

> **!**
>
> **Remember**: the tongue and pulse may indicate the presence of patterns not evident from the clinical manifestations.

tional tendency to be more affected by emotional problems. Case history 28.1 is a good illustration of this.

Case history 28.2 is another example of the importance of pulse and tongue in diagnosis and how these two factors can point to a completely different set of patterns which would not emerge from a superficial examination of symptoms.

Besides giving extremely valuable information for diagnosis, the tongue and pulse are very important also to determine the treatment principle. In fact, they are very important to help us discriminate when a Fullness or Emptiness predominates. For example, in chronic ME (postviral fatigue syndrome), there is

Case history 28.1

A 24-year-old woman complained of chronic aches in her knees, wrists and ankles. She also suffered from chronic tiredness, dizziness and loose stools. Her periods were regular and lasted only 3 days. Apart from this, she had no other symptoms. Her clinical manifestations indicate a deficiency of Blood (tiredness, dizziness, scanty periods) and a Spleen deficiency (tiredness, loose stools). The joint ache may be due to invasion of Cold and Dampness (she lived in a particularly damp area of the British Isles) but it is also aggravated by the underlying Blood deficiency (Liver-Blood not nourishing the sinews).

However, the pulse and tongue indicated totally different patterns. Her pulse was Overflowing on both Front positions and her tongue was very Red, with a redder tip with red points and a Heart crack. Thus, every sign of the pulse and tongue clearly indicated Heart-Fire; she had not related any symptom that would indicate this apart from thirst (which I asked her about after seeing her tongue and feeling her pulse). I

came to the conclusion that she was suffering from severe emotional problems that were probably quite long standing and deriving from her childhood (due to the Heart crack). The acupuncturist who had been treating her and had referred her to me confirmed this. This is therefore a good example of a case when the pulse and tongue throw an entirely different light on the diagnosis; for this reason, the findings of pulse and tongue diagnosis should never be discarded when they do not fit the symptoms and signs. A further confirmation of the accuracy of the diagnosis based on the pulse and tongue was the patient's reaction to the herbal formula prescribed. I totally ignored the presenting symptoms and, only on the basis of the findings from the pulse and tongue, prescribed a variation of the formula Gan Mai Da Zao Tang *Glycyrrhiza-Triticum-Zizyphus Decoction* (which calms the Mind and nourishes the Heart) with the addition of Yuan Zhi *Radix Polygalae tenuifoliae*, Shi Chang Pu *Rhizoma Acori graminei* and Long Chi *Dens Draconis* with good results.

Case history 28.2

A 33-year-old woman had been suffering from abdominal distension and pain for 6 years. Her bowel movements were regular, occurring every day. She was under stress at work. She appeared as a very confident and balanced young professional woman.

Diagnosis: At fist sight, this seems an obvious and simple case of Liver-Qi stagnation deriving from stress at work and probably an irregular diet (these two causes of disease often go together). However, her pulse and tongue showed a totally different story. Her tongue was Red on the sides, and had a deep Heart crack and a sticky-yellow coating. Her pulse was Slippery and quite Overflowing on the Heart position. Her eyes lacked lustre.

The deep Heart crack on the tongue clearly indicates deep-seated and long-standing emotional problems that go beyond just stress at work; this was confirmed by the Overflowing quality of the Heart pulse and the lack of lustre of her eyes. Therefore, the tongue and pulse showed a completely different picture to the image she tried to project: she obviously suffered from deep emotional problems most probably dating back to her childhood or teenage years. I did not feel it appropriate to delve into this during the first consultation but, on asking, she did confirm that she suffered from deep depressions, irregular moods, gloominess, irritability and anxiety.

always a combination of Dampness (or Damp-Heat) with Spleen deficiency; it is therefore important to determine whether we should concentrate on tonifying the Spleen or on resolving Dampness. The tongue and pulse are important to help in determining this: if the tongue has a fairly thick coating and the pulse is Slippery, we should probably concentrate on resolving Dampness.

An even more important case is that of cancer. I usually use Chinese medicine as an adjuvant to Western therapies for cancer. Thus, if a patient is undergoing chemotherapy, I would not treat the cancer but would support the body's Qi and the immune system with herbs to tonify Qi, Blood or Yin. After the end of chemotherapy or after surgery, I assess the tongue and pulse to get an idea of whether the patterns that caused the cancer are still active. In other words, even after surgery to remove a tumour (normally caused by Blood stasis, Phlegm or Toxic Heat, or a combination of these), I assess the situation to determine whether such pathogenic factors are still present and how 'active' they are. The tongue and pulse are important to determine this: if the tongue is Red, with red points and a sticky coating, and the pulse is Rapid and Slippery or Wiry, I assume that, in spite of the surgery, the pathogenic factors are very much active and I therefore administer herbs aimed at expelling such factors, together with anticancer herbs. If, on the other hand, the tongue is not Red and does not have red points or a sticky coating, and the pulse is Weak, Deep and Fine, I dedicate my attention to tonifying the body's Qi and strengthening the immune system.

Case histories 28.3 and 28.4 illustrate the process of interrogation.

Case history 28.3 (Fig. 28.3)

A 37-year-old woman comes in: she is rather thin, pale without 'lustre', she walks slowly and her voice is rather low. As she sits down, we notice that her hair is dry and lifeless and that she looks and sounds in rather low spirits. At this point, a first tentative diagnosis is made already as the thin body, dull-pale complexion, dry hair and low spirits all point to Blood deficiency (this tentative conclusion is illustrated by a triangle): we know that this is all the more likely as Blood deficiency is common in women. However, as mentioned above, we must absolutely keep an open mind and be prepared to acknowledge that the patient does not suffer from Blood deficiency: if we do not keep an open mind, there may be the danger that our whole interrogation is biased, 'forcing' the clinical manifestations into the preconceived pattern of Blood deficiency.

As we ask her about her chief complaint, she reports suffering from premenstrual tension, something that does not directly confirm the diagnosis of Blood deficiency. Since the main complaint is premenstrual tension (illustrated by a double-line box), we

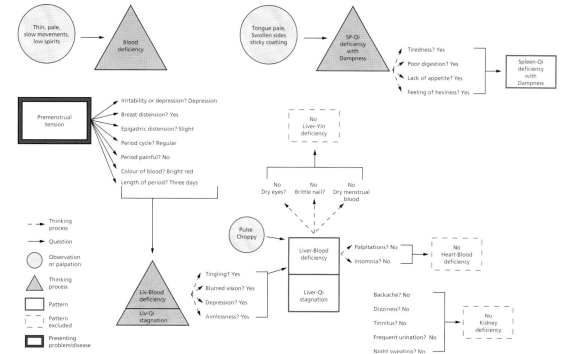

Fig. 28.3 Case history 28.3: process

immediately think of Liver-Qi stagnation first as this is the most common cause of this condition (illustrated by a triangle): however, we also keep in mind that there are other possible causes of premenstrual tension, some Full (such as Phlegm-Fire) and some Empty (such as Liver-Blood deficiency or Kidney deficiency). We therefore start asking questions to confirm or exclude Liver-Qi stagnation. The questions and answers are as follows:

- What are the main manifestations of the premenstrual tension: irritability or depression? She says both, but more depression and crying than irritability. We ask this question to help differentiate a Full (in which irritability predominates) from an Empty (in which depression predominates) condition of premenstrual tension.
- Is there breast distension? Yes. We ask this question to confirm whether or not there is Liver-Qi stagnation: a pronounced feeling of distension indicates Liver-Qi stagnation. In this case, there is a feeling of distension but it is not that pronounced.
- Is there epigastric or abdominal distension? Very little.

- Is the period cycle regular? Yes. We ask this question to confirm whether there is Liver-Qi stagnation or not, as a severe Liver-Qi stagnation may make the period irregular.
- Is the period painful? No, but there is distension. We ask this question because we have ascertained that there is some Liver-Qi stagnation and the next step is to enquire whether this has led to Blood stasis: the absence of menstrual pain tells us that there is no Blood stasis.
- What colour is the menstrual blood? Bright-red. We ask this question as a further aid to confirm or exclude the presence of Blood stasis: the bright-red colour confirms that there is no Blood stasis.
- How many days does the period last? Three days. This confirms that there is Blood deficiency.

At this point, a further picture is tentatively created in our mind: it seems quite clear now that there is some Liver-Qi stagnation causing the premenstrual tension but this is not too pronounced and most probably is secondary to the Liver-Blood deficiency (a situation that is very common in women). This conclusion is illustrated by a single-line box. It remains now to check that there are no other patterns: a very common one in this

situation would be a Kidney deficiency. We therefore ask the following questions:

- Do you ever suffer from backache? No.
- Do you ever suffer from dizziness? Yes.
- Do you ever suffer from tinnitus? No.
- Is your urination too frequent? No.
- Do you ever suffer from night sweating? No.

The absence of backache, tinnitus, frequent urination and night sweating indicates the absence of a Kidney deficiency (this is indicated by a dotted box); although there is some dizziness, in the absence of other Kidney symptoms it must be caused by the Blood deficiency. In order to confirm the diagnosis of Blood deficiency unequivocally, we ask a few more questions about this:

- Do you ever experience some tingling of the limbs? Yes.
- Do you ever experience blurred vision? Yes, sometimes.
- Do you ever feel depressed? Yes.
- Do you ever have a feeling of aimlessness or confusion about what direction to take in life? Yes.

These four further symptoms confirm the deficiency of Liver-Blood unequivocally: the depression, feeling of aimlessness and confusion about life's direction are due to the Ethereal Soul being unrooted in Liver-Blood. Why deficiency of Blood of the Liver and not of other organs? The scanty period, dry hair and blurred vision point to Blood deficiency of the Liver. However, we should check whether there might not be also a Blood deficiency of another organ and especially of the Heart. We therefore ask the following questions:

- Do you ever suffer from palpitations? No.
- Do you suffer from insomnia? No.

The answer to these two questions allows us to exclude the presence of Heart-Blood deficiency (illustrated by a dotted box). Finally, as there is Liver-Blood deficiency, we should check whether this has progressed to Liver-Yin deficiency. We therefore ask the following questions:

- Do you ever suffer from dry eyes? No.
- Dry and brittle nails? No.
- Dry menstrual blood? No.

The negative answer to these three questions tells us that there is no Liver-Yin deficiency (illustrated by a dotted box). Thus, we have established that the main

problem is a deficiency of Liver-Blood giving rise to a secondary stagnation of Liver-Qi; the fact that the Liver-Qi stagnation is secondary is important for the treatment principle as this means that we should concentrate our attention on nourishing Liver-Blood and only secondarily on moving Liver-Qi.

Before concluding the interrogation, we should ask about any other symptoms to make sure that there are no other patterns; we therefore ask about any headache, chest pain, abdominal pain, stools and urine, sleep and sweating: no further symptoms are reported.

It is now time to look at the tongue and feel the pulse. Her tongue is Pale, slightly Swollen, especially on the sides and with a sticky-white coating. Her pulse was Choppy on the left and Weak on the right.

Being Pale, the tongue confirms the Blood deficiency but it also shows other patterns that had not emerged from the interrogation: the swelling on the sides indicates Spleen deficiency and the sticky coating indicates Dampness. A Spleen deficiency with some Dampness is one of the most common conditions in practice and it is therefore not surprising to find it reflected on this patient's tongue. Having noticed this on her tongue we must go back to ask some more questions to confirm that there is a Spleen deficiency with some Dampness. We therefore ask the following:

- Do you feel easily tired? Yes. This tells us that there might be some Spleen deficiency.
- How is your appetite? Poor.
- Do you have any digestive problems? Fullness after eating? A sticky taste? Epigastric pain? The patient reports no epigastric pain but does have some feeling of fullness after eating. This confirms the Dampness.
- Do you ever experience a feeling of heaviness? Yes, slightly. This further confirms the presence of Dampness.

As for the pulse, the Weak quality on the right confirms the Spleen deficiency while the Choppy quality on the left confirms the Blood deficiency.

In conclusion, there is Liver-Blood deficiency, Spleen-Qi deficiency, a secondary stagnation of Liver-Qi and some Dampness; thus, there are two Empty and two Full patterns. The Empty character of the pulse is important in guiding us to the right treatment principle, which in this case must be primarily to nourish Liver-Blood and tonify Spleen-Qi and secondarily to move Liver-Qi and resolve Dampness.

In conclusion, Box 28.4 lists the order I usually follow in my interrogation.

Case history 28.4 (Fig. 28.4)

A 42-year-old woman complains of having suffered benign positional vertigo for the last 20 years. As she comes in, we notice that she is thin, she walks rather slowly, she is quiet, her voice is low and her eyes are slightly dull. These signs derived from observation give us a very first impression of her condition and they clearly point to a deficiency. In addition, the dull-ness of her eyes indicates that emotional problems may be the cause of her condition. As she sits down, we start asking about her symptoms in greater detail. She says that she has been suffering from infrequent attacks of vertigo for the past 20 years and that these got worse and more frequent after the birth of her second daughter two and a half years ago. The aggravation of the symptoms after childbirth leads us to think of a Kidney deficiency as one of the possible

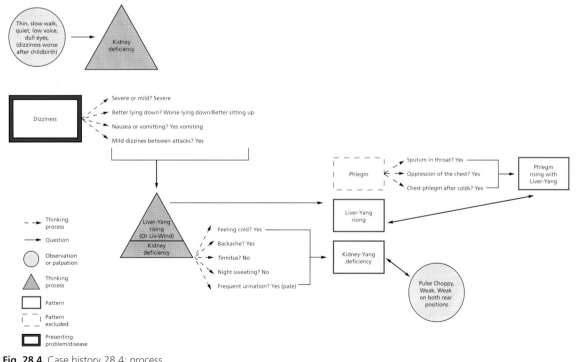

Fig. 28.4 Case history 28.4: process

patterns. During the attacks of vertigo, she suffers from very severe dizziness so that the room seems to be spinning around and she vomits; the attacks usually occur in the mornings and are aggravated by lying down and ameliorated by sitting. The severity of the vertigo clearly indicates that it is due to a Full pattern; therefore, from the few signs and symptoms gleaned from the initial observation and interrogation, we can conclude that there is a mixed condition of Fullness and Emptiness. The severe vertigo could be due to either Liver-Yang rising or Liver-Wind. In between the attacks of severe vertigo she also suffers from bouts of mild dizziness. In contrast to the attacks of severe vertigo, the bouts of mild dizziness must be due to a deficiency, probably of the Kidneys. At this point we have reached some temporary conclusions and we can hypothesize that she suffers from Liver-Yang rising (causing the severe vertigo and possibly vomiting) stemming from a Kidney deficiency (causing the bouts of mild dizziness and also the aggravation of vertigo after childbirth).

We now need to ask about other symptoms and she reports feeling cold in general and suffering from chilblains in winter. In order to confirm or exclude the pattern of Kidney deficiency we ask about backache, tinnitus, night sweating and urination: she does suffer from chronic lower backache and frequent urination with pale urine. Considering the general cold feeling, the backache, the frequent urination, the bouts of mild dizziness and the aggravation after childbirth, we can diagnose the pattern of Kidney-Yang deficiency. We can also deduce that the Kidney deficiency is the underlying condition for the rising of Liver-Yang.

We then ask about her periods, an essential question in all women, and she reports no problems in this area: the periods come regularly, they are not too heavy or too scanty and not painful.

As we know that Phlegm is a frequent cause of dizziness and vertigo, we need to ask questions to confirm or exclude the possibility of the interaction of Phlegm and Liver-Yang rising as a cause of her vertigo. Her body shape does not point to Phlegm as she is thin (Phlegm tends to cause obesity); however, that is not to say that thin people never suffer from Phlegm. We ask her whether she suffers from catarrh

and she does say that she often has to clear her throat in the morning and if she gets a cold, it frequently goes to her chest producing a lot of sputum. She also occasionally suffers from a feeling of oppression of the chest; these symptoms together with the vomiting during the attacks of vertigo point to Phlegm as a concurrent cause of vertigo.

Her tongue has Red sides and apart from that it is fairly normal; the tongue therefore does not show any signs of Phlegm as it is not Swollen and does not have a sticky coating. This does not mean that there is no Phlegm but simply that Phlegm is an accompanying pattern and a further cause of the vertigo secondary to that of Liver-Yang rising. Her pulse is Weak in general, Choppy and Weak on the left and especially Weak on both the Rear positions. The pulse therefore clearly shows only the deficiency patterns of her condition, that is, Kidney-Yang deficiency and Spleen-Qi deficiency, which is at the root of Phlegm. This is a clear example of a case when the pulse and tongue show different aspects of the condition: the pulse shows the underlying deficiency condition whereas the tongue shows Liver-Yang rising. We should not expect the pulse and the tongue always to accord with each other (in this case, we might have expected a Wiry pulse to accord with the Red sides of the tongue) as they often show different aspects of a complex condition.

In conclusion, there are two deficiency patterns: Kidney-Yang deficiency and Spleen-Qi deficiency (which are the Root), and two full patterns: Liver-Yang rising and Phlegm (which are the Manifestation). As far as the severe vertigo is concerned, Liver-Yang rising is primary in relation to Phlegm. The treatment principle in this case would therefore be to treat both the Root and the Manifestation by simultaneously tonifying Kidney-Yang, tonifying Spleen-Qi, subduing Liver-Yang and resolving Phlegm. In this case we treat the Root and the Manifestation simultaneously because the attacks of vertigo are relatively infrequent, coming about every 6 months; had the attacks of vertigo been much more frequent, we should have concentrated on treating the Manifestation, that is, subduing Liver-Yang and resolving Phlegm.

THE 10 TRADITIONAL QUESTIONS

The interrogation is traditionally carried out on the basis of 10 questions. This practice was started by Zhang Jing Yue (1563–1640) but the 10 questions used by subsequent doctors differed slightly from those found in Dr Zhang's book. The 10 questions proposed by Zhang Jing Yue were as follows:

1. Aversion to cold and fever
2. Sweating
3. Head and body
4. The two excretions
5. Food and drink
6. Chest and abdomen
7. Deafness
8. Thirst
9. Previous illnesses
10. Causes of disease.

Besides these questions, Zhang Jing Yue added two more, one regarding women's gynaecological history and the other regarding children, which makes a total of 12 questions.

Although these are usually referred to in Chinese books as 'questions', they rather represent areas of questioning. These varied a lot over the centuries, as different doctors placed the emphasis on different questions.

The most commonly used areas of questioning mentioned in modern Chinese books are 10, as listed in Box 28.5.

BOX 28.5 THE 10 QUESTIONS

1. Aversion to cold and fever
2. Sweating
3. Head and body
4. Chest and abdomen
5. Food and taste
6. Stools and urine
7. Sleep
8. Hearing and tinnitus
9. Thirst and drink
10. Pain

Two areas of questioning are added for women and children, making a total of 12. It must be stressed that not all these questions need be asked in every situation, nor are these the only possible questions since each situation requires an individual approach and other questions may be relevant.

Limitations of the 10 traditional questions

One need not necessarily follow the above order of questioning. In fact, I personally never do because the above order is strongly biased towards an interrogation of a patient suffering from an acute, exterior condition, hence the prominent place afforded to the question about 'aversion to cold and fever' which, in Chinese books, always comes first. In interior conditions, I do ask about sensation of heat or cold to establish or confirm whether there is internal Cold or internal Heat, but usually towards the end of the interrogation.

There is no reason why we should limit our interrogation rigidly to the traditional 10 questions. Each patient is different, with different causes of disease and different patterns of disharmony, and we need to adapt our questions to each patient's unique situation. Moreover, we need to respond to a patient's mental state during an interrogation with sensitivity and flexibility to put a patient at ease, especially during the first consultation. It would be wrong, therefore, to ask the 10 questions routinely without adapting one's approach to the concrete situation. For example, it might well be that a patient bursts into tears as soon as he or she describes his or her main problem and we should react to this situation in a sensitive and sympathetic manner.

The 10 questions, as the basis of the interrogation in Chinese diagnosis, were formulated during the early Qing dynasty in China, thus at a time and in a culture very different than ours. We should therefore not hesitate to change the structure and contents of our interrogation to make it more suitable to our time and culture.

I would add the following to the traditional 10 questions:

- emotions
- sexual symptoms
- energy levels.

In addition, I introduce a separate area of questioning concerning the limbs which traditionally is included under 'body'.

Questions on emotional state

An enquiry about the emotional life of the patient plays a role both in the general enquiry to find the *cause* of the disharmony and in the specific enquiry to find the *pattern* of disharmony. A prevailing emotional state is a clinical manifestation just as any other and it is therefore an important part of the pattern of disharmony. For example, a propensity to anger is a strong indication of Liver-Yang or Liver-Fire rising, sadness often indicates a Lung deficiency, obsessive thinking points to a Spleen pattern, etc.

It may be that, for cultural reasons, there is no specific question regarding the emotional state of the patient among the traditional 10 questions: Chinese patients tend not to talk about their emotions and often express them as physical symptoms as a kind of agreed 'code' between patient and doctor. I list a few examples of the emotional meaning of various symptoms expressed by Chinese patients below:

1. 'Feeling of oppression of chest' (*Xiong Men*) often means that the patient is depressed.
2. 'Intense thirst' often indicates that the patient is angry.
3. 'Tiredness and dizziness' in a woman often means that she is depressed.
4. 'Lack of appetite' often means that the patient is depressed or experiences sexual frustration (the same emotions in a Western patient would be more likely to induce him or her to eat more and 'pick' all the time).
5. 'Insomnia and palpitations' may indicate intense anxiety and fear.
6. 'Bitter pain' may indicate bitter experiences in the patient's life or a state of being embittered.
7. 'Nausea' may indicate that the patient is worried or frustrated or depressed.

Questions about sexual life

Modern Chinese doctors never ask about sexual symptoms owing to the modern Chinese prudery in sexual matters. However, this should always form part of the interrogation as it provides further information on the symptomatology of the patient to arrive at a pattern of disharmony.

Questions on energy levels

An enquiry about energy levels is extremely important as it gives a very simple clue to the presence of a possible Deficiency pattern (excluding the few cases when a person may feel tired from Excess conditions). This question is all the more important since lack of energy is probably one of the main reasons for Western people to consult a practitioner of Chinese medicine.

THE 16 QUESTIONS

Thus, bearing in mind the three new questions on the emotional state, sexual symptoms and energy levels and a different order of questioning, I would therefore propose to revise the traditional 10 questions, making up a total of 16 questions as listed in Box 28.6.

BOX 28.6 THE 16 QUESTIONS

1. Pain
2. Food and taste
3. Stools and urine
4. Thirst and drink
5. Energy levels
6. Head, face and body
7. Chest and abdomen
8. Limbs
9. Sleep
10. Sweating
11. Ears and eyes
12. Feeling of cold, feeling of heat and fever
13. Emotional symptoms
14. Sexual symptoms
15. Women's symptoms
16. Children's symptoms

Apart from adding four questions (on pain, emotional state, sexual symptoms and energy levels), I have changed the order of the traditional 10 questions in accordance with my clinical experience with Western patients and have split some questions into two (for example, 'Food and drink' into 'Food and taste' and 'Thirst and drink').

I have relegated the questions about aversion to cold and fever to twelfth place because they are usually asked towards the end of the interrogation to confirm the Hot or Cold nature of a particular pattern. The prominent place afforded to aversion to cold or fever in the traditional 10 questions is due to historical reasons; in fact, in the times when the traditional 10

questions were formulated, febrile diseases were extremely common in China and would have formed the major part of a doctor's practice.

I have placed the questions on pain in first place in the revised 16 questions because that is by far the most common problem that Western patients present in a modern practice. The question on pain is followed by those about food, bowels, urination and thirst, again because these questions cover a very large area of digestive and urinary problems in the patients we see. The order in which the questions are listed is not necessarily that in which they are asked; for example, in women, the questions about their gynaecological system would be asked fairly early in the interrogation.

The discussion that follows will often list the clinical significance of a given symptom, for example 'night sweating indicates Yin deficiency' or 'thirst indicates Heat'. It should be pointed out that this approach actually contradicts the very essence of Chinese diagnosis and patterns according to which it is the *picture* formed by a number of symptoms and signs, rather than individual symptoms, that matters. No symptom or sign can be seen in isolation from the pattern of which it forms part: it is the landscape that counts, not individual features. Thus it is wrong to say 'night sweating indicates Yin deficiency'; we should say 'in the presence of malar flush, a Red tongue without coating and a dry throat at night, night sweating indicates Yin deficiency, while in the presence of a feeling of heaviness, a sticky taste, a bitter taste, epigastric fullness, night sweating indicates Damp-Heat'. It is only for didactic purposes that we need to list symptoms and signs in isolation with their possible diagnostic significance.

However, after years of practice, in some cases one can deduce the pattern even from an isolated symptom or sign; this is possible because each symptom or sign within a pattern bears within it the 'imprint' of the whole pattern. This can be deduced mostly from observation or hearing/smelling. For example, 'mental restlessness' may be due to Full- or Empty-Heat as indicated above and the diagnosis should be made on the basis of accompanying symptoms. However, an experienced practitioner is able to simply observe the patient and form an idea of whether the 'mental restlessness' derives from Full- or Empty-Heat. It is difficult to describe how this is done, but mental restlessness from Full-Heat manifests with more agitation, it is more 'solid' and the patient is more restless; when mental restlessness is due to Empty-Heat, the patient is restless but in a quieter way, there is a vague feeling of anxiety without knowing why and the patient generally looks more deficient.

Another example would be that of cough, in this case using diagnosis from hearing. Simply by hearing the patient cough, an experienced practitioner can deduce not only whether the cough occurs within a pattern of Phlegm or Dryness, but even whether it is Cold-Phlegm, Damp-Phlegm or Phlegm-Heat.

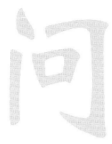

Chapter **29**

PAIN

Chapter contents

INTRODUCTION   253

AREA OF PAIN   255

NATURE OF PAIN   255
  Soreness   255
  Pain with a sensation of heaviness   255
  Distending pain   255
  Pain with a feeling of fullness   256
  Pain with a feeling of emptiness   256
  Pain with a feeling of cold   256
  Burning pain   256
  Colicky pain   256
  Spastic pain   256
  Pain with a distressing feeling   256
  Pain with a sensation of stuffiness   257
  Pushing pain   257
  Pulling pain   257
  Cutting pain   257
  Throbbing pain   257
  Boring pain   257
  Lurking pain   257

TIME OF PAIN   257

FACTORS AFFECTING PAIN   258
  Pressure   258
  Temperature   258
  Food and drink   258
  Bowel movement   258
  Movement and rest   258

ORGAN VERSUS CHANNEL PAIN   259

INTRODUCTION

As mentioned in Chapter 28, I have changed the order of the traditional 10 questions and I assign the first question to pain, but this is not to say that one should always start by asking about pain. The order of questioning should be flexible.

In this chapter I will discuss pain and its diagnostic points in general. Pain in various areas of the body is discussed under the relevant questions; for example, the diagnosis of chest pain will be found under the questions related to 'Chest and abdomen'.

? **WHY** WE ASK

We need to ask about pain because the character, location and timing of pain give a clear indication of the Full or Empty character of the condition and they also clearly indicate various pathogenic factors such as Qi stagnation, Blood stasis, Dampness, and so on.

Obviously, another reason for asking about pain is that it is a very common complaint, and often the one that leads our patients to seek help.

? **WHEN** WE ASK

Obviously we need to ask about pain in great detail when this is the chief complaint. However, even if the patient comes to us for a condition that does not involve pain (e.g. asthma), we should always ask whether the person experiences pain in any part of the body. On the one hand, this may uncover a condition that the patient did not report spontaneously and, on the other hand, an analysis of the character, location

and timing of pain may help us to confirm the original diagnosis; indeed, in some cases an analysis of the pain may also *add* a new dimension to our original diagnosis. For example, a woman may present with a chief complaint of mental depression which we diagnose as being caused by Liver-Qi stagnation; before concluding the interrogation we should ask whether she experiences any pain in any part of the body. If the patient tells us that she suffers from abdominal pain and distension, this would clearly confirm the diagnosis of Liver-Qi stagnation. To carry the example further, if she also suffers from severe period pains, with dark, clotted menstrual blood, this clearly tells us that there is not only Liver-Qi stagnation but also Liver-Blood stasis. Since the Liver-Blood stasis is shown purely by the menstrual pain (e.g. the tongue is not Purple) we would not have known about it if we had not asked about pain.

? HOW WE ASK

When asking about pain, we should ask systematically about the following four aspects:

- location
- nature
- timing
- response to pressure and temperature.

Location of pain

The first obvious question is about the location of the pain. It is important in this respect not to accept automatically the patient's description of the location of the pain. Patients often have their own way of describing a certain location, a common one being 'stomach' when they mean lower abdomen. When the pain is in the abdomen it is particularly important to establish exactly where it is, according to the abdominal areas that are described in Chapter 16, by asking the patient to point to its location. This is even more important in children whose terminology is obviously limited and who often refer to 'tummy ache'.

In channel problems, it is also important to enquire exactly about the location of the pain in order to identify the channel or channels involved. For example, if a patient complains of shoulder pain, we should enquire clearly whether the pain is in the front of (Lung channel), the centre (Large Intestine channel) or the back of the shoulder (Small Intestine channel). However, in channel problems, the identification of the exact location of the pain must be done also with the help of palpation.

Nature of pain

After asking about the location, we should then ask about the nature of the pain. First let the patient describe it spontaneously; do not suggest any special terms. A potential difficulty here is the terminology used by the patient, which will obviously be different from that used in China. With experience, we learn how to 'translate' Western expressions into the Chinese equivalent. For example, 'bloating' indicates 'distension', 'feeling like a weight on the chest' indicates 'feeling of oppression', 'feeling like being pulled down' in the abdomen indicates a 'bearing-down' feeling, and so on. After letting patients describe the nature of the pain, if it is still necessary, we can then ask about the nature of the pain according to the traditional Chinese terminology, which, often, Western patients recognize as a very accurate description of their pain. For example, in cases of abdominal pain, when we ask, 'Is the pain accompanied by a feeling of heaviness?' many patients confirm that that is exactly how it feels.

Timing of pain

After asking about the location and nature of the pain, we should then ask about the exact timing of pain as described below.

Factors affecting pain

Finally, we should ask about the reaction to pressure or temperature. When asking about the reaction of pain to pressure, it is important to formulate the questions in a way that Western patients can understand. Rather than asking, 'Is the pain better or worse with pressure?' (as one might do with a Chinese patient), we should ask something like, 'Does the pain feel better if you rub it or press it, or do you actually dislike its being touched?'

When asking about reaction of the pain to temperature, we should also do it in a way that is readily understandable to Western patients. For example, if a patient complains of joint pain, we should ask whether it feels worse when the weather is cold and rainy. We should also enquire whether the application of heat or cold ameliorates or aggravates the pain.

Chinese medicine offers a detailed classification of pain according to five parameters:

- area of pain
- nature of pain
- time of pain
- factors affecting pain
- organ versus channel pain.

AREA OF PAIN

Localized pain is usually due to Phlegm, Blood stasis, or obstruction by Cold or Dampness, or both.

Moving pain is usually due to Qi stagnation (unless it is due to Wind in the joints).

NATURE OF PAIN

In general, a pain or ache that is mild in nature indicates Deficiency, whereas a sharp, severe pain is due to Fullness. It should be noted that a mild pain is usually dull and that a 'dull' pain may also be intense. For example, a headache from Blood deficiency will be mild in its intensity and dull in nature; however, an occipital headache from invasion of external Cold may be dull in its nature but very intense. Thus when a patient complains of a 'dull' headache, we should clarify whether this is mild (suggesting Deficiency) or intense (suggesting Fullness).

The pain from Fullness is due to the obstruction of the channels by a pathogenic factor. Possible factors are listed in Box 29.1.

BOX 29.1 PATHOGENIC FACTORS CAUSING FULL TYPES OF PAIN

- Exterior pathogenic factor
- Interior Cold or Heat
- Stagnation of Qi
- Stasis of Blood
- Dampness
- Phlegm
- Retention of food

All these pathogenic factors obstruct the circulation of Qi or Blood, or both, and therefore cause pain. There is a well-known saying in Chinese medicine that states:

'Obstruction causes pain; if there is no obstruction there is no pain' (*Bu tong ze tong, tong ze bu tong*). Phlegm does not generally cause pain but it may do so in a few cases.

Deficiency may also cause pain through malnourishment of the channels. In this case, the pain will be mild, more like an ache, and will be clearly alleviated by rest.

There are many different types of pain and the main terms are explained below.

Soreness

This is a dull ache that usually occurs in the four limbs or trunk. It is usually due to a Deficiency condition or to Dampness.

Pain with a sensation of heaviness

This is also a dull ache but accompanied by a sensation of heaviness; this usually occurs in the limbs, head or the whole body. It is typical of Dampness or Phlegm.

Distending pain

This is a pain accompanied by a sensation of distension (bloating). Chinese patients often actually say they have a '*zhang tong*' (i.e. a distending pain). No Western patient will ever use this actual expression but this type of pain is very common in Western patients. In England, they will usually say that they have a pain with a 'bloating' sensation, but very often they will not mention the bloating unless asked. It is therefore very important to elicit the exact symptoms and character of pain with a proper interrogation. A distending pain is typical of Qi stagnation, especially of the Liver. However, it should be noted that other organs may suffer from Qi stagnation too, notably the Stomach, Spleen and Lungs. Thus, a distending pain in the lower abdomen usually indicates Liver- or Spleen-Qi stagnation, in the hypochondrium Liver-Qi stagnation, in the epigastrium Stomach-Qi stagnation, and in the chest Lung-Qi stagnation (although this last one may also be due to the Liver).

A distending pain in the head, such as that experienced during a headache or a migraine, is due to Liver-Yang rising. Anglo-Saxon patients would usually call this pain 'throbbing' rather than 'distending'.

'Distension' is both a symptom and a sign, that is, it indicates the subjective bloating sensation of the

patient, but the bloating may also be felt on palpation when the area feels distended like a drum (this is more easily felt in the epigastrium or lower abdomen). In gynaecology, a distending pain is seen in dysmenorrhoea from Liver-Qi stagnation or premenstrual breast pain and distension also from Liver-Qi stagnation. Pain with distension is usually of a Full nature. Distending pain is treated with warm-pungent herbs that move Qi.

Box 29.2 summarizes the stagnation patterns underlying areas of distending pain.

BOX 29.2 AREAS OF STAGNATION OF QI

- Lower abdomen: stagnation of Liver-Qi
- Hypochondrium: stagnation of Liver-Qi
- Epigastrium: stagnation of Stomach-Qi
- Hypochondrium towards epigastrium: Liver-Qi invading the Stomach
- Chest: stagnation of Lung-Qi or Liver-Qi

Pain with a feeling of fullness

This is an ache or pain accompanied by a sensation of fullness; it usually occurs only in the epigastrium or lower abdomen. A sensation of fullness should be distinguished from distension (bloating). With distension, the patient feels bloated (like a drum) and the area feels like a drum on palpation; with fullness, the patient feels very full as if after a very heavy meal, perhaps also with a slight nausea, and the area feels *hard* rather than distended on palpation. The distension can actually be *seen* (and palpated); fullness cannot be seen but can be felt on palpation.

Typically, pain with a sensation of fullness indicates retention of food and is related to the Stomach and Spleen. Pain with a feeling of fullness is usually of a Full nature. Fullness is treated with digestive herbs.

!

Remember: 'distension' and 'fullness' are not the same. Distension manifests with a bloated feeling, whereas fullness manifests with a full feeling.

Pain with a feeling of emptiness

Pain with a feeling of emptiness indicates either Qi and Blood deficiency or Kidney deficiency and it often occurs in the head.

Pain with a feeling of cold

Pain with a feeling of cold is usually a sharp, stabbing or spastic pain that is clearly accompanied by a pronounced feeling of cold or even shivering and is alleviated by the application of heat. This type of pain usually occurs in the abdomen or limbs and it indicates Full- or Empty-Cold, or Yang deficiency.

Burning pain

Burning pain is accompanied by a burning sensation and it always indicates Heat or Empty-Heat; it may occur in the epigastrium or in the limbs.

Colicky pain

This is a sharp pain of a colicky, cramping nature; it occurs in the epigastrium or, more usually, the lower abdomen. This pain usually indicates Cold in the Intestines, but it may also be due to Blood stasis. In gynaecology, this pain is seen in dysmenorrhoea from Cold in the Uterus. Colicky pain is of a Full nature.

Spastic pain

This is a sharp pain accompanied by spasm (contraction) or a sensation of spasm; it usually occurs in the limbs and is related to the sinews and therefore the Liver. It may be due to Liver-Blood deficiency in conjunction with Liver-Qi stagnation or Liver-Yang rising. In the latter instance, it may also occur on the head. Spastic pain is either of a Full nature or a combination of Deficiency (of Liver-Blood) and Fullness (stagnation of Qi).

Pain with a distressing feeling

This indicates a pain or ache, usually in the epigastrium or chest, accompanied by a restless, undefined, anxious feeling and perhaps palpitations. It is usually due to retention of Phlegm in the epigastrium affecting the Heart. It is also a typical symptom of rebellious Qi in the Penetrating Vessel causing anxiety and palpitations. This type of pain is usually due to a combination of Deficiency (of the Liver, Spleen or Kidneys) and Fullness (rebellious Qi). In gynaecology, this type of pain is seen in menopausal problems.

Pain with a sensation of stuffiness

This is usually a dull ache accompanied by a feeling of 'stuffiness'; it usually occurs in the epigastrium or chest. 'Stuffiness' may be defined as a mild feeling of fullness with an important objective difference on palpation: fullness may be felt on palpation as hardness, whereas with stuffiness the epigastrium feels soft on palpation. A feeling of ache and stuffiness is usually due to a combination of Deficiency (of the Spleen) and Fullness (Heat or Phlegm).

Pushing pain

This is a sharp pain accompanied by a feeling as if something was pushing outwards; it occurs in the hypochondrium or epigastrium and is due to severe Qi stagnation.

Pulling pain

This is a sharp pain accompanied by a sensation as if the skin were being pulled; it occurs only on the head and is due to Liver-Wind. It is of a Full nature (although Liver-Wind itself may derive from a Blood or Yin deficiency).

Cutting pain

This is a very sharp pain that feels like a knife. It usually occurs in the lower abdomen and is due to Blood stasis. It is definitely Full in nature.

Throbbing pain

This pain is usually severe and it feels as if there was a throbbing or pulsation. It usually occurs on the head from Liver-Yang rising. It is of a Full nature (although Liver-Yang may rise from Blood or Yin deficiency).

Boring pain

This is a severe pain that feels like the tip of a knife-blade, a nail or a screw; it is fixed in its location. It is due to Blood stasis and is Full in nature. It may occur in the lower abdomen, epigastrium, hypochondrium, chest or head. In gynaecology, it is seen in dysmenorrhoea from Blood stasis.

Lurking pain

Lurking pain, in Chinese called *Yin Tong*, which means 'latent, hidden or lurking' pain, is not severe, is not acute, is relatively easy to endure but chronic and persistent. It indicates Qi and Blood deficiency or Empty-Cold in the Interior leading to malnourishment of the channels. Lurking pain usually improves with the application of heat; it generally occurs in the abdomen or lower back.

Box 29.3 summarizes the types of pain.

BOX 29.3 TYPES OF PAIN

- Soreness: Deficiency (four limbs or trunk) or Dampness
- Heaviness: Dampness or Phlegm (limbs, head or whole body)
- Distending: Qi stagnation (hypochondrium, epigastrium, lower abdomen, chest, head)
- Fullness: retention of food (epigastrium, lower abdomen)
- Emptiness: Qi and Blood deficiency or Kidney deficiency (head)
- Feeling of cold: Cold or Yang deficiency (abdomen or limbs)
- Burning: Heat or Empty-Heat (epigastrium or limbs)
- Colicky: Cold or Blood stasis (epigastrium, lower abdomen)
- Spastic: Liver-Blood deficiency with Liver-Qi stagnation (limbs, abdomen), Liver-Yang rising (head)
- Distressing: Phlegm or rebellious Qi (chest, epigastrium)
- Stuffiness: Spleen deficiency with Heat or Phlegm (chest, epigastrium)
- Pushing: severe Qi stagnation (hypochondrium, epigastrium)
- Pulling: Liver-Wind (head)
- Cutting: Blood stasis (lower abdomen)
- Throbbing: Liver-Yang rising (head)
- Boring: Blood stasis (head, chest, hypochondrium, epigastrium, lower abdomen)
- Lurking: Qi and Blood deficiency or Empty-Cold in the Interior (abdomen, lower back)

TIME OF PAIN

Daytime pain is usually due to a dysfunction of Qi or Blood.

Pain at night is due to a deficiency of Yin or to Blood stasis.

Intermittent pain is due to either Qi deficiency or Qi stagnation.

Continuous pain is due to Blood stasis.

FACTORS AFFECTING PAIN

The main factors affecting pain are as follows:

- pressure
- temperature
- food and drink
- bowel movement
- movement and rest.

Pressure

Aggravated by pressure This indicates a Full condition (which may be Dampness, Phlegm, Qi stagnation, Blood stasis or retention of food). Aggravation by pressure in Full conditions is common in abdominal pain, stomach ache, menstrual pain and joint pain.

Ameliorated by pressure This indicates Deficiency (e.g. abdominal pain, stomach ache, menstrual pain and joint pain).

Temperature

Alleviated by warmth If a pain is alleviated by the application of heat (such as a hot-water bottle) this indicates that it is due to Cold or Yang deficiency (e.g. backache, joint pain, stomach ache, abdominal pain and menstrual pain). If a pain is alleviated by hot weather, this also indicates that it is due to Cold or Yang deficiency (e.g. backache, joint pain). Similarly if the pain is aggravated by cold.

Alleviated by cold No pain is generally alleviated by the application of cold, except in the case of acute joint sprains. Similarly, no pain is usually alleviated by cold weather.

Food and drink

Aggravated by eating This indicates a Full condition of the Stomach.

Ameliorated by eating This indicates an Empty condition of the Stomach.

Aggravated by drinking cold liquids This indicates a Cold condition of the Stomach.

Aggravated by drinking hot liquids This indicates a Hot condition of the Stomach.

Ameliorated by drinking warm liquids This indicates a Cold condition of the Stomach.

Ameliorated by drinking cold liquids This indicates a Hot condition of the Stomach.

Bowel movement

Ameliorated by a bowel movement This indicates a Full condition of the Intestines.

Aggravated by a bowel movement This indicates an Empty condition of the Intestines or Spleen.

Movement and rest

Ameliorated by movement This indicates stagnation of Qi (e.g. abdominal pain) or Cold (e.g. backache).

Aggravated by movement This indicates a deficiency of Qi or Blood (e.g. backache).

Ameliorated by rest This indicates a deficiency of Qi or Blood (e.g. backache, joint pain and menstrual pain).

BOX 29.4 FACTORS AFFECTING PAIN

Pressure
- Worse with pressure: Full condition
- Better with pressure: Empty condition

Temperature
- Better with warmth: Cold or Yang deficiency
- Better with cold: acute joint sprain

Food and drink
- Worse after eating: Full condition of Stomach
- Better after eating: Empty condition of Stomach
- Worse for drinking cold liquids: Cold condition of Stomach
- Worse for drinking hot liquids: Heat condition of Stomach
- Better for drinking warm liquids: Cold condition of Stomach
- Better for drinking cold liquids: Heat condition of Stomach

Bowel movement
- Better after bowel movement: Full condition of Intestines
- Worse after bowel movement: Empty condition of Intestines or Spleen

Movement and rest
- Better with movement: Qi stagnation or Cold
- Worse with movement: Qi and Blood deficiency
- Better with rest: Qi and Blood deficiency
- Worse with rest: Qi stagnation, Blood stasis, Cold

Aggravated by rest This indicates stagnation of Qi (e.g. joint pain, backache and headache), stasis of Blood (e.g. joint pain, backache and headache) or Cold (e.g. backache).

Box 29.4 summarizes the factors affecting pain.

ORGAN VERSUS CHANNEL PAIN

Besides the above differentiation, another important one is that between pain due to involvement of the internal organs with their respective channels and pain due to involvement of the channels only. There are four possible situations, listed in Box 29.5.

BOX 29.5 CLASSIFICATION OF ORGAN AND CHANNEL PAIN

- Channel pain deriving from a channel pathology only
- Organ and channel pain deriving from an organ pathology
- Organ pain deriving from organ pathology
- Channel pain only deriving from organ pathology

Most pains due to sprains, traumas or Painful Obstruction Syndrome (due to Wind, Cold or Dampness) involve a channel pathology only. The second possibility is that of an organ pathology causing a pain in the organ as well as in its related channel, for example a shoulder pain on the Large Intestine channel associated with Damp-Heat in the Large Intestine causing diarrhoea (Fig. 29.1).

The third possibility is that of an organ pain deriving from an organ pathology. This is of course a very common situation, for example abdominal pain from Dampness in the Intestines, chest pain from Heart-Blood stasis, etc. (Fig. 29.2).

The fourth possibility is that of an organ pathology leading only to a pain in its related channel, for example Damp-Heat in the Large Intestine manifesting only with pain in the arm along the Large Intestine channel. This situation, however, is rather rare (Fig. 29.3).

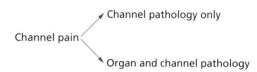

Fig. 29.1 Derivation of channel pain from channel or organ pathology

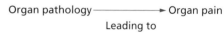

Fig. 29.2 Organ pathology leading to organ pain

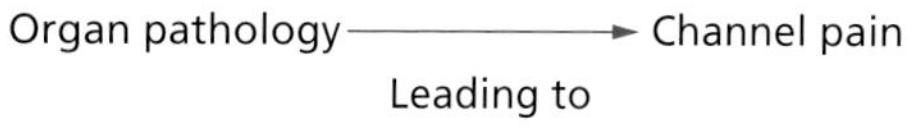

Fig. 29.3 Organ pathology leading to channel pain

Table 29.1 Characteristics of pain from Deficiency, Fullness, Cold and Heat

	Deficiency	Fullness	Cold	Heat
Pressure	Alleviated	Aggravated	—	—
Food	Alleviated	Aggravated	Alleviated by hot food and aggravated by cold food	Alleviated by cold food and aggravated by hot food
Type	Dull, lingering	Sharp	Cramping, spastic	Burning
Temperature	—	—	Alleviated by application of heat	Alleviated by application of cold
Bowel movement	Aggravated	Alleviated	Aggravated	Alleviated
Posture	Better lying down	Better sitting up	—	—
Onset	Slow, gradual	Sudden	—	—
Vomiting	Aggravated	Alleviated	Aggravated	Alleviated
Rest/exercise	Better with rest	Better with exercise	Better with exercise	Worse with exercise

Thus, the two most important diagnostic factors when confronted with pain are:

- whether the pain derives from Deficiency or Fullness
- whether the pain involves the internal organs and channels or the channels only.

Table 29.1 tabulates the characteristics of pain from Deficiency, Fullness, Cold and Heat.

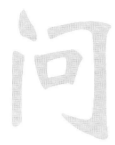

Chapter **30**

FOOD AND TASTE

Chapter contents

INTRODUCTION   261

MAIN PATTERNS OF DIGESTIVE SYMPTOMS   262
  Qi deficiency   262
  Qi stagnation   262
  Qi rebellious   262
  Blood stasis   262
  Dampness   262
  Phlegm   262
  Retention of food   262

FOOD   264

APPETITE   264
  Excessive hunger   264
  Aversion to food   264
  Hunger but no desire to eat   265

TASTE   265

NAUSEA AND VOMITING   266

BELCHING   266

SOUR REGURGITATION   267

INTRODUCTION

The questions regarding reactions to foods, appetite, hunger and taste are aimed primarily at establishing the state of the Stomach and Spleen.

? **WHY** WE ASK

We always need to ask about digestive symptoms because the Stomach and Spleen are the source of Postnatal Qi and therefore a pathology in these two organs eventually affects other organs.

? **WHEN** WE ASK

I always ask about the state of the digestive system before concluding the interrogation of the patient, unless, of course, the presenting problem is a digestive one.

? **HOW** WE ASK

It is important to ask about digestive symptoms in detail. It would not suffice to ask simply 'Do you have any digestive complaints?' We need to ask whether the patient ever experiences any distension, bloating, fullness, pain, heaviness, hiccup, nausea, vomiting, belching, loose stools, diarrhoea, etc.

The Stomach and Spleen are the Root of Post-Heaven Qi and their state affects all the other internal organs; for this reason, it is always necessary to ask questions to assess their state. This is all the more important given the frequency of digestive complaints in Western

patients. The Stomach controls the rotting and ripening of food and for this reason it is compared to a bubbling cauldron in the Middle Burner. The Spleen controls the transformation and transportation (*Yun Hua*) of Qi and it therefore affects the transportation and transformation of food essences in the Middle Burner. Thus, the Stomach and Spleen together are responsible for the proper digestion of food. However, in Chinese medicine, the function of the Stomach and Spleen goes beyond that of digesting food as, in the process of doing so, they are the source of Food Qi (*Gu Qi*), which, in turn, forms the Gathering Qi (*Zong Qi*) and True Qi (*Zhen Qi*). Thus, the Stomach and Spleen are the source of Post-Heaven Qi and an enquiry into the state of these two organs is crucial in every case.

The Stomach and Spleen are particularly important also because they are in the Middle Burner with opposing directions of Qi: Stomach-Qi descends while Spleen-Qi ascends. A normal coordination of these two directions of flow is vital for a proper transformation and transportation of Qi, food essences and fluids; these two organs are at a crucial crossroads in the Middle Burner and an impairment of their movement of Qi has immediate repercussions on Qi, Dampness and Phlegm pathology. In every pathology of the Stomach and Spleen there is some derangement of the proper flow of Qi. For example, when Stomach-Qi rebels upwards rather than descending, it causes symptoms such as hiccup, nausea, vomiting and belching; even when Stomach-Qi is deficient it may fail to descend properly and may cause some of the above symptoms but to a much milder degree. When Spleen-Qi descends rather than ascends, it may cause loose stools or diarrhoea.

MAIN PATTERNS OF DIGESTIVE SYMPTOMS

The main patterns causing digestive symptoms are:

- Qi deficiency
- Qi stagnation
- Qi rebellious
- Blood stasis
- Dampness
- Phlegm
- retention of food.

Qi deficiency

Qi deficiency of the Spleen causes poor appetite, loose stools and slight abdominal distension. Qi deficiency of the Stomach causes poor appetite and slight epigastric discomfort. If there is a pain, it would be slight, dull and better after eating.

Qi stagnation

Qi stagnation causes distension, which affects the epigastrium if the Stomach is primarily involved or the abdomen if the Spleen is primarily involved. If there is a pain, it would be strongly associated with distension. 'Distension' is usually described as 'bloating' by patients in English-speaking countries.

Qi rebellious

Qi rebellious of the Stomach causes belching, hiccup, nausea and vomiting. Qi sinking of the Spleen (i.e. descending rather than ascending) causes loose stools or diarrhoea.

Blood stasis

Blood stasis causes intense, fixed, stabbing pain, which is epigastric in the case of the Stomach, with possible vomiting of blood, and abdominal in the case of the Spleen, with possibly blood in the stools.

Dampness

Dampness causes a feeling of fullness and heaviness in the epigastrium if the Stomach is affected, with a sticky taste and poor appetite, and in the abdomen if the Spleen is affected.

Phlegm

Phlegm causes a feeling of oppression; this usually affects the epigastrium rather than the abdomen and the Stomach more than the Spleen. There is also a sticky taste, nausea and poor appetite.

Retention of food

Retention of food causes a feeling of fullness in the epigastrium if the Stomach is affected and in the abdomen if the Spleen is affected; the latter affects children more

Table 30.1 Differentiation of Stomach and Spleen digestive symptoms according to pattern

Pattern	Stomach	Spleen
Qi deficiency	Slight epigastric discomfort, dull, slight pain improved by eating, poor appetite	Poor appetite, slight abdominal distension, loose stools
Qi stagnation	Epigastric distension	Abdominal distension
Qi rebellious	Hiccup, belching, nausea, vomiting	Loose stools, diarrhoea
Blood stasis	Stabbing, fixed epigastric pain, vomiting of blood	Stabbing, fixed abdominal pain, blood in stools
Dampness	A feeling of fullness and heaviness of the epigastrium, sticky taste, poor appetite	A feeling of fullness and heaviness of the abdomen
Phlegm	A feeling of oppression of the epigastrium, sticky taste, nausea, poor appetite	
Retention of food	A feeling of fullness and pain of the epigastrium, sour regurgitation, nausea, poor appetite	A feeling of fullness and pain of the abdomen

than adults. In the case of the Stomach, there may be sour regurgitation, nausea and poor appetite.

Table 30.1 illustrates the differentiation of symptoms between Stomach and Spleen in the various patterns.

Thus, the five main sensations experienced in the digestive system are a feeling of distension, fullness, oppression, stuffiness and heaviness. Table 30.2 illustrates the pathology and diagnostic manifestation of these five sensations.[1]

Table 30.2 Differentiation of sensations of oppression, distension, fullness, stuffiness and heaviness

Pinyin	Chinese	English	Subjective sensation	Objective finding	Pathology
Men	闷	Oppression, 'tightness'	A feeling of oppression in the epigastrium extending to the chest	No objective finding, purely subjective	Phlegm, severe Qi stagnation, emotional component
Zhang	胀	Distension, 'bloating', 'bursting'	A feeling of distension and bloating in the epigastrium or abdomen	Abdomen feels distended like a drum on palpation	Qi stagnation
Man	满	Fullness	A feeling of fullness (associated with nausea if in the epigastrium)	The abdomen protrudes visibly and is hard on palpation	Dampness, retention of food, accumulation of Phlegm-Fluids (*Tan Yin*), organ pattern of Bright Yang
Pi	痞	Stuffiness ('focal distension' by some authors)	A feeling of stuffiness, a feeling of lump, an uncomfortable and slightly oppressive sensation: usually in the epigastrium or chest	The abdomen feels soft on palpation (which somewhat contradicts the patient's stuffy feeling)	Stomach-Qi deficiency, Stomach-Heat, mixed Deficiency and Excess with secondary Qi stagnation, Damp-Heat injuring Spleen-Yin
Zhong	肿	Heaviness	A feeling of heaviness of the epigastrium or abdomen	No objective finding, purely subjective	Dampness or Phlegm

FOOD

Especially if the patient complains of digestive symptoms, it is imperative to ask about the effect of eating on pain. If a digestive pain is alleviated by eating it means it is of an Empty nature; if it is aggravated by eating, it is of a Full nature.

Food intolerance or allergies are generally due either to Spleen deficiency or Stomach-Heat, depending on the reaction: if the intolerance or allergy manifests with digestive problems and lethargy it may be due to Spleen-Qi deficiency, while if it manifests with skin reactions it may be due to Stomach-Heat.

A feeling of distension after eating indicates Qi stagnation; a feeling of fullness indicates retention of food or Dampness; a feeling of oppression of the epigastrium indicates Phlegm; a feeling of stuffiness (a mild feeling of fullness but the epigastrium is soft on palpation) indicates Heat or Phlegm occurring against a background of Deficiency. A feeling of heaviness of the epigastrium indicates the retention of Dampness or Phlegm.

Digestive problems alleviated by the ingestion of warm liquids or aggravated by cold liquids indicate Cold in the Stomach and Spleen while if they are aggravated by the ingestion of warm liquids and alleviated by cold liquids it means that they are due to Stomach-Heat.

Inability to digest fats indicates Gall-Bladder Dampness.

Box 30.1 summarizes the patterns underlying digestive symptoms.

BOX 30.1 DIGESTIVE SYMPTOMS

- Food intolerance: Spleen deficiency or Stomach-Heat
- Feeling of distension: Qi stagnation
- Feeling of fullness: retention of Food or Dampness
- Feeling of oppression: Phlegm
- Feeling of stuffiness: Deficiency with Heat or Phlegm
- Feeling of heaviness: Dampness or Phlegm
- Improvement on drinking warm liquids, aggravation by cold: Cold in Stomach and Spleen
- Improvement on drinking cold liquids, aggravation by warmth: Stomach-Heat
- Inability to digest fats: Dampness in Gall-Bladder

APPETITE

Symptoms and Signs, Chapter 69

A normal appetite is an indication that the Stomach and Spleen are healthy. For social and historical reasons, lack of appetite is always considered a bad sign in China and always features as a prominent symptom in the pattern of Spleen-Qi deficiency. In the West, lack of appetite is less common and is not usually considered a very important symptom unless, of course, it leads to anorexia. Another cultural difference between Western countries and China is that when Chinese people are under stress they lose their appetite, whereas in the West patients tend to 'pick' constantly, eat more or eat sweets when under stress.

Lack of appetite indicates usually Spleen-Qi deficiency but it may also be due to a Fullness and specifically to Dampness obstructing the Middle Burner; in this case, it will be associated with a feeling of fullness and of mild nausea.

Excessive hunger

Symptoms and Signs, Chapter 69

Excessive hunger usually indicates Stomach-Heat; however, there is an important exception to this rule. In the West, excessive hunger leading to constantly 'picking' is often a sign of emotional stress and frustration rather than actual Stomach-Heat.

Excessive hunger without any desire to eat is due either to Damp-Heat in the Stomach or to Stomach-Yin deficiency with Empty-Heat: Stomach-Heat causes the feeling of hunger, but Dampness in the first instance or Stomach-Yin deficiency in the second instance makes the patient reluctant to eat.

Aversion to food

Symptoms and Signs, Chapter 69

'Aversion to food' is called *Yan Shi* in Chinese and it indicates a strong aversion to eating and to the smell of food. 'Aversion to food' differs from poor appetite in so far as it implies a strong disgust of food. This symptom is obviously seen in food poisoning but, in chronic cases, it may also be seen in retention of food. If aversion to food is accompanied by a very thick, sticky taste, it is due to Dampness in the Middle Burner affecting the Liver, Gall-Bladder, Stomach and Spleen. Aversion to food in pregnancy is due to the Qi of the Penetrating Vessel rebelling upwards.

Hunger but no desire to eat

Symptoms and Signs, Chapter 69

This symptom may seem paradoxical but it does occur occasionally: the patient feels hungry or, more accurately, the Stomach feels hunger pangs but the patient does not want to ingest food. This symptom may be due to two causes: Damp-Heat in the Stomach (the Heat causes hunger but the obstruction of the Middle Burner by Dampness makes the patient reluctant to eat), or the pattern of 'Stomach strong–Spleen weak' (when a Stomach Full condition causes hunger and a Spleen deficiency makes the patient reluctant to eat).

BOX 30.2 APPETITE

Appetite
- Normal appetite: good state of Stomach and Spleen
- Lack of appetite: Spleen-Qi or Stomach-Qi deficiency or Dampness in Middle Burner

Excessive hunger
- Excessive hunger: Stomach-Heat
- Excessive hunger without desire to eat: Damp-Heat in Stomach or Stomach-Yin deficiency with Empty-Heat

Aversion to food
- Food poisoning
- Retention of food
- Dampness in the Middle Burner
- Rebellious Qi of the Penetrating Vessel (in pregnancy)

Hunger but no desire to eat
- Damp-Heat in the Stomach
- 'Stomach strong–Spleen weak' pattern

Box 30.2 summarizes the patterns underlying abnormal appetite symptoms.

TASTE

Symptoms and Signs, Chapter 69

A normal taste sensation depends primarily on the state of the Stomach and Spleen and it reflects a healthy state of these two organs and a normal state of fluids. Thus, a loss of taste sensation often indicates a deficiency of Spleen and Stomach. Loss of the sense of taste accompanied by oversecretion of saliva indicates a deficiency of Stomach and Spleen with retention of Cold in the Stomach. Loss of taste may also be due to retention of Dampness in the Middle Burner.

In most cases, a particular taste indicates a Full rather than an Empty condition of the relevant organ.

A bitter taste indicates either Liver-Fire or Heart-Fire; in the former case, the bitter taste is more or less constant, whereas in the case of Heart-Fire it will be present only in the morning after a bad night's sleep. A bitter taste may also indicate Heat or Damp-Heat in the Gall-Bladder.

!

- **Bitter taste from Liver-Fire**: constant.
- **Bitter taste from Heart-Fire**: in the morning after a bad night's sleep.

A sweet taste indicates either Spleen deficiency or Damp-Heat.

A sour taste indicates retention of food in the Stomach, a disharmony of Liver and Stomach, or Liver- and Stomach-Heat.

A salty taste may indicate a Kidney-Yin deficiency or a severe Kidney-Yang deficiency with fluids rising up to the mouth.

A pungent taste indicates Lung-Heat or Stomach-Heat, or both.

A sticky taste indicates Dampness or Phlegm, usually in the digestive system.

Western patients are often unable to describe the kind of taste they experience: very few report a pungent, sour or salty taste for example. Many patients, when asked, are unable to say whether they experience a sticky taste or not but quite a few report experiencing a 'metallic' taste; I interpret this as a 'sticky' taste. It is due to Dampness.

Box 30.3 summarizes the patterns underlying particular tastes.

BOX 30.3 TASTE

- Loss of sense of taste: Stomach and Spleen deficiency, Dampness in Middle Burner
- Bitter taste: Liver-Fire or Heart-Fire, Heat or Damp-Heat in Gall-Bladder
- Sweet taste: Spleen deficiency or Damp-Heat
- Sour taste: retention of food in the Stomach, disharmony of Liver and Stomach, Liver- and Stomach-Heat
- Salty taste: Kidney deficiency
- Pungent taste: Lung-Heat, Stomach-Heat
- Sticky taste: Dampness

NAUSEA AND VOMITING

Hearing, Chapter 53; Symptoms and Signs, Chapter 69

There are several Chinese terms referring to nausea and vomiting, expressing varying characteristics or degrees of severity. The Chinese term *E Xin* means 'nausea', *Ou* means vomiting accompanied by a sound, *Tu* means vomiting without sound, *Gan ou* indicates short retching with a low sound, and *Yue* indicates long retching with a loud sound (before the Ming dynasty this term indicated 'hiccup'). The two Chinese terms *Ou* and *Tu* are usually used together to indicate vomiting.

Stomach-Qi normally descends; if it ascends it may cause nausea or vomiting, or both. Thus, nausea and vomiting are by definition due to rebellious Stomach-Qi ascending; this is not to say, however, that they are always due to a Full condition as nausea and vomiting may also be due to a Stomach deficiency. The pathological mechanism is different in each case: in Full conditions of the Stomach, Stomach-Qi rebels upwards *actively*, whereas in Empty conditions it fails to descend. Therefore, although nausea and vomiting always involve rebellious Stomach-Qi, this will be combined with various Stomach pathologies of the Full or Empty type such as Stomach-Cold, Stomach-Heat, Stomach-Yin deficiency, etc. This different pathological mechanism explains the different action of the two points Ren-13 Shangwan and Ren-10 Xiawan: the former actively subdues rebellious Stomach-Qi, whereas the latter helps Stomach-Qi to descend.

> **!**
> - In nausea and vomiting from Full conditions, Stomach-Qi *rebels upwards* (Ren-13 Shangwan).
> - In nausea and vomiting from Empty conditions, Stomach-Qi *fails to descend* (Ren-10 Xiawan).

A mild feeling of nausea is usually due to a deficiency of Stomach-Qi, with Stomach-Qi unable to descend. A strong feeling of nausea and vomiting is due to rebellious Stomach-Qi ascending; this may be associated with stagnation, Cold or Heat.

Profuse and loud vomiting of food soon after eating indicates a Full condition of the Stomach; vomiting of fluids with a low sound some time after eating indicates an Empty condition of the Stomach.

Vomiting of sour fluids indicates stagnant Liver-Qi invading the Stomach. Vomiting of bitter fluids indicates Heat in the Liver and Gall-Bladder. Vomiting of thin, watery fluids indicates Cold in the Stomach. Vomiting soon after eating suggests a Heat condition while vomiting some hours after eating suggests a Cold or Empty condition.

Box 30.4 summarizes the patterns underlying nausea and vomiting.

> **BOX 30.4 NAUSEA AND VOMITING**
> - Mild nausea: Stomach-Qi deficiency
> - Severe nausea/vomiting: rebellious Stomach-Qi
> - Vomiting soon after eating: Stomach Full condition
> - Vomiting of fluids: Stomach Empty condition
> - Vomiting of sour fluids: stagnant Liver-Qi invading the Stomach
> - Vomiting of bitter fluids: Heat in the Liver and Gall-Bladder
> - Vomiting of thin, watery fluids: Cold in the Stomach
> - Vomiting immediately after eating: Heat
> - Vomiting some hours after eating: Cold or Empty condition

BELCHING

Hearing, Chapter 53; Symptoms and Signs, Chapter 69

Belching always indicates Stomach-Qi rebelling upwards. This may be due to a purely Full condition, in which case the belching is violent and loud, or it may be due to Deficiency, in which case the belching is mild and with a low sound.

The most common cause of belching is Liver-Qi invading the Stomach and causing Stomach-Qi to rebel upwards; this is accompanied by epigastric and hypochondrial distension.

Retention of food (common in children) may also cause belching, in which case it is accompanied by sour regurgitation and epigastric fullness.

Deficient causes of belching include Stomach- and Spleen-Qi deficiency and Stomach-Yin deficiency; in these cases the belching is mild and its sound is weak.

Box 30.5 summarizes the patterns underlying belching.

> **BOX 30.5 BELCHING**
> - Loud belching: Full condition
> - Quiet belching: Empty condition (Stomach-Qi or Stomach-Yin deficiency)
> - With distension: stagnant Liver-Qi invading the Stomach
> - With sour regurgitation: retention of food

SOUR REGURGITATION

Symptoms and Signs, Chapter 69

Sour regurgitation describes an acidy feeling in the oesophagus which comes up into the mouth. Like belching, it is also a form of rebellious Stomach-Qi. The most common cause is Liver-Qi invading the Stomach and causing Stomach-Qi to rebel upwards.

Retention of food is another possible cause of sour regurgitation. Other causes include Dampness in the Stomach, which may be associated with Heat or with Cold.

Box 30.6 summarizes the patterns underlying sour regurgitation.

BOX 30.6 SOUR REGURGITATION

- With acidity rising: stagnant Liver-Qi invading the Stomach
- With feeling of fullness: retention of food or Dampness in the Stomach

---

NOTES

1. Examples of formulae for the above sensations are Ban Xia Hou Po Tang *Pinellia-Magnolia Decoction* for the sensation of oppression, Chai Hu Shu Gan Tang *Bupleurum Soothing the Liver Decoction* for the feeling of distension, Bao He Wan *Preserving and Harmonizing Pill* for the feeling of fullness (purgation is indicated), Ban Xia Xie Xin Tang *Pinellia Draining the Heart Decoction* for the feeling of stuffiness and Huo Po Xia Ling Tang *Agastache-Magnolia-Pinellia-Poria Decoction* for the feeling of heaviness. The acupuncture extra point Pigen is indicated for the feeling of stuffiness and disharmony of Liver and Spleen. This point is located on the lower back, 3.5 *cun* from the midline, lateral to the inferior border of the spinous process of L1 (i.e. level with BL-22 Sanjiaoshu).

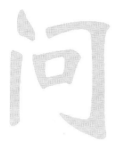

Chapter **31**

STOOLS AND URINE

Chapter contents

INTRODUCTION *269*

STOOLS *270*
  Frequency *270*
  Consistency *271*
  Shape *272*
  Colour *272*
  Odour and sounds *273*
  Abdominal pain related to evacuation *273*

URINE *274*
  Frequency *274*
  Colour *274*
  Amount *275*
  Difficulty in micturition *275*
  Cloudiness *275*
  Incontinence *275*
  Urination at night *275*
  Pain *275*
  Smell *275*

INTRODUCTION

The bowel movement and urination reflect primarily the state of the Yang organs and specifically the Large Intestine, Small Intestine and Bladder. Apart from these organs, other ones also influence defecation and urination: in particular, the Spleen, Liver and Kidneys influence defecation while the Kidneys, Liver, Spleen and Triple Burner influence urination. Defecation and urination generally reflect the state of organs in the Lower Burner and in particular the transportation, transformation and excretion of fluids in the Lower Burner, which is under the control of the Triple Burner.

? **WHY** WE ASK

Questions about bowel movement and urination are important and should always be asked: apart from telling us about the state of the digestive and urinary systems themselves, they serve to establish the Full or Empty and Hot or Cold nature of the condition.

? **WHEN** WE ASK

Unless the presenting problem concerns the functions of urination and defecation, I generally ask about these towards the end of the consultation.

? **HOW** WE ASK

When asking about urination and defecation it is important to be specific: asking 'Are your bowels regular?' may elicit a positive response when the

patient means that he or she evacuates the bowels once every 3 days *regularly*. Similarly, if we ask whether the urination is 'frequent' (by which we mean 'too frequent') the patient might answer affirmatively when it is normal. We should therefore ask precisely how many times patients evacuate their bowels and how many times they urinate in a day (bearing in mind seasonal variations, as urination is generally less frequent in summertime).

As for urination, we should also bear in mind differences between men and women as women have a large bladder and need to urinate less frequently than men. An added difficulty in most Western countries is that many people force themselves to drink a lot of water in the mistaken belief that it flushes the kidneys; this means that the urination will be much more frequent than normal and that the colour of the urine will be paler, making diagnosing from urination more difficult.

STOOLS

Observation, Chapter 20; Hearing and Smelling, Chapter 54; Symptoms and Signs, Chapter 72

When asking about stools we should ask about the following aspects systematically:

- frequency
- consistency
- shape
- colour
- odour and sounds
- abdominal pain related to evacuation.

The bowel movement is an important indicator of the state of the digestive system and specifically of the Large Intestine and Stomach. These two organs are connected within the Bright-Yang system and their pathology is often interconnected. For example, Heat in the Stomach is easily transmitted to the Large Intestine; Stomach-Qi failing to descend may cause constipation, etc. However, other organs also play a role in defecation and especially the Liver, which should assist defecation with its free flow of Qi, the Kidneys, which control the two lower Yin orifices (i.e. the urethra and anus), and the Spleen, which controls the transportation of Qi.

The normal bowel movement should occur at least once a day. The stools should be formed, and not too hard, not dry, and without excessive smell. Evacuation should be easy and effortless.

The Large Intestine, Small Intestine, Stomach, Spleen, Liver, Kidneys and Triple Burner all affect defecation.

Frequency

A normal bowel movement is once or twice a day. Any evacuation that occurs with less frequency than this constitutes constipation. A bowel movement (which may or may not be loose) occurring more than three times a day is considered to be too frequent.

Constipation is the most common disturbance of frequency of evacuation but its clinical significance cannot be separated from the consistency of the stools. Constipation indicates not only the infrequent passage of stools, but also excessive dryness of the stools or difficulty and straining in passing stools.

Acute constipation with thirst and yellow tongue coating indicates acute Heat in the Stomach and Intestines.

Chronic constipation in old people or women may be due to Blood or Kidney deficiency; in this case the stools would be slightly dry and there would be other signs of Blood or Kidney deficiency.

If the stools are bitty, small and difficult to pass, this indicates Liver-Qi stagnation or Heat in the Intestines (if they are also dry); when it is due to Liver-Qi stagnation, it often alternates with diarrhoea or loose stools as so often happens in irritable bowel syndrome.

Constipation with dry stools indicates Heat in the Large Intestine or Yin deficiency and Dryness of the Stomach, Intestines or Kidneys. If there is difficulty in evacuation but the stools are not dry, this indicates Liver-Qi stagnation.

Constipation with abdominal pain that is relieved by the bowel movement indicates retention of food or Dampness in the Intestines; constipation with abdominal pain and distension that is not relieved by the bowel movement indicates Liver-Qi stagnation. Constipation with abdominal pain and a pronounced feeling of cold indicates Cold in the Intestines.

Spleen-Qi deficiency normally causes loose stools but in a few cases a severe Spleen-Qi deficiency may cause constipation because the deficient Spleen-Qi fails

to move and transport. Constipation may also be caused by a so-called 'shut-down' of the Qi mechanism; this happens when there is an impairment of the ascending and descending of Qi in the digestive system, which may be seen, for example, after surgery.

Alternation of constipation and loose stools indicates stagnant Liver-Qi invading the Spleen.

If the stools are not loose but very frequent and the person cannot hold them easily, this indicates deficiency of the Central Qi, that is, the Qi of Stomach and Spleen; it also indicates sinking of Spleen-Qi.

Box 31.1 summarizes patterns underlying constipation and increased frequency.

BOX 31.1 CONSTIPATION

- Acute constipation with yellow tongue coating: Heat in Intestines
- Chronic constipation in women: Blood or Kidney deficiency
- Constipation with dry stools: Heat in the Intestines or Yin deficiency and Dryness
- Small, bitty stools, difficult to pass: Liver-Qi stagnation, Heat in the Intestines
- Difficulty in evacuation, stools not dry: Liver-Qi stagnation
- Constipation relieved by bowel movement: retention of food, Dampness in Intestines
- Constipation with abdominal pain and distension: Liver-Qi stagnation
- Constipation with colicky abdominal pain: Cold in the Intestines
- Alternation of constipation and loose stools: stagnant Liver-Qi invading the Spleen
- Frequent but not loose stools: Spleen-Qi sinking or deficiency of Central Qi

---

Consistency

The normal stool is well formed, not loose, not too dry and floating.

An excessively dry stool indicates either Heat in the Intestines, Blood deficiency (of the Liver) or Yin deficiency (which may affect the Large Intestine, Spleen, Liver or Kidneys).

Loose stools generally indicate a deficiency of the Spleen or Kidneys, or both. A deficiency of the Spleen is by far the most common cause of chronic diarrhoea or loose stools; a Kidney deficiency is a common cause of chronic diarrhoea in the elderly. If the diarrhoea is severe and very watery, this usually indicates Yang deficiency (of the Spleen and/or Kidneys, or both), whereas loose stools usually indicate Spleen-Qi deficiency.

The most common cause of chronic diarrhoea is Spleen-Qi or Spleen-Yang deficiency. Chronic, watery diarrhoea occurring every day in the very early morning is due to Kidney-Yang deficiency and is called 'cock-crow diarrhoea' or 'fifth-hour diarrhoea' (this refers to the ancient Chinese way of measuring time in each 24 hours).

There are, however, also Full causes of diarrhoea and principally Dampness (which could be associated with Heat or Cold) and Cold in the Spleen and Intestines.

The presence of a foul smell with the diarrhoea or loose stools suggests Heat in the Intestines, whereas the absence of smell is either normal or suggestive of Cold.

The presence of pain with the diarrhoea or loose stools suggests Liver-Qi stagnation, Cold or Damp-Heat.

The presence of mucus in the stools indicates Dampness while the presence of blood indicates deficient Spleen-Qi not holding Blood, Damp-Heat or Blood stasis in the Intestines. Acute diarrhoea or loose stools are usually due to invasion of external Dampness, which may be seen in food poisoning; with a foul smell it is due to Damp-Heat, without smell to Damp-Cold.

Undigested food in the stools, stools following blood or diarrhoea with borborygmi indicates Spleen-Qi deficiency; a burning sensation of the anus indicates Damp-Heat in the Intestines.

Sticky stools that necessitate brushing the toilet with a toilet brush every time indicate Dampness in the Intestines.

Case history 31.1 illustrates a pattern underlying diarrhoea.

Case history 31.1

A 25-year-old woman had been suffering from ulcerative colitis for 1 year, after the break-up of a relationship. Her main symptom was diarrhoea with blood and mucus in the stools but without pain. At the time of her consultation, she was taking oral prednisone.

Apart from this she had no other symptoms except that her periods had not yet returned since stopping the contraceptive pill a year and a half previously. Her complexion was dull yellow and her skin was quite greasy.

Her tongue was slightly Pale with a sticky yellow coating and her pulse was Weak on the right and noticeably Wiry on both Rear positions.

Diagnosis: The abdominal symptoms of diarrhoea with mucus and blood and the sticky coating on the tongue clearly indicate Damp-Heat in the Intestines, in this case occurring against a background of Spleen-Qi deficiency as shown by the Pale tongue and the Weak pulse on the right. In intestinal diseases such as ulcerative colitis or Crohn's disease, the pulse is frequently Wiry on both Rear positions.

Box 31.2 summarizes patterns underlying loose stools and diarrhoea.

BOX 31.2 LOOSE STOOLS/DIARRHOEA

- Dry stools: Heat in Intestines, Blood deficiency, Yin deficiency
- Loose stools: Spleen-Qi, Spleen-Yang or Kidney deficiency
- Chronic diarrhoea: Spleen/Kidney deficiency
- Chronic, watery diarrhoea in the early morning: Kidney-Yang deficiency
- Diarrhoea with foul smell: Heat in the Intestines
- Diarrhoea with pain: Liver-Qi stagnation Cold or Damp-Heat
- Diarrhoea with mucus: Dampness in the Intestines
- Diarrhoea with blood: Damp-Heat or Spleen-Qi deficiency
- Acute diarrhoea: external Dampness
- Undigested food in the stools: Spleen-Qi deficiency
- Mucus in stools: Dampness in Intestines
- Burning sensation in the anus: Damp-Heat in the Intestines
- Black or dark stools: Blood stasis
- Blood before stools: Blood-Heat
- Stools before blood: Spleen-Qi deficiency
- Diarrhoea with borborygmi: Spleen-Qi deficiency
- Sticky stools: Dampness in Intestine

Shape

Stools like small pellets indicate Liver-Qi stagnation, or Heat if they are also dry. Long and thin stools like pencils indicate Spleen-Qi deficiency (bear in mind that they could also indicate carcinoma of the bowel) (Fig. 31.1).

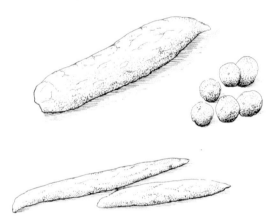

Fig. 31.1 Normal stools, stools like pellets and thin-long stools (Reproduced with permission from Maciocia G 1994 The Practice of Chinese Medicine, Churchill Livingstone, Edinburgh)

Colour

Normal stools are light-brown in colour. Pale-yellow stools indicate Empty-Heat (of the Spleen, Large Intestine or Kidneys). Dark-yellow stools indicate Full-Heat (of the Large Intestine). Dark stools may indicate the presence of occult blood and they generally indicate Heat (of the Large Intestine). Pale, almost white stools indicate Cold in the Large Intestine. Green stools indicate Liver-Qi invading the Spleen. Red stools indicate the presence of fresh blood and this may be due either to Heat in the Large Intestine or to Spleen-Qi deficiency. Greenish-bluish stools indicate the penetration of external Cold into the Large Intestine (common in babies).

Black or very dark stools indicate Blood stasis. Bright-red blood coming before the stools and splash-

ing in all directions indicates Damp-Heat in the Intestines. If the blood comes before the stools and is turbid and the anus feels heavy and painful, this indicates Blood-Heat. If the stools come before the blood and this is watery, it indicates that Spleen-Qi is deficient and is unable to hold Blood.

Box 31.3 summarizes the patterns underlying stool colours.

BOX 31.3 COLOUR OF STOOLS

- Light brown: normal
- Pale yellow: Empty-Heat
- Dark yellow: Full-Heat
- Dark: Heat
- Pale: Cold
- Green: Liver-Qi invading Spleen
- Red: Large Intestine Heat or Spleen-Qi deficiency
- Greenish-bluish: Cold in Large Intestine
- Very dark, black: Blood stasis
- Bright-red blood before stools: Damp-Heat
- Turbid blood before stools: Blood-Heat
- Stools before watery blood: Spleen-Qi deficiency

Odour and sounds

Hearing and Smelling, Chapters 53 and 54

Generally speaking, an absence of smell is either normal or it indicates Cold in the Intestines. A strong, foul smell usually indicates Heat and especially Damp-Heat. A sour smell indicates a disharmony of Liver and Spleen.

Flatulence may be due to Liver-Qi stagnation, to Damp-Heat if there is a foul smell, or to Spleen-Qi deficiency if there is no smell.

Borborygmi with loose stools indicate Spleen deficiency; borborygmi with abdominal distension and without loose stools indicate stagnation of Liver-Qi.

Box 31.4 summarizes patterns underlying odour and sounds.

BOX 31.4 ODOUR OF SOUNDS

- Absence of smell: Cold in the Intestines (or normal)
- Strong, foul smell: Heat or Damp-Heat
- Sour smell: disharmony of Liver and Spleen
- Flatulence: Liver-Qi stagnation, Damp-Heat (if foul smell), Spleen-Qi deficiency (no smell)
- Borborygmi: Spleen-Qi deficiency (with loose stools), Liver-Qi stagnation (with abdominal distension)

Abdominal pain related to evacuation

The feeling of distension before evacuation indicates Liver-Qi stagnation. Abdominal pain before evacuation but not relieved by it also indicates Liver-Qi stagnation. Abdominal pain during evacuation (and generally relieved by it) indicates Dampness in the Large Intestine or retention of food. Abdominal pain during evacuation, which is not relieved by it, generally indicates Cold in the Large Intestine. Abdominal pain after evacuation is normally due to Spleen-Qi deficiency.

Case history 31.2 illustrates a pattern underlying constipation with pain.

Case history 31.2

A 22-year-old woman had been suffering from constipation and abdominal distension and pain for the past 2 years; the abdominal pain was alleviated by the bowel movement. Her complexion was dull, pale and sallow. She also complained of a gradual hair loss on the top of the head, dizziness and itchy skin.

She had been on the contraceptive pill for a long time, having come off it the previous year; her periods failed to return after stopping the contraceptive pill and were only recently beginning to return, albeit with an irregular cycle.

Her tongue was slightly Red on the sides and had a fairly thick, sticky yellow coating and her pulse was Slippery and slightly Wiry.

Diagnosis: This case history is reported here mostly as an example of the importance of the pulse and tongue in diagnosis. In fact, her presenting symptoms clearly reflect Liver-Blood deficiency (gradual loss of hair on top, dizziness, dull, sallow complexion, itchy skin, irregular periods) and Liver-Qi stagnation (abdominal distension and pain). However, the tongue and pulse introduce a completely different dimension to this case history as they clearly reveal the presence of Damp-Heat manifested by the redness on the sides of the tongue and sticky yellow coating and by the Slippery quality of the pulse (the pulse is also slightly Wiry due to Liver-Qi stagnation) (Fig. 31.2).

The condition of Damp-Heat revealed by the pulse and tongue adds to and partially corrects the initial diagnosis: in fact, the alleviation of the abdominal pain after the bowel movement confirms the presence of Damp-Heat which is a 'solid' pathogenic factor that is, so to speak, 'expelled' by the bowel

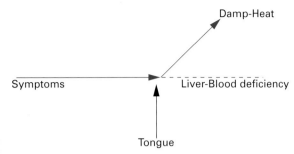

Fig. 31.2 Determining the importance of the tongue in diagnosis

movement. In contrast, abdominal pain due to Liver-Qi stagnation does not usually improve with bowel movement.

The pulse and tongue led me to ask further questions, which I would not have otherwise asked, to confirm or exclude the presence of Damp-Heat: on questioning she did confirm that the abdominal pain was accompanied by a pronounced feeling of fullness and heaviness, which are typical of Dampness.

Box 31.5 summarizes patterns underlying abdominal pain.

BOX 31.5 ABDOMINAL PAIN

- Before evacuation: Liver-Qi stagnation
- During evacuation: Dampness in the Large Intestine or retention of food (relieved by it), Cold in the Large Intestine (not relieved by it)
- After evacuation: Spleen-Qi deficiency

URINE

Observation, Chapter 20; Hearing and Smelling, Chapter 54; Symptoms and Signs, Chapter 73

With regard to urination we should ask about the following aspects systematically:

- frequency
- colour
- amount
- difficulty in micturition
- cloudiness
- incontinence
- urination at night
- pain
- smell.

The urination gives a good indication of the Hot or Cold nature of the condition and also of the state of Kidneys and Bladder.

Frequency

As a general principle, enuresis or incontinence of urine is usually due to Deficiency conditions whereas retention of urine is generally due to a Full condition, but there are exceptions to this rule. For example, severe Qi deficiency of the Lungs and Spleen in the elderly may lead to urine retention.

Frequent urination is generally due to Kidney-Yang deficiency, in which case the urine is pale and abundant; if it is frequent but scanty it indicates Spleen- and Kidney-Qi deficiency.

Nocturnal enuresis in children is due either to a constitutional Kidney deficiency or to Liver-Fire; in the first instance the child will be quiet and listless, while in the case of Liver-Fire the child will be vivacious and prone to fits of anger.

Colour

The colour of the urine gives a good indication of the Hot and Cold condition of the patient. Normal urine is pale yellow. Pale urine indicates Cold in the Bladder or Kidney-Yang deficiency; dark urine indicates Heat in the Bladder or Kidney-Yin deficiency. It should be remembered that the colour of the urine is affected when the person drinks a lot of water (becoming paler than it would otherwise be) and also when the person takes vitamin B, which makes the urine bright yellow.

Blood in the urine indicates either Qi deficiency (of the Spleen and Kidneys), Heat in the Bladder or Kidney-Yin deficiency.

Very dark urine, like soya sauce, indicates a kidney disease such as kidney failure or glomerulonephritis.

BOX 31.6 COLOUR OF URINE

- Pale: Cold in the Bladder or Kidney-Yang deficiency
- Dark: Heat in the Bladder or Kidney-Yin deficiency
- Red (with blood): Qi deficiency, Heat in the Bladder or Kidney-Yin deficiency

---

Box 31.6 summarizes patterns underlying urine colours.

Amount

Copious urination indicates Kidney-Yang deficiency; scanty urination indicates Kidney-Yin deficiency or Heat in the Bladder unless it is due to profuse sweating, repeated vomiting or severe diarrhoea. If the urination is scanty but also frequent, it is normally due to Spleen- and Kidney-Qi deficiency. Copious, clear and pale urination during an exterior invasion of Wind indicates that the pathogenic factor has not penetrated into the Interior (if it had, the urine would be dark).

Difficulty in micturition

Retention of urine from Full patterns may be due to Dampness obstructing the urinary passages, to Blood stasis in the Bladder or to urinary stones. Retention of urine from Empty patterns may be due to Kidney-Yang deficiency, Kidney-Yin deficiency or a deficiency of the Lungs; all these patterns occur mostly in the elderly.

Difficulty in urination (meaning that the micturition is difficult or that it may stop and start) is usually due to Dampness obstructing the urinary passages; a slight difficulty in urination may also be due to Spleen- and Kidney-Qi deficiency. In the elderly, it may be due to Kidney-Yang deficiency; in rare cases, it may be due to Lung-Qi deficiency.

Cloudiness

Turbid urine indicates Dampness in the urinary passages. Urine with small flakes of mucus indicates Damp-Heat in the Bladder.

Incontinence

Incontinence of urine is always due to a deficiency of the Kidneys and sinking of Kidney-Qi; it is common in the elderly and in women after childbirth or after a hysterectomy.

Dribbling of urine after urination indicates the Kidney-Qi is not firm.

Urination at night

Urinating at night indicates Kidney-Yang deficiency. This is due to deficient Yang not controlling Yin at night and therefore fluids leaking out in urination.

> **!**
>
> **Remember**: urination at night is caused by a deficiency of Kidney-Yang, rather than Kidney-Yin.

Pain

Pain and hypogastric distension before urination indicate Liver-Qi stagnation; burning pain during urination indicates Damp-Heat in the Bladder; a dull ache after urination indicates Kidney-Qi deficiency.

Smell

Absence of smell is either normal or indicates Cold in the Bladder; a strong smell indicates Damp-Heat in the Bladder. A sweet smell of the urine may indicate diabetes.

Chapter **32**

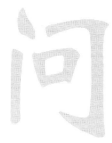

THIRST AND DRINK

Chapter contents

INTRODUCTION *277*

THIRST *278*

DRY MOUTH *279*

PREFERENCE FOR HOT OR COLD DRINKS *279*

ABSENCE OF THIRST *279*

INTRODUCTION

? **WHY** WE ASK

The symptom of thirst (or its absence) reflects the state of the Body Fluids. There are two types of fluid, one called *Jin*, the other called *Ye*. The *Jin* fluids are clear, light and watery and they circulate with the Defensive Qi in the space between skin and muscles; sweat comes from these fluids. The *Ye* fluids are more dense and heavy and they moisten and lubricate the joint spaces and the sense organs. Saliva is an expression of these *Ye* fluids; dryness of the mouth or thirst (these are not the same thing) are therefore symptoms of deficiency of such fluids, either because they are burned by Heat or Empty-Heat, or because there is not enough Yin.

The organ involved most closely with thirst and dry mouth is the Stomach but the Kidneys also exert an influence on saliva. However, Heat or Empty-Heat of any organ may cause thirst or a dry mouth.

? **WHEN** WE ASK

During the time I have been practising, I have never had a patient seek treatment for a problem related to thirst (although in China patients recognize problems related to thirst as being indicative of an imbalance that needs to be treated). However, I will ask almost every patient I see whether they feel particularly thirst, have a dry mouth, etc. I usually do this after I have asked about food and appetite, or when I am trying to establish the Hot or Cold nature of a condition.

I specifically ask about thirst in conditions where a patient has apparent *symptoms* of Heat but I suspect

does not actually have Heat. For example, in cases of rebellious Qi in the Penetrating Vessel, a woman may have a feeling of heat of the face and a red face, but no thirst because there is no actual Heat.

? HOW WE ASK

For cultural reasons, thirst and dry mouth are two symptoms Chinese patients are very aware of; whereas Western patients are somewhat less aware of these symptoms and seldom report them spontaneously. An added difficulty in the West is that more and more people force themselves to drink very frequently in the mistaken belief that this is a beneficial habit that 'flushes the kidneys'. As a result of this habit, such people will seldom feel thirsty even if they suffer from Heat. An added difficulty in England is that tea consumption is very high and this would also stop people from feeling thirsty. The same applies to countries where coffee consumption is high. In the USA, people tend also to drink a lot in general (including water and soda). As a result of these factors, fewer patients will report feeling thirsty than is the case in China even though they do suffer from Heat.

Generally speaking, the preference for hot or cold drinks reflects a condition of Cold or Heat of the Stomach respectively. However, this diagnostic symptom may be rendered invalid by cultural habits in Western countries and especially in the USA, where the consumption of iced drinks is very widespread.

THIRST

Symptoms and Signs, Chapter 70

Generally speaking, thirst indicates Heat, which may be either Full- or Empty-Heat. Thirst is not the same as dry mouth, as the former usually reflects Heat whereas the latter reflects Yin deficiency.

Full-Heat causes intense thirst with desire to drink cold fluids. Full Heat of any organ can cause this symptom, but especially Stomach-Heat, Lung-Heat, Liver-Fire and Heart-Fire.

Empty-Heat causes thirst with desire to drink in small sips, especially in the evening or during the night. This symptom is caused particularly by Empty-Heat of the Stomach, Lungs, Kidneys and Heart.

A particular symptom in Chinese diagnosis is that of 'thirst without desire to drink'. This particular symptom may seem strange but it does occur and Western patients do occasionally report it even spontaneously. Damp-Heat causes thirst but without the desire to drink; this is because Heat causes the thirst but Dampness, obstructing the Middle Burner, makes the patient reluctant to drink.

Thirst with a desire to drink but immediately followed by the vomiting of fluids indicates Phlegm-Heat.

In rare cases, a mild thirst with a desire to sip fluids may be due to severe, chronic Qi deficiency; this is due to the deficient Qi not transporting the fluids to the mouth and causing thirst.

Intense thirst with profuse urination may indicate diabetes (Case history 32.1).

Case history 32.1

A 50-year-old woman had been suffering from type-II, late-onset diabetes which had been diagnosed only 7 weeks before. The first manifestations of it were thirst, frequent urination, vaginal itching and irritation and extreme tiredness. The onset of the diabetes coincided with the stopping of her periods, during which time she suffered from hot flushes, night sweating, urination at night, disturbed sleep, dry eyes and throat at night with desire to sip water and what she described as 'a feeling of adrenaline rushing up and around the chest'. She was overweight, her voice was quite loud and she was generally lively. Her complexion was quite flushed.

Diagnosis: The red complexion and the symptoms she developed after the stoppage of her periods clearly indicate Heat or Empty-Heat. However, this case is an example of a striking contradiction between the symptoms and the tongue: in fact, her tongue was Pale and Swollen. In order to confirm or exclude the presence of Cold or Yang deficiency as manifested by the tongue, I asked about cold feeling and she did confirm that, although she felt hot at night, she also experienced very cold feet and needed to wear socks in bed. This contradiction is very common especially in women of menopausal age and it simply indicates that there is a deficiency of both Kidney-Yin and Kidney-Yang. The deficiency of the Kidneys was also confirmed by the fact that she suf-

fered from chronic lower backache; the symptom of frequent urination experienced with the onset of her diabetes also confirms the Kidney deficiency and it is not by chance that the diabetes developed when her periods stopped and the Kidney energy declined.

Her pulse was Deep, slightly Slippery, Weak on both Rear positions and relatively Overflowing on the Heart position. The Deep and Weak pulse on both Rear positions confirms the Kidney deficiency, while the Slippery quality indicates the presence of Phlegm which is confirmed by her being overweight. The rela-tively Overflowing quality of the Heart pulse is common in menopausal women and, rather than indicating an actual Heart pattern, it reflects a rising of Qi towards the top of the body due to the deficiency of the Kidneys below. It is this rising of Qi that causes the hot flushes and in her case, also the peculiar symptom of 'a feeling of adrenaline rushing up and around the chest'.

The treatment principle in this case is to tonify the Kidneys, strengthen the Penetrating and Directing Vessels, tonify the Spleen and resolve Phlegm.

DRY MOUTH

Symptoms and Signs, Chapter 70

Yin deficiency causes a dry mouth, rather than thirst, especially in the afternoon or evening; also in this case the patient likes to drink in small sips.

Although not common, a dry mouth may also be due to severe, chronic Blood stasis, in which case there would also be a desire to gargle with fluids without swallowing.

> **!**
>
> A dry mouth may be caused by Yin deficiency, rather than Heat. In this case, it would get worse in the afternoon and evening.

PREFERENCE FOR HOT OR COLD DRINKS

Symptoms and Signs, Chapter 70

A patient's preference for hot or cold drinks reflects the Cold or Hot nature of their condition, especially with regard to the Stomach. Stomach-Cold will cause a patient to prefer warm drinks, while Stomach-Heat will cause a patient to desire cold drinks.

A desire to drink warm or hot liquids does not count as 'thirst' and it indicates a Cold pattern of the Stomach, which may include also Cold-Dampness.

ABSENCE OF THIRST

Symptoms and Signs, Chapter 70

Although 'absence of thirst' is not a symptom as such, it is considered in Chinese medicine because it has a particular diagnostic significance. Absence of thirst, that is, if the patient feels seldom thirsty and never has the desire to drink, indicates a Cold pattern. Obviously, this symptom is elicited on interrogation as a patient will not normally report it spontaneously.

> **BOX 32.1 THIRST**
> ___
> - Thirst: Heat
> - Dry mouth: Yin deficiency
> - Thirst with desire to drink cold fluids: Full-Heat
> - Thirst with desire to drink in small sips: Empty-Heat
> - Thirst with no desire to drink: Damp-Heat
> - Thirst with desire to drink, immediately followed by vomiting of fluids: Phlegm-Heat
> - Mild thirst with a desire to sip fluids: Qi deficiency
> - Dry mouth with desire to gargle: Blood stasis
> - Desire to drink warm liquids: Stomach-Cold
> - Desire to drink cold liquids: Stomach-Heat
> - Absence of thirst: Cold
> - Intense thirst with profuse urination: Diabetes

Box 32.1 summarizes the patterns underlying thirst.

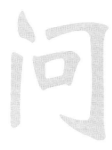

Chapter **33**

ENERGY LEVELS

Chapter contents

INTRODUCTION   *281*

HISTORICAL BACKGROUND   *282*

PATTERNS CAUSING TIREDNESS   *282*

INTRODUCTION

This is not one of the traditional 10 questions of Chinese diagnosis. I have added it to the list of questions because tiredness is one of the most common symptoms reported by Western patients. In my practice, about 12% of patients seek treatment specifically and only for tiredness; and to these should be added all the other patients who come for other symptoms or diseases but who also suffer from chronic tiredness.

? **WHY** WE ASK

It is always essential to ask about level of energy and tiredness because it is such a common complaint: indeed, it is often the main reason that patients seek treatment.

? **WHEN** WE ASK

I generally ask about tiredness quite early during the interrogation and as soon as I suspect a Deficiency pattern.

? **HOW** WE ASK

This is generally quite straightforward and I usually ask whether they 'feel unusually tired' or whether they 'lack energy'. However, when enquiring about tiredness, it is very important to enquire about the patient's lifestyle. Many people have unrealistic expectations about their level of energy. If people in industrialized societies work too much and for far too long, a feeling of tiredness is entirely normal. For example, it is not uncommon for

someone to get up at 6 am, leave home at 6.30 to catch a train, work the whole day under hectic conditions (having a sandwich at the desk for 'lunch') and return home at 9 in the evening; such a schedule is precisely what constitutes 'overwork' in Chinese medicine.

Our level of energy depends also on age. Again, very many people have unrealistic expectations about their desired level of energy and are surprised that they cannot do at 55 what they did when they were 25.

HISTORICAL BACKGROUND

There is no Chinese disease-symptom category called 'tiredness' but there is one called 'exhaustion' (*Xu Lao* or *Xu Sun*). The term *Xu Lao* describes not only a symptom, that is, 'tiredness' (*Lao*) but also its pathology, that is, a deficiency of the body's Qi (*xu*). The term *Xu Lao* was introduced in the 'Prescriptions from the Golden Cabinet' for the first time. It says in Chapter 6: '*When the pulse is big but empty in male patients, it indicates extreme exhaustion from over-exertion.*'[1]

The 'Discussion on the Causes and Symptoms of Diseases' (*Zhu Bing Yuan Hou Lun*, AD610) by Chao Yuan Fang elaborates on the concept of exhaustion by investigating its causes. Dr Chao considers exhaustion to be due to the '6 Excesses' (overexertion leading to depletion of Qi, Blood, Sinews, Bones, Muscles and Essence) and the '7 Injuries'. The '7 Injuries' refer to the damage inflicted on the Internal Organs by various excesses such as:

- overeating injuring the Spleen
- prolonged anger injuring the Liver
- lifting excessive weights or sitting on damp ground injuring the Kidneys
- exposure to cold and drinking cold liquids injuring the Lungs
- exposure to wind, rain, cold and heat injuring the body
- fear, anxiety and shock injuring the Mind.[2]

The 'Simple Questions' in Chapter 23 lists five causes of exhaustion:

- excessive use of the eyes injuring the Heart
- excessive lying down injuring the Lungs
- excessive sitting injuring the Spleen
- excessive standing injuring the Kidneys
- excessive exercise injuring the Liver.[3]

Over the centuries various doctors discussed the treatment of exhaustion according to their particular views and emphases. For example, Li Dong Yuan, author of the famous 'Discussion on Stomach and Spleen' (*Pi Wei Lun*, 1249),[4] considered Stomach and Spleen deficiency to be the main cause of exhaustion. Zhu Dan Xi, author of 'Secrets of Dan Xi' (*Dan Xi Xin Fa*, 1347),[5] placed the emphasis on Kidney- and Liver-Yin deficiency as a cause of exhaustion and advocated nourishing Yin and clearing Heat. Zhang Jie Bin, author of the 'Classic of Categories' (*Lei Jing*, 1624)[6] and the 'Complete Book of Jing Yue' (*Jing Yue Quan Shu*, 1624),[7] advocated tonifying the Kidneys for the treatment of exhaustion.

Zhu Qi Shi (1463–1539) considered the Lungs, Spleen and Kidneys to be the three most important organs to treat in exhaustion. He said in his book 'Discussion on Exhaustion' (*Xu Lao Lun*): '*To treat Exhaustion there are three roots: Lungs, Spleen and Kidneys. Lungs are like the "heaven" of the internal organs, the Spleen is like the "mother" of the body and the Kidneys are like the "root" of life. Treat these three organs to treat Exhaustion.*'[8] Dr Zhu indicated the Spleen and Lungs as the two main organs to treat in cases of chronic tiredness, the Spleen for Yang deficiency and the Lungs for Yin deficiency. Each of these can eventually lead to Kidney-Yang or Kidney-Yin deficiency and Yang deficiency can lead to Yin deficiency, or vice versa. Dr Zhu says: '*To treat Deficiency there are two interconnected systems: either the Lungs or the Spleen. Every [Deficiency] disease boils down to Yang or Yin deficiency. Yang deficiency can lead to Yin deficiency after a prolonged time . . . Yin deficiency can lead to Yang deficiency after a prolonged time . . . In Yang deficiency treat the Spleen, in Yin deficiency treat the Lungs.*'[9]

Thus, tiredness is included in the concept of exhaustion, although the latter is a more serious condition than simple tiredness. However, although exhaustion contemplates only Deficiency causes, tiredness may also be due to Full causes; Dampness, Phlegm and Qi stagnation are common causes of tiredness.

PATTERNS CAUSING TIREDNESS

A chronic feeling of tiredness is usually due to Deficiency. This may be Qi, Yang, Blood or Yin deficiency. In some cases, tiredness may also be due to a Full condition, and especially Dampness, Phlegm or Qi stagnation.

The pulse is an important sign to differentiate Full from Empty types of tiredness: if the pulse is Full

in general (often Slippery or Wiry) it indicates that the tiredness is caused by a Full condition (usually Dampness, Phlegm or Qi stagnation).

> **!**
>
> **Remember**: tiredness is not always due to a condition of *Deficiency*. It can be, and it often is, due to a *Full* condition.

Dampness and Phlegm are 'heavy' and weigh down the body so that the person feels heavy and tired. Qi stagnation may also make a person feel tired; this is not because there is not enough Qi but because, being stagnant, Qi does not circulate properly. This situation is more common in men and it often reflects a state of mental depression. The classic example would be that of a man who seeks treatment primarily for tiredness and whose pulse and tongue reveal no Deficiency at all but only severe Qi stagnation, the pulse being very Wiry and Full on all positions and the tongue being Red on the sides. In such a situation the man feels tired from Qi stagnation and his tiredness is closely linked to a state of mental depression (itself often deriving from repressed anger).

Chronic tiredness associated with a desire to lie down, poor appetite and loose stools indicates Spleen-Qi deficiency, which is probably the most common cause of it; if there are Cold symptoms, it is due to Spleen-Yang deficiency.

Chronic tiredness associated with a weak voice and a propensity to catching colds indicates Lung-Qi deficiency; if there are Cold symptoms, it is due to Lung-Yang deficiency.

Chronic tiredness associated with backache, lassitude, a feeling of cold, depression and frequent urination indicates Kidney-Yang deficiency.

Chronic tiredness associated with slight depression, dizziness and scanty periods indicates Liver-Blood deficiency.

Chronic tiredness associated with anxiety, insomnia, a dry mouth at night and a tongue without coating is due to Kidney-Yin deficiency.

Chronic tiredness associated with a feeling of heaviness of the body and muzziness of the head indicates retention of Dampness.

Chronic tiredness associated with a feeling of oppression of the chest, dizziness and muzziness of the head indicates retention of Phlegm.

Chronic tiredness in an anxious and tense person with a Wiry pulse indicates stagnation of Liver-Qi.

Short-term tiredness with alternating cold and hot feeling, irritability, unilateral tongue coating and a Wiry pulse indicates the Lesser-Yang pattern (either of the Six Stages or of the Four Levels).

Case histories 33.1–33.7 illustrate different patterns causing tiredness.

Case history 33.1

A 56-year-old woman complained of extreme tiredness for the past 3 years since the death of her husband. She said her legs 'felt like lead' and had no motivation to do all the things that needed to be done in the house. She had also been suffering from insomnia, also since her husband's death. She said 'I feel pain inside but the tears don't come'. As she is stoically trying to live through her pain without crying, her grief and depression is probably somatized more, causing more physical symptoms.

Apart from these main two problems she presented with, she had also been suffering from occipital headaches since the birth of her second child 26 years before. On interrogation, it transpired that she also experienced dizziness, hot flushes, urination at night and abdominal distension and heaviness.

Her tongue was slightly Red, Stiff, dry, with a sticky coating and a Heart crack; her pulse was Slippery on the right, Floating-Empty on the left and Weak and Deep on the left Rear position.

Diagnosis: This is a complex combination of patterns. The overwhelming factor is, however, the obvious grief and depression following the death of her husband; the symptom she first complained of was 'tiredness' but, as she went on talking, it was obvious that this was due to a deep depression following the grief caused by her husband's death: hence the lack of motivation and insomnia.

From the point of view of patterns, there is obviously a deficiency of Kidney-Yin evidenced by the urination at night, the headaches stemming from the second birth, the dizziness, the hot flushes, the Red, Stiff and dry tongue, the Floating-Empty quality of the pulse on the left and Weak-Deep Kidney pulse on the left. Accompanying the Kidney-Yin deficiency there is also Heart-Yin deficiency causing the insomnia and manifesting with the deep Heart crack. In addition to these conditions, there is also some Dampness evidenced by the abdominal distension and heaviness and by the sticky tongue coating.

Case history 33.2

An 18-year-old girl had been suffering from tiredness and lassitude for the previous 9 months: this came on gradually and was also accompanied by recurrent sore throats, temporal headaches, a feeling of heaviness, dizziness, a feeling of muzziness of the head, blurred vision, phlegm in the throat and an alternation of hot and cold feeling.

Her tongue was slightly Red on the sides, with red points on the right side and her pulse was generally Wiry.

Diagnosis: This is a very clear example of the Lesser-Yang pattern, not from the Six Stages, but from the Qi level of the Four Levels (called 'Gall-Bladder Heat'). The Gall-Bladder Heat pattern from the Four Levels differs from the Lesser-Yang pattern of the Six Stages in so far as it is characterized by more Heat than Cold and by the presence of Phlegm. This patient's symptoms clearly confirm this as the red points on the right side of the tongue indicate that there is more Heat, while the feeling of heaviness, the feeling of muzziness of the head and the phlegm in the throat indicate the presence of Phlegm.

This is also a good example of tiredness caused not by Deficiency, but by Heat.

Case history 33.3

A 54-year-old man complained of chronic tiredness and lassitude; this was his main presenting complaint. During the interrogation very few other symptoms emerged: in fact the only other symptom of note was the presence of loose stools. There were no other symptoms of Spleen deficiency, nor of Kidney deficiency. This patient looked very quiet and subdued, spoke with a very low voice and walked rather slowly; his facial complexion was quite red.

His tongue was Reddish-Purple in general, and especially on the right side and had a Red tip. His pulse was Wiry in general.

Diagnosis: This is an example of a situation when the demeanour of the patient contradicts the pulse and tongue. His slow walk, low voice and quiet demeanour all indicate Deficiency, while the tongue and pulse clearly indicate the presence of a Full condition. This is also an example when, in the absence of many symptoms, the tongue and pulse become even more important than usual. His tongue indicates Liver-Blood stasis (because it is more Purple on the right side) and his pulse confirms this. Liver-Blood stasis nearly always develops from chronic Liver-Qi stagnation and we can therefore assume that this patient has been suffering from Liver-Qi stagnation for a long time. The most common cause of Liver-Qi stagnation is an emotional problem related to anger, resentment or frustration. In this case, therefore, the chronic tiredness is due, not to a Deficiency, but to a Fullness; the symptom of loose stools, which normally indicates Spleen-Qi deficiency, may be here due to stagnant Liver-Qi invading the Spleen. Thus, although this patient complains primarily of tiredness, it is obvious that he also suffers from mental depression.

Case history 33.4

A 39-year-old man had been suffering from extreme tiredness for many years; the tiredness was accompanied by a feeling of weakness of the limbs and was worse in the morning. When asked whether the tiredness was accompanied by a feeling of heaviness, he said that it was, but only during an acute respiratory infection. He was also prone to frequent colds and upper respiratory infections which affected his sinuses every time, causing a congested feeling in the face and a sticky nasal discharge. Ten years previously he had been experiencing very poor digestion and frequent bouts of diarrhoea; he had been diagnosed as suffering from coeliac disease (from which his father also suffered) and he improved considerably by avoiding gluten. However, he still suffered from an alternation of bouts of loose stools and constipation. On interrogation it transpired that his mouth and lips were frequently dry.

His body type clearly belonged to the Wood element, being tall and thin, but he walked in a slow and slightly awkward way which did not fit in with the Wood body type. He looked fairly relaxed and placid and he spoke slowly and with a soft voice. His complexion was dull-pale yellow but his eyelids, especially the upper ones, were rather red.

His tongue was Red on the sides in the Spleen area, Swollen and had a yellow coating. His pulse was generally Slippery.

Diagnosis: There are clear manifestations of Spleen-Qi deficiency, that is, the tiredness, the feeling of weakness, being prone to frequent colds, the tendency to loose stools and the dull-pale-yellow complexion; the history of coeliac disease (affecting his father as well) indicates that he most probably suffered from a constitutional Spleen deficiency. The Spleen deficiency had obviously given rise to Dampness which is manifesting with the sinus congestion, the feeling of heaviness during acute infections and the Slippery pulse.

There is a third, rather uncommon pattern and that is Spleen-Heat which is causing the tendency to constipation, the dry mouth, dry lips and manifests on the tongue with a Red colour on the sides in the Spleen areas and a yellow coating.

The contrast between his body type, which pertains to Wood, and his prevailing disharmony in the Earth element is a poor prognostic sign; that is, it is better for a Wood type to suffer from a Wood disharmony.

Case history 33.5

A 49-year-old man had been suffering from tiredness and palpitations for the past 18 months. He also complained of irritability and said that all his symptoms became worse in the afternoon.

In the few weeks before the consultation, he had developed a burning sensation on urination. This was a recurrence of a symptom that he had suffered from previously.

His tongue was Swollen and the sides were Red. His pulse was Wiry and Slow.

Diagnosis: In this case, the overall Wiry nature of the pulse points towards the fact that the tiredness is caused by Liver-Qi stagnation rather than Deficiency. Liver-Qi stagnation is also, of course, the reason that the patient often feels irritable. The stagnation has led to some Heat, which is shown on the Red sides of the tongue, and is causing the burning sensation on urination. The Slow quality of the pulse may seem to contradict the symptoms of Heat, but it is due to the long-standing stagnation of Liver-Qi.

Case history 33.6

A 13-year-old boy had been suffering from headaches, night sweating, weakness and tiredness for 3 weeks. These symptoms had an acute onset in springtime and his health and energy before that were good. On closer questioning, his weakness consisted mostly of a feeling of weary limbs and he also complained of an epigastric discomfort which he found difficult to describe; he said that it was like 'a feeling of hunger' and could not decide whether it was hunger or pain. This was also accompanied by a feeling of nausea. In addition, he also experienced ache in the joints, especially of the legs, dizziness, restless sleep and irritability.

His tongue was very slightly Red on the sides and had a sticky-white coating. His pulse was Slippery-Wiry-Rapid (92 b.p.m).

Diagnosis: The essential feature of this boy's condition is its acute onset. If we analyse his symptoms in isolation, many different patterns would emerge: Damp-Heat in the joints (ache in the joints), Liver-Yang rising (headaches, irritability, dizziness), Yin deficiency (night sweating, epigastric discomfort with feeling of hunger), Spleen-Qi deficiency (weakness, tiredness, weary limbs) and Stomach-Qi not descending (nausea). However, if we take the sudden onset into account and consider the symptoms in their totality, it then becomes apparent that this problem is caused by the emergence of Latent Heat in springtime. In this particular case, Latent Heat manifests as Damp-Heat.

Latent Heat occurs when an external pathogenic factor invades the body (in theory in winter but it can happen in any season) without causing apparent symptoms at the time; the pathogenic factor goes into the Interior, turns into Heat and 'lurks' in the Interior to emerge later with a sudden onset in springtime. When it emerges, Latent Heat manifests with symptoms of Interior Heat but with an acute onset; in this boy's case the symptoms of Heat are insomnia, restless sleep, irritability, night sweating, feeling of hunger, Red sides of the tongue and Rapid pulse. The symptoms of Damp-Heat are weary limbs, ache in the joints, sticky tongue coating and a Slippery pulse.

Although the symptoms appear quite complex, the treatment is relatively simple and it should consist in clearing Heat and resolving Damp with a prescription such as Lian Po Yin *Coptis-Magnolia Decoction*.

Case history 33.7

A 20-year-old woman had been suffering from postviral fatigue syndrome for 3 years. Her symptoms were extreme fatigue, swollen glands, a mild, intermittent sore throat, a feeling of tightness of the chest, ache in the muscles, a feeling of muzziness of the head, dizziness, a feeling of heaviness, an alternating feeling of heat and cold, headaches on the temples, blurred vision, tinnitus, thirst, a sticky taste, loose stools and fits of crying. She suffered an acute and severe attack of glandular fever (mononucleosis) when she was 16, which confined her to bed for a long time. On further questioning, she also said that she felt 'a pulsation' in the chest and epigastrium and that she suffered from insomnia.

Her tongue was Red in general and slightly Swollen with a sticky coating, and her pulse was Slippery and Rapid (92).

Diagnosis: There are two main patterns emerging from the numerous symptoms and signs: the first is residual Damp-Heat following the original acute attack of glandular fever and the second is the pattern of Gall-Bladder Heat of the Qi level within the identification of patterns according to the Four Levels. The Gall-Bladder Heat pattern of the Qi level is equivalent to the Lesser-Yang pattern of the Six Stages, the main difference being that it is characterized by more Heat.

The symptoms and signs of Damp-Heat are extreme fatigue, swollen glands, ache in the muscles, intermittent sore throat, feeling of muzziness, feeling of heaviness, sticky taste, thirst, loose stools, a feeling of pulsation in the chest and epigastrium, insomnia, Swollen and Red tongue with sticky coating, Slippery-Rapid pulse. Some of these symptoms are related to the actual Dampness and some to Heat. The symptoms and signs of the Gall-Bladder Heat pattern are alternation of feeling of heat and cold, headaches on the temples, dizziness, blurred vision, tinnitus, insomnia and a Rapid pulse.

Box 33.1 summarizes patterns underlying tiredness.

BOX 33.1 TIREDNESS

- Tiredness with desire to lie down, poor appetite, loose stools: Spleen-Qi or Spleen-Yang deficiency
- Tiredness with weak voice, tendency to catch colds: Lung-Qi or Lung-Yang deficiency
- Tiredness with backache, lassitude, depression, frequent urination: Kidney-Yang deficiency
- Tiredness with slight depression, dizziness: Liver-Blood deficiency
- Tiredness with anxiety, insomnia, dry mouth, Kidney-Yin deficiency
- Tiredness with feeling of heaviness: Dampness
- Tiredness with feeling of oppression of the chest: Phlegm
- Tiredness with anxiety and tenseness: Liver-Qi stagnation

NOTES

1. He Ren 1981 A New Explanation of the Synopsis of Prescriptions from the Golden Cabinet (*Jin Gui Yao Lue Xin Jie* 金匮要略新解), Zhejiang Science Publishing House, Beijing, p. 44. The Synopsis of Prescriptions from the Golden Cabinet was written by Zhang Zhong Jing c. AD200.
2. Chao Yuan Fang AD610 Discussion on Causes and Symptoms of Diseases (*Zhu Bing Yuan Hou Lun* 诸病源候论) cited in Zhang Bo Yu 1986 Chinese Internal Medicine (*Zhong Yi Nei Ke Xue* 中医内科学), Shanghai Science Publishing House, Shanghai, p. 281.
3. 1979 The Yellow Emperor's Classic of Internal Medicine – Simple Questions (*Huang Di Nei Jing Su Wen* 黄帝内经素问), People's Health Publishing House, Beijing, p. 154 First published c. 100BC.
4. Cited in Zhang Bo Yu 1986 Internal Medicine (*Zhong Yi Nei Ke Xue* 中医内科学), Shanghai Science and Technology Publishing House, Shanghai, p. 281.
5. Ibid.
6. Ibid.
7. Ibid.
8. Zhu Qi Shi 1988 Discussion on Exhaustion (*Xu Lao Lun* 虚劳论), People's Health Publishing House, Beijing, p. 19. First published c. 1520.
9. Ibid., p. 21.

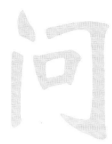

Chapter **34**

HEAD

Chapter contents

INTRODUCTION 287

HEADACHE 288
  Onset 288
  Time 288
  Location 288
  Character of pain 288
  Ameliorating or aggravating factors 289
  Internal and external origin 289

DIZZINESS 295

FAINTING 296

FEELING OF DISTENSION OF THE HEAD 297

FEELING OF HEAVINESS OF THE HEAD 297

FEELING OF MUZZINESS (FUZZINESS) OF THE HEAD 297

BRAIN NOISE 298

FEELING OF COLD OF THE HEAD 298

FEELING OF HEAT OF THE HEAD 299

NUMBNESS/TINGLING OF THE SKIN OF THE HEAD 299

ITCHY SCALP 299

INTRODUCTION

The head is called the 'Fu of the Bright Essence' because it houses the Brain, which is a manifestation of the Sea of Marrow and Marrow itself is a manifestation of Essence; as the Essence is stored in the Kidneys, the head is also under the influence of the Kidneys. The hair on the head is nourished by the Kidneys and Qi and Blood in general and for this reason the hair was said to be the 'abundance of Blood' and the 'glory of the Kidneys'. The head is also called the 'Meeting of all Yang' because all the Yang channels meet in the head where they either end or begin. The head also houses the senses and the Yang channels bring to it clear Yang-Qi, which 'brightens' the senses' orifices and enables a person to have clear sight, hearing, taste and smell.

❓ **WHY** WE ASK

It is important to ask about any problems in the head with practically every patient, first because headache and dizziness are such common complaints and secondly because patients may often forget about some head symptoms unless they are asked. For example, not many patients would volunteer the information of having an itchy scalp or a feeling of heaviness of the head. Problems related to the head often serve to confirm or exclude the presence of Liver patterns (although of course not exclusively Liver patterns). For example, the symptoms of itchiness of the scalp in a patient presenting with a possible Liver disharmony would confirm such disharmony as it may be due to Liver-Blood deficiency, Wind in the skin (also Liver related), Liver-Fire or Damp-Heat in the Liver channel.

? WHEN WE ASK

Questions about the head are obviously particularly important in patients who suffer from headaches; however, they are also important in the elderly and in those suffering from hypertension or tinnitus. In the elderly they have particular importance because head symptoms such as headache, dizziness, feeling of distension of the head, etc. often occur with serious pathologies such as hypertension or may be prodromal signs of Wind-stroke.

I also ask about head symptoms whenever there is Liver-Qi stagnation or Liver-Blood stasis to check whether there may be also Liver-Yang rising or Liver-Fire, which tend to cause symptoms in the head. For example, a woman may complain of premenstrual tension characterized by irritability and breast distension. She may also suffer from premenstrual headaches but may not relate them to the premenstrual phase. The presence of headaches would confirm that there is Liver-Yang rising in conjunction with Liver-Qi stagnation; if we did not ask about the headache, we would never know this. This situation arises especially in Liver disharmonies because in such disharmonies it is common for a patient to suffer from two, three, or even four concomitant Liver patterns.

? HOW WE ASK

I usually ask about any head symptoms whenever this is appropriate during the interrogation.

I especially ask about head symptoms whenever a Liver disharmony emerges to check whether there may be Liver-Yang rising or Liver-Fire.

HEADACHE

Symptoms and Signs, Chapter 55

Headache is one of the most common presenting symptoms in Western patients; Chinese books differentiate first of all between headaches of internal origin and those of external origin, but the latter are not frequently seen in practice.

When asking a patient about headaches it is important to ask systematically about onset, time, location, character of pain and ameliorating or aggravating factors.

Onset

A recent onset and short duration indicate headache from exterior invasion of Wind; a gradual onset with long duration indicates headache from interior causes.

Time

Headache occurring in the daytime usually indicates Qi or Yang deficiency, whereas headache occurring in the evening may be due to Blood or Yin deficiency. Headache starting at night during sleep indicates Blood stasis.

Location

- Occiput: here the location is the Greater-Yang channels (the headache can be from exterior invasion of Wind-Cold if the pain is severe or from interior Kidney deficiency if the pain is dull) (Fig. 34.1).
- Vertex: here the location is the terminal Yin channels (the headache is usually from deficiency of Liver-Blood) (Fig. 34.1).
- Forehead: here the location is the Bright-Yang channels (the headache can be from Stomach-Heat or Blood deficiency) (Fig. 34.2).
- Temples and sides of the head: here the location is Lesser-Yang channels (the headache can be from exterior Wind in the Lesser-Yang or from Liver-Yang rising) (Fig. 34.3).
- Temple, side of head and eye: here the location is the Lesser-Yang channels (the headache is usually from Liver-Yang rising) (Fig. 34.4).
- Behind the eyes: here the location is the Liver channel (the headache cause is either Liver-Yang rising or Liver-Blood deficiency) (Fig. 34.5).
- Whole head: this is caused by exterior invasion of Wind-Heat or Kidney deficiency.

Character of pain

A dull ache usually indicates Deficiency whereas an intense, sharp pain usually indicates Excess. A throbbing and distending pain indicates Liver-Yang rising, a pulling pain indicates Liver-Wind and a fixed, boring pain indicates Blood stasis. A dull ache, with the head

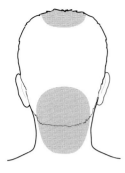

Fig. 34.1 Location of occipital and vertical headache

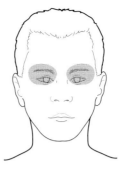

Fig. 34.5 Location of headache behind the eyes

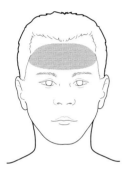

Fig. 34.2 Location of frontal headache

feeling as if it were wrapped in or full of cotton wool, and a sensation of heaviness indicate Dampness or Phlegm. Headache that is experienced 'inside' the head is usually due to a Kidney deficiency (see below).

Ameliorating or aggravating factors

Chronic headaches that are improved by rest are due to Deficiency, whereas if they are improved by exercise they are due to Liver-Fire, Phlegm or Blood stasis. Headaches aggravated by lying down usually indicate Fullness (Liver-Yang rising, Liver-Fire, Phlegm or Blood stasis). If they are ameliorated by lying down they usually indicate Deficiency.

Headaches that are improved by eating usually indicate Deficiency; if they are aggravated by eating they usually indicate Excess, especially Phlegm or retention of food.

Internal and exterior origin

The differentiation of headaches is best done by distinguishing headaches of interior origin from those of exterior origin.

Headaches of internal origin

In headaches of internal origin, it is very important to differentiate between those deriving from Fullness and those deriving from Emptiness. The most common headaches from Fullness include Liver-Yang rising, Liver-Fire, Phlegm, Blood stasis, Liver-Wind, Stomach-Heat and retention of food; the most common headaches from Emptiness include Blood deficiency, Stomach- and Spleen-Qi deficiency and Kidney deficiency.

The headache from Liver-Yang rising manifests with a throbbing pain, which is usually unilateral, often moving from side to side and located behind the eye, on

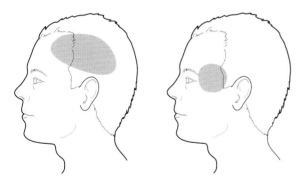

Fig. 34.3 Location of Lesser-Yang headache

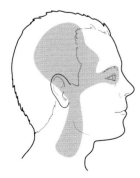

Fig. 34.4 Location of Liver-Yang rising headache

the temples or on the lateral side of the head along the Gall-Bladder channel. It is often accompanied by nausea and vomiting, dizziness, blurred vision, flashing lights and a Wiry pulse.

The headache from Liver-Fire, which is less common, is similar in character to that from Liver-Yang rising but it is accompanied by Liver-Fire symptoms and signs such as intense thirst, bitter taste, red face, dark urine and dry stools.

Another very common type of headache is that from Phlegm obstructing the clear orifices of the head: in this case the headache is dull in nature and the head feels as if it were wrapped in or full of cotton wool and with a pronounced feeling of heaviness, muzziness and blurred vision. Other manifestations include a feeling of nausea, a feeling of oppression of the chest, a Swollen tongue and a Slippery pulse.

A very common type of chronic headache is the one due to a combination of Phlegm and internal Wind. Such a headache has all the characteristics as the one from Phlegm but is characterized by occasional bouts of severe headaches from Wind. Such a pattern is called 'Wind-Phlegm'. However, Phlegm as a cause of headache is frequently also associated with Liver-Yang rising, with the Phlegm being carried upwards by the ascending Liver-Yang; a person suffering from these two patterns will suffer from chronic, dull headaches with a feeling of muzziness and dizzines (caused by Phlegm) punctuated by occasional, acute attacks of severe, throbbing headaches (caused by Liver-Yang rising). Such pattern is also called 'Wind-Phlegm'.

The headache from Blood stasis is characterized by an intense, fixed, boring pain, usually unilateral, and accompanied by a Purple tongue and Wiry pulse. In very chronic, long-standing cases of headache, the Blood stasis type of pain may often be combined with other types; the chronic recurrence of a headache in the same part of the head may by itself cause local Blood stasis. For example, if a patient suffers from a Liver-Yang type of headache for many years occurring always on the right side, this may by itself cause a local stasis of Blood in the head on that side and thus the headache will manifest with symptoms of both Liver-Yang rising and Blood stasis.

The headache from Liver-Wind is characterized by a pulling pain, accompanied by severe dizziness and tremors.

The headache from Stomach-Heat is characterized by an intense frontal pain and is accompanied by epigastric pain, thirst, sour regurgitation and a yellow tongue coating.

The headache from retention of food is characterized by a diffused and intense dull pain on the forehead and is accompanied by nausea, vomiting, sour regurgitation, a feeling of fullness of the epigastrium, a thick and sticky tongue coating and a Slippery pulse.

The headache from Blood deficiency (usually of the Liver or Heart, or both) is characterized by a dull ache, usually on the top of the head, and is accompanied by dizziness, blurred vision, insomnia, palpitations, a Pale tongue and a Choppy pulse.

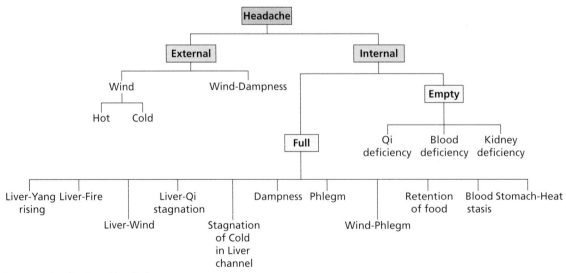

Fig. 34.6 Classification of headaches

The headache from Stomach- and Spleen-Qi deficiency is characterized by a dull frontal ache and is accompanied by tiredness, lassitude, weak limbs, loose stools, poor appetite, a Pale tongue and a Weak pulse.

The headache from Kidney deficiency (which could be Yin or Yang deficiency) is characterized by a dull headache all over the head, accompanied by a feeling of emptiness of the head, dizziness and tinnitus.

Stagnation of Cold in the Liver channel may cause a dull but intense, vertical headache associated with cold feet. However, this headache is rather rare.

Headaches of external origin

External headaches are due to invasion of Wind-Cold, Wind-Heat and Wind-Dampness and they all obviously have an acute onset.

The headache from Wind-Cold is characterized by a severe occipital ache and stiffness and is accompanied by pronounced aversion to cold, fever, sneezing and a Floating-Tight pulse.

The headache from Wind-Heat is characterized by a severe pain as if the head were being cracked open and is accompanied by aversion to cold, fever, sore throat, slight sweating and a Floating-Rapid pulse.

The headache from Wind-Dampness is characterized by a dull headache as if the head were wrapped up and is accompanied by a feeling of heaviness of the head, aversion to cold, fever, slight sweating, nausea and a Floating-Slippery pulse.

Figure 34.6 is a classification of headaches.

Case histories 34.1–34.5 illustrate some different patterns causing headache.

Case history 34.1

A 14-year-old girl had been suffering from recurring headaches since the age of 10 years. The headaches were severe and came approximately every 3 months. The headache was concentrated in the area behind the eyes, was throbbing in character and was accompanied by blurred vision, vomiting, and what she described as 'fuzzy eyes'. Apart from the attacks of severe headaches every 3 months, she also experienced frequent, dull headaches in between.

On interrogation, she said she suffered from chronic tiredness and experienced some tingling of her limbs.

Her tongue was Pale, slightly Swollen and with a sticky coating; her pulse was slightly Slippery.

Diagnosis: The headaches are very clearly of the Liver-Yang type: this is confirmed by the throbbing character of the pain, the location behind the eyes and the vomiting. However, there are two other patterns which are evidenced by very few symptoms. First of all, there is some Liver-Blood deficiency, which is indicated by the chronic tiredness, the Pale tongue and the tingling; Liver-Blood deficiency is obviously

the cause for the rising of Liver-Yang in this case. Secondly, there is also some Phlegm; this is evidenced mostly by the tongue (being Swollen and with a sticky coating) and pulse (being Slippery). The 'fuzzy eyes' could also be interpreted as a sign of Phlegm obstructing the eye orifices.

This is a good example of the importance of tongue and pulse as pointers to a certain pattern even in the absence of symptoms; for this reason, tongue and pulse pictures should never be discounted when they do not appear to accord with the presenting symptoms. For example, in this case of Liver-Blood deficiency with Liver-Yang rising, the tongue 'should' have been Pale and Thin and the pulse might have been Wiry on the left and Weak on the right. Why should the tongue and pulse show a certain pattern and the patient not show any signs of it? This often happens in young people when there is a certain pathogenic factor (in this case Phlegm) but, due to the young age of the person, it has not given rise to clinical manifestations as yet.

The treatment principle in this case should therefore be not only to nourish Liver-Blood and subdue Liver-Yang but also to resolve Phlegm.

Case history 34.2

A 28-year-old woman had been suffering from migraine since the age of 13. She was thin, quite tall and she walked with agility: her body shape was a typical Wood type (see Chapter 1). Her complexion was dull sallow, her hair was dry and her eyes had good *shen*.

The headaches were of a throbbing character and always occurred on the left side of the head, along the Gall-Bladder channel and behind the left eye; they occurred weekly and they were nearly always accompanied by nausea, vomiting and photophobia. The headache was not affected by posture or food intake and, although a headache always occurred with her period, she also suffered from headaches at

other times. The headaches were aggravated by damp and windy weather and also by stress and fatigue. A striking feature of the headaches was that they were markedly better during two pregnancies and markedly worse soon after childbirth both times. She had two children, one 3 years old and one 6 months old. An EEG and CT scan revealed no abnormalities and drugs for migraine produced an aggravation.

The periods were quite normal, coming regularly, with normal amount and colour but rather painful on the first 2 days. Her general health was good with no abnormalities in urination or defecation or sleep.

Diagnosis: Observation of her body type indicates that she is a Wood type: her agile walk accords with this, which is a good sign. As mentioned in the chapter on observation, each Five-Element body type has a characteristic walk and a deviation from this is not a good sign. For example, the Wood type should walk in an agile way and if they walked stiffly it would not be a good sign. Her dull complexion and dry hair suggest Blood deficiency; the normal sparkle of her eyes suggested that she did not suffer from any deep emotional problem.

The marked amelioration during pregnancy and aggravation after childbirth strongly suggests a deficiency of the Kidneys and the disharmony of the Penetrating and Directing Vessels: this is confirmed also by the onset of the headaches soon after menarche (which occurred when she was aged 12½).

We therefore need to confirm the presence of Blood deficiency and Kidney deficiency with further questioning. To confirm or exclude Blood deficiency, we ask about numbness and tingling of the limbs, dizziness, poor memory, insomnia, blurred vision: she did suffer from tingling of her limbs but from none of the other symptoms. However, we can conclude that there is some Blood deficiency from the tingling of her limbs, the dull complexion and the dry hair. As for Kidney deficiency, she had no symptoms of it apart from lower backache, but this symptom together with the onset of the headaches at menarche, the amelioration during pregnancy and the aggravation after childbirth confirms the presence of a Kidney deficiency and the disharmony of the Penetrating and Directing Vessels.

Her tongue was very slightly Pale but Red on the sides, Swollen and with a sticky coating and there was a small, peeled patch on the left side in the breast area; her pulse was generally Weak and Empty at the deep level.

The Pale colour of the tongue and the weakness and emptiness of the pulse confirm Blood deficiency and Kidney deficiency. However, the swelling of the tongue body and the sticky coating point to Phlegm, something that was not apparent from observation nor interrogation: her thin body indicates a tendency to Blood and Yin deficiency whereas Phlegm usually manifests with a tendency to being overweight. Furthermore, she had no other symptoms of Phlegm: there was no dizziness, no blurred vision, no feeling of heaviness of the head, no dull headaches, no expectoration of phlegm. However, in these cases, I never discount the tongue signs and I concluded that, although she had no other symptoms of Phlegm, the tongue signs were clear enough to confirm the presence of Phlegm; this is confirmed by the aggravation of the headaches in damp weather. The simultaneous presence of Liver-Yang rising and Phlegm is a very common cause of chronic headaches.

The character of her headaches points very clearly to Liver-Yang rising: this is confirmed by the throbbing nature of the pain, the nausea and vomiting, the sensitivity to light and the location of the headache on the Gall-Bladder channel. We can therefore conclude that the causes of the rising of Liver-Yang are the Blood and the Kidney deficiency: the former constitutes the Manifestation (*Biao*) and the latter the Root (*Ben*). From the point of view of Deficiency and Excess, the former consists of the Blood deficiency, Kidney deficiency and also Spleen-Qi deficiency, while the latter consists of Liver-Yang rising and Phlegm. We can deduce the presence of Spleen-Qi deficiency from the presence of Phlegm and from the Weak pulse.

The Pale colour of her tongue body can be attributed to any or all of her deficiencies, that is, Blood-Kidney- and Spleen-Qi deficiency. The redness of the sides confirms the rising of Liver-Yang and the swelling of the tongue body and the sticky coating indicate Phlegm. The last aspect of her tongue to interpret is the peeled patch on the left side in what may, under certain circumstances, be the breast area. There are two ways of interpreting the significance of this peeled patch: it could indicate either the very beginning of Yin deficiency (which may develop from Blood deficiency) or a problem in the left breast. This could be a problem in the left breast (such as mastitis) developed after childbirth; however, the patient said that this was not the case. The other possible explanation is that the

peeled patch may indicate a more serious potential problem in the left breast such as a malignant lump.

In this case we need to treat both the Root and Manifestation simultaneously: the Root by nourishing Blood, tonifying Spleen and Kidneys and strengthening the Penetrating and Directing Vessels, and the Manifestation by subduing Liver-Yang and resolving Phlegm.

Case history 34.3

A 50-year-old woman had been suffering from headaches since she was 18 years old. The headaches occurred mostly on the right temple area, were of a throbbing character and were accompanied by blurred vision. The headaches were better during two pregnancies and worse from taking HRT.

She also suffered from insomnia and constipation, her periods had recently become irregular and the menstrual blood had dark clots. Her cheeks were red and her eyes lacked sparkle and looked nervous. Her tongue was Red and slightly Purple, redder on the sides and did not have enough coating; her pulse was Fine and slightly Rapid.

Diagnosis: The headaches are clearly due to the rising of Liver-Yang, indicated by their throbbing character, the location on the temple, the blurred vision, the red cheeks and the insomnia. In this case, Liver-Yang rises from a deficiency of Liver-Yin, which is manifested by the lack of coating on the tongue, the constipation and the blurred vision. The amelioration during the pregnancies and aggravation from taking HRT in this case indicate a Liver disharmony.

The slightly Purple colour of the tongue indicates a tendency to Blood stasis, of which the dark menstrual clots were the only symptom.

Case history 34.4

A 36-year-old man complained of migraine since the age of 11. The attacks came every few months affecting either side of the head along the Gall-Bladder channel, the pain was sharp and throbbing and it was often accompanied by vomiting and blurred vision. In between the severe attacks, he occasionally suffered from a dull occipital headache. He also suffered from high blood pressure for which he took medication, which, however, did not control it well. He also complained of a dry mouth and the interrogation did not reveal any Kidney symptoms.

He was overweight and his complexion was dull and pale with a greasy skin and several small, pale moles on the face; his eyes were very dull and lacking in lustre. His tongue was dark Red with a redder tip, Swollen and with a rootless white coating that looked like salt. Although he was on beta-blockers, which alter the pulse significantly (making it Deep and Slow), his pulse was very Weak on both Rear positions.

Diagnosis: The headaches are clearly due to Liver-Yang rising, which is evidenced by the severity and throbbing nature of the pain, and by the vomiting and blurred vision. In this case, the origin of Liver-Yang rising is in Liver- and Kidney-Yin deficiency: this is apparent from the tongue, which shows a severe Yin deficiency with Empty-Heat. It is unusual, but not infrequent, that there are no other symptoms of Kidney deficiency and the dry mouth is the only symptom of Yin deficiency. Exactly the same pathology that is causing the headaches is also at the root of the hypertension.

His complexion and body shape contradict the above patterns because the complexion is dull and pale (while it should be red or floating red) and the body shape is overweight (whereas Yin deficiency usually causes a person to be thin). This is due to the presence of Phlegm of which he has no other symptoms. However, certain signs do show the presence of Phlegm; these are the swelling of the tongue, the dull-pale complexion, the greasy skin with small pale moles and the overweight body shape. The lack of lustre of the eyes indicates severe emotional problems (which he confirmed having), which may also be causing the complexion to be dull and pale, contradicting the tongue.

Case history 34.5

A 41-year-old woman had been suffering from headaches for over 20 years and they had worsened in the past year. The headaches occurred all over the head and were generally dull in character; occasionally they occurred on the left side of her forehead, in which case they were sharp and throbbing in character.

She also suffered from chilblains, cold hands and feet and tiredness, and she felt cold in general. Occasionally she suffered a visual disturbance consisting in seeing flashing lights. She had had two children, aged 2 and 6 and she had suffered a heavy blood loss after the second childbirth.

Her tongue was slightly Pale on the sides and had a Heart crack. Her pulse was Deep-Weak-Choppy.

Diagnosis: There are symptoms and signs of Liver-Blood deficiency, manifested by the dull headaches, the visual disturbance, the Pale sides of the tongue and the Choppy pulse. This Blood deficiency was obviously aggravated by the haemorrhage after the second childbirth, which explains the aggravation of her headaches. Liver-Blood deficiency has in this case given rise to Liver-Yang rising, which is causing the sharp, throbbing headaches on the left side of the forehead. In addition to this, there are also manifestations of Kidney-Yang deficiency (feeling cold, cold hands and feet, tiredness and the Deep-Weak pulse).

In this case, attention should be paid to treating both the Root and the Manifestation but with special emphasis on treating the Root, that is, nourishing Liver-Blood and tonifying Kidney-Yang.

Box 34.1 summarizes the patterns underlying headache.

BOX 34.1 HEADACHES

Onset
External invasion of Wind: recent onset, short duration
Internal headache: gradual onset, long duration

Time
Qi or Yang deficiency: headache in daytime
Blood or Yin deficiency: headache in the evening
Blood stasis: headache starting at night

Location
Greater-Yang channels: occipital headache
Terminal-Yin channels: headache on vertex
Bright-Yang channels: frontal headache
Lesser-Yang (Gall-Bladder) channel: headache on temples and sides of the head, and eye
Liver channel: headache behind the eyes
External Wind, Kidney deficiency: headache of whole head

Ameliorating factors
Liver-Fire, Phlegm, Blood stasis: headache improved by exercise
Fullness: headache aggravated by lying down
Deficiency: headache ameliorated by lying down or better after eating
Excess: headache worse after eating

Internal
Liver-Yang rising, Liver-Fire: throbbing
Dampness: dull headache with feeling of heaviness
Phlegm: dull headache with feeling of heaviness and dizziness
Blood stasis: intense fixed, stabbing, boring headache
Liver-Wind: headache with pulling pain
Stomach-Heat: intense, frontal headache
Retention of food: severe, dull frontal headache
Blood deficiency: dull headache on vertex
Stomach- and Spleen-Qi deficiency: mild, dull frontal headache
Kidney deficiency: headache with feeling of emptiness of the head

External
External Wind-Cold: acute headache with occipital stiffness
External Wind-Heat: acute, severe headache
External Wind-Dampness: acute, severe, dull headache

DIZZINESS

Symptoms and Signs, Chapter 55

Dizziness is a common complaint, especially in the elderly in whom it often is the main presenting problem.

? **WHY** WE ASK

It is necessary to ask about dizziness particularly with elderly patients because dizziness may be a symptom of Liver-Wind or Phlegm, or both, both of which are pathogenic factors seen in Wind-stroke, to which elderly people are prone. In women, dizziness is often a key symptom to establish the presence of either Liver-Blood deficiency or a Kidney deficiency.

? **WHEN** WE ASK

I generally ask about dizziness in the course of the interrogation to confirm or exclude the presence of Liver-Blood deficiency, Kidney deficiency, Liver-Yang rising or Phlegm in young and middle-aged people or of Liver-Wind in the elderly.

? **HOW** WE ASK

When we ask about dizziness we should make it clear to the patient that, even if this symptom is very sporadic, it still has a clinical significance. Thus, we should ask something like 'Do you ever experience any dizziness, even occasionally?'

Dizziness can be due to four factors, which can be summarized as Wind, Yang, Phlegm and Deficiency. In general a sudden onset of dizziness indicates a Full condition whereas a gradual onset indicates Deficiency.

The dizziness from Wind is very severe and the patient feels as if the ground is moving to the point where he or she loses balance. This is Liver-Wind and is usually seen only in the elderly.

The dizziness from Liver-Yang rising may be also severe but less severe than that from Wind and is accompanied by headache and blurred vision. This is common in patients of all ages.

The dizziness from Phlegm is less severe than in both Liver-Wind and Liver-Yang and is accompanied by a feeling of heaviness and muzziness of the head and nausea.

The dizziness from deficiency of Qi or Blood, or both, is mild. It worsens when the person is tired; it may also be only postural. Dizziness from Deficiency may be due to Blood deficiency (of the Liver or Heart, or both), in which case it is accompanied by blurred vision, poor memory and insomnia, or to Kidney deficiency, in which case it is accompanied by tinnitus.

Of course, dizziness may also occur as a result of a head trauma.

Case history 34.6 illustrates a pattern underlying vertigo.

Case history 34.6

A 42-year-old woman had been suffering from severe vertigo attacks for 20 years. She suffered severe attacks with vomiting every 6 months but she also experienced less severe attacks in between. The attacks occurred usually in the morning, were aggravated by lying down and alleviated by sitting up. These became more frequent after the birth of her second child 2 ½ years previously.

She walked rather slowly, her complexion was dull and sallow, her eyes lacked sparkle and she generally looked very depressed. She had very few other symptoms: she felt cold in general, experienced chilblains in winter, suffered from catarrh and experienced backache.

Her tongue was relatively normal apart from the sides being too Red; her pulse was Weak in general, especially on the left side, and both Kidney positions were very Weak and Deep.

Diagnosis: In this patient, vertigo is caused by a combination of Liver-Yang rising and Phlegm. Apart from the dizziness, Liver-Yang rising is evidenced by the Red sides of the tongue and Phlegm by the catarrh, the vomiting, the aggravation on lying down

and the amelioration when sitting up. Phlegm is causing the more frequent, less severe attacks of dizziness, while Liver-Yang rising is causing the occasional severe attacks.

Apart from these two patterns, there is a Kidney-Yang deficiency and a Spleen-Qi deficiency. The Kidney-Yang deficiency is manifested by the very Weak and Deep pulse on both rear positions, the aggravation of the dizziness after childbirth, the backache and the cold feeling, while the Spleen-Qi deficiency is manifested by the generally Weak pulse and the sallow complexion. Both Spleen-Qi and Kidney-Yang deficiency are obviously the root cause for the formation of Phlegm, while the Kidney deficiency is the cause for Liver-Yang rising. Therefore, Spleen-Qi and Kidney-Yang deficiency are the Root (*Ben*) while Liver-Yang rising and Phlegm are the Manifestation (*Biao*).

Box 34.2 summarizes the patterns underlying dizziness.

BOX 34.2 DIZZINESS

- Internal Liver-Wind: severe vertigo
- Liver-Yang rising: dizziness with headaches with blurred vision
- Phlegm: dizziness and muzziness, worse lying down
- Blood or Qi deficiency: mild dizziness, better lying down
- Kidney deficiency: chronic mild dizziness and tinnitus
- Head trauma: dizziness after accident

FAINTING

Symptoms and Signs, Chapter 55

'Fainting' may range from sudden collapse with total loss of consciousness to mild, transient episodes of 'passing out' but without total loss of consciousness. For example, there are patients who periodically 'pass out' but can still hear people around them.

The most important task is to differentiate Full from Empty causes of fainting. In other words, fainting may occur either because a pathogenic factor obstructs the Mind's orifices or because deficient Qi, Blood or Yin fail to anchor the Mind or Ethereal Soul, or both.

The most common pathogenic factor to cloud the Mind's orifices is Phlegm, which will be manifested by a Swollen tongue with sticky coating and Slippery pulse. Retention of food may also cloud the Mind's orifices, but this is rather more rare and it occurs more in children or in the elderly.

Among the Empty causes of fainting are a deficiency of Blood or Yin of the Heart or Liver, or both, and a deficiency of Kidney-Yang.

Fainting from a Full cause manifests with loss of consciousness, whereas fainting from an Empty cause may manifest with transient episodes of 'passing out' without total loss of consciousness.

Of course, in many cases, there may be a combination of Full and Empty patterns, for example Phlegm with Liver-Blood deficiency.

Case history 34.7 illustrates a pattern of Yin deficiency causing fainting episodes.

Case history 34.7

A 45-year-old woman had been suffering from what she described as 'turns', that is, she had recurrent episodes of fainting but without total loss of consciousness as, during these episodes, she could hear people around her. These episodes were more frequent during or after her periods.

She felt very tired in general and had very little vitality and energy. Her complexion was dull and pale, her tongue was Pale, Swollen and partially peeled with a patchy, sticky coating and her pulse was Weak but slightly Slippery.

Diagnosis: The swelling of the tongue with a sticky coating, and the Slippery pulse, clearly indicate Phlegm clouding the Mind's orifices and causing fainting. The Pale tongue, Weak pulse, dull-pale complexion and the aggravation of the fainting episodes during or after the period indicate a Liver-Blood deficiency. However, even in the absence of other symptoms, the partial peeling of the tongue clearly indicates a condition of Yin deficiency, in this case probably of the Stomach and Liver.

Box 34.3 summarizes patterns underlying fainting.

FEELING OF DISTENSION OF THE HEAD

Symptoms and Signs, Chapter 55

A 'feeling of distension of the head' is characterized by a bursting sensation as if the head were cracking open. The two main causes of this symptom are Liver-Fire blazing and Dampness obstructing the head.

The feeling of distension of the head caused by Liver-Fire is very intense and is accompanied by a headache of a throbbing nature, a dry mouth, bitter taste, a Red tongue with redder sides and a Wiry pulse.

The feeling of distension of the head caused by Dampness is less severe. Dull but intense, it is accompanied by the sensation that the head were wrapped up. The head feels heavy and the patient has nausea, a sticky tongue coating and a Slippery pulse.

Box 34.4 summarizes patterns underlying a feeling of distension of the head.

FEELING OF HEAVINESS OF THE HEAD

Symptoms and Signs, Chapter 55

The symptom of a 'feeling of heaviness of the head' is very common but it is not often reported spontaneously by patients and must be elicited on interrogation. There are five main causes of a feeling of heaviness of the head:

- invasion of Wind-Dampness
- Damp-Heat infusing upwards
- Dampness obstructing the Clear-Yang orifices
- Phlegm obstructing the head
- deficiency of Central Qi.

The feeling of heaviness of the head deriving from invasion of Wind-Dampness has a sudden onset and is due to external Dampness obstructing the head. It is accompanied by other exterior symptoms such as aversion to cold, fever and a Floating pulse.

The feeling of heaviness of the head due to Damp-Heat infusing upwards is quite severe and is accompanied by a dull headache, a red face, a feeling of heat of the head, a sticky taste, a sticky yellow tongue coating and a Slippery-Rapid pulse.

The feeling of heaviness of the head caused by Dampness obstructing the Clear-Yang orifices is quite severe and is accompanied by blurred vision and a feeling of muzziness of the head, nausea, decreased hearing, a sticky tongue coating and a Slippery pulse.

The feeling of heaviness of the head caused by Phlegm is severe and is accompanied by dizziness, a feeling of muzziness of the head, blurred vision, decreased hearing, a feeling of oppression of the chest, nausea, a Swollen tongue with sticky coating and a Slippery pulse.

The feeling of heaviness of the head caused by deficiency of Central Qi (deficiency of Stomach and Spleen) is mild and it is due not to Dampness or Phlegm weighing the head down, as in the previous cases, but to the Stomach and Spleen not nourishing the brain; this being empty, it does not 'sustain' the head, which therefore feels heavy.

Box 34.5 summarizes patterns underlying a feeling of heaviness of the head.

FEELING OF MUZZINESS (FUZZINESS) OF THE HEAD

Symptoms and Signs, Chapter 55

'Muzziness' (or 'fuzziness' in the USA) of the head indicates a feeling of heaviness and cloudiness of the head

accompanied by difficulty in concentration; it is usually worse in the morning. As Phlegm in the head obstructs the orifices, a feeling of muzziness is often accompanied also by a stuffed nose, blurred vision or a sticky taste.

A feeling of muzziness of the head is due either to Dampness (with or without Heat) infusing upwards towards the head, or to Phlegm in the head; if it is caused by Phlegm there will also be dizziness.

Box 34.6 summarizes a feeling of muzziness of the head.

BOX 34.6 FEELING OF MUZZINESS (FUZZINESS) OF THE HEAD

- Damp-Heat: feeling of muzziness of the head with headache and thirst
- Dampness: feeling of muzziness of the head with sticky taste
- Phlegm: severe feeling of muzziness of the head with dizziness

---

!

Dampness and Phlegm in the head both cause a feeling of heaviness and muzziness, but only Phlegm also causes dizziness.

BRAIN NOISE

Symptoms and Signs, Chapter 55

'Brain noise' should be distinguished from tinnitus: the former is experienced inside the head whilst the latter consists of a ringing in the ears. The four main causes of brain noise are:

- deficiency of the Sea of Marrow
- deficiency of Blood of the Heart and Spleen
- Damp-Heat infusing upwards
- Liver-Fire.

The brain noise caused by deficiency of the Sea of Marrow is accompanied by dizziness, poor memory, a weak back and legs; it is due to the deficient Marrow failing to 'fill' the brain.

The brain noise caused by deficiency of Blood of the Heart and Spleen is accompanied by dizziness, palpitations, insomnia, poor memory, a Pale tongue and a Choppy pulse; it is due to Qi and Blood failing to rise to the head to brighten its orifices.

The brain noise due to Damp-Heat infusing upwards is accompanied by a feeling of heaviness of the head, a dull headache, nausea, a sticky yellow tongue coating and a Slippery-Rapid pulse; it is due to Dampness obstructing the head's orifices.

The brain noise due to Liver-Fire is accompanied by irritability, hypochondrial distension, sighing and a Wiry pulse; it is due to Liver-Fire rising to the brain.

Box 34.7 summarizes patterns underlying brain noise.

BOX 34.7 BRAIN NOISE

- Deficiency of the Sea of Marrow: brain noise with dizziness, poor memory, weak back and legs
- Heart- and Spleen-Blood deficiency: brain noise with dizziness, palpitations, insomnia, poor memory, Pale tongue, Choppy pulse
- Damp-Heat: brain noise with feeling of heaviness of the head, dull headache, nausea, sticky yellow tongue coating, Slippery-Rapid pulse
- Liver-Fire: brain noise with irritability, hypochondrial distension, sighing, Wiry pulse

---

FEELING OF COLD OF THE HEAD

Symptoms and Signs, Chapter 55

A feeling of cold of the head is usually experienced on the occiput and, besides an actual feeling of cold, it is characterized by a desire to wear a scarf around the neck and an aversion to being exposed to wind. The two main causes of a feeling of cold of the occiput are stagnation of Cold in the Liver channel and Emptiness and Cold of the Governing Vessel.

The feeling of cold from stagnation of Cold in the Liver channel is characterized by a cold feeling of the occiput, vertical headache, a desire to cover one's head with a scarf, cold hands and feet, a greenish complexion and vomiting.

The feeling of cold of the head from deficiency and Cold of the Governing Vessel is characterized by a cold feeling of the vertex, occiput and upper back, cold limbs, feeling cold in general, a sore and weak back and dull pale complexion.

Box 34.8 summarizes patterns underlying a feeling of cold of the head.

BOX 34.8 FEELING OF COLD OF THE HEAD

- Stagnation of Cold in the Liver channel
- Governing Vessel empty and cold

FEELING OF HEAT OF THE HEAD

Symptoms and Signs, Chapter 55

A 'feeling of heat of the head' includes a subjective feeling of heat and an objective hot feeling of the head to touch. The three main causes of hot feeling of the head are Liver-Fire blazing, Kidney-Yin deficiency with Empty Heat and true Cold–false Heat.

Liver-Fire may cause a feeling of heat of the head and face which is accompanied by irritability, a bitter taste, thirst, a Red tongue with redder sides and a Wiry pulse.

Kidney-Yin deficiency with Empty-Heat may cause a feeling of heat of the head accompanied by dizziness, tinnitus, five-palm heat and a Red tongue with redder tip and no coating.

If there is a feeling of heat in the head with malar flush, sore throat, loose stools, cold limbs and Minute pulse, this may indicate true Cold and false Heat; this condition is quite rare.

Box 34.9 summarizes patterns underlying a feeling of heat of the head.

BOX 34.9 FEELING OF HEAT OF THE HEAD

- Liver-Fire
- Kidney-Yin deficiency with Empty-Heat
- True Cold–false Heat

NUMBNESS/TINGLING OF THE SKIN OF THE HEAD

Symptoms and Signs, Chapter 55

Numbness/tingling is called *Ma Mu: Ma* means 'tingling' while *Mu* means 'numbness'. The two main causes of numbness/tingling of the skin of the head are Blood deficiency and Phlegm. Numbness is more often due to Phlegm, whereas tingling is more often due to Blood deficiency.

Numbness/tingling of the skin of the head due to Blood deficiency is accompanied by dizziness, poor memory, blurred vision, palpitations, insomnia, a Pale tongue and a Choppy pulse; it is due to Liver and Heart-Blood failing to nourish the skin of the head.

Numbness/tingling of the skin of the head due to Phlegm is accompanied by dizziness, blurred vision, nausea, a feeling of oppression of the chest, a Swollen tongue with sticky coating and a Slippery pulse; it is due to Phlegm stagnating in the space between the skin and muscles.

Box 34.10 summarizes patterns underlying numbness and tingling of the head

BOX 34.10 NUMBNESS/TINGLING OF THE SKIN OF THE HEAD

- Blood deficiency: dizziness, blurred vision, poor memory, palpitations, insomnia, Pale tongue, Choppy pulse
- Phlegm: dizziness, blurred vision, nausea, feeling of oppression of the chest, Swollen tongue with sticky coating, Slippery pulse

ITCHY SCALP

Symptoms and Signs, Chapter 55

The most common cause of an itchy scalp is Liver-Blood deficiency and this is especially common in women. An alternative cause is Liver- or Kidney-Yin deficiency, or both. It should not be forgotten that Wind has a drying action on the skin, which may also cause the scalp to be dry and itchy; this is more common in the elderly. Other possible causes of an itchy scalp are Liver-Fire and Damp-Heat in the Liver channel.

Box 34.11 summarizes patterns underlying an itchy scalp.

BOX 34.11 ITCHY SCALP

- Liver-Blood deficiency
- Liver-/Kidney-Yin deficiency
- Internal Wind
- Liver-Fire
- Damp-Heat in Liver channel

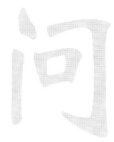

Chapter **35**

FACE

Chapter contents

INTRODUCTION   *301*

FACE   *302*
   Feeling of heat of the face   *302*
   Facial pain   *302*
   Feeling of numbness/tingling of the face   *303*

NOSE   *303*
   Blocked nose   *304*
   Itchy nose   *304*
   Sneezing   *304*
   Runny nose   *305*
   Nose ache   *305*
   Nose pain   *305*
   Dry nostrils   *306*
   Loss of sense of smell   *306*

TEETH AND GUMS   *306*
   Toothache   *306*
   Inflamed gums   *307*
   Bleeding gums   *307*
   Receding gums   *307*

MOUTH AND LIPS   *308*
   Mouth ulcers   *308*
   Cold sores   *309*

TONGUE   *309*
   Itchy tongue   *309*
   Numbness of the tongue   *309*
   Tongue pain   *309*

INTRODUCTION

? **WHY** WE ASK

Energetically, the face is an area of concentration of Yang channels. Pure Yang needs to rise to the face to brighten the orifices so as to promote clear vision, smell, hearing and taste. When clear Yang-Qi fails to ascend to the face, Dampness or Phlegm often accumulate in this area, obstructing the sense orifices and the sinuses. Dampness and Phlegm are extremely common pathogenic factors and, not infrequently, facial symptoms (e.g. sinus problems) are their only manifestation. For this reason, I nearly always ask about facial symptoms to confirm or exclude the diagnosis of Dampness or Phlegm.

Another reason for asking about facial symptoms is to confirm or exclude a diagnosis of Heat or Empty-Heat by asking if the patient has experienced a feeling of heat in the face, which is the main area where Heat or Empty-Heat manifests.

? **WHEN** WE ASK

I generally always ask about any feeling of heat in the face whenever a pattern of Heat or Empty-Heat emerges from the interrogation. It is important to remember that we should ask about feelings of heat in the face even when the patient presents with all the symptoms of Yang deficiency because there are many situations when contradictory Hot and Cold symptoms appear. A common example of this situation is in menopausal women who suffer from hot flushes of the face occurring against a background of a simultaneous Kidney-Yang and Kidney-Yin deficiency,

with a predominance of the former. For other causes of simultaneous hot and cold feeling, see Chapter 43.

I also ask about facial symptoms if I suspect a pattern of Dampness or Phlegm. In such a case I always question the patient about nasal symptoms (e.g. runny or blocked nose), and about facial ache.

? HOW WE ASK

When we ask about feelings of heat in the face, we should make it clear to the patient that, even if this symptom is experienced only occasionally, it has a diagnostic significance. We might therefore ask: 'Do you occasionally feel hot in the face?'

FACE

Feeling of heat of the face

Symptoms and Signs, Chapter 55

It is important to ask if patients suffer from a feeling of heat in the face, even if they feel cold in general. Especially in women, the two symptoms often coexist.

A feeling of heat in the face may be due to either Full- or Empty-Heat of any organ. Full-Heat will manifest with a feeling of heat in the face occurring either mostly in the daytime or throughout the day, whereas Empty-Heat manifests with a feeling of heat in the face occurring mostly in the afternoon and evening. (See Part 5, Chapter 55).

Women

In women, more than men, a feeling of heat in the face is often associated with contradictory Cold symptoms or signs in other parts of the body; for example, women frequently experience a feeling of heat in the face when their feet feel cold or they need to urinate frequently. Women's pathology differs from that of men and a feeling of heat in the face with contradictory Cold symptoms may be due to four main causes.

First of all, it may be due to a simultaneous deficiency of Kidney-Yang and Kidney-Yin with some Empty-Heat – a situation that is very common in menopausal women. In this case, the woman will experience hot flushes and a feeling of heat of the face and other Empty-Heat signs, such as night sweating and five-palm heat, but also Cold symptoms such as cold feet and frequent urination, which derive from Kidney-Yang deficiency. Of course, a simultaneous

deficiency of Kidney-Yin and Kidney-Yang may occur in men too, but it is far more frequent in women; indeed in my experience, especially in women over 40, this situation is the norm rather than the exception.

The second cause of a feeling of heat in the face with contradictory Cold symptoms in women is a deficiency of Blood giving rise to some Empty-Heat; the Blood deficiency may cause some Cold symptoms, especially cold hands, and the Empty-Heat deriving from it may cause a feeling of heat in the face. This pattern (i.e. Empty-Heat from Blood deficiency) occurs only in women.

The third cause of a feeling of heat in the face with contradictory Cold symptoms in women is a disharmony of the Penetrating Vessel. When the Qi of the Penetrating Vessel rebels upwards, it rushes to the face causing a feeling of facial heat and, since it fails to descend to the legs through the descendent branch, it causes cold feet. Again, such pathology of the Penetrating Vessel may occur in men too but it is far more common in women.

The fourth cause of a feeling of heat in the face with contradictory Cold symptoms is Yin Fire. Of course, Yin Fire may occur in men as well as women.

Men

In men, a feeling of heat with contradictory Cold symptoms may be due to three of the above-mentioned causes in women, that is, simultaneous deficiency of Kidney-Yin and Kidney-Yang, rebellious Qi of the Penetrating Vessel and Yin Fire. The first two of these are far less common in men than in women, however.

In men, a feeling of heat in the face with contradictory Cold symptoms in other parts of the body is usually due to coexisting patterns, such as Liver-Fire and Kidney-Yang deficiency.

> **!**
>
> A feeling of heat in the face with contradictory Cold symptoms in women may be caused by:
> - simultaneous deficiency of Kidney-Yin and Kidney-Yang
> - Blood deficiency with Empty-Heat
> - disharmony of the Penetrating Vessel
> - Yin Fire.

Facial pain

Symptoms and Signs, Chapter 55

The five main causes of facial pain are invasion of Wind-Heat, invasion of Wind-Cold, Damp-Heat, Liver-Fire and Qi deficiency with Blood stasis.

The facial pain due to invasion of Wind-Heat is characterized by an acute onset, a severe pain on the cheeks or jaws, a feeling of heat of the face, face feeling hot on palpation, headache, sore throat and an aversion to cold and fever.

The facial pain due to invasion of Wind-Cold is characterized by a spastic pain of the cheeks and jaws with sudden onset, sneezing, runny nose, aversion to cold, fever and a Floating-Tight pulse.

The facial pain due to Damp-Heat is characterized by a severe pain in the cheeks and forehead, and accompanied by red cheeks, greasy skin, a sticky yellow or greenish nasal discharge and a sticky yellow tongue coating.

The facial pain due to Liver-Fire is characterized by pain in the cheeks and forehead, redness of the cheeks, thirst, bitter taste, a Red tongue with redder sides and a Wiry-Rapid pulse.

The facial pain due to Qi deficiency and Blood stasis is characterized by an intense, often unilateral, pain of the cheeks, which is boring in nature and long in duration and accompanied by a dark complexion and a Purple tongue.

Trigeminal neuralgia is, of course, a type of facial pain; it is usually due to Liver-Fire combined with Liver- and Kidney-Yin deficiency.

Box 35.1 summarizes the patterns underlying facial pain.

BOX 35.1 FACIAL PAIN

- Invasion of Wind-Heat: acute onset, severe pain of the cheeks or jaws, feeling of heat of the face, face feels hot on palpation, headache, sore throat, aversion to cold, fever
- Invasion of Wind-Cold: acute onset, spastic pain of cheeks and jaws, sneezing, aversion to cold, dorsum of hands hot, runny nose, Floating-Tight pulse
- Damp-Heat: severe pain in the cheeks and forehead, red cheeks, greasy skin, sticky yellow or greenish nasal discharge, sticky yellow tongue coating
- Liver-Fire: pain in the cheeks and forehead, red cheeks, thirst, bitter taste, Red tongue with redder sides, Wiry-Rapid pulse
- Qi deficiency and Blood stasis: intense, often unilateral pain of the cheeks, boring in nature and long in duration, dark complexion, Purple tongue
- Liver-Fire with Liver- and Kidney-Yin deficiency: trigeminal neuralgia

---

Feeling of numbness/tingling of the face

Symptoms and Signs, Chapter 55

The five main causes of numbness or tingling in the face are invasion of external Wind, internal Liver-Wind, Stomach-Fire, internal Wind with Phlegm and Blood deficiency.

Numbness or tingling in the face caused by invasion of external Wind is characterized by a sudden onset and short duration and is accompanied by deviation of eye and mouth.

Numbness or tingling in the face caused by internal Liver-Wind is accompanied by headache, giddiness, tremors and a Wiry pulse.

Numbness or tingling in the face caused by Stomach-Fire is accompanied by intense thirst, epigastric pain and a yellow tongue coating.

Numbness or tingling in the face caused by internal Wind and Phlegm is accompanied by deviation of the mouth, slurred speech and hemiplegia.

Numbness or tingling in the face caused by Blood deficiency is accompanied by a dull-pale complexion, blurred vision, dizziness, a Pale tongue and a Choppy pulse.

Box 35.2 summarizes the patterns underlying numbness and tingling in the face.

BOX 35.2 FEELING OF NUMBNESS AND TINGLING IN THE FACE

- External Wind: sudden onset, short duration, deviation of eye and mouth
- Internal Liver-Wind: headache, giddiness, tremors, Wiry pulse
- Stomach-Fire: intense thirst, epigastric pain, Yellow tongue coating
- Internal Wind with Phlegm: deviation of the mouth, slurred speech, hemiplegia
- Blood deficiency: dull-pale complexion, blurred vision, dizziness, Pale tongue, Choppy pulse

---

NOSE

The nose was called in Chinese medicine *Ming Tang*, which means 'Bright Hall', signifying that it is an area of concentration of Yang-Qi and a place through which the clear Yang ascends to the head. The Song dynasty's Chen Wu Ze says: '*The nose is the opening of the Lungs through which the five odours are detected; it is the place where the Yin and Yang descend and ascend and*

through which the Clear Qi flows.'[1] The nose is the external orifice of the Lungs and it is therefore closely related to breathing, smell and sound (of the voice). The organs influencing the nose are the Lungs, Kidneys, Spleen, Stomach, Gall-Bladder and Governing Vessel. External Wind-Heat invades the body via the nose and mouth. The nose can reflect pathological changes of many different organs, the balance of Yin and Yang, Heat and Cold, Deficiency and Excess, and stasis of Blood.

Blocked nose

Symptoms and Signs, Chapter 58

Excluding acute invasions of Wind, a blocked nose is usually caused by Dampness stagnating in the nose occurring against a background of Lung- and Spleen-Qi deficiency. In this case, the nose is often also swollen and pale and the problem is intermittent. This is a very common symptom in Western patients and it often leads to chronic sinusitis.

A blocked nose may also be caused by Qi and Blood stagnation, in which case the nose would be swollen, purple and with an uneven surface.

Gall-Bladder Heat may also cause a blocked nose, in which case the nose membranes are red and swollen and there is a sticky yellow nasal discharge.

In a newborn baby, a blocked nose (which may affect its ability to breast-feed) is usually due to invasion of Wind-Cold.

Box 35.3 summarizes the patterns underlying a blocked nose.

BOX 35.3 BLOCKED NOSE

- Lung- and Spleen-Qi deficiency: swollen and pale nose, problem comes and goes
- Qi and Blood stagnation: swollen and purple nose
- Gall-Bladder Heat: nose membranes red and swollen, sticky-yellow nasal discharge
- Invasion of Wind: sudden onset, accompanied by symptoms of Wind-Cold or Wind-Heat

---

Itchy nose

Symptoms and Signs, Chapter 58

Excluding acute invasions of Wind-Heat, itchiness of the nose may be due to Lung-Heat, deficiency of the Defensive Qi and, in children, Nose Childhood Nutritional Impairment.

When the cause is Lung-Heat, the nose is itchy, dry and red. The most common cause of an itchy nose, however, is a deficiency of the Lungs' Defensive Qi causing itchiness of the nose, sneezing and a profuse, watery nasal discharge coming in bouts. This was called in Chinese medicine *Bi Jiu* and it corresponds closely to allergic rhinitis in Western medicine. In my experience, however, the symptoms of allergic rhinitis with itchy nose, sneezing and profuse watery discharge are due also to a deficiency of Kidney-Yang and the Governing Vessel.

In small children, an itchy nose may be a symptom of Nose Childhood Nutritional Impairment. In such cases the itchiness is accompanied by scabs or ulcers on the nose, a watery yellow nasal discharge, dry skin and hot hands and feet, and the child has a tendency to pick his or her nose. This condition is usually caused by irregular feeding and poor-quality breast milk, which leads to Damp-Heat in the nose.

Box 35.4 summarizes the patterns underlying itchy nose.

BOX 35.4 ITCHY NOSE

- Invasion of Wind-Heat: sudden onset, accompanied by symptoms of an external invasion
- Lung-Heat: itchy, dry and red nose
- Deficiency of Lungs' Defensive-Qi system, Kidney-Yang and Governing Vessel: sneezing, profuse, watery nasal discharge coming in bouts
- Nose Childhood Nutritional Impairment: scabs, ulcers, watery yellow nasal discharge, dry skin, hot hands and feet, nose picking

---

Sneezing

Symptoms and Signs, Chapter 58

In acute cases, sneezing is always due to invasion of Wind, which may be either Wind-Cold or Wind-Heat although the former is more common. The sneezing is accompanied by aversion to cold, shivers, fever, body aches and a Floating pulse. Other manifestations depend on whether the cause is Wind-Cold or Wind-Heat.

Chronic sneezing is always a sign of allergic rhinitis which, in Chinese medicine, usually occurs against a background of Lung-Qi deficiency. In my opinion, there will also be a deficiency of the Kidney Defensive-Qi system, as well as of the Governing Vessel. In such cases, sneezing is accompanied by allergy to house-dust mites or pollen, itchy nose, tiredness, sweating,

slight shortness of breath, a Pale tongue and a Weak pulse.

Box 35.5 summarizes the patterns underlying sneezing.

BOX 35.5 SNEEZING

- Invasion of Wind: sudden onset, aversion to cold, shivers, fever, Floating pulse
- Deficiency of Lung-Qi, Kidney Defensive-Qi system and Governing Vessel: allergies, itchy nose, tiredness, sweating, slight shortness of breath, Pale tongue, Weak pulse

---

Runny nose

Observation, Chapter 20; Symptoms and Signs, Chapter 58

A runny nose with an acute onset is due to an invasion of Wind, which may be Wind-Cold or Wind-Heat, but it is especially likely to occur with Wind-Cold. The severity of this symptom reflects directly the severity of the Cold (as opposed to Wind).

A chronic, runny nose with a thick, sticky discharge, which is usually yellow, is generally due to Damp-Heat in the Stomach channel (often corresponding to sinusitis in Western medicine).

A chronic, profusely runny nose with a clear, watery discharge indicates a deficiency of Lung-Qi with Empty-Cold (often corresponding to allergic rhinitis in Western medicine). Such a profuse, watery discharge may also be due to a deficiency of Yang of both the Lungs and Kidneys and of the Governing Vessel (see above).

Box 35.6 summarizes the patterns underlying a runny nose.

BOX 35.6 RUNNY NOSE

- Invasion of external Wind: acute onset
- Damp-Heat in the Stomach channel: chronic, with thick sticky nasal discharge
- Lung-Qi deficiency with Empty-Cold, deficiency of Yang of the Governing Vessel: chronic, with watery white nasal discharge

---

Nose ache

Symptoms and Signs, Chapter 58

Excluding acute invasions of Wind-Heat, nose ache may be due to Phlegm-Heat in the Lungs, Lung-Qi deficiency or Lung- and Spleen-Qi deficiency.

Nose ache due to Phlegm-Heat in the Lungs is accompanied by a sticky yellow nasal discharge, a redness of the nose and a cough with expectoration of sticky yellow phlegm.

When due to Lung-Qi deficiency, the nose ache is accompanied by a watery nasal discharge and spontaneous sweating, a weak voice and an Empty pulse.

Chronic Lung- and Spleen-Qi deficiency with retention of Dampness in the nose may also cause nose ache, in which case there is a sticky white nasal discharge and often loss of the sense of smell.

Box 35.7 summarizes the patterns underlying nose ache.

BOX 35.7 NOSE ACHE

- Acute invasion of Wind-Heat: nose ache with aversion to cold, fever, body aches, Floating pulse
- Phlegm-Heat in the Lungs: nose ache with sticky yellow nasal discharge, red nose, cough with expectoration of sticky yellow phlegm
- Lung-Qi deficiency: dull nose ache, watery nasal discharge, spontaneous sweating, weak voice, Empty pulse
- Lung- and Spleen-Qi deficiency with Dampness: nose ache with sticky nasal discharge, loss of sense of smell

---

Nose pain

Symptoms and Signs, Chapter 55

Excluding acute invasions of Wind-Cold and Wind-Heat, nose pain may be due to Lung-Heat, Damp-Heat, Lung-Yin deficiency with Empty-Heat, or nasal cancer.

Lung-Heat may cause nose pain in acute conditions when the pathogenic factor enters the Qi level; it is accompanied by fever, a red face and nose, a cough with yellow phlegm, thirst and a Rapid-Overflowing pulse. When nose pain is caused by Damp-Heat, it is accompanied by a sticky yellow discharge, cheek pain and a feeling of heaviness and heat in the face. When caused by Empty-Heat of the Lungs, nose pain is dull and accompanied by a dryness and feeling of heat in the nose, with nasal scabs and redness, night sweating, and a Floating-Empty and Rapid pulse. It should be borne in mind that nose pain may also be caused by carcinoma of the nose, in which case the nose pain extends to the head and there is nosebleed with a swelling of the nasal mucosa.

Box 35.8 summarizes the patterns underlying nose pain.

BOX 35.8 NOSE PAIN

- Acute invasion of Wind-Cold: acute nose pain, aversion to cold, fever, sneezing, runny nose with white discharge, Floating-Tight pulse
- Acute invasion of Wind-Heat: acute nose pain, aversion to cold, fever, sticky yellow nasal discharge, sore throat, body aches, Floating-Rapid pulse
- Lung-Heat: acute nose pain after an invasion of external Wind, fever, red face and nose, cough with expectoration of yellow phlegm, thirst, Rapid-Overflowing pulse
- Damp-Heat: nose pain, red cheeks, sticky yellow nasal discharge, cheek pain, feeling of heat in the face and of heaviness of the head
- Lung-Yin deficiency with Empty-Heat: dull nose pain, scabs on the nose, dry nose, malar flush, dry cough, night sweating, Floating-Empty and Rapid pulse
- Cancer of the nose: nose pain extending to the head, nosebleed, swelling of nasal mucosa

---

Dry nostrils

Observation, Chapter 7; Symptoms and Signs, Chapter 58

'Dry nostrils' refers to dryness of the nasal mucosa.

Lung-Yin deficiency with Empty-Heat can cause dryness of the nostrils spreading to the throat. It is accompanied by a dry cough, night sweating and five-palm heat.

Dryness of the nostrils also appears in the Stomach-Heat pattern at the Qi level within the Four Levels identification of patterns, together with fever, thirst and sweating.

Dryness of the nostrils may also be caused by Blood stasis, in which case the nose bridge is dry and purple, there is thirst without desire to swallow, dark rings under the eyes and a dark complexion.

Chronic Lung- and Spleen-Qi deficiency may also cause dryness of the internal mucosa of the nose, a loss of the sense of smell and often a turbid discharge from the eyes.

Box 35.9 summarizes the patterns underlying dry nostrils.

BOX 35.9 DRY NOSTRILS

- Lung-Yin deficiency with Empty Heat: dry nostrils, dry throat, dry cough, night sweating, five-palm heat
- Stomach Heat at the Qi Level: dry nostrils, fever, thirst, sweating
- Blood stasis: dry nostrils and nose bridge, purple nose bridge, dark rings under the eyes, dark complexion, thirst with no desire to swallow
- Lung- and Spleen-Qi deficiency: dry nostrils, loss of sense of smell, turbid discharge from the eyes

---

Loss of sense of smell

Symptoms and Signs, Chapter 58

The most common cause of loss of sense of smell is a deficiency of Lung- and Spleen-Qi with an inability of the clear Qi to rise to the nose. Cases of acute and temporary loss of smell are due to invasion of Wind.

An inability to smell fragrant smells when the nasal mucosa are swollen and dark red is due to Damp-Heat in the nose.

Loss of the sense of smell in the course of a serious illness always indicates a poor prognosis.

Box 35.10 summarizes patterns underlying the loss of sense of smell.

BOX 35.10 LOSS OF SENSE OF SMELL

- Lung-Qi and Spleen-Qi deficiency
- Invasion of external Wind (acute and temporary loss)
- Damp-Heat

TEETH AND GUMS

The teeth are an extension of the bones and as such are governed by the Kidneys while the gums are under the influence of the Stomach. More specifically, the gums of the upper jaw are under the influence of the Large Intestine, and those of the lower jaw are under the influence of the Stomach. The state of the teeth and gums therefore reflects the state of the Kidneys, Stomach and Large Intestine. For example, tooth cavities and loss of teeth may reflect a Kidney deficiency, whereas receding gums may reflect a Stomach deficiency.

Toothache

Symptoms and Signs, Chapter 60

As a general rule, a Full condition causes a toothache that is constant and intense, whereas an Empty condition causes a toothache that comes and goes and is mild. Toothache that is worse in the evening and better in the morning points to Yin deficiency; one that is better in the evening and worse in the morning indicates Yang deficiency. As far as channels are concerned, the upper teeth are influenced by the Large Intestine channel and the lower ones by the Stomach channel.

Excluding external invasions of Wind, which cause an acute and temporary toothache with aversion to cold, toothache may be caused by Stomach-Fire, Toxic

Heat, Heat in the Spleen and Heart, Damp-Heat, 'Wind-Cold in the Brain' or Stomach and Spleen deficiency.

Stomach-Fire is a common cause of toothache, in which the toothache is accompanied by thirst, swollen cheeks, dry stools, mental restlessness, a Red tongue with a dry yellow coating in the centre and a Rapid-Overflowing pulse. When Stomach-Fire combines with Toxic Heat, the toothache is very intense, there may be a fever and the tongue would have a thick, dry yellow coating and red points; this may correspond to a tooth abscess in Western medicine. Toothache may also be caused by Heat in the Spleen and Heart, in which case there may also be bleeding gums, insomnia and mental restlessness.

Damp-Heat in the Stomach is also a frequent cause of toothache; it is usually accompanied by swelling of the gums and a sticky taste in the mouth. The relative importance of the toothache and the gum swelling gives an indication of the prevalence of Heat or Dampness: if the gum swelling predominates over the tooth-ache, Dampness is predominant; if the toothache pre-dominates over the gum swelling, Heat is predominant.

A severe toothache that extends to the head is due to 'Wind-Cold in the Brain' and Blood stasis. Stomach- and Spleen-Qi deficiency may cause a chronic, dull toothache that comes and goes and receding gums; this may be due to excessive consumption of sour foods.

Other teeth symptoms include loose teeth and grind-ing teeth, and other gum symptoms include inflamed gums, bleeding gums and receding gums. For the diag-nostic significance of these symptoms see Part 5, Chapter 60.

BOX 35.11 TOOTHACHE

- Invasion of external Wind: acute toothache with headache and aversion to cold
- Stomach-Fire: intense toothache, thirst, swollen cheeks, dry stools, mental restlessness, Red tongue, Rapid-Overflowing pulse
- Toxic Heat: very intense toothache, very swollen cheeks, fever, Red tongue with red points and thick, dry yellow coating
- Spleen- and Heart-Heat: toothache, bleeding gums, insomnia, mental restlessness
- Damp-Heat in the Stomach: toothache with swelling of the gums and sticky taste
- 'Wind-Cold in the Brain' with Blood stasis: severe toothache extending to the head
- Stomach- and Spleen-Qi deficiency: chronic, dull toothache with receding gums

Box 35.11 summarizes the patterns underlying toothache.

Inflamed gums

Observation, Chapter 8; Symptoms and Signs, Chapter 60

Stomach-Heat is a common cause of inflamed gums; this may be either Full-Heat or Empty-Heat from Stomach-Yin deficiency. Other causes include invasion of external Wind-Heat in acute cases, and two condi-tions that affect children and are characterized by swollen and inflamed gums.

Bleeding gums

Observation, Chapter 8; Symptoms and Signs, Chapter 60

The gums may bleed either from deficient Spleen-Qi not holding Blood, with tiredness, poor appetite and loose stools, or from Heat. This may be Stomach Full- or Empty-Heat, or Empty-Heat from Kidney-Yin deficiency. In Stomach Full-Heat there is a feeling of heat and thirst, in Empty-Heat there is thirst with a desire to drink in small sips, and in Kidney-Yin deficiency there is tinnitus, dizziness, night sweating and a malar flush.

Box 35.12 summarizes the patterns underlying bleeding gums.

BOX 35.12 BLEEDING GUMS

- Deficient Spleen-Qi not holding Blood: bleeding gums, tiredness, poor appetite, loose stools
- Stomach Heat: inflamed, bleeding gums, feeling of heat, thirst
- Stomach Empty-Heat: bleeding gums, dry mouth, desire to drink in small sips
- Kidney-Yin deficiency with Empty-Heat: bleeding gums, dizziness, tinnitus, night sweating, malar flush

Receding gums

Observation, Chapter 8; Symptoms and Signs, Chapter 60

Receding gums may be due to a general deficiency of Qi and Blood, Stomach-Heat or Kidney-Yin deficiency with Empty-Heat. Qi and Blood deficiency is accompa-nied by tiredness poor appetite, loose stools and a pale complexion. In Stomach-Heat there is thirst, a red face and a feeling of heat, while with Kidney-Yin deficiency there is dizziness, a malar flush and night sweating. It should be noted that 'loose teeth' are a prominent symptom of Kidney deficiency patterns; however, teeth

become loose generally because of gum disease. It can therefore be assumed that the Kidneys influence the gums also.

Box 35.13 summarizes the patterns underlying receding gums.

BOX 35.13 RECEDING GUMS

- Qi and Blood deficiency: tiredness, poor appetite, loose stools, pale complexion
- Stomach Heat: receding and inflamed gums, thirst, red face, feeling of heat
- Kidney-Yin deficiency with Empty-Heat: receding gums, dizziness, tinnitus, malar flush, night sweating

---

MOUTH AND LIPS

The mouth and lips are related to the Spleen. Chapter 37 of the 'Spiritual Axis' says: *'The mouth and lips are the orifice of the Spleen.'*[2] Chapter 17 of the same book says: *'The Spleen opens into the mouth. When the Spleen is harmonized the mouth can distinguish the five flavours.'*[3]

The mouth and lips are primarily influenced by the Stomach and Large Intestine channels; the Liver channel wraps around the lips and so do the Penetrating and Directing Vessels. Internally, other channels flow to the inside of the mouth and the tongue and, in particular, the Heart Connecting channel, the Kidney Main and Divergent channel and the Spleen main channel.

The saliva is mostly under the control of the Stomach, Spleen and Kidneys and a normal moisture of the mouth indicates a normal state of the Body Fluids.

Mouth ulcers

Observation, Chapter 8; Symptoms and Signs, Chapter 60

Recurrent mouth ulcers are a relatively common symptom and the most important differentiation is that between ulcers deriving from a Full condition and those deriving from an Empty condition. As a general rule, mouth ulcers that recur very frequently or are even almost permanent indicate a Full condition, whereas ulcers that come and go usually indicate an Empty condition.

The most common cause of ulcers is Heat. Full-Heat should be differentiated from Empty-Heat: in general mouth ulcers from Full-Heat are very painful and with

a red rim around them, whereas those from Empty-Heat are less painful and with a pale rim around them.

Mouth ulcers should be further differentiated according to their location: ulcers on the gums are due to Full-Heat or Empty-Heat of the Stomach or Large Intestine (the Stomach if on the lower gum and the Large Intestine if on the upper gum); ulcers on the tongue are usually related to the Heart channel, especially if they occur on the tip; ulcers on the inside of the cheeks are usually related to the Stomach channel. In women, and especially in pregnancy or after childbirth, a disharmony of the Directing Vessel may cause mouth ulcers; typically these occur on the floor of the mouth under the tongue.

The most common cause of mouth ulcers is Stomach-Heat in which case the ulcers have a red rim around them, they are inside the cheeks or on the lower gums and are associated with thirst, epigastric pain and a yellow tongue coating in the centre. Another common type of mouth ulcer is that from Kidney-Yin deficiency with Empty-Heat, in which case the ulcers have a pale rim around them and are aggravated by overwork and lack of sleep; other symptoms and signs would include a dry throat at night, night sweating and a Red tongue without coating.

Mouth ulcers may also arise from a severe Stomach- and Spleen-Qi deficiency and a deficiency of the Original Qi: the depletion of the Original Qi (after a chronic illness or from overwork) creates the conditions for the pathological arousal of the Minister Fire, which flows upwards to the mouth causing mouth ulcers. These ulcers are intermittent, have pale rims, are aggravated by overwork and are associated with other manifestations of Qi deficiency. For the diagnostic significance of other types of mouth ulcers see Part 5, Chapter 60.

BOX 35.14 MOUTH ULCERS

- Stomach Full-Heat: very painful, red-rimmed ulcers on the gums or on the inside of the cheeks
- Stomach Empty-Heat: pale-rimmed ulcers on the lower gums
- Large Intestine Full- or Empty-Heat: ulcers on the upper gum
- Heart-Fire or Heart Empty-Heat: ulcers on the tip of the tongue
- Disharmony of Directing Vessel: ulcers in pregnancy under the tongue
- Kidney-Yin deficiency or Original-Qi deficiency: pale-rimmed ulcers aggravated by overwork

Box 35.14 summarizes the patterns underlying mouth ulcers.

Cold sores

Observation, Chapter 8; Symptoms and Signs, Chapter 60

Cold sores are generally related to the Stomach channel and reflect Full-Heat, Empty-Heat or Qi deficiency. When due to Stomach-Heat, the cold sores appear suddenly and cause a burning pain; when due to Stomach Empty-Heat, they come in bouts, recurring over many years; when due to Qi deficiency, they occur in bouts over a long period of time, are usually pale in colour and are aggravated by overwork.

(For other signs related to the lips, see Part 5, Chapter 60.)

TONGUE

Itchy tongue

Symptoms and Signs, Chapter 60

Itchy tongue is generally due to Heat and this can be either external Heat in the form of Wind-Heat or Heart-Heat, which may be Full or Empty.

Numbness of the tongue

Symptoms and Signs, Chapter 60

Numbness of the tongue may be due to Heart-Blood deficiency or to Spleen-Qi deficiency. In Full conditions, numbness of the tongue may be due to Phlegm obstructing the orifices, to Liver-Wind or to chronic Blood stasis.

Tongue pain

Symptoms and Signs, Chapter 60

Pain of the tongue is always due to Heat and the most common cause is Heart-Fire or Heart Empty-Heat. Liver-Fire or Phlegm-Fire in the Heart may also cause tongue pain.

NOTES

1. Cited in Ma Zhong Xue 1989 Great Treatise of Chinese Diagnostic Methods (*Zhong Guo Yi Xue Zhen Fa Da Quan* 中国医学诊法大学) Shandong Science Publishing House, Jinan p. 56.
2. 1981 Spiritual Axis (*Ling Shu Jing* 灵枢经), People's Health Publishing House, Beijing, p. 78. First published c. 100BC.
3. Ibid, p. 50.

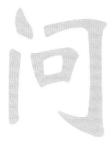

Chapter **36**

THROAT AND NECK

Chapter contents

INTRODUCTION   *311*

CHANNELS INFLUENCING THE THROAT AND NECK   *312*

THROAT   *312*
  Sore throat   *312*
  Dry throat   *313*
  Itchy throat   *313*
  Hoarse voice   *313*
  Feeling of obstruction in the throat   *314*
  Swollen and red tonsils   *314*

NECK   *315*
  Goitre   *315*
  Painful or stiff neck   *316*

INTRODUCTION

Chinese medicine talks about the 'throat' in general without distinguishing the pharynx (related to both respiratory and digestive systems) from the larynx (pertaining to the respiratory system). There are, however, signs that the ancient Chinese doctors were aware of such a differentiation. For example, even as early as 100BC, the 'Spiritual Axis' said in Chapter 69: *'The throat is the passage for food and drink; the throat is also where Qi goes up and down.'*[1] It is interesting that the Chinese text uses two different terms in this sentence: *Yan-hou* for the passage of food and *Hou-long* for the passage of Qi; both are translated as 'throat' in modern texts.

Bearing in mind the dual function of the throat in respect of respiratory and digestive systems, one can generally differentiate two broad types of throat problems: one related to the respiratory system and in Chinese medicine to the Lungs and Kidney channels, the other related to the digestive system and in Chinese medicine to the Stomach and Large Intestine channels (see next section). In adults, chronic sore throats are more commonly related to the Lung and Kidney channels, and in children more commonly to the Stomach and Large Intestine channels.

With regard to Heat and Cold, the throat is prone only to Heat (whether Full or Empty) and does not have any Cold patterns.

? **WHY** WE ASK

I generally ask about throat symptoms to confirm either a pattern of Heat (because the throat is an area of concentration of Heat) or a pattern of Qi stagnation.

I usually ask about neck symptoms to confirm the presence of a Liver pattern such as Liver-Qi stagnation or Liver-Yang rising, which, barring invasion of external Cold, comprise the most common causes of chronic neck ache.

? **WHEN** WE ASK

It is useful to ask about throat symptoms when there is Heat (Full or Empty) or Qi stagnation. If no earlier mention of throat symptoms has been made, I generally ask about them towards the end of the consultation. I always ask about the throat when I suspect a pattern of rebellious Qi of the Penetrating Vessel.

? **HOW** WE ASK

I usually ask patients whether they experience a feeling of tightness in the throat or a sensation of having a lump in the throat. If the patients speak of discomfort in the neck, it is important to ask them to point clearly to the area involved: the sides of the neck are influenced by the Gall-Bladder channel and often Liver patterns, while the back of the neck is influenced by the Bladder channel (see below).

CHANNELS INFLUENCING THE THROAT AND NECK

The throat and the front of the neck form an area in which practically all channels converge (see Fig. 10.1 on p. 109). With the single exception of the Bladder channel, 11 of the 12 channels course either through the front or the side of the throat. Of the eight Extraordinary Vessels, six go through the centre or the side of the throat; the exceptions are the Governing Vessel and the Girdle Vessel. Thus, being influenced by so many channels and therefore Internal Organs, the throat reflects clearly conditions of Yin–Yang, Heat–Cold and Deficiency–Excess and is an important diagnostic area. The throat is influenced particularly by the Lungs, Stomach, Large Intestine, Liver, Kidneys and Directing Vessel channels.

THROAT

Sore throat

Symptoms and Signs, Chapter 59

Both acute and chronic sore throat are due to Heat, which may be Full or Empty; however, we should always check this symptom with the findings from observation, especially in acute cases. A redness of the pharynx confirms the presence of Heat, especially Full-Heat.

When diagnosing sore throat, the first thing to establish is whether it is of external or internal origin, and the clinical significance of this symptom will therefore be analysed according to this distinction.

Sore throat of external origin

A sore throat of external origin has a sudden onset and short duration. In external invasions of Wind a sore throat generally points to Wind-Heat rather than Wind-Cold, especially if it is very severe. Other symptoms would include aversion to cold, a fever (or body hot to touch), headache, sneezing and a Floating-Rapid pulse.

Sore throat of internal origin

A sore throat from internal origin is usually due to Heat, which may be Full or Empty. In general, the sore throat from Full-Heat is very severe and the throat is red and swollen, whereas that from Empty-Heat is less severe, worse in the evening and associated with dryness. However, a chronic sore throat may also arise from a long-standing Yin deficiency, without Empty-Heat.

In adults, the most common chronic sore throat is that from Kidney- or Lung-Yin deficiency, or both, with Empty-Heat; this sore throat is not very severe, is worse in the evening, and is associated with dryness of the throat and other Yin deficiency manifestations. A chronic sore throat may also be caused simply by Qi and Yin deficiency without Empty-Heat; in this case the sore throat is mild, it comes in bouts, caused or aggravated by overwork, and is associated with other Qi and Yin deficiency manifestations.

In some cases patients complain of a 'sore throat' that comes and goes according to the emotional state; if there is no redness inside the throat and there are no other signs of Heat, this may be due to stagnation of Qi (of the Liver or Lungs) from emotional problems.

In children, external Wind-Heat has a stronger tendency than Wind-Cold to cause interior Heat. If not cleared properly after the initial stages, it is very likely to give rise to residual pathogenic factors. When a child presents with a recurrent, chronic sore throat, the two most common causes are either residual Heat in the Lung channel following an invasion of Wind-Heat or an accumulation of Heat in the Stomach and Large Intestine channels due to retention of food. In the case of residual Heat in the Lung channel, the child will present with a history of repeated invasion of Wind-Heat, which has usually been treated with antibiotics; other manifestations may include a cough, thirst, a feeling of heat, red cheeks and disturbed sleep. In the case of sore throat from accumulation of Heat in the Stomach and Large Intestine channels, there will be no history of repeated invasions of Wind-Heat, but rather one of successive digestive upsets such as vomiting and regurgitation of food; other manifestations may include abdominal pain, constipation, epigastric pain and disturbed sleep.

Box 36.1 summarizes the patterns underlying sore throats.

> **BOX 36.1 SORE THROAT**
>
> - Invasion of external Wind-Heat: sore throat with acute onset, with aversion to cold, fever or hot body, Floating-Rapid pulse
> - Full-Heat in Stomach and Intestines: severe sore throat with swelling and redness
> - Kidney-/Lung-Yin deficiency with Empty-Heat: chronic mild sore throat with dryness
> - Severe Qi and Yin deficiency: chronic, intermittent mild sore throat aggravated by overwork
> - Residual Heat in Lung channel or Heat in Stomach and Large Intestine channel: recurrent, chronic sore throat in children with a history of Wind invasion or digestive upset
> - Qi stagnation (Liver or Lungs): chronic 'sore throat' that comes and goes, without redness

Dry throat

Symptoms and Signs, Chapter 59

Excluding external invasions of Wind-Heat which may cause a dry throat, the most common cause of chronic dryness of the throat is a deficiency of Yin of the Lung or Kidneys, or both. In fact, in these situations, a dry throat is an important symptom confirming the diagnosis of Yin deficiency. A chronic dryness of the throat from Full-Heat may be related to the Stomach channel, but this is much less common than the former type.

Chronic dryness of the throat may also be related to the Liver and Gall-Bladder channels and be caused by Heat in the Liver and Gall-Bladder or by the Lesser Yang syndrome within the Six Stages or the Gall-Bladder Heat pattern at the Qi level within the Four Levels.

Box 36.2 summarizes the patterns underlying dry throat.

> **BOX 36.2 DRY THROAT**
>
> - External invasion of Wind-Heat
> - Lung-Yin deficiency
> - Kidney-Yin deficiency
> - Stomach-Heat
> - Heat in Liver and Gall-Bladder
> - Lesser Yang pattern (Six Stages)
> - Gall-Bladder Heat (Four Levels)

Itchy throat

Symptoms and Signs, Chapter 59

Itchiness of the throat with sudden onset is always related to invasion of Wind, which may be Wind-Cold, Wind-Heat or Wind-Dryness. Chronic itchiness of the throat is usually due to Lung-Yin deficiency or Lung Dryness; in this case the itchy feeling of the throat is worse in the evening and is associated with a desire to drink water in small sips.

Hoarse voice

Hearing, Chapter 53; Symptoms and Signs, Chapter 59

In acute cases, hoarse voice is due either to external invasion of Wind-Heat or to Lung-Heat, which may develop from such an invasion. In invasions of external Wind the presence of a hoarse voice by itself indicates Wind-Heat rather than Wind-Cold because the throat is a place where Heat easily accumulates. In such cases, a hoarse voice is accompanied by a sore throat, aversion to cold, fever, a Red tongue in the front or sides and a Floating-Rapid pulse.

A hoarse voice may also occur with acute Lung-Heat after an invasion of Wind-Heat. In such a case, the hoarse voice will be accompanied by a sore throat, a feeling of blockage of the throat, cough with scanty yellow sputum, chest pain, a Red tongue with dry yellow coating and an Overflowing-Rapid pulse.

In chronic cases, by far the most common cause of a hoarse voice is a deficiency of Yin of both Lungs and

Kidneys. In such cases, a hoarse voice is accompanied by a dry throat at night, an itchy throat, weak voice, dizziness, tinnitus, night sweating, a tongue without coating and a Floating-Empty pulse. This pattern is more common in the elderly.

A less common cause of a chronic hoarse voice (also in the elderly) is an accumulation of Phlegm and Blood stasis in the throat, in which case there will also be a sore throat, a feeling of obstruction of the throat, thickening of the vocal chords, nodules on the vocal chords, a swelling of the throat, a Purple tongue and a Wiry pulse.

Box 36.3 summarizes the patterns underlying a hoarse voice.

BOX 36.3 HOARSE VOICE

- Invasion of Wind-Heat: sore throat, sudden onset, aversion to cold, fever, Red tongue, Floating-Rapid pulse
- Lung-Heat: sore throat, feeling of blockage of the throat, cough with scanty yellow sputum, chest pain, Red tongue with a dry yellow coating, Overflowing-Rapid pulse
- Lung- and Kidney-Yin deficiency: dry throat at night, itchy throat, weak voice, dizziness, tinnitus, night sweating, tongue without coating, Floating-Empty pulse
- Phlegm and Blood stasis in the throat: sore throat, feeling of obstruction of the throat, thickening of the vocal chords, nodules on the vocal chords, swelling of the throat, Purple tongue, Wiry pulse

---

Feeling of obstruction in the throat

Symptoms and Signs, Chapter 59

The feeling of obstruction in the throat may be compared to having a piece of meat lodged in the throat; it cannot be swallowed down or coughed up, but there is no redness, no pain and no swelling of the throat. It is commonly referred to as the Plum Stone Syndrome, although the first reference to this syndrome in the 'Discussion of Cold Induced Diseases' mentions a piece of meat rather than a plum stone.

This symptom is nearly always caused by a stagnation of Qi due to emotional problems; modern Chinese textbooks always relate this to stagnation of Liver-Qi and to emotional problems such as anger, repressed anger or frustration, but it may also be due to Lung-Qi stagnation and failure of Lung-Qi to descend caused by emotions such as worry, sadness or grief. Whatever the emotion or the channel involved, when due to Qi stagnation the feeling of a foreign body in the throat comes and goes according to the emotional state of the patient.

A feeling of obstruction in the throat may be due also to rebellious Qi of the Penetrating Vessel. In such a case, it would be accompanied by symptoms throughout the course of this channel such as abdominal fullness or pain, or both, menstrual irregularities in women, tightness of the chest, anxiety and palpitations.

However, stagnation of Qi and rebellious Qi of the Penetrating Vessel are not the only possible causes of a feeling of obstruction in the throat. This symptom may also be caused by deficiency of Yin of the Lung or Kidneys, or both. In this case, the feeling of a foreign body in the throat is less severe than in the previous case, it is worse in the evening and is aggravated by overwork.

Box 36.4 summarizes the patterns underlying a feeling of obstruction in the throat.

BOX 36.4 FEELING OF OBSTRUCTION IN THE THROAT

- Liver- or Lung-Qi stagnation: severe, comes and goes according to mood
- Rebellious Qi in the Penetrating Vessel: worse in pregnancy or before menstruation, with abdominal fullness/ pain, chest tightness, anxiety, palpitations
- Lung-/Kidney-Yin deficiency: mild, worse in the evening, aggravated by overwork

---

Swollen and red tonsils

Observation, Chapter 10; Symptoms and signs, Chapter 59

The tonsils are influenced by the Lung, Stomach and Large Intestine channels and are prone to Heat or Toxic Heat.

Acute conditions

In acute conditions, redness and swelling of the tonsils may occur with an invasion of Wind-Heat; indeed, this sign always indicates that the pathogenic factor is Wind-Heat rather than Wind-Cold. However, swelling and redness of the tonsils with an invasion of Wind also indicate that there is Toxic Heat of external origin (this is an important diagnostic differentiation in the choice of herbs as we will need to address the Toxic Heat).

Chronic conditions

In chronic conditions, redness and swelling of the tonsils indicates either Heat (which may be Full or Empty) or Toxic Heat. These may affect the Stomach or

Case history 36.1

A 24-year-old woman complained of chronic tonsillitis suffering two or three bouts each year since the age of 5. Six weeks prior to the consultation she had had her tonsils removed and she had been much worse since then, suffering from sore throat, tiredness, swollen glands, headaches, thirst, a feeling of heaviness and a congested feeling in the sinuses. Her pulse was Slippery on the whole, but Weak on the right. Her tongue was Red in the front, slightly Thin and with a sticky yellow coating.

Diagnosis: This is a typical example of residual pathogenic factor and specifically Toxic Heat in the throat. This is an unusual case as the residual pathogenic factor stems from an operation, whereas it normally develops after a febrile disease. Toxic Heat is manifested by the swollen glands, the sore throat, a feeling of heaviness, the headache, the Slippery pulse and the Red tongue with a thick, sticky yellow coating. Obviously, Toxic Heat is only the acute, recent cause of her problem and there is an underlying deficiency of Stomach and Spleen, probably stemming from the chronic tonsillitis which she had

suffered from since childhood. The deficiency of Stomach and Spleen is manifested by the tiredness and Weak pulse.

Treatment principle: This is a very good example of a condition characterized by a mixture of Deficiency and Excess: the residual Toxic Heat is an Excess, acute condition and it constitutes the Manifestation (*Biao*), whereas the deficiency of Stomach and Spleen is an Empty, chronic condition and it constitutes the Root (*Ben*). In such cases, one should have a clear idea about the priorities of treatment, that is, whether one should treat the Excess, acute condition first or the deficient, chronic condition first. The pulse, tongue and severity of the symptoms are important guidelines to assist us in choosing the proper treatment principle. In this case, it is clear that the residual Toxic Heat should be eliminated first because the symptoms are acute, the pulse is Slippery and the tongue has a thick, sticky yellow coating.

Treatment: The prescription used was a variation of the formula Li Yan Cha *Benefiting the Throat Tea*, which is specific for eliminating Toxic Heat from the throat.

Large Intestine channels. In children, chronic tonsillitis is nearly always related to residual Heat or Toxic Heat (following repeated invasions of Wind-Heat, especially if treated with antibiotics). In adults, chronic tonsillitis is often due to Empty-Heat in the Lung or Stomach channel, or both.

Case history 36.1 illustrates a pattern underlying chronic tonsillitis.

Box 36.5 summarizes patterns underlying swollen and red tonsils.

NECK

Goitre

Observation, Chapter 10; Symptoms and Signs, Chapter 59

A discussion of goitre is relevant in interrogation as well as observation when there is a past history of it, or

---

> **BOX 36.5 SWOLLEN AND RED TONSILS**
>
> **Acute**
> - Invasion of Wind-Heat with Toxic Heat
>
> **Chronic**
> - Stomach and Large Intestine Heat
> - Stomach and Large Intestine Empty-Heat
> - Toxic Heat in Stomach and Large Intestine
> - Residual Heat or Toxic Heat
> - Empty-Heat of Lung and Stomach channels

when the patient has had a goitre but has undergone an operation to remove it.

Goitre is always by itself a sign of Phlegm. Very frequently, the pathology of Phlegm is combined with Qi stagnation in the throat; this is not always related to the Liver but may be related to the Lungs and Stomach too. In such cases, it is accompanied by irritability,

depression, and variation in the goitre size according to mood. In chronic cases, there is always an underlying deficiency of Qi or Yin, or both, which may cause the goitre to go up and down.

Goitre is closely related to the Liver and Lung channel and Liver-Fire combined with Phlegm is a frequent cause of it. Finally, in chronic cases, Phlegm may also combine with Blood stasis to cause goitre. In case of Liver-Fire and Blood stasis the goitre would be hard; in all other cases, it would feel soft to palpation.

Box 36.6 summarizes the patterns underlying goitre.

BOX 36.6 GOITRE

- Phlegm: large, soft goitre
- Qi stagnation with Phlegm: soft goitre with irritability, depression, goitre size varying according to mood
- Yin deficiency with Phlegm: small soft goitre of variable size, tiredness
- Liver-Fire with Phlegm: hard goitre, irritability
- Liver-Blood stasis with Phlegm: hard goitre, Purple tongue

Painful or stiff neck

Symptoms and Signs, Chapter 62

The most common cause of a painful or stiff neck is retention of Wind and Dampness in the muscles of the neck; this is a type of Painful Obstruction Syndrome. It is very common in cold and damp climates and varies with the weather.

Another common cause of a painful or stiff neck is Liver-Qi stagnation and this is usually due to stress, frustration and resentment being held in. It comes and goes according to the mood and is not affected by the weather. Liver-Yang rising or Liver-Wind may also cause a stiff or painful neck and this is more common in the elderly; it is often, but not necessarily, associated with hypertension.

A less common cause of a stiff or mildly painful neck is a Kidney deficiency, being due to Kidney-Yang not nourishing the Bladder channel in the neck. This causes only chronic stiff neck and again is seen usually only in the elderly.

Invasion of external Wind-Cold causes an acute stiff neck with all the other characteristic symptoms of external invasions such as sudden onset, aversion to cold and sneezing.

Box 36.7 summarizes the patterns underlying painful or stiff neck.

BOX 36.7 PAINFUL OR STIFF NECK

- Wind and Dampness in the muscles of the neck: pain and stiffness, reacting to weather
- Liver-Qi stagnation: comes and goes according to the mood, not reacting to weather
- Liver-Yang rising: intense stiffness, dizziness, propensity to outbursts of anger, Wiry pulse, often with hypertension (in elderly)
- Liver-Wind: stiffness, tremor, often with hypertension (in elderly)
- Kidney deficiency: chronic, more common in the elderly
- Invasion of Wind-Cold: sudden onset, acute, accompanied by aversion to cold and sneezing

---

NOTES

1. 1981 The Yellow Emperor's Classic of Internal Medicine – Spiritual Axis (*Ling Shu Jing* 灵枢经), People's Health Publishing House, Beijing, p. 125. First published c. 100BC.

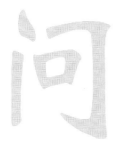

Chapter **37**

BODY

Chapter contents

INTRODUCTION *317*

ACHES IN THE WHOLE BODY *317*

PAIN IN THE JOINTS *318*

LOWER BACKACHE *318*

NUMBNESS/TINGLING *319*

ITCHING *319*

LOSS OF WEIGHT *319*

OBESITY *319*

INTRODUCTION

Questions about the body concern mostly pain and numbness. Chest and abdomen are discussed in Chapter 38 and limbs in Chapter 39.

? **WHY** WE ASK

Apart from the question regarding lower backache, which I ask every time I suspect a Kidney deficiency, questions about the body concern mostly symptoms affecting the whole body which do not pertain to any specific area, such as pain, numbness or itching of the whole body or loss of weight or obesity.

? **WHEN** WE ASK

Apart from the question about backache, I generally ask questions about the body only if relevant. In particular, the question about gain or loss of weight is important to give us an idea of the state of Blood and Yin and of the Stomach and Spleen.

? **HOW** WE ASK

The questions about the body concerning numbness, pain or itching are self-explanatory.

ACHES IN THE WHOLE BODY

Symptoms and Signs, Chapter 68

By 'aches in the whole body', I refer to aching or pain in most of the joints and muscles; it is not a common

symptom. The most important distinction is that according to onset. Aching or pain in the whole body with sudden onset is due to invasion of external Wind and it is therefore accompanied by aversion to cold, shivers, fever and a Floating pulse.

In chronic conditions, the most common cause of aches in the whole body is deficiency of Qi and Blood. In this case, it is accompanied by pronounced lassitude and it is ameliorated by rest.

Aches in the muscles of the body and especially the limbs are usually due to retention of Dampness in the muscles and are frequently seen in ME (postviral fatigue syndrome); in this case, the muscle ache is accompanied by a pronounced feeling of heaviness of the limbs and body. Aches in all the muscles with a hot sensation of the body on palpation are due to Stomach-Heat.

Pain in the arms and shoulders experienced only when walking is due to Liver-Qi stagnation.

In women after childbirth, pain in the whole body is due to Blood deficiency if it is dull or to Blood stasis if it is severe and stabbing.

Box 37.1 summarizes the patterns underlying aches in the whole body.

BOX 37.1 ACHES IN THE WHOLE BODY

- Invasion of external Wind: aching with aversion to cold, shivers, fever, Floating pulse
- Deficiency of Qi and Blood: aching with lassitude, ameliorated by rest
- Retention of Dampness in the muscles: aching with feeling of heaviness of the limbs and body
- Stomach-Heat: aching with hot sensation of the body
- Liver-Qi stagnation: pain in the arms and shoulders when walking
- Blood deficiency: dull pain after childbirth
- Blood stasis: severe, stabbing pain after childbirth

PAIN IN THE JOINTS

Symptoms and Signs, Chapter 68

Pain in the joints is due to invasion of Wind, Dampness or Cold in the channels of the joints. Joint ache from Wind moves from joint to joint; joint pain from Dampness is fixed and is characterized by swelling and numbness; joint pain from Cold is fixed, usually in one joint only and the pain is intense.

In chronic cases, any of the above pathogenic factors can transform into Heat, Dampness is formed

and Damp-Heat accumulates in the joints causing chronic pain. Severe stabbing pain in the joints may be due to Blood stasis.

Box 37.2 summarizes the patterns underlying joint pain.

BOX 37.2 JOINT PAIN

- Invasion of Wind: pain wandering from joint to joint
- Invasion of Dampness: pain with swelling and feeling of heaviness/numbness
- Invasion of Cold: severe pain in single joint
- Damp-Heat: chronic pain, swelling, redness
- Blood stasis: severe, stabbing pain, rigidity

LOWER BACKACHE

Symptoms and Signs, Chapter 67

Acute pain in the lower back is due either to sprain or to invasion of Cold. If it is due to sprain, the pain is intense, with pronounced stiffness, and is improved by rest and aggravated by movement; this pain is due to local stagnation of Qi and Blood. If the pain is due to invasion of Cold, it is worse with rest, usually worse in the mornings, and is alleviated by gentle movement. Chronic lower backache is due to a Kidney deficiency, in which case the backache is alleviated by rest and aggravated by overwork and excessive sexual activity. In many cases of chronic lower backache, there is a combination of the above three factors; for example an underlying Kidney deficiency (causing a chronic dull ache) predisposes the patient to invasion of Cold or to sprain and therefore to periodic acute attacks.

Pain of the lower back extending to the upper back is usually due to a combination of Kidney deficiency and Liver-Qi stagnation.

Box 37.3 summarizes patterns underlying lower backache.

BOX 37.3 LOWER BACKACHE

- Sprain: acute lower backache ameliorated by rest, aggravated by movement
- Invasion of Cold: acute lower backache aggravated by rest, ameliorated by movement
- Kidney deficiency: chronic lower backache ameliorated by rest, aggravated by overwork or sexual activity
- Kidney deficiency and Liver-Qi stagnation: chronic lower backache extending to the upper back

NUMBNESS/TINGLING

Symptoms and Signs, Chapter 68

Numbness or tingling may be due to three main causes: Blood deficiency, Phlegm or internal Wind. With Blood deficiency, there is numbness or tingling of both arms or legs or only hands or feet; this is more common in women. Phlegm may cause numbness or tingling in one or both limbs usually accompanied by a feeling of heaviness. Internal Wind usually causes unilateral numbness in a limb; if it affects the first three fingers in an old person this may indicate the possibility of impending Wind-stroke.

Box 37.4 summarizes the patterns underlying numbness and tingling of the body.

BOX 37.4 NUMBNESS/TINGLING

- Blood deficiency: both limbs, more in women
- Phlegm: with feeling of heaviness
- Internal Wind: usually unilateral

ITCHING

Symptoms and Signs, Chapter 68

The three main causes of itching are generally Wind, Dampness or Heat; these three pathogenic factors cause intense itching. Blood deficiency may also cause itching, which would be less intense than the three above-mentioned pathogenic factors.

Itching caused by Wind is very intense and it occurs either in different parts of the body, moving from one place to another, or in the whole body. The itching due to Wind may be accompanied by a rash but it may also occur without any external skin signs. Itching caused by Wind may also be accompanied by dry skin because Wind itself has a drying effect. In itching caused by Wind the patient has an irresistible desire to scratch; the skin may break and bleed but it heals soon after scratching.

Itching caused by Dampness is more localized, and usually occurs only in specific places such as the axilla, the genital region or the hands or feet. It is accompanied by the appearance of vesicles and the skin breaks after scratching, oozing a fluid that may be white or yellow according to whether the Dampness is associated with Cold or Heat. Itching caused by Damp-Heat is more intense and is characterized by the appearance of yellow vesicles or pustules. In severe, chronic cases the pustules may fester and ooze pus and blood.

Itching caused by Blood-Heat is usually accompanied by a red rash and it may occur either locally or in the whole body.

Itching caused by Blood deficiency is less intense, the skin is dry and scaly and the itching is worse at night.

Itching caused by Toxic Heat is very intense and is accompanied by the appearance of furuncles or festering ulcers which ooze pus and blood. Toxic Heat in the skin is often a complication of chronic eczema when the skin becomes infected.

Under certain circumstances itching can be a normal manifestation that occurs during healing of wounds or ulcers.

Box 37.5 summarizes the patterns underlying itching.

BOX 37.5 ITCHING

- Wind: intense generalized itching, possibly moving, with rash or dry skin
- Dampness: localized itching, damp skin, vesicles
- Blood-Heat: itching with a red rash
- Blood deficiency: mild generalized itching with dry skin, worse at night
- Toxic Heat: intense itching with pustules, ulcers or eczema
- Itching during healing of wounds or ulcers: normal

LOSS OF WEIGHT

The two most common causes of loss of weight are Blood or Yin deficiency; other causes include Stomach- and Spleen-Qi deficiency, Stomach-Heat and Liver-Fire. Although Stomach- and Spleen-Qi deficiency normally tend to make a person overweight because they lead to Dampness and Phlegm, in severe cases (such as in anorexia) they may lead to loss of weight because the body is not nourished by the Food Essences.

OBESITY

Symptoms and Signs, Chapter 68

When not due purely to overeating, obesity is generally caused by retention of Damp-Phlegm occurring against a background of Spleen-Qi or Kidney-Yang deficiency, or both.

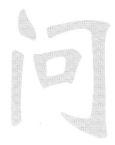

Chapter **38**

CHEST AND ABDOMEN

Chapter contents

CHEST   *321*
  Cough   *322*
  Chest pain   *323*
  Pain in the ribs   *324*
  Feeling of oppression of the chest   *324*
  Feeling of heat in the chest   *325*
  Palpitations   *325*

ABDOMEN   *326*
  Sensations   *326*
  Areas of abdominal pain   *327*

Interrogations in relation to diagnoses of the chest and abdomen are discussed separately below.

CHEST

The chest, or thorax, refers to the part of the body enclosed by the ribs and breast bone. From the Chinese point of view, there is a difference between the front part of the chest, which is under the influence of the Heart and Lungs, and the sides of the chest, which are under the influence of the Liver and Gall-Bladder. The front of the chest is also the area where the Gathering Qi (*Zong Qi*) is concentrated (see Fig. 12.1, p. 121).

? **WHY** WE ASK

It is necessary to ask about chest symptoms because some of them occur frequently in practice. In particular, symptoms often manifest themselves in the chest; for example, a feeling of oppression may be felt there, or palpitations, which often derive from emotional stress.

Patients do not often volunteer information on chest symptoms unless we ask. For example, in my experience, few patients will actually describe experiencing a 'feeling of oppression' in the chest.

In addition, both the tongue and the pulse frequently reflect a pathology of the chest: a Purple area in the tongue's chest area (see Fig. 23.10 on p. 206), for example, or a pulse that is Weak and Deep on both Front positions.

? **WHEN** WE ASK

Chest symptoms often reflect very common pathologies such as Liver-Qi stagnation, Phlegm in the chest

and Heart-Blood deficiency. Therefore, I specifically ask about chest symptoms quite early in the interrogation as patients are describing their symptoms.

? **HOW** WE ASK

It is important to be sensitive when asking questions regarding the chest because people often fear that if we ask about the chest we suspect a heart pathology. Besides this, some typical Chinese expressions are not used by Western patients and we should therefore phrase the question in a way that is understandable to the patient. For example, few patients will actually use the expression 'feeling of oppression of the chest'; they will probably describe a 'feeling of tightness of the chest' or say a feeling was 'like having a weight on the chest'.

'Palpitations' is another example of the importance of asking questions in a way that the patient can understand. Most people think that palpitations are synonymous with tachycardia, that is, the heart beating faster than normal. We should therefore explain to the patient that 'palpitations' simply means an uncomfortable sensation of being aware of one's heartbeat.

Cough

Observation, Chapter 20; Hearing, Chapter 53; Symptoms and Signs, Chapter 63

When a patient presents with a cough, we must first of all establish whether it is an acute or a chronic cough. By 'acute' we mean a cough that had a sudden onset and may continue for a few days or weeks. By 'chronic', we mean either a cough that began insidiously without a previous invasion of Wind and persisted for months or years, or one that began with an exterior invasion of Wind and persisted for months or years.

An acute cough may have any of three causes. First, it may be an acute cough in the very beginning stages of an invasion of Wind, when the pathogenic factor is still on the Exterior. Secondly, it may be an acute cough with the pathogenic factor (such as Heat or Phlegm-Heat) in the Interior following an external invasion. Thirdly, it may be an acute cough caused by a residual pathogenic factor (such as Dryness or Phlegm) following an external invasion. In the first case the cough will be accompanied by signs of the external invasion such as aversion to cold, fever, sore throat, a runny nose and a Floating pulse. Heat or Phlegm-Heat in the Lungs produces a barking cough with yellow mucus, feelings of heat and thirst, and an Overflowing-Rapid pulse. In residual Dryness with Phlegm in the Lungs, the cough is dry with difficult expectoration of scanty sputum after repeated bouts of coughing, and a tickling sensation in the throat.

A chronic cough is generally due either to chronic retention of Phlegm in the Lungs (which may be combined with Dampness, Heat or Dryness), or to deficiency of Qi or Yin, or both, of the Lungs.

A very common type of chronic cough is one due to Damp-Phlegm in the Lungs, which is characterized by the expectoration of profuse, white sputum which is easy to expectorate, a feeling of oppression of the chest, a Swollen tongue with a sticky coating and a very Slippery pulse. When Phlegm combines with Heat in the Lungs the cough has a louder sound and is characterized by the expectoration of yellow sputum, a feeling of oppression of the chest, a feeling of heat and a Red and Swollen tongue with a sticky yellow coating and a Slippery-Rapid pulse.

A common type of chronic cough in the elderly is that due to Dry-Phlegm in the Lungs which is characterized by a chronic, dry cough with a weak sound and the occasional, difficult expectoration of scanty sputum, a dry throat and a Swollen tongue with a dry coating.

A chronic cough due to a deficiency of Lung-Qi or Lung-Yin is characterized by a slight, dry cough with a weak sound, dry throat in the evening accompanied by the signs of Qi or Yin deficiency, such as night sweating, and a tongue without coating.

Case history 38.1 illustrates a pattern underlying chronic cough.

Case history 38.1

A 48-year-old woman had been suffering from a persistent cough for 6 months: she felt she had some phlegm in the throat but this was difficult to expectorate so that the cough was often dry. When she did expectorate some sputum, this was thick, sticky and white. She also complained of breathlessness and a feeling of tightness and oppression of the chest. A chest specialist had diagnosed bronchiectasis.

She was thin and slightly built and she had experienced loss of weight for the past 2 years. Her complexion was very dull and sallow. She also suffered from a general cold feeling, cold hands and feet, constipation and a yellow vaginal discharge.

Her tongue-body colour was normal but the tongue body was Swollen; the back of the tongue had a rootless, yellow coating but no 'spirit'. Her pulse was Weak in general, especially in both the Rear positions, but also slightly Slippery.

Diagnosis: The cough with expectoration of thick, sticky white sputum, together with the breathlessness and feeling of tightness and oppression of the chest, indicate the presence of Damp-Phlegm in the Lungs, which is confirmed by the swelling of the tongue body and the Slippery pulse. The general cold feeling, cold hands and feet, constipation and Weak Rear pulse positions also indicate Kidney-Yang deficiency, which obviously contributed to the formation of Phlegm. The Kidney deficiency is also evidenced by the absence of 'spirit' on the root of the tongue. Besides Damp-Phlegm in the Lungs, there is also Damp-Heat in the Lower Burner, which causes the yellow vaginal discharge.

The loss of weight which occurred in the previous 2 years and the rootless tongue coating point to the beginning of a situation of Kidney-Yin deficiency, which may sometimes develop from Kidney-Yang deficiency.

The treatment should concentrate first on resolving Damp-Phlegm and stimulating the descending of Lung-Qi and secondly on tonifying the Kidneys.

Box 38.1 summarizes the patterns underlying cough.

Chest pain

Observation, Chapter 16; Symptoms and Signs, Chapter 63

Here 'chest' indicates the front of the chest. A pain in this area is usually due to either the Heart or Lung channel and it always denotes a Full condition (even though this may itself derive from an underlying Empty condition).

Chest pain can be differentiated according to its character. A fixed, pricking, stabbing or needle-like pain indicates Blood stasis. Chest pain accompanied by a feeling of distension of the chest itself and the hypochondrium indicates Qi stagnation and is usually accompanied by sighing and irritability. An intermittent, chronic chest pain that comes and goes also indicates Blood stasis but suggests an underlying Empty condition of Qi or Yang deficiency.

A stabbing or pricking chest pain indicates Blood stasis affecting the Heart channel (especially if it radiates down the left arm) and this often occurs against a background of Heart-Yang deficiency; it falls into the category of Chest Painful Obstruction Syndrome.

BOX 38.1 COUGH

Acute
* External invasion of Wind: acute cough, aversion to cold, fever, sore throat, runny nose, Floating pulse
* Heat or Phlegm-Heat in the Lungs: acute, barking cough with expectoration of yellow mucus, feeling of heat, thirst, Overflowing-Rapid pulse
* Residual dryness and Phlegm in the Lungs: acute, dry cough with difficult expectoration of scanty sputum after repeated bouts of dry coughing, tickling sensation in throat.

Chronic
* Damp-Phlegm in the Lungs: chronic cough with easy expectoration of profuse, white sputum, feeling of oppression of the chest, Swollen tongue with sticky coating, Slippery pulse
* Phlegm-Heat in the Lungs: loud chronic cough with expectoration of profuse yellow or greenish sputum, feeling of heat, feeling of oppression of the chest, Red and Swollen tongue with sticky yellow coating, Slippery-Rapid pulse
* Dry-Phlegm in the Lungs: chronic dry cough with occasional, difficult expectoration of scanty sputum, dry throat, Swollen tongue with a dry coating
* Lung-Qi deficiency: chronic, slight cough with weak sound, weak voice, Empty pulse
* Lung-Yin deficiency: chronic, dry cough, dry throat in the evening, night sweating, tongue without coating

Chest pain accompanied by cough with expectoration of profuse yellow sputum is due to Phlegm-Heat in the Lungs and this may be seen in acute lung conditions, such as bronchitis, pneumonia or pleuritis.

A chest pain in a large area of the chest together with a cough, breathlessness and a red face indicates Lung-Heat. Chest pain extending to the hypochondrial region may be due to Damp-Heat in the Liver and Gall-Bladder channel, in which case it may be accompanied by feeling of heaviness and a sticky taste.

Pain in the heart region on the left side of the chest indicates either Heart-Blood stasis or Phlegm obstructing the Heart channel.

Chest pain extending to the upper back is usually due to Phlegm or Blood stasis.

Box 38.2 summarizes the patterns underlying chest pain.

BOX 38.2 CHEST PAIN

- Heart-Blood stasis: fixed, stabbing or pricking chest pain
- Liver-Qi stagnation: distending chest and hypochondrial pain
- Blood stasis with underlying Empty condition: intermittent chronic chest pain
- Phlegm-Heat in the Lungs: chest pain with cough and profuse, yellow sputum
- Lung-Heat: chest pain with cough and breathlessness, red face
- Damp-Heat in Liver and Gall-Bladder: chest and hypochondrial pain with feeling of heaviness and sticky taste
- Phlegm obstructing the Heart: pain in the left side of the chest
- Phlegm or Blood stasis: chest pain extending to the upper back

---

Pain in the ribs

Symptoms and Signs, Chapter 63

'Pain in the ribs' refers to pain on the lateral aspect of the rib cage above the hypochondrial area.

The most common patterns causing pain in the ribs are Liver-Qi stagnation, Blood stasis and Damp-Heat in the Gall-Bladder. The characteristic symptoms of these patterns are listed in Box 38.3.

BOX 38.3 PAIN IN THE RIBS

- Liver-Qi stagnation: pain in the ribs with a pronounced feeling of distension
- Blood stasis: severe, stabbing pain
- Damp-Heat in the Liver and Gall-Bladder: pain in the ribs with a feeling of oppression and heaviness

---

Feeling of oppression of the chest

Symptoms and Signs, Chapter 63

A feeling of oppression of the chest is the translation of the Chinese term *Xiong Men*. Western patients, at least in Anglo-Saxon countries, would seldom use this term and report this symptom as a feeling of tightness, discomfort in the chest, or the sensation of having a weight on the chest.

A feeling of oppression of the chest accompanied by slight breathlessness, sighing, a cough and expectoration of phlegm indicates retention of Phlegm in the Lungs, which is the most common cause of this symptom. A feeling of oppression of the chest without a cough and without expectoration of phlegm, and accompanied by slight breathlessness, sighing and a feeling of a lump in the throat, indicates stagnation of Lung-Qi with Lung-Qi failing to descend; this is usually caused by emotional problems such as sadness or worry. Although a feeling of a lump in the throat is usually related to Liver-Qi stagnation, stagnation of Lung-Qi caused by emotional problems is a very frequent cause of this symptom together with a feeling of oppression of the chest.

Another very common cause of a feeling of oppression of the chest is rebellious Qi of the Penetrating Vessel, which is more common in women. However, before diagnosing rebellious Qi of the Penetrating Vessel, we should check whether the feeling of oppression of the chest is accompanied by other relevant symptoms such as abdominal distension or fullness, pain or fullness around the umbilicus, or epigastric tightness.

In a few cases, a severe stagnation of Liver-Qi from emotional problems may also cause a feeling of oppression of the chest.

Box 38.4 summarizes the patterns underlying a feeling of oppression of the chest.

BOX 38.4 FEELING OF OPPRESSION OF THE CHEST

- Phlegm in the Lungs: slight breathlessness, sighing, cough with expectoration of phlegm
- Stagnation of Lung-Qi: sighing, feeling of lump in the throat, slight breathlessness without cough or expectoration
- Rebellious Qi of the Penetrating Vessel: abdominal distension/fullness, epigastric tightness, pain/fullness around umbilicus
- Severe Liver-Qi stagnation: depression, irritability

Feeling of heat in the chest

Symptoms and Signs, Chapter 63

Excluding external invasions of Wind-Heat, a feeling of heat in the chest is due to Full- or Empty-Heat of the Lung or Heart channels. If there is a feeling of heat in the chest, accompanied by thirst, insomnia, palpitations, agitation and a Red tip of the tongue, this indicates Heart-Fire; if there is a feeling of heat in the evening, dry mouth at night, insomnia, night sweating and five-palm heat, it is due to Heart Empty-Heat.

A feeling of heat in the chest accompanied by a cough, hot hands, a red face and expectoration of yellow mucus is due to Lung-Heat; if it is accompanied by night sweating, a feeling of heat in the afternoon, five-palm heat, a dry throat at night and a dry cough it indicates Lung Empty-Heat.

BOX 38.5 FEELING OF HEAT IN THE CHEST

- Invasion of external Wind-Heat: aversion to cold, fever, sore throat
- Heart-Fire: thirst, insomnia, palpitations, agitation, Red tip of the tongue
- Heart Empty-Heat: insomnia, night sweating, feeling of heat in the evening, dry mouth at night, five-palm heat
- Lung-Heat: cough, hot hands, red face
- Lung Empty-Heat: dry cough, feeling of heat in the afternoon, night sweating, dry throat at night, five-palm heat

---

Box 38.5 summarizes the patterns underlying a feeling of heat in the chest.

Palpitations

Symptoms and Signs, Chapter 63

When we ask patients about palpitations it is important to explain to them the meaning of this symptom, as most patients mistakenly identify 'palpitations' with tachycardia, that is, the pulse beating faster than normal. In reality, palpitations are not related to the rate or speed of the pulse but simply indicate a subjective and uncomfortable sensation of being aware of one's heartbeat.

Palpitations are a symptom that is always related to the Heart and may appear in any of the Heart patterns.

Palpitations with an acute onset may be due to external stimuli such as a fright or an overwhelming emotional upset, in which case they are called 'fright palpitations' (*Jing Ji*).

Palpitations that extend upwards towards the chest and throat and downwards towards the umbilicus and abdomen are called *Zheng Chong*, which I translate as 'panic palpitations' (literally it means 'panic and anxiety'). This type of palpitations is due to rebellious Qi in the Penetrating Vessel affecting the Heart and is considered more severe than ordinary palpitations.

Case history 38.2 illustrates a pattern underlying palpitations.

Case history 38.2

A 44-year-old woman had been suffering from palpitations for 8 years. 'Palpitations' was just a subjective symptom of a feeling of her heart thumping in her chest and was not associated with tachycardia. The palpitations were always worse before her period. She also complained of nausea and an epigastric pain, which was experienced just under the sternum, a sticky taste and a feeling of lump in the throat. She experienced a dry mouth occasionally, and occasionally suffered from tinnitus.

Her periods were basically normal, coming every 4 weeks, lasting 6 days and they were not painful. The only problem associated with the periods was premenstrual tension.

Her complexion was dull and sallow without lustre and her eyes were very dull and lacked lustre to an extreme degree.

Her tongue was of a normal colour, except for a Red tip. It had a Heart crack and, although it could not be defined as being peeled, the coating was not sufficient. Her pulse was Fine on the right and Floating-Empty on the left.

Diagnosis: The aggravation of the palpitations before the period, together with the nausea, epigastric pain under the sternum and the feeling of lump in the throat, indicate a condition of rebellious Qi in the Penetrating Vessel, as this vessel flows through the stomach, connects with the heart, traverses the chest and goes over the throat (on its way to the face).

However, the pulse, being Fine on the right, and the dull-sallow complexion clearly show a condition of Blood deficiency, while the Floating-Empty nature of the pulse on the left side and the insufficient coating on the tongue show the beginning of Yin deficiency (of the Liver, Kidneys and Heart). In this

case, therefore, the condition of rebellious Qi in the Penetrating Vessel is secondary to the condition of Blood and Yin deficiency; in other words, the Qi of the Penetrating Vessel rebels upward *because* there is a deficiency of Blood and Yin. In fact, the Penetrating Vessel is the Sea of Blood and it is therefore easily affected by Blood deficiency. The treatment principle in this case, therefore, should be to nourish Blood and Yin (of the Heart and Liver) primarily and to subdue rebellious Qi in the Penetrating Vessel secondarily.

The Heart crack and the very dull appearance of the eyes indicate a disturbed Mind and a strong propensity to emotional problems.

ABDOMEN

Abdomen here refers to the area of the trunk between the diaphragm and the symphysis pubis (see Fig. 16.7, p. 145).

? **WHY** WE ASK

Abdominal symptoms are so frequent that it is absolutely crucial to ask about them in every case, even if the patient presents with a problem in an entirely different area, (e.g. headaches). The abdomen readily reflects extremely common patterns such as Qi stagnation, Blood stasis and Dampness.

? **WHEN** WE ASK

If the patient does not come specifically to consult about abdominal symptoms, I generally ask about these immediately after asking about digestive problems (related to the Stomach).

? **HOW** WE ASK

It is important to be clear about the area involved because patients are often vague about the location of their abdominal symptoms. For example, someone might refer to the whole abdomen as the 'stomach'. We should therefore always make sure we ask the patient to point to the area involved.

In the case of pain, we should first let patients describe the abdominal pain in their own words; only then can we ask systematically about the reaction of pain to pressure, application of heat and food or drinks in order to establish the Full or Empty and the Hot or Cold character of the pain. When asking about the reaction of their abdominal pain to 'pressure', instead of simply asking 'Is it better with pressure or not?', which the patient would not really understand, we should ask, 'When you have the pain, do you like to press the area of pain with your hands, or do you dislike being touched?' We should then ask about the reaction of the abdominal pain to exposure to heat or cold and to ingestion of hot or cold drinks.

Besides this, there is also a terminology problem since few patients will actually use the term 'distension' (often described as 'bloating' in English), and even fewer the term 'stuffiness'. The exact meaning of these symptoms is described below.

The discussion of abdominal symptoms will be centred first on the four most common sensations experienced in the abdomen, which are:

- distension
- pain
- fullness
- stuffiness.

After this, the various abdominal symptoms will be discussed according to areas (see Fig. 16.7 on p. 145), which are:

- the area under the xyphoid process (*Xin Xia*)
- the epigastrium
- the hypochondrium
- the umbilical area
- the central-lower abdominal area
- the right-lateral and left-lateral lower abdominal area.

Sensations
Distension
Observation, Chapter 16; Symptoms and Signs, Chapter 71

A feeling of abdominal distension or 'bloating' is an extremely common symptom. The following patterns

most commonly cause distension of the abdomen (in order of frequency):

- Qi stagnation – severe distension
- Spleen-Qi deficiency – mild distension
- Damp-Phlegm.

Besides the subjective feeling of bloating, distension is also characterized by an objective, distended, drum-like feeling on palpation.

> **!**
>
> **Remember**: distension is a subjective feeling of bloating but it is also an objective sign of the abdomen, i.e. the abdomen feels distended like a drum on palpation.

Pain

Symptoms and Signs, Chapter 71

Abdominal pain can be due to a very wide variety of conditions, some Full and some Empty. By definition, the abdominal pain from a Full condition is severe, whereas that from an Empty condition is mild. Among the Full conditions that may cause abdominal pain are:

- Qi stagnation
- Blood stasis
- Dampness
- Retention of food
- Cold.

Among the Empty conditions are:

- Spleen-Qi deficiency
- Empty-Cold
- Kidney deficiency.

(For a detailed discussion of the patterns causing abdominal pain in its various areas, see Part 5, Chapter 71.)

Abdominal pain is one of the most common presenting symptoms in practice. When diagnosing such pain, it is important to refer to the basic principles, which allow us to differentiate Fullness from Emptiness and Heat from Cold. Abdominal pain that is alleviated by pressure indicates Deficiency, whereas if it is aggravated by pressure or if the patient dislikes being touched in the area this indicates Fullness. Abdominal pain that is alleviated by the application of heat (such as a hot-water bottle) or by the ingestion of warm drinks indicates a Cold condition, and the same if it is aggravated by exposure to cold or ingestion of cold drinks. Abdominal pain that is aggravated by exposure to heat or by the ingestion of warm drinks indicates a Heat condition, and the same if it is alleviated by exposure to cold (which is very rare even in Heat conditions) or by the ingestion of cold drinks.

Fullness

Symptoms and Signs, Chapter 71

A feeling of fullness in the abdomen is usually caused by Dampness or retention of food. Subjectively the patient feels full as if having had a large meal and there is a very slight feeling of nausea; objectively the abdomen feels hard on palpation.

> **!**
>
> A subjective feeling of fullness is mirrored by an objective hardness of the abdomen on palpation.

Stuffiness

'Stuffiness' is a translation of the Chinese term *Pi* (although this term has a broader meaning than simply 'feeling of stuffiness'). A feeling of stuffiness in the abdomen is characterized by a subjective mild feeling of fullness, together with an objective soft feeling of the abdomen on palpation. This symptom is usually due to either Dampness or Heat occurring against a background of Deficiency.

> **!**
>
> A feeling of stuffiness is characterized by the contradiction between a subjective feeling of fullness and an objective, soft feeling to the abdomen on palpation.

Areas of abdominal pain

Before establishing the Full or Empty and Hot or Cold nature of the condition according to the abdominal symptoms, it is important to ask the patient to identify clearly the location of the problem, which is most commonly pain. Patients are often vague about the location of the pain and we should ask them to pay attention and be exact. This difficulty is particularly evident in children who are often unable to identify the exact location of the abdominal pain.

The regions of the abdomen in Chinese medicine are as follows (see Fig. 16.7 on p. 145):

- Area under the xyphoid process: this is the small area immediately below the xyphoid process extending approximately 50 mm (2 inches) and bordered by the ribs. It is influenced by the Heart and Stomach channels and the Penetrating Vessel.
- Epigastric: this is the area between the xyphoid process and the umbilicus but excluding the hypochondrial area. It is related to the Stomach and Spleen channels.
- Hypochondrial: these are the two areas below the rib cage. This area is influenced by the Liver and Gall-Bladder channels.
- Umbilical: this is the area around the umbilicus. It is influenced by the Spleen, Liver, Kidney and Small Intestine channels.
- Central-lower abdominal (*Xiao Fu*): this is the area between the umbilicus and the symphysis pubis. This area is influenced by the Liver, Kidney, Bladder and Large Intestine channels and by the Directing Vessel; in women, it is also influenced by the Uterus.
- Right-lateral-lower abdominal and left-lateral-lower abdominal (*Shao Fu*): these are the lateral areas of the lower abdomen. This area is influenced by the Liver and Large Intestine channels, and by the Penetrating Vessel.

The diagnosis of abdominal problems, and especially abdominal pain, is much more complex than with those of the epigastric region because of the large number of channels involved. In women, it is even more complex because the lower abdomen can reflect problems of all the above channels as well as those of the Uterus and gynaecological system. In practice it is therefore often difficult in women to differentiate whether an abdominal pain is of intestinal or gynaecological origin. This difficulty exists also in Western medicine. In Chinese medicine, however, the distinction is less important than it is in Western medicine as there is often an overlap between a pathology of the Intestines and one of the gynaecological system. For example, in women stasis of Blood in the lower abdomen may cause painful periods and an abdominal pain of intestinal origin at the same time.

Here I will discuss the most common patterns and conditions differentiated according to their location (i.e. the area under the xyphoid process, epigastrium, hypochondrium, umbilical area, central-lower abdomen, right-lateral lower abdomen and left-lateral lower abdomen). (For the differentiation of various abdominal symptoms, see Part 5, Chapter 71.)

Area under the xyphoid process
Symptoms and Signs, Chapter 71

The area under the xyphoid process extends approximately 50 mm (2 inches) from the xyphoid process and is bordered by the ribs. It is influenced by the Stomach, Heart and Penetrating Vessel channels and its symptomatology often reflects emotional problems. In fact, this is an area that is very easily and frequently affected by emotional problems due to worry, fear, sadness or grief. The symptoms related to this area may include a feeling of tightness, distension, oppression, stuffiness and palpitations depending on the channel and pathology involved.

The Penetrating Vessel has a strong influence on this area causing a feeling of tightness; however, a pathology of the Penetrating Vessel can be diagnosed only if the feeling of tightness in this area is associated with other abdominal or chest sensations, such as lower abdominal fullness or pain, epigastric distension or pain and chest oppression or tightness. A typical symptom of the Penetrating Vessel in the area below the xyphoid is characterized by a feeling of 'urgency', anxiety and palpitations in that area. Occasionally, Western patients will describe this Penetrating Vessel symptomatology in different and unusual ways; for example, in England, a patient may describe a feeling of 'butterflies' in this area, of 'heart cascading', 'as if the stomach was having an argument with itself' or 'adrenaline rushing up and down the chest'. All these are symptoms related to rebellious Qi in the Penetrating Vessel along its course in the abdomen and chest and affecting the Heart and the region under the xyphoid process.

In the absence of other Penetrating Vessel symptoms along its course, symptoms in the area under the xyphoid are usually related to the Stomach or Heart. The symptoms in this area should be closely integrated with palpation: a hardness on palpation indicates a Full condition whereas a softness indicates an Empty condition.

A feeling of oppression in the area under the xyphoid process usually indicates Phlegm or severe stagnation of Qi in the Heart and Stomach channel. A feeling of fullness in this area indicates retention of

food in the Stomach affecting the Heart; a feeling of stuffiness in this area (i.e. the patient feels full but the area is soft on palpation) indicates Stomach and Spleen deficiency with Heart-Heat. A feeling of distension in this area indicates stagnation of Qi in the Stomach.

On the pulse, this area can be felt on the distal end of the right Middle position, by placing the finger on the Stomach position and rolling it distally very slightly.

Box 38.6 summarizes patterns underlying pain in the area under the xyphoid process.

BOX 38.6 AREA UNDER THE XYPHOID PROCESS

- Rebellious Qi in the Penetrating Vessel: tightness and distension with anxiety and palpitations
- Phlegm or severe Qi stagnation: feeling of oppression
- Retention of food: feeling of fullness
- Stomach and Spleen deficiency with Heart-Heat: feeling of stuffiness
- Stomach-Qi stagnation: feeling of distension

Epigastrium

Symptoms and Signs, Chapter 71

This refers to the area between the xyphoid process and the umbilicus, but excluding the hypochondrial area. The epigastrium is closely related to the Stomach and Spleen channels and it reflects primarily Stomach patterns, such as Cold in the Stomach, Stomach-Heat, Stomach-Fire, Damp-Heat in the Stomach, Stomach deficient and cold, Stomach-Yin deficiency, etc.

In a patient presenting with an epigastric problem (which is usually pain or distension) it is important to integrate questions about the character of the epigastric pain with those about thirst, taste, nausea, belching and sour regurgitation.

The upper part of the epigastrium (i.e. the area just below the xyphoid process) is influenced also by the Heart channel and in Chinese medicine there is often an overlap and an interaction between the Stomach and the Heart channels in certain patterns. For example, rebellious Stomach-Qi causing nausea and vomiting is often associated with rebellious Heart-Qi, that is, Heart-Qi not descending so that the patient may have epigastric pain, nausea, vomiting, belching, sour regurgitation but also palpitations and a discomfort that extends from the epigastrium to the sternum area.

However, epigastric pain is not always related to the Stomach channel and in some cases the Chinese diagnosis of epigastric pain should be integrated with a Western diagnosis. For example, when the Large Intestine is affected by stagnation of Qi and there is severe flatulence in the transverse colon, this may cause an epigastric pain; in this case it would be wrong to attribute the problem to the Stomach channel simply because it occurs in the epigastric area. Of course, in such a case there would be other symptoms such as lower abdominal pain, constipation and small stools, which would point to the Large Intestine.

There are many types of epigastric pain, as follows:

- A spastic epigastric pain that is ameliorated by the application of heat and the ingestion of warm drinks indicates Full-Cold in the Stomach.
- Epigastric pain with a pronounced feeling of fullness indicates retention of food, which is more common in children.
- A distending epigastric pain radiating to the right or left hypochondrium indicates rebellious Liver-Qi invading the Stomach; this is a very common type of epigastric pain.
- Burning epigastric pain denotes Stomach-Heat.
- Burning epigastric pain with a feeling of heaviness, nausea and a feeling of oppression of the chest indicates Phlegm-Heat in the Stomach.
- Burning epigastric pain with a feeling of heaviness, a sticky taste and a sticky yellow tongue coating denotes Damp-Heat in the Stomach.
- A severe, stabbing epigastric pain indicates Blood stasis in the Stomach.
- A chronic, intermittent, dull ache that is ameliorated by the application of heat and the ingestion of warm drinks, and is aggravated by overwork, indicates Stomach deficient and cold.
- A chronic, intermittent, dull, slightly burning epigastric pain with a dry mouth indicates Stomach-Yin deficiency.

Feelings of pain, distension, tightness or oppression of the epigastrium may also be caused by rebellious Qi in the Penetrating Vessel. However, such epigastric sensations point to a Penetrating Vessel pathology only when they are associated with other abdominal symptoms such as pain or distension in the lower abdomen or umbilical pain.

Interrogation about epigastric symptoms should be closely integrated with investigation of the tongue and pulse.

Epigastrium manifestation on the tongue

On the tongue, the epigastric area is reflected either in the centre or on the sides around the centre (see Fig. 23.3 on p. 205). An examination of the coating in this area is essential to distinguish Full from Empty conditions as a Full condition will be reflected by a thick coating in this area and an Empty condition by a rootless coating or the absence of coating. The coating in this area also closely reflects the Hot or Cold nature of Stomach problems: a white coating indicates Cold while a yellow (including brown) coating indicates Heat. The thickness of the coating reflects the intensity of the pathogenic factor: the thicker the coating, the more intense is the pathogenic factor.

To summarize, when examining the coating in the Stomach area of the tongue, we should establish systematically first whether there is a coating or not, secondly the colour of the coating and thirdly the thickness of the coating. Some Stomach pathologies are reflected in the central section of the tongue on the sides; for example, Stomach-Heat often manifests with a redness in these areas. Cracks in the central area are a very clear reflection of Stomach-Yin deficiency; these may be small horizontal or vertical cracks or a wide, midline crack in the central area. While small cracks in this area develop gradually from dietary irregularities, a wide central midline Stomach crack may be heredi-tary and indicate a tendency to develop Stomach-Yin deficiency.

Epigastrium manifestation on the pulse

With regard to the pulse, the right Middle position of course reflects closely Stomach disharmonies. The most common pulse qualities in this position are Slippery, Soggy, Floating-Empty and Wiry. A Slippery pulse in the Stomach/Spleen position indicates retention of Dampness in the Stomach and Spleen; a Soggy quality indicates Dampness occurring against a background of Stomach and Spleen deficiency; a Floating-Empty pulse in this position indicates Stomach-Yin deficiency; a Wiry pulse in this position denotes Stomach-Qi stagnation, which may occur by itself or as a consequence of Liver-Qi stagnation in which case the pulse would be Wiry in both Middle positions. An interesting aspect of the Stomach pulse is its upper part, which is felt by rolling the finger distally (towards the fingers) very slightly. This corresponds to the oesophagus and if the pulse is Tight in this area it indicates rebellious Stomach-Qi or stagnation of food in the upper part of the Stomach, which is often due to eating too fast or eating when under pressure at work.

Case history 38.3 illustrates a case of deficiency and rebellious Liver-Qi causing epigastric pain.

Case history 38.3

A 42-year-old woman complained of indigestion, belching, acidity, sour regurgitation and epigastric distension. She had been suffering from this problem for several years. Her appetite was normal, there was no nausea and her stools were normal. Her complexion was dull and pale.

Her tongue was Pale on the sides, slightly Swollen and very slightly lacking a coating in the centre. Her pulse was Weak and Choppy.

Diagnosis: The digestive symptoms clearly suggest the condition of rebellious Liver-Qi invading the Stomach and preventing Stomach-Qi from descending, which causes the belching and sour regurgitation. However, the tongue and pulse show predominantly Deficiency and in particular, deficiency of Spleen-Qi (Weak pulse), a slight Stomach-Yin deficiency (lack of coating in the centre) and a Liver-Blood deficiency (Pale sides and Choppy pulse). In conditions of rebellious Liver-Qi invading the Stomach and Spleen, one can distinguish two situations: one when the primary problem is a disharmony of the Liver channel caused by emotional problems and the other when the primary problem is a weakness of the Stomach and Spleen, which 'allow' themselves to be invaded by the Liver. In this case, the latter situation clearly applies. This distinction is important to determine the appropriate treatment principle because, in the first situation, the primary aim is to subdue rebellious Liver-Qi and the secondary one to tonify the Stomach and Spleen; in the second situation, the primary aim is to tonify the Stomach and Spleen and the secondary one to subdue rebellious Liver-Qi.

Box 38.7 summarizes the patterns underlying epigastric pain.

BOX 38.7 EPIGASTRIC PAIN

- Cold in the Stomach: spastic pain ameliorated by heat
- Retention of food: pain with feeling of fullness
- Rebellious Liver-Qi invading the Stomach: Distending pain radiating to the right or left hypochondrium
- Stomach-Heat: burning, redness in centre of tongue
- Phlegm-Heat in the Stomach: burning pain with feeling of heaviness and feeling of oppression of chest
- Damp-Heat in the Stomach: pain with feeling of heaviness and sticky taste, sticky yellow tongue coating
- Blood stasis in the Stomach: severe, stabbing pain
- Stomach deficient and cold: chronic, intermittent, dull ache ameliorated by heat and warm drinks, aggravated by cold
- Stomach-Yin deficiency: chronic, intermittent burning pain, dry mouth
- Rebellious Qi in the Penetrating Vessel: distension, tightness and pain radiating to abdomen/umbilicus/chest, anxiety

---

Hypochondrium

Symptoms and Signs, Chapter 71

Most patients are not familiar with the word 'hypochondrium'. Therefore when I ask patients about symptoms in this area, I simply point to it. The hypochondrial area includes the ribs and the area immediately below them on both sides; this area is influenced by the Liver and Gall-Bladder channels and it is important to note that the left hypochondrial area may also reflect Liver disharmonies. Again, when patients report abdominal problems in this area, it is important to identify the location exactly. If any pain is located only in the hypochondrial region, it is definitely related to the Liver or Gall-Bladder channels, or both; if the pain starts in the hypochondrial region and radiates towards the centre of the epigastrium, it indicates rebellious Liver-Qi invading the Stomach; if the pain starts in the centre of the epigastrium and radiates towards either the right or left hypochondrium, it indicates a primary deficiency of the Stomach with a secondary stagnation of Liver-Qi.

Case history 38.4 illustrates a pattern underlying hypochondrial pain.

Case history 38.4

A 49-year-old woman had been suffering from recurrent bouts of pain and discomfort in the right hypochondrium for the past 7 years. The pain was sometimes sharp in nature and radiated to her shoulder.

The patient also suffered from a feeling of muzziness in her head, lacked concentration and sometimes had difficulty finding her words. She had occasional dizzy spells in the mornings and also suffered from blurred vision and floaters. She often felt tired and her joints would ache, especially her left hip where she had had pain for a long time.

The patient suffered from insomnia and often woke up between 3 am and 4 am. She used to suffer from colitis, with abdominal pain, mucus and blood in the stools and diarrhoea. This had been helped by acupuncture although she still had loose stools.

She suffered from premenstrual breast distension and irritability. Her periods were becoming scantier and her left breast hurt after her period. She had several breast lumps.

The tongue body was slightly Pale-Purple, with Red points and slightly Red sides. It was Swollen with teethmarks and had a sticky coating. Her pulse was Deep-Weak-Choppy and the left Front position was relatively Overflowing.

Diagnosis: The hypochondrial pain is caused by Liver-Qi stagnation. Other symptoms of Liver-Qi stagnation are the premenstrual breast distension and irritability. Evidence of the long-standing and severe nature of the stagnation is shown by the tongue having a slightly Purple colour.

The feeling of muzziness in the head, lack of concentration, difficulty in finding words, breast lumps and dizzy spells in the morning point towards the presence of Phlegm. This is confirmed by the Swollen tongue body and the sticky tongue coating.

The underlying Deficiency which has led to the development of Phlegm is predominantly one of Spleen- and Kidney-Yang. This is causing the loose stools and tiredness and is reflected in the pulse, which is Deep and Weak, and on the tongue, which is Swollen with teethmarks.

There is also a deficiency of Liver-Blood, manifesting with blurred vision, floaters, the periods becoming scantier, the Choppy quality of the pulse and the Pale colour of the tongue. The pain in the left breast occurring *after* the period indicates that, although it is due to Liver-Qi stagnation, there is an underlying Blood deficiency. Ache in the joints is normally due to Painful Obstruction Syndrome with Wind, Dampness or Cold; however, in women, ache in the joints without swelling is often caused simply by deficient Blood failing to nourish the sinews, as is the case in this patient.

Box 38.8 summarizes the patterns underlying hypochondrial pain.

BOX 38.8 HYPOCHONDRIAL PAIN

- Liver and Gall-Bladder channels: hypochondrial pain or distension
- Stagnant Liver-Qi invading the stomach: hypochondrial pain radiating to centre
- Stomach deficiency with secondary Liver-Qi stagnation: epigastric pain radiating to right or left hypochondrial region

---

Umbilical area

Symptoms and Signs, Chapter 71

The umbilical area is influenced by the Kidney and Liver channels and by the Directing and Penetrating Vessel. Pain in this area is more common in children than in adults.

The most common patterns causing umbilical pain are:

- Cold in the abdomen
- Qi stagnation
- Blood stasis
- retention of food (more common in children).

Central-lower abdominal area

Symptoms and Signs, Chapter 71

The central-lower abdominal area is influenced by many different channels: the Kidney, Liver, Bladder, Small Intestine, Directing Vessel, Penetrating Vessel and the Uterus itself. Pain in this area is therefore often difficult to diagnose because of the involvement of so many different channels; and the difficulties are compounded in women because of the influence of the Uterus on this area.

The most common patterns causing problems in this area are:

- stagnation of Qi – producing a pronounced feeling of distension or distending pain
- stasis of Blood – producing a fixed, severe and stabbing pain
- Dampness – producing a feeling of heaviness.

Apart from identifying the pattern, it is of course necessary to identify the channel involved and this is done according to the accompanying symptoms. In the case of the Bladder, there will be some urinary symptoms; in the case of the Uterus, there will be some menstrual irregularities; in the case of the Small Intestine, there will be borborygmi, loose stools or constipation; in the case of the Liver, there will be a pronounced distension and a clear correlation of the abdominal problem with the emotional state.

Case history 38.5 illustrates a pattern of Blood stasis and Deficiency causing central-lower abdominal pain.

Case history 38.5

A 31-year-old woman complained of abdominal pain following a dilatation and curettage operation on her uterus. Ten months previously she had had an exploratory laparoscopy for a suspected ovarian cyst; she developed complications after this operation with an infection of the scar and a haematoma in the abdomen. Three months after that she had a termination of pregnancy; as she developed complications, she was advised to have a dilatation and curettage of her womb. Following these procedures she developed a constant, sharp lower abdominal pain, pain on intercourse and mid-cycle bleeding, and her menstrual blood became dark with clots. Before all this happened, her periods were painful but not dark and without any mid-cycle bleeding.

Apart from the above problem, she also complained of a pronounced tiredness and, on interrogation, it transpired that she suffered from floaters in the afternoon, tingling of her limbs, poor memory and dizziness. She also complained of lower backache, which she attributed to riding, and the occasional tinnitus. She felt cold in general and suffered from cold hands and feet. She occasionally also suffered from a slight pain in the chest with a feeling of palpitations and breathlessness, for which she used an inhaler.

Her complexion was rather pale and the *shen* of her eyes was bright. Her voice sounded clear but with a very subtle tone of sadness to it. Her tongue was Pale in general with paler sides, Swollen, with a Stomach crack and a rootless coating on the root. Her pulse was Weak and Choppy and particularly Weak on both Rear positions; the Heart position was also particularly Choppy.

Diagnosis: In diagnosis, we must differentiate the diagnosis of her present, acute problem (abdominal pain, dyspareunia and mid-cycle bleeding following the dilatation and curettage) from that of her underlying condition. The present problem of abdominal pain is clearly due to Blood stasis; this is clearly shown by the sharpness of the pain and the darkness of the menstrual blood with clots. The tongue does not show any Blood stasis (as it is not Purple) owing to the relatively short duration of this problem.

The underlying condition is characterized primarily by three problems:

1. Blood deficiency (Pale tongue, floaters, tiredness, tingling, poor memory and dizziness): there is Blood deficiency of the Liver but also of the Heart, as is evidenced by the palpitations, breathlessness and the Choppy pulse on the Heart position.
2. Stomach and Spleen deficiency with some affliction of the Intestines: the Spleen deficiency

is manifested clearly by the swelling of the sides of the tongue and the tiredness. The Stomach deficiency is manifested by the Stomach crack and the rootless coating: the fact that the rootless coating is on the root of the tongue shows that there is an intestinal pathology. It was only after I pointed this out to her that she told that she had also just been diagnosed as suffering from intestinal parasites.

3. Kidney-Yang deficiency: this is manifested by lower backache, feeling cold, cold feet and hands and occasional tinnitus.

As for possible aetiology, I ventured to say that in my opinion the main origin of the problem was emotional. I based this primarily on the Choppiness of the pulse (especially on the Heart pulse) and its lack of wave, which is usually due to sadness. As I told her that I thought sadness was the main origin of the problem, she confirmed this by saying that she had been repeatedly sexually abused as a child. I think this was the emotional cause for the Blood deficiency (especially of the Heart) and also of the Kidney deficiency as the sexual abuse was obviously accompanied by fear, which injured the Kidneys. Besides being sexually abused she was also frequently beaten across the lower back; I think that that, rather than riding, was the cause of the lower backache.

Treatment: In treatment, one must concentrate on the present, acute problem of Blood stasis in the abdomen with a formula to invigorate Blood and eliminate stasis such as Sheng Hua Tang *Generating and Transforming Decoction*; this is a formula for abdominal pain from Blood stasis after childbirth. The termination and dilatation and curettage are somewhat energetically equivalent to childbirth (without, of course, the pronounced depletion of Qi and Blood that follows childbirth).

Box 38.9 summarizes the patterns underlying pain in this area.

Right-lateral lower abdominal area

Symptoms and Signs, Chapter 71

This area is influenced primarily by the Large Intestine and Liver channels and by the Penetrating Vessel. As a rule of thumb, problems in this area are caused by the gynaecological system more often than by the Large

---

BOX 38.9 CENTRAL-LOWER ABDOMINAL PAIN

- Bladder Damp-Heat: pain with frequent and difficult urination
- Blood stasis or Damp-Heat in the Uterus: pain during the periods, menstrual irregularities
- Damp-Heat in the Small Intestine: pain with borborygmi and loose stools or constipation
- Liver-Qi stagnation: distending pain aggravated by emotional stress

Intestine. For example, in women, pain in this area is very often due to ovarian cysts.

The most common patterns causing pain in this area are:

> • stagnation of Qi – producing distension or distending pain, or both
> • stasis of Blood – producing a fixed, severe, stabbing pain with a feeling of mass
> • Dampness – accompanied by a feeling of heaviness
> • Cold – producing a severe, spastic pain that is alleviated by the application of heat.

Left-lateral lower abdominal area

Symptoms and Signs, Chapter 71

This area is influenced by the Large Intestine, Liver and Spleen channels and by the Penetrating Vessel. As a rule of thumb, compared with the right-lower abdominal region, problems in this area are often caused by the pathology of the Large Intestine. The most common patterns causing problems in this area are the same as those of the right-lateral lower abdominal area, that is:

> • stagnation of Qi – producing distension or distending pain, or both
> • stasis of Blood – producing a fixed, severe, stabbing pain with a feeling of mass

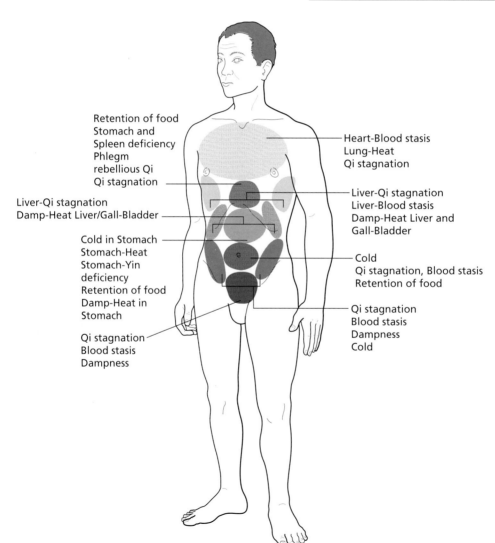

Retention of food
Stomach and
Spleen deficiency
Phlegm
rebellious Qi
Qi stagnation

Liver-Qi stagnation
Damp-Heat Liver/Gall-Bladder

Cold in Stomach
Stomach-Heat
Stomach-Yin
deficiency
Retention of food
Damp-Heat in
Stomach

Qi stagnation
Blood stasis
Dampness

Heart-Blood stasis
Lung-Heat
Qi stagnation

Liver-Qi stagnation
Liver-Blood stasis
Damp-Heat Liver and
Gall-Bladder

Cold
Qi stagnation, Blood stasis
Retention of food

Qi stagnation
Blood stasis
Dampness
Cold

Fig. 38.1 Main patterns in the chest and abdomen by area

- Dampness – accompanied by a feeling of heaviness
- Cold – producing a severe, spastic pain that is alleviated by the application of heat.

Figure 38.1 summarizes the most common patterns affecting each area of the chest and abdomen.

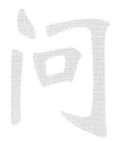

Chapter **39**

LIMBS

Chapter contents

INTRODUCTION *337*

WEAKNESS OF THE LIMBS *338*

DIFFICULTY IN WALKING (ATROPHY/FLACCIDITY OF LIMBS) *338*

FEELING OF DISTENSION OF THE LIMBS *338*

FEELING OF HEAVINESS OF THE LIMBS *339*

MUSCLE ACHE IN THE LIMBS *339*

NUMBNESS/TINGLING OF THE LIMBS *339*

GENERALIZED JOINT PAIN *339*

TREMOR OF LIMBS *340*

UPPER LIMBS *341*
   Pain and inability to raise the shoulder *341*
   Pain in the elbow *342*
   Pain in the hands *342*
   Cold hands *342*
   Hot hands *343*
   Itchy hands *343*
   Numbness/tingling of the hands *343*
   Oedema of the hands *343*

LOWER LIMBS *343*
   Pain in the hip 343
   Pain in the thigh *344*
   Pain in the knees *344*
   Weak knees *344*
   Cramps in the calves *344*
   Cold feet *344*
   Pain in the feet *344*
   Oedema of the feet *345*
   Pain in the soles *345*
   Burning sensation in the soles *345*

INTRODUCTION

This chapter deals with symptoms that may occur either in the arms or in the legs, or in all four limbs. Apart from the obvious influence of each channel on the limb it traverses, the four limbs are influenced primarily by the Spleen and Stomach in general.

? **WHY** WE ASK

Generally speaking, questions about the four limbs are asked only when the patient presents with a problem specific to them. The main exceptions to this are when a patient presents with symptoms of Blood deficiency, in which case I always ask about numbness of the limbs, or when a patient has symptoms of Dampness, in which case I ask about any feeling of heaviness in the limbs.

? **WHEN** WE ASK

I generally ask about problems in the limbs when the patient presents with a specific problem such as oedema, numbness or weakness of the limbs.

I also ask about the limbs in three other situations. When I suspect a Stomach-Qi deficiency I ask about weakness of the limbs, when I suspect a Kidney deficiency I ask about weakness of the knees, and when I suspect Phlegm or a Blood deficiency I ask about numbness or tingling of the limbs.

? **HOW** WE ASK

When we ask about the limbs, we should make it clear that we mean all four limbs – that is, whether the

patient has a problem such as weakness, heaviness or numbness of all limbs.

WEAKNESS OF THE LIMBS

Symptoms and Signs, Chapters 64 and 66

The three most common causes of weakness of the limbs are Stomach-Qi deficiency, a general Qi and Blood deficiency and a deficiency of Kidney-Yang. The Stomach carries the food essences to the four limbs and for this reason a weakness of Stomach-Qi is the most common cause of a feeling of weakness of the limbs. The Kidneys carry food essences and Blood to the legs; a weakness of the limbs in the elderly is more likely to be due to a Kidney deficiency.

Box 39.1 summarizes the patterns underlying weakness of the limbs.

BOX 39.1 WEAKNESS OF LIMBS

- Stomach-Qi deficiency
- Qi and Blood deficiency
- Kidney-Yang deficiency

DIFFICULTY IN WALKING (ATROPHY/FLACCIDITY OF LIMBS

Observation, Chapter 18; Symptoms and Signs, Chapter 64

Atrophy or flaccidity of the limbs causes a difficulty in walking; the most common example of this in Western patients is multiple sclerosis.

In the beginning stages, atrophy or flaccidity of the limbs is often due to a Stomach- and Spleen-Qi deficiency, failing to carry food essences to the limbs. In later stages, atrophy or flaccidity of the limbs, or both, is often due to a Yin deficiency of the Liver and Kidneys or a Yang deficiency of the Spleen and Kidneys.

Atrophy or flaccidity of the limbs in children is due to a deficiency of Kidney-Essence. A general deficiency of Qi and Blood may also cause atrophy or flaccidity of the limbs.

BOX 39.2 DIFFICULTY IN WALKING

- Stomach- and Spleen-Qi deficiency
- Liver- and Kidney-Yin deficiency
- Spleen- and Kidney-Yang deficiency
- Qi and Blood deficiency
- Deficiency of Kidney-Essence (in children)

Box 39.2 summarizes the patterns underlying difficulty in walking.

FEELING OF DISTENSION OF THE LIMBS

Symptoms and Signs, Chapter 64

The five most common causes of a feeling of distension of the limbs are:

- Qi stagnation
- Qi stagnation with Dampness
- Blood stasis from Qi deficiency
- Wind-Phlegm
- Dampness in the muscles.

Qi stagnation causes a feeling of distension of the limbs, particularly in the hands and feet.

If the feeling of distension of the limbs is accompanied by a swelling under the skin and a sallow complexion, then it is due to Qi stagnation with Dampness. It should be noted that this swelling is not real oedema and finger pressure does not leave a dip in the skin. This type of distension and swelling of the limbs is very common in women suffering from premenstrual syndrome.

If the feeling of distension of the limbs is aggravated by overexertion and the lower legs have a purple colour, it is due to Blood stasis deriving from Qi deficiency.

If the feeling of distension of the limbs is accompanied by numbness, tingling, a feeling of heaviness and tremor, it is due to Wind-Phlegm.

A feeling of distension of the limbs may also be due to retention of Dampness in the muscles, which may

---

BOX 39.3 FEELING OF DISTENSION OF THE LIMBS

- Qi stagnation: feeling of distension especially in hands and feet
- Qi stagnation with Dampness: feeling of distension with swelling, sallow complexion
- Blood stasis from Qi deficiency: feeling of distension with weakness, purple colour of legs, aggravated by overwork
- Wind-Phlegm: feeling of distension, numbness, tingling, feeling of heaviness, tremor
- Dampness: feeling of distension and heaviness

---

be associated with Cold or Heat; in this case, there would also be a feeling of heaviness of the limbs.

Box 39.3 summarizes the patterns underlying a feeling of distension of the limbs.

FEELING OF HEAVINESS OF THE LIMBS

Symptoms and Signs, Chapters 64 and 66

Patients quite often spontaneously report a sensation of heaviness of the limbs although they may not necessarily use such terms. They often say that their legs 'feel like lead'.

A feeling of heaviness of the limbs is more frequently experienced in the legs. A feeling of heaviness of the legs is always due to Dampness in the Lower Burner. The Dampness may be combined with Heat or Cold, and it may be Full or Empty. The feeling of heaviness from Full-Dampness is more pronounced than that from Dampness associated with Spleen-Qi deficiency.

When the Spleen-Qi deficiency is associated with Stomach-Qi deficiency, the feeling of heaviness is frequently experienced in all four limbs rather than just the legs. Similarly, when Phlegm causes a feeling of heaviness, it is experienced in all four limbs.

MUSCLE ACHE IN THE LIMBS

Symptoms and Signs, Chapter 64

Muscle ache in the limbs is nearly always due to retention of Dampness in the space between skin and muscles. This may be a Full or an Empty condition (associated with Spleen-Qi deficiency) and the Dampness may or may not be combined with Heat. If it is combined with Heat, the ache is more intense. In addition to the ache, there is a pronounced feeling of heaviness of the limbs. In a few cases, muscle ache in the limbs may be due to Liver-Blood deficiency, in which case it would be very mild and associated with tingling.

Muscle ache in the limbs is a common symptom in postviral fatigue syndrome.

NUMBNESS/TINGLING OF THE LIMBS

Symptoms and Signs, Chapter 64

'Numbness' here includes tingling in the limbs. Generally speaking, a feeling of numbness/tingling may be due to:

- Wind
- Phlegm
- Dampness or Damp-Heat
- stagnation of Qi and Blood.

Blood deficiency usually causes tingling, whereas Phlegm and Wind tend to cause more numbness: with Wind, the numbness is often unilateral. However, these are only general rules.

Blood deficiency is a common cause of numbness/tingling of the limbs in younger people, especially women. In the elderly, a numbness of the limbs is very often caused by Wind or Wind-Phlegm obstructing the channels and, in the case of Wind, the numbness is often unilateral. Dampness or Damp-Heat may also cause numbness of the limbs and especially of the legs. In a few cases, numbness may be caused by stagnation of Qi and Blood in the limbs, in which case it is relieved by exercise.

Box 39.4 summarizes the patterns underlying numbness/tingling of the limbs.

BOX 39.4 NUMBNESS/TINGLING OF THE LIMBS

- Blood deficiency: more tingling, common in women
- Wind: more numbness, often unilateral, common in the elderly
- Phlegm: more numbness, with feeling of heaviness
- Dampness or Damp-Heat: numbness especially of legs, with swelling
- Stagnation of Qi and Blood: with pain, relieved by exercise

---

GENERALIZED JOINT PAIN

Pain in multiple joints is generally due to Wind (Wind Painful Obstruction Syndrome) combined with Dampness or Cold, or both. If the site of the pain moves, affecting different joints every day, this strongly indicates Wind. A severe pain indicates Cold, whereas swelling of the joints indicates Dampness. In chronic conditions, Dampness frequently combines with Heat and causes swelling, redness and heat of the joints.

Generalized joint pain may also be caused by Qi stagnation; in this case, the pain is alleviated by gentle exercise. Blood stasis may also cause generalized joint pain; in this case, the pain is intense and often worse at night. Finally, a general deficiency of Qi and Blood may cause a dull, mild joint ache that improves with rest.

Case history 39.1 illustrates a pattern underlying generalized joint pain.

Case history 39.1

A 50-year-old woman had been suffering from osteoarthritis for the past year. There had been a sudden onset of the condition after the patient had suffered a severe shock. The pain, which was stabbing in nature, had first affected the elbow, shoulder and neck; however, it spread to all the other joints after the patient was put in neck traction. The joints were not swollen. The patient said she felt like she 'was being crushed inside'. The pain was alleviated by taking a hot bath and made worse by damp or cold weather and stress.

She had had four children. During her first pregnancy, she suffered from repeated kidney infections; during her third pregnancy she developed asthma; during her fourth pregnancy she developed a pre-eclampsia condition with high blood pressure. Her blood pressure had remained high ever since and she was on medication for this.

The patient had a tendency towards constipation and said that she had no energy. She started taking hormone replacement therapy (HRT) 5 years previously, after suffering from hot flushes, lethargy and mood swings. She had continued to suffer from recurrent kidney infections since her first pregnancy.

The tongue body was Reddish-Purple, Swollen and with cracks in the Stomach and Spleen area. The tongue coating was very thin. The pulse was Slippery in general and Weak in both Rear positions.

Diagnosis: The widespread and moving joint pain, which is aggravated by exposure to damp and cold weather, indicates Painful Obstruction Syndrome from Wind and Cold. Wind is indicated by the moving pain, while Cold is indicated by the intensity of the pain and its aggravation from exposure to cold. The absence of swelling of the joints indicates that there is no pronounced Dampness.

The stabbing joint pain is caused by Blood stasis in the channels which was brought on by the sudden shock the patient experienced just prior to the onset of the symptoms. Being put in neck traction, with the consequent restriction of movement, would have only exacerbated the Blood stasis. Blood stasis is obvious from the Purple colour of the tongue body and the stabbing nature of the joint pain. The hypertension is caused by Kidney deficiency and retention of Phlegm, which itself has come about as a result of the long-standing Kidney deficiency and which is evidenced by the Swollen tongue and Slippery pulse.

There is an underlying Kidney deficiency, which is predominantly a deficiency of Kidney-Yin. This probably originated during her first pregnancy at the age of 16 when she suffered from kidney problems, and was exacerbated by her third pregnancy which was when she developed asthma, and further aggravated during the fourth pregnancy when she developed a pre-eclampsia condition. Other signs and symptoms of Kidney-Yin deficiency are the hot flushes the patient suffered before going on HRT, the tendency towards constipation, and the lack of tongue coating.

I interpreted the expression she used 'feeling like being crushed inside' as strongly suggestive of the emotional origin (shock) of her problem.

Box 39.5 summarizes the patterns underlying generalized joint pain.

BOX 39.5 GENERALIZED JOINT PAIN

- Wind: pain moving from joint to joint
- Cold: severe pain
- Dampness: dull ache with swelling of joints
- Damp-heat: chronic ache and swelling of joints
- Qi stagnation: pain in the joints that is alleviated by exercise
- Blood stasis: severe pain, often worse at night
- Qi and Blood deficiency: generalized mild ache that is better with rest

---

TREMOR OF THE LIMBS

Observation, Chapters 4 and 18; Symptoms and Signs, Chapter 64

A tremor of the limbs always indicates Liver-Wind; we should therefore establish the source of Liver-Wind and whether it is Full- or Empty-Wind. The root cause of Liver-Wind may be Heat during an acute febrile disease, Liver-Fire, Liver-Yang rising, a deficiency of Yin of the Liver or Kidneys, or both, and Liver-Blood deficiency. The last two types of Wind are of the Empty type, whereas all the others are of the Full type.

Full Wind is characterized by pronounced tremors or convulsions (during an acute febrile disease), vertigo, unilateral numbness and a Wiry pulse. Empty-Wind is

Case history 39.2

A 45-year-old man had been suffering from a fine tremor of his right arm for 3 years. He had seen a neurologist who excluded the diagnosis of Parkinson's disease. This patient had very few other symptoms, complaining only of a feeling of heat in the head, cold hands and feet, floaters, an occasional itch in the left eye and occasional heat and dryness in both eyes. His skin was also rather dry and he had been suffering from myopia from the age of 8.

His body type was a mixture of Metal and Wood. His tongue was slightly Thin, Red on the sides and not enough coating in the centre. His pulse was slightly Wiry on the left and Weak on the right, most of all on the Lung position.

Diagnosis: The tremor of the arm is an unmistakable sign of Liver-Wind and we should establish the

root pattern giving rise to Wind. In this case, it is Liver-Blood and Liver-Yin deficiency. The symptoms of Liver-Blood deficiency are floaters, itch of the left eye, dry skin, myopia from childhood, Weak pulse on the right, while dryness of the eyes and the lack of coating on the tongue indicate Liver-Yin deficiency. There are also some symptoms of Liver-Yang rising (feeling of heat in the head and eyes, Red sides of the tongue) and of Liver-Qi stagnation (cold hands and feet). The Wiry pulse may be related to any of the Full Liver patterns. In Liver disharmonies, it is not unusual to have a combination of several different patterns.

There are no symptoms or signs corresponding to the weakness of the Lung pulse, which is not unusual for this organ. When the Lung pulse is the weakest of all the pulse positions, I usually relate this to emotional problems due to sadness and grief.

Case history 39.3

A 45-year-old woman had been suffering from a fine tremor of the left arm for 1 year. She also experienced numbness and tingling of the left arm. She had very few other symptoms, except for her periods being quite scanty.

Her tongue was Pale and slightly Thin and her pulse was Fine and Wiry.

Diagnosis: This is a clear example of Empty-Wind deriving from Blood deficiency. The Blood deficiency is evident from the Pale and Thin tongue and Fine pulse, while the Wind is evident from the Wiry pulse and obviously the tremor of the arm.

characterized by fine tremors or tics, mild dizziness, tingling and a Choppy or Fine and slightly Wiry pulse.

The tongue indicating Liver-Wind may be Moving, Deviated or Stiff.

Case histories 39.2 and 39.3 illustrate tremor caused by Liver-Wind.

Box 39.6 summarizes the patterns of Liver-Wind.

BOX 39.6 LIVER-WIND

- Full type: pronounced tremors, convulsions, vertigo, unilateral numbness of a limb, Wiry pulse
- Empty type: fine tremors, tics, mild dizziness, tingling of limbs, Choppy or Fine and slightly Wiry pulse

---

UPPER LIMBS

Pain and inability to raise the shoulder

Symptoms and Signs, Chapter 65

Inability to raise the shoulder, which is nearly always accompanied by pain in the shoulder, is a

very common complaint, especially after the age of 40.

The most common cause of inability to raise the shoulder is chronic retention of Cold in the joint owing to successive exposures to cold and damp weather; this syndrome falls under the category of Painful Obstruction Syndrome. In this case the pain is worse with rest and better with exercise, aggravated by exposure to cold and alleviated by exposure to heat and by wearing warm clothes.

Another common cause of this problem is sprain of the shoulder joint, which leads to local stagnation of Qi and Blood; in this case the pain is better with gentle exercise and worse with rest.

In old people, chronic inability to raise the shoulder is often due to local Blood stasis and this may be a consequence of chronic retention of Cold or repetitive strain. In this case, the inability to raise the shoulder is very pronounced and there is severe pain and stiffness that are worse at night.

In rare cases, an inability to raise the shoulder accompanies Chest Painful Obstruction Syndrome, in

which case the patient suffers from chest pain, breathlessness and palpitations.

Box 39.7 summarizes the patterns underlying pain and inability to raise the shoulder.

BOX 39.7 PAIN AND INABILITY TO RAISE THE SHOULDER

- Cold in the joint: Painful Obstruction Syndrome pain better with exercise, worse with rest, aggravated by cold, ameliorated by warmth
- Stagnation of Qi and Blood: pain better with exercise, worse with rest
- Local Blood stasis: severe pain and stiffness, worse at night
- General Blood stasis: Chest Painful Obstruction Syndrome (Chest *Bi*) with breathlessness, palpitations

---

Pain in the elbow

Symptoms and Signs, Chapter 65

Pain in the elbow is usually due either to retention of Cold or to local stagnation of Qi and Blood due to repetitive strain injury. In the case of retention of Cold, the pain is severe and is aggravated by exposure to cold and alleviated by the application of heat. In the case of stagnation of Qi and Blood, the pain is aggravated by rest and slightly ameliorated by movement.

Box 39.8 summarizes patterns underlying elbow pain.

BOX 39.8 PAIN IN THE ELBOW

- Retention of Cold: severe pain aggravated by cold and ameliorated by warmth
- Stagnation of Qi and Blood: pain ameliorated by exercise

Pain in the hands

Symptoms and Signs, Chapter 65

Pain in the hands may be of a Full or Empty nature: in Full conditions the pain is severe, whereas in Empty conditions it is dull.

The three most common causes are retention of Cold, Dampness or Wind (or a combination of these) in the hands; this falls under the category of Painful Obstruction Syndrome. When the hand pain is due to Cold, it is intense, aggravated by exposure to cold and alleviated by application of heat. When it is due to Dampness, there is swelling of the fingers. When due

to Wind, the pain in the hands is usually associated with pain in other joints.

Pain in the hands may also be due to Liver-Qi stagnation, in which case it may be accompanied by pain in the feet. In chronic cases, Qi stagnation will lead to Blood stasis and this may cause a severe pain in the fingers, which is worse at night, and a pronounced stiffness in them.

Blood deficiency may cause a dull ache in the hands. This is due to deficient Blood not reaching the hands and causing a minor local stagnation; it is more common in women. Yang deficiency may also cause a dull ache in the hands, similar to Blood deficiency, and, in addition, the hands have a pronounced cold feeling.

Box 39.9 summarizes the patterns underlying hand pain.

BOX 39.9 PAIN IN THE HANDS

- Severe hand pain aggravated by cold: Cold Painful Obstruction Syndrome
- Hand pain with swelling: Damp Painful Obstruction Syndrome
- Pain in the hands and other joints: Wind Painful Obstruction Syndrome
- Hand pain with swelling and heat: Damp-Heat in the joints
- Pain in the hands and feet: Liver-Qi stagnation
- Severe pain in the hands and fingers that is worse at night and with stiffness: Blood stasis
- Dull ache in the hands: Blood deficiency
- Dull ache in the hands ameliorated by heat, cold hands: Yang deficiency

---

Cold hands

Symptoms and Signs, Chapter 65

Cold hands are due to three possible causes: Yang deficiency (the most common one), Blood deficiency and Qi stagnation.

Yang deficiency causing cold hands is most commonly of the Spleen, Lungs or Heart; it is ameliorated by the application of heat. Blood deficiency, especially of the Heart, may also cause cold hands; it is accompanied by palpitations and dizziness, and is more frequent in women. Liver-Qi stagnation may also cause cold hands but in conjunction with cold feet; this is called the 'Four Rebellious Syndrome' in which the 'four rebellious' indicate cold hands and feet. The famous formula Si Ni San *Four Rebellious Powder* is used for this pattern. An important difference between cold limbs due to Yang deficiency and cold limbs due to Qi stagna-

tion is that in the former case the whole limb will be cold, whereas in the latter case only the hands and feet, particularly the fingers and toes, are cold.

In the case of deficiency of Yang or Blood, the cold feeling is due to deficient Yang-Qi or Blood not reaching the extremities; in the case of Liver-Qi stagnation, Qi does not reach the extremities because it stagnates in the body.

Box 39.10 summarizes the patterns underlying cold hands.

BOX 39.10 COLD HANDS

- Dull ache in the hands ameliorated by heat, cold hands: Yang deficiency
- Cold hands with palpitations and dizziness: Heart-Blood deficiency
- Cold fingers and toes: Liver-Qi stagnation

Hot hands

Symptoms and Signs, Chapter 65

To diagnose the significance of hot hands, we must first of all differentiate between exterior and interior syndromes. In exterior syndromes due to invasion of Wind, the dorsum of the hands feels hot to the touch while the patient feels cold, and an aversion to cold, in general. The acute onset, simultaneous subjective cold feeling of the patient (to the point of shivering) and the objective feeling of heat in the dorsum of the hands characterize the initial stages of an invasion of Wind.

In interior conditions, hot hands are due to either Full- or Empty-Heat usually of the Lungs, Heart or Stomach. In Full-Heat the whole hand feels hot, whereas in Empty-Heat especially the palms feel hot.

Box 39.11 summarizes the patterns underlying hot hands.

BOX 39.11 HOT HANDS

- Hot dorsum of the hands with acute onset and aversion to cold: invasion of external Wind
- Chronic hot dorsum of the hands: Full-Heat (Lungs, Heart or Stomach)
- Chronic hot palms: Empty-Heat (Lungs or Heart)

Itchy hands

Symptoms and Signs, Chapter 64

A common cause of itchiness of the hands is Dampness, which may be associated with Heat. With Dampness, the itchiness of the hands is associated with a swelling of the fingers and often small, white vesicles; with Damp-Heat the itching is more intense and is associated with swelling and redness of the fingers.

Another possible cause of itchiness of the hands is Blood deficiency leading to Wind in the skin.

Box 39.12 summarizes the patterns underlying itchy hands.

BOX 39.12 ITCHY HANDS

- Dampness: with white vesicles
- Damp-Heat: intense itching
- Blood deficiency with Wind in the skin: mild itching

Numbness/tingling of the hands

Symptoms and Signs, Chapter 65

When asking patients about numbness, it is important to explain to them that this includes any feeling of tingling (in Britain often called 'pins and needles').

Causes of numbness or tingling of the hands include:

- Blood deficiency
- Phlegm
- Qi and Blood stagnation
- Wind.

Blood deficiency is a common cause of numbness/tingling of the hands, especially tingling. Phlegm may also cause numbness/tingling of the hands and especially numbness. Another less common cause of numbness/tingling of the hands is chronic Qi and Blood stagnation. Unilateral numbness or tingling of the first three fingers in an old person may indicate the possibility of impending Wind-stroke.

Oedema of the hands

Observation, Chapter 18; Symptoms and Signs, Chapters 64 and 65

Oedema of the hands may be due to Lung-Yang deficiency or Spleen-Yang deficiency; in this case the oedema is pitting. If the oedema is not pitting it is due to Qi stagnation.

LOWER LIMBS

Pain in the hip

Symptoms and Signs, Chapter 66

The most common cause of hip pain is invasion of Cold and Dampness in the hip joint, in which case the pain

is unilateral, severe in nature and with marked rigidity of the joint.

In the elderly, hip pain is often due to chronic stagnation of Qi and stasis of Blood affecting the Gall-Bladder channel.

Pain in the thigh

Symptoms and Signs, Chapter 66

Pain in the thigh may be due to retention of Dampness in the muscles which may be associated with Heat or Cold; in this case, the pain radiates to the groin.

Chronic thigh pain may also be due to Qi deficiency with Blood stasis, or to Kidney-Yang deficiency.

Pain in the knees

Symptoms and Signs, Chapter 66

The most common cause of pain in the knees is invasion of Cold and this falls under the category of Painful Obstruction Syndrome. Invasion of Cold in the knee causes a severe pain, which is usually unilateral, and rigidity. Cold is often associated with Dampness, in which case the knee is also swollen. When Dampness is retained for a long time it may transform into Damp-Heat, in which case the knee is painful, swollen and hot.

Another common cause of pain in the knee is sprain due to working conditions, which usually causes local stagnation of Qi and Blood. It is ameliorated by gentle exercise.

Dull knee ache which improves with rest, has a gradual onset and is associated with weakness of the knees is due to Kidney deficiency.

Box 39.13 summarizes the patterns underlying knee pain.

BOX 39.13 PAIN IN THE KNEES

- Invasion of Cold: severe pain with rigidity, usually unilateral
- Damp-Cold: pain and swelling
- Damp-Heat: pain, swelling and hot to the touch
- Stagnation of Qi and Blood: better with exercise
- Kidney deficiency: chronic ache of gradual onset, better with rest

---

Weak knees

Symptoms and Signs, Chapter 66

The most common cause of weak knees is a deficiency of the Kidneys. A chronic deficiency of Stomach and Spleen may also cause a weakness of the knees.

Cramps in the calves

Symptoms and Signs, Chapter 66

The most common cause of cramps in the calves is Liver-Blood deficiency. This symptom is more common in the elderly and it frequently occurs at night. If the cramps are very severe and are accompanied by numbness of the legs, this may indicate the presence of Empty-Wind stemming from Liver-Blood deficiency.

Cramps in the calves may also be caused by a combination of Wind and Phlegm in the limbs and this generally occurs only in patients over 70 years of age. If cramps in the calves are accompanied by pain, this indicates that, in addition to Liver-Blood deficiency, there is also Liver-Blood stasis.

Cold feet

Symptoms and Signs, Chapter 66

The most common cause of cold feet is Kidney-Yang deficiency; indeed, this symptom is a relatively important one to diagnose a Kidney-Yang deficiency. Another possible cause of cold feet, especially in women, is Liver-Blood deficiency.

Obstruction of Phlegm in the Lower Burner may also cause the feet to be cold.

Pain in the feet

Symptoms and Signs, Chapter 66

By 'pain in the foot', we mean a localized pain, usually unilateral, without swelling or redness. It is therefore different from the pain in the joints due to invasion of Wind, Cold or Dampness causing Painful Obstruction Syndrome. Pain in the foot may occur on the dorsum, the sides or the soles and the three most common causes of it are a Kidney deficiency (which may be of Yin or Yang), Blood deficiency and Dampness or Phlegm.

Dampness produces pain with swelling, and in Damp-Heat there is also redness and Heat. Phlegm causes a pain with numbness and tingling. A pain in the ball of the foot which is aggravated by walking if the patient is overweight is due to Damp-Phlegm.

Pain that is due to Blood deficiency is a chronic pain with tingling.

When the pain extends from the side of the foot towards the sole, it is usually due to Kidney-Yang deficiency; if due to Kidney-Yin deficiency it is accompanied by a feeling of heat of the soles, and is worse at night.

In addition, a severe pain may be due to Cold.

Box 39.14 summarizes the patterns underlying foot pain.

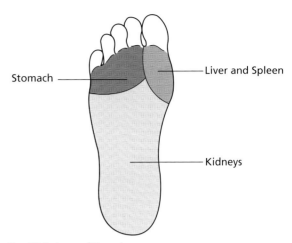

Fig. 39.1 Areas of the sole

Oedema of the feet

Observation, Chapters 18 and 19; Symptoms and Signs, Chapters 64, 66, 68

Oedema of the feet is usually due to Kidney-Yang deficiency; in this case the oedema is pitting. If the oedema is not pitting, it is due to Qi stagnation. Oedema is discussed in more detail in Chapter 18.

Pain in the soles

Symptoms and Signs, Chapter 66

We can differentiate three distinct areas of the sole (Fig. 39.1): the ball of the foot, which pertains to the Stomach channel; the area under the big toe, which pertains to the Liver and Spleen channels, and the rest of the sole, which pertains to the Kidney channel. Therefore a pain in the ball of the foot is often due to a Stomach-Qi deficiency with invasion of Dampness in the limbs or to Stomach-Heat, while a pain below the big toe is often due to Liver-Fire or Dampness in the Spleen.

A pain in the sole proper is generally due to a Kidney deficiency (Yin or Yang), also with invasion of Dampness.

Burning sensation in the soles

Symptoms and Signs, Chapter 66

A burning sensation of the soles may be due to Full-Heat of the Liver or Stomach. If it is in the Liver, only the area under the big toe will feel hot; if it is in the Stomach, the ball of the foot will feel hot.

However, the most common cause of burning sensation in the soles proper is a deficiency of Kidney-Yin, usually with Empty-Heat; in such a case, the burning sensation is worse in the evening and at night.

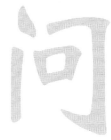

Chapter 40

SLEEP

Chapter contents

INTRODUCTION   *347*

INSOMNIA   *348*

EXCESSIVE DREAMING   *349*

SOMNOLENCE   *349*

INTRODUCTION

Sleep disturbances are very common in Western patients; when asking a patient about a sleep problem, it is important to clarify whether there is difficulty in falling or staying asleep, waking up early in the morning or excessive dreaming.

? WHY WE ASK

It is essential to ask every patient about their sleep because this gives an indication of the state of the Mind (*Shen*) and Ethereal Soul (*Hun*). A disturbance of the Mind or Ethereal Soul, or both, is of course extremely common in Western patients whose lives are generally subject to a considerable amount of stress.

The length of sleep needed varies according to age and, in general, it gradually decreases in one's lifetime, being highest in babies and lowest in the elderly. We should therefore take age into account when judging whether the patient's sleep is adequate or not.

? WHEN WE ASK

I ask about sleep and dreaming early on in the consultation in every case. Even if a patient does not apparently present with any problems of that kind, I always ask about sleep and dreaming to get an idea of the state of the Mind and Ethereal Soul.

? HOW WE ASK

It is important to be specific when asking about sleep and dreaming; it will not suffice to ask 'Do you sleep

well?' I generally ask patients whether they fall asleep easily, whether they wake up during the night and whether they dream excessively. The last symptom is difficult to define as we all dream: dreaming seems to be an essential part of sleep, performing a function that is still the subject of debate and disagreement. What, therefore, constitutes 'excessive' dreaming in Chinese medicine? I personally think this can be defined either as having many dreams, to the point of feeling exhausted in the morning because of them, or as having unpleasant dreams which leave one tired and slightly disturbed in the morning or even wake one up during the night.

If the patient dreams excessively, I then ask whether there is any recurrent dream. Apart from a modern psychological interpretation of dreams according to the theories of Freud, Jung and others, I always try to interpret recurrent dreams in terms of Chinese medicine. The 'Simple Questions' has a long list of dreams with their significance in Chinese medicine and these are listed in Part 5, Chapter 81. For example, recurrent dreams of water usually indicate a Kidney deficiency (while in Jungian psychology water is a symbol of the unconscious).

INSOMNIA

Symptoms and Signs, Chapter 81

In general, sleep depends on the state of Blood and Yin, especially of the Heart and Liver, although the Blood and Yin of other organs also influences sleep. During the night Yin energy predominates and the Mind and the Ethereal Soul should be anchored in the Heart-Blood and Liver-Blood respectively (Fig. 40.1).

A sleep disturbance may be due to the Mind or the Ethereal Soul not being anchored in the Heart-Blood

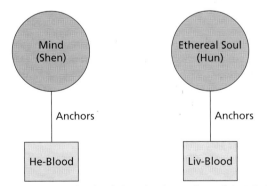

Fig. 40.1 Heart-Blood and Liver-Blood as anchors of the Mind and Ethereal Soul

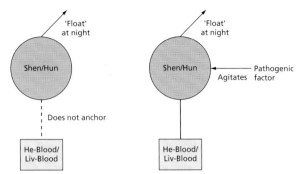

Fig. 40.2 Pathology of insomnia

(or Heart-Yin) or the Liver-Blood (or Liver-Yin) respectively; this can happen either because there is not enough Blood or Yin to anchor the Mind or the Ethereal Soul, or both, or because a pathogenic factor (such as Heat) agitates them. The former is an Empty type of sleep disturbance, the latter a Full type. In both cases, the Mind or the Ethereal Soul is said to 'float' at night causing insomnia (Fig. 40.2).

In general, in Deficiency, a difficulty in falling asleep indicates a Blood deficiency of the Heart, Spleen or Liver, whereas difficulty in staying asleep and a tendency to wake up during the night indicate a Yin deficiency. Of course, waking up during the night may also be due to a Full condition such as Heat, Fire, Phlegm-Fire or retention of food.

> **!**
>
> A difficulty in falling asleep generally indicates a deficiency of Blood or Yin; waking during the night generally indicates Yin deficiency with Empty-Heat.

When diagnosing sleep disturbances it is important to distinguish, first, a Full from an Empty condition and, secondly, a Heart from a Liver pattern. Full conditions are characterized by very restless sleep with a feeling of heat, agitation and excessive dreaming; Empty conditions are characterized by not being able to fall or stay asleep without any of the above symptoms. A Liver pattern causing insomnia is characterized by excessive dreaming and, compared with a Heart pattern, a more severe restlessness.

However, the Heart and Liver are not the only organs that may cause insomnia: the Stomach, Spleen, Kidneys and Gall-Bladder may all play a role in insomnia. For example, a deficiency of Spleen-Blood often accompanies a deficiency of Heart-Blood and con-

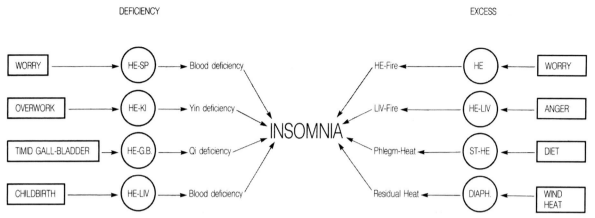

DEFICIENCY   EXCESS

Fig. 40.3 Aetiology and pathology of insomnia (Reproduced with permission from Maciocia G 1994 The Practice of Chinese Medicine, Churchill Livingstone, Edinburgh)

tributes to causing insomnia (the famous formula Gui Pi Tang *Tonifying the Spleen Decoction* treats insomnia from these patterns). Kidney-Yin, like Liver-Yin, also needs to anchor the Mind and the Ethereal Soul at night; therefore a deficiency of Kidney-Yin, with or without Empty-Heat, is also a frequent cause of insomnia.

A deficiency of the Gall-Bladder may cause someone to wake up early in the morning without being able to fall asleep again.

A less common cause of insomnia is residual Heat in the diaphragm, which may occur after an invasion of Wind-Heat; this is obviously an acute type of insomnia with recent onset.

For a detailed description of the patterns causing insomnia see Part 5, Chapter 81. Figure 40.3 illustrates the aetiology and pathology of insomnia differentiated into the main Empty and Full patterns.

The main patterns appearing in insomnia are summarized in Box 40.1.

Other doctors define 'excessive dreaming' as waking up with an unpleasant feeling from dreaming; by implication, from a Chinese perspective, 'normal' dreaming is not remembered in the morning.

'Excessive dreaming' was called *Ye You*, which means 'wandering at night', or *Meng You*, which means 'wandering in one's dream', or *Meng Xing*, which means 'moving in one's dream': all these terms are a clear reference to the wandering of the Ethereal Soul at night when we dream too much.

With the exception of Heart and Gall-Bladder deficiency, excessive dreaming is usually caused by a Full condition, generally of the Liver or Heart, such as Liver-Fire, Heart-Fire or Phlegm-Fire in the Heart. Full conditions of the Stomach also frequently cause excessive dreaming, especially Phlegm-Fire in the Stomach and retention of food.

The main patterns causing excessive dreaming are summarized in Box 40.2.

EXCESSIVE DREAMING

Symptoms and Signs, Chapter 81

Excessive dreaming is another common sleep disturbance, which is usually due to a pathogenic factor agitating the Ethereal Soul; this may be either a pathogenic factor such as Fire or Phlegm-Fire, or such a one as Empty-Heat deriving from Yin deficiency.

'Excessive dreaming' is difficult to define because dreaming is a normal, physiological aspect of sleep. From the perspective of Chinese medicine it can be defined as a level of dreaming, whether pleasant or unpleasant, that makes the sleeper restless or wakes the patient up; it also includes nightmares, especially when they are recurrent.

SOMNOLENCE

Interrogation, Chapter 44; Symptoms and Signs, Chapter 81

Somnolence means dozing off frequently in the daytime or early evening. Some Chinese books also add that the patient wakes up as he or she breathes out and then dozes off again. 'Somnolence' also includes some people's physiological need of sleeping a longer time than normal, which, in adults, is approximately 7–8 hours.

Somnolence may be due to Deficiency, usually of Qi or Yang, or both, or to Excess, such as Dampness or Phlegm. The most common situation is a combination of Deficiency (of the Spleen or Kidneys, or both) and a Full condition consisting of Dampness or Phlegm.

BOX 40.1 INSOMNIA

- Heart-Blood deficiency: insomnia with difficulty in falling asleep, palpitations, Pale tongue, Choppy or Fine pulse
- Deficiency of Qi and Blood of the Spleen and Heart: insomnia with difficulty in falling asleep, palpitations, tiredness, Pale tongue, Choppy pulse
- Heart-Yin deficiency: insomnia with difficulty in falling asleep, palpitations, tongue without coating, Floating-Empty pulse
- Liver-Blood deficiency: insomnia with difficulty in falling asleep, dreaming, dizziness, blurred vision, Pale tongue, Choppy or Fine pulse
- Liver-Yin deficiency: insomnia with difficulty in falling asleep, dreaming, dizziness, blurred vision, dry eyes, tongue without coating, Floating-Empty pulse
- Heart- and Kidney-Yin deficiency: insomnia with difficulty in falling asleep, dizziness, tinnitus, tongue without coating, Floating-Empty pulse
- Heart- and Kidney-Yin deficiency with Heart Empty-Heat: insomnia, waking up frequently during the night with a dry mouth, dreaming, anxiety, night sweating, dizziness, tinnitus, Red tongue without coating, Floating-Empty and Rapid pulse
- Liver-Yin deficiency with Empty-Heat: insomnia with difficulty in staying asleep, blurred vision, dry eyes, Red tongue without coating, Floating-Empty and slightly Rapid pulse
- Gall-Bladder deficiency: easily awakened at night and easily startled with difficulty in going back to sleep, or apt to wake up early in the morning, depression, timidity, hypochondrial discomfort, palpitations
- Liver-Fire: insomnia, excessive dreaming, restless sleep, propensity to outbursts of anger, headaches, Red tongue with redder sides and dry yellow coating, Wiry-Rapid pulse
- Phlegm-Fire harassing the Stomach/Heart: restless sleep, insomnia, dream-disturbed sleep, sputum in throat, Red tongue with redder tip and a sticky yellow coating, Slippery-Overflowing-Rapid pulse
- Heart-Fire: restless sleep, dream-disturbed sleep, palpitations, agitation, Red tongue with redder tip and yellow coating, Overflowing-Rapid pulse
- Residual Heat in the diaphragm: restless sleep, preference for sleeping propped up, inability to fall asleep, mental restlessness, a feeling of oppression of the diaphragm, red points in the front or around the centre of the tongue, slightly Rapid pulse
- Full-Heat (Heart, Liver or Stomach), Phlegm-Fire (Stomach and/or Heart): restless sleep with excessive dreaming
- Retention of food: restless sleep with abdominal fullness

BOX 40.2 EXCESSIVE DREAMING

- Liver-Fire: excessive dreaming, nightmares, restless sleep, headaches, Red tongue with redder sides and dry yellow coating, Wiry-Rapid pulse
- Heart-Fire: excessive dreaming, restless sleep, palpitations, insomnia, Red tongue with redder tip and yellow coating, Overflowing-Rapid pulse
- Phlegm-Fire harassing the Heart: excessive dreaming, restless sleep, insomnia, waking up from nightmares, palpitations, agitation, sputum in throat, Red tongue with redder tip and a sticky yellow coating, Slippery-Overflowing Rapid pulse
- Phlegm-Fire in the Stomach: excessive, agitated dreams, restless sleep, burning epigastric pain, insomnia, Red tongue with a sticky yellow or dark-yellow (or even black) coating, Stomach crack with a rough, sticky yellow coating inside it, Slippery-Rapid and slightly Overflowing pulse on the Right-Middle position
- Heart-Yin deficiency with Empty-Heat: dream-disturbed sleep, insomnia, Red tongue with redder tip and without coating, Floating-Empty and Rapid pulse
- Liver-Yin deficiency with Empty-Heat: dream-disturbed sleep, insomnia, blurred vision, dry eyes, Red tongue without coating, Floating-Empty and slightly Rapid pulse
- Heart- and Kidney-Yin deficiency with Empty-Heat: dream-disturbed sleep, palpitations, dizziness, tinnitus, Red tongue with redder tip without coating, midline Heart crack, Floating-Empty and Rapid pulse, or Deep-Weak on both Rear positions and relatively Overflowing on both Front positions
- Heart and Gall-Bladder deficiency: excessive dreaming, waking up easily from dreaming, absentmindedness, emotionally unstable, anxiety and palpitations

societies) then somnolence is not a pathological symptom.

For a detailed description of the patterns causing somnolence, see Part 5, Chapter 81.

Box 40.3 summarizes the patterns underlying somnolence.

BOX 40.3 SOMNOLENCE

- Spleen-Yang deficiency: somnolence, desire to lie down, loose stools, Pale tongue, Weak pulse
- Kidney-Yang deficiency: somnolence, listlessness, backache, dizziness, tinnitus, Pale-Swollen tongue, Deep-Weak pulse
- Dampness: somnolence after eating, feeling of heaviness, sticky coating, Slippery pulse
- Phlegm: somnolence after eating and in the morning, muzziness of the head, dizziness, Swollen tongue with sticky coating, Slippery pulse

Of course, when a patient complains of somnolence, one should first of all enquire about the patient's working hours: if the person works very long hours (a very common occurrence in Western industrialized

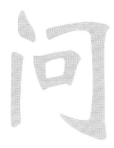

Chapter **41**

SWEATING

Chapter contents

INTRODUCTION   *351*

CLINICAL SIGNIFICANCE OF SWEATING   *352*
   Exterior patterns   *352*
   Interior patterns   *352*

PATHOLOGY OF SWEATING   *352*

CLASSIFICATION OF SWEATING   *353*
   Area of body   *353*
   Time of day   *353*
   Condition of illness   *353*
   Quality of sweat   *353*

ABSENCE OF SWEATING   *353*

INTRODUCTION

Excessive sweating is always considered a symptom requiring the doctor's attention in Chinese medicine. In order to define 'excessive sweating' we should bear in mind that under certain circumstances sweating is a normal physiological process. For example, it is normal to sweat during exercise, after eating spicy foods, in very hot weather and when under emotional strain.

❓ **WHY** WE ASK

Daytime spontaneous sweating is not a crucial area of questioning for various reasons. First of all, it is a symptom that only Chinese patients are particularly aware of and which they therefore often report spontaneously. Western patients report this symptom quite rarely. In terms of clinical significance as part of a pattern, daytime spontaneous sweating is seldom a crucial manifestation that clinches a diagnosis.

An exception to this occurs when we see a patient during an acute invasion of Wind, in which case we should always ask whether there is sweating or not. The presence of sweating indicates that the pathogenic factor is either Wind-Heat or Wind-Cold but with the prevalence of Wind (Wind Attack Pattern of the Greater-Yang Pattern) and that the patient's Upright Qi is relatively weak. Conversely, absence of sweating during an invasion of external Wind generally indicates that Cold predominates over Wind and that the patient's Upright Qi is strong.

Night sweating is quite different in so far as Western patients are more aware of this symptom; in particular, in menopausal women this is a major symptom that is definitely reported by the patient. Night sweating is clinically significant to clinch the diagnosis of

Yin deficiency (although it should be remembered that other patterns may cause night sweating, e.g. Damp-Heat, Stomach-Heat, etc.).

? **WHEN** WE ASK

I ask about daytime sweating mostly to confirm a diagnosis of Lung-Qi deficiency and about night sweating to confirm a diagnosis of Yin deficiency. If night-time sweating appears without any manifestation of Yin deficiency, then we need to think again and check whether this symptom is being caused by Damp-Heat or other less common patterns.

? **HOW** WE ASK

When asking about daytime sweating, I generally ask, 'Do you tend to sweat abnormally even in the absence of exercise?' In the case of night-time sweating, the question is easier and I simply ask, 'Do you tend to sweat at night sometimes?' We should, however, exclude night sweating that is simply caused by too heavy a blanket and too hot a bedroom.

CLINICAL SIGNIFICANCE OF SWEATING

Evaluation of symptoms of sweating must be made by considering if it is part of an exterior or interior pattern.

Exterior patterns

In exterior patterns, spontaneous sweating indicates either invasion of Wind-Cold with the prevalence of Wind, which is due to a disharmony of Nutritive and Defensive Qi, or invasion of Wind-Heat. In invasion of Wind-Cold with the prevalence of Wind, the deficient Nutritive Qi fails to hold fluids in the space between skin and muscles, the pores are open and the patient sweats slightly. It is important to note that this is not a profuse, spontaneous sweating and the patient may not be aware of it unless we ask. In exterior patterns, slight sweating may also occur during invasions of Wind-Heat, Wind-Dampness or Summer-Heat.

In the course of acute febrile diseases, when the pathogenic factor penetrates into the Interior there is often profuse sweating, such as at the Bright-Yang stage of the Six Stages or the Qi level of the Four Levels.

Interior patterns

In interior patterns, spontaneous sweating is due to Qi or Yang deficiency, or to Full-Heat if it occurs in daytime and to Yin deficiency or Damp-Heat if it occurs at night. In Qi or Yang deficiency it is usually a deficiency of Lungs or Heart; in Full-Heat it is usually Heat (or Damp-Heat) in the Heart, Liver, Lungs or Stomach.

> **!**
>
> Night sweating is *not* always due to Yin deficiency.

Box 41.1 summarizes the patterns causing sweating in interior conditions.

> **BOX 41.1 SWEATING IN INTERIOR CONDITIONS**
>
> **Daytime sweating**
> - Qi deficiency (of Lungs/Heart)
> - Yang deficiency (of Lungs, Heart or Kidneys)
> - Collapse of Yang or Yin
> - Liver-Fire
> - Heart-Fire
> - Lung-Heat
> - Stomach-Heat
> - Damp-Heat in the Stomach and Spleen
> - Phlegm-Heat in the Lungs
> - Phlegm-Heat in the Heart
> - Phlegm-Heat in the Stomach
>
> **Night sweating**
> - Yin deficiency (of any organ)
> - Yin deficiency with Empty-Heat
> - Damp-Heat in Stomach and Spleen
> - Deficiency of Qi and Blood of the Heart

PATHOLOGY OF SWEATING

Daytime sweating involves loss of fluids from the space between skin and muscles where the Defensive Qi circulates; sweating at night (called *Dao Han* in Chinese, which literally means 'thief sweating') involves loss of fluids from the bone level and is often called 'steaming from the bones'. Therefore the fluids lost during night sweating are more precious than those lost during

daytime sweating: the fluids lost during daytime sweating are simply Body Fluids (*Jin-Ye*), whereas those lost during night sweating are nutritive Yin Essences. However, both daytime and night-time sweating start a pathological vicious circle because they can derive from a deficiency but also aggravate that deficiency. In fact, daytime sweating injures Qi (the pores are called 'Qi holes') while night sweating injures Yin.

Old Chinese books say that night-time sweat tastes sweet (because it is a Yin Essence), while sweat lost in daytime tastes salty.

Besides daytime and night-time sweating, there are two other types of sweating: sweating from collapse (*Jue Han*); and shiver sweating (*Zhan Han*).

Sweating from collapse occurs during collapse of Yang or collapse of Yin: the sweat from collapse of Yin is oily, whereas that from collapse of Yang pours out in watery and dilute drops.

Shiver sweating is seen usually in acute, febrile diseases and is characterized by a bout of shivering followed by sweating. If the fever abates after sweating, and the pulse is quiet and the body feels cold to the touch, this means that the pathogenic factor has been expelled and the Upright Qi has prevailed; but if after sweating there is restlessness and the pulse is Rapid it indicates that the pathogenic factor has prevailed and the Upright Qi has been severely weakened.

CLASSIFICATION OF SWEATING

Observation, Chapter 20; Symptoms and Signs, Chapter 76

One must distinguish sweating according to the area of body, time of day, conditions and quality of sweat.

Area of body

The significance of body areas may be summarized as:

- **only on head**: Heat or Damp-Heat in the Stomach, Heat in the Upper Burner, deficient Yang floating upwards, retention of food
- **only on hands and feet**: deficiency of Qi or Yin of the Lungs or Heart and Kidneys; it could also be due to Heat in the Lungs or Heart and Kidneys
- **oily sweat on forehead**: collapse of Yin
- **only on nose**: Damp-Heat in the Lungs or Stomach, or both

- **only on arms and legs**: Stomach and Spleen deficiency
- **only on hands**: deficiency of Qi or Yin of the Lungs or Heart, or Heat in the Lungs or Heart
- **whole body**: Lung-Qi deficiency
- **on palms, soles and chest**: Yin deficiency (called five-palm sweat).

Time of day

The significance of time of day may be summarized as:

- **in daytime**: Yang deficiency
- **at night-time**: Yin deficiency (in some cases it can also be from Damp-Heat).

Condition of illness

The conditions of illness are:

- **profuse cold sweat during a severe illness**: collapse of Yang
- **sweat on forehead, like pearls, not flowing**: collapse of Yang, danger of imminent death.

Quality of sweat

The different qualities of sweat are:

- **oily**: severe Yin deficiency
- **yellow**: Damp-Heat.

ABSENCE OF SWEATING

Symptoms and Signs, Chapter 76

Absence of sweating is also a symptom in Chinese medicine. In exterior invasions of Wind, it is always important to ask about sweating: the absence of sweating indicates invasion of Wind-Cold with the prevalence of Cold and this corresponds to the Greater-Yang stage within the Six Stages identification of patterns. The Greater-Yang stage is always caused by the invasion of Wind-Cold, of which there are two types: one with the prevalence of Cold (in which there is no sweating), the other with the prevalence of Wind (in which there is sweating).

In other exterior conditions, absence of sweating usually indicates Cold or Cold-Dampness in the superficial layers of the body (the space between skin and muscles).

In interior conditions, absence of sweating indicates a 'tight' and excessively closed state of the space between the skin and muscles (*Cou Li*). This renders the person more prone to fever when invaded by a pathogenic factor and it also indicates that the person is more prone to Full than Empty conditions.

For a more detailed description of various types of sweating, see Part 5, Chapter 76.

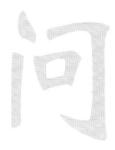

Chapter **42**

EARS AND EYES

Chapter contents

EARS   *355*
  Tinnitus   *356*
  Deafness   *357*
  Earache   *357*
  Itchy ears   *357*

EYES   *357*
  Eye pain   *358*
  Itchy eyes   *359*
  Feeling of distension of the eyes   *360*
  Streaming eyes   *360*
  Dry eyes   *360*
  Blurred vision   *360*

EARS

The ears are the orifices of the Kidneys and for this reason tinnitus and deafness are often due to a Kidney deficiency. However, the ears are also influenced by many other organs including the Liver, Heart, Lungs and Gall-Bladder. In addition, although the Spleen is not directly related to the ears, Dampness or Phlegm (deriving from Spleen-Qi deficiency) may also affect the ears.

? **WHY** WE ASK

I generally ask about any ear symptoms under three main circumstances: when there is a Kidney deficiency, Liver-Yang rising or Phlegm. In the last of these, Phlegm obstructs the orifices and may cause tinnitus or deafness.

? **WHEN** WE ASK

I usually ask about any ear symptoms towards the end of the consultation, primarily to confirm a pattern of Kidney deficiency, Liver-Yang rising or Phlegm.

? **HOW** WE ASK

When asking about tinnitus it is important to express this symptom in terms patients can understand. I generally ask them whether they experience any 'ringing in the ears'. It is important to let the patient understand that even an occasional ringing in the ears has clinical significance.

In general terms, the ears may be affected by a pathology of Deficiency (usually of the Kidneys but also of Lung and Heart) causing tinnitus, hardness of hearing or deafness, or by one of Fullness, usually due to Heat or Phlegm.

The main deficiency patterns affecting the ear are:

- Kidney deficiency (or Yin or Yang) causing tinnitus or deafness, or both
- Lung-Qi deficiency causing tinnitus
- Heart-Blood deficiency causing tinnitus.

The main Full patterns affecting the ears are:

- Liver-Yang rising causing tinnitus and deafness
- Liver-Fire causing tinnitus and deafness
- Phlegm in the head causing tinnitus
- Damp-Heat in the Gall-Bladder causing earache.

Tinnitus

Symptoms and Signs, Chapter 57

Tinnitus is caused either by a failure of Qi to rise to the ears (Empty type) or by an excess of Qi in the ears (Full type). In order to differentiate between the Empty types and the Full types, we need to consider the onset, the pitch, the duration and the reaction to pressure of the tinnitus.

A sudden onset suggests a Full condition, which may be internal such as Liver-Fire or Liver-Wind, or external such as Heat in the Lesser Yang. A gradual onset suggests an Empty condition, which may be due to a deficiency of the Kidneys, Lung or Heart.

A loud, high-pitched, ringing noise like a whistle indicates Liver-Yang rising, Liver-Fire or Liver-Wind, whereas a low-pitched noise like rushing water indicates a Kidney deficiency.

Tinnitus of short duration is usually due to an external invasion of Wind-Heat affecting the Lesser Yang channels. Chronic tinnitus of long duration is due to either a Kidney deficiency or a Liver pathology (Liver-Yang rising, Liver-Fire, or Liver-Wind).

If the tinnitus is aggravated by pressing one's hands on the ears, this suggests a Full condition; if it is alleviated it suggests an Empty condition.

Case history 42.1 illustrates a pattern of tinnitus caused by Yin deficiency.

Box 42.1 summarizes the patterns underlying tinnitus.

> **BOX 42.1 TINNITUS**
>
> - Lesser-Yang Heat pattern: tinnitus of sudden onset and alternation of chills and fever
> - Liver-Fire or Liver-Yang rising: tinnitus of sudden onset with headache
> - Liver-Fire, Liver-Wind or Liver-Yang rising: high-pitched tinnitus
> - Kidney deficiency: low-pitched tinnitus
> - Liver-Fire, Liver-Yang rising or Liver-Wind: chronic, severe tinnitus
> - Kidney deficiency: chronic, mild, intermittent tinnitus
> - Deficiency of Heart- and Lung-Qi: chronic, mild, intermittent tinnitus with palpitations and weak voice

Case history 42.1

A 56-year-old woman had been suffering from tinnitus for 3 years. The onset had been slow and gradual and the ear noise was low in pitch. She also suffered from poor memory, lack of concentration, blurred vision, dizziness and hot flushes (flashes). On asking her, it transpired that she also experience a dry mouth, anxiety and palpitations. Her urine was dark. She also said that she startled easily.

She also experienced occasionally a dull ache in the chest, with the pain sensation extending up to the neck like a 'steel band'.

Her periods had stopped 2 years previously. Her tongue was Red, with a redder tip, entirely without coating and dry. Her pulse was Weak on both Rear positions and very slightly Wiry but Fine on the left.

Diagnosis: This patient presents with very clear manifestations of Kidney-Yin deficiency (dark urine, tinnitus, dizziness, blurred vision, hot flushes) and Heart-Yin deficiency (poor memory and concentration, palpitations, anxiety and propensity to be startled). The condition of Yin deficiency is shown very clearly by the absence of coating, and the redness of the tongue (combined with the lack of coating) clearly indicates Empty-Heat. I interpreted the dull ache in the chest extending to the neck as a symptom of rebellious Qi of the Penetrating Vessel, a common complicating factor in menopausal problems. The Wiry quality of the pulse on the left supports this diagnosis.

Deafness

Symptoms and Signs, Chapter 57

The diagnostic criteria of deafness or hardness of hearing are similar to those of tinnitus: an acute onset points to Fullness, whereas a gradual onset points to Deficiency. The main Excess causes of deafness or hardness of hearing are Liver-Fire, Liver-Yang rising and Phlegm-Fire affecting the Liver channel.

The main Empty cause of deafness or hardness of hearing is a Kidney deficiency (the most common cause in the elderly). However, the Kidneys are not the only organ that influences the ears; hardness of hearing may also be caused by Heart-Blood, Heart-Yin, Lung- or Heart-Qi deficiency, or deficiency of the Gathering Qi (*Zong-Qi*) or Yang-Qi. In all these cases, hardness of hearing is due to Qi or Blood not flowing upwards to the ears.

Box 42.2 summarizes the patterns underlying deafness.

BOX 42.2 DEAFNESS

- Kidney deficiency: dizziness, tinnitus, backache
- Liver-Yang rising: dizziness, tinnitus, headache
- Liver-Fire: tinnitus, thirst, bitter taste
- Phlegm-Fire in the Liver channel: dizziness, tinnitus, sputum in throat, headache
- Heart- and Kidney-Yin deficiency: dizziness, palpitations, insomnia
- Lung- and Heart-Qi deficiency: palpitation, shortness of breath, weak voice
- Heart-Blood deficiency: palpitations, poor memory, insomnia

---

Earache

Symptoms and Signs, Chapter 57

With the exception of Qi and Blood stagnation, earache is usually due to Heat; this can be an invasion of Wind-Heat affecting the Lesser-Yang channels (which is very common in children, and accompanied by aversion to cold and fever), Damp-Heat in the Liver and Gall-Bladder channel or Liver-Fire. A yellow discharge from the ear may accompany an invasion of Wind-Heat or Damp-Heat in the Liver and Gall-Bladder. Earache from Liver-Fire is accompanied by headache, a red face and a bitter taste in the mouth. The chronic earache from Qi and Blood stagnation is not common and is usually seen only in the elderly.

BOX 42.3 EARACHE

- Wind-Heat in Lesser Yang channels: aversion to cold, fever, yellow discharge
- Damp-Heat in Gall-Bladder: ear discharge
- Liver-Fire: headache, red face, bitter taste in mouth
- Qi and Blood stagnation: chronic earache (in the elderly)

Box 42.3 summarizes the patterns underlying earache.

Itchy ears

Symptoms and Signs, Chapter 57

In acute cases, itchiness in the ears is due to invasion of Wind-Heat in the Lesser-Yang channels. In chronic cases, it is due either to Blood deficiency leading to internal Wind or to Kidney-Yin deficiency with Empty-Heat.

Box 42.4 summarizes the patterns underlying itchy ears.

BOX 42.4 ITCHY EARS

- Wind-Heat in the Lesser-Yang channels: acute
- Blood deficiency leading to Wind: chronic
- Kidney-Yin deficiency with Empty-Heat: chronic

EYES

The eyes are the orifice of the Liver, but this does not mean that all eye problems are related to the Liver. In fact, other organs affect the eyes and notable among these are the Heart, Kidneys and Gall-Bladder.

The Heart influences the eyes as both its Main and Connecting channels go to the eyeballs (see Fig. 6.1 on p. 77). For this reason, many eye problems are due to Heart-Heat deriving from emotional problems.

The Kidneys nourish and moisten the eyes in a similar way to the Liver, and eye problems in the elderly are very frequently due to a Kidney deficiency.

The Gall-Bladder channel also goes through the eyes and it may cause eye problems, usually in conjunction with Liver-Fire or Liver-Yang rising.

❓ **WHY** WE ASK

The questions regarding the eyes are somewhat more important than those regarding the ears, first because

eye problems are more common and secondly because some eye symptoms often clinch a diagnosis. For example, the symptom of dry eyes often clinches the diagnosis of Liver-Yin deficiency (although it may also be caused by Kidney-Yin deficiency).

? WHEN WE ASK

I ask about eye symptoms early during the interrogation in conjunction with questions aimed at identifying a particular pattern. For example, if a patient displays symptoms of Liver-Blood deficiency, I would ask about blurred vision and floaters immediately; I would then ask about dry eyes to find out whether the Liver-Blood deficiency has progressed to a deeper level of Liver-Yin deficiency.

Questions regarding blurred vision, floaters, dry eyes and red/painful/itchy eyes are important and I ask them in nearly every case.

? HOW WE ASK

'Blurred vision' is not an expression most patients are familiar with. I generally ask them whether their vision is sometimes 'not clear or somewhat obfuscated', stressing that the condition at issue is quite apart from their being short sighted or not. 'Floaters' is another expression most patients are not familiar with and I generally ask whether they ever see 'black or white spots floating in the field of vision'.

Eye pain

Symptoms and Signs, Chapter 61

Full or Empty character of eye pain

Table 42.1 and Figure 42.1 summarize the Full and Empty characteristics of eye pain.

Radiation of pain

Eye pain should also be differentiated according to its radiation. If the pain radiates to the occiput, the Greater-Yang channels are affected; if it radiates to the sides of the head and the outer corners of the eyes, the Lesser-Yang channels are affected; if it radiates to the nose and teeth, the Bright-Yang channels are affected; if it radiates to the top of the head, the Liver channel is affected.

Eye pain of internal or external origin

Eye pain can first be differentiated into internal and external types (Fig. 42.1); secondly internal eye pain can be differentiated into Full and Empty as indicated in Table 42.1.

Table 42.1 Full and Empty characteristics of eye pain

	Full/Yang	Empty/Yin
Onset	Sudden	Gradual
Time	Day	Night
Time of day	Morning	Afternoon
Constancy	Chronic and persistent	Chronic on and off
Swelling	With swelling	Without swelling
Intensity	Severe, unbearable	Dull, mild
Inflammation	Inflamed, red and hot	Not red, not hot
Pressure	Worse with pressure	Better with pressure
Temperature	Worse with heat, better with cold	Worse with cold, better with heat
Irritability	Pain with irritability (Liver)	Pain without irritability (Yang deficiency)
Character of pain	Pain like needles	Mild pain
Food	Worse after eating	Better after eating, worse when hungry
Two excretions (urination and defecation)	Redness, excretions affected	No redness, excretions not affected
Eyeball movement	With moving eyeballs	Eyeballs not moving

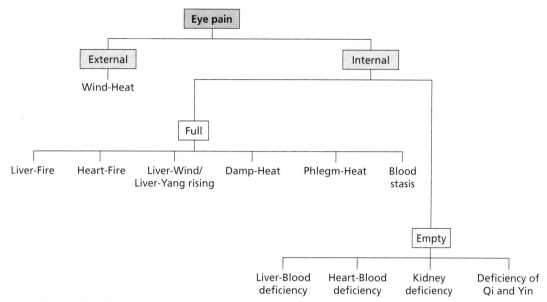

Fig. 42.1 Differentiation of eye pain

Eye pain of external origin is mostly due to invasion of Wind-Heat and is characterized by a sudden onset, sticky eyelids and streaming eyes, with an aversion to cold and a fever.

Eye pain from a Full condition is often accompanied by swelling and redness.

Box 42.5 summarizes the patterns underlying eye pain.

BOX 42.5 EYE PAIN

Full
- Wind-Heat: acute onset, sticky and streaming eyes, aversion to cold, fever
- Liver-Fire: red eyes, thirst, bitter taste, Wiry pulse
- Liver-Yang rising: headache, eye distension
- Heart-Fire: red eyes, palpitations, anxiety
- Liver-Wind: vertigo
- Damp-Heat: sticky eyelids, sticky yellow tongue coating
- Phlegm-Heat: sticky eyelids, feeling of oppression of the chest, dizziness
- Blood stasis: bulging eyes, dark complexion, Purple tongue

Empty
- Liver-Blood deficiency: dizziness, blurred vision
- Heart-Blood deficiency: insomnia, poor memory, palpitations
- Kidney deficiency: dizziness, tinnitus
- Deficiency of Qi and Yin: slightly hot and painful eyes, mild pain, desire to shut eyes, red eyes, tiredness, dry eyes

---

Itchy eyes

Symptoms and Signs, Chapter 61

Excluding invasions of external Wind, itchy eyes are usually caused either by Liver-Fire or by a deficiency of Liver-Blood giving rise to Liver-Wind. Itchy eyes in allergic rhinitis are a separate pathology which is not Liver-related, but is related to external Wind as the reaction caused by the invasion of allergens mimics that of invasion of external Wind.

Box 42.6 summarizes the patterns underlying itchy eyes.

BOX 42.6 ITCHY EYES

- Liver-Fire: intensely itchy and red eyes
- Liver-Blood deficiency leading to Wind: intense itchiness and tic of the face
- External Wind: acute

Feeling of distension of the eyes

Symptoms and Signs, Chapter 61

A feeling of distension of the eyes is often associated with emotional problems affecting the Liver, causing Liver-Qi stagnation and Liver-Fire.

Streaming eyes

Observation, Chapter 6; Symptoms and Signs, Chapter 61

Streaming eyes may be due to Heat of the Full or Empty type. In particular, it may be due to Full-or Empty-Heat of the Lung or Stomach.

Other causes of streaming eyes include external Wind-Heat, Liver-Fire and Liver-Blood deficiency associated with Liver-Heat. In some cases, streaming eyes may be due to Liver-Blood deficiency and general Qi deficiency or to Kidney-Yang deficiency: these two types of streaming eyes are called 'cold streaming'.

Box 42.7 summarizes the patterns underlying streaming eyes.

BOX 42.7 STREAMING EYES

- Lung-Heat: cough
- Lung Empty-Heat: dry cough
- Stomach-Heat: epigastric pain, thirst
- Stomach Empty-Heat: epigastric pain, thirst with desire to sip
- External Wind-Heat: aversion to cold, fever
- Liver-Fire: red eyes, bitter taste
- Liver-Blood deficiency with some Heat: blurred vision, red eyes
- Liver-Blood deficiency: blurred vision
- Kidney-Yang deficiency: backache, abundant clear urine
- General Qi deficiency: tiredness, loose stools, weak voice

Dry eyes

Symptoms and Signs, Chapter 61

The most common causes of dry eyes are severe Liver-Blood deficiency or Liver-Yin deficiency. In the elderly, dry eyes are often due to Liver- and Kidney-Yin deficiency; in some cases Lung-Yin deficiency is also involved. Dry eyes with acute onset may be due to invasion of Wind-Heat, in which case they would also be red.

Box 42.8 summarizes the patterns underlying dry eyes.

BOX 42.8 DRY EYES

- Liver-Yin deficiency: blurred vision
- Liver- and Kidney-Yin deficiency: dizziness, tinnitus
- Lung-Yin deficiency: dry cough
- External Wind-Heat: acute onset, red eyes, aversion to cold, fever

---

Blurred vision

Symptoms and Signs, Chapter 61

'Blurred vision', called *Mu Xuan* in Chinese, indicates not only blurring of vision and floaters but also includes a slight dizziness.

Although blurred vision is a relatively common complaint, when asked whether they suffer from it most patients will either answer negatively or not know what we mean. Thus, this question should be asked in a different way, such as 'Do you have any problems with your vision?' or 'Is your vision sometimes unclear?'

First of all, it should be remembered that the eyes are under the control not only of the Liver but also of the Gall-Bladder and Kidneys; especially in the elderly, a Kidney deficiency is often at the root of eye problems and blurred vision.

Among the Deficiency types, the most common causes of blurred vision are Liver-Blood or Liver-Yin deficiency. If blurred vision is associated with dryness of the eyes, this suggests either Liver-Yin deficiency or Liver- and Kidney-Yin deficiency, which is common in the elderly.

Blurred vision may also be due to Excess patterns such as Gall-Bladder Heat, Liver-Yang rising (a common feature in migraine), Liver-Fire and Phlegm. Phlegm, in particular, is not often recognized as a possible cause of blurred vision; however, it may cause a blurring of vision with muzziness and dizziness because it obstructs the clear orifices of the head, including the eyes (for the same reason, Phlegm may cause tinnitus).

Box 42.9 summarizes the patterns underlying blurred vision.

BOX 42.9 BLURRED VISION

- Liver-Blood deficiency: floaters, dizziness
- Liver-Yin deficiency: dry eyes
- Kidney-Yin deficiency: dizziness, tinnitus
- Gall-Bladder Heat: eye pain, red eyes
- Liver-Yang rising: headache
- Liver-Fire: red, painful eyes
- Phlegm: dizziness, muzziness

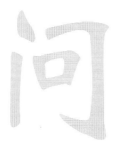

Chapter **43**

FEELING OF COLD, FEELING OF HEAT AND FEVER

Chapter contents

INTRODUCTION   *361*

FEELING OF COLD   *362*
  Feeling of cold in interior conditions   *363*
  Feeling of cold in exterior conditions   *365*
  How to distinguish between external and internal causes of feeling of cold   *366*

SIMULTANEOUS FEELING OF COLD AND FEVER IN EXTERIOR CONDITIONS   *367*
  Wind-Cold and Wind-Heat   *369*
  Summer-Heat   *370*
  Damp-Heat   *370*
  Dry-Heat   *370*

ALTERNATING FEELING OF COLD AND FEELING OF HEAT   *370*

FEELING OF HEAT FROM INTERNAL CAUSES   *371*

INTERIOR FEVER   *372*
  Acute fever   *372*
  Chronic fever   *374*

FIVE-PALM HEAT   *376*

CONTRADICTORY FEELINGS OF COLD AND HEAT IN INTERNAL CONDITIONS   *376*
  Simultaneous deficiency of Kidney-Yin and Kidney-Yang   *376*
  Blood deficiency with Empty-Heat   *376*
  Disharmony of the Penetrating Vessel   *376*
  Yin Fire   *376*

INTRODUCTION

Questions about feeling of cold or heat and fever are generally asked towards the end of the interrogation to establish the Hot or Cold nature of a pattern.

? **WHY** WE ASK

We should always ask all our patients about feelings of cold or heat; the clinical significance, however, varies in internal and external conditions. In internal conditions (which constitute the overwhelming majority of most practices) the distinction between feelings of cold and feelings of heat simply tells us about the Cold or Hot nature of the prevailing pattern.

In external conditions (e.g. when a patient presents with an acute cold or influenza) questions about feelings of cold or heat are needed primarily to establish, first of all, whether it is indeed an external condition and whether the pathogenic factor is on the Exterior or Interior.

The patient's cold or hot feeling should never be discounted, even when it contradicts the tongue or pulse, or both. For example, a patient may have a clearly Red tongue but always feel cold: although the sign of a Red tongue is very important, we should not discount the cold feeling and should investigate further to find the cause of this discrepancy.

? **WHEN** WE ASK

As mentioned above, questions about feelings of cold and heat should always be asked routinely in all patients.

In **internal conditions**, questions about a patient's feeling cold or hot are often asked towards the end of the consultation to confirm the existence of a Cold or Hot pattern. Often questions about feelings of cold or heat also help us to detect the constitutional tendency of a patient to Cold or Hot conditions. For example, patients may not have significant symptoms of Yang deficiency and Cold but, on asking, may say that they always feel cold, need to wear more clothes than other people, etc.; this symptom should never be discounted because it indicates an underlying tendency to Yang deficiency and Cold patterns.

In **external conditions**, questions about feelings of cold and heat are crucial and should always be asked in detail to establish whether the pathogenic factor has gone into the Interior or whether it is still on the Exterior. If we see a patient every day in the course of an acute, exterior condition, as we should, we should carefully ask about feelings of cold and heat every day to establish the exterior or interior nature of the pattern.

? **HOW** WE ASK

In China, the questions about feeling of cold and feeling of heat coincide almost exactly with the terminology of Chinese medicine, which makes it very easy for Chinese doctors. With Western patients, it is a little more difficult and we need to make sure that we ask patients about feelings of cold and heat in a way that they can readily understand.

In interior conditions, for feelings of cold we should simply ask, 'Do you feel cold in general?', 'Do you have a tendency to feel cold?' or 'Do you notice that you feel colder than other people?'. For feelings of heat we should ask questions such as, 'Would you say you feel hot in general?', 'Do you sometimes feel unusually hot?' or 'Do you want to open the window when everyone else wants it closed?' If patients answer affirmatively to one of the above questions about feelings of heat, then we should go on to ask more specifically about when they tend to feel hot in order to establish whether it is Full- or Empty-Heat. We therefore ask questions such as 'Do you tend to feel hotter in the afternoon or evening?'

Terminology

Before discussing the various causes of feeling cold, or feeling of hot and feverish, I would like to clarify some

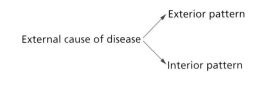

points regarding terminology, particularly with regard to fever.

The *cause* of disease in feeling of cold, feeling of heat or fever may be **external** (e.g. external Wind) or **internal**; thus, the cause of disease simply refers to the origin of the pathogenic factor.

The *pattern* (or *syndrome*) refers to the location of the pathogenic factor, which may be on the **Interior** or **Exterior**: this is decided *not* according to the origin of the pathogenic factor but on the basis of the clinical manifestations. In other words, an external cause of disease (e.g. external Wind) may cause both an exterior pattern and an interior pattern (Fig. 43.1).

An external cause of disease is, for example, external Wind: this causes initially an exterior pattern; if the pathogenic factor is not expelled, however, it goes on to cause an interior pattern. An internal cause of disease (such as Liver-Fire) causes an interior pattern by definition.

With regard to fever, we should not confuse a fever from an external cause with an exterior fever: an external cause may cause an exterior fever initially and later, if the pathogenic factor is not expelled, it will cause an interior fever.

FEELING OF COLD

Symptoms and Signs, Chapter 82

There are four different degrees of 'cold feeling' which apply both to interior and exterior conditions. In ascending order of severity with their clinical significance these are:

- 'aversion to wind' (*Wu Feng*, literally 'loathing or disliking wind')
- 'fear of cold' (*Wei Han*)
- 'aversion to cold' (*Wu Han*, literally 'loathing or disliking cold')
- 'shivers' (*Han Zhan*).

Aversion to wind means that the patient has goose pimples, dislikes going out in the wind and wants to stay indoors.

Fear of cold means that the patient feels quite cold, wants to stay indoors and close to a source of heat, and wants to cover up.

Aversion to cold means that the patient feels very cold, wants to stay indoors and likes to wrap up in bed with many blankets.

Shivers means that the patient feels extremely cold, shivers and wants to be covered up in bed under a heap of blankets.

The symptoms of feeling cold should be clearly differentiated between interior and exterior patterns.

Feeling of cold in interior conditions

In internal diseases, questions about feeling cold serve to establish the Cold nature of the presenting patterns. Cold may be Full or Empty. Whether it is Full or Empty, it always manifests with a feeling of cold.

If a person feels easily cold and experiences cold limbs, this clearly indicates either Full-Cold or Empty-Cold deriving from Yang deficiency. In patients with chronic diseases, Empty-Cold is more common than Full-Cold.

Full-Cold is characterized by an intense feeling of cold and shivers; the body also feels cold to the touch. Various parts of the body may feel particularly cold depending on the location of the Cold: if it is in the Stomach the limbs and epigastrium will feel cold, if in the Intestines the legs and lower abdomen are cold, if in the Uterus the lower abdomen feels cold. Full-Cold has usually a sudden onset and may last only a few months at the most because Cold will inevitably injure Yang and lead to Yang deficiency and therefore Empty-Cold.

Box 43.1 summarizes the clinical manifestations of Full-Cold.

Yang deficiency of any organ may cause a cold feeling or cold limbs, or both. It could be due especially to a deficiency of Yang of the Heart, Lungs, Spleen, Kidneys and Stomach. The cold feeling is both subjective and objective, that is, the patient feels easily and frequently cold and the limbs or other parts of the body will feel cold to the touch.

A deficiency of Yang of the Lungs or Heart, or both, will manifest especially with cold hands (Fig. 43.2), a deficiency of Spleen-Yang with cold limbs and abdomen (Fig. 43.3) and that of Kidney-Yang especially with cold legs, knees, feet and back (Fig. 43.4). A deficiency of Stomach-Yang will manifest with cold epigastrium and cold limbs in a similar way to Spleen-Yang deficiency (Fig. 43.3).

Box 43.2 summarizes the clinical manifestations of Empty-Cold.

There are however, other causes of cold limbs (as opposed to a general cold feeling). One is Qi stagnation: when Qi stagnates it may fail to reach the hands and feet and these become cold (Fig. 43.5). This is called the 'Four Rebellious Syndrome', in which the 'Four Rebellious' indicate cold hands and feet; the famous formula Si Ni San *Four Rebellious Powder* is used for this pattern. An important difference between cold in the

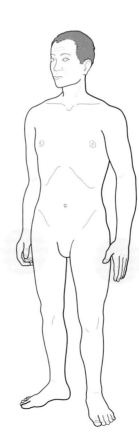

Fig. 43.2 Lung- and Heart-Yang deficiency

BOX 43.1 CLINICAL MANIFESTATIONS OF FULL-COLD

- Intense feeling of cold and shivers
- Body feels noticeably cold and relatively hard to touch
- Pain
- Full pulse
- Sudden onset

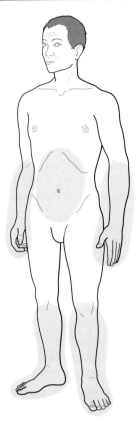

Fig. 43.3 Spleen-Yang deficiency

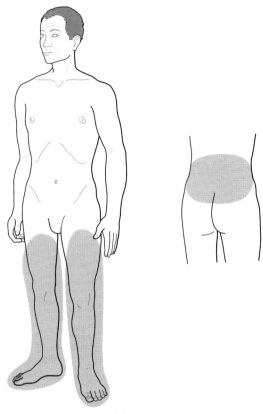

Fig. 43.4 Kidney-Yang deficiency

BOX 43.2 CLINICAL MANIFESTATIONS OF EMPTY-COLD

- Mild, persistent cold feeling or tendency to feeling cold
- Body feels mildly cold to touch
- No pain
- Weak pulse
- Slow, gradual onset

---

limbs due to Yang deficiency and that due to Qi stagnation is that in the former case the whole limb will be cold whereas in the latter case only the hands and feet, and especially the fingers, are cold.

Besides this, cold limbs may also derive in women from Blood deficiency; this is due to the deficient Blood not reaching the extremities. In cases of Heart-Blood deficiency only the hands and chest will be cold (Fig. 43.6), whereas in cases of Liver-Blood deficiency the feet will be cold (Fig. 43.7).

We should bear in mind that, even if patients feel cold in general, they may have a feeling of heat in a specific part of their body, (e.g the face) and we should therefore always remember to ask about specific parts of the body after we have asked about the general

feeling. A very common example of this, especially in women, is a general cold feeling with occasional episodes of feeling hot in the face.

!

When patients feels cold in general, remember to ask then whether they feel hot in any particular part of the body.

Box 43.3 summarizes the patterns underlying a cold feeling and cold limbs in interior conditions.

BOX 43.3 FEELING OF COLD IN INTERIOR CONDITIONS

- Yang Deficiency of Heart/Lungs: cold hands, sweaty hands
- Spleen-Yang/Stomach-Yang deficiency: cold limbs and abdomen
- Kidney-Yang deficiency: cold legs, knees, feet, back
- Qi stagnation: cold hands and feet, and especially the fingers
- Heart-Blood deficiency: cold hands and chest
- Liver-Blood deficiency: cold feet

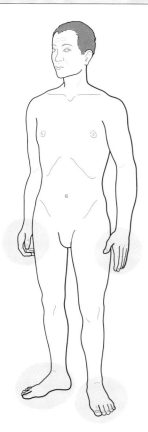

Fig. 43.5 Cold hands and feet from Qi stagnation

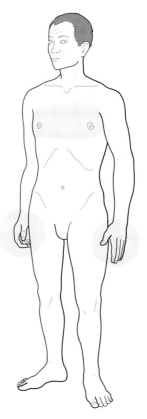

Fig. 43.6 Heart-Blood deficiency

Feeling of cold in exterior conditions
External invasions

In external invasions, a feeling of cold or shivers serves to establish whether the pathogenic factor is in the Exterior or in the Interior. In fact, when the pathogenic factor is on the Exterior, the patient feels cold, shivers and dislikes the idea of going out (often referred to as 'aversion to cold'). The cold feeling may or may not be accompanied by an actual fever, but it will be associated with heat in the skin, that is, the patient feels cold and shivers but his or her skin feels hot to the touch.

The areas that are usually touched to gauge this are the dorsum of the hands and the forehead. It should be stressed that the feeling of cold and fever (or body feeling hot to the touch) are *simultaneous* and not alternating: thus, if a patient feels cold in the morning without a fever and without body feeling hot to the touch and has a fever in the evening, this would correspond to the Lesser-Yang syndrome and would *not* constitute the beginning stage of an invasion of Wind. Figure 43.8 differentiates the manifestations of cold feeling in exterior and interior conditions.

In exterior syndromes, the presence of a cold feeling and shivering is a determining factor in diagnosing that the pathogenic factor is still on the Exterior and that the pattern is therefore an 'Exterior' one. As soon as the cold feeling disappears and the patient feels hot, this is a certain sign that the pathogenic factor is in the Interior and it has transformed into Heat. One can see these signs very clearly in small children: when the pathogenic factor is on the Exterior, the child will tend to go to bed and cover himself or herself with lots of blankets. As the pathogenic factor enters the Interior (usually changing into Heat), the child throws the blankets off.

Box 43.4 summarizes the clinical manifestations of interior and exterior pathogenic factors.

BOX 43.4 INTERIOR VERSUS EXTERIOR PATHOGENIC FACTOR

- Pathogenic factor on the Exterior: feeling of cold, shivers, dislike of going out, possibly a fever, patient is hot to the touch (especially forehead and dorsum of the hand)
- Pathogenic factor in the Interior: cold feeling disappears, patient feels *only* hot

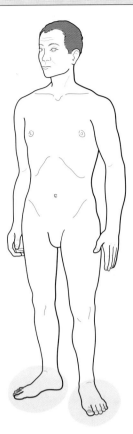

Fig. 43.7 Liver-Blood deficiency

How to distinguish between external and internal causes of feeling of cold

The distinction between a cold feeling from an invasion of external Wind and a cold feeling from internal Cold (which may be Full or Empty) is fairly easy as the accompanying symptoms are quite obvious. During an external invasion with the pathogenic factor still on the Exterior, the patient feels cold, dislikes the idea of going out, shivers, and may have a fever, and the dorsum of the hand feels hot; in addition, there will be sneezing, a cough, a nasal discharge, a sore throat, a headache, body aches and a Floating pulse.

When the patient suffers from interior Cold, there are none of the above symptoms. Another distinction between a cold feeling in exterior syndromes and one in interior syndromes is that in the former case the cold feeling is *not* alleviated by covering oneself, while in the latter case it is. In fact patients who feel cold and shiver from an invasion of exterior Wind will want to go to bed and cover up with blankets, but this will not alleviate the cold feeling and shivering. If a patient suffers from internal Cold, this will be alleviated by covering oneself. Table 43.1 summarizes the differentiation between external and internal Cold.

Wind-Cold versus Wind-Heat

In exterior patterns, both Wind-Cold and Wind-Heat cause a cold feeling and shivering; it is a common misconception that this is not the case with Wind-Heat. Since the cold feeling is caused by the obstruction of Defensive Qi by Wind (whether it is Wind-Cold or Wind-Heat) in the space between skin and muscles, the cold feeling and shivering are present also in invasions of Wind-Heat, albeit to a lesser degree than in Wind-Cold. This will be explained in greater detail below.

Table 43.1 Differentiation between external and internal Cold	
External invasion of Cold	**Internal Cold**
Feels cold, shivers, dislikes going out, fever, sneezing, cough, sore throat, nasal discharge	Feels cold, none of the symptoms associated with an external invasion is present
Cold feeling *not* alleviated by wrapping up in clothes and blankets	Cold feeling *is* alleviated by wrapping up warm

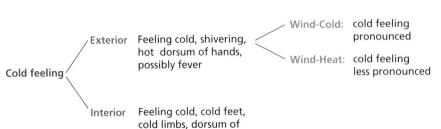

Fig. 43.8 Cold feeling in exterior and interior conditions

Differentiation of pathology of a feeling of cold from external or internal causes

The pathogenesis of a cold feeling in exterior patterns is different from that in interior patterns. In exterior patterns, the cold feeling is due to the fact that the external Wind obstructs the space between skin and muscles where the Defensive Qi circulates; as Defensive Qi warms the muscles, its obstruction by Wind causes the patient to feel cold and shiver (even if the pathogenic factor is Wind-Heat). Thus, Defensive Qi is not necessarily weak but only obstructed in the space between skin and muscles.

In interior patterns, the cold feeling is usually due either to a Yang deficiency and a failure of Yang Qi to warm the muscles and limbs (in case of Empty-Cold) or to Cold obstructing the flow of Yang Qi to the muscles and limbs (in case of Full-Cold).

SIMULTANEOUS FEELING OF COLD AND FEVER IN EXTERIOR CONDITIONS

First of all, we should define 'fever'. 'Fever' does not indicate an actual raised temperature (as measured by a thermometer) but an objective emanation of heat from the patient's body felt on palpation (especially on the forehead and dorsum of hands). This is discussed in more detail below.

A simultaneous feeling of cold and fever indicates the invasion of an exterior pathogenic factor and that this factor is still on the Exterior. The simultaneous presence of a cold feeling or shivers with a fever, or both, usually indicates an acute invasion of Wind and it denotes that the pathogenic factor is still on the Exterior: as long as there is a feeling of cold the pathogenic factor is on the Exterior. The clinical situations when the pathogenic factor is on the Exterior are described in the Greater-Yang pattern within the Six Stages from the 'Discussion of Cold-induced Diseases' (*Shang Han Lun*) and the Defensive-Qi level within the Four Levels described by the School of Warm Diseases (*Wen Bing*) of the Qing dynasty (see Part 6). As mentioned above, it is important to stress that the feeling of cold and fever (or body feeling hot to the touch) are simultaneous and not alternating (Fig. 43.9).

Although it is the simultaneous occurrence of cold feeling and fever that defines an exterior pattern due to invasion of exterior Wind, I shall discuss the pathology of cold feeling and fever in more detail separately.

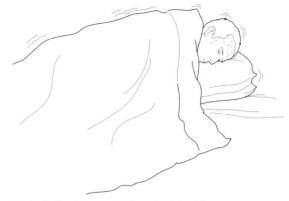

Fig. 43.9 Simultaneous feeling of cold and fever

The aetiology and pathology of Wind-Heat can be used as a blueprint to explain the aetiology and pathology of Summer-Heat, Damp-Heat and Dry-Heat.

The pathogenic factors discussed are:

- Wind-Heat
- Wind-Cold
- Summer-Heat
- Damp-Heat
- Dry-Heat.

Before discussing the above pathogenic factors, we should first discuss the pathology and clinical manifestation of 'feeling of cold' and 'fever'.

Cold feeling ('aversion to cold') in exterior patterns

In exterior patterns, as explained above, the cold feeling is due to the fact that the external Wind obstructs the space between the skin and muscles (called *Cou Li*) where the Defensive Qi circulates; and Defensive Qi is not necessarily weak but only *obstructed*. Also, since the cold feeling is caused by the obstruction of Defensive Qi by Wind (whether it is Wind-Cold or Wind-Heat) in the space between the skin and muscles, the cold feeling and shivering are present also in invasions of Wind-Heat, albeit to a lesser degree than in Wind-Cold.

As mentioned above, there are four different degrees of 'cold feeling' in Exterior conditions: 'aversion to wind', 'fear of cold', 'aversion to cold' and 'shivers'. The clinical significance of these four degrees of feeling of cold in the context of exterior invasions is listed in Box 43.5.

Thus, generally speaking, there are three aspects to the 'cold feeling' in invasions of exterior Wind: the

---

BOX 43.5 DEGREES OF FEELING COLD

- **Aversion to wind**: the patient has goose pimples, dislikes going out in the wind and wants to stay indoors
- **Fear of cold**: the patient feels quite cold, wants to be indoors near sources of heat and wants to cover up
- **Aversion to cold**: the patient feels very cold and wants to stay indoors but covering up or staying in bed under blankets does not relieve the cold feeling
- **Shivers**: the patient feels extremely cold and shivers but covering up or staying in bed under blankets does not relieve the cold feeling

---

!

'Fever' does not necessarily indicate a raised temperature: it indicates that the patient's forehead and dorsum of hands feel hot to the touch. The patient may or may not have an actual fever.

---

patient feels cold, has 'waves' of shivers and is reluctant to go out and wants to stay indoors near sources of heat. Except in mild cases, the cold feeling is not relieved by covering oneself.

In conclusion, a feeling of cold in exterior invasions is due to the obstruction of Defensive Qi in the space between skin and muscles and it indicates that the pathogenic factor is on the Exterior; as soon as the feeling of cold goes, the pathogenic factor is in the Interior.

Fever in exterior patterns

As for 'fever' it is important to understand that the Chinese term *Fa Shao* does not necessarily indicate what we mean by fever. 'Fever' is a sign in modern Western medicine, not in old Chinese medicine. In old China, there were obviously no thermometers and the symptom *Fa Shao* described in the old texts does not necessarily mean that the patient has an actual fever. It literally means 'emitting burning heat' and it indicates that the patient's body feels hot, in severe cases almost burning to the touch; the areas touched are usually the forehead and especially the dorsum of the hands (as opposed to the palms, which tend to reflect more Empty-Heat).

In fact, it is a characteristic of *Fa Shao* (so-called 'fever') in the exterior stage of invasions of Wind that the dorsum of the hands feels hot compared with the palms and the upper back feels hot compared with the chest.[1] This objective hot feeling of the patient's body may or may not be accompanied by an actual fever. Indeed, in fevers of internal origin, there may even be cases when the patient has an actual low-grade fever and the body feels cold to the touch.

Thus, it is important to remember that, in the context of exterior conditions from invasions of Wind, 'fever' indicates the *objective* hot feeling of the patient's body (with or without an actual raised body temperature) and *not* a feeling of heat; in fact, as described above, the patient feels cold.

Simultaneous fever and feeling of cold

When the symptom of shivers and feeling cold occurs simultaneously with the objective sign of the patient's body feeling hot to the touch (or having an actual fever), this indicates an acute invasion of external Wind and it denotes that the pathogenic factor is still on the Exterior. In particular, it is the symptoms of shivering and feeling cold that indicate that the pathogenic factor is on the Exterior: the moment the patient does not feel cold any longer but feels hot and, if in bed, throws off the blankets, this means that the pathogenic factor is in the Interior and it has turned into Heat.

Pathology of fever

The fever, or hot feeling of the body in external invasions of Wind, is due to the struggle between the body's Qi (Upright Qi) and the external pathogenic factor. Thus, the strength of the fever (or hot feeling of the body) reflects the intensity of this struggle; this depends on the relative strengths of the external pathogenic factor and the Upright Qi. The stronger the external pathogenic factor, the higher is the fever (or hot feeling of the body); likewise, the stronger the Upright Qi, the higher is the fever (or hot feeling of the body). Thus the fever will be highest when both the external pathogenic factor and the Upright Qi are strong.

The relative strength of the pathogenic factor and the Upright Qi is only one factor which determines the intensity of the fever (or hot feeling of the body). Another is simply the constitution of a person: a person with a Yang constitution (i.e. with predominance of Yang) will be more prone to a higher fever (or hot feeling of the body).

!

The intensity of fever in exterior conditions is related to the struggle between the Upright Qi and the external pathogenic factor and has nothing to do with whether the pathogenic factor is Wind-Cold or Wind-Heat.

Degrees of fever

Thus, there are three possible degrees of fever (or hot feeling of the body); the patterns underlying these are listed in Box 43.6.

BOX 43.6 DEGREES OF EXTERIOR FEVER

- **Strong pathogenic factor and strong Upright Qi**: high fever (or hot feeling of the body)
- **Strong pathogenic factor with weak Upright Qi or vice versa**: medium fever (or hot feeling of the body)
- **Weak pathogenic factor and weak Upright Qi**: low fever (or hot feeling of the body) or no fever

---

Wind-Cold and Wind-Heat

Factors determining the development of Wind-Cold or Wind-Heat

The constitution of a person is the main factor which determines whether a person who falls prey to an invasion of Wind develops Wind-Cold or Wind-Heat. Were it not so, in cold northern countries nobody should fall prey to invasions of Wind-Heat, which is not the case. This is also the reason why, in children, invasions of Wind-Heat are far more prevalent than Wind-Cold: this is because children are naturally Yang in nature compared with adults. There are, however, also new, artificial factors which may predispose a person to invasions of Wind-Heat when succumbing to Wind, such as living in very dry, centrally heated places,

working in hot conditions (e.g. cooks, metal workers), etc.

Clinical manifestations of Wind-Heat and Wind-Cold

Although a fever is more likely to occur in invasions of Wind-Heat, the differentiation between Wind-Heat and Wind-Cold is not made on the basis of the intensity of aversion to cold and fever (or a hot feeling of the body). Other factors such as the tongue and other symptoms help us to differentiate between Wind-Cold and Wind-Heat. These are listed in Table 43.2.

Wind-Cold: differentiation between 'Attack of Wind' and 'Attack of Cold'

So far we have talked about Wind-Cold in general but the 'Discussion of Cold-induced Diseases' differentiates between two types of Wind-Cold invasions: one with prevalence of Wind, called 'Attack of Wind', and the other with prevalence of Cold, called 'Attack of Cold'. The Attack of Wind is described in Clause 2 of the 'Discussion of Cold-induced Diseases': *The Greater-Yang pattern with fever, sweating, aversion to wind and a Floating and Slowed-down pulse is called Attack of Wind*.[2] It may seem strange that the pulse is Slowed-down in this pattern as Wind is a Yang pathogenic factor that moves and opens. However, it is also true that Wind may cause stiffness (as in occipital stiffness in Wind-Cold invasions), rigidity and paralysis; thus it is quite

---

Table 43.2 Differentiation between Wind-Cold and Wind-Heat manifestations

		Wind-Cold	Wind-Heat
Pathology		Wind-cold obstructing the space between skin and muscles	Wind-Heat obstructing the space between skin and muscles and impairing the descending of Lung-Qi
Symptoms and signs	Fever	Slight	High
	Shivers	Pronounced	Slight
	Aches	Pronounced	Slight
	Thirst	No	Yes
	Urine	Clear	Slightly dark
	Headache	Occipital	Deep inside, severe
	Sweating	If sweating, in top part, head	Slight sweating
	Sore throat	Itchy throat	Very sore throat
	Tongue	No change	Slightly red on the sides/front
	Pulse	Floating-Tight	Floating-Rapid
Treatment		Pungent-warm herbs to cause sweating	Pungent-cool herbs to release the Exterior

Table 43.3 Differentiation between Attack of Cold and Attack of Wind in Wind-Cold

	Wind-Cold – Attack of Cold	Wind-Cold – Attack of Wind
Common manifestations	Aversion to cold, occipital stiffness, Floating pulse	
Other symptoms	Pronounced aversion to cold, body aches, no sweating, pulse Floating-Tight	Aversion to wind, fever, slight sweating, pulse Floating-Slow
Treatment	Release the Exterior by causing sweating (Ma Huang Tang)	Release the Exterior by adjusting the space between skin and muscles and regulating Defensive and Nutritive Qi (Gui Zhi Tang)

possible for the Attack of Wind of external Wind-Cold to cause a Slowed-down pulse (which is less slow than the Slow pulse). The commentary to Clause 2 confirms that *Huan* in this case means a 'moderate and slow (Chi) pulse'.[3]

Clause 3 describes the Attack of Cold: '*The Greater-Yang pattern with fever or no fever, aversion to cold, body aches, retching and Tight pulse on both Yin and Yang, is called Attack of Cold.*'[4]

In Attack of Wind, the patient's Nutritive Qi is more deficient than in the Attack of Cold and this causes a slight sweating. Other symptoms are tabulated in Table 43.3.

Apart from Wind-Heat and Wind-Cold, simultaneous shivers and fever may also occur with invasions of Summer-Heat, Damp-Heat and Dry-Heat.

Summer-Heat

Summer-Heat is a type of Wind-Heat and therefore manifests with a simultaneous feeling of cold and fever. The clinical manifestations usually are: fever (or hot feeling of the body), shivers, no sweating, headache, a feeling of heaviness, an uncomfortable sensation in the epigastrium, irritability, thirst, tongue Red in the front or sides with a sticky white coating, and a Soggy and Rapid pulse.

The tongue coating is white because the pathogenic factor is on the Exterior.

Damp-Heat

Damp-Heat from external origin also manifests with a simultaneous feeling of cold and fever at its very beginning stages. The clinical manifestations are usually

fever that is worse in the afternoon, body hot to touch, aversion to cold, shivers, swollen glands, headache, a feeling of heaviness, a feeling of oppression of the epigastrium, sticky taste, thirst with no desire to drink, sticky white tongue coating, and a Soggy-Slow pulse.

The pulse is Slow because of the obstructive influence of Dampness. The tongue coating is white because the pathogenic factor is on the Exterior.

Dry-Heat

Dry-Heat is a type of Wind-Heat and therefore manifests with a simultaneous feeling of cold and fever. The clinical manifestations usually are: fever, slight aversion to cold, shivers, slight sweating, dry skin, nose, mouth and throat, dry cough, sore throat, Dry tongue with thin white coating, and a Floating-Rapid pulse.

The tongue coating is white because the pathogenic factor is on the Exterior.

ALTERNATING FEELING OF COLD AND FEELING OF HEAT

An alternating feeling of cold and feeling of heat (or fever) should not be confused with the *simultaneous* feeling of cold and fever which characterizes invasions of external Wind. There are two main differences. First, in alternating feeling of cold and feeling of heat, the feeling of heat is a subjective feeling of the patient, whereas in the simultaneous aversion to cold and fever of external invasions the feeling of heat is an objective feeling of heat on palpation of the patient's forehead and hands. Secondly, in alternating feeling of cold and feeling of heat, the cold and hot sensations alternate

Case history 43.1

An 18-year-old girl complained of an acute illness manifesting with alternation of shivers and feeling of heat, swollen glands, sore throat, headache, lethargy and a feeling of heaviness of the head. These symptoms had started 3 weeks before the consultation. Her tongue was Red with red points in the front with a thin yellow coating. Her pulse was Floating in general, especially on both Front positions and slightly Slippery on the right side.

Diagnosis: This is a very clear case of acute invasion of Wind-Damp-Heat still at the exterior level at the time of consultation. It is still at the exterior level because she still experiences shivers. Together with the typical symptoms of Wind-Heat, there is also acute, exterior Dampness manifesting with swollen glands, a feeling of heaviness of the head and the Slippery quality on the right side of the pulse.

---

whereas in aversion to cold and fever, they are simultaneous.

Alternating feeling of cold and feeling of heat occurs also in external invasions, but only those affecting the Lesser-Yang channels (whereas aversion to cold and fever occurs in external patterns affecting the Greater-Yang channels). This symptom is a chief symptom of the Lesser-Yang pattern within the Six Stages (Chapter 105) or of the Gall-Bladder Heat pattern within the Four Levels (Chapter 104). The latter is also a Lesser-Yang-type of pattern but with the prevalence of heat rather than cold. This is reflected in the patient's sensations in that the feeling of heat is predominant over the feeling of cold.

> !
> - 'Feeling of heat' in alternating cold and hot feeling is subjective.
> - 'Feeling of heat' (or fever) in simultaneous aversion to cold and fever is objective, i.e. the patient's body feels hot to the touch.

Case history 43.1 illustrates a pattern causing alternating feeling of heat and feeling of cold.

FEELING OF HEAT FROM INTERNAL CAUSES

A subjective feeling of heat may be caused by Full-Heat or Empty-Heat of any organ. In Full-Heat, the feeling of heat is somewhat more intense than in Empty-Heat; another difference is that in Empty-Heat, the feeling of heat tends to be more marked in the afternoon or evening. Also, Empty-Heat is characterized by a feeling

of heat especially in the Yin areas of the body, and particularly in the chest, palms and soles. Of course, the differentiation between Full-Heat and Empty-Heat is done on the basis of other manifestations such as thirst, complexion and most of all the tongue, which will be Red with a coating in Full-Heat and Red without coating in Empty-Heat. The main differentiating manifestations of Full-Heat and Empty-Heat are shown in Box 43.7.

With Full-Heat, the organs that are most often involved are the Liver, Heart, Stomach and Lungs; with Empty-Heat, the organs that are most often involved are the Kidneys, Heart, Stomach and Lungs.

We should bear in mind that, in some cases, a person may feel hot in general but simultaneously experience cold feet, for example. Therefore, when a patient replies

---

BOX 43.7 DIFFERENTIATION BETWEEN FULL-HEAT AND EMPTY-HEAT

Full-Heat
- Usually a more intense heat
- Generalized over the body or in the face
- Not related to time of day
- Intense thirst
- Pronounced irritability
- Complexion red all over
- Red tongue with thick, dry yellow coating
- Overflowing-Rapid pulse

Empty-Heat
- Less intense heat
- Often on chest, soles and palms
- Worse in afternoon and evening
- Dry mouth with a desire to sip drinks
- Vague anxiety
- Redness on the cheekbones
- Red tongue without coating
- Floating-Empty and Rapid pulse

affirmatively to the question 'Do you have a tendency to feel hot in general?', our questioning should not stop there; rather it should continue in order to ascertain whether there is any cold feeling in any particular parts of the body. For a discussion on the clinical significance of simultaneous (and contradictory) hot and cold feelings in internal conditions, see below.

> **!**
>
> When a patient feels hot in general, remember to ask about any possible cold feeling in a particular part of the body (and vice versa).

INTERIOR FEVER

Symptoms and Signs, Chapter 82

By 'fever' is meant the situation when the patient has a fever but no simultaneous cold feeling or shivers; thus, we are now discussing interior fevers, which, it should be remembered, may be of external or internal origin. An interior fever of external origin is one caused by an exterior pathogenic factor (such as Wind-Heat, Wind-Cold or Damp-Heat) which has penetrated into the Interior and caused a fever; an interior fever of internal origin stems from an internal disharmony such as interior Heat, Yin deficiency, Qi or Blood deficiency and Blood stasis (Figs 43.10 and 43.11).

In some of the patterns discussed, there may not be an actual fever but only a feeling of heat: the pathology and pathogenesis of interior fever or feeling of heat is the same. Generally speaking, acute fevers are characterized by an actual fever, (i.e. raised body temperature), whereas chronic 'fevers' may be characterized simply by a feeling of heat without a rise in body tem-

perature. Thus, contrary to the situation in exterior syndromes when 'fever' indicates an objective hot feeling of the body, in chronic interior syndromes with fever of internal origin, 'fever' may indicate a subjective feeling of heat.

There are three degrees of interior fever (or hot body sensation); these are listed in Box 43.8.

> **BOX 43.8 DEGREES OF INTERIOR FEVER**
>
> - **Slight fever** (*Wei Re*): the fever is very low and the body is only slightly hot: the patient may not be aware of having a fever
> - **Fever** (*Fa Re*): the body temperature is raised (or the body feels quite hot to the touch): the patient is aware of the fever and has a feeling of heat
> - **Strong fever** (*Zhuang Re*): the fever is very high, the body is very hot to the touch, the patient has an intense feeling of heat and throws off bedclothes

Acute fever

When discussing fevers of internal origin, it is important to differentiate between acute and chronic fever. Acute interior fevers usually develop from the acute stage of an invasion of external Wind: both Wind-Cold and Wind-Heat may lead to an interior fever. Thus, the fever discussed here is primarily an acute fever deriving from external causes but at the interior stage. In such acute fevers the identification of patterns according to the Four Levels provides the best framework of interpretation and is clinically more relevant than the identification of patterns according to the Six Stages. However, there may be other acute interior fevers that are of internal origin, for example from Damp-Heat in the Liver and Gall-Bladder (febrile episode of cholecys-

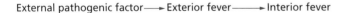

External pathogenic factor ⟶ Exterior fever ⟶ Interior fever

Pathogenic factor penetrates into the Interior

Fig. 43.10 Relationship between external pathogenic factor and interior fever

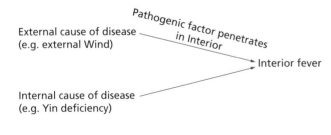

External cause of disease (e.g. external Wind)

Pathogenic factor penetrates in Interior

Internal cause of disease (e.g. Yin deficiency)

Interior fever

Fig. 43.11 External and internal causes of interior fevers

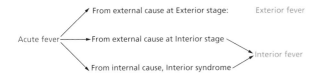

Fig. 43.12 Origin of acute fevers

titis), or Damp-Heat in the Bladder (cystitis with fever) (Fig. 43.12).

The Four Levels

The Four Levels patterns are discussed in Chapter 104. Within the Four Levels, the Defensive-Qi level is the only Exterior one and therefore there is simultaneous fever and shivering with a cold feeling. At the other three levels (Qi, Nutritive Qi and Blood), Heat is in the Interior and the fever is interior. The identification of patterns according to the Four Levels describes the symptomatology of invasions of Wind-Heat. However, fever, to a lesser degree, may be present also in invasions of Wind-Cold, for which the identification of patterns according to the Six Stages is used.

The three interior levels, Qi, Nutritive-Qi and Blood levels, within the Four Levels represent three different depths of penetration of the Heat, the Qi being the most superficial (or rather least deep) and Blood the deepest. At the Qi level, the Upright Qi is still strong and it engages in a fight with the pathogenic factors leading to a high fever and acute, strong manifestations characterized by restlessness, high fever, profuse sweating, etc. At the Nutritive-Qi and Blood levels, the Upright Qi is injured, the Heat has injured the fluids and there is Yin deficiency. These levels are usually characterized by a fever at night and by the Mind being affected, causing delirium, severe mental restlessness and, in severe cases, coma. At the Blood level, internal Wind can develop and bleeding occurs. At the Blood level and, to a lesser extent, at the Nutritive-Qi level, there are maculae.

The tongue is an important and objective sign to differentiate the Qi level from the Nutritive-Qi level and the Blood levels: at the Qi level the tongue is Red and has a thick coating, whereas at the Nutritive-Qi and Blood levels the tongue is dark Red and has no coating.

The clinical manifestation of the Four Levels in fever is summarized in Box 43.9.

The clinical manifestations of the Defensive-Qi level, which causes a simultaneous feeling of cold and fever, have already been discussed above. The detailed clinical manifestations of the main patterns appearing at the Qi, Nutritive-Qi and Blood levels are described below.

Heat in the Lungs (Qi level)

Clinical manifestations Fever, cough with yellow sputum, sweating, thirst, a feeling of oppression or pain of the chest, Red tongue with sticky yellow coating and Rapid-Overflowing pulse.

This is one of the patterns appearing at the Qi level within the Four Levels; it is characterized by acute, interior Lung-Heat. From a Western perspective, it could correspond to acute bronchitis, pneumonia or pleurisy. In this case there is an actual fever as well as an objective hot feeling of the patient's body.

Phlegm-Heat in the Lungs (Qi level)

Clinical manifestations Fever, cough with abundant sticky yellow sputum, thirst, sweating, a feeling of oppression of the chest, nausea, Red tongue with sticky yellow coating and Rapid-Slippery pulse.

This is one of the possible patterns appearing at the Qi level within the Four Levels; it is characterized by acute, interior Lung-Heat with Phlegm.

Heat in Bright Yang – channel pattern

Clinical manifestations Fever, sweating, intense thirst, Big or Overflowing pulse and Red tongue with yellow coating.

This corresponds to acute, interior Heat in the Stomach channel and its manifestations are described by the Stomach-Heat level within the Four Levels or the Bright-Yang channel pattern within the Six Stages. This pattern is often summarized in a nutshell as the 'four big', that is, high fever, intense thirst, profuse sweating and Overflowing or Big pulse.

BOX 43.9 THE FOUR LEVELS IN A NUTSHELL

- **Defensive-Qi level**: fever, aversion to cold
- **Qi level**: fever, feeling of heat, thirst
- **Nutritive-Qi level**: fever at night, mental confusion, maculae
- **Blood level**: fever at night, mental confusion, maculae, bleeding

Heat in Bright Yang – organ pattern

Clinical manifestations Fever, abdominal pain and fullness, dry stools, constipation, thirst, Red tongue with a thick, dry yellow, brown or black coating and Deep-Full-Rapid pulse.

This is the Dry-Heat in the Intestines level within the Four Levels and is the same as the Bright Yang – organ pattern within the Six Stages.

Damp-Heat in the Stomach and Intestines

Clinical manifestations Fever, thirst with no desire to drink, loose stools, abdominal pain, a feeling of heaviness, Red tongue with sticky yellow coating and Slippery-Rapid pulse.

This is Damp-Heat in the Stomach and Intestines level within the Four Levels.

Heat at Nutritive-Qi level

Clinical manifestations Fever at night, thirst, dry mouth with no desire to drink, mental restlessness, delirium, aphasia, coma, Red tongue without coating, Fine-Rapid pulse.

This is Heat at the Nutritive-Qi level within the Four Levels.

Heat at Blood level

Clinical manifestations Fever at night, thirst, mental restlessness, bleeding, convulsions, tremor, Red tongue without coating, Fine-Rapid pulse.

This is Heat at the Blood level within the Four Levels.

In addition to the above interior patterns with internal fever of the Four Levels, two commons patterns from interior Heat which may give rise to an acute, internal fever are Damp-Heat in the Gall-Bladder and Liver (as in acute cholecystitis) and Damp-Heat in the Bladder (as in acute cystitis).

Damp-Heat in the Gall-Bladder and Liver

Clinical manifestations Fever, bitter and sticky taste, hypochondrial pain which may extend to the right shoulder and scapula, irritability, a feeling of oppression of the chest, nausea, vomiting, dark urine, tongue with Red sides and sticky yellow tongue coating and Wiry-Slippery-Rapid pulse.

Damp-Heat in the Bladder

Clinical manifestations Fever, burning of urination, difficult urination, scanty and dark urine, blood in the urine, mental restlessness, sticky yellow tongue coating on the root of the tongue and Slippery-Rapid pulse.

Chronic fever

Chronic interior fevers may be due to Deficiency or Excess. Yin deficiency is a common and obvious cause of chronic interior fever, but Qi and Blood deficiency may also cause it. Among the Full causes of internal fever are stagnant Liver-Qi turned into Heat and Blood stasis. Thus, there are five main causes of chronic interior fever:

- Empty-Heat from Yin deficiency
- Qi deficiency
- Blood deficiency
- stagnant Liver-Qi turned into Heat
- Blood stasis.

Empty-Heat from Yin deficiency

Clinical manifestations Low-grade fever or feeling of heat in the afternoon or evening, five-palm heat, malar flush, thirst with desire to drink in small sips, dry mouth and throat at night, mental restlessness, night sweating, insomnia, dream-disturbed sleep, dry stools, dark-scanty urination, a thin red line on the inside of the lower eyelid, Red tongue without coating and with cracks, and Fine-Rapid pulse.

These are the general symptoms of Empty-Heat deriving from Yin deficiency; they may arise from the Lungs, Heart, Stomach, Spleen, Liver and Kidneys. Other accompanying symptoms (or more accentuated symptoms) according to the organ involved are listed in Box 43.10.

BOX 43.10 CLINICAL MANIFESTATIONS OF EMPTY-HEAT FROM YIN DEFICIENCY

- Lungs: dry throat, dry cough, malar flush
- Heart: insomnia, mental restlessness, dream-disturbed sleep, malar flush, Red tip of the tongue
- Spleen: dry lips, dry stools
- Liver: dry eyes, red eyes, dream-disturbed sleep, Red sides of the tongue
- Kidneys: dizziness, tinnitus
- Stomach: dry mouth, bleeding gums

Qi deficiency

Clinical manifestations Low-grade fever or feeling of heat that is aggravated by overwork, dizziness, tired-

ness, depression, muscular weakness, spontaneous sweating, shortness of breath, loose stools, poor appetite, weak voice, Pale tongue and Weak or Empty pulse.

This fever is caused by a severe deficiency of Qi, usually of the Spleen, Stomach and Lungs, and a deficiency of the Original Qi. This situation was described by Li Dong Yuan in the famous classic 'Discussion on Stomach and Spleen' (*Pi Wei Lun*) (see Bibliography). He said that overwork and irregular diet weaken the Qi of the Stomach and Spleen and the Original Qi, which resides in the Lower Field of Elixir (*Dan Tian*); here it shares a place with the (physiological) Minister Fire. If the Minister Fire is stirred by overwork and emotional problems, it becomes pathological, 'displaces' the Original Qi in the Lower Field of Elixir and it rises upwards causing a low-grade fever or a feeling of heat (Fig. 43.13).

Li Dong Yuan called this pathological Minister Fire a 'thief' of the Original Qi; the Heat generated by the pathological Minister Fire is called 'Yin Fire' and it is neither Full- nor Empty-Heat, although it is more similar to the latter. Li Dong Yuan said that this Yin Fire is treated not by clearing it with bitter-cold herbs but by tonifying the Original Qi with sweet-warm herbs: as the Minister Fire and the Original Qi share the same

place, tonifying the Original Qi will automatically displace and subdue the pathological Minister Fire.

The representative prescription to subdue Yin Fire is Bu Zhong Yi Qi Tang *Tonifying the Centre and Benefiting Qi Decoction*, within which Ren Shen *Radix Ginseng* tonifies the Original Qi.

This condition of Yin Fire and feeling of heat deriving from Qi and Blood deficiency is very common nowadays and is frequently seen in chronic cases of ME (CFIDS, postviral fatigue syndrome) and other modern autoimmune diseases, such as lupus or rheumatoid arthritis.

Blood deficiency

Clinical manifestations Low-grade fever or feeling of heat in the afternoon, dizziness, tingling, blurred vision, poor memory, tiredness, depression, scanty periods, palpitations, dull and pale complexion, pale lips, Pale-Thin tongue and Fine or Choppy pulse.

This fever is caused by a severe depletion of Blood and by Empty-Heat resulting from it; it is more common in women and it may occur after childbirth.

Stagnant Liver-Qi turned into Heat

Clinical manifestations Chronic low-grade fever or feeling of heat that comes and goes according to the emotional state (it comes when the person is upset), volatile mood, irritability, a feeling of oppression and distension of the chest and hypochondrium, dry throat, sighing, a bitter taste, irregular periods, premenstrual tension, Red tongue with redder sides and thin-yellow coating and Rapid-Wiry pulse.

This is due to Liver-Heat generated by chronic Liver-Qi stagnation and is usually caused by chronic emotional problems.

Blood stasis

Clinical manifestations Low-grade fever or feeling of heat in the afternoon or evening, dry mouth, abdominal pain, dry skin and nails, dark complexion, purple lips, Purple tongue and Choppy or Firm pulse.

This is chronic Blood stasis and it is usually related to the Liver. The manifestations of dryness are due not to Yin deficiency but to Blood stasis. Due to the interactions and interchange between Blood and Body Fluids, when Blood stagnates for a long time, it cannot interchange with the Body Fluids and these fail to moisten the body. Fever from chronic Blood stasis is frequently seen in cancer.

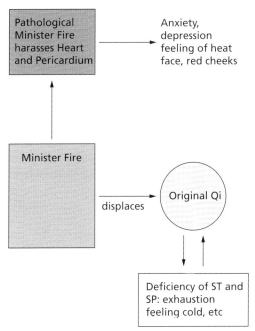

Fig. 43.13 Pathology of Yin Fire

FIVE-PALM HEAT

This is a feeling of heat in the palms, soles and chest, which is also sometimes called five-centre heat or five-heart heat; this may or may not be accompanied by an actual fever. It is usually accompanied by mental restlessness, night sweating and insomnia. This is frequently seen in practice; however, it may sometimes manifest only in the soles and palms, or palms and chest.

Yin deficiency of any organ may cause five-palm heat: Lungs, Heart, Liver, Spleen, Kidneys, Stomach. However, there are other, less common, possible causes of five-palm heat: these include Blood deficiency, Latent Heat in the Lesser Yin and Liver-Fire.

In Blood deficiency, the five-palm heat is experienced mainly in the afternoon and is accompanied by other symptoms of Blood deficiency. This occurs almost exclusively in women.

Latent Heat in the Lesser Yin is characterized by Heat in the Kidneys and is frequently seen in ME (postviral fatigue syndrome). The main manifestations are a low-grade fever or feeling of heat in the afternoon or evening, feeling cold in the morning, dizziness, tinnitus and night sweating.

Liver-Fire may also cause five-palm heat although not frequently; this symptom will be accompanied by other manifestations of Liver-Fire.

Box 43.11 summarizes the patterns underlying five-palm heat.

BOX 43.11 FIVE-PALM HEAT

- Yin deficiency of any organ: this is the most common pattern
- Blood deficiency: more common in women and occurs more frequently in the afternoon
- Latent Heat in the Lesser Yin: occurs more frequently in the evening with low-grade fever
- Liver-Fire: severe five-palm heat with a sudden onset (not common)

CONTRADICTORY FEELINGS OF COLD AND HEAT IN INTERNAL CONDITIONS

Contradictory hot and cold feelings are very common especially in women and especially those over the age of 40. This is due to four possible causes:

- simultaneous deficiency of Kidney-Yin and Kidney-Yang
- Blood deficiency with Empty-Heat
- disharmony of the Penetrating Vessel
- Yin Fire.

Simultaneous deficiency of Kidney-Yin and Kidney-Yang

A simultaneous deficiency of Kidney-Yin and Kidney-Yang is very common in women over the age of 40; indeed, it is probably more the norm than the exception. Kidney-Yin and Kidney-Yang have a common root and, especially after 40, a deficiency of one often involves also a deficiency of the other, albeit in different degrees. Thus, when there is a deficiency of both Kidney-Yang and Kidney-Yin with a predominance of the latter there will be dizziness, tinnitus, night sweating, malar flush, five-palm heat and a feeling of heat, but possibly also cold feet; when there is a predominance of Kidney-Yang deficiency there will be dizziness, backache, tinnitus, frequent urination, a pronounced feeling of cold and cold feet, but possibly also a feeling of heat in the afternoon.

Blood deficiency with Empty-Heat

Blood deficiency may also cause some Empty-Heat and therefore contradictory hot and cold symptoms. In fact, Blood deficiency may cause cold hands, but when Empty-Heat arises from it in chronic cases there may be a feeling of heat in the face.

Disharmony of the Penetrating Vessel

Contradictory hot and cold symptoms may be caused by a disharmony of the Penetrating Vessel. When this vessel is deficient (which involves a Kidney deficiency), a deficiency of Qi in its descending branch may cause cold feet while the ascending rebellious Qi may cause a feeling of heat in the face.

Yin Fire

Finally, Yin Fire may cause a person to feel cold in general and experience occasional feeling of heat in the face. The pathology of Yin Fire has already been explained above.

Box 43.12 summarizes the patterns underlying contradictory feeling of heat and cold.

> **BOX 43.12 CONTRADICTORY FEELING OF COLD AND FEELING OF HEAT**
>
> - Simultaneous deficiency of both Kidney-Yin and Kidney-Yang: cold feet, feeling of heat and five-palm heat or heat in afternoon
> - Blood deficiency with Empty-Heat: cold hands, heat in face
> - Disharmony of the Penetrating Vessel with rebellious Qi: cold feet, heat in face
> - Yin Fire: cold in general, low-grade fever or feeling of heat

NOTES

1. Deng Tie Tao, Practical Chinese Diagnosis (*Shi Yong Zhong Yi Zhen Duan Xue* 实用中医诊断学), Shanghai Science Publishing House, Shanghai, 1988, p. 90.
2. Shang Han Lun Research Group of the Nanjing College of Chinese Medicine, An Explanation of the 'Discussion of Cold-induced Diseases' (*Shang Han Lun Yi Shi* 伤寒论详释), Shanghai Science Publishing House, Shanghai, 1980, p. 351.
3. Ibid., p. 351.
4. Ibid., p. 354.

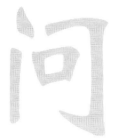

Chapter **44**

MENTAL–EMOTIONAL SYMPTOMS

Chapter contents

INTRODUCTION *379*

DEPRESSION *380*
  Definition of depression *380*
  Diagnosis of depression *381*
  Depression in Chinese medicine *381*
  Patterns in depression *382*

FEAR/ANXIETY *384*

IRRITABILITY/ANGER *385*

WORRY/OVERTHINKING *386*

SADNESS/GRIEF *387*

EXCESS JOY *388*

MENTAL RESTLESSNESS *388*

INTRODUCTION

? **WHY** WE ASK

The area of questioning surrounding the emotions experienced by the patient is one of the most important, if not *the* most important one. Emotional causes of disease play a very prominent role in the aetiology and clinical manifestations of most of our patients. Therefore we should always ask patients about their emotional life. However, some patients may regard an enquiry about their emotional life as an intrusion and we should be sensitive about this.

The emotional state of the patient reflects of course the state of their Mind and Spirit and the findings from interrogation need to be carefully integrated with those gleaned from observation, particularly observation of the lustre (*shen*) of the eyes. In addition, the state of the patient's Mind and Spirit is an important prognostic factor.

? **WHEN** WE ASK

Enquiry about a patient's emotional life must be closely integrated with observation (especially of the eyes, complexion and tongue), with palpation (of the pulse) and with hearing (voice).

If the emotional condition is not the presenting problem, I generally ask about a patient's emotional life towards the end of the consultation to try to find the cause of the disease. In many cases, the emotional state of the patient is the main presenting problem; for example, patients may come to us because they are depressed or anxious. In other cases, the emotional state of the patient is the underlying cause of physical

symptoms; for example, a patient may complain of tiredness and digestive symptoms when frustration and resentment may be the cause of the condition.

Unless the patient comes specifically seeking help for an emotional state such as depression, irritability or anxiety, I generally ask about the patient's emotions when the pattern emerging from the interrogation, together with observation of the eyes and tongue and palpation of the pulse, strongly points to an emotional cause of disease. For example, if the Lung pulse is somewhat full and the patient looks sad, I may try and find out whether sadness or grief has been experienced that has not been expressed (the fullness of the Lung pulse would indicate this).

If the Heart pulse is Overflowing and there is a Heart crack on the tongue, I may enquire whether the patient has suffered from a shock. If the Lung pulse is particularly Weak and without wave and the eyes lack lustre, I may explore whether events in the patient's life have caused sadness or grief. If the pulse is Wiry on all positions I ask the patient whether some life situation is causing frustration, anger or resentment. If the Heart pulse is Choppy, the complexion dull, the eyes lustreless and the voice weak and weepy, I will try and determine whether the patient is sad.

There are two main reasons why I ask a patient to confirm what I suspect from observation, palpation and hearing. First, it engages patients more with the treatment and, by making them aware of a possible emotional cause of their symptoms, it may further their healing process. Secondly, even if the eyes lack lustre, there is a deep Heart crack on the tongue and the pulse is Sad, this may be caused by a severe physical illness such as cancer, or a treatment such as chemotherapy (which may weaken even the strongest of Spirits).

It is important to be sensitive when asking about the emotional state of the patient (if this is not the presenting problem) and often it is observation that gives us a clue about the emotional state, in which case I would ask the patient about it. For example, a patient may come in complaining of tiredness and premenstrual breast distension: if the eyes of the patient lack lustre, I would suspect emotional stress to be the cause of the problem and I would circumspectly ask the patient about it.

It is important to mention, however, that in most cases of treating emotional symptoms, or symptoms which are caused by emotional problems, observation should take precedence over what a patient verbally reports. It is most often when we see beyond what a patient is telling us that we find the true cause of a disease.

? HOW WE ASK

As mentioned above, we must use great sensitivity when asking patients about their emotions.

First of all, we should ask only if they appear willing to talk about their emotions and respect their wish if they do not want to do so. If I suspect that emotional stress is the cause of a problem I ask questions like 'Have you suffered any shock in the past?', 'Do you tend to feel irritable about some situation?' or 'Do you sometimes feel sad?', etc.

Of course, if the patient comes to us specifically for an emotional condition, the questioning is conducted differently as the patient will openly volunteer the information.

DEPRESSION

Symptoms and Signs, Chapter 79

Depression is a very common symptom in Western patients, even though some patients may not admit to being depressed and others may not even recognize that they are depressed.

Definition of depression

'Depression' is a modern Western term which indicates a change in mood ranging from a very mild feeling of despondency to the most abject depression and despair. In mild depression the change in mood varies and is not permanent, whereas in severe depression the change in mood is fixed and persists over a period of months or years. Severe depression is also accompanied by characteristic changes in behaviour, attitude, thinking efficiency and physiological functioning. Of course, it is normal to experience a temporary feeling of depression following adverse life events such as bereavement. In distinguishing a normal reaction from pathological depression a quantitative judgement has to be made. If the precipitant seems inadequate, or the depression appears too severe or too long lasting, the condition may be regarded as abnormal. In addition, the severity and incapacity in depressive illness differ qualitatively as well as quantitatively from depressed feelings that are part of normal experiences.

Depression is twice as common in women as in men and its onset increases towards middle age. The main symptoms of depression are depressed mood, loss of interest, self-esteem or motivation, fatigue, anxiety, insomnia and loss of appetite. In very severe cases, the patient never comes out of an extremely depressed mood, is unable to experience any pleasure at any time, is in utter despair and may be suicidal. A major depressive syndrome has the following characteristics:

- very depressed mood most of the day nearly every day
- markedly diminished interest or pleasure in all or almost all activities most of the day, nearly every day
- significant weight loss (or gain), decrease (or increase) in appetite
- insomnia or sleepiness
- psychomotor agitation or retardation every day
- fatigue nearly every day
- feelings of worthlessness or guilt (which may be delusional) nearly every day (not merely self-reproach or guilt about being ill)
- diminished ability to think or concentrate, indecisiveness nearly every day
- recurrent thoughts of death, recurrent suicidal ideation without a specific plan or a suicide attempt or a specific plan for committing suicide.

In addition to the above manifestations, a major depressive syndrome is also defined by the absence of the following: an organic factor, a normal reaction to bereavement, delusions or hallucinations in the absence of mood symptoms, schizophrenia, delusional disorder, psychotic disorder.[1]

Diagnosis of depression

Asking patients about feelings of depression should always be part of our questions about the patient's emotional state and it should be carried out with sensitivity and tact. In fact, some patients will not want to admit to being depressed, some will admit to being depressed but do not necessarily want to talk about it, and others may not even realize that they are in a state of depression. These patients will often complain only of physical symptoms such as extreme tiredness, lack of motivation and feeling cold, preferring not to face up to the fact that they may be depressed. In China this is more the norm than the exception as Chinese patients will seldom complain of feeling 'depressed' and somatization of their feelings of depression into bodily symptoms is often seen.

Signs of depression   In patients who are not aware of being depressed, Chinese diagnosis often enables us to recognize the true condition of the patient's mental–emotional state. In fact there are certain signs that point to mental depression as the root cause of the patient's problems and these are:

- the complexion
- the eyes
- the tongue
- the voice
- the pulse.

The complexion of a severely depressed person will lack lustre and will tend to be greyish or greenish; the eyes will also lack sparkle (*shen*); the tongue has a Red tip and may have a deep Heart crack; and the voice will be low and lacking vitality.

The pulse in a depressed person varies according to whether the condition is primarily Full or Empty. In Full conditions, the pulse feels very Wiry or Wiry and Slippery, whereas in Empty conditions (especially when sadness and grief prevail) the pulse is Weak or Choppy, often Short and nearly always lacks a 'wave' (Sad pulse). Interestingly, very often the pulse of a depressed person may point to the true cause of the problem being repressed anger; in fact, in some cases, a depressed patient may display many signs pointing to an Empty condition (low voice, dull complexion, slow movements) while the pulse is very Wiry. This usually indicates that the patient's depression is due to repressed anger. Vice versa, a pulse that is Choppy, Short or Sad indicates that sadness or grief is the prevalent emotion at the root of the depression.

Depression in Chinese medicine

In Chinese medicine, mental depression was called *Yin Yu*, which means 'gloominess' or 'depression' or, *Yu Zheng*, which means 'depression pattern'. *Yu* has the double meaning of 'depression' and 'stagnation', which implies that, according to this theory, mental depression is always caused by a stagnation.

In fact, the 'Simple Questions' in Chapter 71 mentions the Five Stagnations of Wood, Fire, Earth, Metal

and Water.[2] The 'Essential Method of Dan Xi' (*Dan Xi Xin Fa*, 1347) describes six stagnations of Qi, Blood, Dampness, Phlegm, Heat and Food. It says: '*When Qi and Blood are harmonized, no disease arises. If they stagnate diseases arise. Many diseases are due to stagnation . . . stagnation makes things accumulate so that they cannot flow freely, they would like to rise but cannot, they would like to descend but cannot, they would like to transform but cannot . . . thus the 6 Stagnations come into being.*'[3]

The 'Complete Book of Jing Yue' (*Jing Yue Quan Shu*, 1624) gives stagnation an emotional interpretation and talks about Six Stagnations of anger, pensiveness, worry, sadness, shock and fear. This confirms that all emotions can lead to stagnation of Qi. It says: '*In the 6 Stagnations, stagnation is the cause of the disease. In emotional stagnation, the disease [i.e. the emotion] is the cause of the stagnation.*'[4]

Patterns in depression

Chinese books normally ascribe mental depression to Liver-Qi stagnation in its various manifestations including Liver-Qi stagnation turning into Heat and Liver-Qi stagnation with Phlegm. In the later stages of mental depression, Empty patterns appear. Thus, although in Chinese medicine stagnation and depression are almost synonymous, Empty patterns may also cause depression.

In severe depression, the Liver is always involved owing to its housing the Ethereal Soul (*Hun*). The Ethereal Soul is responsible for our life's dreams, plans, ideas, projects, relationship with other people, etc. The Ethereal Soul was often described as 'the coming and going of the Mind (*Shen*)': this means that the Ethereal Soul assists the Mind in giving it the capacity to have dreams, plans, ideas, projects, etc. In this sense, the Ethereal Soul gives the Mind 'movement', outward projection and ability to form relationships with other people, hence its 'coming and going' described above. On the other hand, the Mind guides and controls the Ethereal Soul and, most of all, integrates the activity of the Ethereal Soul within the overall psychic life of the person.

Thus, if the 'movement' of the Ethereal Soul is lacking (either through its lack of activity or through overcontrol of the Mind), the person is depressed; if the 'movement' of the Ethereal Soul is excessive (either through its overactivity or through lack of control by the Mind), the person may display manic behaviour (bearing in mind that the latter may vary in intensity

and seriousness from full-blown bipolar disease to much less severe manifestations that are relatively common also in mentally healthy individuals).

When a person is severely depressed, the Ethereal Soul is not 'coming and going' enough, and therefore the person lacks dreams, has lost faith in the future, does not know which direction to take in life and has a feeling of loss, isolation and separation. From this point of view, many Liver (and other organs) patterns, and not just Liver-Qi stagnation, may cause depression. When the Ethereal Soul 'comes and goes' too much, the person may develop manic behaviour; in this case, the person has lots of dreams, projects and ideas but nothing comes to fruition because of the chaotic state of the Ethereal Soul and the lack of control of this by the Mind.

Figure 44.1 illustrates the two states of the Ethereal Soul: when it 'comes and goes' too much; and when it does not 'come and go' enough.

Essential to the proper movement of the Ethereal Soul is its restraint by the Mind. The Mind (*Shen* of the Heart) needs to restrain the Ethereal Soul (but not too much) and integrate the material coming from it into the totality of the psyche. If the Mind controls and restrains the Ethereal Soul too much, depression ensues; if the Mind fails to control and restrain the Ethereal Soul, manic behaviours may result (Fig. 44.2).

The lack of 'movement' of the Ethereal Soul and hence depression may be due to pathogenic factors inhibiting the Ethereal Soul (e.g. Liver-Qi stagnation),

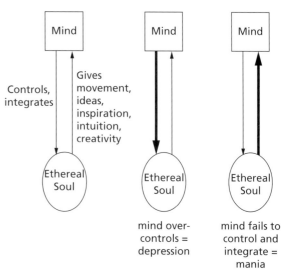

Fig. 44.1 The 'coming and going' of the Ethereal Soul

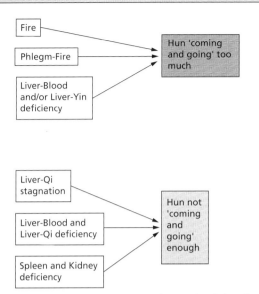

Fig. 44.2 Relationship between the Mind and the Ethereal Soul

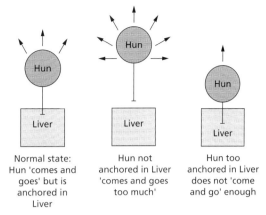

Fig. 44.3 Patterns leading to excessive and deficient movement of the Ethereal Soul

or to a deficiency of the Liver, Spleen or Kidneys not stimulating the Ethereal Soul. The excessive movement of the Ethereal Soul and hence manic behaviour may be due to pathogenic factors overstimulating the Ethereal Soul (e.g. Fire or Phlegm-Fire), or to the lack of anchoring of this Soul from a deficiency of Liver-Blood or Liver-Yin, or both. Note that Liver-Blood deficiency may lead to lack of movement of the Ethereal Soul when it is combined with Liver-Qi deficiency (itself associated with deficiency of Gall-Bladder Qi); otherwise, deficient Liver-Blood fails to house the Ethereal Soul and this leads to excessive movement.

Box 44.1 summarizes patterns relating to 'movement' of the Ethereal Soul.

BOX 44.1 'MOVEMENT' OF THE ETHEREAL SOUL

Lack of movement of the Ethereal Soul
- Liver-Qi stagnation
- Liver-Blood and Liver-Qi deficiency
- Spleen and Kidney deficiency

Excessive movement of the Ethereal Soul
- Fire
- Phlegm-Fire
- Liver-Blood/Liver-Yin deficiency

Figure 44.3 illustrates the Liver patterns leading to excessive and to deficient movement of the Ethereal Soul.

When diagnosing the prevailing patterns in depressed patients, it is important to differentiate between Full and Empty conditions; as the mood of depressed patients is the same in both cases, the main differentiating signs are the pulse and the tongue. In Full conditions causing depression, the pulse is usually Wiry or Slippery and Wiry, while in Empty conditions it is Choppy, Short or Sad. As depression is often accompanied by anxiety, this is obviously more pronounced in Full than in Empty conditions.

The main Full patterns accompanying depression are:

- Liver-Qi stagnation
- stagnant Liver-Qi turning into Heat
- Liver-Qi stagnation with Qi-Phlegm
- Phlegm-Fire harassing the Mind
- Blood stasis
- Gall-Bladder Heat.
- diaphragm Heat.

The main Empty patterns accompanying depression are:

- Spleen- and Heart-Blood deficiency
- Heart-Yang deficiency
- Liver-Blood deficiency
- Kidney- and Heart-Yin deficiency with Empty-Heat
- Kidney-Yang deficiency.

For a detailed description of these patterns, see Part 5, Chapter 79.

Box 44.2 summarizes the clinical manifestations of these patterns.

BOX 44.2 DEPRESSION

- Liver-Qi stagnation: depression, moodiness, irritability
- Stagnant Liver-Qi turning into Heat: depression, irritability, Red tongue
- Liver-Qi stagnation with Qi-Phlegm: depression, moodiness, feeling of a lump in the throat
- Phlegm-Fire harassing the Mind: depression, anxiety, agitation, expectoration of phlegm, Swollen tongue
- Heart-Blood stasis: depression, agitation, Purple tongue
- Gall-Bladder Heat: depression, irritability, bitter taste, hypochondrial fullness
- Diaphragm Heat: depression, anxiety, feeling of stuffiness in the chest following an invasion of Wind-Heat
- Spleen- and Heart-Blood deficiency: depression, insomnia, palpitations, tiredness
- Heart-Yang deficiency: depression, palpitations, cold hands
- Liver-Blood deficiency: depression, lack of sense of direction, sadness
- Kidney- and Heart-Yin deficiency with Heart Empty-Heat: depression, anxiety, night sweating, palpitations, Red tongue without coating
- Kidney-Yang deficiency: depression, lack of motivation, lack of will-power, feeling cold, frequent urination

---

FEAR/ANXIETY

Symptoms and Signs, Chapter 79

A chronic feeling of anxiety (occurring on its own without depression) is very common in Western patients. A feeling of anxiety includes emotional states akin to the emotions of fear and worry (two of the seven emotions) in Chinese medicine. It may be accompanied or caused by deficiency (usually of Blood or Yin), by Excess (usually Heat) or by a combination of Deficiency and Excess (usually Yin deficiency with Empty-Heat).

The main patterns in anxiety are listed in Box 44.3.

BOX 44.3 PATTERNS IN ANXIETY

Empty
- Deficiency of Blood
- Deficiency of Yin

Full
- Heat

Full/Empty
- Yin deficiency with Empty-Heat

When there is a deficiency of Blood or Yin, the Mind and Ethereal Soul lose their 'residence' in the Heart-Blood and Liver-Blood respectively and the person becomes anxious and sleeps badly. Conversely, pathogenic factors such as Qi stagnation, Blood stasis, Heat or Phlegm-Heat may 'agitate' the Mind and Ethereal Soul and lead to anxiety and insomnia. In some cases, of course, the Mind and Ethereal Soul are restless both from a deficiency (e.g. Yin deficiency) and a pathogenic factor (e.g. Empty-Heat). Figure 44.2 illustrates graphically the two causes of anxiety, that is, a Deficiency leading to the Mind's not being 'anchored' (Fig. 44.2, bottom) or a pathogenic factor 'agitating' the Mind (Fig. 44.2, top).

As a general rule, the degree of anxiety or fear depends on whether it is caused by an Empty or a Full condition: in Empty conditions it is mild whereas in Full conditions it is severe.

It is usually easy to see whether patients are anxious: they look restless, their voice may be quivering, they may fidget, talk a lot (in the case of a Full condition) or be very quiet (in the case of an Empty condition), and may be very anxious about receiving acupuncture. In a few cases, however, a state of anxiety may not be apparent in patients who make a brave attempt to hide their true state. In fact, those who are in a constant state of fear may initially appear to be calm and grounded. In these cases, the tongue, pulse and eyes may reveal the patient's state of anxiety or fear. The tongue may have a Red tip, often with a deep Heart crack, the pulse may be Wiry (in case of a Full condition) or Floating-Empty (in case of an Empty condition) and Rapid, and the eyes may look 'unstable' and lack control (see Part 1, Chapter 6).

Case history 44.1 illustrates a pattern underlying panic attacks.

Case history 44.1

A 39-year-old woman had been suffering from panic attacks for the past 6 years. During the attacks her throat would become tense, she felt as if she were unable to swallow, she became slightly breathless, had palpitations and felt hot. They occurred every day and became worse after eating lunch. It was interesting to note that when the patient was describing the attacks she repeatedly mentioned the word 'throat'.

The patient also mentioned that she suffered from night sweats. Her periods were unproblematic but she did become aggressive premenstrually.

The tongue body was Swollen, slightly peeled on the root and very slightly Red on the sides and tip. Her pulse was very Weak in the left Rear position and Overflowing in the left Front position.

Diagnosis: The panic attacks are caused by rebellious Qi in the Penetrating Vessel. The clinical manifestations displayed by this patient are fairly typical of the Penetrating Vessel's pathology of Qi rebelling upwards along its pathway. The Penetrating Vessel flows up through the abdomen and chest, along the line of the Kidney channel and flowing through the Heart on its way up to the throat and face. It therefore influences the Heart and chest area and, in this case, is causing the symptoms of palpitations and breathlessness. The symptoms associated with the syndrome of Qi rebelling upwards in the Penetrating Vessel were called *Li Ji*, which literally means 'internal urgency', and it indicates a state of anxiety and panic, as in this case.

The tension in the throat and difficulty in swallowing are caused by the Qi of the Penetrating Vessel rebelling upwards. The feeling of heat is caused by the Qi of the Penetrating Vessel rushing up to the face: this is reflected in the Overflowing quality of the pulse on the left Front position and the Weak quality on the left Rear position. This pulse reflects clearly the deficiency of the Penetrating Vessel in the Lower Burner and the subsequent rushing upwards of the rebellious Qi to the face. It should be remembered that the pulse positions reflect not only the organs but also the areas of the body and their respective channels; in this case there is Emptiness below (the lower abdomen) and Fullness above (throat and face) making the pulse Weak in the third position and Overflowing in the first.

However, in this case, the pulse is reflecting also a pathology of the relevant organs. The Weak pulse on the left Rear position indicates a Kidney deficiency, predominantly of Kidney-Yin, as evidenced by the peeling of the root of the tongue and the night sweating. The Overflowing quality on the left Front position indicates Heart-Heat, which is evidenced also by the Red tip of the tongue.

The swelling of the tongue indicates the presence of Phlegm but the patient has no symptoms of this at present; such cases highlight the preventative value of tongue diagnosis and I would therefore resolve Phlegm even in the absence of symptoms.

The fact that, when describing her symptoms, the patient repeatedly and emphatically said the word 'throat' may indicate that the origin of her condition is an emotional one and that she had felt unable to express herself, leading to a feeling of restriction in the throat area.

For a detailed description of the patterns accompanying anxiety and fear, see Part 5, Chapter 79.

Box 44.4 summarizes the main patterns and their clinical manifestations.

IRRITABILITY/ANGER

Symptoms and Signs, Chapter 79

Irritability is a common emotional complaint. It includes feeling irritable frequently, flying off the handle easily, feeling frustrated, and similar emotional states. Of the traditional seven emotions, irritability is akin to 'anger' but it encompasses a broader range of emotional states and is generally not so intense. A propensity to anger is generally due to Liver patterns, whereas irritability may be caused by many different patterns affecting most organs.

In particular, the patterns that may cause irritability include:

- Qi stagnation
- Blood stasis
- Liver-Yang rising
- Blood deficiency
- Yin deficiency (with or without Empty-Heat)
- Heat (including Damp-Heat)
- Empty-Heat.

BOX 44.4 FEAR/ANXIETY

Empty
- Heart-Blood deficiency: mild anxiety, insomnia, palpitations
- Heart-Yin deficiency: anxiety that is worse in the evening, palpitations, night sweating
- Liver-Blood deficiency: mild anxiety, depression, insomnia
- Liver-Yin deficiency: mild anxiety, depression, insomnia, tongue without coating
- Kidney-Yin deficiency: anxiety that is worse in the evening, lack of will-power, dizziness, tinnitus
- Deficiency of Qi of the Heart and Gall-Bladder: mild anxiety, insomnia, timidity

Full
- Heart-Fire: severe anxiety, palpitations, Red tongue with coating
- Heart-Blood stasis: severe anxiety, palpitations, Purple tongue
- Phlegm-Fire harassing the Mind: severe anxiety, manic behaviour, Swollen tongue
- Liver-Qi stagnation: anxiety, depression, irritability, hypochondrial distension
- Liver-Fire: severe, anxiety, headache, thirst, Red tongue, Wiry pulse
- Liver-Yang rising: anxiety, headache, dizziness
- Rebellious Qi of the Penetrating Vessel: anxiety, panicky feeling, feeling of constriction of the throat, palpitation, tightness of the chest, abdominal fullness, Firm pulse
- Diaphragm-Heat: anxiety and feeling of stuffiness in the region under the heart following an invasion of Wind-Heat

Full/Empty
- Kidney- and Heart-Yin deficiency with Heart Empty-Heat: anxiety that is worse in the evening: dizziness, tinnitus, palpitations
- Heart-Yin deficiency with Empty-Heat: anxiety that is worse in the evening, palpitations, Red tongue without coating

---

BOX 44.5 EXAMPLES OF PATIENTS' EXPRESSIONS IN PATTERNS CAUSING IRRITABILITY

- Liver-Qi stagnation: *'I feel extremely irritable before my periods and take it out on my family.'*
- Lung-Qi stagnation: *'I feel this lump in the throat, I am on edge and feel like bursting into tears.'*
- Liver-Blood stasis: *'I seethe with resentment.'*
- Heart-Blood stasis: *'My mind is constantly judging and I feel resentful.'*
- Liver-Yang rising: *'I fly off the handle easily.'*
- Liver-Fire: *'I explode into a rage.'*
- Heart-Fire: *'I feel irritable, impatient and angry.'*
- Lung-Heat: *'I feel frustrated, weepy and irritable.'*
- Stomach-Heat: *'I feel often angry and obsessive.'*
- Liver-Blood deficiency: *'I feel lost, overwhelmed and on edge and I can't cope.'*
- Kidney-Yin deficiency: *'I feel helpless, unmotivated and on edge in the evening.'*
- Heart-Blood deficiency: *'I feel sad and on edge, and I can't cope.'*
- Kidney-Yin deficiency with Empty-Heat: *'I feel hot and bothered.'*
- Heart-Yin deficiency with Empty-Heat: *'I feel sad and hot and bothered.'*
- Damp-Heat: *'I feel heavy, yucky and irritable.'*

WORRY/OVERTHINKING

Many patients complain of a propensity to worry and overthinking and, even if it is not the presenting condition, many people profess to it when asked. The emotion of worry is related to the Spleen, and overthinking is more akin to the Lungs. Worry describes a condition when the patient is prone to imagining the worst possible outcome in a certain situation, for example a mother who imagines that her son has been in an accident when he is late home. Overthinking describes a state where the patient is unable to empty the mind of repetitive thoughts, which may be of a relatively trivial nature. Molehills may become mountains in these patients' minds when an apparently insignificant issue develops into a cause of great concern.

A propensity to worry and overthinking is most commonly caused by, and may in turn cause, an Empty condition. A deficiency of Spleen-Qi or Spleen-Blood, or both, is the most commonly seen pattern leading to worry and overthinking. However, deficiency of Heart-Qi, Lung-Qi, Heart-Yin, or of Heart- or Liver-Blood, or both, may also lead to excessive worrying.

Therefore, irritability may be due to Full or Empty causes; in general, the irritability from Empty causes is mild and somewhat vague, whereas that due to Full causes is more intense. The interrogation, therefore, should first of all try to establish the Full or Empty character of the irritability. In Empty conditions, the patient may say 'I get easily annoyed', or 'Things that did not use to get to me, now do', etc. In Full conditions, the patient may say something like 'I feel always irritable', 'I feel so on edge that I take it out on my children', etc.

Box 44.5 links examples of patterns that may cause irritability and examples of patients' expressions.

There are also cases where overthinking is caused by a mixed or Full condition, namely stagnation of Lung-Qi or Yin deficiency and Empty-Heat. Worry from a Full condition (such as Lung-Qi stagnation) is usually more intense and consuming than that from an Empty condition, which a patient may describe as more 'lurking in the background'.

Box 44.6 summarizes patterns underlying worry and overthinking.

BOX 44.6 WORRY/OVERTHINKING

- Heart- and Spleen-Qi deficiency: worry, slightly obsessive thinking, slight depression, overthinking, Pale tongue, Empty pulse
- Lung-Qi deficiency: worry, depression, Pale tongue, Empty pulse
- Heart-Blood deficiency: worry, depression, Pale and Thin tongue, Choppy or Fine pulse
- Liver-Blood deficiency: worry which increases after the period in women, Pale tongue, Choppy or Fine pulse
- Heart-Yin deficiency: worry, insomnia, dream-disturbed sleep, poor memory, anxiety, propensity to be startled, mental restlessness, uneasiness, 'feeling hot and bothered', Floating-Empty pulse, especially on the left Front position
- Lung-Qi stagnation: worry, mild irritability, depression, a feeling of a lump in the throat, tongue slightly Red on the sides in the chest areas, pulse very slightly Tight on the right Front position
- Heart-Yin deficiency with Empty-Heat: worry, especially in the evening, anxiety, propensity to be startled, mental restlessness, uneasiness, 'feeling hot and bothered', Red tongue, redder on the tip, no coating, Floating-Empty and Rapid pulse

---

SADNESS/GRIEF

'Sadness', which pertains to the Lungs, must be distinguished from a 'lack of joy', which pertains to the Heart. Sadness is an emotional state that weakens the Lungs and usually manifests with Lung-related symptoms such as a pale complexion, a weepy and weak voice. Lack of joy, on the other hand, is not an actual emotional state but a certain lack of vitality deriving from Heart deficiency; this manifests not with a sad demeanour, but with a flatness and lack of 'fire'.

A patient may report a feeling of sadness, or may be unaware of it. A Full or Empty quality on the Lung pulse is usually the most reliable indication of whether sadness is involved in a presenting condition. I find that a Full Lung pulse often indicates sadness which has been held on to for a long time by the patient, who may be totally unaware of its presence. When the Lung pulse is Weak or Empty, I find the patient more likely to report feeling sad.

Sadness depletes Lung- and Heart-Qi; however, with time, the deficiency of Qi in the chest may also give rise to some stagnation of Qi in the chest. This stagnation is associated with the Lungs and Heart and not the Liver. It manifests with a slight feeling of tightness of the chest, experiencing the sadness in the chest, sighing and slight palpitations.

The most likely Empty patterns giving rise to sadness are a deficiency of Lung-Qi and Heart-Qi, Liver-Blood or Heart-Blood. When sadness is due to an Empty condition it is often accompanied by frequent crying. Sadness from Liver-Blood deficiency is more common in women and becomes worse after the period or after childbirth. Sadness with a feeling of lump in the throat may be due to Lung-Qi stagnation.

Grief is akin to sadness and usually derives from loss, separation or bereavement. Like sadness, it depletes Lung- and Heart-Qi but, with time, it may also give rise to some stagnation of Qi in the chest causing similar symptoms to the ones mentioned above for sadness.

Case history 44.2 illustrates a pattern of grief underlying chest pain.

Case history 44.2

A 57-year-old woman presented with the main complaint of pain in the chest. As she was speaking, I observed that her eyes were quite lustreless and lacking in *shen*. This always points to an emotional origin of the problem. I asked her how long she had had the chest pain and she replied that it had started after her husband's death a few years before.

Her tongue was Swollen with a red tip and her pulse was slightly Slippery but very slightly Tight on the Lung position.

Diagnosis: This is a very good example of the effect of grief. The grief from her husband's death had caused initially a deficiency of the Heart and Lungs; with time, this had caused some stagnation of Qi in these two organs. The stagnation of Heart-Qi manifested with a red tip of the tongue while the stagnation of Qi in both

Heart and Lungs caused the chest pain. As this condition was long-standing, the depletion and simultaneous stagnation of Lung-Qi had disrupted the movement and transformation of Qi and fluids, giving rise to some Phlegm in the chest which contributed to the chest pain. The Phlegm was indicated by the swelling of the tongue and the Slippery pulse.

This patient had an interesting emotional reaction to the treatment which is worth reporting. I used a simple treatment needling PE-6 Neiguan on one side, LU-7 Lieque on the other, Ren-12 Zhongwan and ST-40 Fenglong. A few days after the treatment she went to the graveyard to visit her husband's grave for the first time since his death and she cried. She had obviously repressed her grief for many years and this

had caused the stagnation of Qi of the Heart and Lungs in the chest. Another emotional reaction a few days after the treatment was that for the first time she experienced anger at work. This is also interesting as, just as there is a controlling relationship between Wood and Metal, there is one between their allied emotions (i.e. anger and sadness/grief). Obviously the release of Qi stagnation in Metal had stopped excessive control of Metal over Wood and led to an explosion of anger. Moreover, each emotion can counteract another across the reverse Controlling (*Ke*) cycle of the Five Elements; that is, anger (Wood) counteracts sadness (Metal), joy (Fire) counteracts fear (Water), pensiveness (Earth) counteracts anger (Wood), etc.

Box 44.7 summarizes the patterns underlying sadness and grief.

BOX 44.7 SADNESS/GRIEF

- Lung- and Heart-Qi deficiency: sadness, crying, depression, Pale tongue, Empty pulse
- Liver-Blood deficiency: sadness, crying, worse after the period or childbirth (women), mental confusion, aimlessness, Pale tongue, Choppy or Fine pulse
- Heart-Blood deficiency: sadness, crying, depression, Pale and Thin tongue, Choppy or Fine pulse
- Lung-Qi stagnation: sadness with feeling of a lump in the throat, mild irritability, depression, tongue slightly Red on the sides in the chest areas, pulse very slightly Tight on the right Front position

---

EXCESS JOY

Of course, few patients will report feeling excessively joyful! A normal state of joy is obviously not a cause of disease. Several emotional states are included under the term of 'excess joy'. First, it includes the sudden state of extreme elation deriving from joyful news. This makes Qi rise and it expands the Heart. Secondly, excess joy can be interpreted as a life characterized by excessive excitement and stimulation. This also causes Qi to rise and may lead to Heart-Fire. Thirdly, excess joy is seen in certain mental conditions such as hypomania or manic behaviour.

The negative effect of excess joy can be easily observed in young children. Every mother knows that

a period of extreme playfulness, hyperactivity and laughing is frequently followed by tears.

A Full pattern of the Heart is most likely to cause excess joy. Phlegm-Fire harassing the Heart may cause the most severe cases of excess joy; that seen in mental diseases such as bipolar disorder is a typical example of this. However, Phlegm-Fire does not necessarily *always* cause severe symptoms. It may be seen relatively frequently in milder forms when it causes excessive and inappropriate laughter, bouts of excess joy and hyperactivity. Heart-Fire may also cause a permanently elated mood.

> **!**
>
> Phlegm-Fire harassing the Heart does not always manifest with severe mental symptoms.

Empty-Heat of the Heart may also lead to excess joy and a feeling of being driven and not being able to stop.

Box 44.8 summarizes the patterns underlying excess joy.

MENTAL RESTLESSNESS

'Mental restlessness' is a translation of the term *Fan Zao*, which literally means 'vexation and restlessness'. It also includes restless legs. The term *Fan Zao* encompasses two different symptoms: *Fan* (vexation) is due to Full-Heat and pertains to the Lungs, whereas *Zao* (rest-

---

BOX 44.8 EXCESS JOY

- Phlegm-Fire harassing the Heart: excess joy, mental confusion, excessive and inappropriate laughter, mental restlessness, Red tongue with redder swollen tip, Heart crack with a sticky yellow coating inside it, Slippery-Rapid or Slippery-Overflowing-Rapid pulse
- Heart-Fire: Excess joy, permanently elated mood, excessive laughter, mental restlessness, feeling of agitation, Red tongue with redder tip and yellow coating, Overflowing-Rapid pulse
- Heart Empty-Heat: excess joy, permanently elated feeling as if being driven, anxiety, propensity to be startled, mental restlessness, uneasiness, 'feeling hot and bothered', Red tongue, redder on the tip, no coating, Floating-Empty and Rapid pulse

---

lessness) is due to Empty-Heat and pertains to the Kidneys. *Fan* is Yang whereas *Zao* is Yin.

A patient is unlikely to use the term 'mental restlessness' but may describe having 'difficulty in concentration', 'not being able to focus on one thing for any length of time' or 'not being able to sit still and do nothing'.

Yin deficiency with Empty-Heat may cause a vague feeling of mental restlessness which worsens in the evening. Phlegm-Heat in the Stomach or Heart, or both, or Heart-Fire, will cause a more intense feeling which may be accompanied by mental confusion. Mental restlessness may also be caused by Lung-Heat, in which cause it will be accompanied by worry and other Lung symptoms such as breathlessness or cough.

Box 44.9 summarizes the patterns underlying mental restlessness.

BOX 44.9 MENTAL RESTLESSNESS

- Yin deficiency with Empty-Heat: vague mental restlessness, restless legs, Red tongue without coating, Floating-Empty and Rapid pulse
- Phlegm-Heat in the Stomach and Heart: mental restlessness, mental confusion, agitation, rash behaviour, tendency to hit or scold people, shouting, depression, manic behaviour, tongue Red in the centre with a sticky yellow coating and a Stomach/Heart crack with a rough, sticky yellow coating inside it, Slippery-Rapid pulse
- Heart-Fire: pronounced mental restlessness, agitation, Red tongue with redder tip and yellow coating, Overflowing-Rapid pulse
- Lung-Heat: mental restlessness, worry, Red tongue with yellow coating, Overflowing-Rapid pulse

---

NOTES

1. Jamison K R 1993 Touched with Fire – Manic-Depressive Illness and the Artistic Temperament. The Free Press, New York, pp. 261–262.
2. 1979 The Yellow Emperor's Classic of Internal Medicine – Simple Questions (*Huang Di Nei Jing Su Wen* 黄帝内经素问), People's Health Publishing House, Beijing, p. 492. First published c. 100BC.
3. Cited in Zhang Bo Yu 1986 Internal Medicine (*Zhong Yi Nei Ke Xue* 中医妇科学), Shanghai Science Publishing House, Shanghai. p. 121.
4. Ibid., p. 121.

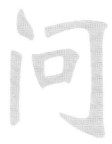

Chapter **45**

SEXUAL SYMPTOMS

Chapter contents

INTRODUCTION *391*

MEN *392*
  Impotence *392*
  Lack of libido *392*
  Premature ejaculation *393*
  Nocturnal emissions *393*
  Tiredness and dizziness after ejaculation *393*

WOMEN *393*
  Lack of libido *393*
  Headache soon after orgasm *394*

INTRODUCTION

An enquiry about the sexual life of the patient should always form part of the interrogation. This is not one of the traditional 10 questions from Chinese books, partly for cultural reasons. In fact, starting from the Ming period and especially during the Qing dynasty, Chinese medicine was heavily influenced by the prevalent Confucian morality, which condemned any talk or display of sexuality.

? **WHY** WE ASK

Questions about sexual symptoms are asked primarily to ascertain the state of the Kidneys. In fact a Kidney deficiency is at the basis of many sexual symptoms such as impotence, premature ejaculation or frigidity.

In men, apart from asking about any sexual problems such as impotence, it is important to establish whether any of their symptoms is aggravated by sexual activity or if they feel excessively tired after sexual activity. An aggravation of a symptom after sexual activity always indicates a Qi deficiency, often of the Kidneys. A Kidney deficiency is indicated also if a man feels especially tired after sexual activity and particularly if the tiredness is accompanied by dizziness, backache, weak knees, etc.

However, it should not be forgotten that other organs play a role in the origin of sexual symptoms and particularly the Liver and the Heart. The Heart, in particular, plays an important role in sexual desire and in the achievement of a normal erection in men.

? WHEN WE ASK

I generally ask about sexual symptoms when the patient presents with a clear Kidney- or Heart-deficiency pattern. I also ask about sexual symptoms when the patient is clearly under emotional stress and I suspect that this may be due to sexual problems such as impotence in men or failure to achieve an orgasm in women.

? HOW WE ASK

For obvious reasons, the practitioner needs to be particularly tactful when asking about sexual symptoms, especially when the practitioner and patient are of the opposite sex. In some cases, when I feel instinctively that the patient would not appreciate such questions, I do not ask them.

An enquiry about sexual activity in men is important not only for diagnostic reasons but also to be able to advise them about appropriate levels of sexual activities according to Chinese medicine.[1] There are significant differences between the sexual physiology of men and of women that are not often taken into account when advising patients about the desirable frequency of sexual activity: the Chinese caution about 'excessive sexual activity' is more relevant to men than to women. In fact, the *Tian Gui*, a direct manifestation of Essence (*Jing*), is sperm in men and menstrual blood in women: quite simply, because men lose sperm but women do not obviously lose menstrual blood during intercourse, sexual activity may potentially be weakening for men (when it is too frequent) but not so much for women.

MEN

The sexual symptoms discussed are:

- impotence
- lack of libido
- premature ejaculation
- nocturnal emissions
- tiredness and dizziness after ejaculation.

(The symptoms and signs related to men's sexual system are in Chapter 75 of Part 5.)

Impotence

Symptoms and Signs, Chapter 75

Impotence is by far the most common sexual complaint in men and the first cause that would come to mind would be a Kidney deficiency and especially a Kidney-Yang deficiency. This is a common cause of impotence, especially in older men, in which case it is accompanied by a feeling of cold, backache, weak knees, dizziness, tinnitus and poor memory, and abundant and clear urine.

In young men, however, it is my experience that impotence is more often related to a Heart pattern, such as Heart-Blood deficiency or Heart-Fire, and anxiety. In a few cases, impotence may also be caused by Damp-Heat in the Liver channel.

> **!**
>
> Impotence in young men is caused more frequently by a Heart pattern than by a Kidney deficiency.

Box 45.1 summarizes patterns underlying male impotence.

> **BOX 45.1 IMPOTENCE**
>
> - Kidney (especially Kidney-Yang) deficiency: impotence, feeling of cold, backache, abundant clear urine, weak knees, dizziness, tinnitus, poor memory
> - Heart-Blood deficiency: impotence, dizziness, palpitations, Choppy pulse
> - Heart-Fire: impotence, palpitations, insomnia, dream-disturbed sleep, Rapid-Overflowing pulse
> - Damp-Heat in the Liver channel: impotence, heaviness of the scrotum, urethral discharge, sticky yellow coating

Lack of libido

Symptoms and Signs, Chapter 75

Lack of libido in men is usually related to a deficiency of Qi or Yang, most frequently of the Kidneys; however, other organs may be relevant and a severe Qi deficiency of such organs as Spleen, Heart or Lungs may also cause lack of libido. In my experience, a deficiency of the Heart is a more common cause of lack of libido than deficiency of the Kidneys. Among Full conditions, Liver-Qi stagnation may also cause lack of libido. Dampness in the Lower Burner may also cause lack of libido.

Box 45.2 summarizes patterns underlying lack of libido in men.

BOX 45.2 LACK OF LIBIDO IN MEN

- Kidney-Yang deficiency
- Deficiency of Qi of the Heart, Lungs or Spleen
- Heart-Blood deficiency
- Liver-Qi stagnation
- Dampness

Premature ejaculation

Symptoms and Signs, Chapter 75

Premature ejaculation is usually related to a Kidney pattern and Kidney-Qi especially may not be firm. It may also be due to a Heart pattern such as Heart-Qi or Heart-Blood deficiency.

Box 45.3 summarizes patterns underlying premature ejaculation.

BOX 45.3 PREMATURE EJACULATION

- Kidney-Qi not firm
- Kidney-Yang deficiency
- Heart-Qi or Heart-Blood deficiency

Nocturnal emissions

Symptoms and Signs, Chapter 75

'Nocturnal emissions' indicates ejaculation during sleep; this symptom always has 'pride of place' among Kidney-deficiency symptoms in Chinese books. In the West, this symptom is relatively rare and it is not even considered a 'symptom' unless it occurs very frequently (e.g. once a week or more).

There are cultural reasons why this symptom always has a prominent place among Kidney-deficiency symptoms in Chinese books. In ancient times ejaculation during sleep, especially if with sexual dreams, was considered to be due to the man having intercourse with female ghosts at night; such ghosts were considered very dangerous because they robbed men of their vital Essence.

In general, nocturnal emissions without sexual dreams are due purely to a deficiency (usually of the Kidneys), while nocturnal emissions with sexual dreams are usually due to Heat (which may be Full or Empty). Thus, Empty-Heat arising from a Kidney deficiency may cause nocturnal emissions with dreams; Full-Heat, particularly of the Liver or Heart, or both, may also cause this symptom.

> **!**
>
> Nocturnal emissions without dreams are due to a Kidney-Yin deficiency whereas nocturnal emissions with dreams are due to Heat (Full or Empty).

Tiredness and dizziness after ejaculation

Symptoms and Signs, Chapter 75

A pronounced feeling of tiredness and dizziness after ejaculation is nearly always due to a deficiency of the Kidneys.

WOMEN

The sexual symptoms discussed are as follows:

- lack of libido
- headache soon after orgasm.

Lack of libido

Symptoms and Signs, Chapter 89

Lack of libido or an inability to reach an orgasm in women is usually related to a Kidney or Heart deficiency.

Generally, sexual desire depends on the state of Kidney-Yang and the Minister Fire: a deficient Minister Fire may cause a lack of sexual desire (and conversely, Fire of the Liver or Heart, or both, and Empty-Heat deriving from Kidney-Yin deficiency may cause an excessive sexual desire).

The Heart plays an important role in sexual arousal and orgasm in women. During sexual arousal, there is an arousal of the (physiological) Minister Fire of the Kidneys, which goes up towards the Heart and Pericardium; it is this upward flow of the Minister Fire towards the Heart that causes a flushed face and an increased heart rate. Thus, a lack of sexual desire is often due to a deficient Minister Fire and therefore Kidney-Yang.

During orgasm, the Minister Fire that was rising during sexual arousal is suddenly discharged downwards; this downward movement of the Minister Fire is controlled by the Heart (whose Qi naturally descends). Hence an inability to reach an orgasm may be due to a Heart deficiency.

Of course, a woman's inability to reach an orgasm depends also on the man's performance during the

sexual act. According to Daoist sexual alchemy, men pertain to Fire and Fire flares up easily and is easily extinguished; women pertain to Water and Water is 'slow to boil and slow to cool down'. It is for this reason that the ancient Daoist sex manuals were aimed primarily at men so that they would be skilled in the art of sexual foreplay. Therefore, when considering a woman's inability to reach an orgasm we should keep in mind the possibility that this is due to her partner's lack of skill rather than her own deficiency pattern.

BOX 45.4 LACK OF LIBIDO IN WOMEN

- Kidney-Yang deficiency
- Heart-Yang deficiency
- Heart-Blood deficiency

Box 45.4 summarizes patterns underlying lack of libido in women.

Headache soon after orgasm

Symptoms and Signs, Chapter 89

A headache soon after orgasm usually indicates rebellious Qi of the Penetrating Vessel. It may also indicate Heart-Fire.

NOTES

1. See Maciocia G 1998 The Foundations of Chinese Medicine. Churchill Livingstone, Edinburgh, pp. 137–139.

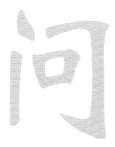

Chapter **46**

WOMEN'S SYMPTOMS

Chapter contents

INTRODUCTION   *395*

THE GYNAECOLOGICAL HISTORY   *396*

BREAST SYMPTOMS   *397*
  Breast lumps   *397*
  Premenstrual breast distension   *398*

MENSTRUATION   *398*
  Amount of bleeding   *399*
  Colour   *400*
  Consistency   *400*
  Cycle   *400*
  Menarche   *401*
  Menopause   *401*
  Pain   *401*
  Premenstrual symptoms   *404*
  Other symptoms occurring around menstruation   *405*

PREGNANCY AND CHILDBIRTH   *406*
  Fertility   *406*
  Miscarriage and abortion   *408*
  Childbirth   *408*
  Lactation   *408*

VAGINAL DISCHARGE   *409*

INTRODUCTION

❓ **WHY** WE ASK

In women patients, an enquiry about gynaecological symptoms is absolutely essential, as such questions are often crucial to reach a diagnosis in women, even for non-gynaecological problems. For example, if a woman suffers from lower abdominal pain and we are uncertain as to the cause, if her periods are painful and the menstrual blood is dark and with clots this indicates conclusively that the abdominal pain is due to Blood stasis.

❓ **WHEN** WE ASK

Unless a woman presents specifically with a gynaecological complaint, I generally ask about her gynaecological history towards the end of the consultation. An enquiry into the gynaecological history even in post-menopausal women gives us an idea of the general condition of Qi and Blood. For example, a woman may have suffered throughout her life from heavy periods that were caused by Blood-Heat; if she comes to us after the menopause and we suspect that she might suffer from Blood-Heat but we are uncertain because the symptoms are quite mild, an enquiry into her menstrual history would help to confirm this diagnosis.

❓ **HOW** WE ASK

When asking about a woman's gynaecological history, we should always start from the beginning by enquiring about the conditions of her cycle 2 years after

menarche (because it is common for the cycle to be irregular for the first 2 years before it settles down).

We should ask systematically first about the actual menstrual cycle and, secondly, about all other events in a woman's gynaecological history.

Regarding the menstrual cycle, we should ask about: the age of menarche, the cycle, the amount of bleeding, the colour of menstrual blood, and whether there are clots, pain, and any premenstrual symptoms.

With regard to other gynaecological events, we should ask specifically about: childbirth, abortion, miscarriage, use of contraceptives (the Pill, uterine coil), or of hormone replacement therapy, the presence of pelvic inflammatory disease, whether there have been any gynaecological surgical interventions (such as dilatation and curettage, laser treatment, hysteroscopy, colposcopy, laparoscopy, etc.).

THE GYNAECOLOGICAL HISTORY

Women's gynaecological history may sometimes be complicated; for example, a woman may have used the contraceptive pill or the coil for some years, or she may have had two children with possibly one or more miscarriages or terminations in between. In such cases, it is useful to draw a diagram illustrating clearly the ages at which such events occurred. As an illustration, Figure 46.1 shows the gynaecological history of a woman whose menarche occurred at 14 and who had an abortion at 18, a child at 24 and 28, an ovarian cyst at 36 and the menopause at 52.

If the woman's cycle is irregular and characterized by discharges or mid-cycle pain or discharge, it is also

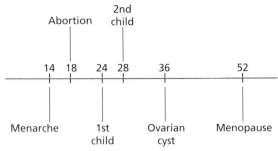

Fig. 46.1 Diagram of gynaecological history

useful to draw a diagram illustrating clearly at what part of the cycle such events take place. As a way of illustration, Figure 46.2 shows the menstrual cycle of a woman whose period lasts 7 days and who experiences mid-cycle pain and premenstrual tension with breast distension.

Some women may complain of prolonged menstrual bleeding whereas, in fact, they may suffer from mid-cycle bleeding. Case history 46.1 illustrates this.

Gynaecological events affecting diagnosis

Some gynaecological events (e.g. colposcopy) have a certain effect on the woman's physiology which we need to take into account when diagnosing; others make diagnosing practically impossible, (e.g. the Pill).

The answers to questions regarding regularity of cycle, amount of bleeding, colour of menstrual blood, pain, etc., are unreliable if the woman is on the Pill or has an intrauterine device. The Pill regularizes the periods, makes them usually scanty and less painful, and often prevents clotting; the intrauterine device

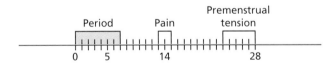

Fig. 46.2 Diagram of menstrual cycle

Case history 46.1

A 42-year-old woman complained of 'almost constant menstrual bleeding'. She said that her period would last for 3 weeks and she would then have a week without bleeding before the next period began.

However, on closer interrogation it emerged that what she described as 'bleeding' was in fact a dark vaginal discharge. The diagnostic interpretation and treatment were therefore obviously different from what would be suggested by prolonged bleeding.

generally makes the periods heavier and more painful. In such cases, it is important to ask the patient what her menstrual cycle was like before she began using these forms of contraception.

BREAST SYMPTOMS

The breasts in women are influenced primarily by the Stomach channel, which controls the main tissues of the breast and the lactiferous ducts; the Liver channel influences the nipple but also, together with the Gall-Bladder channel, the lateral side of the breast. The Penetrating Vessel also influences the lactiferous ducts and the connective tissues of the breast, which, in Chinese medicine, would be classified as 'Membranes' (*Huang*). The Muscle channels of the Gall-Bladder, Heart and Pericardium flow over the breast. (See Fig. 46.3 and also Fig. 12.1 on p. 121 illustrating the channels coursing through the breast.)

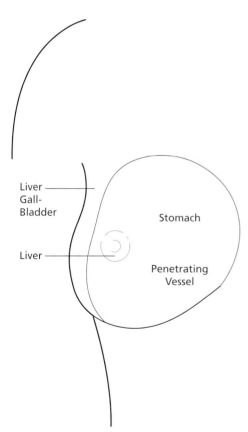

Fig. 46.3 Organs influencing areas of the breast

The Penetrating Vessel originates from the Uterus and connects with the breasts and this relationship can be seen in the linkage that exists between menstrual blood and breast milk: breast milk is a transformation of menstrual blood that occurs after childbirth and the Penetrating Vessel, being the Sea of Blood, is therefore, after childbirth, the source of breast milk. Many breast pathologies, including breast lumps, especially in women over the age of 40, nearly always occur against a background of 'disharmony' of the Penetrating Vessel, which means either a deficiency or stasis of Blood in this vessel.

Breast lumps

Observation, Chapter 12; Palpation, Chapter 51; Symptoms and Signs, Chapter 88

A common pathology of the breasts in women is the development of lumps.

Relatively soft, movable, painless, multiple lumps with distinct edges usually indicate fibrocystic disease, which, from the Chinese point of view, is due to Phlegm.

A single, movable, relatively hard lump with distinct edges usually indicates a fibroadenoma, which, from the Chinese point of view, is due to a combination of Phlegm and Blood stasis.

A single, painless, immovable lump with indistinct edges may indicate carcinoma of the breast which, from the Chinese point of view, is usually due to a combination of Phlegm, Qi stagnation and Blood stasis.

The age of the patient may give a rough indication of which is the most likely of these three pathologies

---

BOX 46.1 BREAST LUMPS

Chinese medicine differentiation
- Relatively soft, movable, painless multiple lumps with distinct edges: Phlegm
- Single, movable, relatively hard lump with distinct edges: Phlegm with Blood stasis
- Single, not movable, relatively hard lump with indistinct edges: Phlegm with Qi stagnation and Blood stasis

Western medicine differentiation
- Soft, movable, painless, multiple lumps with distinct edges: fibrocystic disease
- Single movable, relatively hard lump with distinct edges: fibroadenoma
- Single, not movable, relatively hard lump with indistinct edges: carcinoma

because fibroadenomas are more common between the ages of 20 and 30, cysts between 30 and 50 and carcinoma from 50 onwards; of course, these are only general statistical indications which always have exceptions in practice.

Box 46.1 summarizes patterns underlying breast lumps.

Premenstrual breast distension

Observation, Chapter 12; Symptoms and Signs, Chapter 88

One of the most common presenting breast symptoms is premenstrual breast distension, which is a very typical sign of Liver-Qi stagnation. Although Liver-Qi stagnation affecting the breasts is a very common condition, stagnation of Lung-Qi also has an important influence on the breasts in women. Emotional problems such as sadness, grief and worry affect the Lungs and may impair the circulation of Qi in the chest and therefore in the breasts as well. For this reason, many breast pathologies in women, including breast lumps, may be due to stagnation of Lung-Qi rather than Liver-Qi and to the above-mentioned emotions rather than anger or repressed anger. In particular, some modern Chinese doctors relate breast pathologies to the emotional stress deriving from separation such as widowhood, breaking up of relationships, divorce, death of one's children or bereavement at a young age from the death of one's spouse. Liver-Qi stagnation is accompanied by irritability and a Wiry pulse, whereas in Lung-Qi stagnation there is sadness and a Weak pulse.

If the breasts become also swollen, uncomfortable and noticeably larger before the period, this also indicates also Liver-Qi stagnation but combined with Phlegm, in which case the tongue is swollen. If the breasts are distended and noticeably painful before the periods, with a Purple tongue, this indicates Liver-Blood stasis. A slight feeling of distension of the breasts after the periods, with a Choppy pulse, is usually due to Liver-Blood deficiency.

Case history 46.2 illustrates a pattern underlying breast distension.

Box 46.2 summarizes the patterns underlying breast distension.

MENSTRUATION

When asking about menstruation, we should ask about the following aspects systematically:

- amount of bleeding
- colour
- consistency
- cycle
- menarche
- menopause
- pain
- premenstrual symptoms
- other symptoms occurring around menstruation.

Case history 46.2

A 36-year-old woman had been suffering from premenstrual swelling and pain of both breasts, but worse on the left, with a lump on the edge of the left breast which came up before the period and disappeared afterwards. She had been suffering from this problem for approximately 8 years. She suffered no other menstrual irregularity as her periods came regularly and were not too heavy or scanty and not painful.

On interrogation, it transpired that she also suffered from tiredness, floaters, weakness, dizziness, palpitations, loose stools and anxiety in the evening.

Her tongue was slightly Pale and Swollen on the sides and had a sticky coating. Her pulse was Fine and slightly Wiry.

Diagnosis: The breast pathology itself shows a clear condition of Liver-Qi stagnation because the swelling of the breast is clearly premenstrual; however, the breast lump, the pronounced swelling and the pain indicate that there is also Phlegm. This is Qi-Phlegm and the lump comes and goes because of the Qi stagnation. Liver-Qi stagnation occurs against a background of Liver-Blood deficiency of which there are clear manifestations (tiredness, floaters, dizziness, Pale sides of the tongue, Fine pulse). There is also some Heart-Blood deficiency indicated by the palpitations and the anxiety in the evening. Finally, there is an underlying Spleen-Qi deficiency indicated by the weakness and the loose stools; the Spleen-Qi deficiency has given rise to Phlegm.

BOX 46.2 PREMENSTRUAL BREAST DISTENSION

- Liver-Qi stagnation: pronounced distension, irritability, Wiry pulse
- Lung-Qi stagnation: slight breast distension, sadness, Weak pulse
- Liver-Qi stagnation with Phlegm: swollen and painful breasts, Swollen tongue
- Liver-Blood stasis: painful breasts, Purple tongue
- Liver-Blood deficiency: mild breast distension, Choppy pulse

---

When asking questions about the menstrual cycle, I always ask the woman how her periods were about 2 years after the menarche (remember that it is normal for the period to be somewhat irregular for 2 years after menarche). This is important because it gives us an idea of the woman's *constitutional* menstrual cycle, eliminating the influence of subsequent gynaecological events (e.g. pregnancy, childbirth, miscarriage, abortion, contraception, etc).

For example, a woman may have suffered heavy blood loss during childbirth and therefore develop a Blood deficiency which makes her periods scanty. The scanty period in this case shows not her constitutional menstrual cycle but the consequence of a definite cause of disease. By asking her about her menstruation 2 years after menarche, we formulate an idea of the constitutional state of her gynaecological system.

Case history 46.3

A 42-year-old woman had been suffering from heavy periods for 15 years: the periods came regularly, they lasted 7 days, they were not painful and the menstrual blood was dark with clots. The heaviest flow was in the first 3 days of the period. A month before her consultation a scan revealed the presence of fibroids in the uterus.

Her body build was robust, her eyes had good lustre indicating good Spirit and her general energy was good. She was rather overweight and her complexion was sallow. She had no other symptoms, apart from occasionally mucus in the stools. Questions investigating a possible Kidney deficiency revealed no symptoms of it. On palpation, her abdomen felt quite soft and the fibroids could not be palpated. Her tongue had a normal colour but was very Swollen. Her pulse was Slippery, Full and slightly Overflowing.

Amount of bleeding

Symptoms and Signs, Chapter 84

The loss of blood during menstruation can vary between 30 and 80 ml. A period is defined as 'heavy' if the loss of blood is either profuse or prolonged. It is important to ask how many days the period lasts because a period that lasts more than 5 days is normally considered excessive in Chinese medicine, while one that lasts under 4 days is normally considered scanty. While most women would describe as abnormal a period that either lasts too long or is too heavy, they would not use the same term for a period that is too short or too scanty. In other words, many women would say that their period is 'normal' when it lasts 3 days or even less or when the bleeding is very light.

A heavy loss of blood is due to Qi deficiency, Blood-Heat, Blood Empty-Heat, Liver- and Kidney-Yin deficiency or Blood stasis. If the period is scanty, this denotes Blood deficiency. Cold in the Uterus or Liver-Blood stasis.

> **!**
>
> In my experience, there is strong bias among practitioners to attribute heavy periods always to Qi deficiency. This is not so and, in my experience, about half the cases are due to Blood-Heat and half to Qi deficiency.

Case history 46.3 illustrates a pattern underlying heavy periods.

Diagnosis: Her body build, the good Spirit and general energy indicate a good constitution, although being overweight indicates Phlegm. The presence of Phlegm is confirmed by the presence of occasional mucus in the stools, her being overweight, the swelling of the tongue and the Slippery pulse; the fibroids could also be partly due to Phlegm. The dark menstrual blood with clots and the presence of the fibroids themselves indicates Blood stasis localized in the Uterus and not severe enough to turn the tongue Purple. In this case, we can therefore conclude that the fibroids are due to a combination of both Phlegm and Blood stasis; the softness of her abdomen on palpation indicates that Phlegm is the predominant pathogenic factor in the formation of the fibroids.

The two major causes of heavy menstrual flow are usually Qi deficiency or Blood-Heat and in this case it is due to Blood-Heat; there are not many signs of this because the tongue is not Red, but it is shown prima-

rily by the Overflowing pulse. On the other hand, there are no signs of a Spleen or Kidney deficiency even though the Spleen must be deficient for Phlegm to form. In her case, there are probably not many symptoms of deficiency because of her good constitution, which is also shown by the Full pulse; this, while it does indicate the presence of pathogenic factor also indicates that the Upright Qi has not been severely affected.

In this case, it is necessary to treat her three main conditions (i.e. Phlegm, Blood-Heat and Blood stasis) simultaneously and the treatment principle is therefore to resolve Phlegm, cool and invigorate Blood and stop bleeding.

Box 46.3 summarizes the patterns underlying abnormal amounts of bleeding.

BOX 46.3 AMOUNT OF BLEEDING

Heavy
- Qi deficiency
- Blood-Heat
- Blood Empty-Heat
- Liver- and Kidney-Yin deficiency
- Liver-Blood stasis

Scanty
- Blood deficiency
- Cold in the Uterus
- Liver-Blood stasis

Colour

Observation, Chapter 20; Symptoms and Signs, Chapter 84

The colour of the menstrual blood varies slightly during the period. In general, it is usually dark red, being lighter at the beginning, deep red in the middle, and pinkish at the end of the period. Box 46.4 summarizes the main areas of questioning and patterns with regard to colour.

BOX 46.4 COLOUR OF MENSTRUAL BLOOD

- Blood-Heat: dark red or bright red
- Blood deficiency: pale
- Stasis of Blood: blackish, very dark
- Full-Cold: purplish
- Empty-Cold: brownish like soya-bean sauce and dilute
- Empty-Heat in Blood: scarlet red

Consistency

Observation, Chapter 20; Symptoms and Signs, Chapter 84

The normal flow does not coagulate and there are no clots; the blood is neither dilute nor thick. Box 46.5 summarizes the main areas of questioning and patterns with regard to the consistency of menstrual blood.

BOX 46.5 CONSISTENCY OF MENSTRUAL BLOOD

- Stasis of Blood or Cold in the Uterus: clotted, with dark, dull clots
- Heat: clotted, with dark but fresh-looking clots
- Stasis of Blood: large clots
- Cold in the Uterus: small dark clots, but blood not dark
- Blood or Yin deficiency: watery
- Dampness or Damp-Heat in the Uterus: sticky

Cycle

Symptoms and Signs, Chapter 84

The length of the cycle is ideally 28 days, but it may vary from this norm. The regularity of the cycle is somewhat more important than its absolute value; thus, if the cycle is consistently of 32 days, this can be deemed normal and would not be considered as 'late periods'. Moreover, an occasional deviation from a regular cycle should not be considered abnormal as the menstrual cycle is influenced by many factors such as travelling, emotional stress, etc.

There are several main areas of questioning with regard to the cycle. Periods that are always early (i.e. more than 7 days early) may be due to Qi deficiency, Blood-Heat or Empty-Heat in the Blood from Blood or Yin deficiency. Periods that are always late (i.e. more than 7 days late) may be due to Blood deficiency, stasis of Blood or stasis of Cold. Periods that are irregular (sometimes late, sometimes early) may be due to stagnation of Liver-Qi, stasis of Liver-Blood, Spleen deficiency or Kidney deficiency. Periods that stop and start, or that start or end with a brownish discharge, may be due to Liver-Blood stasis. If there is mid-cycle bleeding then this may be due to Damp-Heat, especially if there is also some pain, Qi deficiency, or Liver- and Kidney-Yin deficiency.

Amenorrhoea may be due to severe Blood deficiency (as often happens in women athletes), Blood stasis or Cold in the Uterus.

Box 46.6 summarizes the patterns underlying menstrual cycle irregularites.

BOX 46.6 CYCLE IRREGULARITIES

- Always early: Qi deficiency, Blood-Heat, Blood Empty-Heat, Liver- and Kidney-Yin deficiency
- Always late: Blood deficiency, Liver-Blood stasis, Cold in the Uterus
- Irregular: Liver-Qi stagnation, Liver-Blood stasis, Spleen deficiency, Kidney deficiency
- Hesitant start: Liver-Blood stasis
- Starting or ending with brownish discharge: Liver-Blood stasis
- Mid-cycle bleeding: Damp-Heat, Qi deficiency, Liver- and Kidney-Yin deficiency
- Amenorrhoea: severe Blood deficiency, Blood stasis, Cold in the Uterus

---

Menarche

The age of menarche ranges between 10 and 16, with a mean at 12.8. Menarche tends to occur at a younger age in industrialized countries compared with developing, agricultural societies.

Early menarche (i.e. before about 13) may indicate Blood-Heat, whereas late menarche (after about 16) may indicate Blood or Kidney deficiency, or both, or Cold in the Uterus.

Menopause

Symptoms and Signs, Chapter 89

By menopause is meant the period of time during which levels of oestrogen decline sharply, menstruation stops and a woman becomes infertile. From the Chinese point of view, the menopause is due to a natural, physiological decline of Kidney-Essence and it is therefore not a gynaecological 'disease'. It requires therapeutic intervention only when the manifestations of this transitional period become uncomfortable or distressing.

!

The menopause is *not* a 'disease'.

The main manifestations which usually bring a woman to seek treatment are hot flushes, sweating and vaginal dryness. Strictly speaking, these three are the only symptoms which are directly related to a decline of hormone levels. However, many other symptoms may appear owing to the decline of Kidney-Essence and other allied patterns. These may be headaches, depression, anxiety, irritability, crying, poor memory, clumsiness, insomnia, tiredness, dry skin and hair.

It is a common misconception that menopausal symptoms are always due to Kidney-Yin deficiency because they are characterized by hot flushes. Although the hot flushes will obviously be more intense if there is a Kidney-Yin deficiency, they also occur in woman suffering from Kidney-Yang deficiency because, especially during the menopausal years, a Kidney deficiency nearly always includes a deficiency of both Yin and Yang. This very frequently gives rise to contradictory hot and cold symptoms. For example, a menopausal woman suffering from Kidney-Yin deficiency may experience severe hot flushes, night sweating, dryness of the vagina and skin, but she may also suffer from cold feet. Vice versa, a menopausal woman suffering from Kidney-Yang deficiency may experience cold feet and a cold feeling in general, frequent urination but also hot flushes.

There are two other patterns associated with a Kidney deficiency in the menopausal years which are particularly common; these are Liver-Yang rising (causing headaches) and Heart-Yin deficiency with Empty-Heat (causing insomnia, anxiety, agitation and poor memory).

Finally, menopausal symptoms may be aggravated by pre-existing patterns, the main one being Phlegm. This may aggravate the hot flushes and also worsen the mental–emotional symptoms associated with the menopause.

!

Menopausal symptoms occur against a background of Kidney-Yang as often as Kidney-Yin deficiency.

Pain

Symptoms and Signs, Chapter 84

Apart from a slight discomfort, normally the menstrual period should be almost painless. The main areas of questioning with regard to menstrual pain are as follows.

Time of pain

Pain before the period may be caused by stagnation of Qi or stasis of Blood; the latter is typically relieved by the onset of the period. Pain during the period is generally due to Blood-Heat or Blood stasis. If there is pain

after the period then this may be a result of Blood deficiency.

Nature of pain

Severe, stabbing pain indicates a stasis of Blood. Severe, cramping pain, which is eased by application of heat such as a hot-water bottle, is caused by stasis of Cold.

Case history 46.4

A 15-year-old girl had been suffering from severe abdominal pain for just over a year, beginning 18 months after menarche. The pain was on the right side of her abdomen and she described it as a continuous, dull ache. However, it would become sharp and stabbing in nature during her period and also at other times. The pain was relieved by the application of heat.

Three months before she came for treatment, the patient had had an ovarian cyst removed from her left side and one on her right side had been drained. She had also had recurrent attacks of oral and genital ulcers since the age of 9. These had been relieved by treatment with steroids. On questioning, the patient revealed that she was prone to constipation, specifically that she had infrequent bowel actions.

Her tongue body was Swollen and slightly Red on the sides. It had a white-sticky coating, particularly in the Gall-Bladder area, and was peeled in the centre. Her pulse was Wiry on the right and slightly Wiry on the left, where it was also Empty at the Deep level.

Diagnosis: The stabbing nature of the abdominal pain, together with its alleviation by the application of heat, seems to suggest Cold in the Uterus as the main cause. The abdominal pain began shortly after menarche, which also would suggest the presence of Cold in the Uterus as this is a very common pathogenic factor in young girls suffering from dysmenorrhoea. The Wiry quality of the pulse seems also to confirm the presence of stagnation. However, this initial hypothesis is not confirmed by the other clinical manifestations.

Ovarian cysts are usually characterized by Dampness, which is the case in this patient, as the presence of Dampness is confirmed by the swelling of the tongue and the sticky coating.

The recurrent oral and genital ulcers are caused by Damp-Heat in the Girdle and Directing Vessels. A disharmony of the Girdle Vessel is a frequent cause of the accumulation of Dampness in the genital system, especially in women: a disharmony of this Vessel is

A mild pain can indicate either Blood-Heat or deficiency of Blood; a dragging feeling in the lower abdomen accompanying mild pain is due to sinking of Qi. A feeling of heaviness in the lower abdomen with pain, or pain on ovulation, may be caused by Damp-Heat.

Case histories 46.4–46.6 illustrate some patterns underlying menstrual pain.

confirmed by the distribution of the tongue coating in the Gall-Bladder areas (Fig. 46.4) This disharmony of the Directing Vessel is shown clearly by the distribution of oral and genital ulcers as this vessel starts from Ren-1, flows through the external genitalia and, on the face, it wraps around the mouth. In this case, Dampness is combined with Heat, which is evident from the redness of the sides of the tongue.

Therefore, we can conclude that the abdominal pain is caused by Damp-Heat and not by Cold as it would appear on first impression. The long-standing retention of Dampness in the Lower Burner (it started when she was aged 9) also led to Qi and Blood stasis and therefore the aggravation of the pain during the period. From a Western medicine point of view, recurrent oral and genital ulcers, which are inflammatory and non-infectious, are known as Behçet's disease.

The peeling of the central area of the tongue indicates Stomach-Yin deficiency, which was probably caused by Heat injuring Yin. The pulse being Empty at the Deep level confirms the Yin deficiency; however, it is Empty on the left side (rather than the right side as it would be expected in Stomach-Yin deficiency) and this may be due to a deficiency of Liver-Yin. This is all the more likely owing to the disharmony of the Girdle Vessel, which affects the Gall-Bladder and Liver channels.

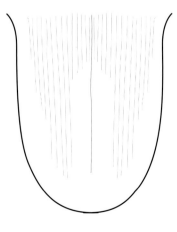

Fig. 46.4 Patient's tongue

Case history 46.5

A 49-year-old woman had been suffering from menstrual flooding for 11 years. Since the birth of her second child, when she was 35, her cycle had been irregular, varying in length between 17 and 45 days; the period lasted 7 days in total, was painful, the menstrual blood had clots and she had a brown discharge for 1 day after the period. Her periods had been painful also in the years following the menarche at 12. Her gynaecological history was rather complicated as she had been on the contraceptive pill from the age of 18 to 30, she had a miscarriage at 30, the first child at 31, another miscarriage at 34, a second child at 35 and the periods became very heavy at 38. In complicated histories such as these it is helpful to draw two diagrams, one outlining the main gynaecological events of her life and the other depicting the menstrual cycle (Figs 46.5 and 46.6).

Apart from the gynaecological problem, she has also had difficulty in controlling her bladder and also her bowel since the second pregnancy.

Her pulse was slightly Overflowing and Rapid and very Weak on both Rear positions; her tongue was Red and slightly Purple.

Diagnosis: The menstrual flooding is caused by Blood-Heat, which is evidenced by the Red tongue and Overflowing-Rapid pulse. There is also some Blood stasis indicated by the painful period, menstrual clots, irregular cycle and slightly Purple tongue. There is, thirdly, an underlying Kidney deficiency, which is indicated by the weakness of the pulse in both Rear positions and by the fact that the menstrual flooding started after the second childbirth and that she had two miscarriages.

The treatment principle is therefore to cool Blood, stop bleeding, invigorate Blood and tonify the Kidneys. In gynaecological problems, it is often appropriate to apply different treatment principles in each phase of the menstrual cycle. There are four phases in the menstrual cycle, the first being the period itself during which Blood is moving, the second being the postmenstrual phase during which there is a relative Blood deficiency, the third being ovulation during which the Penetrating and Directing Vessels are active and the fourth being the premenstrual phase during which Liver-Qi moves. In this case, we can therefore cool and invigorate Blood during the premenstrual phase and the period itself and tonify the Kidneys after the period for about 2 weeks.

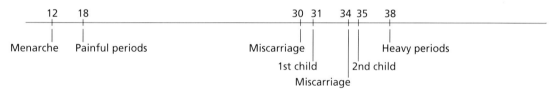

Fig. 46.5 Diagram of gynaecological events

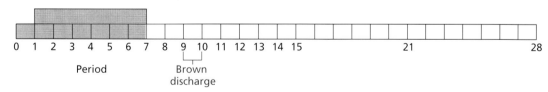

Fig. 46.6 Diagram of menstrual cycle

Case history 46.6

A 28-year-old woman had been suffering from painful periods ever since the menarche. The periods came regularly and lasted 9 to 10 days; the menstrual blood was dark with occasional clots. The pain was stabbing in nature at times but at other times it was a

dull, deep ache rather than a pain and with a pronounced feeling of heaviness: she said 'my whole lower body feels thick, heavy and stodgy', which was clearly her way of expressing what, in Chinese medicine, is called 'a feeling of heaviness'. The pain was situated in the central-lower abdominal area and was alleviated by a hot bath. Recently, she had been expe-

riencing pain on intercourse which was sharp in nature and also located in the central-lower abdominal area. Apart from painful periods, she had also been experiencing a dull, mid-cycle ache on the right-lower abdominal area for the past 2 years; this ache was also accompanied by a dark-brown discharge. She also suffered from premenstrual tension, manifesting with irritability and distension of the breasts and abdomen. On the basis of an internal examination and an ultrasound scan, she had been diagnosed as suffering from endometriosis.

Other symptoms elicited from interrogation included cold limbs, occasionally a feeling of heat in the face, palpitations, anxiety and tightness of the chest.

The tongue was Red on the tip and the pulse was slightly Slippery in general and slightly Tight on the left rear position.

Diagnosis: The stabbing character of the pain and the dark colour of the menstrual blood with clots clearly indicates Blood stasis which most probably derives from Cold in the Uterus. We can deduce the presence of Cold in the Uterus from the alleviation of the pain by a hot bath and also by the history: in fact, if the periods are painful from the time of menarche, the most common aetiological factor is invasion of the Uterus by external Cold owing to playing games wearing shorts in cold and damp weather. In this case, therefore, Cold in the Uterus obstructs the circulation of blood and causes Blood stasis.

In addition to Blood stasis, there is also a clear pattern of Dampness in the Lower Burner, which is manifested by the occasional dull ache during the periods, the pronounced feeling of heaviness and the mid-cycle pain. There is also some Liver-Qi stagnation causing the premenstrual symptoms.

An occasional feeling of heat in the face, cold limbs, palpitations, anxiety and tightness of the chest can all be explained as manifestations of rebellious Qi in the Penetrating Vessel. In fact, given these symptoms and the menstrual symptoms, we can say that all her symptoms reflect a disharmony of the Penetrating Vessel.

The main treatment principle is therefore simply to regulate the Penetrating Vessel by warming the Uterus, invigorating Blood and resolving Dampness from the Lower Burner.

Box 46.7 summarizes the patterns underlying menstrual pain.

BOX 46.7 MENSTRUAL PAIN

Time of pain
- Pain before the period: stagnation of Qi or stasis of Blood (the latter is typically relieved by the onset of the period)
- Pain during the period: Blood-Heat or Blood stasis
- Pain after the period: Blood deficiency

Nature of pain
- Severe, stabbing pain: stasis of Blood
- Severe, cramping pain, eased by application of heat (such as a hot-water bottle): stasis of Cold
- Mild pain: Blood-Heat or deficiency of Blood
- Dragging feeling in the lower abdomen with mild pain: sinking of Qi
- Feeling of heaviness in the lower abdomen with pain: Damp-Heat
- Pain on ovulation: Damp-Heat

Premenstrual symptoms

Symptoms and Signs, Chapter 85

The most common cause of premenstrual tension is Liver-Qi stagnation which manifests with irritability, depression and moodiness, a tendency to crying, impatience and a Wiry pulse; these emotional states are often accompanied by abdominal or breast distension.

However, many other patterns may cause premenstrual tension. Liver-Fire or Heart-Fire, or both, may cause premenstrual tension manifesting with a propensity to outbursts of anger, irritability and agitation, together with shouting, anxiety, insomnia and dream-disturbed sleep. Phlegm-Fire harassing upwards may also cause premenstrual tension manifesting with similar symptoms, as well as mental confusion and hyperactivity; with Phlegm-Fire there is also premenstrual breast swelling and pain.

Premenstrual tension may also be caused by Deficiency, and primarily Liver-Blood deficiency, Liver- and Kidney-Yin deficiency, Spleen- and Kidney-Yang

deficiency, and Spleen-Qi deficiency with Dampness. In Deficiency premenstrual tension manifests primarily with depression, crying, lack of motivation, feelings of heaviness, tiredness and lassitude, and only a mild irritability.

> **!**
>
> Premenstrual tension is *not* always due to Liver-Qi stagnation.

Nausea or vomiting before the period denotes stagnant Liver-Qi invading the Stomach, whereas premenstrual constipation with bitty stools and abdominal distension indicates stagnant Liver-Qi invading the Intestines and Spleen. It is always important to ask whether there is a change in bowel movements around period time because such changes reflect the state of the Yang organs in a woman. Loose stools or constipation are frequent symptoms appearing at period time. Constipation at period time may be due to stagnant Liver-Qi invading the Intestines, Liver-Blood deficiency (with dry stools) or Kidney-Yang deficiency (with infrequent movements), whereas loose stools may be due to Spleen-Qi deficiency, stagnant Liver-Qi invading the Spleen (with abdominal distension) or Kidney-Yang deficiency (with diarrhoea).

Headaches before the period indicate Liver-Qi stagnation or Liver-Yang rising. Distension of the breasts denotes Liver-Qi stagnation, but if the breasts become very swollen and painful this may denote Phlegm (which, in premenstrual problems, usually combines with Qi stagnation). Acute breast pain may be due to Toxic Heat in the breast, such as happens in acute mastitis after childbirth.

Retention of water with oedema before the period indicates Spleen-Yang or Kidney-Yang deficiency, or both.

Box 46.8 summarizes patterns underlying premenstrual symptoms.

Other symptoms occurring around menstruation

Symptoms and Signs, Chapter 85

Headaches that occur during the period are usually due to Liver-Yang rising or Liver-Fire blazing, occurring against a background of Blood-Heat. Headaches

---

BOX 46.8 PREMENSTRUAL SYMPTOMS

- Irritability, depression, moodiness, propensity to outbursts of anger/crying, abdominal/breast distension, impatience, Wiry pulse: Liver-Qi stagnation
- Propensity to outbursts of anger, irritability, mental restlessness, shouting, feeling of agitation, anxiety, insomnia: Liver- and Heart-Fire
- Mental restlessness, anxiety, insomnia, dream-disturbed sleep: Heart-Fire
- Mental restlessness, anxiety, insomnia, hyperactivity, dream-disturbed sleep, mental confusion: Phlegm-Fire harassing upwards
- Weepiness, crying, depression, mild irritability: Liver- Blood deficiency with secondary Liver-Qi stagnation
- Weepiness, crying, depression, lack of motivation, insomnia: Liver- and Kidney-Yin deficiency
- Weepiness, crying, depression, lack of motivation, tiredness, lassitude: Spleen- and Kidney-Yang deficiency
- Weepiness, tiredness, lassitude, feeling of heaviness, swollen breasts: Spleen-Qi deficiency with Dampness and secondary Liver-Qi stagnation
- Nausea, vomiting: Liver-Qi invading the Stomach
- Constipation with bitty stools and abdominal distension: Liver-Qi invading the Intestines
- Constipation with dry stools: Liver-Blood deficiency
- Constipation with infrequent bowel movement: Kidney-Yang deficiency
- Loose stools: Spleen-Qi deficiency
- Loose stools with abdominal distension: stagnant Liver-Qi invading the Spleen
- Diarrhoea: Kidney-Yang deficiency
- Headaches, Liver-Yang rising or Liver-Qi stagnation
- Breast distension and pain: Liver-Qi stagnation and/or Phlegm
- Breast pain (acute): severe Liver-Qi stagnation or Toxic Heat
- Oedema: Spleen- and Kidney-Yang deficiency

---

occurring after the period indicate Liver-Blood deficiency.

Constipation during the period may be due to Liver-Fire, whereas constipation after the period is due to Blood or Kidney deficiency.

Insomnia during the period indicates Blood-Heat, often with Liver-Fire or Heart-Fire, or both. Insomnia after the period denotes Blood deficiency.

Diarrhoea after the period indicates Spleen-Yang or Kidney-Yang deficiency, or both.

Box 46.9 summarizes the patterns underlying other miscellaneous symptoms occurring around menstruation.

BOX 46.9 OTHER SYMPTOMS OCCURRING AROUND MENSTRUATION

- Headaches
  —during the period: Liver-Yang rising or Liver-Fire blazing
  —after the period: Liver-Blood deficiency
- Constipation
  —during the period: Liver-Fire
  —after the period: Blood deficiency, Kidney deficiency
- Insomnia
  —during the period: Blood-heat, Liver-Fire, Heart-Fire
  —after the period: Liver-Blood deficiency
- Diarrhoea: Spleen/Kidney-Yang deficiency

PREGNANCY AND CHILDBIRTH

Fertility

Symptoms and Signs, Chapters 86 and 89

Infertility can be due to many different deficient or excess conditions. These are:

- Blood deficiency
- Kidney deficiency
- stasis of Blood
- Cold in the Uterus
- Damp-Phlegm.

A slight feeling of nausea in the first 3 months of pregnancy is normal; persistent vomiting during the first 3 months of pregnancy, or even continuing over the following months, is a pathological sign which usually indicates rebellious Qi in the Penetrating Vessel affecting the Stomach channel. This can occur against a background of Stomach deficiency or Stomach-Heat.

Oedema during pregnancy indicates Kidney-Yang deficiency. High blood pressure denotes a Kidney deficiency with Liver-Yang rising: this may herald a pre-eclampsia state which is also characterized by headache, dizziness and blurred vision. A full eclampsia state manifests with convulsions which, from a Chinese perspective, indicate the development of Liver-Wind from Liver and Kidney deficiency.

An aggravation or an amelioration of certain symptoms by pregnancy both indicate a Kidney deficiency. Most people think that pregnancy is a weakening event in a woman's life: in my opinion this is not so and a pregnancy can be weakening only if there is a pre-existing Kidney deficiency and the woman does not look after herself. If any pre-existing Kidney deficiency is not very severe and the woman looks after herself during pregnancy, this event may actually strengthen the Kidneys (because menstruation itself is moderately weakening and therefore its cessation can increase Blood and strengthen the Kidneys). For this reason, an aggravation of certain symptoms during pregnancy indicates that the Kidneys have been weakened by it, while an amelioration indicates that the Kidneys have been strengthened. Common examples of diseases that may get better or worse during pregnancy are asthma, migraine and rheumatoid arthritis.

> **!**
> Pregnancy is not necessarily-weakening to a woman's organism. It may have a neutral effect or it may even have a strengthening effect.

Case histories 46.7–46.9 illustrate some patterns underlying problems with fertility.

Case history 46.7

A 45-year-old woman had been trying to conceive for 7 years; she did have an 18-year-old child. Her periods were scanty lasting only 2 or 3 days, she suffered from premenstrual tension and from abdominal distension *after* the period; she also suffered from constipation and a dragging feeling in the lower abdomen during the periods. Other symptoms elicited from interrogation included backache, occasional dizziness, frequent urination and nocturia. She also suffered from insomnia and anxiety. She was slightly overweight and her eyes lacked sparkle to a severe degree.

She had seen a gynaecologist and had had various tests and the Western medicine diagnosis was endometriosis and ovarian cysts.

Her tongue was slightly Pale and, although it had a sticky yellow coating in the centre and root, it was Peeled on the sides and the front; her pulse was Slippery in general, slightly Moving on the left Front and Middle positions, Weak on both Rear positions and Rapid (112 b.p.m.).

Diagnosis: This patient presents with a complex picture of patterns. There is definitely Dampness as evidenced by her being overweight, the dragging feeling in the abdomen, the sticky tongue coating and the Slippery pulse. Dampness is associated with Heat because the tongue coating is yellow. Another pattern is that of Kidney deficiency, which is manifested by the backache, dizziness, frequent urination, nocturia, scanty periods and Weak pulse on both Rear positions.

The lack of sparkle in the eyes and the Moving and Rapid pulse suggest the presence of a Heart pattern, which is probably due to shock. This is confirmed by the insomnia and the anxiety; the tongue is slightly Pale but also Peeled in the front and we can therefore conclude that there is deficiency of both Qi and Yin of the Heart. The premenstrual tension indicates Liver-Qi stagnation but this is not a major problem in this case as it is secondary to the Kidney deficiency; this is confirmed by the fact that abdominal distension occurs after rather than before the period.

Case history 46.8

A 39-year-old woman had suffered from excessive body hair since the onset of puberty at the age of 15. She had recently been diagnosed with polycystic ovary syndrome after an ultrasound scan. Her menstrual cycle was 5 weeks long, the period lasted 5–6 days and she had a white, jelly-like vaginal discharge at mid-cycle.

She often felt tired and her sleep was not good, regularly waking up early in the morning. She had a tendency towards constipation and suffered from haemorrhoids. Her hands and feet were often cold. Her mouth tended to be dry and she had catarrh in her throat.

The tongue was Swollen with Red sides and red points on the tip and with a sticky yellow coating. The pulse was Deep-Weak and Slow (60 b.p.m.) overall, the right Front and left Rear positions being especially Weak.

Diagnosis: Excessive body hair and polycystic ovary syndrome often go hand in hand and, in this case, are caused by Phlegm, which has developed as a result of an underlying Kidney-Yang deficiency. While in Western medicine the excessive growth of body hair

is explained by an imbalance between oestrogen and testosterone (with excessive levels of the latter), in Chinese medicine it is due to a disharmony of the Penetrating Vessel: the Penetrating Vessel is the Sea of Blood and a disharmony may cause the Blood to promote the growth of body hair excessively. The Penetrating Vessel disharmony is also indicated by the onset of the problem at puberty, which is a time when the Directing and Penetrating Vessels are in a state of transition and change and are therefore susceptible to disharmonies.

The presence of Phlegm is confirmed by the Swollen tongue, the mid-cycle vaginal discharge and the ovarian cysts themselves. The symptoms of tiredness, constipation and cold extremities are due to the Kidney-Yang deficiency, which is shown by the pulse being Deep-Weak and Slow, especially in the left Rear position.

The swelling and the redness of the sides of the tongue body, the sticky-yellow tongue coating and the red points on the tip indicate Phlegm-Heat affecting probably the Lungs and Heart, but she has hardly any symptoms of this apart from the dry mouth and the phlegm in the throat.

Case history 46.9

A 41-year-old woman had been trying to conceive for over a year without success. During that year she did become pregnant once, but the pregnancy was ectopic and she had to have her right tube removed. She had already had a child two and a half years previously. She also complained of feeling tired, exhausted, with low motivation and lack of libido. Her sleep was disturbed and she occasionally experienced floaters and night sweating.

Her periods were quite normal, being regular, lasting 5 days and being not too heavy or too scanty and not painful. She had a past history of abdominal

pain caused by pelvic inflammatory disease, causing dyspareunia (pain on intercourse) which had improved with acupuncture.

Her tongue was practically normal, being only very slightly Pale on the sides and with a slightly Red tip with red points. Her pulse was Wiry in general and slightly Slippery and noticeably Full at the Middle level.

Diagnosis: This case history is presented here as an example of the importance of the pulse in diagnosis. On first analysis, it would appear that this patient suffers from a Kidney deficiency which is causing her to be infertile, tired, exhausted, lacking in motivation and libido. However, further questioning aimed

at confirming or excluding the Kidney deficiency did not reveal any backache, dizziness or tinnitus. Moreover, she did conceive once resulting in an ectopic pregnancy, which normally indicates an obstruction of the Lower Burner from Dampness, Phlegm, stagnation of Qi or stasis of Blood; therefore, if she is infertile, it is probably more from a Full condition than from a Kidney deficiency. Furthermore, the pulse and the tongue do not show a deficiency of the Kidneys or any other organ.

The Wiry pulse clearly indicates severe stagnation of Qi, probably deriving from emotional problems, which is confirmed by the Red tip with red points on the tongue. Therefore we can conclude that her exhaustion, lack of motivation and lack of libido are due more to mental depression than to a Kidney deficiency. Moreover, the Full quality of the Middle level of the pulse (corresponding to Blood) confirms a condition of Blood stasis in the Uterus. Her past history of pelvic inflammatory disease and dyspareunia confirms this diagnosis.

The treatment principle in this case therefore should be to move Qi, pacify the Liver, invigorate Blood and calm the Mind.

Miscarriage and abortion

It is important to ask about miscarriages and abortion as they weaken a woman's body. There is a saying in Chinese gynaecology that states: 'Miscarriage is more serious than childbirth.' It is easy to understand why this should be so: during a miscarriage there is a heavy loss of blood; moreover, from a mental–emotional point of view, it means a great loss to the woman with ensuing sadness and grief, which are often underestimated.

Abortion is also weakening but to a lesser degree because there is not the loss of blood that occurs during a spontaneous miscarriage.

Miscarriage before 3 months indicates a Kidney deficiency, whereas miscarriage after 3 months denotes sinking of Spleen-Qi, Liver-Blood stasis or Blood-Heat.

Childbirth

Symptoms and Signs, Chapter 87

There are several main areas of questioning with regard to the conditions of labour. Nausea and heavy bleeding after labour may be caused by exhaustion of the Penetrating Vessel. Sweating with fever after labour is due to exhaustion of Qi and Blood.

Postnatal depression is caused by Liver-Blood and Heart-Blood deficiency. Postnatal psychosis indicates a stasis of Blood in the Uterus and Heart.

Lactation

Symptoms and Signs, Chapter 87

Breast milk not flowing (agalactia) after childbirth may be due to Blood deficiency, Stomach and Spleen deficiency or Liver-Qi stagnation. Spontaneous flow of milk after childbirth may be due to Spleen-Qi deficiency, Stomach-Heat or Liver-Fire.

Mastitis after childbirth is due to Toxic Heat in the Stomach channel.

Box 46.10 summarizes patterns underlying pregnancy- and childbirth-related problems.

BOX 46.10 PREGNANCY AND CHILDBIRTH

Fertility and pregnancy
- Infertility: Blood deficiency, Kidney deficiency, Blood stasis, Cold in the Uterus, Damp-Phlegm
- Severe morning sickness: rebellious Qi of the Penetrating Vessel, Stomach deficiency or Stomach-Heat
- Oedema during pregnancy: Kidney-Yang deficiency
- High blood pressure during pregnancy: Kidney deficiency with Liver-Yang rising
- Eclampsia: Liver-Wind
- Miscarriage:
  —before 3 months: Kidney deficiency
  —after 3 months: sinking of Spleen-Qi, Liver-Blood stasis, Blood-Heat

Childbirth and lactation
- Nausea and heavy bleeding: exhaustion of the Penetrating Vessel
- Sweating and fever after labour: exhaustion of Qi and Blood
- Postnatal depression: Liver-Blood and Heart-Blood deficiency
- Postnatal psychosis: stasis of Blood in the Uterus and Heart
- Agalactia: Blood deficiency, Stomach and Spleen deficiency, Liver-Qi stagnation
- Spontaneous milk flow: Spleen-Qi deficiency, Stomach-Heat, Liver-Fire
- Mastitis: Toxic Heat in Stomach channel

VAGINAL DISCHARGE

Observation, Chapter 20; Hearing and Smelling, Chapter 54; Symptoms and Signs, Chapter 89

By 'vaginal discharge' is meant an abnormal discharge and not the normal transparent, egg-white-like secretion occurring during ovulation. Vaginal discharge must be differentiated according to colour, consistency and smell. An increase in vaginal secretions mid-cycle and during pregnancy is normal.

Box 46.11 summarizes patterns underlying abnormal vaginal discharge.

BOX 46.11 VAGINAL DISCHARGE

Colour
- White: Cold from Spleen- or Kidney-Yang deficiency or from exterior Cold-Dampness
- Yellow: Heat, usually Damp-Heat in the Lower Burner
- Greenish: Damp-Heat in the Liver channel
- Red and white: Damp-Heat
- Yellow, red with white pus after menopause: Toxic Heat

Consistency
- Watery: Cold-Dampness, Deficiency condition
- Thick: Damp-Heat, Excess condition

Smell
- Fishy: Cold
- Leathery: Heat

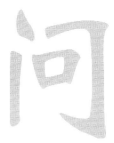

Chapter **47**

CHILDREN'S SYMPTOMS

Chapter contents

INTRODUCTION *411*

MOTHER'S PREGNANCY *411*

CHILDBIRTH *412*

POSTPARTUM PROBLEMS *412*

CHILDHOOD DISEASES *412*

DIGESTIVE SYMPTOMS *412*

IMMUNIZATIONS *412*

RESPIRATORY SYMPTOMS AND EARACHE *412*
  Coughs and wheezing *413*
  Earache *413*
  Chronic catarrh *413*

SLEEP *413*

SLOW DEVELOPMENT *413*

INTRODUCTION

The interrogation of children, especially young children, obviously needs to be carried out with the help of the child's parents or other relatives. In older children (over the age of 5 years), although we still need the help of the parents in describing the child's symptoms and signs, it is important to listen carefully to the child as well. When asking children about their symptoms, we should obviously avoid the use of difficult medical terms such as 'abdomen' and use colloquial terms such as 'tummy'.

Most of the questions related to adults discussed in the previous chapters apply to children as well (e.g. digestive system and taste, thirst, defecation, urination, etc.). There are, however, several questions which pertain only to children and these are the mother's pregnancy, childbirth, postpartum problems, immunizations and childhood diseases. In addition to the above areas of questioning, questions about the child's digestive system, respiratory symptoms, earache, and sleep are also important and have a slightly different significance to that in adults.

MOTHER'S PREGNANCY

The period in the womb is extremely important in influencing the constitution of the baby. Many factors affect the baby and its constitution in the gestation period. Emotional shocks to the mother can affect the child's nervous system and the Heart. The consumption of alcohol and recreational drugs and smoking obviously affect the child's constitution adversely.

When a baby cries a lot at night and vomits frequently, this may be due to what the Chinese called

'womb Heat', which itself may be due either to the pregnant mother's consumption of excessively hot foods or, more commonly, to her suffering from shock during pregnancy. Prenatal shock may also manifest with a bluish tinge on the baby's forehead and chin.

The influence of pregnancy events on the baby's health is discussed also in Chapter 48.

CHILDBIRTH

The conditions of childbirth also have an important influence on the baby's constitution. Premature cutting of the umbilical cord, induction or a Caesarean birth can all affect the baby's constitution adversely and in particular may cause a Lung deficiency. Therefore if a baby or very young child suffers from a Lung deficiency, this may be due to the above mentioned conditions in childbirth.

POSTPARTUM PROBLEMS

The main question to ask is about breast feeding: lack of breast feeding or too short breast feeding often adversely affects a baby's digestive system causing either a Stomach deficiency or retention of food in the Stomach. Giving solid food to babies too early (before 6 months of age) is a very common cause of retention of food in babies and children.

CHILDHOOD DISEASES

We should always ask parents about their child's childhood diseases. A history of several childhood diseases with rashes (e.g. measles, chickenpox, German measles) suggests the child's tendency to Heat. Whooping cough has a weakening effect on the child's lungs and this may cause a weak Lung constitution and the tendency to develop Lung patterns later in life.

DIGESTIVE SYMPTOMS

Symptoms and Signs, Chapter 90

Digestive symptoms are very common in children owing to the Stomach and Spleen being inherently weak at birth; the younger the child, the more common are digestive symptoms. The two most

common causes of abdominal pain in children are retention of Cold in the Stomach and Intestines and stagnation of Qi in the Intestines. In babies, retention of food (called Accumulation Disorder in babies) is very common and it manifests with vomiting of milk and with colic.

IMMUNIZATIONS

A full discussion on immunizations is beyond the scope of this book. To understand the effect of immunizations from a Chinese perspective it is necessary to refer to the theory of the Four Levels (see Part 6). When a pathogenic factor invades the body, it enters the Defensive-Qi level first and, if not expelled, progresses through the Qi, Nutritive-Qi and Blood levels. The Four Levels represent four different energetic layers of penetration of Heat, the Defensive-Qi level being the most superficial and the Blood level the deepest.

From a Chinese perspective, therefore, immunizations basically consist in injecting a 'pathogenic factor' (i.e. the live or attenuated germ) directly at the Blood level. This may cause Latent Heat to develop at the Blood level, which may cause problems to the child both in the short term and in the long term.

In the short term, Latent Heat may cause a skin rash, insomnia and a temporary change in the child's character. The long-term effects of immunizations are more difficult to establish and are the subject of great controversy. However, if immunizations lead to Latent Heat at the Blood level, it is quite possible that they may have serious long-term effects. These include brain damage, possibly autism, asthma, chronic cough, allergies and skin diseases later in life.

The effect of immunizations from the Chinese perspective is discussed also in Chapter 48.

> **!**
>
> Immunizations are a common cause of Latent Heat in children, which may persist into adulthood.

RESPIRATORY SYMPTOMS AND EARACHE

Symptoms and Signs, Chapter 90

Questions concerning cough, wheezing, breathlessness or earache are always important in the child's

interrogation because children are very prone to invasions of Wind, which may cause the above symptoms.

Coughs and wheezing

Symptoms and Signs, Chapter 90

A history of repeated bouts of cough and wheezing nearly always indicates a residual pathogenic factor (usually Lung Phlegm-Heat) following invasions of external Wind. These give rise to a residual pathogenic factor when the Wind is not cleared properly, when antibiotics are used too frequently or when the child has a weak constitution. In such cases the child will suffer from a chronic cough or wheezing, or both, and will be prone to frequent respiratory infections.

Earache

Symptoms and Signs, Chapter 90

A history of chronic earache also indicates the presence of a residual pathogenic factor, which, in this case, is usually Damp-Heat in the Gall-Bladder channel. This is also the result of frequent, acute ear infections usually treated by the repeated administration of antibiotics, which only makes matters worse by promoting the development of a residual pathogenic factor.

BOX 47.1 INFLUENCES ON CHILDREN AND CHILDREN'S SYMPTOMS

- Mother's pregnancy: 'womb Heat', prenatal shock
- Childbirth: Lung deficiency
- Postpartum problems: Stomach deficiency, retention of food in the Stomach
- Childhood diseases: rashes (tendency to Heat), weak Lung constitution after whooping cough
- Digestive symptoms: retention of Cold in Stomach and Intestines, stagnation of Qi in Intestines, Accumulation Disorder
- Cough and wheezing: invasions of Wind, residual pathogenic factor
- Earache: residual pathogenic factor, usually Damp-Heat in Gall-Bladder
- Chronic catarrh: Phlegm
- Disturbed sleep: retention of food and Stomach-Heat (babies), Liver-Fire, Stomach-Heat or retention of food (older children)
- Immunizations: Latent Heat
- Slow development (Five Retardations): congenital weakness of Liver, Kidney, Stomach, Heart

---

Chronic catarrh

The condition of chronic catarrh is very common in children and this is the consequence of a residual pathogenic factor after repeated invasions of Wind combined with a Spleen deficiency, leading to the formation of Phlegm. A child with this condition will have a constantly runny nose or a blocked nose, cough and glue ear.

SLEEP

We should always ask about sleep in babies and children because not only does it give us an indication of the state of the Mind but also a disturbance of sleep often reflects the presence of certain pathogenic factors.

Disturbed sleep with crying in babies is often due to retention of food and Stomach-Heat, in which case the baby will cry out loudly. If the baby cries relatively quietly during the night, it may be due to a prenatal shock.

Disturbed sleep in older children may be due to the same factors as in adults but the most common ones are Liver-Fire, Stomach-Heat and retention of food.

SLOW DEVELOPMENT

Slow development in children was summarized in ancient China as the 'Five Retardations'. These consist in slow development in standing, walking, teeth growth, hair growth and speech.

Slow development is caused primarily by congenital weakness of the Liver and Kidneys with the Kidneys affecting standing, teeth growth and hair growth and the Liver affecting standing and walking. Among postnatal causes, the Stomach influences walking and the Heart speech. Figure 47.1 illustrates the influence of prenatal and postnatal deficiencies on the Five Retardations.

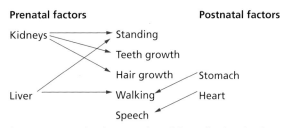

Fig. 47.1 Prenatal and postnatal conditions affecting the Five Retardations

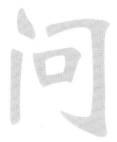

Chapter **48**

DIAGNOSING THE CAUSES OF DISEASE

Chapter contents

INTRODUCTION   415

INTERACTIONS BETWEEN CAUSES OF DISEASE   416
  Interaction of trauma with climate   416
  Interaction of hereditary weak constitution with
    diet   416
  Interaction of emotional problems at puberty with
    overwork   416
  Interaction of weak Heart constitution and emotional
    problems   417

THE FIVE STAGES OF LIFE   417
  Childhood   417
  Adolescence   417
  Young adulthood   417
  Middle age   418
  Old age   418

THE CAUSES OF DISEASE   418
  Heredity   418
  Emotions   420
  Overwork   427
  Diet   427
  Climate   428
  Trauma   428
  Drugs including immunizations   429
  Excessive sexual activity   430

INTRODUCTION

As mentioned earlier, the identification of the possible causes of patients' disharmony is linked to general enquiries about their emotional life, working life, diet, past history of shocks or traumas, family history and environmental influences. I usually begin by carrying out a specific interrogation to identify the patterns of disharmony *before* delving into these aspects of a patient's life. It is important not to confuse the general interrogation to find the *causes* of disease with the specific interrogation to identify the *patterns* of disharmony.

Identifying the causes of disease is not easy and therefore not always possible, but to try to do so is important as it is only by finding the causes of disease that we can help the patient to eliminate or minimize them if at all possible. Even if the patient can do nothing about a particular cause that is rooted in the past (such as an earlier accident), its identification is still important in order that we may channel our advice to the patient along the right lines. For example, there is no point in delving deeply into a patient's emotional life if the cause of the problem is a past accident; vice versa, there is no point in tinkering with a patient's diet or suggesting strict dietary prohibitions if the cause of the problem is clearly emotional.

One of the strengths of Chinese medicine, when compared with some branches of modern complementary medicine that consider a particular cause of disease to the exclusion of all others, is precisely that it contemplates many different causes of disease without a particular emphasis on one or another.

Traditionally the causes of disease were differentiated according to three broad categories: external (due to climate), internal (due to emotions), and

miscellaneous. Nowadays, this classification is no longer relevant (not least because some of the most important causes of disease are in the 'miscellaneous' group) and we need not follow it. The main causes of disease, listed in approximate order of their importance and frequency are:

- heredity
- emotions
- overwork
- diet
- climate
- trauma
- drugs including immunizations
- 'recreational' drugs
- excessive sexual activity.

I find that, when identifying a cause or causes of disease, it is helpful to divide a person's life into five distinct ages (see below). Because each cause of disease is more prevalent during a certain period of life, establishing when the cause arose helps us to identify the disease. There seldom is only one cause of disease; nearly always a disease results from the combination of at least two causes. Usually one cause occurs at a certain point of the patient's life, then, some years later, another cause intervenes and the combination of the two triggers a disharmony (Fig. 48.1). Some examples will be given below.

INTERACTIONS BETWEEN CAUSES OF DISEASE

Interaction of trauma with climate

A trauma to a knee that occurred at a young age when the patient was playing sports may heal without any apparent consequence but when, years later, the patient is then subject to invasion of Cold and Dampness (when he goes out walking in the rain and remains in wet clothes for the whole day), he may develop Painful Obstruction Syndrome in that knee. A previous trauma, in fact, often explains the unilaterality of a particular joint problem.

Interaction of hereditary weak constitution with diet

A girl is born with a weak Stomach and Spleen constitution, which appears to improve after the age of 7, as often happens. When the girl reaches 14 she becomes a vegetarian. Her diet now consists mainly of cheese and salads; this interacts with the pre-existing weak Stomach and Spleen constitution to cause Spleen-Qi deficiency and possibly also Blood deficiency.

Interaction of emotional problems at puberty and overwork

A girl suffers deep emotional traumas around the time of puberty, owing to family conflicts. These have no apparent effect until she is an older woman. At the age

(a)

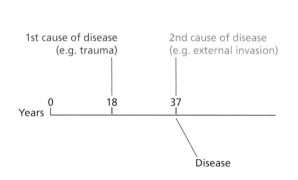

(b)

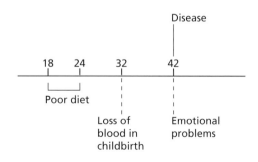

Fig. 48.1 Interaction of causes of disease: (a) trauma followed by external invasion; (b) poor diet, childbirth problems followed by emotional problems

of 27 she is working very hard and for very long hours; the emotional problems at puberty (which affect the Directing and Penetrating vessels) interact with the overwork later in life to cause gynaecological problems, possibly endometriosis.

Interaction of weak Heart constitution and emotional problems

A child is born with a weak Heart constitution manifesting with a nervous disposition, restlessness in sleep and a deep Heart crack on the tongue. At a later age, the young man suffers deep emotional stress owing to relationship difficulties; the interaction of a pre-existing weak Heart constitution and the subsequent emotional problems causes serious Heart patterns and possibly severe anxiety and depression.

THE FIVE STAGES OF LIFE

The patient's life can be differentiated into five stages:

- childhood (from birth to puberty)
- adolescence (from puberty to about 20 years)
- young adulthood (from 20 to 40)
- middle age (from 40 to 60)
- old age (from 60 onwards).

Of course, the above age limits are intended only as a guideline and individual cases may differ from them according to individual body conditions. For example, a 38-year-old person who is in very poor health could be included in the middle-aged group, whereas a youthful and healthy 42-year-old person could be included in the young adulthood age. The following are the main characteristics and possible aetiology and pathology of these five ages.

Childhood

During early childhood there are only three possible causes of disease, that is, weak hereditary constitution, irregular feeding and climate. Therefore, if a patient has been suffering from a particular complaint since early childhood, this can be due to one of these three causes. We can eliminate climate as a cause because it does not usually cause long-lasting consequences (unless there is a residual pathogenic factor), so the problem can therefore be due only to heredity or irreg-

ular feeding. An example of such a problem is early-onset atopic disease (asthma and eczema), which is usually due to a hereditary weakness of the Lungs' and Kidneys' Defensive-Qi systems.

A new possible cause of disease in young children is immunizations, which are often the cause of chronic infections, sleep problems or hyperactivity.

Older children's main causes of disease are primarily diet, climate, emotions and traumas. For example, if a patient has been suffering from persistent headaches since childhood, this could be due either to a trauma to the head or to irregular diet as a child. The emotional life of a child is quite different from that of an adult and a child's emotional problems are largely the reflection of the family's emotional state.

Adolescence

Adolescence is a very vulnerable period of life both on a physical and on an emotional level, especially for girls. Taking a careful history will often reveal the onset of a particular problem during adolescence. For example, if a girl has been suffering from headaches since the onset of the menarche (which can be established only with very careful questioning) this most probably indicates Liver-Blood deficiency (resulting in Liver-Yang rising) as the main cause of the problem. This, in turn, is most probably due to dietary irregularity or an injudicious vegetarian diet.

Skin problems from this age may also be due to the aggravation of Blood deficiency with the onset of the menarche. If a young woman has been suffering from painful periods ever since their onset, this almost certainly points to invasion of Cold in the Uterus during early adolescence when the Uterus is in a particularly vulnerable state.

Adolescence is also a vulnerable time from the emotional point of view and deep emotional problems in a young adult often stem from that time.

Young adulthood

Many events characterize the early young adulthood, for example leaving home, change of diet, sexual activity, and infections.

Leaving home often coincides with a deterioration in the young person's dietary habits characterized by irregular meals, eating 'fast foods', and often becoming vegetarian. When practised without a proper understanding

of nutrition, a vegetarian diet may lead to Blood deficiency, especially in girls. Therefore, digestive problems later in life often have their root in the early 20s.

Young adulthood is also the time of emotional stress deriving from work, relationships and unresolved family situations. The pulse reflects the emotional cause of disease quite accurately. For example, if the Lung pulse is somewhat full and the patient looks sad, it may be due to sadness or grief which has not been expressed (the fullness of the Lung pulse would indicate this). If the Lung pulse is particularly Weak and without wave and the eyes lack lustre, I may enquire whether events in the patient's life have caused sadness or grief.

If the Heart pulse is Overflowing and there is a Heart crack on the tongue, I may ask if the patient has suffered from a shock. If the Heart pulse is Choppy, the complexion dull, the eyes lustreless and the voice weak and weepy, it often indicates long-standing sadness.

If the pulse is Wiry on all positions, I may enquire whether there is some situation in the patient's life that is causing frustration, anger or resentment.

The pulse, complexion and eyes often point to the true emotion underlying the disease, sometimes even contradicting the patient's own perception. For example, a patient complained of various symptoms which she attributed to the anger she felt at having suffered sexual abuse as a teenager. Her therapist had also identified anger as a cause of her symptoms. However, her very pale complexion, sad eyes and Weak pulse without wave, especially on the Lung position, showed a different picture; in other words, all the signs pointed to sadness and grief as the predominant emotions. I therefore asked her how she felt about her past experiences and she confirmed that those were the predominant emotions.

Another case showed almost the opposite situation. A young woman complained of premenstrual tension and depression; she looked quite sad and her voice was somewhat weepy. However, her pulse was not weak but somewhat full; in particular, it was Moving, especially on the Heart position. I asked her if she had suffered a shock during childhood and she burst into tears, telling me about sexual abuse suffered from an uncle.

Middle age

The main causes of disease in middle age are emotions, overwork and diet.

The emotional state of middle age may take two opposite directions: some people have been able to resolve the emotional problems of their youth and have settled into a way of life that pays attention to the needs of the Self; for others, middle age is a time of crisis and emotional turmoil when every aspect of their life is questioned. Most people overcome this crisis to achieve a better emotional balance.

Overwork is probably the most important cause of disease in middle age. This comes about because middle age is a time when people usually reach the peak of their profession, which imposes the heaviest demands. Unfortunately, this comes at a time when our energy is naturally declining and Kidney-Qi begins to decline too. Most people make unreasonable demands on their own bodies; they expect their energy to be the same as when they were in their 30s or even 20s, and have no idea about the need for rest; they think it is 'normal' to get up at 6.30 in the morning, catch a train at 7.30, work all day under conditions of stress, eat a sandwich at their desk for lunch without any interruption from work, and return home at 9 in the evening. This constitutes 'overwork' and is a major cause of Kidney deficiency in the Western world.

Old age

Old age is a time when causes of disease have a lesser impact than in any other period of life. Generally speaking, past causes of disease are already well entrenched and usually no new causes of disease play a role. This is not because diet or emotional problems do not affect the elderly but because any cause of disease at this time of one's life inevitably has its roots in the distant past; for this reason, a change in habits is somewhat less important in the elderly than at any other time of life, particularly with regard to diet. For example, if an 85-year-old man suffers from Phlegm due to a lifelong excessive consumption of greasy foods, a change in diet at this late time of life will have little impact on his organism (although it may still be advisable for him to make these changes). Of course, that is not to say that other changes in life's habits do not have an impact on a person's health: for example, it is never too late to explore the root of one's emotional problems or to take up exercise.

THE CAUSES OF DISEASE

Heredity

The constitutional body condition inherited from our parents depends on three factors:

1. The parents' health in general
2. The parents' health at the time of conception
3. The conditions of the mother's pregnancy.

Any of these factors can affect the body condition and become a cause of disease later in life. If the parents' Qi and Essence are weak, the child's resulting Pre-Heaven Essence will also be weak. Similarly, if the mother conceives in later life, this can result in a Kidney or Liver deficiency starting during childhood.

Even though the parents' general health may be good, if it is poor at the time of the child's conception (perhaps through overwork, excessive sexual activity, excessive consumption of alcohol, or use of certain medications or drugs such as cannabis or cocaine), this will result in the child's having a weak constitution. In this case, the weakness will affect not the Kidneys or Liver, but any of the other organs (i.e. Spleen, Lungs or Heart), depending on what particular condition is negatively affecting the parents' health. For example, if a parent has been overworking at the time of conception, his or her poor health may cause hereditary Spleen weakness in the child; excessive consumption of alcohol or the use of drugs or certain medicines may cause a hereditary weakness of the child's Heart or Liver.

The mother's condition during the pregnancy can affect the fetus. For example, an accident to the mother can cause headaches later in the child. A shock during pregnancy can cause a baby to cry during sleep or a child to suffer nightmares (this will also manifest with a bluish tinge on the forehead and chin).

The clinical manifestations of a poor constitution in each of a child's organs are indicated below. Possible causes arising during pregnancy for each such constitution will be given, but we must obviously bear in mind that the manifestation may result from a constitutional weakness in one or both parents and not necessarily from what happened during pregnancy.

Weak-Spleen constitution

Manifestations of this constitution include flaccid muscles alongside the spine, digestive problems, vomiting, diarrhoea and a sallow complexion; the child may be quiet, with a thin body, or fat if there is Phlegm when newborn but becoming thinner after 1 month.

The cause of a weak Spleen constitution is usually to be found in improper diet or the mother's overworking during pregnancy.

Weak-Lung constitution

Manifestations of this constitution include a white complexion, fear, shyness, proneness to colds, whooping cough, asthma and eczema, a thin chest, a 'special' Lung pulse (Fig. 48.2) and Lung cracks on tongue.

In pregnancy, the causes of this constitution are usually emotional upsets to the mother, especially sadness or grief. Of course, smoking during pregnancy also affects the baby's Lungs negatively.

Weak-Heart constitution

Manifestations of this constitution include a bluish tinge on the forehead, fear, crying at night, and a Heart crack on the tongue; the child may be tense, with a hot body, red eyes, red cheeks (or the opposite, i.e. very pale) and a Red tip of the tongue.

In pregnancy, this constitution may be caused by the mother's suffering a shock.

Weak-Liver constitution

Manifestations of this constitution include myopia or headaches from an early age; the child may be

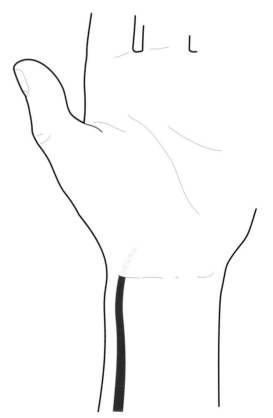

Fig. 48.2 Special Lung pulse

very tense with a sinewy body, nocturnal enuresis, restless sleep, twitching in sleep, screaming during sleep, feeding a lot as a baby, hungry as a child, short-tempered, a Wiry pulse and a Red tongue with coating.

In pregnancy, this constitution may be caused by the mother's emotional stress and anger.

Weak-Kidney constitution

Manifestations of this constitution include nocturnal enuresis; the child may be listless or timid, with lassitude, a thin body, slow development in babyhood, atopic asthma and eczema, headaches from an early age, frequent urination and generally feel cold.

In pregnancy, this constitution may be caused by the mother's overworking.

Emotions

Emotions are mental stimuli which influence our affective life. Under normal circumstances, they are not a cause of disease. Indeed, 'emotions' should be more appropriately called 'feelings' and feelings are a natural expression of human life. Without feelings, we would not be human. Hardly any human being can avoid being angry, sad, aggrieved, worried, or afraid at some time in his or her life. For example, the death of a relative provokes a very natural feeling of grief. It is only when such feelings take over our life inappropriately and disturb our psyche and body that they become pathological; when this happens, feelings have turned into 'moods'.

Moods often arise precisely when feelings are suppressed; for example, if a certain situation makes us angry and we recognize the anger we can deal with it and perhaps even come to the conclusion that part of the anger was a projection of our own 'Shadow'. In such a case, the anger is a normal feeling that will probably not have pathological consequences. But if we fail to recognize our anger, this will be driven to deeper levels of our psyche and turn into a 'mood' that possesses us. We 'possess' feelings, but moods possess us.

Thus, emotions (or 'feelings') become causes of disease only when they are excessive, prolonged, suppressed, or unrecognized, in which case they turn into moods. For example, hardly anyone can avoid being angry sometimes, but a temporary state of anger does not lead to disease. However, if a person is constantly angry about a certain situation in life for many years,

or, even worse, if the anger is not recognized, this emotion will definitely disturb the Mind and Spirit and cause disease.

In Chinese medicine, 'emotions' (the term here signifies causes of disease, not normal feelings) are mental stimuli which disturb the Mind and Spirit and, through these, alter the balance of the Internal Organs and the harmony of Qi and Blood. For this reason, emotional stress is an internal cause of disease which injures the Internal Organs directly. Conversely, and this is a very important feature of Chinese medicine, the state of the Internal Organs affects our emotional state. For example, if Liver-Yin is deficient (perhaps from dietary factors) and causes Liver-Yang to rise, this may result in a person becoming irritable all the time. Vice versa, if a person is constantly angry about a certain situation or with a particular person, this may cause Liver-Yang to rise.

The 'Spiritual Axis' in Chapter 8 clearly illustrates the reciprocal relationship between the emotions and the Internal Organs. It says: *'The Heart's fear, anxiety and pensiveness injure the Mind . . . the Spleen's worry injures the Intellect . . . the Liver's sadness and shock injure the Ethereal Soul . . . the Lung's excessive joy injures the Corporeal Soul . . . the Kidney's anger injures the Will-Power . . .'.*[1] On the other hand, further on it says: *'If Liver-Blood is deficient there is fear, if it is in excess there is anger . . . if Heart-Qi is deficient there is sadness, if it is in excess there is manic behaviour . . .'*[2] These two passages clearly show that, on the one hand, emotional stress injures the Internal Organs and, on the other hand, disharmony of the Internal Organs causes emotional imbalance.

The emotions taken into consideration in Chinese medicine have varied over the years. From a Five-Element perspective, the 'Yellow Emperor's Classic'[3] considered five emotions, each one affecting a specific Yin organ:

- anger affecting the Liver
- joy affecting the Heart
- pensiveness affecting the Spleen
- worry affecting the Lungs
- fear affecting the Kidneys.

However, these are not by any means the only emotions discussed in the 'Yellow Emperor's Classic'. In other passages sadness and shock are added, giving seven emotions:

- anger affecting the Liver
- joy affecting the Heart
- worry affecting the Lungs and Spleen
- pensiveness affecting the Spleen
- sadness affecting the Lungs and Heart
- fear affecting the Kidneys
- shock affecting the Kidneys and Heart.

Other doctors considered other emotions such as grief, love, hatred and desire (craving).

Finally, and interestingly, there is one last emotion which is not usually mentioned in Chinese medicine, and that is guilt. Yet, in my opinion, guilt is very pervasive in Western patients and definitely an emotional cause of disease.

Thus, the list of emotions could be expanded as follows:

- anger (and frustration and resentment) affecting the Liver
- joy affecting the Heart
- worry affecting the Lungs and Spleen
- pensiveness affecting the Spleen
- sadness (and grief) affecting the Lungs
- fear affecting the Kidneys
- shock affecting the Kidneys and Heart
- love affecting the Heart
- hatred affecting the Heart and Liver
- craving affecting the Heart
- guilt affecting the Kidneys and Heart.

The effect of each emotion on a relevant organ should not be interpreted too restrictively. There are passages from the 'Yellow Emperor's Classic' that attribute the effect of emotions to organs other than the ones just mentioned. For example, the 'Spiritual Axis' in Chapter 28 says: *'Worry and pensiveness agitate the Heart'*.[4] The 'Simple Questions' in Chapter 39 says: *'Sadness agitates the Heart . . .'*[5]

Furthermore, all emotions, besides affecting the relevant organ directly, affect the Heart indirectly because the Heart houses the Mind. It alone, being responsible for consciousness and cognition, can recognize and feel the effect of emotional tension.

Fei Bo Xiong (1800–1879) put it very clearly when he said:

The seven emotions injure the 5 Yin organs selectively, but they all affect the Heart. Joy injures the Heart . . . Anger injures the Liver, the Liver cannot recognize anger but the Heart can, hence it affects both Liver and Heart. Worry injures the Lungs, the Lungs cannot recognize it but the Heart can, hence it affects both Lungs and Heart. Pensiveness injures the Spleen, the Spleen cannot recognise it but the Heart can, hence it affects both Spleen and Heart.[6]

Yu Chang in 'Principles of Medical Practice' (1658) says: *'Worry agitates the Heart and has repercussions on the Lungs; pensiveness agitates the Heart and has repercussions on the Spleen; anger agitates the Heart and has repercussions on the Liver; fear agitates the Heart and has repercussions on the Kidneys. Therefore all the five emotions [including joy] affect the Heart'.*[7] Chinese writing clearly bears out the idea that all emotions affect the Heart since the characters for all seven emotions are based on the 'heart' radical.

The way that all emotions afflict the Heart also explains why a Red tip of the tongue, indicating Heart-Fire, is so commonly seen even in emotional problems related to other organs.

The first effect of emotional stress on the body is to impair the proper circulation and direction of Qi. Qi is non-substantial and the Mind, with its mental and emotional energies, is the most non-material type of Qi. It is therefore natural that emotional stress affecting the Mind impairs the circulation of Qi first of all.

Each emotion is said to have a particular effect on the circulation of Qi. The 'Simple Questions' in Chapter 39 says: *'Anger makes Qi rise, joy slows down Qi, sadness dissolves Qi, fear makes Qi descend . . . shock scatters Qi . . . pensiveness knots Qi . . .'*[8] Dr Chen Yan in 'A Treatise on the Three Categories of Causes of Diseases' (1174) says: *'Joy scatters, anger arouses, worry makes Qi unsmooth, pensiveness knots, sadness makes Qi tight, fear sinks, shock moves.'*[9]

Again, this should not be taken too literally as, in certain cases, emotional pressure may have a different effect on Qi from the one outlined above. For example, fear is said to make Qi descend and it may cause enuresis, incontinence of urine or diarrhoea, since the Kidneys control the two lower orifices (urethra and anus). This is certainly true in cases of extreme and sudden fear, which may cause incontinence of urine or diarrhoea, or in the case of children when anxiety about a certain family situation may cause enuresis. However, the effect of fear on Qi depends also on the state of the Heart. If the Heart is strong, it will cause Qi

to descend, but if the Heart is weak, it will cause Qi to rise in the form of Empty-Heat. This is more common in old people and in women. In such cases, fear and anxiety may weaken Kidney-Yin and give rise to Empty-Heat of the Heart with such symptoms as palpitations, insomnia, night sweating, a dry mouth, red face and a Rapid pulse.

Box 48.1 summarizes the relationships between the seven emotions and the Internal Organs.

BOX 48.1 EMOTIONS AND THE INTERNAL ORGANS

- Anger: Liver
- Joy: Heart
- Worry: Lungs and Spleen
- Pensiveness: Spleen
- Sadness: Lungs and Heart
- Fear: Kidneys
- Shock: Kidneys and Heart

Let us now discuss the effects of each emotion individually.

Anger

The term 'anger', perhaps more than any other emotion, should be interpreted very broadly to include several other allied emotional states, such as resentment, repressed anger, feeling aggrieved, frustration, irritation, rage, indignation, animosity, or bitterness.

Any of these emotional states can affect the Liver, if they persist for a long time, causing stagnation of Liver-Qi or Blood, rising of Liver-Yang or blazing of Liver-Fire. The effect of anger on the Liver depends, on the one hand, on the person's reaction to the emotional stimulus and, on the other hand, on other concurrent factors. If the anger is bottled up it will cause stagnation of Liver-Qi, whereas if it is expressed it will cause Liver-Yang rising or Liver-Fire blazing. In women, stagnation of Liver-Qi may easily lead to stasis of Liver-Blood. Those who also suffer from some Kidney-Yin deficiency (perhaps from excessive sexual activity) may develop Liver-Yang rising. Those who, on the other hand, have a tendency to Heat (perhaps from excessive consumption of hot foods) will tend to develop Liver-Fire blazing.

Anger (intended in the broad sense outlined above) makes Qi rise and many of the symptoms and signs will manifest in the head and neck, such as headaches, tinnitus, dizziness, red blotches on the front part of the neck, a red face, thirst, a bitter taste and a Red tongue with red sides.

The 'Simple Questions' in Chapter 39 says: *'Anger makes Qi rise and causes vomiting of blood and diarrhoea.'*[10] It causes vomiting of blood because it makes Liver-Qi and Liver-Fire rise and diarrhoea because it induces Liver-Qi to invade the Spleen.

Anger does not always manifest outwardly with outbursts of fury, irritability, shouting, a red face, etc. Some individuals may carry anger inside them for years without ever manifesting it. In particular, long-standing depression may be due to repressed anger or resentment. A person who is very depressed may look subdued and pale, walk slowly and speak with a low voice – all signs which one would associate with a depletion of Qi and Blood deriving from sadness or grief. However, when anger rather than sadness is the cause of disease, the pulse and tongue will clearly show it: the pulse will be Full and Wiry and the tongue will be Red with redder sides and with a dry yellow coating. This type of depression is most probably due to long-standing resentment, often harboured towards a member of that person's family.

In some cases anger can affect other organs, especially the Stomach. This can be due to stagnant Liver-Qi invading the Stomach. Such a condition is more likely to occur if one gets angry at mealtimes, which may happen if family meals become occasions for regular rows. It also happens when there is a pre-existing weakness of the Stomach, in which case the anger may affect only the Stomach without even affecting the Liver.

If one regularly gets angry an hour or two after meals, then the anger will affect the Intestines rather than the Stomach. This happens, for example, when one goes straight back to a stressful and frustrating job after lunch. In this case, stagnant Liver-Qi invades the Intestines and causes abdominal pain, distension and alternation of constipation with diarrhoea.

Finally, anger, like all other emotions, also affects the Heart. This organ is particularly prone to be affected by anger also because, from a Five-Element perspective, the Liver is the mother of the Heart and often Liver-Fire is transmitted to the Heart giving rise to Heart-Fire. Anger makes the Heart full with blood rushing to it. With time, this leads to Blood-Heat affecting the Heart and therefore the Mind. According to Dr J. H. F. Shen, anger tends to affect the Heart particularly when the person does a lot of jogging or exercising; this is because excessive exercise dilates the heart, which is

then more prone to be affected by the transmission of Fire from the Liver to the Heart.

In some cases, anger disguises other emotions such as guilt. Some people may harbour guilt inside for many years and be unable or unwilling to recognize it; they may then use anger as a mask for their guilt. Moreover, there are some families in which everyone is perpetually angry. This happens more in Mediterranean countries such as Italy, Spain or Greece. In these families, anger is used as a mask to hide other emotions such as guilt, fear or dislike of being controlled, or to conceal weakness or an inferiority complex. When this is the case, it is important to be aware of this situation as one needs to treat not the anger but the underlying psychological and emotional condition.

Box 48.2 summarizes the effects of anger.

BOX 48.2 ANGER

- Affects the Liver (and Heart)
- Makes Qi rise
- Expressed anger causes Liver-Yang rising or Liver-Fire blazing
- Repressed anger causes Liver-Qi stagnation
- Anger at mealtimes affects Stomach
- Anger after eating affects Intestines
- Anger may disguise guilt

Joy

A normal state of joy is not in itself a cause of disease; on the contrary, it is a beneficial mental state which favours a smooth functioning of the Internal Organs and their mental faculties. The 'Simple Questions' in Chapter 39 says: *'Joy makes the Mind peaceful and relaxed, it benefits the Nutritive and Defensive Qi and it makes Qi relax and slow down.'*[11] On the other hand, in Chapter 2 the same book says: *'The Heart . . . controls joy, joy injures the Heart, fear counteracts joy.'*[12]

What is meant by 'joy' as a cause of disease is obviously not a state of healthy contentment but one of excessive excitement and craving, which can injure the Heart. This happens to people who live in a state of continuous mental stimulation (however pleasurable) or excessive excitement – in other words, a life of 'hard playing'.

As indicated above, inordinate craving is an aspect of the emotion 'joy' and it stirs up the Minister Fire, which overstimulates the Mind.

Joy, in the broad sense indicated above, makes the Heart larger. This leads to excessive stimulation of the Heart, which, in time, may lead to Heart-related symptoms and signs. These may deviate somewhat from the classical Heart patterns. The main manifestations would be palpitations, overexcitability, insomnia, restlessness and talking a lot; the tip of the tongue would be red. The pulse would typically be Slow, slightly Overflowing but Empty on the left Front position.

Joy may also be marked out as a cause of disease when it is sudden; this happens, for example, on hearing good news unexpectedly. In this situation, 'joy' is akin to shock. Fei Bo Xiong in 'Medical Collection from Four Families from Meng He' says: *'Joy injures the Heart . . . [it causes] Yang Qi to float and the blood vessels to become too open and dilated . . .'*[13] In these cases of sudden joy and excitement the Heart dilates and slows down and the pulse becomes Slow and slightly Overflowing but Empty. One can understand the effect of sudden joy further if one thinks of situations when a migraine attack is precipitated by the excitement of suddenly hearing good news. Another example of joy as a cause of disease is that of sudden laughter triggering a heart attack; this example also confirms the relationship existing between the Heart and laughter.

Finally, one can also get an idea of the effects of joy as an emotion by considering children, in whom overexcitement usually ends in tears.

Box 48.3 summarizes the effects of joy.

BOX 48.3 JOY

- Affects the Heart
- Makes Qi slow down
- Joy is a state of excessive excitement/craving
- Joy makes the heart larger

Worry

Worry is one of the most common emotional causes of disease in our society. The extremely rapid and radical social changes that have occurred in Western societies in the past decades have created a climate of insecurity and anxiety in all spheres of life. Of course, there are also people who, because of a pre-existing disharmony of the Internal Organs, are very prone to worry, even about very minor incidents in life. For example, many people appear to be very tense and worry a lot. On close interrogation about their work and family life, often nothing of note emerges. They simply worry excessively about trivial everyday activities and they tend to do everything in a hurry and be pressed for time. This may be due to a constitutional weakness of the Spleen, Heart or Lungs, or a combination of these.

Worry knots Qi, which means that it causes stagnation of Qi, and it affects both the Lungs and the Spleen: the Lungs because when one is worried breathing is shallow, and the Spleen because this organ is responsible for thinking and ideas. Worry is the pathological counterpart of the Spleen's mental activity in generating ideas.

In a few cases, worry may also affect the Liver as a result of the stagnation of the Lungs; in a Five-Element sense this corresponds to Metal insulting Wood. When this happens, the neck and shoulders will tense up and become stiff and painful.

The symptoms and signs caused by worry will vary according to whether they affect the Lungs or the Spleen. If worry affects the Lungs it disturbs the breathing and the Corporeal Soul (*Po*); this will cause an uncomfortable feeling in the chest, slight breathlessness, anxiety, tensing of the shoulders, sometimes a dry cough and a pale complexion. The right Front pulse position (of the Lungs) may feel slightly Tight or Wiry, indicating the knotting action of worry on Qi.

If worry affects the Spleen it may cause poor appetite, a slight epigastric discomfort, some abdominal pain and distension, tiredness and a pale complexion. The right Middle pulse position (Spleen) will feel slightly Tight but Weak. If worry affects the Stomach as well (which happens if one worries at mealtimes), the right Middle pulse may be Weak-Floating.

Box 48.4 summarizes the effects of worry.

BOX 48.4 WORRY

- Affects the Lungs, Heart and Spleen
- Knots Qi
- It may also affect the Liver and Stomach
- It affects breathing and the Corporeal Soul (*Po*)

Pensiveness

Pensiveness is very similar to worry in its character and effect. It consists in brooding, constantly thinking about certain events or people (even though not worrying), nostalgic hankering after the past and generally thinking intensely about life rather than living it. In extreme cases, pensiveness leads to obsessive thoughts. In a different sense, pensiveness also includes excessive mental work in the process of one's work or study.

Pensiveness affects the Spleen and, like worry, it knots Qi. It will therefore cause similar symptoms to those outlined above. The only difference will be that the pulse of the right side not only will feel slightly Tight, but will have no wave. One can feel the normal pulse as a wave under the fingers moving from the Rear towards the Front position. The pulse without wave lacks this flowing movement from Rear to Front position and it is instead felt as if each individual position were separate from the others (see Fig. 50.1 on p. 477). In the case of pensiveness, the pulse will lack a wave only on the right Middle position. A pulse without wave in the Front and Middle position indicates Sadness.

Box 48.5 summarizes the effects of pensiveness.

BOX 48.5 PENSIVENESS

- Affects the Spleen and Heart
- It knots Qi
- In severe cases it leads to obsessive thoughts
- 'Pensiveness' include also excessive mental work

Sadness and grief

Sadness includes the emotion of regret, as when someone regrets a certain action or decision in the past and the Mind is constantly turned towards that time. Sadness and grief affect the Lungs and Heart. In fact, according to the 'Simple Questions', sadness affects the Lungs via the Heart. It says in Chapter 39: '*Sadness makes the Heart cramped and agitated; this pushes towards the lungs' lobes, the Upper Burner becomes obstructed, Nutritive and Defensive Qi cannot circulate freely, Heat accumulates and dissolves Qi.*'[14] According to this passage then, sadness primarily affects the Heart, and the Lungs suffer in consequence since they are both situated in the Upper Burner. The Lungs govern Qi and sadness and grief deplete Qi. This is often manifested on the pulse as a Weak quality on both left and right Front positions (Heart and Lungs). In particular, the pulse on both Front positions is Short and has no wave, that is, it does not flow smoothly towards the thumb. Other manifestations deriving from sadness and grief include a weak voice, tiredness, pale complexion, slight breathlessness, weeping and a feeling of oppression in the chest. In women, deficiency of Lung-Qi from sadness or grief often leads to Liver-Blood deficiency and amenorrhoea.

Although sadness and grief deplete Qi, and therefore lead to deficiency of Qi, they may also, after a long time, lead to stagnation of Qi, because the deficient Lung- and Heart-Qi fail to circulate properly in the chest.

As mentioned before, each emotion can affect other organs apart from its 'specific' one. For example, the 'Spiritual Axis' in Chapter 8 mentions injury of the Liver from sadness rather than anger: *'When sadness affects the Liver it injures the Ethereal Soul; this causes mental confusion . . . the Yin is damaged, the tendons contract and there is hypochondrial discomfort.'*[15] This shows how organs can be affected by emotions other than the one 'specific' to them. In this case, sadness can naturally affect the Ethereal Soul and therefore Liver-Yin. Sadness has a depleting effect on Qi and it therefore, in some cases, depletes Liver-Yin leading to mental confusion, depression, lack of a sense of direction in life and inability to plan one's life.

Finally, some doctors consider that grief which is unexpressed and borne without tears affects the Kidneys. According to them, when grief is held in without weeping, the fluids cannot come out (in the form of tears) and they upset the fluid metabolism within the Kidneys. This would happen only in situations when grief had been felt for many years.

Box 48.6 summarizes the effects of sadness and grief.

BOX 48.6 SADNESS AND GRIEF

- Affect the Lungs and Heart
- Deplete Qi
- In time, they may also lead to stagnation of Qi
- Sadness may also affect Liver-Blood in women
- Unexpressed grief without tears affects the Kidneys

Fear

'Fear' includes both a chronic state of fear and anxiety, and a sudden fright. It depletes Kidney-Qi and makes Qi descend. The 'Simple Questions' in Chapter 39 says: *'Fear depletes the Essence, it blocks the Upper Burner, which makes Qi descend to the Lower Burner.'*[16] Examples of Qi descending are nocturnal enuresis in children and incontinence of urine or diarrhoea in adults, following a sudden fright.

Situations of chronic anxiety and fear will have different effects on Qi depending on the state of the Heart. If the Heart is strong, it will cause Qi to descend, but if the Heart is weak, it will cause Qi to rise in the form of Empty-Heat. This is more common in women and in old people of either sex as fear and anxiety weaken Kidney-Yin and give rise to Empty-Heat of the Heart with such symptoms as palpitations, insomnia, night sweating, a dry mouth, a malar flush and a Rapid pulse.

If a person has a tendency to a constitutional weakness of the Heart (manifested with a midline crack on the tongue extending all the way to the tip), fear will affect the Heart rather than the Kidneys.

There are, however, other causes of fear that are not related to the Kidneys. Liver-Blood deficiency and a Gall-Bladder deficiency can also make the person fearful.

Box 48.7 summarizes the effects of fear.

BOX 48.7 FEAR

- Affects the Kidneys and Heart
- Makes Qi descend (in theory)
- May also make Qi ascend (in my opinion)

Shock

Mental shock scatters Qi and affects the Heart and Kidneys. It causes a sudden depletion of Heart-Qi, makes the Heart smaller and may lead to palpitations, breathlessness and insomnia. This is often reflected in the pulse with the Moving quality, that is, a pulse that is short, slippery, shaped like a bean, rapid and gives the impression of vibrating as it pulsates.

Shock also 'closes' the Heart or makes the Heart smaller. This can be observed in a bluish tinge on the forehead and a Heart pulse which is Tight and Fine.

Shock also affects the Kidneys because the body draws on the Kidney-Essence to supplement the sudden depletion of Qi. For this reason, shock can cause such symptoms as night sweating, a dry mouth, dizziness, or tinnitus.

Box 48.8 summarizes the effects of shock.

BOX 48.8 SHOCK

- Affects Kidneys, Spleen and Heart
- Suspends Qi, causes a sudden depletion of Heart-Qi
- Makes heart smaller or 'closes' it

Love

'Love' here means not normal love, such as that of a mother towards her child or that between two lovers, but rather the condition when love becomes an obsession or when it is misdirected, as when a person loves someone who is persistently hurtful. In this context, 'love' indicates a rather obsessive love for a particular person, a misdirected emotion focusing on someone who persistently hurts the lover, whether physically or mentally, or narcissistic love. Obsessive jealousy would

also fall under this broad category. In these senses, love becomes a cause of disease.

'Love' in the sense outlined above affects the Heart and quickens Qi. This will be felt on the left Front position (Heart) with an Overflowing quality, and the pulse will also be rapid. It may cause such symptoms and signs as palpitations, a red tip of the tongue, a red face, insomnia and mental restlessness.

Box 48.9 summarizes the effects of 'love'.

BOX 48.9 'LOVE'

- Affects the Heart
- Quickens Qi
- Consists of:
  —obsessive love
  —misdirected love (towards a person who hurts us)
  —jealousy and possessiveness
  —narcissistic love

Hatred

Hatred is quite similar to anger but differs from it in so far as it indicates a 'cold' and calculating malice rather than the uncontrollable and spontaneous outbursts that are typical of anger. When harboured for many years, hatred is a very damaging and destructive emotion. It affects the Heart and Liver and it knots and slows down Qi. It can be felt on the pulse of the left-hand side with a Wiry but Slow quality. The symptoms and signs caused by hatred include chest pain, hypochondriac pain, insomnia, headache and palpitations. These manifestations include pain in some part of the body as, when hatred is felt for many years, it turns inwards to injure only the person feeling it.

Box 48.10 summarizes the effects of hatred.

BOX 48.10 HATRED

- Affects the Liver and Heart
- Similar to anger
- Knots and slows down Qi

Craving

'Desire' means excessive craving. The inclusion of this as a cause of disease reflects the Buddhist influence on Chinese medicine, which began during the Tang dynasty. The ultimate cause of disease according to Buddhist thought is desire, that is, clinging to external objects or other people and always wanting more. This excessive craving, which is one aspect of the emotion of 'joy' in Chinese medicine, causes the Minister Fire to blaze upwards and harass the Mind. By this is meant a state of constant craving which is never satisfied. This can include craving for material objects or recognition.

Craving affects the Heart and it scatters Qi. Craving also affects the Pericardium by stirring the Minister Fire. In disease, Minister Fire refers to a pathological Empty-Fire arising from the Kidneys; it affects the Pericardium and therefore the Mind.[17] If the Mind is calm, settled and content, the Pericardium follows its direction and there is a happy and balanced life. If the Mind is weak and dissatisfied, the Pericardium follows the demands of the craving and the person constantly desires new objects or new marks of recognition, which, however, even when attained, are never satisfying and leave the person more frustrated. It is for these reasons that both Daoism and Buddhism put the emphasis on reducing craving to prevent the arousal of Minister Fire, which stirs the Mind.

Craving will cause Heart-Fire or Heart Empty-Heat depending on the underlying condition of the person. If there is a tendency to Yin deficiency, which is common in people who tend to overwork, it will lead to Heart Empty-Heat. This will cause palpitations, a malar flush, a dry throat, insomnia and mental restlessness.

Box 48.11 summarizes the effects of craving.

BOX 48.11 CRAVING

- Affects the Heart and Pericardium
- Scatters Qi
- Akin to 'joy'

Guilt

Guilt is an extremely common emotion and a cause of disease in the West. A feeling of guilt may derive from the transgression of social or religious taboos or from having done something wrong which is later regretted. People who are prone to blame themselves for everything that goes wrong may also suffer an unjustified and subjective sense of guilt.

Guilt affects the Heart and Kidneys and it causes Qi either to stagnate or to sink. It may cause stagnation of Qi in the chest, epigastrium, or abdomen, and its clinical manifestations include an uncomfortable feeling in the chest, epigastric or abdominal pain and distension and a Fine pulse. The tongue will have a red tip and the pulse will be vibrating as it pulsates. The eyes will look unstable and often flap shut while a person is talking.

If it affects the Kidneys, guilt may cause Qi to sink giving rise to urinary problems such as a slight incontinence, dribbling of urine and a bearing-down feeling in the hypogastrium.

In some cases, guilt may also arise from the repression of anger. When anger is repressed and not recognized, it may turn inwards and cause an attitude of self-punishment and guilt. When guilt results from repressed anger, the pulse will be Wiry.

Box 48.12 summarizes the effects of guilt.

BOX 48.12 GUILT

- Affects the Kidneys and Heart
- May cause sinking or stagnation of Qi

Overwork

By 'overwork' I mean not physical work but the habit of working long hours every day without adequate rest, usually accompanied by irregular eating for many years. As stated earlier, someone who 'overworks' leaves home perhaps at 7 in the morning, catches a train to work, works under stressful conditions through the lunch hour (eating a sandwich at the desk), and returns home at about 9 in the evening. When such a routine is carried out for many years, it constitutes what I call 'overwork'. It is an extremely common cause of disease in Western patients about which they need to be educated. Most people who follow such a routine at work are surprised when I suggest to them that they work too much and that their working habits might have something to do with their illness.

Overwork as defined above is probably the most common cause of Yin deficiency in the patients we see. It depletes primarily Kidney-Yin but also Liver- and Stomach-Yin, depending on the circumstances. In women, it is likely to injure Liver-Yin as well as Kidney-Yin; on the other hand, when overwork is associated with an irregular diet (as it often is), it injures Stomach-Yin.

Diet

Diet influences our health in two main ways: first through our choice of foods, and secondly through our eating habits.

Choice of foods

Our choice of foods can become unbalanced in four main ways: eating too much cold food, eating too much hot food, eating too much greasy food, and not eating enough.

Eating too much cold food

'Cold' food includes raw fruit, raw vegetables and cold drinks. Patients are often surprised to be told that an excessive consumption of such foods might be detrimental as this advice runs counter to the prevailing view of 'healthy' eating, that is, eating lots of fruit and salads in order to secure the maximum intake of vitamins and minerals. It is true that raw foods are rich in vitamins and minerals and a small consumption of such foods is not detrimental and indeed healthy. It becomes detrimental from the point of view of Chinese medicine only when the mainstay of someone's diet is exclusively raw fruit and vegetables.

Excessive consumption of cold foods (including cold drinks) injures the Spleen and leads to internal Cold in the body. This will cause a pale complexion, loose stools, tiredness, a feeling of cold, and abdominal pain.

Eating too much hot food

'Hot' foods include red meat (especially lamb, beef and game), spices and alcohol. Excessive consumption of hot foods causes Heat in the Internal Organs and will manifest with a red complexion, a feeling of heat, thirst, insomnia, mental restlessness and a Red tongue.

Eating too much greasy food

'Greasy' foods include all dairy foods, bananas and peanuts. In addition, this category includes foods cooked in animal fats, and fried or deep-fried foods. Sugar is also a 'greasy' food.

Greasy foods lead to the formation of Dampness or Phlegm, or both, and an excessive consumption of such foods is extremely common in Western countries, especially in the USA and Northern European countries.

Not eating enough

In affluent countries, 'not eating enough' is due to following a restrictive diet, often aimed at slimming, and may also result from following a vegetarian diet injudiciously, especially in women. Many young girls become vegetarian and, not having a good knowledge of food combining, they tend to eat a lot of salads and cheese, which injure the Spleen and lead to Dampness. Such girls will tend to be pale and suffer from tiredness, digestive problems, loose stools and menstrual problems; the tongue will be Pale and the pulse Choppy.

Box 48.13 summarizes the effects of diet.

BOX 48.13 DIET – CHOICE OF FOODS

- Too much cold food: injures Spleen and leads to Cold
- Too much hot food: leads to Heat
- Too much greasy food: leads to Dampness and Phlegm
- Not eating enough: leads to Qi and Blood deficiency

Eating habits

Chinese medicine places stress not only on the range of foods eaten but also, and as important as what foods we eat, on the way that we eat. We may eat a very balanced diet with exclusively organic foods but if our eating habits are chaotic this will lead to disease.

Chinese medicine stresses the importance of routine and regularity in one's diet. It also stresses the importance of having a short break after eating at lunchtime. Unfortunately, most people who work full-time have very irregular eating habits, which may include any of the following:

- eating in a hurry
- eating standing up
- eating at one's desk while working
- having business lunches
- eating without routine (e.g. a very large business lunch one day, followed by skipping lunch the next)
- eating late in the evening.

Such eating habits injure Stomach-Qi initially and then Stomach-Yin. One of the clearest signs of this, apart from digestive problems, is a tongue with a Stomach crack or scattered Stomach cracks and without coating.

Climate

Invasion of external pathogenic factors is an important cause of disease in Painful Obstruction Syndrome (*Bi*). The main external pathogenic factors are Wind, Dampness and Cold. Once in the body, any of these pathogenic factors can turn into or combine with Heat.

Wind   Wind is characterized by soreness and pain of muscles and joints, limitation of movement, with the pain moving from joint to joint. In acute cases the pulse would be Floating and slightly Rapid. An important characteristic of Wind is that the pain moves from joint to joint on different days and it may also come and go quickly.

Dampness   Dampness is characterized by pain, soreness and swelling in muscles and joints with a feeling of heaviness and numbness of the limbs, the pain being fixed in one place and aggravated by damp weather. In acute cases the pulse would be Slow and slightly Slippery.

Cold   Cold is characterized by a severe pain in a joint or muscle with limitation of movement, usually unilateral. In acute cases the pulse is Tight.

Heat   Heat originates from any of the previous three types when the exterior pathogenic factor turns into Heat in the Interior and gives rise to Heat Painful Obstruction Syndrome. This happens especially with an underlying deficiency of Yin. Heat is characterized by pain and redness, swelling and heat in the joints (which feel hot to the touch), limitation of movement and severe pain. In acute cases there is thirst, a fever which does not abate after sweating and a Slippery and Rapid pulse. This syndrome is characterized not just by Heat, but Damp-Heat. In fact, Dampness is the primary aspect of this syndrome and Heat the secondary one.

The diagnosis of external pathogenic factors is based on two main factors: the acute onset of the problem and a sensitivity of pain to weather changes.

Besides affecting the joints, climatic pathogenic factors can also affect the Internal Organs directly. This happens when external Cold invades the Stomach (causing acute epigastric pain and vomiting), the Intestines (causing acute abdominal pain and diarrhoea) or the Uterus (causing acute dysmenorrhoea).

Box 48.14 summarizes the climatic factors affecting joints.

BOX 48.14 CLIMATIC FACTORS AFFECTING JOINTS

Wind: pain moving from joint to joint
Cold: severe pain in one joint
Dampness: dull ache and swelling of joints
Damp-Heat: ache, swelling and redness of joints

Trauma

By 'trauma' is meant physical trauma. Accidents cause local stagnation of Qi. If the trauma is severe, it also causes local Blood stasis.

The diagnosis of trauma is obvious from the history, except when the trauma occurred several years before

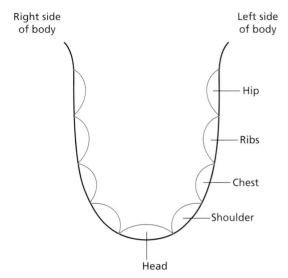

Right side of body

Left side of body

— Hip

— Ribs

— Chest

—Shoulder

Head

Fig. 48.3 Body areas reflected on the tongue

and the patient has either forgotten it or not related it to the presenting problem.

If the trauma causes local Blood stasis, this may manifest on the tongue with a single purple spot which (when compared with points) is relatively large. The tongue reflects also areas of the body and the location of the purple spot points to the site of the trauma, which may also be very old (Fig. 48.3).

Thus, for example, a small purple spot on the right side of the tip may indicate a trauma to the right side of the head.

Drugs including immunizations
Medicinal drugs

Obviously medicinal drugs are an important cause of disease in Western patients. A discussion of the side-effects of drugs is beyond the scope of this book. It should be noted, however, that with few important exceptions (such as chemotherapy and steroids), the side-effects of drugs are relatively short lived (once they are stopped) compared with other causes of disease. For example, an antidepressant will have some well-known side-effects but these will stop when the drug is discontinued and will not cause lasting damage. It is different with the other causes of disease such as heredity, emotional stress or diet. For example, an emotional problem dating back to a person's child-hood will have long-lasting effects even after the person has recognized the problem and taken steps to face it and resolve it. Likewise, if a person eats irregu-

larly for some years, the effects of this may be very long lasting even a considerable time after the diet has been rectified.

Immunizations

Immunizations, in my opinion, lead to the formation of Latent Heat. Latent Heat is formed when a pathogenic factor invades the body without causing apparent symptoms; the pathogenic factor penetrates the Interior, turns into Heat and 'lurks' in the Interior for some time. After some time (usually weeks or months), the Heat emerges in the form of Latent Heat with symptoms such as sudden weariness, tired limbs, insomnia, thirst, irritability, Red tongue and Rapid pulse. It should be stressed that the fact that the Latent Heat emerges does not mean that it is being expelled but simply that it is manifesting after lurking in the Interior for some time.

In order to understand the effect of immunizations we need to refer to the theory of the Four Levels. According to this theory, an external pathogenic factor invades the body passing through four energetic levels: the Defensive-Qi, Qi, Nutritive-Qi and Blood levels. (See Fig. 104.2 on p. 959.)

The Defensive-Qi level is an exterior level, that is, at this stage the pathogenic factor is on the Exterior of the body. At the Qi level, the pathogenic factor turns into interior Heat. The three levels, Qi, Nutritive-Qi and Blood, are all interior and all characterized by interior Heat but at three different energetic layers, Qi being the most superficial and Blood the deepest. With an immunization, it is as if the 'pathogenic factor' (i.e. the vaccine) were injected directly at the Blood level. Once there, it 'lurks', turns into Heat and emerges later as Latent Heat.

It is of course impossible to prove, but my impression is that many modern autoimmune diseases, some cancers (such as leukemia) and AIDS manifest as Latent Heat and their growing incidence may partly be due to immunizations.

Recreational drugs

The ill-effects of 'recreational' drugs such as cocaine, heroin, LSD and Ecstasy are well known. However, so-called 'soft' drugs such as cannabis also have a pro-found impact on our health. Regular smoking of cannabis over a long period has definite neurological actions on the brain affecting memory and concentra-tion negatively.[18] It is my experience that these effects are permanent in long-term users even after they stop

using the drug. Long-term use of the drug may also cause loss of brain substance; cannabis also impairs cell division by lymphocytes in tissue culture.[19]

In my experience, long-term users display a certain lack of centredness and a weak Stomach and Spleen.

Excessive sexual activity

By 'sexual activity' is meant ejaculation in men and orgasm in women. Excessive sexual activity may weaken the Kidneys because sperm is a direct emanation of the Kidney-Essence (sexual activity not culminating in ejaculation does not deplete the Kidneys). It is difficult to define what is 'excessive' because it depends on the age and health of the person. A very rough guide to the recommended frequency of ejaculation in healthy men is to divide the man's age by five (e.g. every 8 days in a 40-year-old man). It should be stressed that this period should be extended if the man is in poor health and especially if he suffers from a Kidney deficiency.

Excessive sexual activity weakens the Kidney-Essence and may cause backache, dizziness, tinnitus, poor memory and concentration, and weak knees.

I have so far referred to men deliberately because, in my opinion, the effect of sexual activity in women is quite different from that in men. Sperm in men is an emanation of the Kidney-Essence; the equivalent in women is menstrual blood. Sperm and menstrual blood constitute the 'Tian Gui' essence which arrives at puberty. Quite simply, men lose sperm during orgasm but women do not lose menstrual blood; therefore, sexual activity and orgasm in women are not weakening to the Kidneys. A cause of disease in women equivalent to excessive ejaculation in men would be a heavy loss of blood after childbirth or a heavy monthly blood loss in a woman suffering from menorrhagia. Some people say that the increased fluid lubrication in the vagina during sexual arousal and orgasm is equivalent to ejaculation in men. I tend to disagree with this view because, in my opinion, such fluids are part of Body Fluids rather than an emanation of the Kidney-Essence.

Finally, it should be mentioned that lack of sexual activity may also be a cause of disease but only when sexual desire is present. If sexual desire is totally absent, then lack of sexual activity has no health repercussions. Sexual desire makes the Minister Fire rise upwards; with orgasm this Fire is discharged downwards. When sexual desire is unfulfilled, the Minister Fire rises up without being discharged during orgasm and it affects the Heart, causing Heart-Fire or stagnation of Heart-Qi.

NOTES

1. 1981 Spiritual Axis (*Ling Shu Jing* 灵枢经), People's Health Publishing House, Beijing, p. 24. First published c. 100 BC.
2. Ibid., p. 24.
3. 1979 The Yellow Emperor's Classic of Internal Medicine – Simple Questions (*Huang Di Nei Jing Su Wen* 黄帝内经素问), People's Health Publishing House, Beijing, pp. 36–42. First published c. 100BC.
4. Spiritual Axis, p. 67.
5. Simple Questions, p. 221.
6. Fei Bo Xiong et al 1985 Medical Collection from Four Families from Meng He (*Meng He Si Jia Yi Ji* 孟河四家医集), Jiangsu Science Publishing House, Nanjing, p. 40.
7. Yu Chang 1658 Principles of Medical Practice, cited in Wang Ke Qin 1988 Theory of the Mind in Chinese Medicine (*Zhong Yi Shen Zhu Xue Shuo* 中医神主学说), Ancient Chinese Medical Texts Publishing House, Beijing, p. 34.
8. Simple Questions, p. 221.
9. Chen Yan 1174 A Treatise on the Three Categories of Causes of Diseases (*San Yin Ji Yi Bing Zheng Fang Lun* 三因极一病证方论), cited in Wang Ke Qin 1988 Theory of the Mind in Chinese Medicine (*Zhong Yi Shen Zhu Xue Shuo* 中医神主学说), Ancient Chinese Medical Texts Publishing House, Beijing, p. 55.
10. Simple Questions, p. 221.
11. Ibid., p. 221.
12. Ibid., p. 38.
13. Medical Collection from Four Families from Meng He, p. 40.
14. Simple Questions, p. 221.
15. Spiritual Axis, p. 24.
16. Simple Questions, p. 222.
17. For this reason 'Minister Fire' refers both to the physiological or pathological Fire of the Kidneys and to the Pericardium. This accounts for the assignment of the right Rear position on the pulse variously to the Kidney-Yang by some doctors, or to the Pericardium by others.
18. Lawrence D R 1973 Clinical Pharmacology, Churchill Livingstone, Edinburgh, p. 14.29.
19. Ibid., pp. 14.30 and 14.31.

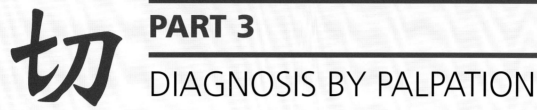

PART 3

DIAGNOSIS BY PALPATION

Part contents

49 Pulse diagnosis *433*
50 Pulse qualities *465*
51 Palpation of parts of the body *509*
52 Palpation of channels *525*

INTRODUCTION

Diagnosis by palpation includes palpation of the pulse, chest and abdomen, various parts of the body, channels and points. The two most important parts of diagnosis by palpation are the pulse and the abdomen.

Pulse diagnosis developed to a very high level of sophistication in Chinese medicine, benefiting from an unbroken continuous tradition for over 2000 years. The first systematic elements of pulse diagnosis are found in the Yellow Emperor's Classic of Internal Medicine. It is possible that, in later centuries (from the Song dynasty onwards) when Confucian morality prevailed, pulse diagnosis was developed in preference to abdominal diagnosis as it was considered improper for male physicians to palpate the body of women.

Diagnosis by palpation of channels and points is very important especially for acupuncturists as palpation and needling of tender points merges diagnosis and therapy in one.

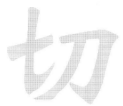

Chapter **49**

PULSE DIAGNOSIS

Chapter contents

INTRODUCTION   433

THE 'NINE REGIONS' OF THE PULSE FROM THE 'YELLOW EMPEROR'S CLASSIC OF INTERNAL MEDICINE'   434

THE PULSE IN THE 'CLASSIC OF DIFFICULTIES'   435

THE THREE SECTIONS OF THE PULSE   436

ASSIGNMENT OF PULSE POSITIONS TO ORGANS   438
  Organ positions on the pulse   438
  Reconciling different pulse arrangements   443

THE THREE LEVELS   445

METHOD OF PULSE TAKING   446
  Time   446
  Levelling the arm   446
  Equalizing the breathing   447
  Placing the fingers   447

FACTORS AFFECTING THE PULSE   449
  Season   449
  Gender   450
  Age   450
  Body build   450
  Menstruation   451
  Pregnancy   451
  Fan Guan Mai and Xie Fei Mai   451

ATTRIBUTES OF THE NORMAL PULSE   451
  Spirit   451
  Stomach-Qi   451
  Root   452

GUIDELINES FOR INTERPRETING THE PULSE   454
  Feeling the pulse as a whole with three fingers   454
  Feeling the spirit, Stomach-Qi and root   454
  Feeling the three positions together first and then individually   454

Feeling the three levels   455
Feeling the overall quality of the pulse, if there is one   456
Feeling the pulse quality, strength and level of each individual position by rolling and pushing the fingers   456
Counting the pulse rate   457

CLINICAL APPLICATION OF PULSE DIAGNOSIS   457
  The pulse is often crucial in clinching a diagnosis   457
  The pulse is essential to distinguish Deficiency from Excess   457
  The pulse is essential to determine the treatment principle   458
  The pulse in emotional problems   458
  The pulse as an indicator of an organ problem   459
  The pulse as an indicator of a heart problem   459
  The pulse does not necessarily reflect all the aspects of a disharmony   461
  The pulse indicates disharmonies beyond the presenting patterns   461
  The pulse can indicate an underlying Deficiency in the absence of symptoms   461
  The pulse in cancer   462

INTEGRATION OF PULSE AND TONGUE DIAGNOSIS   463
  Qi and Blood   463
  Time factor   463
  When the pulse is Rapid and the tongue is not Red   463
  When the pulse is Slow and the tongue is Red   463
  Pulse diagnosis adds detail to tongue diagnosis   463

LIMITATIONS OF PULSE DIAGNOSIS   464
  It is subjective   464
  It is subject to short-term influences   464

INTRODUCTION

Pulse diagnosis is the most difficult of the Chinese diagnostic arts: it is a very complex subject which must involve a deep level of understanding and a great deal

of skill. An essential diagnostic tool for all practitioners of Chinese medicine, pulse diagnosis is truly an 'art'; it has more right to that title than any other of the Chinese diagnostic skills. To acquire the skills of good pulse diagnosis requires great patience and to become proficient takes years of practice. It is a study that has no end: one will continue to develop one's skills and understanding of pulse diagnosis throughout a lifetime of practice.

What is one feeling when taking the pulse? Basically, we are feeling the pulsation of Qi through the pulsation of Blood. Qi is a subtle energy and cannot be 'felt' (except by expert practitioners of Qi Gong) or 'measured'; we therefore use the radial artery to feel the pulsation of the blood to give us an idea of the state of Qi. This is made possible by the strong link between Qi and Blood: Qi is the commander of Blood and Blood is the mother of Qi. Thus, through the pulsation of Blood, we can feel the state of Qi. That we use pulse diagnosis to feel the state of Qi is also shown by the fact that the pulse is felt on the radial artery where the Lung channel flows; because the Lungs govern Qi, that particular artery tells us about the state of Qi.

Pulse diagnosis is important for two reasons: it helps to identify the internal organ affected or the prevailing pattern and it reflects the whole complex of Qi and Blood.

The pulse identifies organ and pattern disharmony

Within the general picture of a disharmony, the pulse may be considered to be a manifestation like any other (e.g. thirst, dizziness, red face, etc.). The unique significance of pulse diagnosis, however, is that it, by itself, allows us to diagnose a pattern, even in the absence of other symptoms. For example, dizziness indicates a

Kidney deficiency only if it occurs together with other Kidney-deficiency symptoms, such as tinnitus, lower backache and night sweating. However, a Deep-Weak Kidney pulse on both Rear positions by itself unequivocally indicates a Kidney deficiency.

In addition, the pulse may also indicate, by itself, a pattern with some certainty. For example, dizziness may be caused by Phlegm and, in order to diagnose this, it should be accompanied by other symptoms or signs of Phlegm such as a feeling of oppression in the chest, a feeling of muzziness in the head, a Swollen tongue, etc. However, a Slippery pulse by itself indicates Phlegm (excluding of course the case of pregnancy).

The pulse gives us an idea of the state of Qi and Blood as a whole

Another way in which the pulse differs from other clinical manifestations is that it gives a picture of the body as a whole, of the state of Qi and Blood, of the state of Yin and Yang organs, of the state of parts of the body, and of the constitution of an individual. No other clinical manifestation can do that and only the tongue comes anywhere near so doing.

THE 'NINE REGIONS' OF THE PULSE FROM THE 'YELLOW EMPEROR'S CLASSIC OF INTERNAL MEDICINE'

The practice of feeling the pulse on the radial artery was described in the 'Classic of Difficulties' (c. AD 100); before that, the pulse was taken on nine different arteries: three in the head, three on the hands and three in the legs, as described in Chapter 20 of the 'Simple Questions': *'There are three areas in the body, each area is*

Table 49.1 The nine regions of the pulse from the 'Simple Questions'					
Area	Location	Region	Point	Organ or body part	Alternative
Upper	Head	Upper	Taiyang	Qi of head	
		Middle	ST-3 Juliao	Qi of mouth	
		Lower	TB-21 Ermen	Qi of ears and eyes	
Middle	Hand	Upper	LU-8 Jingqu	Lungs	
		Middle	LI-4 Hegu	Centre of thorax	
		Lower	HE-7 Shenmen	Heart	
Lower	Leg	Upper	LIV-10 Wuli	Liver	LIV-3 Taichong
		Middle	KI-3 Taixi	Kidneys	
		Lower	SP-11 Jimen	Spleen and Stomach	ST-42 Chongyang

divided into three which makes nine regions: these are used to determine life and death [i.e. prognosis], and in them, 100 diseases manifest, Deficiency and Excess are regulated and the pathogenic factors can be expelled.'[1]

The 'nine regions' are the arteries where the pulse is felt and which reflect the state of the Upper, Middle and Lower Burners; each of these three areas is divided into three regions identified with Heaven, Person and Earth to indicate Upper, Middle and Lower regions as indicated in Table 49.1.

Although this method of taking the pulse on nine different arteries and in nine different places was superseded by that of taking only the pulse of the radial artery, feeling the pulses of the nine regions may still be useful in clinical practice to confirm the Emptiness or Fullness of a particular area. For example, in a patient suffering from hypertension caused by the rising of Liver-Yang, it may be useful to check the pulses of the upper regions to determine the degree and severity of this pathology (the stronger, harder and fuller the pulses of the upper regions, the more severe is the rising of Liver-Yang).

Another example of the use of the pulses of the nine regions is in patients with circulatory problems in the legs; in this case, it may be useful to feel the pulses of the lower regions to establish the degree of severity of this problem (the weaker and emptier the pulses of the lower regions, the poorer is the circulation of Qi in the lower legs). Furthermore, this method may be particularly important if taking the pulse of a patient whose arm or leg has been amputated; in such a case the three pulses of the radial artery of the missing limb may be replaced by the nine regions from the 'Simple Questions'.

THE PULSE IN THE 'CLASSIC OF DIFFICULTIES'

The 'Classic of Difficulties' (AD100) established for the first time the practice of taking the pulse at the radial artery; this pulse was variously called *Qi Kou* ('Portal of Qi'), *Cun Kou* ('Portal of Inch [Front pulse position]') and *Mai Kou* ('Portal of Pulse'). The 'Classic of Difficulties' says:

The 12 main channels have their own arteries but the pulse can be taken only at the Portal of Inch [LU-9 position] reflecting the life and death of the 5 Yin and 6 Yang organs . . . The Portal of Inch is the beginning and end point

of the energy of the 5 Yin and 6 Yang organs and that is why we can take the pulse at this position only.[2]

The last part of this statement is interesting since the description of the pulse of the Portal of Inch as the 'beginning and end point of the energy of the 5 Yin and 6 Yang organs' seems to imply an understanding of the circulation of blood as a closed circuit.

There are two main reasons why the pulse is felt at the 'Qi Portal' position on the radial artery by the wrist in correspondence with the Lung channel. First of all, the Lungs govern Qi and this channel is therefore the best to gauge the state of Qi in the body. In fact, Chapter 1 of the 'Classic of Difficulties' says:

Twelve channels have places where a pulse can be felt and yet one selects only the Inch Portal to determine the state of the 5 Yin and 6 Yang organs, why is this? The Inch Portal constitutes the great meeting place of the vessels, it is the place where the pulse of the Hand Greater Yin [Lungs] beats . . . the Inch Portal is the beginning and end of the 5 Yin and 6 Yang organs and therefore only the Inch Portal is used [for diagnosis].[3]

Secondly, Postnatal Qi and Blood are derived from food and water entering the Stomach. The Stomach extracts the essences of food, which go to the Lungs; from the Lungs, they go to the skin and the five Yin and six Yang organs and to all the arteries in the body; this is a reason why LU-9 Taiyuan is the Gathering point of all blood vessels. The 'Simple Questions' says in Chapter 11:

The Yellow Emperor asked: why is it that one can tell the state of the 5 Yin organs only from the Qi Portal? Chi Po replied: the Stomach is the Sea of Food and Drink and the great origin of the 6 Yang organs. The five flavours enter the mouth and are stored in the Stomach which nourishes the Qi of the 5 Yin organs; the Qi Portal is the Greater Yin. The flavours of the 5 Yin and 6 Yang organs are all derived from the Stomach and then transformed to become visible at the Qi Portal.[4]

Chapter 21 of the same text says:

The Qi of food enters the Stomach, Food-Qi goes to the Heart and its refined part enters the vessels, the Qi of the vessels flows into the 12 channels and the Qi of the channels reaches the Lungs. The Lungs govern all vessels and their refined essence goes to the skin and body hair. The body hair and vessels combine together and Qi is transmitted to the 6 Yang organs whose Qi is manifested and nourishes the four Yin organs [apart from the Heart]. When Qi is in balance, the Qi Portal becomes the Inch Portal [i.e. the pulse position] from which the state of the body can be determined.[5]

Thus, the section of radial artery on the Lung channel can tell us about the state of Qi and Blood of the whole body (Box 49.1).

> **BOX 49.1 WHY THE PULSE IS FELT ON THE RADIAL ARTERY (LUNG CHANNEL)**
>
> • The Lungs govern Qi
> • The Lungs receive the Food-Qi from the Stomach

Dr J. H. F. Shen has an interesting further idea why the pulse is felt at the radial artery by the wrist. He compares the blood flowing in the radial artery by the wrist with a sea wave and the metacarpal bone of the thumb with a cliff: because the wave of blood in the radial artery crashes against the cliff and is pushed back, we can feel the pulse here. If the blood did not encounter this obstacle, it would flow through undeflected and we would not be able to interpret it in the same way (Fig. 49.1).

THE THREE SECTIONS OF THE PULSE

The three pulse sections are as follows:

Inch (*Cun*)	Front
Gate (*Guan*)	Middle
Foot (*Chi*)	Rear

The second chapter of the 'Classic of Difficulties' explains how its author arrived at feeling the pulse at the three positions called Inch or Front, Gate or Middle and Foot or Rear (Cun, Guan and Chi):

The Foot and Inch sections of the pulse are the meeting point of the channels. The distance from the Gate position [LU-8, level with the radial apophysis] to the Foot position in the elbow represents the Foot-Interior and it reflects the Yin energies. The distance from the Gate position to the point Fish Margin [the thenar eminence] is the Foot-Exterior and it reflects the Yang energies. Hence, the distance of 1 inch is separated from the distance of 1 foot [from the Gate position to the elbow crease], so that the distance of 1 foot is represented by 1 inch. Hence the Yin energies are reflected within that 1-inch section of the foot-long section and the Yang energies are reflected within a 9-fen [nine-tenths of an inch] section of the Inch section. The total length of the Foot and Inch section extends over 1 inch and 9 fen; hence one speaks of Foot and Inch sections.[6]

In other words, the distance from the Gate-Guan (or Middle) position of the pulse (on LU-8 Jingqu) to the crease of the elbow measures one Chinese foot and reflects the Yin energies; the distance from the Gate-Guan position to the crease of the wrist is 9 *fen* (nine-tenths of an inch) and reflects the Yang energies. However, a 1-inch section is separated from the 1-foot distance from the Gate-Guan position to the elbow crease to represent the Yin energies; in other words,

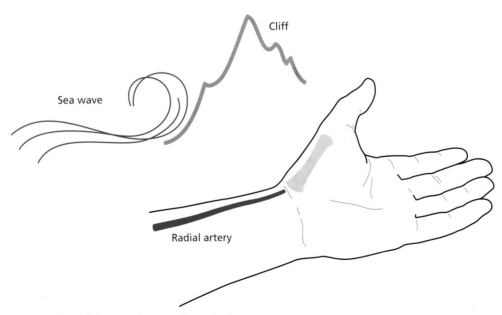

Fig. 49.1 The radial artery pulse according to Dr Shen

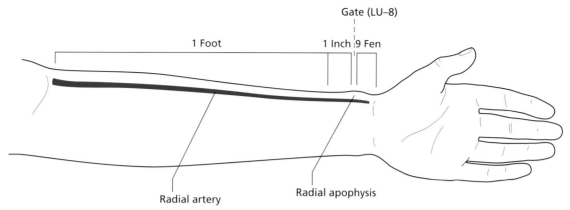

Fig. 49.2 Inch, Gate and Foot pulse sections from the 'Classic of Difficulties'

this 1-inch section is representative of the 1-foot section (Fig. 49.2).

The 'Pulse Classic' says something similar:

From the Fish Margin [the thenar eminence] to the prominent bone [the radial styloid process] moving one inch backwards [proximally], in the middle of this is the Inch Portal. From the Inch to the Foot, it is called Chi Ze and this position is called Foot. The position behind the Inch and in front of the Foot positions, is called Gate position: this is the boundary between the emerging Yang [at the Inch position] and submerging Yin [at the Foot position]. Emerging Yang occupies three divisions [positions] and submerging Yin also occupies three divisions [positions]. Yang originates at the Foot position and moves [or manifests] in the Inch position; Yin originates in the Inch position and moves [or manifests] in the Foot position. The Inch position governs the Upper Burner including the skin and hair up to the hands; the Gate position governs the Middle Burner including the abdomen and back; the Foot position governs the Lower Burner including the lower abdomen up to the feet.[7]

The 'Classic of Difficulties' says in Chapter 3: 'In front [i.e. distal] of the Gate position Yang moves, the pulse here is 9 fen long and superficial . . . behind [i.e. proximal to] the Gate position Yin moves, the pulse here is 1 cun long and is deep.'[8]

Thus, three sections of the pulse are identified: the Inch-*Cun* (Front) section reflecting the Yang energies, and the Gate-*Guan* (Middle) section and the Foot-*Chi* (Rear) section reflecting the Yin energies, (Box 49.2).

Three different types of finger pressure are applied to each section, making up the 'nine regions', which share the same name with but have a different

---

BOX 49.2 THE THREE POSITIONS OF THE PULSE

- The Inch-*Cun* (Front) position reflects the Yang energies
- The Gate-*Guan* (Middle) and Foot-*Chi* (Rear) positions reflect the Yin energies

---

meaning from those of the 'Simple Questions' listed above. This was the revolution brought to pulse diagnosis by the 'Classic of Difficulties': the same information that could be gained by feeling the pulse on nine separate arteries in the head, hands and legs, could now be gained by feeling the pulse at the radial artery only.

Chapter 18 of the 'Classic of Difficulties' describes the three different pressures applied to the pulse:

There are three sections, Inch, Gate and Foot, and three pressures, superficial, middle and deep [which makes] 9 regions. The Upper section pertains to Heaven and reflects diseases from the chest to the head; the Middle section pertains to Person and reflects diseases from the diaphragm to the umbilicus; the Lower section pertains to Earth and reflects diseases from the umbilicus to the feet. [One must] examine [these sections] before needling.[9]

This passage establishes clearly the principle, adopted by all successive doctors, that the Inch section of the pulse corresponds to the Upper Burner and diseases from the chest upwards, the Gate section to the Middle Burner and diseases from the diaphragm to the umbilicus, and the Foot section to the Lower Burner and diseases from the umbilicus to the feet (Fig. 49.3).

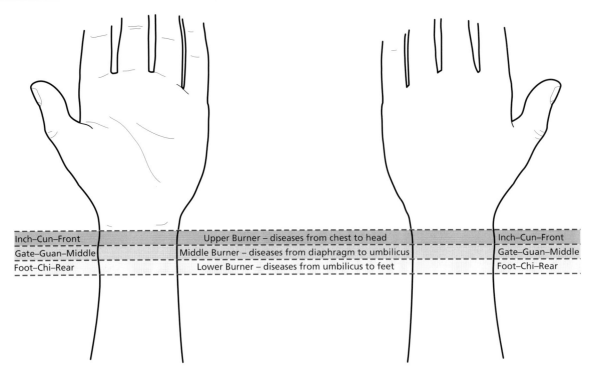

Inch–Cun–Front	Upper Burner – diseases from chest to head	Inch–Cun–Front
Gate–Guan–Middle	Middle Burner – diseases from diaphragm to umbilicus	Gate–Guan–Middle
Foot–Chi–Rear	Lower Burner – diseases from umbilicus to feet	Foot–Chi–Rear

Fig. 49.3 Correspondence of three sections to the Three Burners

ASSIGNMENT OF PULSE POSITIONS TO ORGANS

I shall discuss the assignment of pulse positions to organs by examining the various pulse arrangements over the ages, and then trying to reconcile the discrepancies between the various arrangements.

Organ positions on the pulse

Besides attributing the three sections of the pulse to the Three Burners, Chinese pulse diagnosis goes much further in assigning each pulse position to the Qi of a particular organ. Through the centuries, Chinese doctors have disagreed over such assignment and many different opinions exist. Table 49.2 summarizes the assignment of pulse positions to various organs, according to six representative major classics:

- 'The Yellow Emperor's Classic of Internal Medicine' (*Huang Di Nei Jing*), c. 100BC
- 'The Classic of Difficulties' (*Nan Jing*), c. AD100
- 'The Pulse Classic' (*Mai Jing*) by Wang Shu He, c. AD280

- 'The Study of the Pulse from Pin Hu Lake' (*Pin Hu Mai Xue*) by Li Shi Zhen, 1564
- 'The Complete Works of Jing Yue' (*Jing Yue Quan Shu*) by Zhang Jing Yue, 1624
- 'The Golden Mirror of Medicine' (*Yi Zong Jin Jian*) by Wu Qian, 1742.

It is worth reporting the actual passages concerning the correlation between organs and pulse positions from some of the classics to show how such correlation has never been so simple and mechanical as what tends to be taught today, that is, that we feel the 'Yang organs at the superficial level and Yin organs at the deep level'.

Classic of Difficulties (Nan Jing, AD100)

Chapter 18 of the 'Classic of Difficulties' explains the correspondence of pulse positions to organs (or channels) in accordance with the five Elements in a rather complex statement:

The Hand Greater Yin [Lungs] and the Hand Bright Yang [Large Intestine] pertain to Metal; the Foot Lesser Yin [Kidneys] and Foot Greater Yang [Bladder] pertain to Water. Metal generates Water, Water flows downwards and cannot ascend. Therefore, these are felt at the position below

Table 49.2 Assignment of organs to pulse positions by different authors

	Left			Right		
	Front	Middle	Rear	Front	Middle	Rear
Nei Jing	Heart, Shanzhong	Liver, diaphragm	Kidney, abdomen	Lung, centre of thorax	Stomach, Spleen	Kidney, abdomen
Nan Jing	Heart, Small Intestine	Liver, Gall-Bladder	Kidney, Bladder	Lung, Large Intestine	Spleen, Stomach	Pericardium, Triple Burner
Mai Jing	Heart, Small Intestine	Liver, Gall-Bladder	Kidney, Bladder	Lung, Large Intestine	Spleen, Stomach	Kidney, Bladder/Triple Burner/Uterus
Pin Hu Mai Xue	Heart	Liver	Kidney	Lung	Spleen, Stomach	Ming Men
Jing Yue Quan Shu	Heart, Pericardium	Liver, Gall-Bladder	Kidney, Bladder/ Large Intestine	Lung, Shanzhong	Spleen, Stomach	Kidney, Triple Burner/Ming Men/ Small Intestine
Yi Zong Jin Jian	Shanzhong, Heart	Gall-Bladder, Liver	Bladder/ Small Intestine, Kidney	Centre of Thorax, Lung	Stomach, Spleen	Large Intestine, Kidney

the Gate position [i.e. Foot position]. The Foot Terminal Yin [Liver] and the Foot Lesser Yang [Gall-Bladder] pertain to Wood; Wood generates the Fire of the Hand Greater Yang [Small Intestine] and Hand Lesser Yin [Heart]. Fire blazes upwards and cannot descend. Hence, the Hand Greater Yang [Small Intestine] and Hand Lesser Yin [Heart] correspond to the position above the Gate [i.e. the Inch position]. The Fire of the Hand Heart Master [i.e. Pericardium] and Lesser Yang [Triple Burner] generates the Earth of Foot Greater Yin [Spleen] and Foot Bright Yang [Stomach], Earth governs the Centre and its position is therefore the central one. This is in accordance with the Five-Element Mother–Child mutual generating and nourishing relationship.[10]

Thus, the 'Classic of Difficulties' assignment of organs to pulse positions follows strictly the Generating cycle of the Five Elements as follows (Fig. 49.4):

Left	Right
Small Intestine/Heart	Lungs/Large Intestine
Gall-Bladder/Liver	Spleen/Stomach
Bladder/Kidneys	Pericardium/Triple Burner

It is interesting to note that this strict assignment of organs to pulse positions according to the Five Elements and the assignment of the right Foot (Rear) position to the Pericardium and Triple Burner would suggest that the 'Classic of Difficulties' assigns channels rather than organs to the pulse positions. Thus, the arrangement of pulse positions in the 'Classic of Difficulties' is seen clearly from the acupuncturist's

perspective rather than the herbalist's and this would confirm that the two main pulse arrangements, that is, one with the Small Intestine and Large Intestine on the Front and the other with them on the Rear position, reflect the different perspectives of the acupuncturist and herbalist, as discussed in more detail below.

Pulse Classic (Mai Jing, AD280)

The 'Pulse Classic' discusses the correspondence of pulse positions to organs (or channels) in Chapter 7. It says:

The Heart position is assigned to the left Cun [which is] distal to the Gate position. The Heart is the Hand Lesser Yin and is exteriorly–interiorly related to the Hand Great Yang, i.e. the Small Intestine. The Liver position is assigned to the left gate position. The Liver is the Foot Terminal Yin and is exteriorly–interiorly related to the Foot Lesser Yang, i.e. the Gall-Bladder. The Kidneys position is assigned to the left Foot position which is proximal to the Gate position. The Kidneys are the Foot Lesser Yin which is exteriorly– interiorly related with the Foot Greater Yang, i.e. the Bladder. The Lungs position is assigned to the right Cun position, distal to the Gate position. The Lungs are the Hand Greater Yin and are exteriorly–interiorly related to the Hand Bright Yang, i.e. the Large Intestine. The Spleen position is assigned to the right Guan position. The Spleen is the Foot Greater Yin which is exteriorly–interiorly related to the Foot Bright Yang, i.e. the Stomach. The Kidneys position is assigned to the right Foot position, proximal to the Gate position. The Kidneys are the Foot Lesser Yin which is exteriorly–interiorly related to the Foot

(a)

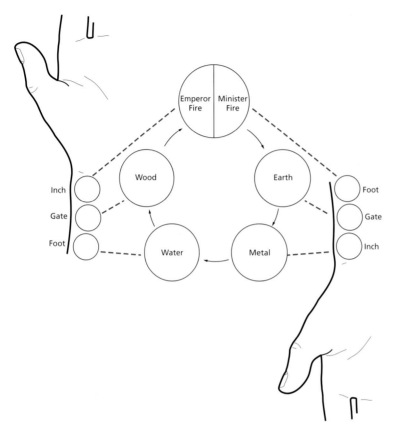

(b)

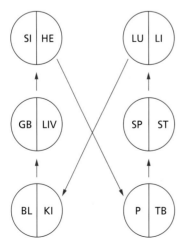

Fig. 49.4 (a) Five-Element influence on correspondence between organs and (b) pulse position in the 'Classic of Difficulties'

Greater Yang, i.e. the Bladder. The Kidneys and Bladder meet in the Lower Burner at a point to the right of Guan Yuan [Ren-4]: to the left of this point are the Kidneys, to the right the Uterus also called Triple Burner.[11]

The last part of this statement is of note as it seems to assign both left and right Rear positions to the Kidneys and Bladder, while the Rear position reflects also the Uterus and Triple Burner. Most authors translate the end of the above passage as meaning that the left Rear position corresponds to the Kidneys and the right Rear one to the Uterus and Triple Burner; I personally think that 'right' and 'left' at the end of the above passage refer to right and left of Ren-4 Guanyuan. In conclusion, the pulse arrangement from the 'Pulse Classic' is:

Left	Right
Small Intestine/Heart	Lungs/Large Intestine
Gall-Bladder/Liver	Spleen/Stomach
Bladder/Kidneys	Kidneys/Uterus/Triple Burner/Bladder

The association between Uterus and Triple Burner is interesting as it confirms the statement from Chapter 66 of the 'Classic of Difficulties', according to which the Original Qi stems from the space between the two kidneys (and therefore also the Uterus in women) and

it spreads to the five Yin and six Yang organs via the intermediary of the Triple Burner.

The 'Study of the Pulse from Pin Hu Lake' (Pin Hu Mai Xue, 1564)

The 'Study of the Pulse from Pin Hu Lake' assigns only the Yin organs to the pulse positions:

'The Heart and Liver are on the left and Lungs and Spleen on the right. The Kidneys and Gate of life [Ming Men] are at the Foot position on left and right.'[12]

The 'Golden Mirror of Medicine' (Yi Zong Jin Jian, 1742)

The 'Golden Mirror of Medicine' by Wu Qian assigns the pulse positions to the organs as follows:

Left	Right
'External'/'Internal'	'Internal'/'External'
Shanzhong/Heart	Lungs/Centre of thorax
Gall-Bladder/Liver	Spleen/Stomach
Bladder, Small Intestine/Kidneys	Kidneys/Large Intestine

Figure 49.5 is a reproduction of the diagram from the original text and Figure 49.6 is a translation of the same.[13]

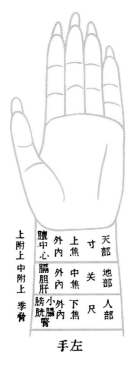
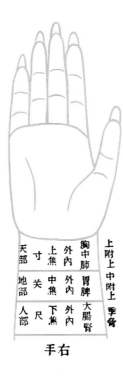

Fig. 49.5 Pulse diagram from the 'Golden Mirror of Medicine'

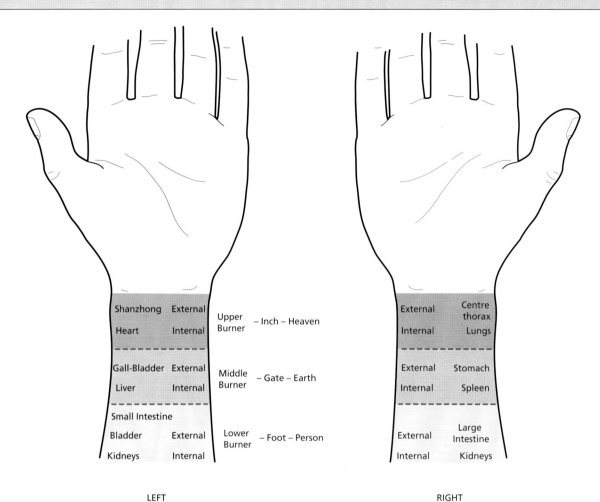

LEFT   RIGHT

Fig. 49.6 Translation of pulse diagram from the 'Golden Mirror of Medicine'

The diagram from the 'Golden Mirror of Medicine' clearly shows that 'external' and 'internal' mean distal and proximal respectively: this means that the Yang and Yin organs within each position are felt at the distal and proximal ends respectively. This is discussed in greater depth below.

Modern China

The most common pulse assignment in modern China is as follows:

Left	Right
'External'/'Internal'	*'Internal'/'External'*
Pericardium/Heart	Lungs
Gall-Bladder/Liver	Spleen/Stomach
Small Intestine/	Kidney-Yang/Large
Bladder/Kidney-Yin	Intestine

Such assignment of pulse positions to organs is something that I have deduced from the various teachers I learned with in China as modern books do not usually present this information in a clear form. This is probably due to the fact that there has been considerable disagreement on this over the centuries and modern books tend therefore to gloss over this. For example, 'Chinese Acupuncture and Moxibustion' of 1987 does not even give any assignment of pulse positions to organs.[14] Other texts often overlook the assignment of the Small and Large Intestine organs as this is the subject of more disagreement: for example, the 'Fundamentals of Chinese Medicine' (a translation of a Chinese text) of 1985 says: *'The right Inch pulse is associated with the Lungs, and the right Barrier pulse is associated with the Stomach and Spleen. The left Inch pulse is associated with the Heart, and the left Barrier pulse is associated with the Liver and Gall-Bladder.*

The Kidney and Bladder are reflected in both Cubit pulses.'[15]

Reconciling different pulse arrangements

Although different pulse assignments may seem contradictory, there is a common thread running through them. It is generally agreed that the Front position reflects the Upper Burner, the Middle position the Middle Burner and the Rear position the Lower Burner. Generally, the main discrepancies occur with the assignment of the Yang organs and especially the Small and Large Intestine. Indeed, many doctors do not assign the Yang organs to the pulse at all (the 'Yellow Emperor's Classic of Internal Medicine' does not).

Yin and Yang organ as reflected on the pulse

The commonly held assumption that the superficial level reflects the state of the Yang organs and the deep level that of the Yin organs has never been the only one in Chinese medicine. In fact, the different levels (or different places) where the Yang and Yin organs are felt

are often described as *wai* (external) and *nei* (internal) and 'external' and 'internal' may be interpreted in three ways:

> • 'external' meaning superficial and 'internal' meaning deep level
> • 'external' meaning lateral and 'internal' meaning medial
> • 'external' meaning distal and 'internal' meaning proximal.

The first interpretation is by far the most common today but it is important to realize that it is not the only one and also that the three interpretations are not mutually exclusive. Indeed, Dr J. H. F. Shen often uses the second and third interpretations when reading the pulse; this will be discussed later. Figure 49.7 illustrates the three different ways of interpreting 'external' and 'internal'.

In any case, the relationship between Yin and Yang organs as reflected on the pulse needs to be interpreted dynamically and not mechanically; we should not simply assign the superficial level to the Yang organs and the deep level to the Yin ones, for example on the

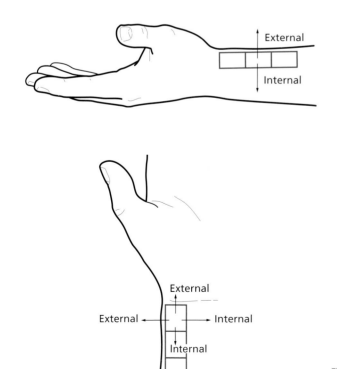

Fig. 49.7 Meanings of 'external' and 'internal' in pulse taking

left Middle position the Gall-Bladder on the superficial level and the Liver on the deep level. As the relationship between the paired Yin and Yang organs is very close (except for the Small Intestine/Heart and Large Intestine/Lung, which will be discussed shortly), each individual pulse position should be first analysed as a whole, paying attention to the intensity and the level of the pulse, rather than mechanically feeling the 'Gall-Bladder' on the superficial level and the 'Liver' on the deep level as two separate entities.

Each pulse position can reflect different phenomena in different situations. For example, let us consider the left Middle position (Liver and Gall-Bladder): in a state of health, the Liver and Gall-Bladder will be balanced or, to put it differently, Yin and Yang within the Liver/Gall-Bladder sphere are balanced. In this case, the pulse will be relatively soft and smooth and not particularly superficial or deep and the Gall-Bladder influence on the pulse will not be felt. But if Liver-Yang is in excess and rises upwards affecting the Gall-Bladder channel (causing severe temporal headaches), the rising Qi will be reflected on the pulse, which will be Wiry (harder than normal) and more superficial (it will be felt pounding under the finger). In interpreting this pulse we can say that Liver-Yang is rising or, to put it differently, that the Gall-Bladder Qi is in excess.

The acupuncturist's and herbalist's perspectives in pulse diagnosis

One of the possible explanations for the different pulse arrangements is the therapeutic approach of the practitioner, that is, the acupuncturist or the herbalist. Given that the pulse reflects the Qi of both organ and channel, acupuncturists working on the channels would naturally assign the Small Intestine and Large Intestine to the same positions as the Heart and Lungs respectively to which their channels are paired. Herbalists, on the contrary, would give more importance to the Internal Organs rather than the channels and therefore assign the Small and Large Intestine to the Rear positions, that is, the Lower Burner where their organs are located.

Small and Large Intestine channels versus organs in pulse diagnosis

The Small and Large Intestine are probably the subject of the widest discrepancies in pulse diagnosis because they are sometimes placed on the Front and sometimes on the Rear position. This discrepancy may be explained by the fact that the connection between these two organs and their channels is somewhat looser than that of other organs. In fact, the Small and Large Intestine organs are in the Lower Burner while their channels are in the arms (the organs of the Upper Burner have their channels in the arm, whereas the organs of the Middle and Lower Burner have their channels in the legs). Furthermore, the functions of the intestinal organs do not correspond closely to those of their channels; in fact, although the arm points of the Small and Large Intestine can of course be used for intestinal problems, their chief clinical application is to treat problems of the neck, shoulders, face and head as well as external invasions of Wind.

Thus, the same pulse quality in the specific example of the Front position could mean two different things in different situations. For example, if the right Front position (Lung) is quite superficial, slightly big and slightly Rapid, this could indicate an emotional upset affecting the Lungs. Here, the pulse reflects the state of the Lungs. But on another occasion exactly the same type of pulse may indicate something quite different when, for example, the patient has an acute, large, purulent tooth abscess. In such a case, the pulse reflects the state of the Large Intestine channel (where the abscess is) rather than a problem with the Lung organ. On the other hand, problems with the Large Intestine *organ* (rather than channel) more often manifest on the Rear position of the pulse and often on both sides. For example, in patients suffering from ulcerative colitis nearly always the Rear position of both sides is very Wiry, reflecting the Heat and stagnation in the Large Intestine. Thus, from these two examples (tooth abscess and ulcerative colitis) we can see how the contradictory assignments of the Large Intestine to the right Front and right Rear positions can *both* be right.

Clinical significance of pulse diagnosis irrespective of organ positions

We should not make too much of the different pulse positions assumed by different doctors and we should not view the relationship between pulse positions and organs mechanically. In fact, it would be perfectly possible to make a good, clinically significant pulse diagnosis without referring to the Internal Organs at all. This is because the pulse gives us an idea of the relative strength of Qi in the Three Burners, at the three levels and on left and right sides.

The pulse essentially reflects the state of Qi in the different Burners and at different energetic levels which are dependent on the pathological condition. We need

to interpret the pulse dynamically rather than mechanically. The most important thing is to appraise how Qi is flowing, what is the relationship between Yin and Yang on the pulse (i.e. is there Deficiency or Excess of Yin or Yang), at what level is Qi flowing (i.e. is the pulse superficial or deep), and whether the body's Qi is deficient and whether there is an attack by an external pathogenic factor.

> !
> The pulse gives us clinically relevant information, even without reference to organ positions.

Clinical interpretation of the pulse in acute versus chronic conditions

The clinical relevance of the assignment of pulse positions to organs differs in acute and chronic conditions. In acute conditions, especially in fevers, after operations, during infections, etc., the assessment of the individual pulse positions is somewhat less important than that of its overall quality and rate. For example, if a person suffers a severe invasion of Wind, the pulse will be Floating in all the positions and, of course, this does not indicate a pathology in each of the organs corresponding to those positions.

The pulse as a reflection of Heart-Qi

Although each pulse position can be assigned to a particular Internal Organ or channel, we should not lose sight of the fact that the pulse as a whole reflects the state of Heart-Qi and Heart-Blood: the Heart governs Blood and the blood vessels and it is therefore natural that a disharmony of the Heart may reflect on the pulse *as a whole*. The influence of the Heart on the pulse as a whole is particularly manifest when the pulse is extremely Weak, Fine or Choppy, or, conversely, Overflowing, in *all* positions, and also when it is very Slow or very Rapid.

Furthermore, any irregularity of the pulse (Knotted, Hasty, Hurried, Intermittent) always indicates a Heart disharmony, whatever the other Internal Organs that may be involved. Frequently, but by no means always, the above pulse qualities may indicate not only a Heart disharmony in the Chinese sense, but possibly also a heart problem in a Western sense. For example, a congenital heart defect may manifest with one of the above qualities.

The clinical significance of pulse diagnosis in heart problems is discussed further below.

> !
> Independently of positions, the pulse as a whole reflects Heart-Qi.

THE THREE LEVELS

When feeling the pulse one should apply three different pressures to feel three different levels of energy: the superficial level is felt with a very light pressure and corresponds to Qi, Yang and the Yang organs, the deep level is felt with a heavy pressure and corresponds to Yin and the Yin organs; and the middle level is felt in between the two levels with a moderate pressure and corresponds to Blood.

The clinical significance of the three levels is summarized in Table 49.3.

The correlation that relates the superficial level to Qi and Yang, the middle level to Blood and the deep level to Yin is clinically important. This distinction, is after all, implicit in many of the pulse qualities; for example, when we say that a pulse is Weak we mean that it is weak at the superficial level and it therefore indicates deficiency of Yang; when we say that a pulse is Floating-Empty we mean that it is weak at the deep level and it therefore indicates Yin deficiency; when we say that a pulse is Hollow we mean that it is empty at the middle level and it therefore indicates deficiency of Blood.

The above three examples all refer to a deficiency of energy at the three levels. Of course, the pulse can also be too strong at each of those levels. For example, a Floating pulse is too superficial and it therefore indicates 'Excess of Yang', which may be external (as Wind is a Yang pathogenic factor) or internal; a Firm pulse is by definition full, strong and hard at the middle and deep levels and it may therefore indicate Blood stasis or

Table 49.3 Correspondence of three levels of the pulse to Yang and Yin energies (Li Shi Zhen)

Level	Energy	Yin or Yang	Organs
Superficial	Qi/Yang	Yang organs	Lungs and Heart
Middle	Blood		Stomach and Spleen
Deep	Yin	Yin organs	Liver and Kidneys

Table 49.4 Clinical significance of the pulse strength at the three levels

Level	Weak	Strong
Superficial	Yang or Qi deficiency (Deep, Weak, Soggy, Hidden)	Excess of Yang, invasion of external pathogenic factor (Floating, Big, Overflowing, Wiry)
Middle	Blood deficiency (Choppy, Leather, Hollow, Scattered)	Blood-Heat or Blood stasis (Firm, Wiry, Slippery, Big, Overflowing)
Deep	Yin deficiency (Floating-Empty, Leather, Scattered)	Internal Cold or internal Heat, stasis in the Yin organs (Deep, Full, Slippery, Wiry, Firm, Tight)

Blood-Heat; a Deep and Full pulse indicates the presence of a pathogenic factor in the Interior and therefore in the Yin energy. The clinical significance of the strength of the pulse at each level is summarized in Table 49.4, which also indicates the pulse qualities corresponding to each level.

Another way of interpreting the three levels is that given by Li Shi Zhen, who correlates the superficial, middle and deep levels with the energy of Lungs and Heart, Stomach and Spleen, and Liver and Kidneys respectively (Table 49.3). This means that, according to his theory, the whole of the superficial level (irrespective of positions) reflects the state of the Lung and Heart, the whole of the middle level reflects the state of the Stomach and Spleen, and the whole of the deep level (irrespective of position) reflects the state of the Liver and Kidneys; this thinking is certainly clinically useful especially when the pulse displays the same quality in all positions. For example, if the pulse is Empty at the deep level in all positions, we can certainly deduce that there is a deficiency of Yin of the Liver and Kidneys; that does not mean to say, of course, that other organs may not have Yin deficiency but if, say, there was a deficiency of Yin of the Lungs, the pulse would be Empty at the deep level only in the Lung position. The idea that the three different levels can be correlated to the energy of different organs is actually very old and is present in both the 'Classic of Difficulties' and the 'Pulse Classic'.

The 'Pulse Classic' (*Mai Jing*) says:

Initially one should apply the pressure [equivalent to] 3 soya beans and [this level corresponds to] skin and hair and to the energy of the Lungs; with the pressure equivalent

to 6 soya beans, it corresponds to blood vessels and the energy of the Heart; with the pressure equivalent to 9 soya beans it corresponds to the muscles and the energy of the Spleen; with the pressure equivalent to 12 soya beans it corresponds to the sinews and the energy of the Liver; finally, pressing down to the bone and then releasing the pressure, if the pulse comes fast, it corresponds to the energy of the Kidneys.[16]

Wang Shu He (author of the 'Pulse Classic') obviously relied here on the description in the 'Classic of Difficulties' which has a passage that is almost identical in Chapter 5.[17]

It should be noted that some pulse qualities (Wiry, Slippery, Big, Overflowing, etc.) manifest of course at more than one level.

METHOD OF PULSE TAKING

There are four aspects to the method of taking the pulse:

- time
- levelling the arm
- equalizing the breathing
- placing the fingers.

Time

In theory the best time to take the pulse is in the early morning when the Yin is calm and the Yang has not yet stirred; it is also the time when the pulse is not affected by work, eating, emotions, etc. The 'Simple Questions' explains why the early morning is the best time to take the pulse: *'Normally the pulse should be taken in the morning when Yin Qi has not stirred yet [not yet decreased after the night], Yang Qi is not yet dispersed [not yet emerged after the night], the patient has not eaten yet, the main channels are not yet full, the Connecting channels are balanced, and Qi and Blood are balanced.'*[18] Obviously this is not possible in clinical practice and we should therefore bear in mind the various factors that could affect the pulse in the short term, that is, hurrying at work, hurrying to get to the clinic, having just had a meal or being in a state of hunger, an emotional upset, etc.

Levelling the arm

The patient's arm should be horizontal and should not be held higher than the level of the heart. If the patient is lying down, the arm should be resting on the couch;

(a)

(b)

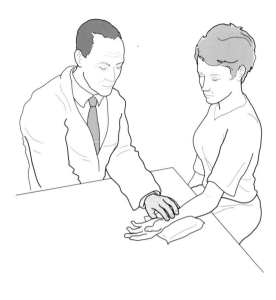

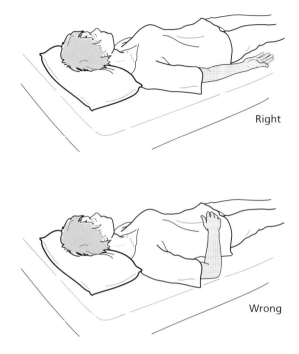

Right

Wrong

Fig. 49.8 Patient's arm position when taking the pulse: (a) sitting; (b) lying down

it should *not* be bent, resting on the patient's body (Fig. 49.8). If the patient is sitting, the arm should be resting comfortably on the table. In China, this is the most common way of taking the pulse, using a small soft cushion for the patient to rest his or her wrist on.

Equalizing the breathing

Traditionally, equalizing the breathing was necessary to determine whether the pulse was Slow or Rapid, by relating it to the practitioner's breathing cycle: if the patient's pulse beats three times or less per practitioner's breathing cycle, it is Slow; if it beats five times or more, it is Rapid. This method is not used nowadays because we can make use of a watch to count the rate of a pulse; however, 'equalizing the breathing' is still a useful procedure because it facilitates the practitioner's necessary relaxation and concentration.

Placing the fingers

Placing the fingers involves five aspects, as follows:

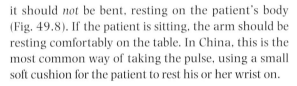

- placing the fingers
- arranging the fingers
- regulating the fingers

- using the fingers
- moving the fingers
  —lifting
  —pressing
  —searching
  —pushing
  —rolling.

Placing the fingers

Placing the fingers means that the practitioner's three fingers (index, middle and ring fingers) are placed simultaneously on the radial artery to make an initial assessment of the strength, level and quality of the pulse. To assess individual positions, it may be necessary to lift two of the fingers slightly, while interpreting the pulse with the third finger. Usually, one feels the pulse of the patient's right arm with one's left hand and vice versa (Fig. 49.9) and the index, middle and ring fingers are placed on the Front, Middle and Rear positions respectively.

Arranging the fingers

Arranging the fingers means that the practitioner should either spread the fingers slightly or press them

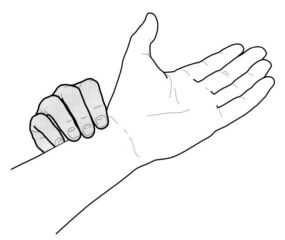

Fig. 49.9 Placing the fingers when taking the pulse

close together according to the size of the patient's arm. For example, when feeling the pulse of a
10-year-old child, we should press our fingers closer
together to feel the three positions; the younger the
child, the closer together our fingers should be and, in
a baby under a year old, we feel the three positions with
a single finger (by rolling it proximally and distally to
feel the Rear and Front positions respectively). When
taking the pulse of a very tall man, we should spread
the fingers out slightly to feel the three positions.

Regulating the fingers

Regulating the fingers means that the practitioner
should place the fingertips on the three positions,
allowing for the different length of the fingers. In other
words, the middle finger, being the longest, is slightly
contracted. To feel the pulse, the pads rather than the
tips of the fingers are used (Fig. 49.10).

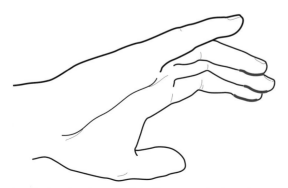

Fig. 49.10 Using the pads of the fingers to take the pulse

Using the fingers

Using the fingers means that the practitioner should
bear in mind the subtle difference in sensitivity
between the three fingers. Generally, the ring finger is
slightly more sensitive than the others and we should
take this into account when comparing the different
strengths of the three positions; however, the difference in sensitivity is very small and not too important
in clinical practice.

Moving the fingers

Moving the fingers means that the fingers should be
moved in various directions when feeling the pulse. It is
a common misconception that the pulse is felt by
keeping the fingers absolutely still for a long time; in

> **!**
>
> Remember: the pulse is not felt with the fingers totally still
> but moving the fingers in four ways:
> 1. Lifting (upwards)
> 2. Pressing (downwards)
> 3. Pushing (from side to side)
> 4. Rolling (proximal–distal).

BOX 49.3 THE FIVE MOVEMENTS

- **Lifting**: this consists of gently lifting the fingers to
  check the strength of the pulse at the superficial level
  and therefore whether the pulse is Floating, normal or
  deficient at that level.
- **Pressing**: this consists of gently pressing the fingers
  downwards to check the strength of the pulse at the
  middle and deep levels and therefore whether the pulse
  is Deep, normal or deficient at these levels: this is
  necessary to determine whether the pulse is Deep,
  Hollow, Hidden or empty at the deep level.
- **Searching**: this consists of not moving the fingers but
  keeping them still to count the rate of the pulse, to
  decide whether it is Slow, Rapid or normal.
- **Pushing**: this consists of gently moving the fingers from
  side to side (lateral-medial) in each position (Fig. 49.11).
  This movement is necessary to interpret many pulse
  qualities, such as Slippery, Wiry, Leather, Tight, Choppy,
  Fine, Minute, etc. One can only identify these pulse
  qualities by moving the fingers in this way in order to
  feel *around* the pulse: it is only by feeling round the
  pulse that we can determine its shape.
- **Rolling**: this consists of moving the fingers back and
  forth (proximal-distal) in each position (Fig. 49.12): this
  movement is necessary to determine whether the pulse
  is Short, Long or Moving or to read the pulse of a child
  under 1 year old.

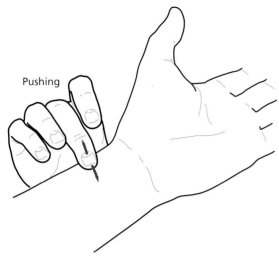

Fig. 49.11 Pushing the fingers from side to side

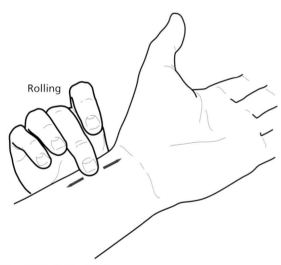

Fig. 49.12 Rolling the fingers

fact, the fingers are kept still only when counting the rate of the pulse to decide whether it is Slow, Rapid or normal. The movements are five (Box 49.3).

FACTORS AFFECTING THE PULSE

There is no such thing as a 'standard' normal pulse. A person's pulse varies according to many factors, all of which should be taken into account.

The following factors affect the pulse:

> - season
> - gender
> - age
> - body build
> - menstruation
> - pregnancy
> - *Fan Guan Mai* and *Xie Fei Mai*.

Season

The pulse varies considerably according to the seasons (Box 49.4), becoming relatively Wiry in the spring, Overflowing in the summer, Soft in the autumn and Deep in the winter.

> **BOX 49.4 SEASONAL PULSES**
>
> - Spring: slightly Wiry
> - Summer: superficial, Overflowing
> - Autumn: soft
> - Winter: Deep

In spring the pulse should be slightly Wiry, straight and relatively Long. It was traditionally described as 'feeling like the tender tip of a bamboo pole'.

In summer the pulse should be more superficial than in other seasons. It should feel round, slightly Slippery, coming forcefully and disappearing quickly. It was traditionally described as feeling like a hook or 'a string of pearls'. In late summer, the pulse should be relatively soft, light and relaxed and was traditionally described as 'feeling like the steps of a chicken'.

In autumn, the pulse should again be relatively soft, superficial, light and relaxed. It was traditionally described as 'feeling like a group of seedlings sprouting together'.

In winter, the pulse should be deeper than at other seasons and should feel relatively hard and round like a stone.

The normal seasonal pulses have been described in slightly different ways in various passages from the classics. The 'Classic of Categories' by Zhang Jing Yue (1624) describes the pulse in springtime as round and Slippery, in summertime as Overflowing and Big, in the autumn as Floating and like a hair and in wintertime as Deep and like a stone.[19] It also says that '*In Springtime the pulse is floating like a fish swimming in the waves; in Summertime it is at the skin level, flooding and*

full; in the Autumn it is under the skin and like a hibernating worm about to move; in Wintertime it is at the level of the bones and like a hidden hibernating worm'.[20]

The 'Simple Questions' in Chapter 19 describes the normal seasonal pulses as follows: 'In springtime the pulse is like a bowstring . . . in summertime like a hook . . . in the autumn floating . . . and in wintertime like a storage place.'[21]

The 'Simple Questions' describes the normal pulses in each season by comparing them with various instruments for measuring such as a ruler, the carpenter's square, the steelyard arm (the arm of a weighing scale) and the counterpoise weight: 'In springtime the pulse should be like a ruler, in summertime like a [carpenter's] square, in the autumn like the arm of a steelyard and in wintertime like a counterpoise [weight].'[22] The analogy between the seasonal pulses and the measuring instruments highlights the idea of balance and harmony of the pulse with the changing seasons. The modern commentary explains that in springtime the pulse should be light, supple and Slippery, in summertime Overflowing and relatively Rapid, in the autumn superficial and relatively soft like hair and in wintertime like a stone and Deep.

Gender

Men's pulses are relatively stronger than women's in general. There are two other differences between men's and women's pulses. First, the left-side pulse is rather stronger than the right-side pulse in men and vice versa in women; this is only a very slight difference (some authors say it is about 8%). The 'Pulse Classic' (Chapter 7) says: 'The left side [of the pulse] is big in men, the right side is big in women.'[23] Li Shi Zhen also discusses the differences between left and right: 'In men the left pulse should be stronger, in women the right pulse should be stronger.'[24]

Secondly, in men, the Front position is relatively stronger than the Rear one and vice versa in women (Box 49.5). The 'Classic of Difficulties' (Chapter 19) says: 'In men the pulse [is found] above the Middle position, in women below the Middle position. Thus, men's pulse is usually weak on the Rear position while women's pulse is strong on the Rear position: this is normal.'[25] Li Shi Zhen says something similar in his book 'The Study of the Pulse from Pin Hu Lake': 'There are differences in the Rear position in men and women: in women, the Yang [i.e. the Front position] is weak and the Yin [i.e. the Rear position] is strong.'[26] Qing dynasty's Chen Jia Yuan says:

Men have less Yin and more Yang, women have less Yang and more Yin. South corresponds to Fire and man, the two Front pulse positions correspond to South and the original Yang, hence they are big and overflowing while the two Rear positions are weak and soft. Women correspond to North, and so the two Front pulse positions are fine and weak while the two Rear positions are big.[27]

Box 49.5 summarizes gender differences in the pulse according to the classics.

> ### BOX 49.5 DIFFERENCES BETWEEN THE PULSES OF MEN AND WOMEN
>
> - The left side is slightly stronger in men, the right in women
> - The Front positions are slightly stronger in men, the Rear in women (not verified in my practice)

It is interesting to note that this situation is hardly ever encountered in practice as women's pulses are more commonly weak on the Rear position, perhaps indicating a decline of hereditary Kidney strength compared with previous generations. In my practice, from a database of more than 2500 patients, I have found that 22% of women have a very weak pulse on both Rear positions, as opposed to 4.6% of men.

> **!**
>
> Contrary to what the classics say, the Rear positions are usually weaker in women than in men.

Age

The pulse varies considerably with age, especially in its rate, being faster in small children and slower in old people (see Chapter 50). Most Chinese books also say that the pulse is naturally weaker in old people; I do not find this to be true in practice as in many cases, the pulse of the elderly is often Full and Wiry. This is because old people frequently suffer from Liver-Wind or Phlegm.

Body build

The pulse should naturally be stronger, larger and longer in robust, large people and weaker, smaller and shorter in small, frail people. Thus, a pulse that would be judged to be too weak and short in a robust man might be normal in a small, thin woman. The 'Pulse Classic' says:

When diagnosing from the pulse one must take into account whether the patient is large, small, tall or short and whether their nature is placid or nervous. If the pulse, whether slow, rapid, big, small, long or short, accords with the patient's nature, it is normal; if it does not accord with it, it is abnormal. The three pulse positions tend to be of equal size. For example in a small-size person, or a woman, or a thin person the pulse is small and soft.[28]

Menstruation

In the week preceding the onset of the period, the pulse is slightly Slippery, especially on the right Rear position. When the period arrives, the pulse loses its Slippery quality and becomes relatively Weak and maybe a bit slower.

Pregnancy

The pulse becomes Slippery during pregnancy; this quality is therefore normal in pregnancy. The more advanced the pregnancy, the more Slippery is the pulse. It is also normal for the Front and Rear pulses to become stronger in pregnancy.

Fan Guan Mai and Xie Fei Mai

Fan Guan Mai

The radial artery is displaced in a small percentage of people (about 5%) so that it lies on the dorsal rather than the inner aspect of the arm (Fig. 49.13). This anatomical abnormality was called *Fan Guan Mai* in Chinese, meaning 'pulse on the opposite gate'. In such cases (which usually occur on one side only) we cannot

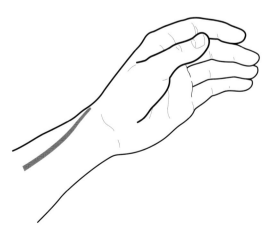

Fig. 49.13 *Fan Guan Mai* pulse

interpret the pulse properly and we should therefore refer to the pulses of the nine regions on the head, hand and feet. Thus, whenever the pulse cannot be felt at all, or can be felt only very faintly, we should always check the dorsal aspect of the arm to see if the artery is displaced, lest we deduce wrongly that the pulse is very weak and almost non-existent.

Xie Fei Mai

In a few individuals, the pulse runs from the Rear position obliquely towards the Front position. This pulse was called *Xie Fei Mai*, which means Oblique-Flying Pulse. Like the Fan Guan Mai, it is due to an irregularity of the radial artery which makes it difficult to read and interpret the pulse properly.

Box 49.6 summarizes the factors affecting the pulse.

BOX 49.6 FACTORS AFFECTING THE PULSE

- Season
- Gender
- Age
- Body build
- Menstruation
- Pregnancy
- *Fan Guan Mai* and *Xie Fei Mai*

ATTRIBUTES OF THE NORMAL PULSE

The normal pulse has three attributes: 'spirit', 'Stomach-Qi' and 'root'.

Spirit

The Chinese word used here is *shen*, which is of course used very frequently in the context of diagnosis to indicate a favourable condition, a good prognosis. The word *shen* is used in the context of tongue diagnosis, facial and eye diagnosis. In the context of pulse diagnosis, a pulse has 'spirit' when it is soft and gentle but with strength. It also has 'spirit' when it is regular in rate and 'orderly' in quality. A pulse without 'spirit' is too hard, not soft, not gentle, perhaps irregular and maybe also changing quality frequently.

Stomach-Qi

The pulse has Stomach-Qi when it is relatively slow (Slowed-down, i.e. four beats per breathing cycle), gentle, calm and relatively soft.

We feel the pulse on the radial artery along the Lung channel to gauge the state of Qi and Blood of all the organs; however, the Qi of the organs cannot reach the Lung channel without the force of Stomach-Qi. As a Chinese textbook says, '*The food essences enter the Stomach, Food-Qi goes to the Heart and the excess enters the blood vessels. The Qi of the blood vessels flows in the twelve channels which are all under the control of the Lungs.*'[29] This means that Lung-Qi reflects the Qi of all the channels and blood vessels and for this reason we can feel the pulse on the radial artery along the Lung channel, but Lung-Qi relies on the motive force and nourishment of Stomach-Qi to reach the channels and blood vessels.

The Stomach has an important influence on the pulse as it is from the Stomach that the motive force for the beating of the Heart comes. Also, the beating of the left ventricle that can be felt below and to the left of the left nipple is, in Chinese medicine, the beating of *Xu Li*, that is, the Great Connecting channel of the Stomach. The Stomach is the Source of Post-Heaven Qi, the Sea of Food, the source of Postnatal Qi and Blood and it therefore gives 'body' to the pulse; for this reason, a pulse that is not soft, too hard, not gentle and not Slowed-down means that it has no Stomach-Qi.

It is important not to confuse the quality of having 'Stomach-Qi' with the actual Stomach pulse as the former applies to all pulse positions. Moreover, it is important to stress that 'not having Stomach-Qi' does not necessarily imply a deficiency: 'not having Stomach-Qi' can apply both to Deficient- and to Full-type pulses. Thus, for example, a Wiry pulse by definition lacks Stomach-Qi because it is too hard; conversely, a Soggy pulse also lacks Stomach-Qi because it is too soft.

> **!**
>
> Remember: a pulse may lack 'Stomach-Qi' by being too soft (Empty) or too hard (Full).

Root

The normal pulse should have a 'root'; this has two meanings. First, it means that the pulse on the Kidney position should be normal; secondly, the pulse at the deep level (corresponding to Liver and Kidneys in Li Shi Zhen's configuration described above) should be normal. Thus, a pulse 'without root' is either very weak on the Kidney positions or very empty at the deep level.

In a few cases, however, obstruction of the Lower Burner or the Uterus by Cold may cause the Kidney pulse to be very weak or almost imperceptible. This is due to Cold obstructing the Lower Burner and preventing the blood coming through to the Rear position of the pulse; it would be wrong to interpret this pulse as having 'no root' because, once Cold is removed, the Kidney pulse returns to normal. Thus, if the Kidney pulse is very weak, one should always bear in mind the possibility that this might be due to obstruction of the Lower Burner by Cold and check the symptoms and signs to exclude this.

To summarize, the normal pulse has 'spirit', which indicates good Heart-Qi, Stomach-Qi, which indicates good Stomach-Qi, and a root, which indicates good Kidney-Qi; these three aspects correspond to the Three Treasures: Spirit, Qi and Essence (*Jing–Qi–Shen*) (Table 49.5).

Table 49.5 Normal pulse attributes

Normal pulse attributes	Organ	Vital substance
Spirit	Heart	Spirit (*Shen*)
Stomach-Qi	Stomach	Qi
Root	Kidneys	Essence (*Jing*)

I would add that the normal pulse also has a fourth quality and that is a 'wave'. This is a clear, smooth, wave-like movement from the Rear towards the Front position; such a pulse indicates good Stomach- and Heart-Qi. The pulse 'without wave' lacks the smooth, wave-like flow and may be pathological either because it has no wave or because its wave movement is excessively long. Many pulse qualities actually depict a pulse without wave (e.g. Short, Choppy, Scattered, Weak, Soggy), whereas others depict a pulse with an excessive wave (e.g. Wiry, Long, Overflowing, Big). The pulse lacking a wave often reflects the presence of emotional problems due to sadness and grief, while the pulse with an excessive wave often reflects emotional problems due to anger.

Passages from both the 'Pulse Classic' and the 'Classic of Difficulties' seem to describe the attribute of a normal pulse with wave even though they do not mention this word. For example, the 'Pulse Classic' says:

The position behind the Inch and in front of the Foot position is the Gate position; this is the boundary between the emerging Yang [at the Inch position] and submerging Yin [at the Foot position]. Emerging Yang occupies three divi-

(a)

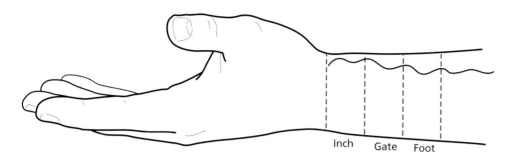

Inch   Gate   Foot

(b)

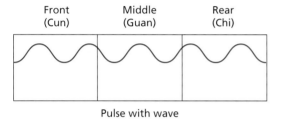

Front   Middle   Rear
(Cun)   (Guan)   (Chi)

Pulse with wave

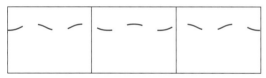

Pulse without wave

Fig. 49.14 Wave-like flow of Qi in the pulse

sions [positions] and submerging Yin also occupies three divisions [positions]. Yang originates at the Foot position and moves [or manifests] towards the Inch position; Yin originates in the Inch position and moves [or manifests] towards the Foot position.[30]

This passage clearly implies the notion of a wave of Qi, in its Yin and Yang qualities, moving in the pulse from the Inch to the Rear and from the Rear to the Inch position (Fig. 49.14).

The 'Classic of Difficulties' in Chapter 3 has a similar concept in a passage that describes the pulse lacking a wave (Fig. 49.14b) or having an excessive wave:

In front of the Gate position, Yang moves and the pulse should extend in 9 fen and be near the surface; if it exceeds 9 fen, it is in excess and if it is shorter than 9 fen, it is deficient . . . Behind the Gate position, Yin moves and the pulse should extend to 1 cun and be at the deep level. If it exceeds 1 cun, it is in excess, while if it is less than 1 cun, it is deficient.[31]

This passage essentially describes Long and Short pulse qualities and a pulse having an excessive wave or lacking one respectively.

Box 49.7 summarizes the attributes of a normal pulse.

GUIDELINES FOR INTERPRETING THE PULSE

When taking the pulse, I recommend assessing the aspects in the following order.

1. Feel the pulse as a whole with three fingers to get an initial idea of its overall strength or weakness.
2. Feel whether the pulse has spirit, Stomach-Qi and root.
3. Feel the three positions first with three fingers and then individually by gently lifting two of the fingers and feeling with the third.
4. Feel the three levels by constantly lifting and pressing the fingers, searching for them.
5. Feel the overall quality of the pulse, if there is one.
6. Feel the pulse quality, strength and level of each individual pulse position by rolling and pushing the fingers as described above.
7. Count the pulse rate.

It is a good idea to train oneself to assess the above aspects of the pulse in a rational order; for example, when taking the pulse one should never immediately concentrate on a particular quality of a specific organ position without first assessing the pulse as a whole. Each of the above aspects of pulse taking has its own clinical significance.

Feeling the pulse as a whole with three fingers

Feeling the pulse as a whole with three fingers gives us an initial idea of the overall strength or weakness of the pulse; this gives us an initial assessment of the patient's constitution and the strength of his or her body's Qi. It also enables us to appraise whether the pulse matches the person's body build.

Feeling the spirit, Stomach-Qi and root

Feeling the spirit, Stomach-Qi and root of the pulse gives us an idea of the state of the Mind, Stomach-Qi and Kidneys. Stomach-Qi is particularly important as it gives us an immediate idea of whether the pulse is normal or not: any pulse that is either too soft or too hard and full immediately tells us that Stomach-Qi is lacking.

Feeling the three positions together first and then individually

Feeling the three positions together first is important to give us an idea of the overall strength or weakness of the pulse and also to compare the relative strengths of the left and right pulses. After feeling the three positions together with the three fingers, we should feel each position individually, gently lifting two of the fingers and feeling with the third. At this stage, this is done not so much to feel the state of the Internal Organs related to each position but more to get an idea of the distribution and balance of Qi among the three positions and therefore the Three Burners.

It is important to remember that the feeling of strength or weakness in the three pulse positions reflects the state and distribution of Qi in the Three Burners, irrespective of the individual organs; in other words, we can get a good idea of the strength or weakness of Qi and its 'rebelliousness' (flowing in the wrong direction) by carefully feeling and assessing the flow of Qi in the three pulse positions initially ignoring the organs associated with those positions. To put it differently, we must remember that the three pulse positions reflect parts of the body as well as organs. The 'Simple Questions' confirms this in Chapter 17 when it says: *'When the upper [position] of the pulse is strong [it means that] Qi is rushing upwards; when the lower [position] of the pulse is strong [it means that] Qi is distended [below].'*[32]

At this stage, we can get an initial idea of the relative strength of Qi and Blood in the Three Burners. For example, if the pulse is very weak on both Rear positions and relatively overflowing on both Front positions, this may indicate that Qi is rebelling upwards and that this upward rebellion is most probably due to a deficiency of Qi and Blood in the Lower Burner so that Qi is not 'anchored' in the Lower Burner and rebels upwards towards the Upper Burner.

Feeling the three levels

One feels the three levels by constantly lifting and pressing down the fingers to 'search' for them. It is a good idea to search for the middle level in two different ways: first by gently pressing down from the superficial level, and then by pressing all the way down to the deep level and slowly lifting the fingers to stop at the middle level.

Feeling the three levels is essential to give us an idea of the state of Qi/Yang, Blood and Yin and also of the level of Qi in the body. For example, if the pulse is Floating-Empty, this means two things: first, that Qi is weak at the deep level and in relative excess at the superficial level; secondly, that there is a Yin deficiency with a relative Yang excess. These are not two different phenomena but simply two different ways of interpreting the same clinical situation and expressing its pathology.

Integrating the three positions (corresponding to the Three Burners) with the three levels, we form a three-dimensional picture of the Qi in the body in a similar way that Western medicine does with CT (computerized tomography), MRI (magnetic resonance imaging) and PET (positron emission tomography) scans (Fig. 49.15). This picture is clinically relevant even without referring to the correspondence of positions to organs at all. The relative strength of Qi in each Burner and at each level is clinically significant even without referring to the organs at all and it is actually a good exercise when reading the pulse not to get too 'fixated' on the assignment of each position to a particular organ. In other words, an assessment of Qi in the three positions and three levels gives us a dynamic picture of the distribution and balance of Qi in the body which is necessary *before* we analyse each position in its relation to a particular organ.

Figure 49.16 shows how the pulse reflects the energy in the Three Burners, at the three levels and on the left and right sides.

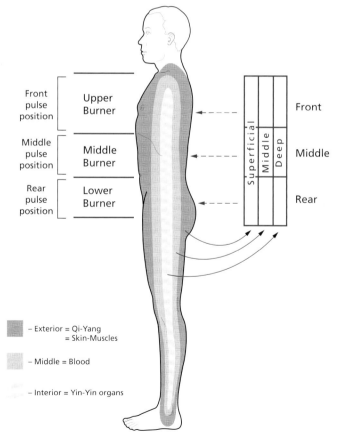

Front pulse position — Upper Burner

Middle pulse position — Middle Burner

Rear pulse position — Lower Burner

Superficial — Middle — Deep

Front

Middle

Rear

– Exterior = Qi-Yang
= Skin-Muscles

– Middle = Blood

– Interior = Yin-Yin organs

Fig. 49.15 Relationship between the three positions and Three Burners and between the three levels and the three energetic layers

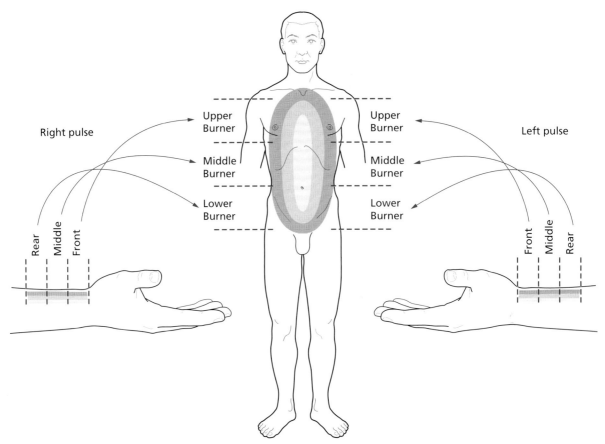

Fig. 49.16 Relationship between the three positions and Three Burners, between the three levels and the three energetic layers and between the left and right pulse and the left and right side

Feeling the overall quality of the pulse, if there is one

The next step is to try to feel if the pulse has an overall quality, remembering that a pulse's 'quality' can be felt only by 'rolling' and 'pushing' the fingers as described above. The pulse does not always have an overall quality; for example, it may be slightly Overflowing in the Heart position but very Weak in the Spleen/Stomach position. In contrast, a pulse may feel very clearly and very definitely Wiry in all positions, giving a strong indication of a Liver disharmony (or Phlegm).

If a pulse has a clear, overall quality, this generally means that the disharmony of the patient is fairly simple; for example, if all the pulse positions are Wiry, this indicates a Liver disharmony (or Phlegm) and no other disharmonies. In contrast, if a pulse has several different qualities in different positions, this indicates that the patient suffers from a complex disharmony characterized by both Deficiency and Excess conditions in various organs.

Feeling the pulse quality, strength and level of each individual position by rolling and pushing the fingers

The next step consists in feeling the pulse quality, strength and level of each individual position by gently lifting two fingers while the third concentrates on a particular position. It is important to note that to assess each individual position the finger is constantly moving, searching, exploring the shape and level of pulse; this is done by 'rolling' the finger distally and medially, 'pushing' the finger medially and laterally, and 'lifting and pressing' the finger to feel the level of the pulse. Rolling tells us whether the pulse in that position is Short, Long, Choppy, Moving or without

wave; pushing tells us whether the pulse in that position is Choppy, Slippery, Wiry, Weak, Scattered, Big, Overflowing, Fine, Minute, etc.; lifting and pressing tells us whether the pulse in that position is Floating, Deep, Weak, Soggy, Floating-Empty, Hidden, Leathery, or Firm.

Counting the pulse rate

Finally, counting of the pulse rate is carried out. As mentioned above, in past times this was done by referring the pulse rate to the breathing rate of the practitioners. Nowadays, we simply count the pulse rate with a watch. This is of course crucial to diagnosing pulse qualities that reflect irregularities of the pulse rate and rhythm (e.g. Slow, Rapid, Slowed-Down, Hurried, Moving, Knotted, Hasty, Intermittent).

CLINICAL APPLICATION OF PULSE DIAGNOSIS

Pulse diagnosis is an essential part of Chinese diagnosis for many reasons. Two aspects could be singled out as being the most important features of pulse diagnosis: first, apart from giving us indications about prevailing disharmonies, it also reflects the constitution of a person; secondly, when expertly applied, pulse diagnosis can give us a very detailed and accurate picture of the state of Qi in all organs and all parts of the body.

The following are some examples of the clinical application of pulse diagnosis.

The pulse is often crucial in clinching a diagnosis

The pulse is often crucial in clinching a diagnosis. A common example of the value of the pulse in clinching the diagnosis is when a person (usually a man) presents complaining of tiredness, sluggishness and general listlessness. He may speak with a low voice and the general first impression would be that a Deficiency is the cause of the problem. However, if the pulse is Wiry on both sides (as often happens in such patients), this clearly points to Liver-Qi stagnation as the cause of the problem; in such a case, the pulse is often the only symptom pointing to a Full condition, and specifically Liver-Qi stagnation, as the cause of the problem.

Case history 49.1 is an illustration of the value of the pulse in clinching a diagnosis.

The pulse is essential to distinguish Deficiency from Excess

Distinguishing Deficiency from Excess is one of the most useful aspects of pulse diagnosis. In many cases, the patient presents with a mixture of Deficiency and Excess; indeed, this, rather than a pure Deficiency or pure Excess condition, is probably the most common situation in practice.

Postviral fatigue syndrome is a good example of this situation: practically all patients suffering from this condition suffer from retention of Dampness together with a deficiency of the Spleen, Stomach, Lungs or Kidneys, or a mixture of these. However, the

Case history 49.1

A 65-year-old woman complained of an acute pain in the ribs on the left-hand side. She had seen her doctor and an orthopaedic surgeon who had ordered X-rays, which showed no abnormality. Both the doctor and the surgeon treated this as a musculoskeletal problem.

When asking her about her symptom I was also somewhat puzzled as she had no symptoms of a Liver or Gall-Bladder pattern that might explain the rib pain. I was also puzzled as to why, if this was indeed a musculoskeletal problem, it should start suddenly without a fall or any other apparent cause. However,

her pulse told a completely different story: it was very Rapid (over 100), Overflowing and Slippery. In particular, the right Front position (Lung position) was very Overflowing. This pulse clearly indicated that, far from being a simple musculoskeletal problem, she had a serious internal organ problem and, although one cannot conclusively diagnose cancer, I suspected there was a serious disease in the left lung causing the rib pain. I thought this would be either pleurisy or a carcinoma.

I insisted that she went back to the doctor for further tests. An MRI scan and blood tests showed that she had carcinoma of the left lung and spine.

combination of a Deficient and an Excess condition is never 50–50: one aspect is always predominant and it is often not easy to determine this from the symptoms and signs. For example, a patient suffering from postviral fatigue syndrome will experience extreme fatigue and poor appetite (symptoms of Deficiency) but also muscle aches and a feeling of heaviness (symptoms of Fullness, in this case Dampness). In such a situation, the pulse is absolutely crucial in clinching whether the Deficiency or the Excess predominates: if the pulse is on the whole weak, this means that the Deficiency predominates; if the pulse is on the whole of the full type, this means that the Excess predominates. Thus, in this case, the pulse is the single most important aspect of diagnosis to make this differentiation.

The important implication of this is that the pulse therefore determines the choice of treatment principle: if it is weak on the whole, we should concentrate on tonifying the Upright Qi; if it is of the full type on the whole, we should concentrate on expelling pathogenic factors (in this case, resolve Dampness).

The pulse is essential to determine the treatment principle

The pulse is essential to determine the treatment principle in complex conditions of mixed Deficiency and Excess. The example of postviral fatigue syndrome was given above. Another example could be a situation of Liver-Blood deficiency leading to Liver-Yang rising; this situation is very common in women and it is often the cause of menstrual problems such as premenstrual tension or menstrual headaches. The symptoms themselves may not help us to determine whether the deficiency of Liver-Blood or the rising of Liver-Yang predominates. The pulse can help us to differentiate this very clearly: if it is Choppy or Fine, the deficiency of Liver-Blood predominates and we should therefore nourish Blood; if it is Wiry, the rising of Liver-Yang predominates and we should therefore subdue Liver-Yang.

The pulse in emotional problems

In many situations, the pulse reflects emotional problems clearly. A few examples will be given here.

When a person is affected by sadness, grief or worry, the Heart pulse may become slightly and relatively Overflowing; it is important to note that this is not the true Overflowing pulse, but it is nevertheless slightly Overflowing *in relation to* the other positions. Often the pulse may be quite Weak or Choppy on the whole, but a careful feeling of the Heart position reveals that it is very slightly Overflowing compared with the rest of the pulse. This Heart-pulse quality is quite subtle and may be easily missed; besides being more superficial compared with the other pulse positions, the Heart pulse also feels somewhat 'round' and very slightly Slippery. This is a sure sign that the patient is deeply affected by emotional problems such as sorrow, sadness or grief affecting the Heart. When all the other pulses are weak but the Heart pulse is relatively Overflowing as described, this usually indicates that the person is suffering from sadness and bears the emotional strain in silence.

Another good example of a clear reflection of emotional stress by the pulse is the situation when a patient may appear very depressed, walk slowly and talk with a low voice – all of which lead us to assume that he or she suffers from a Deficiency; however, very often (and more commonly in men), the pulse of these people is extremely Wiry and Full in all positions. This is an absolutely reliable indication that that person is not really depressed but angry, or, to put it differently, may be depressed because of repressed anger.

A Rapid pulse is another indication of emotional stress. Usually the person is under great stress and suffers from fear, anxiety, guilt or the consequence of shock. Case history 49.2 is an illustration of this point.

Case history 49.2

A 28-year-old woman complained of tiredness, nausea and dizziness. She had no other symptoms and she seemed quite healthy. Emotionally she appeared to be quite happy and she spoke with a cheerful, ringing voice, smiling frequently. All the indications were, therefore, that she suffered from a simple deficiency of the Spleen and possibly Blood as many women do. However, the pulse showed a completely different picture: it was Fine and very Rapid (over 100). Her tongue had a red tip. I had the feeling that she had long-standing, repressed emotional problems and I suspected shock was the main cause of them. When I asked her whether she had suffered a shock some years before she burst into tears and said that she had been sexually abused from the age of 6 to 9.

Of course, we should exclude other causes of a Rapid pulse such as an infection, a true Heat pattern or Blood Heat. In the absence of clear Heat symptoms and signs, a Rapid pulse usually indicates the above-mentioned emotional problems.

A pulse without wave indicates that the person suffers from sadness or grief, which may also be indicated by a very Weak Lung pulse. A Full Lung pulse may indicate that the person suffers either from worry or from unexpressed grief. If both Front positions (Lungs and Heart) are Weak and Short, they indicate long-standing emotional problems deriving from sadness or grief. A Moving pulse often indicates shock; it should be noted that the pulse may retain this quality many years after the original shock.

Box 49.8 summarizes the pulse qualities in emotional problems.

BOX 49.8 THE PULSE IN EMOTIONAL PROBLEMS

- Heart pulse slightly Overflowing: sadness, grief or worry
- All pulses Wiry and Full: repressed anger or frustration
- Rapid pulse: fear, guilt or shock
- Pulse without a wave: sadness or grief
- Weak Lung pulse: sadness or grief
- Full Lung pulse: worry or unexpressed grief
- Both Front positions Weak and Short: long-standing sadness or grief
- Moving pulse: shock

The pulse as an indicator of an organ problem

When all the pulse positions are very weak and deep except for one, this usually indicates that the organ corresponding to that position is 'diseased'. This often points to an actual organic disease in a Western medical sense (rather than a Chinese pattern of disharmony), but it is by no means an absolute rule. For example, if the pulse is Weak, Choppy and Deep in all positions except in the Heart position, this may simply indicate deep emotional problems as described above, but it may also indicate an actual heart problem; the latter is all the more likely if the Heart pulse feels Slippery and Fine, and particularly if Slippery in its medial and lateral sides.

A Floating quality on the Heart pulse also often indicates a problem with the heart itself, especially if it is Floating-Hollow on the lateral and medial sides of the pulse position (which may indicate high blood pressure). A Floating-Weak-Hollow quality indicates that the heart is dilated; this occurs often in people who jog for long distances every day. A Floating-Tight-Hollow quality may indicate hardening of the arteries.

The pulse as an indicator of a heart problem

Just as Heart-Qi is reflected on the pulse as a whole, irrespective of positions, the condition of the heart (in the Western sense) is also reflected on the whole pulse, not only at the left Front position. We should always remember that when we feel the pulse we feel the radial artery, which is a blood vessel, and that the Heart governs all blood vessels; thus, by definition, the general feeling of the radial artery reflects the condition of the Heart in a Chinese sense and also of the heart in a Western medical sense.

For example, when the whole pulse is Wiry, Slippery, Overflowing and Hurried and feels very hard, aortic aneurysm may be suspected.

If the pulse is Hurried (i.e. very rapid and agitated) and generally Full, this often indicates a heart problem such as tachycardia (in all its various types, e.g. supraventricular tachycardia, junctional tachycardia or broad-complex tachycardia). Similarly, any irregu-

larity of the pulse (Knotted, Hasty, Intermittent) may indicate a heart conduction problem such as atrial fibrillation (when it is rapid and irregular, i.e. Hasty), sick sinus syndrome, Wolff–Parkinson–White (WPW) syndrome or Lown–Ganong–Levine (LGL) syndrome.

If the pulse is extremely Slow, this may also indicate a heart problem such as sick sinus syndrome or atrioventricular block (unless, of course, it is due to intense, regular exercise such as in athletes).

If the pulse is Minute or Scattered, this may indicate the possibility of heart failure. The medial and lateral aspects of the Heart pulse may reflect problems of the valves such as mitral stenosis, mitral regurgitation or mitral prolapse; in such cases, these aspects of the Heart pulse (felt by rolling the finger medially and laterally very slightly) feel Slippery or Tight. (See Fig. 50.2 on p. 500.)

> **!**
>
> Remember: the pulse as a whole may reflect a heart pathology.

Case histories 49.3–49.5 illustrate the use of the pulse in diagnosing heart conditions.

Case history 49.3

A 45-year-old woman complained of extreme tiredness, something she had been suffering from for over 20 years. She also complained of poor memory, floaters, tinnitus, frequent urination and occasional dribbling of urine. She also suffered from constipation and her periods had stopped 6 months previously.

As a child, she had suffered from frequent bouts of bronchitis and pneumonia. She had received acupuncture treatment for 5 years and Chinese herbs for about 2; these treatments did produce some improvement but it never lasted.

Her tongue was slightly Red on the sides and Swollen and her pulse was Deep, very Weak, Choppy, Fine and Slow (52).

Three main patterns emerge from an analysis of the clinical manifestations: Liver-Blood deficiency (stoppage of the periods, floaters, tiredness, Choppy pulse), Kidney-Yang deficiency (tinnitus, frequent urination, dribbling of urine, tiredness, constipation, Deep-Weak-Slow pulse), and Heart-Blood deficiency (poor memory, Choppy pulse). However, the fact that the pulse is very Weak, Choppy and Fine in *all* positions and also that it is very Slow clearly indicates that the main problem probably lies in the Heart, and specifically a severe deficiency of Qi and Blood of the Heart. This deficiency may be congenital or may have been induced by the frequent bouts of bronchitis and pneumonia during her childhood. I advised this patient to have her heart examined by a cardiologist; she did this and the cardiologist did say that the pericardium membrane was enlarged and showed signs of inflammation.

The principle of treatment in this case, therefore, should be not only to nourish Liver-Blood and tonify Kidney-Yang, but also to tonify the Qi and Blood of the Heart.

Case history 49.4

A 60-year-old man sought treatment for a frozen shoulder. On taking his pulse, I noticed that it was very Full, Slippery, Wiry, very Overflowing and Rapid. The combination of these qualities to such a degree clearly indicated not only a Heart disharmony but also the possibility of a problem in the heart or blood vessels; however, he had no symptoms of heart problems (no hypertension, no chest pain, no arrhythmia). Although he came to me for treatment of his shoulder problem, I tried to encourage him to see a cardiologist, which he did and he was found to have an aneurysm of the aorta for which he needed an operation.

Case history 49.5

A 25-year-old woman complained of painful periods with clear symptoms of Cold in the Uterus (spastic pain, feeling cold during the period, menstrual blood with small dark clots, Pale tongue, Slow pulse). However, a striking feature of her pulse (for her age) was its Slowness (48) and its stopping at irregular intervals: such pulse quality (Slow and stopping at irregular intervals) is called Knotted. This indicated the possibility, not only of a Heart disharmony, but of an actual heart problem and she was advised to see a cardiologist who indeed diagnosed a conduction problem in the heart.

The pulse does not necessarily reflect all the aspects of a disharmony

As for the tongue, we should not expect the pulse to reflect *all* the aspects of a disharmony. For example, if a woman suffers from Liver-Qi stagnation causing very clear symptoms of premenstrual tension with distension of the breasts and abdomen and irritability, the pulse may not be Wiry if the Liver-Qi stagnation occurs against a background of Liver-Blood deficiency; in such a case, the pulse may be Weak and Choppy reflecting the Liver-Blood deficiency but not the Liver-Qi stagnation. The opposite may also occur: in the above example, the pulse may be Wiry if the Liver-Qi stagnation is intense, in which case the pulse quality reflects only this pattern and not the Liver-Blood deficiency.

In the elderly, the pulse is frequently of the full type, often being Wiry or Slippery, or both; this happens because old people suffer frequently from chronic Phlegm, Blood stasis or internal Wind, all of which may make the pulse Wiry and hard. However, very many old people suffering from such patterns also frequently suffer from Yin deficiency (which may be apparent from a lack of tongue coating); the Wiry and Full quality of the pulse masks the Yin deficiency, which does not show on the pulse.

The pulse indicates disharmonies beyond the presenting patterns

When the pulse indicates disharmonies beyond the presenting patterns it raises the important issue of integration of pulse diagnosis with symptom diagnosis. In the majority of cases, the pulse and clinical manifestations accord with each other; for example, if a patient displays all the symptoms of Phlegm, the pulse is most likely Slippery. In other cases, as mentioned above, the pulse reflects only one aspect of a disharmony. There are cases, however, when the pulse seems to be at variance with the clinical manifestations, or at least unrelated to them. The tendency in modern China (according to my experience) is to give more importance to the clinical manifestations; if the pulse does not accord with them it is simply ignored. I personally disagree with this approach as I think that the pulse is always clinically significant and should never be discarded as a diagnostic sign.

Many examples could be given of situations when the pulse seems to be unrelated to the clinical manifestations (not necessarily contradicting them); for example, the patient has symptoms of Phlegm but the pulse is not Slippery, the patient has *no* symptoms of Phlegm but the pulse is Slippery, the patient appears to be an exuberant, Yang type of person but the pulse is very Weak and Deep; the patient has no symptoms of any Liver disharmony but the pulse is Wiry (or vice versa), etc.

In such cases, apart from the above-mentioned situation when the pulse reflects one aspect of a disharmony and the clinical manifestations another, a pulse that is seemingly unrelated to the presenting clinical manifestations simply reflects the existence of a disharmony that has not *yet* caused symptoms.

A common example relates to the Lung pulse: a woman may present with clinical manifestations of Liver-Qi stagnation causing premenstrual tension or other menstrual irregularities and the pulse is slightly Wiry but the position that most stands out is that of the Lung being extremely Weak and Deep. What are we to make of this? Since all the clinical manifestations and the Wiry pulse point to a Liver disharmony shall we ignore the Lung position? In my opinion, this should never be done. In this example, the weakness of the Lung position simply indicates that this patient suffers from Lung-Qi deficiency without symptoms of it *yet*; the weakness of the Lung position should never be ignored also because, after all, a Weak Lung pulse is reflective of Lung-Qi deficiency as much as a weak voice and chronic cough. In such a case, I would definitely pay attention to the weakness of the Lung pulse and tonify the Lungs (in addition to treating the Liver disharmony).

To give another example relating to a full rather than empty-type of pulse, it happens frequently that a person has no symptoms of Phlegm but the pulse is clearly Slippery; barring the cases when a Slippery pulse may indicate health (or of course pregnancy), this definitely indicates that the patient is suffering from Phlegm even though there are no manifestations of it.

Incidentally, this characteristic applies to tongue diagnosis too: the tongue also can show disharmonies beyond the presenting manifestations. A good example is a central Stomach crack on the tongue indicating a tendency to Stomach-Yin deficiency even in the absence of any digestive symptoms.

The pulse can indicate an underlying Deficiency in the absence of symptoms

When the pulse is Weak in a certain position, it definitely indicates Deficiency of that particular organ whether there are symptoms of Deficiency or not. It is

precisely for this reason that pulse diagnosis allows us to give preventive treatment before the onset of clinical manifestations.

A weakness of the Kidney pulse (often on both sides) is the most common example of this situation. There are very many patients (especially women) who have a very Weak pulse on both Rear positions without any symptoms of Kidney deficiency; however, as mentioned above, a Weak and Deep pulse on both Rear positions reflects a Kidney deficiency as much as tiredness, backache, dizziness and tinnitus do. Indeed, this is precisely one reason why pulse diagnosis is so important: it points to a certain disharmony unequivocally, which is more than isolated symptoms do. In the example just mentioned above, if the patient suffered only from dizziness we could not diagnose a Kidney deficiency because this symptom may be due to many other disharmonies (Blood deficiency, Phlegm, Liver-Yang rising, etc.), but the weakness of the pulse on both Rear positions points unequivocally to a Kidney deficiency.

The pulse in cancer

There is no specific pulse quality or pulse picture that allows us to diagnose cancer unequivocally. Generally speaking, in advanced cancer two opposite pulse pictures may emerge: either the pulse becomes extremely Weak, Choppy, Fine and Deep or it becomes Full, Slippery, Overflowing and Rapid.

Although the pulse cannot be used to diagnose cancer, it is very important to determine the prognosis and the treatment principle.

As for *prognosis*, if a patient has cancer the prognosis is poor if the pulse has either of the pictures described above (i.e. it is either very Deep, Weak, Choppy and Fine, or very Full, Slippery, Overflowing and Rapid). If the pulse in addition is particularly Rapid and Overflowing this may indicate the presence of Toxic Heat, which is never a good sign in cancer or in cancer patients who have undergone Western treatment.

As for the *treatment principle*, the pulse is very important indeed. Generally speaking, cancer patients will undergo some treatment in the form of surgery, radiotherapy or chemotherapy, or a combination of these. At the end of these treatments, our role is to stimulate the immune system to prevent a recurrence. From the point of view of Chinese medicine, we have to assess the condition of the patient as if the cancer were still present. In fact, Western treatments may remove the cancer surgically, by radiotherapy or chemotherapy,

but they do not remove the patterns that were at the root of the cancer; the most common patterns seen are Phlegm, Blood stasis, Toxic Heat and Dampness.

We should therefore assess the patient's condition very carefully to determine whether Deficiency or Excess predominates, that is, whether the above pathogenic factors are relatively weak and the main problem is a deficiency of the Upright Qi or whether the above pathogenic factors are still quite strong. In the former case, the aim is to tonify the Upright Qi primarily and expel pathogenic factors secondarily; in the latter case the aim is to expel pathogenic factors primarily and tonify the Upright Qi secondarily. The pulse is crucial in making this distinction and choosing the appropriate treatment principle: if the pulse is primarily Weak, Fine, Choppy or Empty, we need to concentrate our attention on tonifying the Upright Qi; if the pulse is of the full type, Slippery, Wiry, Tight or Firm, we need to concentrate on expelling pathogenic factors (which may be to resolve Phlegm, invigorate Blood, resolve Dampness or clear Toxic Heat).

> **!**
>
> In cancer patients after surgery, the pulse is crucial in determining whether there is still an active pathogenic factor and therefore in determining the treatment principle.

For example, let us assume that a woman suffering from a malignant breast tumour comes to us after undergoing a lumpectomy and ensuing radiotherapy. We should assess her condition carefully as if she still had the tumour because the surgery and radiotherapy have removed the tumour but not the pattern at the root of its formation. The patterns appearing in breast cancer are usually Phlegm or Blood stasis, or both, in differing combinations; of course, there is often also Qi stagnation but this cannot cause a tumour by itself, whereas Phlegm and Blood stasis can.

When presented with such patients we should therefore not assume in all cases that we must tonify the Upright Qi to prevent a recurrence: we must choose the treatment principle according to the clinical manifestations bearing in mind that we cannot rely on an examination of the tumour as this has been removed. In the presence of a tumour we would palpate it to decide whether it is caused by Phlegm (in which case it is relatively soft and painless) or by Blood stasis (in which case it is hard and probably painful). A decision on the choice of treatment principles relies a lot on the pulse: if this is of the empty type, we should concentrate our attention on

tonifying the Upright Qi; if it is of the full type (Slippery, Wiry, Tight) we should concentrate on expelling pathogenic factors (resolve Phlegm or invigorate Blood, or both). If the pulse in addition is also Rapid and Overflowing this may indicate the presence of Toxic Heat and we need to clear Heat and resolve Toxin (in herbal medicine this is done by using herbs from the category which clear Toxic Heat, many of which have also an anticancer effect).

INTEGRATION OF PULSE AND TONGUE DIAGNOSIS

There are many ways in which the integration of pulse and tongue diagnosis is crucial in clinical practice.

Qi and Blood

The pulse and tongue are quite complementary in so far as the pulse reflects more the state of Qi while the tongue that of Blood; of course this is a generalization (because the pulse can reflect the state of Blood, e.g. when it is Choppy), but it is a useful one nevertheless.

This distinction can be useful in patients suffering from emotional problems. For example, a Wiry and Full pulse often indicates a Liver pattern deriving from emotional stress and if the tongue-body colour is normal this tells us that the emotional problem is not long standing; if the tongue is Red this indicates that the emotional problem is more long standing and more severe.

Time factor

The pulse is more influenced by short-term factors than is the tongue. For example, a period of overwork, an emotional upset and physical exercise can all change the pulse in the short term but not the tongue.

For this reason, the tongue is a good indicator of the length of a problem; for example, an Overflowing Heart pulse indicates that the person is under emotional stress and if the tongue is Red with a redder tip this indicates that this problem is long standing.

Another example is that of Blood stasis. A Choppy or Firm pulse may point to Blood stasis and if the tongue is Purple this indicates that the problem is of long duration. Another good example is that of Yin deficiency. A Floating-Empty pulse indicates Yin deficiency and we can tell exactly the stage of Yin deficiency by observing the degree of absence of coating on the tongue.

When the pulse is Rapid and the tongue is not Red

A Rapid pulse indicates Heat and this should be mirrored by a Red tongue. In practice, quite often the pulse is Rapid but the tongue is not Red.

Shock may be an explanation of this discrepancy because it often makes the pulse Rapid but it does not cause redness of the tongue.

Another explanation of this discrepancy is in cases when a person constantly pushes himself or herself into working too much and too long hours; this causes the heart to become dilated and then the Heart pulse is often Overflowing but Empty and the pulse Rapid.

When the pulse is Slow and the tongue is Red

The most common explanation of this discrepancy is the practice of intense exercise, especially jogging or running; this makes the pulse Slow. Because the Slowness is due to the exercise and not to a true Cold pattern, the tongue is not Pale and may be Red from other reasons.

Another possible explanation of a contradiction between a Slow pulse and a Red tongue (and one that should always be kept in mind) is heart disease. A very Slow pulse may often indicate some irregularities in heart conduction, especially if the pulse is also irregular.

Pulse diagnosis adds detail to tongue diagnosis

The pulse often adds detail to the findings from tongue diagnosis. For example, a sticky yellow coating with red points on the root of the tongue indicates Damp-Heat in the Lower Burner but it does not tell us whether this is in the Bladder, Intestines or Uterus. The pulse would add detail to the information gleaned from the tongue because Damp-Heat in the Bladder would manifest with a Slippery-Wiry quality on the left Rear position, Damp-Heat in the Intestines with the same quality on both Rear positions, while Damp-Heat in the Uterus would manifest with the same quality on the Uterus position just proximal to the left Rear position.

Another field in which the pulse adds detail to the tongue is that of Heart patterns. When the tongue has a deep central crack, this indicates the tendency to Heart patterns from emotional problems. However, it may also indicate the hereditary tendency to actual

heart problems. If the Heart pulse is Full and hard on the lateral and medial positions of the Heart position (rolling the finger laterally and medially very slightly), this indicates the possibility of an actual heart disease.

Another situation in which the pulse adds detail to the findings from the tongue is when the tongue is Purple, indicating Blood stasis. If the whole tongue is Purple, this does not help us to pinpoint the organ affected; the Wiry quality of the pulse in one or other organ position helps us to pinpoint which organ is particularly affected by Blood stasis.

LIMITATIONS OF PULSE DIAGNOSIS

The main drawbacks of pulse diagnosis are its subjectivity and its being readily affected by short-term changes.

It is subjective

More than any other element of Chinese diagnosis, pulse diagnosis is rather subjective, at least compared with other elements of diagnosis such as looking. For example, there can be little disagreement over whether a face is red or a tongue very Red; such signs can also be seen objectively by different observers. If, however, a pulse is described as being Wiry, this is a purely subjective interpretation on the part of the practitioner; it is impossible to 'show' other observers how the pulse is Wiry and, moreover, another practitioner might describe the same pulse as Slippery.

It is subject to short-term influences

The pulse is easily and quickly influenced by short-term factors, at least when compared with the tongue. For example, if a person has a sudden emotional upset, this may make the pulse rapid but it will not change the tongue in the short term. Likewise, the pulse is obviously affected by exercise, becoming rapid, whereas the tongue is not affected by it. If a person works very hard for a week with little sleep the pulse will reflect this, immediately becoming quite weak and deep, but a single week would not bring about a change in the tongue-body colour (though there are some situations, such as in acute febrile diseases, when the tongue-body colour does change rapidly).

For these reasons, the integration of tongue and pulse diagnosis, as discussed above, is absolutely crucial.

NOTES

1. 1979 The Yellow Emperor's Classic of Internal Medicine – Simple Questions (*Huang Di Nei Jing Su Wen* 黄帝内经素问), People's Health Publishing House, Beijing, p. 130. First published c. 100BC.
2. Nanjing College of Traditional Chinese Medicine 1979 A Revised Explanation of the Classic of Difficulties (*Nan Jing Jiao Shi* 难经校释), People's Health Publishing House, Beijing, pp. 1–2. First published c. AD100.
3. Ibid., p. 2.
4. Simple Questions, p. 78.
5. Ibid., p. 139.
6. Classic of Difficulties, pp. 4–5.
7. Fuzhou City People's Hospital 1988 'A Revised Explanation of the Pulse Classic (*Mai Jing Jiao Shi* 脉经校释), People's Health Publishing House, Beijing, p. 7. The 'Pulse Classic' was written by Wang Shu He and was first published in AD280.
8. A Revised Explanation of the Classic of Difficulties, p. 6.
9. Ibid., p. 46.
10. Ibid., pp. 45–46.
11. A Revised Explanation of the Pulse Classic, pp. 18–19.
12. Cheng Bao Shu 1988 An Annotated Translation of the Study of the Pulse from Pin Hu Lake (*Pin Hu Mai Xue Yi Zhu* 濒湖脉学译注) Ancient Chinese Medical Texts Publishing House, Beijing, pp. 3–4. 'The Study of the Pulse from Pin Hu Lake' was first published in 1564.
13. Wu Qian 1977 Golden Mirror of Medicine (*Yi Zong Jin Jian* 医宗金鉴), People's Health Publishing House, Beijing, Vol. 2, p. 909. First published in 1742.
14. Cheng Xin Nong 1987 Chinese Acupuncture and Moxibustion, (*Zhong Guo Zhen Jiu* 中国针灸学), Foreign Languages Press, Beijing, 1987.
15. Bejing/Nanjing/Shanghai College of Chinese Medicine, 'Fundamentals of Chinese Medicine', translated by N. Wiseman and A. Ellis, Paradigm Publications, Brookline, Massachusetts, USA, 1985.
16. A Revised Explanation of the Pulse Classic, p. 15.
17. A Revised Explanation of the Classic of Difficulties, p. 12.
18. Simple Questions, p. 98.
19. Zhang Jing Yue 1982 Classic of Categories (*Lei Jing* 类经), People's Health Publishing Company, Beijing, p. 561. The Classic of Categories was first published in 1624.
20. Ibid., p. 131.
21. Simple Questions, pp. 118–119.
22. Ibid., p. 101.
23. A Revised Explanation of the Pulse Classic, p. 16.
24. An Annotated Translation of the Study of the Pulse from Pin Hu Lake, p. 4.
25. A Revised Explanation of the Classic of Difficulties, p. 50.
26. An Annotated Translation of the Study of the Pulse from Pin Hu Lake, p. 4.
27. Chen Jia Yuan 1988 'Eight Secret Books on Gynaecology' (*Fu Ke Mi Shu Ba Zhong* 妇科秘书八种), Ancient Chinese Medicine Texts Publishing House, Beijing, p. 153. Chen's book, written during the Qing dynasty (1644–1911), was entitled 'Secret Gynaecological Prescriptions' (*Fu Ke Mi Fang* 妇科秘方).
28. Pulse Classic, p. 14.
29. Guang Dong College of Chinese Medicine 1979, 'Diagnosis in Chinese Medicine' (*Zhong Yi Zhen Duan Xue* 中医诊断学), Shanghai Science Publishing House, Shanghai, p. 178.
30. A Revised Explanation of the Pulse Classic, p. 7.
31. A Revised Explanation of the Classic of Difficulties, p. 6.
32. Simple Questions, p. 98.

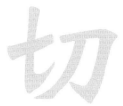

PART 3

Chapter **50**

PULSE QUALITIES

Chapter contents

INTRODUCTION *465*

FEELING AND IDENTIFYING THE PULSE QUALITY *466*

THE EIGHT BASIC PULSE QUALITIES *467*
  Floating *467*
  Deep *469*
  Slow *470*
  Rapid *472*
  Empty *474*
  Full *475*
  Slippery *476*
  Choppy *477*

EMPTY-TYPE PULSES *479*
  Weak *479*
  Fine *480*
  Minute *480*
  Soggy (Weak-Floating) *481*
  Short *481*
  Hollow *482*
  Leather *482*
  Hidden *483*
  Scattered *484*

FULL-TYPE PULSES *485*
  Wiry *485*
  Tight *486*
  Overflowing *487*
  Big *488*
  Firm *489*
  Long *490*
  Moving *490*

PULSES WITH IRREGULARITIES OF RATE OR RHYTHM *491*
  Knotted *491*
  Hasty *492*
  Hurried *492*
  Intermittent *493*
  Slowed-Down *494*

THREE NON-TRADITIONAL PULSE QUALITIES *494*
  Irregular *494*
  Stagnant *495*
  Sad *495*

CLASSIFICATION OF PULSE QUALITIES *496*
  The eight basic groups of pulse qualities *496*
  The different aspects for the classification of pulse
    qualities *497*
  Classification of pulse qualities according to Qi,
    Blood and Body Fluids patterns *497*
  Classification of pulse qualities according to the
    Eight Principles *497*
  Classification of pulse qualities according to the
    Six Stages patterns *498*
  Classification of pulse qualities according to the
    Four Levels patterns *498*
  Classification of pulse qualities according to the
    Triple Burner patterns *498*

TERMINOLOGY *498*

THE PULSE POSITIONS IN DETAIL *499*
  Left Front position (Heart) *500*
  Left Middle position (Liver) *501*
  Left Rear position (Kidney) *502*
  Right Front position (Lungs) *503*
  Right Middle position (Stomach and Spleen) *504*
  Right Rear position (Small Intestine and Kidneys) *506*

PULSE QUALITIES INDICATING DANGEROUS
CONDITIONS *506*

THE INFLUENCE OF DRUGS ON THE PULSE *507*

INTRODUCTION

The pulse 'qualities' described in Chinese books over the centuries have varied but they have been standardized today into 28 or 29 qualities. In theory, there is no

special reason why we should be restricted to using only those terms; for example, there is no 'Hard' pulse quality, but this is a term that often comes to mind when feeling a particular pulse. However, it is important to train oneself to use the set terminology of pulse qualities in order to establish a common ground of communication among practitioners and between teachers and students; for example, a practitioner or student might describe a pulse as 'squidgy' in his or her own terminology (in fact, the term 'squidgy' describes the Soggy pulse quite well) but this would not be much use to other practitioners or students.

It cannot be stressed strongly enough that the pulse qualities, with their description and clinical significance, should be memorized. Only by memorizing the pulse qualities can students then communicate with the clinical teacher; only when both the students and the clinical teacher are clear as to what a Wiry pulse feels like and means, can they communicate with each other, and students correlate the theoretical description of a Wiry pulse with their own feeling of the pulse.

FEELING AND IDENTIFYING THE PULSE QUALITY

It should be stressed that the pulse 'quality' can be felt and identified only if we move the fingers constantly by 'rolling' them distally and proximally, 'pushing' them medially and laterally, and 'pressing' down and releasing upwards as described in the previous chapter. We cannot feel and identify the pulse quality if we keep the fingers absolutely still because the fingers need to feel, probe and explore the shape and size of the pulse and this can be done only by moving the fingers in all four directions around a given pulse position (i.e. distally, proximally, medially and laterally). For example, we can deduce that a pulse is Long or Short only if we gently roll the finger distally; we can deduce that a pulse is Slippery only if we feel 'around' it by moving the fingers medially and laterally; we can deduce that a pulse is Floating-Empty only if we press the fingers down and then release them to explore its depth.

Table 50.1 The 29 pulse qualities

No.	English	Pinyin	Literal translation	Chinese
1	Floating	*Fu*	Floating	浮
2	Deep	*Chen*	Deep (sinking)	沉
3	Slow	*Chi*	Slow, tardy	迟
4	Rapid	*Shu*	Several (in succession)	数
5	Empty	*Xu*	Empty	虚
6	Full	*Shi*	Solid	实
7	Slippery	*Hua*	Slippery	滑
8	Choppy	*Se*	Rough	涩
9	Weak	*Ruo*	Weak, feeble	弱
10	Fine	*Xi*	Thin, slender	细
11	Minute	*Wei*	Minute, tiny	微
12	Soggy	*Ru (Ruan)*	Immerse, moist, (soft)	濡
13	Short	*Duan*	Short	短
14	Hollow	*Kou*	Hollow	芤
15	Leather	*Ge*	Leather	革
16	Hidden	*Fu*	Hide, lie prostrate	伏
17	Scattered	*San*	Break-up, disperse, dispel	散
18	Wiry	*Xian*	Bowstring	弦
19	Tight	*Jin*	Tight, taut	紧
20	Overflowing	*Hong*	Big, vast, flood	洪
21	Big	*Da*	Big	大
22	Firm	*Lao*	Firm, fastened, prison	牢
23	Long	*Chang*	Long	长
24	Moving	*Dong*	To move	动
25	Knotted	*Jie*	Tie, knot, knit	结
26	Hasty	*Cu*	Hurried, urgent, short of time	促
27	Hurried	*Ji*	Fast, rapid, urgent	疾
28	Intermittent	*Dai*	Take the place of	代
29	Slowed-down	*Huan*	Slow, delay, postpone	缓

> **!**
>
> Remember: the pulse qualities cannot be felt by keeping the fingers absolutely still. The fingers must feel all around the pulse position, i.e. distally, proximally, medially, laterally and at different levels.

> **BOX 50.1 THE EIGHT BASIC PULSE QUALITIES**
>
> - Floating = Exterior
> - Deep = Interior
> - Rapid = Heat
> - Slow = Cold
> - Full = Excess
> - Empty = Deficiency
> - Slippery = Phlegm or Dampness
> - Choppy = Blood deficiency

The pulse qualities discussed are as illustrated in Table 50.1. The order in which I have arranged these 29 pulse qualities is different from that traditionally used in Chinese books. The first 8 qualities are the traditional, basic ones, that is, Floating, Deep, Slow, Rapid, Empty, Full, Slippery and Choppy. The other 21 qualities are arranged in three groups:

- from 9 to 17: empty-type qualities
- from 18 to 24: full-type qualities
- from 25 to 29: qualities denoting rate or rhythm of pulse.

In addition to the above 29 traditional qualities, I shall also discuss three new qualities, mostly owed to Dr Shen's experience: Irregular, Stagnant, and Sad.

For each pulse quality, I shall discuss the following:

- pulse description
- clinical significance
- combinations
- differentiation from similar pulses
- clinical significance in each position according to Li Shi Zhen.

I have paired the eight basic qualities (Floating/Deep, Slow/Rapid, Full/Empty and Slippery/Choppy) each with its opposite. These pulse qualities are considered to be the eight basic ones because they correspond closely to the eight principles; that is, Floating and Deep correspond to Exterior and Interior, Slow and Rapid to Cold and Heat, and Full and Empty to Excess and Deficiency. The Slippery and Choppy qualities are added to this group of eight basic qualities because they are extremely common, the former indicating Phlegm or Dampness and the latter Blood deficiency. These two pulse qualities are paired also because to a certain extent they are at different ends of a scale in terms of how they feel under the finger.

Box 50.1 summarizes the eight basic pulse qualities.

THE EIGHT BASIC PULSE QUALITIES

Floating

Pulse description

This pulse is felt on very light pressure; in extreme cases it is felt with no pressure at all. As its name implies, it has a 'floating' quality and it is relatively resistant to pressure. We can think of a large plank of wood in water: we can push it down with some resistance but it comes back up. In other words, there is a difference between a pulse that is felt clearly on the surface (as it should be if Yang-Qi is normal) and a pulse that is Floating: the Floating pulse is more resistant to finger pressure than a pulse that is normal at the superficial level. Especially in summertime, it is normal for the pulse to be relatively more superficial but that does not make it a Floating pulse. Bearing in mind the three levels of the pulse as discussed in the previous chapter, the Floating pulse is felt very clearly (and somewhat excessively) on the superficial level, which corresponds to the Qi and Yang energies.

The traditional description of a Floating pulse was like 'feathers being ruffled by the wind'. The 'Classic of Difficulties' in Chapter 18 says: *'When the pulse is Floating, it is felt moving above the muscle.'*[1]

Clinical significance

Generally speaking, the Floating pulse indicates the presence of a pathogenic factor on the Exterior of the body: it is therefore associated with exterior symptoms caused by invasion of Wind. Indeed, the presence of aversion to cold, fever (or being hot to the touch) and a Floating pulse is enough to diagnose an invasion of an external pathogenic factor. Thus the Floating pulse is one of the main clinical signs of invasion of Wind. In fact, the 'Discussion of Cold-induced Diseases' says: *'A Floating pulse, stiffness and pain of the neck and aversion to cold are signs of the Greater-Yang pattern [invasion of Wind].'*[2]

The reason that the pulse becomes floating in invasions of external pathogenic factors is that when the body is attacked by external evils the Defensive Qi is attracted to the surface of the body and the space between skin and muscles, to fight the external pathogenic factors. Thus, the increased Yang-Qi on the surface of the body is reflected in a more Yang pulse (i.e. Floating). However, if the patient has weak Defensive Qi and does not react well to the invasion of pathogenic factors, the pulse may not be Floating.

The Floating pulse is not found only in exterior conditions but also occurs in interior ones. I shall therefore discuss the clinical significance of the Floating pulse, distinguishing between exterior and interior conditions; this will be done under 'Combinations'.

Under the following conditions, a Floating pulse is normal and does not indicate a pathology:

> • in an underweight person
> • in very hot weather.

Box 50.2 summarizes the clinical significance of a Floating pulse.

BOX 50.2 FLOATING PULSE: SUMMARY OF CLINICAL SIGNIFICANCE

- Invasion of external Wind
- Yin deficiency (interior conditions)
- Organ disease (interior conditions)
- Stomach prolapse (interior conditions)

Combinations

The clinical significance of the Floating pulse combined with other pulses must be differentiated according to interior or exterior conditions.

Exterior conditions

In exterior conditions the pulse should be Floating by definition and is clearly accompanied by exterior symptoms such as an aversion to cold and the presence of fever. The Floating pulse of exterior conditions can be combined with other qualities as follows.

Floating-Full   This indicates an External-Full condition, found when the patient has a strong Defensive Qi.

Floating-Weak   This indicates an External-Empty condition, found when the patient has a weak Defensive Qi that does not react properly to the invasion of external pathogenic factors.

Floating-Slow   This indicates an invasion of Wind-Cold with a prevalence of Wind.

Floating-Tight   This indicates an invasion of Wind-Cold with a prevalence of Cold.

Floating-Empty   This indicates an invasion of Summer-Heat; it is more floating than the Floating-Empty pulse from Yin deficiency.

Floating-Slippery   This indicates an invasion of Wind-Damp or Wind complicated by Phlegm.

Interior conditions

The Floating pulse can be found in interior conditions and it is, indeed, relatively common. In interior conditions, exterior symptoms such as an aversion to cold and the presence of fever are obviously absent. Thus, if we feel a Floating pulse, we should first establish whether the patient's condition is exterior or interior; this is easily done because an exterior condition presents with an acute onset of aversion to cold, fever, body aches, sore throat, etc. In the absence of such symptoms the condition is interior and we must therefore interpret the significance of the Floating pulse differently.

The Floating quality of the pulse in interior conditions is not as pronounced as in exterior ones; in exterior conditions the pulse is clearly floating like a piece of wood in water as described above and is rather resistant to pressure, whereas in interior conditions the Floating quality of the pulse is less pronounced and is not so resistant to pressure.

!

The Floating quality of the pulse in interior conditions is not as pronounced as in exterior ones.

A Floating pulse in an interior condition associated with an emptiness at the deep level of the pulse generally indicates a potentially serious problem often with severe Blood, Yin or Essence deficiency. Thus, a relatively Floating pulse that is Empty at the deep level in interior conditions may be associated with anaemia, chronic asthma, cirrhosis of the liver or cancer.

In addition, if the pulse is generally Weak and Deep but Floating in one particular position, there may be a problem (often organic rather than just energetic) with the organ corresponding to that position. For example, if the pulse is generally Weak and Deep in all positions except in the Heart position, where it is Floating, this may indicate heart disease.

The Floating pulse without strength in interior conditions may also be associated with prolapse of the stomach, in which case the pulse would also be Fine or Soggy.

Box 50.3 summarizes Western conditions that may be indicated by a Floating pulse.

BOX 50.3 WESTERN DISEASES POTENTIALLY INDICATED BY A FLOATING PULSE

- Floating-Empty: anaemia, chronic asthma, cirrhosis of the liver, cancer
- Floating in one position but Deep-Weak in all others: potential disease in that organ
- Floating-Fine or Floating-Soggy: prolapse of the stomach

If, in the absence of exterior symptoms, the pulse is Floating in all positions and, although it feels relatively hard on the superficial level, it disappears on pressure, this indicates that the person is overworking and pushing himself or herself to the limit; Dr Shen calls this condition 'Qi wild'.

The clinical significance of the Floating pulse in interior conditions needs to be interpreted according to its combinations as follows.

Floating-Empty   This is a relatively common pulse in interior conditions and it indicates Yin deficiency. The Floating-Empty pulse is felt clearly and easily on the superficial level with very light pressure but, with a deeper pressure, the pulse feels empty. However, the Floating-Empty pulse is not as floating as the Floating pulse of exterior conditions.

The emptiness of the pulse at the deep level clearly reflects the deficiency of Yin. On the other hand, its floating quality at the superficial level reflects the rising Yang that derives from Yin deficiency. The Floating-Empty pulse reflects a relatively advanced condition of Yin deficiency when this gives rise to Floating Yang and possibly Empty-Heat. There are of course other pulse qualities that may indicate Yin deficiency such as Fine, Leather or Minute.

Floating-Choppy   This indicates severe Blood deficiency. What is the difference in the clinical significance between a Choppy pulse (which also indicates Blood deficiency) and a Floating-Choppy pulse? The latter indicates a more serious condition of Blood deficiency to such an extent that there is some Empty-Heat associated with it. Thus a woman with a Floating-Choppy pulse who is suffering from Blood deficiency may experience a feeling of heat in the face owing to Empty-Heat arising from Blood deficiency; this occurs only in women.

Floating-Hollow   This pulse appears after a haemorrhage. If it is also Rapid, however, it may indicate a forthcoming haemorrhage.

Floating-Short   This indicates severe deficiency of Qi.

Floating-Rapid   This indicates a serious condition of severe exhaustion (*Xu Lao*). Of course, this applies only if the Floating-Rapid pulse occurs in interior conditions; in the presence of exterior symptoms, of course, it indicates an invasion of Wind-Heat and its clinical significance is therefore completely different.

Floating-Slippery-Rapid   This indicates long-term retention of Phlegm-Heat usually in the Lungs and is seen in chronic bronchitis.

Floating-Weak   This indicates Yin deficiency.

Differentiation of similar pulse qualities

Soggy   The Soggy pulse is soft, without strength, difficult to feel at the superficial level and comparable with wet cotton wool, whereas the Floating pulse is easily felt at the superficial level and, although it decreases in strength when pressed harder, it is not as soft as the Soggy pulse. However, in interior conditions, the combined Floating-Weak pulse feels very similar to the Soggy pulse.

Clinical significance in each position (Li Shi Zhen)

Front position   This indicates invasion of external Wind with dizziness and headache, or invasion of Wind-Heat with mucus in the chest.

Middle position   This indicates deficiency of the Spleen with excess of the Liver.

Rear position   This is seen in difficulty in urination and defecation.

Deep
Pulse description

The Deep pulse can be felt only at the middle and deep levels, and especially the latter. It feels as if it were sunken underneath the muscle. It was also described in the old books as 'a stone in the water'.

The depth at which the pulse is felt needs to be correlated with the body build of the patient; obviously, in obese patients, the pulse will be deeper. Thus the description of the Deep pulse is relative: what feels deep in a thin person may be normal in an obese person.

Clinical significance

This pulse quality indicates simply that the condition is an interior one. A further interpretation of the clinical significance of this pulse must be based on the differentiation between a Deep-Full and a Deep-Weak pulse.

Deep-Full

The Deep-Full pulse denotes the presence of a pathogenic factor in the Interior: this could be Cold, Heat, retention of food, stagnation of Qi or Blood, or accumulation of Water, depending on the combination with other pulse qualities.

Deep-Weak

The Deep-Weak pulse quality indicates Yang deficiency and it is very common.

Box 50.4 summarizes the clinical significance of a Deep pulse.

BOX 50.4 DEEP PULSE: SUMMARY OF CLINICAL SIGNIFICANCE

- Pathogenic factor in the Interior (Deep-Full)
- Yang deficiency (Deep-Weak)

Combinations

Deep-Weak   A very common pulse quality, this indicates Yang deficiency. This pulse is felt at the deep level with moderate pressure and it feels weak.
Deep-Wiry   This indicates stasis of Blood and a possible pathology of the Penetrating Vessel.
Deep-Wiry-Slow   This indicates Blood stasis deriving from Cold, or stagnation of Cold in the Liver channel.
Deep-Slow   This denotes interior Cold.
Deep-Rapid   This indicates interior Heat.
Deep-Soggy-Slow   This denotes Dampness in the Interior, frequently with oedema.

Differentiation of similar pulses

Hidden   The Hidden pulse, essentially the same as the Deep pulse, is an extreme case of it. The Deep pulse is sunken underneath the muscle and can be felt clearly with strong pressure, whereas the Hidden pulse is sunken near the bone and is difficult to feel even with strong pressure.
Firm   The Firm pulse is a type of Deep pulse in so far as it can be felt only at the deep level. It is essentially a pulse that is Wiry at the deep level (the Wiry pulse is felt at all levels).

Clinical significance in each position (Li Shi Zhen)

Front position   This indicates Phlegm or Phlegm-Fluids stagnating in the chest.
Middle position   This indicates pain from Cold in the Middle Burner.
Rear position   This is seen in white spermatorrhoea and diarrhoea or lumbago from Kidney deficiency and abdominal pain.

Slow
Pulse description

In antiquity, the pulse was defined as slow in relation to the breathing cycles of the doctor. Thus a pulse was described as slow if it beat three times or less during the time it takes the doctor to breathe in and out, and as rapid if it beat five times or more during the same time. Obviously this method relies on the doctor's being in good health: it would not work if the doctor suffered from asthma! Although this method is not used any longer, the concentration on one's own breathing focuses and relaxes the doctor's mind.

In modern times, the definition of a Slow or Rapid pulse is related to the pulse rate, which must be correlated to the age of the patient as follows:

Age	Rate
0–1	120/140
1–3	110
4–10	84/90
11–15	78/80
16–35	76
36–50	72/70
50+	68

Any pulse rate below the above values is therefore a Slow pulse. Of course these values should not be adhered to rigidly: for example, a pulse rate of 74 b.p.m. in the 16–35 years age range would be only very slightly slow and have no clinical significance.

Clinical significance

A Slow pulse almost always indicates a Cold pattern. A different interpretation of a Slow pulse is that it denotes a problem in the Yin organs, as opposed to the

Rapid pulse, which indicates a problem in the Yang organs; however, this is a broad generalization and it is not that clinically relevant. The 'Classic of Difficulties' in Chapter 9 says, *'Rapid pulse indicates problems in the Yang organs, the Slow pulse problems in the Yin organs'.*[3]

The clinical significance of the Slow pulse depends on whether it is Full or Empty: a Slow and Full pulse indicates Full-Cold, whereas a Slow and Empty pulse indicates Empty-Cold deriving from Yang deficiency. A condition of Full-Cold can last only a relatively short time (a matter of weeks or months) as interior Cold will eventually injure Yang and lead to Yang deficiency and therefore Empty-Cold. For this reason, in clinical practice Empty-Cold is more common than Full-Cold because we generally see patients with chronic conditions.

If the pulse is very slow, beating only twice for each breath cycle, it is called a Harmful pulse; if it beats only once per each breath, it is called the Destroyed pulse. Both these pulses, and especially the second one, indicate extreme depletion of the Internal Organs and are always associated with serious conditions.

Common Cold conditions manifesting with a Slow pulse

Common conditions which present with a Slow pulse are Stomach-Qi deficiency, Spleen-Yang deficiency, Heart-Yang deficiency, Kidney-Yang deficiency, deficiency of Gathering Qi (*Zong Qi*), Lung-Yang deficiency, Cold in the Stomach, Cold in the Uterus, abdominal masses, Cold-Phlegm and Damp-Cold.

A Slow pulse in chronic conditions may also indicate a deficiency of the Original Qi (*Yuan Qi*).

Box 50.5 summarizes the clinical significance of a Slow pulse.

BOX 50.5 CONDITIONS COMMONLY MANIFESTING WITH A SLOW PULSE

- Stomach-Qi deficiency
- Spleen-Yang deficiency
- Heart-Yang deficiency
- Kidney-Yang deficiency
- Deficiency of Gathering Qi (*Zong Qi*)
- Lung-Yang deficiency
- Cold in the Stomach
- Cold in the Uterus
- Abdominal masses
- Cold-Phlegm
- Damp-Cold

Contradictory manifestations characterized by a Slow pulse and Heat symptoms

Very occasionally the Slow pulse occurs in combination with Heat symptoms; one of the reasons for this contradiction may be Damp-Heat as the Dampness itself may slow the pulse down.

Of course, a contradiction between a Slow pulse and Heat symptoms may simply be due to the coexistence of Cold and Heat patterns. For example, the combination of Kidney-Yang deficiency with Damp-Heat in the Bladder is relatively common. Another possible common combination is that of Kidney-Yang deficiency with Liver-Yang rising.

In menopausal women, a simultaneous deficiency of Kidney-Yin and Kidney-Yang is very common; if the Kidney-Yang deficiency is more pronounced the pulse may be Slow, but the Kidney-Yin deficiency will cause some Empty-Heat signs such as hot flushes and night sweating.

In the context of acute febrile diseases of the Warm-Disease type, the pulse can be Slow with the pattern of Damp-Heat at the Defensive-Qi level.

A Slow pulse with Heat symptoms may also indicate the condition of True Cold and False Heat, but this is quite rare. Yet another possible explanation of a Slow pulse with Heat symptoms is when the Heat is so intense that it obstructs the circulation of Qi and makes the pulse Slow; however, this is also quite rare.

Box 50.6 summarizes conditions with contradictory pulse and Heat symptoms.

BOX 50.6 SITUATIONS GIVING RISE TO CONTRADICTORY SLOW PULSE AND HEAT SYMPTOMS

- Damp-Heat
- Coexistence of Cold and Heat patterns
- Simultaneous deficiency of Kidney-Yin and Kidney-Yang (with predominance of the latter)
- Damp-Heat at the Defensive-Qi level in Warm diseases
- True Cold and false Heat
- Intense Heat obstructing the circulation of Qi

The Slow pulse and jogging

Dr Shen relates a Slow pulse always to a Heart disharmony and poor circulation and, paradoxically, it is often seen in people who jog a lot: according to Dr Shen, excessive jogging (in his opinion more than 4 miles a day) leads to a dilation of the blood vessels which eventually becomes permanent and therefore

slows the circulation down so that the pulse becomes Slow.

A Slow pulse is relatively common in Western patients who are joggers. Indeed, when we feel a Slow pulse, the first question we should ask is whether the patient jogs regularly. However, this is not necessarily a 'false' sign that should be discounted because it reflects the fact that excessive jogging injures Yang and leads to internal Cold. Therefore, although the Slow pulse should be taken into consideration, it is important also to bear in mind that it may be 'disguising' the presence of Heat.

Situations which may cause a Slow pulse without involving Heat

The following life situations may cause a Slow pulse:

- old age
- childbirth
- excessive consumption of fatty and sweet foods.

A Slow pulse of course appears when a patient is on beta blockers; in this case it is a false sign and can be ignored.

Combinations

Slow-Floating   This indicates invasion of exterior Wind-Cold with a prevalence of Wind.
Slow-Deep   This indicates interior Cold (which may be Full or Empty according to whether the pulse is Full or Empty).
Slow-Slippery   This denotes Cold Phlegm or Damp-Cold.
Slow-Choppy   This indicates Blood deficiency and interior Cold deriving from it. (A Slow-Slippery pulse indicates a pathology of Qi, whereas a Slow-Choppy pulse indicates a pathology of Blood.)
Slow-Weak   This denotes Empty-Cold with Yang deficiency.
Slow-Full   This denotes internal Cold and is often seen in chronic, painful conditions.
Slow-Wiry   This indicates accumulation of Phlegm-Fluids or stagnation of Cold in the Liver channel.
Slow-Deep-Weak   This may indicate Heart-Yang deficiency with symptoms of cold limbs, cold feeling, sweating and depression.
Slow-Tight-Overflowing   This indicates that the blood vessels are dilated: in a young person this is often due to excessive jogging, whereas in the elderly it may indicate hardening of the blood vessels.

Differentiation of similar pulses

Slowed-Down   This pulse has four beats per breathing cycle, whereas the Slow pulse has three beats or less.
Knotted   This pulse is slow and it stops at irregular intervals, whereas the Slow pulse is regular.

Clinical significance in each position (Li Shi Zhen)

Front position   This indicates Deficiency and Cold in the Upper Burner.
Middle position   This is seen in pain from Cold in the Middle Burner.
Rear position   This is seen in backache and leg ache with a feeling of heaviness from Kidney deficiency.

Rapid
Pulse description

The Rapid pulse has six beats or more to each breathing cycle; in modern clinical practice a pulse is defined as being Rapid when it beats more times than the values indicated under the Slow pulse above. For example, a pulse rate of 82 b.p.m. in the age range 16–35 indicates a Rapid pulse.

Clinical significance

The Rapid pulse always indicates Heat, which may be Full or Empty according to whether the pulse is Full or Empty. Typical examples of a pulse that is Rapid and of the Full-type are Rapid-Wiry, indicating Liver-Fire, or Rapid-Slippery, indicating Phlegm-Fire.

Examples of a pulse that is Rapid and of the Empty-type are Rapid-Fine, indicating Yin deficiency with Empty-Heat, or Rapid and Floating-Empty, also indicating Yin deficiency with Empty-Heat. It is important to stress that, in Yin deficiency, a Rapid pulse indicates the presence of Empty-Heat rather than Yin deficiency itself; this is manifested by the pulse being either Fine or Floating-Empty. This is equivalent to the situation in tongue diagnosis when, in Yin deficiency, a Red tongue body indicates the presence of Empty-Heat rather than the presence of Yin deficiency itself, which would be manifested by the absence of coating.

> **!**
>
> Yin deficiency is indicated by a Floating-Empty pulse; it is only when it is also Rapid that Empty-Heat is indicated.

As mentioned above under the Slow pulse, the 'Classic of Difficulties' relates the Rapid pulse to problems of the Yang organs, and the Slow pulse to problems of the Yin organs. Of course, this is a broad generalization which suffers from exceptions (e.g. Liver-Fire may manifest with a Rapid pulse).

Common conditions which present with a Rapid pulse include Stomach-Heat, Heat in the Intestines, Lung-Heat, Liver-Fire, Heart-Fire, Yin deficiency with Empty-Heat, Phlegm-Heat, Damp-Heat and invasion of Wind-Heat. The Rapid pulse is also seen in the Lilium Syndrome described in Chapter 3 of the 'Synopsis of Prescriptions from the Golden Cabinet'.[4]

Box 50.7 summarizes the common clinical manifestations of a Rapid pulse.

BOX 50.7 COMMON CONDITIONS MANIFESTING WITH A RAPID PULSE

- Stomach-Heat
- Heat in the Large Intestine
- Lung-Heat
- Liver-Fire
- Heart-Fire
- Yin deficiency with Empty-Heat
- Phlegm-Heat
- Damp-Heat
- Invasion of Wind-Heat
- Lilium Syndrome

In fevers, whether of internal or external origin, the pulse should be Rapid; if it is not, this is a serious sign.

!

In fevers, if the pulse is not Rapid this is a bad sign.

However, there are a few situations when a Rapid pulse does not indicate Heat because the clinical manifestations do not point to Heat. When we feel a Rapid pulse, it is important to check this against the tongue and the inside of the lower eyelids: in true conditions of Heat, the tongue will be Red and the inside of the lower eyelids will also be red.

The following are examples of situations when the Rapid pulse does not correspond to Heat.

- **The pulse can become Rapid following an emotional upset**, such as a shock or an outburst of anger. Thus if we see a patient whose clinical manifestations do not point to Heat and the pulse is Rapid, we should always ask whether they have had an emotional upset recently (within hours or days). The 'Simple Questions', in Chapter 17, says, '*A Rapid pulse may indicate that a person has suffered a sudden fright and the pulse will revert back to normal in three to four days.*'[5]
- **The pulse can become Rapid when a person suffering from Qi and Blood deficiency works very hard, pushing himself or herself to the limit.** In such a case the pulse becomes Rapid manifesting an attempt by the body's Qi to cope with such demands: Dr J. H. F. Shen describes this situation as 'Qi wild' when the pulse is also Overflowing. The 'Complete Book of Jing Yue' confirms this by saying that one of the causes of a Rapid pulse may be exhaustion (*Xu Lao*).[6] If the pulse is Rapid and Big but also Empty, this may indicate severe exhaustion of Essence and Blood which occur also without Empty-Heat.
- **The pulse can become Rapid in advanced cases of cancer**, even in the absence of a Heat pattern. In a patient suffering from cancer this is often a bad sign indicating a poor prognosis and, potentially, a rapid spread of the cancer.
- **The pulse can become Rapid in extreme Qi deficiency**, again reflecting an attempt by the body's Qi to cope with its demands.
- **The pulse can become Rapid in Yin Fire.** The concept of Yin Fire was introduced by Li Dong Yuan in his famous 'Discussion on Stomach and Spleen' (*Pi Wei Lun*, 1249). According to Li Dong Yuan irregular diet, overwork and emotional stress weaken the Stomach and Spleen and the Original Qi (*Yuan Qi*). When the Original Qi declines, the Minister Fire becomes pathological and rises from the space between the Kidneys to harass the Heart and Pericardium; Li Dong Yuan called this Yin Fire (not to be confused with Empty-Heat). The pathological Minister Fire (i.e. Yin Fire) 'displaces' the Original Qi because they both occupy the same space in between the Kidneys; for this reason Li Dong Yuan says that the Yin Fire is a 'thief' of the Original Qi. Thus

in this kind of pathology there may be some Cold symptoms and signs arising from a deficiency of the Original Qi (such as cold feet, a feeling of cold and a Pale tongue) and some Heat manifestations from the rising of the Yin Fire (such as a feeling of heat in the face and a Rapid pulse). Arousal of the Yin Fire is treated not by clearing Heat but by tonifying the Original Qi with sweet and warm herbs; the representative formula for this is Bu Zhong Yi Qi Tang *Tonifying the Centre and Benefiting Qi Decoction* (*Tonify Qi and Ease the Muscles* in the *Three Treasures*).

As Yin Fire derives from a deficiency of the Original Qi, if the latter predominates, the pulse may be Slow rather than Rapid.

- **A Rapid pulse may also simply indicate nervous tension without any Heat.** This is usually found in people who are constitutionally nervous: these patients will most probably have a Heart crack on the tongue.

Box 50.8 summarizes those situations when a Rapid pulse does not correspond to Heat.

BOX 50.8 SITUATIONS WHEN THE PULSE IS RAPID FOR REASONS OTHER THAN HEAT

- Emotional upset
- Severe Qi and Blood deficiency from overwork
- Cancer
- Extreme Qi deficiency
- Yin Fire
- Nervous tension

The following factors may also cause the pulse to become temporarily Rapid in the absence of Heat: vigorous physical exercise, heavy meals, alcohol, smoking, tea, coffee, fright, emotional upsets, certain herbs such as Ma Huang *Ephedrae sinicae* or Ren Shen *Radix Panax Ginseng* and anaemia.

Combinations

Rapid-Full   This indicates the presence of Full-Heat from Excess of Yang.

Rapid-Empty   This indicates Empty-Heat from deficiency of Yin.

Rapid-Floating   This denotes invasion of external Wind-Heat.

Rapid-Deep   This indicates interior Heat.

Rapid-Overflowing   This indicates Full-Heat usually in the Stomach, Lungs or Heart.

Rapid-Fine   This denotes Empty-Heat from Yin deficiency.

Rapid-Floating-Empty   This indicates Empty-Heat from Yin deficiency.

Rapid-Wiry   This indicates Liver-Fire.

Rapid-Slippery   This denotes Phlegm-Heat.

Rapid-Deep-Full   This indicates interior Fire in the Stomach and the Intestines.

Rapid-Wiry-Big   This indicates Blood-Heat. According to Dr Shen, this pulse may be seen when there is too much glucose or cholesterol in the blood.

Differentiation of similar pulses

Hasty   The Hasty pulse is rapid and stops at irregular intervals, whereas the Rapid pulse is regular.

Hurried   The Hurried pulse beats seven to eight times per breath cycle, it is regular and it gives the sensation of being hurried and anxious. It feels extremely agitated and urgent.

Moving   The Moving pulse is rapid and short, it is shaped like a bean and gives the impression of vibrating rather than pulsating. The Rapid pulse is simply rapid and does not have any of the above attributes.

Clinical significance in each position (Li Shi Zhen)

Front position   This is found in sore throat, tongue or mouth ulcers, vomiting of blood, cough and lung abcess.

Middle position   This indicates Stomach-Fire if on the right Middle position, and Liver-Fire if on the left Middle position.

Rear position   This indicates the need to nourish the Yin and clear Fire.

Empty
Pulse description

The Empty pulse has no strength and disappears with a light pressure, feeling empty; it is soft but also *relatively* big and distended at the superficial level.

Clinical significance

The Empty pulse indicates Qi deficiency at its beginning or middle stages; in chronic Qi deficiency, the Empty pulse will usually become Weak (see below). Since most of the patients we see suffer from chronic conditions, the classic Empty pulse is relatively rare. When discussing the clinical significance of the

'Empty' pulse, it is important to be precise about one's terminology: there is a difference between the classic 'Empty' pulse as defined above, indicating purely Qi deficiency, and an empty-type pulse, which encompasses a broad range of deficient pulses, such as Weak, Fine, Choppy, etc. It is therefore important, especially in training clinics, not to use the word 'Empty' in a loose sense but only to indicate a precise pulse quality.

> **!**
>
> Remember: do not confuse the specific 'Empty' pulse quality with a generic, loosely defined 'empty-type' of pulse.

The Empty pulse is most common on the Lung position and in chronic conditions it may indicate Lung exhaustion (*Fei Xu Lao*).

If the pulse is Empty and relatively Floating and without strength in all three positions, especially of the left, it indicates Blood deficiency.

If the pulse is Empty and slightly Rapid in acute exterior syndromes, it indicates invasion of Summer-Heat.

Box 50.9 summarizes the clinical significance of an Empty pulse.

BOX 50.9 EMPTY PULSE: SUMMARY OF CLINICAL SIGNIFICANCE

- Qi deficiency
- Blood deficiency (slightly Floating)
- Summer-Heat (slightly Rapid)

Combinations

Empty-Floating without strength   This indicates Blood deficiency.

Empty-Rapid   In exterior syndromes this may denote invasion of Summer-Heat. In interior syndromes it may indicate the rising of Yin Fire from a deficiency of Original Qi as described above under the Rapid pulse.

Differentiation of similar pulses

Weak   The Weak pulse is slightly deeper than the Empty pulse and therefore requires a slightly harder finger pressure and it lacks the relatively big and distended quality of the Empty pulse; it is also softer than the Empty pulse.

Choppy   The Choppy pulse is deeper than the Empty pulse, it lacks its relatively big and distended quality, it

is weaker than the Empty pulse and it lacks a wave. By contrast, the Empty pulse has a wave. The Choppy pulse also feels 'jagged', whereas the Empty pulse feels quite rounded.

Hollow   The Hollow pulse is empty only at the middle level and can be felt at the superficial and deep levels; the Empty pulse is empty at the superficial level and is softer than the Hollow pulse.

Soggy   The Soggy pulse is soft and without strength but also slightly floating, whereas the Empty pulse is bigger and not floating.

Clinical significance in each position (Li Shi Zhen)

Front position   This indicates deficient Blood not nourishing the Heart.

Middle position   This is found in abdominal distension, retention of food and Qi stagnation.

Rear position   This indicates Atrophy or Painful Obstruction Syndrome from steaming of the bones injuring Essence and Blood with deficiency in the Lower Burner.

Full

Pulse description

The Full pulse feels hard, full and long; it is felt easily at all levels and it has a springy quality resistant to finger pressure.

Clinical significance

The Full pulse simply indicates the presence of a Full pattern; its precise clinical significance can be deduced only from its combination with other qualities. When discussing the clinical significance of the 'Full' pulse, it is important to be precise about terminology: there is a difference between the classic 'Full' pulse as defined above, indicating purely a Full condition, and a full-type pulse, which encompasses a broad range of full pulses, such as Wiry, Slippery, Tight, Big, Overflowing, etc. It is therefore important, especially in training clinics, not to use the word 'Full' in a loose sense but only to indicate a precise pulse quality.

A proper identification of the Full pulse is essential to determine the correct principle of treatment in chronic conditions which are usually characterized by the simultaneous presence of Full and Empty patterns. In such cases, we must have a clear idea in mind as to what our treatment strategy should be, that is, tonify

the body's Qi or expel pathogenic factors. When we are confronted by these alternative treatment strategies, the pulse quality is extremely important in our deciding which one to choose; if the pulse is Full it is usually better to concentrate our attention on expelling pathogenic factors, even if the condition is chronic. Postviral fatigue syndrome is a case in point. In this condition there is nearly always Deficiency, usually of Qi, and Excess, usually of Dampness, and I often base my decision whether to tonify Qi or resolve Dampness on the pulse quality: if it is Full or of the full type, I start by resolving Dampness rather than tonifying Qi. The same principle applies to any chronic conditions manifesting with simultaneous Deficiency and Excess.

Box 50.10 summarizes the common conditions presenting with a Full pulse.

BOX 50.10 COMMON CONDITIONS MANIFESTING WITH A FULL PULSE

- Heart-, Stomach- or Liver-Fire
- Retention of Food
- Phlegm
- Full Cold
- Stagnation of Qi/Blood

Combinations

Full-Rapid   This indicates Full-Heat.
Full-Slow   This indicates Full-Cold.
Full-Tight   This denotes Full-Cold.
Full-Slippery   This indicates Phlegm.
Full-Long   This indicates Heat.
Full-Wiry   This indicates a Full Liver pattern.

Differentiation of similar pulses

Overflowing   The Overflowing pulse is large, long and relatively floating and it decreases in strength when pressed heavily. The Full pulse is not so long, not so floating and does not decrease in strength when pressed heavily.

Clinical significance in each position (Li Shi Zhen)

Front position   This is found in invasion of Wind-Heat in the head and face, sore throat, stiff tongue and a feeling of fullness in the chest.
Middle position   This is found in Heat in the Spleen, abdominal distension and fullness.
Rear position   This is found in backache, abdominal pain and constipation.

Slippery
Pulse description

The Slippery pulse feels slippery or 'oily': it is rounded, 'slips' or slides under the finger and flows smoothly. In ancient times, it was described as feeling like 'pearls rolling in a basin' or 'raindrops rolling on a lotus leaf'. Students can get a good idea of what a Slippery pulse is by feeling the pulse of a pregnant woman in an advanced stage of pregnancy; most probably, the pulse will be very Slippery (if it is not, this is a bad sign).

Clinical significance

The Slippery pulse indicates primarily Phlegm or retention of food; it may also indicate Blood stasis. Generally speaking, the Slippery pulse is full by definition indicating the presence of Phlegm; however, it may also be combined with empty-type pulses reflecting the simultaneous deficiency of Qi and the presence of Phlegm (which usually derive from Qi deficiency).

Although the Slippery pulse is traditionally associated with Phlegm, it may also be seen in cases of chronic Dampness; for example, it is very common in chronic cases of postviral fatigue syndrome with clear manifestations of Dampness.

It is normal for the pulse to become Slippery during pregnancy and, indeed, it indicates a healthy pregnancy. Conversely, if the pulse is not Slippery during pregnancy, it is not a good sign and it may indicate impending problems; in such cases, the woman should be treated even in the absence of symptoms. In particular, there are certain pulse qualities which are undesirable during pregnancy, such as Choppy, Choppy-Wiry, Fine, Weak, Leather and Hollow, all of which may indicate the possibility of miscarriage.

According to some Chinese sources, a Slippery pulse that is Slowed-Down and relatively soft indicates health.

Common conditions manifesting with a Slippery pulse include a whole range of diseases characterized by Phlegm in all of its manifestations (i.e. Phlegm-Heat, Cold-Phlegm, Damp-Phlegm, Wind-Phlegm, etc.). In the organs, Phlegm can be retained primarily in the Lungs, Stomach and Heart (non-substantial Phlegm misting the Mind). Phlegm in the Lungs is extremely common and a good example of a Slippery pulse is that felt in a patient with acute or chronic bronchitis.

Conditions other than Phlegm, such as Damp-Heat or retention of food, may also lead to a Slippery pulse.

According to Dr Shen, when a Slippery quality is felt only in one position, it does not necessarily indicate Dampness or Phlegm. For example, he attributes the following clinical significance to a Slippery quality in individual positions:

- Lungs: Phlegm
- Stomach: excessive acidity
- Bladder: disturbance of bladder function
- Heart: heart-valve problem
- Liver: disturbance of liver function
- Gall-Bladder: gallstones
- Kidney: kidney infection.

Box 50.11 summarizes the clinical significance of a Slippery pulse.

BOX 50.11 SLIPPERY PULSE: SUMMARY OF CLINICAL SIGNIFICANCE

- Phlegm
- Retention of food
- Blood stasis
- Dampness (chronic)
- Pregnancy

Combinations

Slippery-Floating   This indicates Wind-Phlegm.
Slippery-Deep   This indicates Phlegm or retention of food.
Slippery-Rapid   This indicates Damp-Heat or Phlegm-Heat.
Slippery-Slow   This indicates Damp-Cold or Cold-Phlegm (it is often seen in diarrhoea).
Slippery-Big   This denotes Phlegm-Heat with the predominance of Heat.
Slippery-Short   This indicates Dampness or Phlegm against a background of Qi deficiency.
Slippery-Weak   This indicates Dampness or Phlegm against a background of Qi deficiency.
Li Shi Zhen summarizes the combinations of Slippery pulses as follows:

- Slippery-Floating: Wind-Phlegm
- Slippery-Deep: Phlegm with retention of food
- Slippery-Rapid: Phlegm-Fire
- Slippery-Slow: retention of food.

Differentiation of similar pulses

Moving   The Moving pulse is rounded like the Slippery pulse but it is also short, is shaped like a bean and gives the impression of vibrating rather than pulsating.
Soggy   The Soggy pulse is very slightly slippery, as well as being soft and relatively floating. The Slippery pulse is much fuller than the Soggy pulse and is not soft.

Clinical significance in each position (Li Shi Zhen)

Front position   This is found in Phlegm in the chest or diaphragm, vomiting, vomiting of sour fluids, stiff tongue and cough.
Middle position   This indicates retention of food or Heat in the Spleen and Liver.
Rear position   This is found in diabetes, diarrhoea, hernia and Painful Urination Syndrome.

Choppy
Pulse description

The Choppy pulse feels rough, 'jagged' and short. It flows without a 'wave', the normal pulse flows from the Rear position to the Front with a smooth and continuous movement like a sea wave. The Choppy pulse lacks this continuous movement between the three positions and does not feel like a wave; this is an important difference from a normal pulse as the Choppy pulse is felt within each position separately (Fig. 50.1).

For this reason, when deciding whether or not a pulse is Choppy, it is important to feel the pulse with three fingers to detect the presence or absence of the wave between the three positions. However, this does not mean that the pulse may not be Choppy in one position only.

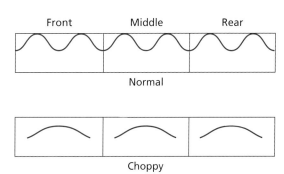

Fig. 50.1 The Choppy pulse quality in relation to a wave

> **!**
>
> The Choppy pulse must be felt with three fingers simultaneously.

There are many other ways of describing the Choppy pulse. First, it appears to be flowing vertically up and down rather than horizontally. It also gives the impression of coming and going, of being stagnant and not flowing properly. One description is 'the throb of the beat arrives but not all at once; it falls away but not immediately'. Another characteristic of the Choppy pulse is that it may appear to change quality and strength as we feel it.

In ancient times it was described as 'a knife scraping bamboo' or 'raindrops in the sand'. Some Chinese books describe this pulse as a 'three-five pulse' meaning that it changes rate frequently, sometimes beating three times and sometimes five times per respiration. Other authors say that the Choppy pulse combines three qualities: it is Slow, Fine and Short.

Box 50.12 summarizes these descriptions of a Choppy pulse.

BOX 50.12 DESCRIPTIONS OF THE CHOPPY PULSE QUALITY

- Rough, jagged and short
- Without a wave
- Gives the impression of flowing vertically rather than horizontally
- Gives the impression of coming and going
- Stagnant, not flowing properly
- The throb of the beat arrives but not all at once: it falls away but not immediately
- It may change quality and strength as we feel it
- Knife scraping bamboo
- Raindrops in the sand
- Changes rate frequently
- It is a combination of three qualities: Slow, Fine and Short

---

Clinical significance

The Choppy pulse indicates a deficiency of Blood or Essence. It may also indicate loss of Body Fluids occurring after profuse sweating, vomiting or diarrhoea. In a pregnant woman, a Choppy pulse is always a bad sign, at the beginning of term indicating the possibility of miscarriage and towards the end of term indicating the possibility of eclampsia. In men, a Choppy pulse indicates deficiency of Essence, which may derive from excessive sexual activity.

Besides Blood deficiency, the Choppy pulse may also indicate Blood stasis but only when this occurs against a background of deficiency of Qi or Blood.

Generally speaking, the Choppy pulse is, of course, by definition of the empty type. However, although the Choppy pulse is short, rough, jagged and lacking a wave, it can also be relatively Full. The word 'relatively' is important in the description of this pulse combination, as the Choppy-Full pulse is not nearly as full as the Full pulse. The Choppy and relatively Full pulse often indicates Blood stasis rather than Blood deficiency, frequently deriving from emotional problems.

The Choppy pulse generally indicates the patterns of Blood deficiency (especially in women), Essence deficiency (especially in men) and Blood stasis. Common conditions presenting with these patterns and a Choppy pulse include heart disease, Chest Painful Obstruction Syndrome, many menstrual disorders, postnatal disorders such as depression, and cancer.

Box 50.13 summarizes the clinical significance of a Choppy pulse.

BOX 50.13 CHOPPY PULSE: SUMMARY OF CLINICAL SIGNIFICANCE

- Blood deficiency
- Essence deficiency
- Body Fluids deficiency
- Blood stasis

Combinations

Choppy-Weak This indicates depletion of both Qi and Blood.

Choppy-Minute This indicates extreme Blood deficiency.

Choppy-Soggy This denotes Qi and Blood deficiency with some Dampness and is very common.

Choppy-Floating This indicates an invasion of external Wind occurring against a background of Qi and Blood deficiency.

Choppy-Deep This indicates chronic Blood deficiency.

Choppy-Full This may indicate Blood stasis.

Choppy-Knotted This indicates Blood stasis deriving from Yang deficiency and internal Cold.

Choppy-Fine This indicates deficiency of Body Fluids.

Differentiation of similar pulses

Weak The Weak pulse is deep, weak and soft but it has a wave; the Choppy pulse is rough, jagged, not so soft and lacks a wave.

Minute The Minute pulse is very fine, almost blurred, whereas the Choppy pulse is not so fine.

Fine The Fine pulse is thin but well defined and with a wave. The shape of the Choppy pulse is less well defined and it lacks a wave.

Clinical significance in each position (Li Shi Zhen)

Front position This is found in Heart-Qi deficiency and pain in the chest.

Middle position This is found in Stomach and Spleen deficiency and hypochondrial distension.

Rear position This is found in injury of Essence and Blood, Painful Urination Syndrome, constipation and blood in the stools.

EMPTY-TYPE PULSES

Weak

Pulse description

As the Weak pulse cannot be felt at the superficial level it is, by definition, Deep. It feels soft and without strength. When discussing the clinical significance of the 'Weak' pulse, it is important to be precise about one's terminology: there is a difference between the classic 'Weak' pulse as defined above, indicating purely Yang deficiency, and a weak-type pulse that encompasses a broad range of deficient pulses, such as Empty, Fine, Choppy, Soggy, etc. It is therefore important, especially in training clinics, to use the word 'Weak' not in a loose sense but only to indicate a precise pulse quality.

> **!**
>
> The Weak pulse is not just 'weak' but a precise pulse quality: it is extremely common.

Clinical significance

The Weak pulse indicates Yang deficiency; it is a very common pulse in chronic conditions, more so than the Empty pulse. However, it may also indicate Blood deficiency or deficiency of the Original Qi.

If the pulse is relatively Floating at the middle level and very Weak at the deep level, this indicates severe deficiency of Blood with collapse of the blood vessels.

According to Dr Shen, we can differentiate the Weak pulse at the superficial, middle or deep level. A Weak quality at the superficial level indicates Yang deficiency and it may be due to overwork; if the pulse becomes

Weak at the superficial level in the short term, this indicates lack of sleep. A Weak quality at the middle level indicates Blood deficiency, whereas a Weak quality at the deep level indicates Yin deficiency.

Common conditions presenting with a Weak pulse are Yang deficiency, Blood deficiency and deficiency of the Original Qi. These patterns, presenting with a Weak pulse, are common in many digestive diseases, menstrual disorders, profuse sweating, nocturnal emissions and haemorrhages.

Box 50.14 summarizes the clinical significance of a weak pulse.

> **BOX 50.14 WEAK PULSE: SUMMARY OF CLINICAL SIGNIFICANCE**
>
> - Yang deficiency
> - Blood deficiency
> - Deficiency of Original Qi
> - Yin deficiency (deep level)

Combinations

Weak-Choppy This indicates Blood deficiency.

Weak-Fine This indicates severe Blood deficiency.

Weak-Slow This indicates Yang deficiency.

Weak-Rapid This indicates bleeding from Qi deficiency.

Weak-Soggy This denotes Yang deficiency with some Dampness.

Weak-Floating This indicates Qi deficiency.

Differentiation of similar pulses

Empty The Empty pulse is soft, relatively big and can be felt at a superficial level, whereas the Weak pulse is thinner and can be felt only at the middle and deep levels.

Choppy The Choppy pulse is rough, jagged and lacks a wave. The Weak pulse is softer but it has a wave.

Fine The Fine pulse is thin but distinct, while the Weak pulse is soft and has no distinct shape.

Soggy The Soggy pulse is soft and weak but also relatively floating, whereas the Weak pulse is not at all floating and cannot be felt on the superficial level.

Clinical significance in each position (Li Shi Zhen)

Front position This indicates Yang deficiency.

Middle position This indicates Stomach and Spleen deficiency.

Rear position This denotes decline of Yang-Qi, or exhaustion of Yin-Essence.

Fine

Pulse description

The Fine pulse is thin and thread-like but it is clear and straight, although soft. It feels like a fine line under the finger.

Clinical significance

The Fine pulse indicates primarily a severe deficiency of Blood but also of Qi. The 'Simple Questions' in Chapter 17 says: '*The Fine pulse indicates Qi deficiency*'.[7] Compared with the Choppy pulse, the Fine pulse indicates a more severe deficiency of Blood. It may also indicate Yin deficiency.

The Fine pulse is obviously of the empty type by definition but it may be combined with full-type qualities, such as Wiry or Tight. The Fine pulse with strength indicates Dampness.

A Fine and Weak pulse in very young people indicates a constitutional deficiency of Original Qi.

The Fine pulse is a very common pulse quality, mostly appearing in Blood or Yin deficiency, or both. Diseases commonly presenting with this pulse include digestive diseases, diarrhoea and menstrual disorders.

Box 50.15 summarizes the clinical significance of a Fine pulse.

BOX 50.15 FINE PULSE: SUMMARY OF CLINICAL SIGNIFICANCE

- Blood deficiency
- Qi deficiency
- Yin deficiency
- Dampness (Fine with strength)
- Deficiency of the Original Qi (Fine and Weak in the very young)

Combinations

Fine-Rapid This indicates Yin deficiency with Empty-Heat.

Fine-Wiry This indicates Liver-Qi stagnation or Liver-Yang rising occurring against a background of Blood deficiency.

Fine-Tight This indicates Empty-Cold occurring against a background of Blood deficiency.

Fine-Choppy This indicates severe Blood or Essence deficiency.

Fine-Deep This indicates retention of Dampness, as often seen in Painful Obstruction Syndrome.

Fine-Weak This indicates severe Blood deficiency and it is often seen in night sweating.

According to Dr Shen, a Fine-Weak pulse in a middle-aged person means that he or she has overworked or overexercised between the ages of 15 and 20.

Differentiation of similar pulses

Choppy The Choppy pulse is rough, and jagged, lacks a wave and is rather indistinct. The Fine pulse is thin but clear and distinct and has a wave.

Minute The Minute pulse is nothing but an extreme case of Fine pulse; it is simply thinner than the Fine pulse.

Weak The Weak pulse is softer and less well defined than the Fine pulse. It is also missing at the superficial level, whereas the Fine pulse can be felt at the superficial level.

Clinical significance in each position (Li Shi Zhen)

Front position This is found in chronic vomiting.

Middle position This is found in abdominal distension and Stomach and Spleen deficiency.

Rear position This is found in Cold in the Lower Burner, diarrhoea and nocturnal emissions.

Minute

Pulse description

The Minute pulse is very thin, almost blurred; it is basically an extreme case of a Fine pulse. It is almost imperceptible under the finger.

Clinical significance

The Minute pulse indicates severe deficiency of Blood, Essence or Yin; it may also indicate deficiency of the Original Qi. It is only seen in chronic conditions and it indicates a poor prognosis; it is often seen in cancer.

Common conditions which present with a Minute pulse include haemorrhages, spontaneous sweating, nocturnal emissions, chronic diarrhoea, menstrual diseases, collapse of Yang and chronic vomiting.

Box 50.16 summarizes the clinical significance of a Minute pulse.

BOX 50.16 MINUTE PULSE: SUMMARY OF CLINICAL SIGNIFICANCE

- Severe Blood deficiency
- Severe Yin deficiency
- Severe Essence deficiency
- Deficiency of the Original Qi

Combinations

Minute-Rapid   This indicates Yin deficiency with Empty-Heat.

Minute-Slow   This indicates severe Qi and Blood deficiency with internal Cold.

Minute-Choppy   This indicates exhaustion of Blood.

Minute-Soggy   This indicates Qi and Blood deficiency with some Dampness.

Minute-Deep   This indicates Yin deficiency.

Minute-Wiry   This indicates Liver-Yang rising occurring against a background of severe Blood deficiency.

Differentiation of similar pulses

Fine   The Minute pulse is nothing but an extreme case of Fine pulse; it is simply thinner than the Fine pulse.

Weak   The Weak pulse is deep and soft but not so thin and imperceptible as the Minute pulse.

Clinical significance in each position (Li Shi Zhen)

Front position   This is found in breathlessness and palpitations.

Middle position   This is found in abdominal distension and fullness, and Stomach and Spleen deficiency.

Rear position   This is found in deficiency of Blood, exhaustion of Essence, diabetes and abdominal pain.

Soggy (Weak-Floating)

Pulse description

The Soggy (also called Weak-Floating) pulse can only be felt at the superficial level; it is relatively floating but weak and soft like wet cotton-wool or wet bread. It disappears when a stronger pressure is applied. In Chinese it is called *ru*, which means 'sodden', but also *ruan*, which means 'soft'.

   In my previous books, I call this pulse quality 'Weak-Floating', which describes well its characteristic of being weak, soft but also slightly floating.

Clinical significance

The Soggy pulse indicates chronic Qi deficiency with retention of Dampness. It is a relatively common pulse quality in chronic conditions with Dampness, such as postviral fatigue syndrome. The Soggy pulse also indicates Stomach-Qi deficiency.

   Common conditions presenting with a Soggy pulse are digestive disorders, chronic fatigue syndrome, asthma, nocturnal emissions and diarrhoea.

Box 50.17 summarizes the clinical significance of a Soggy pulse.

> ### BOX 50.17 SOGGY PULSE: SUMMARY OF CLINICAL SIGNIFICANCE
> * Chronic Qi deficiency with Dampness

Combinations

Soggy-Fine   This indicates severe Spleen-Qi deficiency with chronic retention of Dampness.

Soggy-Choppy   This indicates exhaustion of Blood.

Soggy-Floating   This denotes deficiency of Defensive Qi.

Soggy-Wiry   This denotes Dampness with Liver-Qi stagnation.

Soggy-Rapid   This indicates Damp-Heat.

Differentiation of similar pulses

Empty   The Empty pulse feels soft but relatively big and floating, whereas the Soggy pulse is thinner, weaker, softer and less floating.

Weak   The Weak pulse is soft and can be felt only at the deep level, whereas the Soggy pulse is also soft but can be felt at the superficial level.

Clinical significance in each position (Li Shi Zhen)

Front position   This is found in decline of Yang-Qi with incessant sweating.

Middle position   This denotes deficiency of Central Qi.

Rear position   This denotes injury of Essence and Blood, deficient Cold in the Lower Burner; warm and tonify the true Yin to bring about an improvement.

Short

Pulse description

The Short pulse does not fill a pulse position. Within each position it can be felt in the centre but it tapers off at the head and tail. The Short pulse is more commonly felt in the Front and Middle positions, especially the former.

Clinical significance

The Short pulse indicates severe deficiency of Qi, especially of the Lungs and Heart.

   Common patterns which present with a Short pulse are Lung-Qi deficiency, Heart-Qi deficiency, Stomach-Qi deficiency and deficiency of Qi and Blood.

Box 50.18 summarizes the clinical significance of a Short pulse.

BOX 50.18 SHORT PULSE: SUMMARY OF CLINICAL SIGNIFICANCE

- Severe deficiency of Qi (of Lungs, Heart or Stomach)
- Deficiency of Qi and Blood

Combinations

Short-Floating This indicates Lung-Qi deficiency.
Short-Choppy This denotes Heart-Qi deficiency.
Short-Rapid This indicates severe Heart-Blood deficiency with Empty- Heat.
Short-Slow This indicates Yang deficiency with internal Cold.
Short-Deep This indicates accumulation in the Interior with Spleen deficiency.
Short-Hasty This indicates stagnation of Qi with non-substantial Phlegm or retention of food.

Differentiation of similar pulses

Moving The Moving pulse is short, shaped like a bean, rapid and gives the impression of vibrating rather than pulsating. The Short pulse shares with the moving pulse only the characteristic of being short, but none of the others.
Empty The Empty pulse is soft and relatively floating and, like the Short pulse, indicates Qi deficiency. The Short pulse is neither soft nor floating.
Weak The Weak pulse is soft and can be felt only at the middle and deep levels but is not short. The Short pulse can be felt at all levels.
Hidden The Hidden pulse is very deep and difficult to feel but it occupies its normal pulse position, whereas the Short pulse does not fill its pulse position.

Clinical significance in each position (Li Shi Zhen)

Not given by Li Shi Zhen.

Hollow
Pulse description

The Hollow pulse can be felt at the superficial and deep levels but not at the middle one; it is, as its name implies, hollow like an onion stalk. This pulse also feels quite solid on the sides of the fingers when rolling the fingers from side to side.

Clinical significance

The Hollow pulse indicates loss of Blood and it appears after a haemorrhage. It should be stressed that this indicates a pathological haemorrhage and not, for example, the normal menstrual bleeding. It may also appear after a profuse loss of Body Fluids from sweating, vomiting or diarrhoea. If the pulse is Hollow and Rapid, it may indicate a *forthcoming* haemorrhage. The Hollow pulse is not common.

Box 50.19 summarizes the clinical significance of a Hollow pulse.

BOX 50.19 HOLLOW PULSE: SUMMARY OF CLINICAL SIGNIFICANCE

- Loss of blood
- Loss of Body Fluids

Combinations

Hollow-Floating This indicates injury of Qi and Yin.
Hollow-Rapid This indicates Yin deficiency with Empty-Heat or an impending haemorrhage.
Hollow-Empty-Soggy This indicates loss of Essence or depletion of Blood.
Hollow-Knotted This indicates Yang deficiency or Blood stasis.
Hollow-Slow This indicates loss of Blood and injury of the Upright Qi.

Differentiation of similar pulses

Choppy The Choppy pulse is generally empty, rough and without a wave, whereas the Hollow pulse has a definite shape and a wave but is empty only at the middle level.
Empty The Empty pulse is relatively superficial and soft and disappears with a relatively light pressure. The Hollow pulse is neither superficial nor soft; it disappears with a stronger pressure but it has more shape than the Empty pulse.

Clinical significance in each position (Li Shi Zhen)

Not given by Li Shi Zhen.

Leather
Pulse description

The Leather pulse can be felt at a superficial level, stretched like the skin of a drum and empty at the deep

level; it feels hard on the outside but empty inside, like a drum.

Clinical significance

The Leather pulse indicates severe deficiency of Blood, Essence or Yin. It also indicates Qi floating upwards because it is not rooted by Blood.

Common patterns presenting with a Leather pulse include depletion of Blood or Yin, or both, and these may appear in habitual miscarriage, menorrhagia and nocturnal emissions. In my experience, the Leather pulse is frequently felt in advanced cases of multiple sclerosis.

Box 50.20 summarizes the clinical significance of a Leather pulse.

BOX 50.20 LEATHER: SUMMARY OF CLINICAL SIGNIFICANCE

- Severe deficiency of Blood
- Severe deficiency of Essence
- Severe deficiency of Yin
- Qi floating upwards

Combinations

Leather-Rapid This indicates severe deficiency of Yin with Empty-Heat.
Leather-Slow This indicates severe Blood deficiency with Blood stasis.
Leather-Choppy This denotes severe Blood deficiency.

Differentiation of similar pulses

Choppy The Choppy pulse is rough, jagged and lacks a wave but is not felt clearly at the superficial level. The Leather pulse, which like the Choppy pulse also indicates Blood deficiency, feels relatively hard at the superficial level; at the deep level, it is more empty than the Choppy pulse.
Hollow The Hollow pulse is empty in the middle and can be felt clearly at the superficial and deep levels, whereas the Leather pulse cannot be felt at the deep level. Another difference is that the Leather pulse feels relatively hard and stretched at the superficial level, which the Hollow pulse does not.
Floating-Empty The Floating-Empty pulse and the Hollow pulse share the common characteristic of being empty at the deep level. However, the Floating-Empty pulse is relatively soft at the superficial level, or

at least much softer than the Leather pulse, which feels hard and stretched at the superficial level.
Wiry The Leather pulse has a slightly Wiry quality on the surface but it disappears on pressure, whereas the Wiry pulse is Wiry at all levels and does not disappear on pressure. The Leather pulse, although hard on the superficial level like the Wiry pulse, feels more 'flat' on the superficial level than the Wiry pulse.

Clinical significance in each position (Li Shi Zhen)

Not given by Li Shi Zhen.

Hidden
Pulse description

The Hidden pulse is simply an extreme case of a Deep pulse: it is deeper than the Deep pulse and can be felt only with a very strong pressure at a very deep level near the bone.

Clinical significance

The clinical significance of the Hidden pulse is similar to that of the Deep pulse: it simply means that the condition is an interior one and its clinical significance depends on its association with other qualities, especially the Full or Empty ones.

However, the Hidden quality always indicates a 'blockage' in the Interior, especially when it is of the full type; 'blockage' in this case means that a pathogenic factor is lodged deep in the interior of the body. It is 'locked' inside and it is difficult to expel. For example, depending on its association with other qualities, the Hidden pulse could indicate 'blocked' stagnation of Qi, 'blocked' Blood stasis, 'blocked' Heat in the Interior, 'blocked' Cold, 'blocked' chronic pain, 'blocked' Phlegm and 'blocked' retention of food. The most important distinction to make is whether the Hidden pulse is of the full or empty type.

When the Hidden pulse is also of the empty type, it indicates severe Yang deficiency.

!

The Hidden pulse often indicates that a pathogenic factor is 'blocked' deep inside the body. Examples of such pathogenic factors are Qi stagnation, Blood stasis, Heat, Cold, Phlegm or retention of food.

Common conditions presenting with a Hidden pulse include digestive diseases, Blood stasis, abdominal masses, heart disease and vomiting.

According to Dr Shen, the Hidden pulse in apparently healthy people indicates a lifestyle of overindulging in drugs and sexual activity. He pinpoints the age to which this lifestyle refers according to the degree of the Hidden pulse: if the pulse is very Hidden it indicates that that lifestyle occurred between 10 and 15; if slightly less Hidden, between 15 and 20; if even less Hidden, over 20.

> **!**
>
> According to Dr Shen, the Hidden pulse in a seemingly healthy person may indicate overindulgence in drugs and excessive sexual activity in the past.

Box 50.21 summarizes the clinical significance of a Hidden pulse.

> **BOX 50.21 HIDDEN PULSE: SUMMARY OF CLINICAL MANIFESTATIONS**
>
> - Pathogenic factor (blockage) in the Interior (Hidden-Full)
> - Severe Yang deficiency (Hidden-Weak)

Combinations

Hidden-Full   This indicates Qi and Blood stagnation, retention of food or internal Cold or internal Heat according to whether the pulse is Slow or Rapid.

Hidden-Empty   This indicates severe Yang deficiency with internal Cold.

Hidden-Rapid   This indicates interior Heat, which may be Full- or Empty-Heat according to whether the pulse is full or empty.

Hidden-Slow   This indicates interior Cold.

Differentiation of similar pulses

Deep   The Deep and Hidden pulses are not significantly different because the Hidden pulse is simply an extreme case of Deep pulse.

Short   The Hidden pulse is very deep and difficult to feel but it occupies its normal pulse position, whereas the Short pulse does not fill its pulse position.

Clinical significance in each position (Li Shi Zhen)

Front position   This is seen in retention of food in the chest, stagnation of Qi, retching, and an uncomfortable sensation in the heart region.

Middle position   This is seen in abdominal pain, feeling of heaviness of the body, and weakness.

Rear position   This is seen in severe hernia pain.

Scattered

Pulse description

The Scattered pulse feels as if it were 'broken' into many tiny dots instead of flowing smoothly. It is relatively superficial but it disappears easily with pressure.

Clinical significance

The Scattered pulse indicates a severe and advanced stage of Qi and Blood deficiency and particularly of Kidney-Qi and of the Original Qi; it is a pulse that always indicates a serious condition.

In pregnancy, the Scattered pulse indicates the likelihood of an imminent miscarriage, while before delivery it indicates that the labour may be long and difficult. After childbirth it indicates severe depletion of Blood and the woman should be treated, even in the absence of symptoms, to prevent collapse of Blood.

Common conditions presenting with a Scattered pulse include heart disease, digestive disorders, miscarriage, and asthma.

Box 50.22 summarizes the clinical significance of a Scattered pulse.

> **BOX 50.22 SCATTERED PULSE: SUMMARY OF CLINICAL SIGNIFICANCE**
>
> - Severe Qi-Blood deficiency
> - Severe Kidney-Qi deficiency
> - Severe deficiency of Original Qi

Combinations

Scattered-Slow   This indicates severe Qi and Yang deficiency

Scattered-Rapid   This denotes severe Blood deficiency with Empty-Heat.

Scattered-Floating   This indicates severe deficiency of the Original Qi with floating of Yang or with Yin Fire.

Differentiation of similar pulses

Empty   The Empty pulse and the Scattered pulse share the characteristic of being relatively superficial and of disappearing when more pressure is applied. The Empty pulse has more shape and flows more smoothly than the Scattered pulse; although obviously

empty, the Empty pulse has much more 'body' than the Scattered pulse. In addition the Scattered pulse, unlike the Empty pulse, feels as if it were broken into tiny dots.

Choppy The Choppy pulse and the Scattered pulse share the characteristic of feeling 'rough' and not flowing smoothly. However, the Choppy pulse has more shape than the Scattered pulse.

Fine The Fine pulse is simply thinner than normal but it can be felt clearly and flows relatively smoothly, whereas the Scattered pulse does not flow smoothly and has no clear shape.

Minute The Minute pulse is extremely thin but can be felt clearly and flows relatively smoothly, whereas the Scattered pulse does not flow smoothly and has no clear shape.

Clinical significance in each position (Li Shi Zhen)

Front position In the left Front it denotes anxiety and palpitations; in the right Front it is found in sweating.

Middle position In the left Middle it denotes Phlegm-Fluids in the limbs, and in the right Middle twitching of legs and oedema.

Rear position This denotes decline of Original Qi.

FULL-TYPE PULSES

Wiry

Pulse description

The Wiry pulse feels superficial and hard: it can be felt very clearly at every level. At the superficial level it 'hits' the finger with its force. It is often compared with the taut string of a musical instrument and if we try to push it down, it 'springs' back up. This is a common pulse in clinical practice and one that is relatively easy to distinguish; because it is superficial, hard and springy, it manifests itself easily without the practitioner having to concentrate on interpreting it.

Clinical significance

The Wiry pulse is extremely common. The chief clinical significance of the Wiry pulse is that it indicates any of the Full type of Liver disharmonies (e.g. Liver-Qi stagnation, Liver-Blood stasis, Liver-Yang rising, Liver-Fire, Liver-Wind).

A Wiry pulse may also indicate the presence of chronic Phlegm and it is usually seen in old people. Finally the Wiry pulse may also indicate chronic pain, even if that pain does not derive from a Liver dishar-

mony; for example, if a patient has been suffering from chronic sciatica on the Bladder channel, the left Rear pulse position may become Wiry.

> **!**
>
> The Wiry pulse does not denote Liver disharmonies only: it may also indicate long-standing retention of Phlegm.

The Wiry pulse is of the full type by definition but it may be seen in Empty conditions as well combining with empty-type pulse qualities; for example, a relatively common clinical finding is that of a pulse that is Fine in general but also Wiry on the left in a patient suffering from Blood deficiency and Liver-Yang rising. A Wiry but relatively Weak pulse, or a pulse that is Wiry on the left and Weak on the right, indicates Stomach and Spleen deficiency with stagnation of Cold or rebellious Liver-Qi invading the Stomach; such patterns manifest with sour regurgitation, nausea, vomiting, epigastric pain, hiccup and belching.

It is normal for the pulse to be relatively Wiry in spring. The 'Simple Questions' in Chapter 19 says: *'Spring is the season of the Liver, it pertains to East and Wood. Everything grows during this season; when the Qi of the Spring arrives the pulse should be relatively soft, weak, light, slippery and long, all of which explain why it is called Wiry. The opposite of this indicates disease.'*[8]

Common conditions that present with a Wiry pulse are menstrual pain, premenstrual tension, depression, anxiety, chronic Phlegm, chronic pain and mental illness.

Box 50.23 summarizes the clinical significance of a Wiry pulse.

> **BOX 50.23 WIRY PULSE: SUMMARY OF CLINICAL MANIFESTATIONS**
>
> - Liver disharmony (Full type)
> - Phlegm
> - Chronic pain

Combinations

Wiry-Rapid This indicates Liver-Fire.

Wiry-Slow This indicates stagnation of Cold in the Liver channel or rebellious Liver-Qi invading the Stomach.

Wiry-Slippery This indicates the simultaneous presence of a Full Liver pattern and Phlegm: this is a relatively common pulse combination.

Wiry-Long This indicates stagnation of Liver-Qi or stasis of Liver-Blood.

Wiry-Deep This indicates chronic Phlegm.

Wiry-Fine This indicates a Full Liver pattern (often Liver-Yang or Liver-Wind) occurring against a background of Blood deficiency.

Wiry-Tight This indicates Blood stasis.

Wiry-Big This indicates Liver-Fire or Liver-Yang rising.

Wiry-Overflowing This denotes Liver-Fire.

Differentiation of similar pulses

Tight The Tight pulse and the Wiry pulse share the common characteristic of feeling hard under pressure and being 'springy'. The two main differences are that the Tight pulse is thicker than the Wiry pulse and feels like a rope rather than the string of a musical instrument, and that the Wiry pulse is more superficial than the Tight pulse and it hits the finger more forcefully.

Firm The Firm pulse can be felt only at the middle and deep levels and feels hard. The Wiry pulse also feels hard but it is more springy and can be felt clearly at the superficial level as well. In other words, the Firm pulse is a pulse that is Wiry but only at the middle and deep levels.

Leather The Leather pulse has a slightly Wiry quality on the surface but it disappears on pressure, whereas the Wiry pulse is Wiry at all levels and does not disappear on pressure. The Leather pulse, although hard on the superficial level like the Wiry pulse, feels more 'flat' on the superficial level than the Wiry pulse.

Clinical significance in each position (Li Shi Zhen)

Front position This occurs in headaches, Phlegm in chest and diaphragm.

Middle position In the left Middle it is seen in alternation of chills and fever, and abdominal masses; in the right Middle it denotes Cold in Stomach and Spleen, and chest and abdominal pain.

Rear position This denotes hernia pain and stiffness of the legs.

Tight

Pulse description

The Tight pulse is hard and feels like a rope being twisted; it is strong and has a springy feeling when the pressure is released, although not as springy as the Wiry pulse.

Clinical significance

In general the Tight pulse indicates Cold and can be found in many different conditions.

In external invasions of Wind, the Floating-Tight pulse indicates the invasion of Wind-Cold with the prevalence of Cold (Greater-Yang pattern – prevalence of Cold within the identification of patterns according to the Six Stages).

In internal conditions a Tight pulse indicates Cold and usually Full-Cold, although it can be combined with an empty type of pulse quality in conditions of Empty-Cold.

Like the Wiry pulse it may indicate chronic pain, usually from Cold. The Tight pulse is also frequently seen in asthma when this condition is associated with Cold in the Lungs.

The Tight pulse is also frequently seen in digestive disorders characterized by the presence of Cold or retention of food in the Stomach and Spleen, or both, with nausea, vomiting and diarrhoea.

The Tight pulse is frequently combined with a Slippery pulse in the presence of Cold-Phlegm.

The Tight pulse may also indicate Cold in the Blood.

Common conditions presenting with a Tight pulse include chronic pain, digestive disorders, invasion of Cold, menstrual pain, diarrhoea from Cold, asthma and arteriosclerosis.

Box 50.24 summarizes the clinical significance of a Tight pulse.

BOX 50.24 TIGHT PULSE: SUMMARY OF CLINICAL MANIFESTATIONS

- Internal Cold
- Invasion of external Wind-Cold
- Chronic pain
- Cold in the Blood

Combinations

Tight-Floating This indicates invasion of Wind-Cold with the prevalence of Cold.

Tight-Deep This indicates internal Full-Cold.

Tight-Full This indicates chronic pain from Cold.

Tight-Fine This denotes Empty-Cold occurring against a background of Stomach and Spleen deficiency.

Tight-Overflowing This indicates ulcers or carbuncles.

Tight-Choppy This is seen in chronic Painful Obstruction Syndrome from Cold.

Tight-Slippery   This denotes Cold Phlegm and is common in asthma.

Tight-Firm   This indicates Blood stasis from Cold.

Differentiation of similar pulses

Wiry   The Tight pulse and the Wiry pulse share the common characteristic of feeling hard pressure and being 'springy'. The two main differences are that the Tight pulse is thicker than the Wiry pulse and feels like a rope rather than the string of a musical instrument, and that the Wiry pulse is more superficial than the Tight pulse and it hits the finger more forcefully.

Firm   The Firm pulse is Full, Wiry and can be felt only at the middle and deep level. The Tight pulse can be felt at all levels. The Tight pulse feels more 'knotted' (like a rope) than the Firm pulse.

Clinical significance in each position (Li Shi Zhen)

Front position   There is a difference between left and right Front positions (Li Shi Zhen does not expand on this).

Middle position   This is seen in severe chest and abdominal pain.

Rear position   This denotes syndrome from excess Cold, Running Piglet syndrome, or hernia pain.

Overflowing

Pulse description

The Overflowing pulse feels large under the finger, very superficial and broad; as its name implies, it is often described as feeling like a river flooding its banks because the pulse goes beyond its natural boundary in all directions.

Clinical significance

The Overflowing pulse indicates Heat and it is nearly always rapid as well. Although the Overflowing pulse is full by definition, to interpret its clinical significance we need to distinguish an Overflowing pulse with strength from one without strength.

Although, according to the theory, an Overflowing pulse indicates Heat by definition, there are situations where it may be due to other causes, especially when it is found in only one position, and some of these are described below. For example, an Overflowing quality on the Heart pulse may indicate emotional problems, not necessarily manifesting with Heat. Therefore, when we feel an Overflowing pulse, it is important to check this against the tongue and the inside of the lower eyelids: in true conditions of Heat, the tongue will be Red and the inside of the lower eyelids will also be red.

Overflowing with strength

The Overflowing pulse with strength always indicates Full-Heat, which may affect the Liver, Heart, Lungs or Stomach; in this case it is also rapid.

In the course of an acute febrile disease, the Overflowing pulse with strength is seen with Heat in the Stomach at the Qi level. In this case the Overflowing quality indicates that the Heat is overflowing from the main channels into the Connecting channels; in such a case, if the pulse is very Overflowing and very rapid this indicates that the Heat is close to progressing to the Nutritive-Qi or Blood level and the possible development of macules. Thus, in the course of an acute febrile disease, an Overflowing quality often indicates that the condition is changing and progressing to the next level.

The Overflowing pulse quality is frequently felt in individual positions only and in such cases it usually indicates Heat in that particular organ. However, its clinical significance in such cases may be slightly different, often indicating severe emotional problems. For example, if the pulse is Overflowing only on the Heart position, this definitely indicates that the patient is suffering from severe emotional problems affecting the Heart. If the pulse is Overflowing only on the Liver position, it indicates that the person is suffering from repressed anger, resentment or frustration. If it is Overflowing on the Lung position it indicates that the patient is suffering from long-term unexpressed sadness and grief.

It is important to stress that, when the pulse is Overflowing only in one position, it may be 'Overflowing' only in relation to the other positions. For example, the pulse may be Weak in general and quite difficult to feel but the pulse of the Heart position stands out as being more superficial and larger than the others: we would therefore interpret this Heart pulse as being 'Overflowing' but it would not be as overflowing as the classic Overflowing pulse.

> **!**
>
> The Overflowing pulse on individual positions indicates either Heat in that particular organ (tongue Red and pulse Rapid) or severe emotional problems related to that particular organ (Heart, Liver, Lungs).

Overflowing without strength

The Overflowing pulse without strength feels large, superficial and flooding but it disappears when more pressure is applied and it has no strength at the deep level. Its strength indicates Yin deficiency with Empty-Heat and exhaustion of Body Fluids. In this respect, its clinical significance is the same as the Floating-Empty pulse but it indicates a more severe stage of it and more intense Empty-Heat.

The pulse may also be Overflowing without strength and Floating, which indicates a condition of severe Yin deficiency, intense Empty-Heat and Qi rising to the top.

According to Dr Shen, an Overflowing-Hollow pulse is frequently seen in hypertension and diabetes; in the former condition, the pulse is Overflowing and Hollow more in the Front and Middle positions, whereas in the latter more so in the Middle and Rear positions.

Common conditions that present with an Overflowing pulse include mental illness, febrile diseases and severe emotional problems.

Box 50.25 summarizes the clinical significance of an Overflowing pulse.

BOX 50.25 OVERFLOWING PULSE: SUMMARY OF CLINICAL SIGNIFICANCE

- Full-Heat (Overflowing with strength)
- Stomach-Heat pattern at Qi Level
- Heat in a particular organ
- Yin deficiency with Empty-Heat and exhaustion of Body Fluids (Overflowing without strength)

Combinations

Overflowing-Floating   This indicates invasion of Wind-Heat with intense Heat; this condition would progress very rapidly to the Qi level.

Overflowing-Floating without strength   This denotes severe Yin deficiency with Empty-Heat.

Overflowing-Deep   This indicates internal Heat.

Overflowing-Slippery   This indicates Phlegm-Heat with prevalence of Heat.

Overflowing-Soft   This indicates Yin deficiency with exhaustion of Body Fluids and Empty-Heat.

Overflowing-Tight   This indicates Chest Painful Obstruction Syndrome or blood in the stools with constipation.

Overflowing-Hollow-Rapid with strength   This indicates imminent bleeding.

Overflowing-Hollow-Weak   This indicates a previous haemorrhage.

Differentiation of similar pulses

Big   The Big pulse is very similar to the Overflowing pulse in so far as they are both superficial, large and beyond the pulse boundary. The Big pulse, however, is 'rounder' than the Overflowing pulse, has more shape and is not necessarily rapid.

Full   The Full pulse simply indicates that the pulse is full and relatively hard, whereas the Overflowing pulse is larger than its boundary, more superficial and relatively softer.

Long   The Long pulse extends beyond the pulse positions lengthwise and is not superficial. The Overflowing pulse extends beyond the pulse positions in all directions and is superficial.

Clinical significance in each position (Li Shi Zhen)

Front position   In the left Front this denotes Heart-Fire blazing upwards; in the right Front it is found in a feeling of heaviness in the chest.

Middle position   This indicates Liver-Yang rising, or Stomach and Spleen deficiency.

Rear position   This denotes exhaustion of Kidney-Essence, or deficiency of Yin with blazing Fire.

Big
Pulse description

The Big pulse is large, broad, overflowing from its boundary and full. It is very similar to the Overflowing pulse but it has more shape and is not necessarily rapid.

Clinical significance

The Big pulse generally indicates Heat and its clinical significance is similar to that of the Overflowing pulse. When we feel a Big pulse, it is important to check this against the tongue and the inside of the lower eyelids: in true conditions of Heat, the tongue will be Red and the inside of the lower eyelids will also be red. We need to differentiate the Big pulse with strength from the Big pulse without strength.

Big with strength

The Big pulse with strength indicates internal Heat which may occur in the Heart, Liver, Lungs or Stomach. In acute febrile diseases, it indicates Heat in the Stomach at the Qi level.

Common patterns presenting with a Big pulse with strength are acute febrile diseases at the Qi level, Liver-

Fire, Heart-Fire, Heat in the Intestines and Phlegm-Fire and these appear in conditions such as acute chest infections, intestinal infections or heart disease.

Big without strength

The Big pulse without strength indicates Yin deficiency with Empty-Heat or severe depletion of Blood. The 'Simple Questions' in Chapter 17 says: '*The Big pulse indicates deficiency of Yin and excess of Yang with Empty-Heat.*'[9]

Common patterns presenting with a Big pulse without strength are severe Blood deficiency, Yin deficiency with Empty-Heat and Blood deficiency with Liver-Yang rising. This pulse frequently appears in menstrual disorders and diabetes.

Box 50.26 summarizes the clinical significance of a Big pulse.

BOX 50.26 BIG PULSE: SUMMARY OF CLINICAL MANIFESTATIONS

- Full-Heat (Big with strength)
- Heat in the Stomach at Qi level (febrile disease)
- Yin deficiency with Empty-Heat (Big without strength)

Combinations

Big-Deep   This indicates internal Heat.
Big-Wiry   This indicates Liver-Fire.
Big-Soggy   This denotes Empty-Heat with Dampness.
Big-Overflowing   This indicates Stomach-Heat.
Big-Full   This indicates severe Qi stagnation.

Differentiation of similar pulses

Overflowing   The Big pulse is very similar to the Overflowing pulse in so far as they are both superficial, large and going beyond the pulse boundary. The Big pulse, however, is 'rounder' than the Overflowing pulse, has more shape and is not necessarily rapid.

Full   The Full pulse simply indicates that the pulse is full and relatively hard, whereas the Big pulse is larger than its boundary, more superficial and relatively softer.

Long   The Long pulse extends beyond the pulse positions lengthwise and is not superficial. The Big pulse extends beyond the pulse positions in all directions and is superficial.

Clinical significance in each position

This is the same as for the Overflowing pulse.

Firm

Pulse description

The Firm pulse is felt only at the deep level; it feels hard and it combines the qualities of Full, Wiry and Long. It is basically a pulse that is Wiry only at the middle and deep levels (the Wiry pulse can be felt clearly at all levels).

Clinical significance

The Firm pulse generally indicates internal Cold often causing chronic pain. It may also indicate accumulation in the Interior, stagnation of Qi or stasis of Blood. It is a pulse quality that is associated with abdominal masses or abdominal pain and it may also indicate Blood stasis deriving from Cold.

A pulse that is Firm on all three positions of the right or on both Middle positions of left and right indicates a pathology of the Penetrating Vessel.

The Firm pulse quality is relatively common.

Common conditions presenting with a Firm pulse include Chest Painful Obstruction Syndrome, convulsions, abdominal masses, abdominal pain, menstrual diseases, and arteriosclerosis.

Box 50.27 summarizes the clinical significance of a Firm pulse.

BOX 50.27 FIRM PULSE: SUMMARY OF CLINICAL SIGNIFICANCE

- Internal Cold
- Accumulation in the Interior
- Stagnation of Qi
- Blood stasis
- Stagnation in the Penetrating Vessel

Combinations

Firm-Tight   This indicates internal Cold possibly with oedema.
Firm-Slow   This indicates internal Cold and Blood stasis.
Firm-Choppy   This denotes Blood stasis.

Differentiation of similar pulses

Wiry   The Wiry pulse and the Firm pulse share similar characteristics of being hard, full and long. The main difference is that the Wiry pulse is felt clearly at all levels, whereas the Firm pulse is felt only at the middle and deep levels.

Tight   The Tight pulse and the Firm pulse share similar characteristics of being hard and full. The main difference is that the Tight pulse is felt clearly at all

levels, whereas the Firm pulse is felt only at the middle and deep levels.

Full   The Full pulse can be felt at all levels, whereas the Firm pulse can be felt only at the deep level.

Hidden   The Hidden pulse is sunken beneath the muscles near the bone and is very difficult to feel, whereas the Firm pulse can be felt clearly at the middle and deep levels.

Clinical significance in each position (Li Shi Zhen)

Not given by Li Shi Zhen.

Long
Pulse description

The Long pulse is simply longer than normal, that is, it extends lengthwise beyond the pulse boundary. In order to judge whether a pulse is Long, normal or Short, it is important to roll the finger back and forth (distally and proximally) on each position.

Clinical significance

The Long pulse usually indicates Heat. It may also indicate a Liver disharmony of the Full type with rebellious Qi (e.g. Liver-Yang rising or rebellious Qi in the Penetrating Vessel).

The Long pulse may also indicate Phlegm. The 'Simple Questions' in Chapter 18 says: *'If the Liver pulse is relatively soft and feels like the tip of a long bamboo pole, it indicates a harmonious state of the Liver . . . If the Liver pulse is Full and Slippery and feels like moving along a long bamboo pole, it indicates Liver disease.'*[10]

If the pulse is Long, relatively soft, Slowed-down, neither Floating nor Deep, neither Rapid nor Slow, neither Full nor Empty, it is a sign of health.

Common conditions that present with a Long pulse are Liver disease, hypochondrial pain, mental illness, rebellious Qi in the Penetrating vessel and haemoptysis.

According to Dr Shen, if the pulse is Long on one side and Short on the other, it indicates a serious problem. Usually the side displaying the Long quality is also Wiry, Fine and Rapid. For example, if the left-side pulse is Long-Wiry-Fine-Rapid and the right-side Short, this indicates that the person is extremely nervous and suffers from a Liver and Heart disharmony. If the right-side pulse is Long, Weak on the Lung position, Fine-Tight on the Middle and Rear positions and Short on the left side, it indicates a Stomach disharmony and general deficiency of Qi.

Box 50.28 summarizes the clinical significance of a Long pulse.

BOX 50.28 LONG PULSE: SUMMARY OF CLINICAL SIGNIFICANCE

- Heat
- Liver disharmony (Full type)
- Phlegm
- Health (relatively soft, Slowed-down, neither Floating nor Deep, neither Rapid nor Slow, neither Full nor Empty)

Combinations

Long-Rapid   This indicates internal Heat.

Long-Slow   This indicates stagnation of Qi.

Long-Floating   This indicates invasion of external Wind-Heat.

Long-Deep   This indicates internal Heat.

Long-Wiry   This indicates a Liver disharmony of the Full type.

Long-Slippery   This indicates Phlegm-Heat.

Long-Overflowing   This indicates excess of Yang and Heat.

Long-Firm   This indicates internal accumulation.

Long-Overflowing-Hollow   This may indicate hypertension or diabetes, according to Dr Shen.

Differentiation of similar pulses

Overflowing   The Long pulse extends beyond the pulse positions lengthwise and is not superficial. The Overflowing pulse extends beyond the pulse positions in all directions and is superficial.

Clinical significance in each position (Li Shi Zhen)

Not given by Li Shi Zhen.

Moving
Pulse description

The Moving pulse is short, Slippery, rapid and it gives the impression of 'shaking' or 'vibrating' instead of pulsating. It is shaped like a bean without head or tail. The Moving pulse is felt more frequently on the Front and Middle positions.

Clinical significance

The Moving pulse generally reflects severe emotional problems and particularly shock, fright or severe anxiety. In cases of shock, the pulse can remain Moving for years afterwards.

The Moving pulse may also indicate severe deficiency of Qi and Blood, often manifesting with cramps in the legs. The Moving pulse with strength may also indicate Qi stagnation.

Box 50.29 summarizes the clinical significance of a Moving pulse.

BOX 50.29 MOVING PULSE: SUMMARY OF CLINICAL SIGNIFICANCE

- Shock
- Severe deficiency of Qi and Blood
- Qi stagnation

Combinations

Moving-Rapid This indicates Heat occurring against a background of severe emotional problems.
Moving-Slippery This indicates severe deficiency of Qi and Phlegm.
Moving-Full This indicates chronic pain.
Moving-Empty This indicates severe depletion of Blood.
Moving-Weak This indicates shock.

Differentiation of similar pulses

Short: The Moving pulse is short by definition but in addition it is also rapid, shaped like a bean, somewhat Slippery and giving the impression of 'shaking' rather than pulsating.
Slippery The Moving pulse is Slippery by definition but in addition it is also Short, rapid, shaped like a bean, somewhat Slippery and giving the impression of 'shaking' rather than pulsating.

Clinical significance in each position (Li Shi Zhen)

Not given by Li Shi Zhen.

PULSES WITH IRREGULARITIES OF RATE OR RHYTHM

Knotted
Pulse description

The Knotted pulse quality refers to the rhythm of the pulse: it denotes a pulse that is Slow and that stops at irregular intervals.

Clinical significance

The Knotted pulse indicates internal Cold with stagnation of Qi and Blood and it always indicates a Heart disharmony (although, of course, the rate and rhythm of the pulse are the same in all positions). It is frequently seen in heart disease, such as coronary heart disease, angina pectoris, rheumatic heart disease, etc. A Knotted pulse can also come on after surgery. In young people, a Knotted pulse may indicate a constitutional deficiency of the Original Qi or a severe deficiency of Yang due to excessive physical work or excessive sexual activity during puberty.

We need to differentiate between the Knotted pulse with strength and the Knotted pulse without strength.

Knotted with strength

The Knotted pulse with strength may indicate several conditions as follows:

- severe Qi stagnation from Cold
- chronic Phlegm stagnating in the Interior in old people
- retention of food
- severe Qi stagnation from emotional problems
- Blood stasis
- abdominal masses.

Knotted without strength

The Knotted pulse without strength may indicate a constitutional deficiency of the Original Qi, a deficiency of Kidney-Essence, possibly from excessive sexual activity, or a severe deficiency of Yang.

Common conditions presenting with a Knotted pulse include heart disease, coronary heart disease, angina pectoris and rheumatic heart disease.

Box 50.30 summarizes the clinical significance of a Knotted pulse.

BOX 50.30 KNOTTED PULSE: SUMMARY OF CLINICAL SIGNIFICANCE

- Severe Qi stagnation from Cold
- Chronic Phlegm stagnating in the Interior (old people)
- Retention of food
- Severe Qi stagnation from emotional problems
- Blood stasis
- Deficiency of Original Qi (without strength)
- Deficiency of Kidney-Essence (without strength)
- Severe deficiency of Yang
- Heart disease

Combinations

Knotted-Choppy This indicates Blood stasis and may point to coronary heart disease.

Knotted-Slippery This indicates chronic retention of Phlegm and may point to rheumatic heart disease.
Knotted-Floating This indicates invasion of Cold in the Channels.
Knotted-Deep This indicates accumulation in the Interior.
Knotted-Wiry This indicates a disease of the arteries or hypertension.

Differentiation of similar pulses

Intermittent The Intermittent pulse stops at *regular* intervals and may be rapid, slow or of normal rate, whereas the Knotted pulse is always slow and stops at *irregular* intervals.
Slow The Slow pulse and the Knotted pulse are both slow but the Knotted pulse stops at irregular intervals.

Clinical significance in each position

This is not applicable as an abnormality in the speed or rate of the pulse will be the same in all positions.

Hasty
Pulse description

The Hasty pulse quality refers to the rhythm of the pulse: it denotes a pulse that is Rapid and stops at irregular intervals.

Clinical significance

The Hasty pulse indicates internal Heat and it is always related to a Heart disharmony (although, of course, the rate and rhythm of the pulse are the same in all positions). The Hasty pulse may also indicate retention of food or Phlegm occurring against a background of internal Heat, or stagnation of Qi or Blood.

The Hasty pulse without strength indicates severe depletion of the Original Qi and a separation of Yin and Yang; this always indicates a serious condition, more so than the Knotted pulse without strength.

The Hasty pulse may also indicate rebellious Qi from anger.

Common conditions which present with a Hasty pulse are mental illness, chronic bronchitis with Phlegm-Heat and heart disease.

Box 50.31 summarizes the clinical significance of a Hasty pulse.

Combinations

Hasty-Overflowing This indicates Heat in the Stomach.

> **BOX 50.31 HASTY PULSE: SUMMARY OF CLINICAL SIGNIFICANCE**
>
> - Heat
> - Retention of food with Heat
> - Phlegm with Heat
> - Severe stagnation of Qi and Blood
> - Severe depletion of Original Qi (without strength)
> - Separation of Yin and Yang
> - Rebellious Qi from anger

Hasty-Slippery This indicates long-standing retention of Phlegm-Heat.
Hasty-Wiry This indicates Liver-Fire and Heart-Fire.
Hasty-Slippery-Wiry This indicates Heart-Fire, Liver-Fire and Phlegm-Heat.
Hasty-Floating This indicates Heat in the Bright Yang.
Hasty-Fine without strength This indicates collapse of Heart-Qi.

Differentiation of similar pulses

Intermittent The Intermittent pulse stops at regular intervals and may be rapid, slow or of normal rate, whereas the Hasty pulse is always rapid and stops at irregular intervals.
Rapid The Rapid pulse and the Hasty pulse are both rapid but, whereas the Rapid pulse is regular, the Hasty pulse stops at irregular intervals.

Clinical significance in each position

This is not applicable as an abnormality in the speed or rate of the pulse will be the same in all positions.

Hurried
Pulse description

The Hurried pulse is rapid by definition, beating at least eight times for each breath cycle, and it gives the impression of being hurried, anxious, agitated and urgent.

Clinical significance

The Hurried pulse generally indicates severe deficiency of Yin with intense Empty-Heat; it always indicates a serious condition.

The Chinese name for this pulse quality, *Ji*, is the same as in *Li Ji*, that is, the symptomatology of rebellious Qi in the Penetrating Vessel. Literally, *Ji* means

'urgency' and in the context of this pathology, *Li Ji* indicates a feeling of energy rising from the abdomen to the throat, accompanied by a feeling of restlessness and anxiety. In severe cases of this pathology, the pulse could be Hurried.

Box 50.32 summarizes the clinical significance of a Hurried pulse.

BOX 50.32 HURRIED PULSE: SUMMARY OF CLINICAL SIGNIFICANCE

- Deficiency of Yin with Empty-Heat
- Severe rebellious Qi of the Penetrating Vessel

Combinations

Hurried-Floating   This indicates severe Empty-Heat arising from Yin deficiency.
Hurried-Deep   This indicates a condition of rebellious Qi in the Penetrating Vessel.
Hurried-Floating-Empty   This denotes severe Yin deficiency.
Hurried-Slippery   This indicates Empty-Heat from Yin deficiency with Phlegm.
Hurried-Overflowing   This indicates severe Empty-Heat arising from Yin deficiency.

Differentiation of similar pulses

Hasty   The Hasty pulse is Rapid and stops at irregular intervals. The Hurried pulse is more rapid than the Rapid pulse and it gives the impression of being agitated and urgent.
Rapid   The Hurried pulse is a form of the Rapid pulse. It differs from it in so far as it is more rapid and it conveys the impression of being extremely agitated, urgent and hurried.

Clinical significance in each position

This is not applicable as an abnormality in the speed or rate of the pulse will be the same in all positions.

Intermittent
Pulse description

The Intermittent pulse stops at regular intervals: it may be slow, rapid or of normal rate. After stopping, it gives the impression of taking a long time to start again. In order to establish whether or not a pulse is Intermittent, it is important to count the beats for a long time because it may stop only once in every 50 beats.

Clinical significance

The Intermittent pulse indicates always a Heart disharmony but also the severe depletion of other Yin organs. The 'Simple Questions' in Chapter 17 says: '*The Intermittent pulse indicates depletion of Qi.*'[11] The Intermittent pulse is seen most frequently in severe deficiency of Heart-Qi and Spleen-Qi.

The shorter the interval at which it stops, the greater the number of Yin organs are diseased. According to Chapter 5 of the 'Spiritual Axis', if the pulse halts every 50 beats, one Yin organ is diseased; if it halts every 40 beats, two Yin organs are diseased; if it halts every 30 beats, three Yin organs are diseased; if it halts every 20 beats, four Yin organs are diseased; and if it halts every 10 beats, all the Yin organs are diseased.[12] If the pulse stops regularly after less than 4 beats, this indicates a serious condition.

The Intermittent pulse may also indicate shock. Strangely, old Chinese books say that an Intermittent pulse at around a hundred days of pregnancy is normal.

Common conditions which present with an Intermittent pulse include heart disease, Chest Painful Obstruction Syndrome and some menstrual disorders.

Box 50.33 summarizes the clinical significance of an Intermittent pulse.

BOX 50.33 INTERMITTENT PULSE: SUMMARY OF CLINICAL SIGNIFICANCE

- Heart disharmony
- Shock
- Disease in Yin organs

Combinations

Intermittent-Slow   This indicates exhaustion of the Original Qi.
Intermittent-Rapid   This indicates internal Heat occurring against a background of a Heart disharmony.
Intermittent-Overflowing   This indicates the location of the disease in the Connecting channels.
Intermittent-Fine-Deep   This denotes severe Spleen-Qi deficiency, possibly with chronic diarrhoea.
Intermittent-Fine-Minute   This indicates exhaustion of Body Fluids.
Intermittent-Knotted   This indicates heart disease occurring against a background of Heart-Yang deficiency.

Differentiation of similar pulses

Knotted The Knotted pulse is slow and stops at irregular intervals, whereas the Intermittent pulse may be slow, rapid or of normal rate and stops at regular intervals.

Hasty The Hasty pulse is rapid and stops at irregular intervals, whereas the Intermittent pulse may be slow, rapid or of normal rate and stops at regular intervals.

Clinical significance in each position

This is not applicable as an abnormality in the speed or rate of the pulse will be the same in all positions.

Slowed-Down
Pulse description

The Slowed-Down pulse has four beats per breath cycle: it is therefore neither rapid nor slow.

Clinical significance

If the patient has no symptoms and the pulse is neither Floating nor Deep and neither Full nor Empty, the Slowed-Down pulse indicates health. In fact, the Slowed-Down quality indicates the presence of Stomach-Qi, which is one of the three attributes of the normal pulse, as described above.

In pathological conditions, when combined with other pulse qualities, it usually indicates Dampness occurring against a background of Stomach and Spleen deficiency.

Common conditions which present with a Slowed-Down pulse include stroke with Phlegm, Wind Painful Obstruction Syndrome, vomiting and hiatus hernia.

Box 50.34 summarizes the clinical significance of a Slowed-Down pulse.

BOX 50.34 SLOWED-DOWN PULSE: SUMMARY OF CLINICAL SIGNIFICANCE

- Dampness with Stomach- and Spleen-Qi deficiency
- Health (if neither Floating nor Deep and neither Full nor Empty)

Combinations

Slowed-Down-Soggy This indicates Dampness with Spleen-Qi deficiency.

Slowed-Down-Slippery This indicates Cold-Dampness.

Slowed-Down-Fine This indicates deficiency of Qi and Blood.

Slowed-Down-Floating This indicates weakness of the Defensive Qi.

Slowed-Down-Deep This indicates weakness of the Nutritive Qi.

Slowed-Down-Choppy This indicates Blood deficiency.

Slowed-Down-Big without strength This indicates Yin deficiency.

Differentiation of similar pulses

Slow The Slow pulse beats three times or less per breath cycle, while the Slowed-Down pulse beats four times per breath cycle.

Clinical significance in each position

This is not applicable as an abnormality in the speed or rate of the pulse will be the same in all positions.

THREE NON-TRADITIONAL PULSE QUALITIES

Irregular
Pulse description

The Irregular pulse stops at irregular intervals but it is neither Slow nor Rapid. The traditional pulse qualities of Knotted and Hasty also describe an irregular pulse but only when it is Slow or Rapid respectively. In order to decide whether the pulse is Irregular, it is necessary to feel it for a long time because the pulse may stop only after many beats. Furthermore, it would be advisable not to diagnose an Irregular pulse during the first consultation because the pulse may become Irregular only for a definite time; this happens when the patient has had a shock or has suffered emotional stress.

Clinical significance

An Irregular pulse always indicates a Heart disharmony, which may be Deficiency such as Heart-Qi or Heart-Blood deficiency or Excess such as Heart-Blood stasis. As mentioned above, a pulse may be Irregular only for a certain time when the patient has suffered a shock or a deep emotional upset. Conversely, a person with an Irregular pulse is easily frightened and is prone to suffer from shock.

A person with an Irregular pulse should not work overlong hours, should not lift heavy things and should abstain from excessive sexual activity (especially if male).

Box 30.35 summarizes the clinical significance of an Irregular pulse.

> **!**
>
> A person with an Irregular pulse should not work too long hours, should not do heavy lifting and should abstain from excessive sexual activity.

BOX 50.35 IRREGULAR PULSE: SUMMARY OF CLINICAL SIGNIFICANCE

- Heart-Qi deficiency
- Heart-Blood deficiency
- Heart-Blood stasis
- Shock

Combinations

Irregular-Floating   This indicates severe Heart-Qi deficiency from overwork.
Irregular-Deep   This denotes Heart-Blood stasis.
Irregular-Full   This also denotes Heart-Blood stasis.
Irregular-Empty   This indicates severe Heart-Qi deficiency.
Irregular-Choppy   This indicates severe Heart-Blood deficiency.
Irregular-Slippery   This indicates Heart-Qi deficiency with Phlegm.

Differentiation of similar pulses

Intermittent   The Intermittent pulse stops at regular intervals, whereas the Irregular pulse stops at irregular intervals.
Knotted   The Knotted pulse is a form of Irregular pulse in so far as it stops at irregular intervals but it is Slow. Unlike the Knotted pulse, the Irregular pulse has a normal rate.
Hasty   The Hasty pulse is a form of Irregular pulse in so far as it stops at irregular intervals but it is Rapid. Unlike the Hasty pulse, the Irregular pulse has a normal rate.

Clinical significance in each position

This is not applicable as an abnormality in the speed or rate of the pulse will be the same in all positions.

Stagnant
Pulse description

The Stagnant pulse feels reluctant to come, as if being suppressed, and seems unlikely to last; it does not flow smoothly and does not have a 'wave'.

Clinical significance

The Stagnant pulse nearly always indicates deep emotional problems, pent-up feelings, resentment and depression. It also appears when the patient is on certain drugs and especially tranquillizers.

Box 50.36 summarizes the clinical significance of a Stagnant pulse.

BOX 50.36 STAGNANT PULSE: SUMMARY OF CLINICAL SIGNIFICANCE

- Deep emotional problems
- Pent-up feelings
- Resentment
- Drugs especially tranquillizers

Combinations

Stagnant-Weak   This indicates severe emotional problems occurring against a background of Qi and Blood deficiency.
Stagnant-Choppy   This indicates severe emotional problems occurring against a background of Heart-Blood deficiency; the patient is usually very depressed.
Stagnant-Full   This indicates pent-up emotions, bottled-up resentment and depression occurring against a background of Liver-Qi stagnation.

Differentiation of similar pulses

Choppy   The Choppy pulse lacks a 'wave' and is weak and empty by definition. The Stagnant pulse also lacks a 'wave' but in addition it feels reluctant to come and suppressed.
Sad   The Sad pulse, like the Stagnant pulse, lacks a 'wave' but it is also Short, which the Stagnant pulse is not.

Clinical significance in each position

Front position   This denotes Heart- and/or Lung-Qi stagnation from sadness, grief or depression.
Middle position   This denotes Liver-Qi stagnation from pent-up anger or resentment, or tranquillizers.
Rear position   This denotes Qi stagnation in the Intestines.

Sad
Pulse description

The Sad pulse does not flow smoothly and lacks a wave and is also Short and rather weak. It is found either in all positions or, if in individual positions, only in the

Front or Middle positions; in other words, the pulse can never have a Sad quality only on the Rear position. (See Fig. 50.1 on p. 477.)

Clinical significance

The Sad pulse always indicates emotional problems, especially from sadness and grief; it is a pulse that is frequently seen in bereaved patients. One can gauge roughly the duration of the emotional problem according to how many positions are affected. If the pulse is Sad only on the Front position, the problem is recent (about 6 months in duration); if it is Sad on the Front and Middle positions the problem is of about a year's duration; if it is Sad all over, this indicates the patient has been sad for a very long time, possibly the whole life.

If the person suffering from the above emotional problems has a good constitution, the pulse will display only the Sad quality and no others; if the person has a weak constitution, emotional problems will eventually affect one or more organs and this will be reflected in the relevant pulse positions (e.g. Weak Lung pulse, Weak Stomach pulse, Wiry Liver pulse, etc.).

Box 50.37 summarizes the clinical significance of a Sad pulse.

BOX 50.37 SAD PULSE: SUMMARY OF CLINICAL SIGNIFICANCE

- Emotional problems from sadness or grief

Combinations

Sad-Full   This indicates emotional problems from grief affecting the Lungs.
Sad-Empty   This indicates emotional problems from sadness affecting particularly the Heart.
Sad-Rapid   This indicates emotional problems from grief and worry.
Sad-Slow   This indicates emotional problems from deep sadness affecting the Heart.
Sad-Choppy   This denotes Heart-Blood deficiency deriving from sadness.
Sad-Fine   This denotes Heart-Blood deficiency deriving from sadness.

Differentiation of similar pulses

Choppy   The Choppy pulse, like the Sad pulse, lacks a 'wave' but it is also weak and empty by definition. The Sad pulse is not necessarily weak or empty and it is also Short.

Clinical significance in each position

Front position   This denotes Heart- or Lung-Qi deficiency, or both, from recent sadness (about 2 years' duration).
Middle position   This denotes Liver- and Heart-Blood deficiency from long-term sadness. The pulse cannot have the Sad quality in the Middle position only so that, in this case, it will have this quality in the Middle and Front positions.
Rear position   A pulse does not usually have a Sad quality in the Rear position.

CLASSIFICATION OF PULSE QUALITIES

Pulse qualities can be classified in various ways, each of which helps to shed more light on their nature.

The eight basic groups of pulse qualities

Floating pulses

Floating – Hollow – Leather – Soggy – Overflowing

Deep pulses

Deep – Hidden – Firm

Slow pulses

Slow – Knotted

Rapid pulses

Rapid – Hasty – Hurried – Overflowing – Moving

Slippery pulses

Slippery – Soggy – Moving

Choppy pulses

Choppy – Scattered

Empty pulses

Empty – Weak – Soggy – Fine – Minute – Scattered – Short – Choppy

Full pulses

Full – Wiry – Tight – Big – Overflowing – Long

Of course, the same pulse quality may appear in more than one category according to different aspects, for example Overflowing appears in the Floating and the Full categories.

The different aspects for the classification of pulse qualities

It may help us to understand the nature of pulse qualities if we realize that they reflect different aspects of the pulse; for example, Slow and Rapid clearly refer to an irregularity of the rate of the pulse, whereas Knotted, Hasty and Intermittent refer to an irregularity of the rhythm.

According to depth

Floating – Deep – Hidden – Firm – Leather

According to rate

Slow – Rapid – Slowed-down – Hurried – Moving

According to strength

Empty – Full – Weak – Scattered

According to size

Big – Overflowing – Fine – Minute

According to length

Long – Short – Moving

According to shape

Slippery – Choppy – Wiry – Tight – Moving – Hollow – Firm

According to rhythm

Knotted – Hasty – Intermittent

Of course, some pulse qualities escape such classification because they are defined according to more than one aspect. The following pulse qualities are good examples:

- The Soggy pulse is defined according to depth (it is floating), size (it is thin) and strength (it is soft).
- The Leather pulse is defined according to strength (it is empty at the deep level) and depth (it is relatively superficial).
- The Firm pulse is defined according to depth (it is deep), strength (it is full) and shape (it is wiry).
- The Scattered pulse is defined according to strength (it is weak), depth (it is relatively floating) and shape (it is 'broken up').

Classification of pulse qualities according to Qi, Blood and Body Fluids patterns

Having discussed the pulse qualities and their clinical significance one by one, it may be helpful to summarize them by grouping them according to the main patterns.

Qi deficiency

Empty – Short – Scattered

Yang deficiency

Deep – Weak – Hidden

Blood deficiency

Choppy – Fine – Scattered

Yin deficiency

Fine – Minute – Leather

Qi stagnation

Wiry

Blood stasis

Wiry – Choppy – Slippery – Firm

Phlegm

Slippery – Wiry

Dampness

Soggy – Slippery

Classification of pulse qualities according to the Eight Principles

Yin–Yang

Yang deficiency Weak, Slow, Deep
Yin deficiency Fine, Minute, Floating-Empty, Leather
Collapse of Yang Hidden, Slow, Scattered
Collapse of Yin Minute, Rapid

Exterior–Interior

Exterior Floating

- Cold: Floating-Tight
- Heat: Floating-Rapid
- Deficient: Floating-Slow-Weak
- Excess: Floating-Full-Tight

Interior   Deep

- Cold: Deep-Slow
- Heat: Deep-Rapid
- Deficient: Deep-Weak
- Excess: Deep-Full

Heat–Cold

Heat   Rapid, Hasty, Hurried, Big, Overflowing
Cold   Slow, Knotted, Tight

Deficiency–Excess

Deficiency   Empty, Weak, Choppy, Fine, Minute, Soggy, Short, Hollow, Leather, Hidden, Scattered:

- deficiency of Qi: Empty, Soggy
- deficiency of Yang: Weak, Hidden
- deficiency of Blood: Choppy, Fine
- deficiency of Yin: Fine, Minute, Leather, Floating-Empty

Excess   Full, Slippery, Wiry, Tight, Overflowing, Big, Firm, Long:

- stagnation of Qi: Wiry
- Blood stasis: Wiry, Choppy, Firm, Slippery

Classification of pulse qualities according to the Six Stages patterns

This is illustrated in Table 50.2.

Classification of pulse qualities according to the Four Levels patterns

This is illustrated in Table 50.3

Table 50.3 Pulses of the Four Levels Patterns		
Defensive Qi	Wind-Heat	Floating-Rapid
	Damp-Heat	Soggy-Slow
	Dry-Heat	Floating-Rapid
	Summer-Heat	Soggy-Rapid
Qi	Lung-Heat	Slippery-Rapid
	Stomach-Heat	Overflowing-Rapid
	Intestines Dry-Heat	Deep-Full-Rapid
	Gall-Bladder-Heat	Wiry-Rapid
	Damp-Heat in Stomach and Spleen	Soggy-Rapid
Nutritive Qi	Heat in Nutritive-Qi Level	Fine-Rapid
	Heat in Pericardium	Fine-Rapid
Blood	Heat Victorious moving Blood	Wiry-Rapid
	Heat Victorious stirring Wind	Wiry-Rapid
	Empty Wind agitating in the Interior	Fine-Rapid
	Collapse of Yin	Minute-Rapid
	Collapse of Yang	Hidden-Slow-Scattered

Classification of pulse qualities according to the Triple Burner patterns

This is illustrated in Table 50.4

TERMINOLOGY

In order to facilitate cross-reference with other authors, Table 50.5 indicates the terminology of pulse qualities used by myself and six authors.

Table 50.2 Pulses of the Six Stages Patterns			
Greater Yang	Channel	Prevalence of Cold	Floating-Tight
		Prevalence of Wind	Floating-Slow
	Organ	Accumulation of Water	Floating-Rapid
		Accumulation of Blood	Deep-Fine-Rapid
Bright Yang	Channel	Overflowing-Rapid	
	Organ	Deep-Full-Slippery-Rapid	
Lesser Yang	Wiry		
Greater Yin	Deep-Weak-Slow		
Lesser Yin	Cold transformation	Deep-Weak-Slow	
	Heat transformation	Fine-Rapid	
Terminal Yin	Wiry		

Table 50.4 Pulses of the Triple Burner Patterns

Upper Burner	Wind-Heat in the Lung Defensive-Qi portion	Floating-Rapid
	Heat in the Lungs (Qi level)	Rapid-Overflowing
	Heat in the Pericardium (Nutritive-Qi level)	Fine-Rapid
Middle Burner	Heat in Bright Yang	Overflowing-Rapid
	Damp-Heat in the Spleen	Soggy-Rapid
Lower Burner	Heat in the Kidneys	Floating-Empty and Rapid
	Liver-Heat stirs Wind	Wiry-Fine-Rapid
	Liver-Empty Wind	Deep-Fine-Rapid

THE PULSE POSITIONS IN DETAIL

I shall now discuss the various pulse qualities appearing at each pulse position and their clinical significance. This information is derived primarily from Dr J. H. F. Shen and secondarily from my own experience. As indicated above, Dr Shen places the Large Intestine on the left and the Small Intestine on the right Rear position: most other authors reverse this.

Table 50.5 Pulse terminology of different authors

Maciocia	Seifert[a]	Kaptchuk[b]	Yang[c]	Cheng[d]	Flaws[e]	Wiseman[f]
Floating	Floating	Floating	Floating	Superficial	Floating	Floating
Deep	Deep	Sinking	Deep	Deep	Sunken	Deep
Slow	Slow	Slow	Slow	Slow	Slow	Slow
Rapid	Rapid	Rapid	Rapid	Rapid	Rapid	Rapid
Empty	Empty	Empty	Vacuous	Deficiency type	Vacuous	Vacuous
Full	Full	Full	Replete	Excess type	Replete	Replete
Slippery	Slippery	Slippery	Slippery	Rolling	Slippery	Slippery
Choppy	Choppy	Choppy	Choppy	Hesitant	Choppy	Rough
Weak	Weak	Frail	Weak	Weak	Weak	
Fine	Thin	Thin	Fine	Thready	Fine	Thin
Minute	Minute	Minute	Faint		Faint	
Soggy	Soft	Soggy	Soft	Soft	Soggy	Soggy
Short	Short	Short			Short	Short
Hollow	Hollow	Hollow	Scallion-stalk		Scallion-stalk	
Leather	Leather	Leather	Drumskin		Drumskin	
Hidden	Hidden	Hidden	Hidden		Deep-lying	
Scattered	Scattered	Scattered	Dissipated		Scattered	
Wiry	Stringy	Wiry	Bowstring	String-taut	Bowstring	Wiry
Tight	Tight	Tight	Tight	Tense	Tight	
Overflowing	Flooding	Flooding	Surging	Surging	Surging	Surging
Big		Big				
Firm	Firm	Confined			Confined	
Long	Long	Long			Long	Long
Moving	Moving	Moving	Stirring		Stirring	
Knotted	Knotted	Knotted	Bound	Knotted	Bound	Slow-irregularly interrupted
Hasty	Hasty		Skipping	Abrupt	Skipping	Rapid-irregularly interrupted
Hurried		Hurried				
Intermittent	Intermittent	Intermittent	Interrupted	Regularly intermittent	Regularly interrupted	Regularly interrupted
Slowed-down	Retarded	Moderate	Moderate		Moderate	

a Garry Seifert 1985 'Li Shi Zhen Pulse Diagnosis', published by Garry Seifert, Haymarket, NSW, Australia.
b Ted Kaptchuk 1983 'The Web that has no Weaver', Congdon and Weed, NY.
c Yang Shou Zhong (translator) 1997 'The Pulse Classic' (*Mai Jing*), Blue Poppy Press, Boulder, CO, USA.
d Cheng Xin Nong 1987 'Chinese Acupuncture and Moxibustion', Foreign Languages Press, Beijing.
e B. Flaws (translator) 1998 'The Lakeside Master's Study of the Pulse' by Li Shi Zhen, Blue Poppy Press, Boulder, CO, USA.
f N. Wiseman and A. Ellis (translators) 1985 'Fundamentals of Chinese Medicine', Paradigm Publications, Brookline, MA, USA.

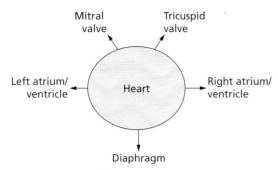

Fig. 50.2 Structure of left Front pulse position

Left Front position (Heart)

The structure of the left Front position is illustrated in Figure 50.2.

The left Front position corresponds to the Heart and Pericardium, or to the Heart and Small Intestine in the Five-Element arrangement of the pulses.

Emotional stress frequently causes abnormal qualities at this position and I shall discuss the most frequent qualities one by one. This discussion assumes that a particular pulse position has a quality that is different from the rest of the pulse. For example, the discussion of the Overflowing quality on the left Front position applies if such quality is found only at this position; if all the pulse positions were Overflowing, the interpretation would of course be different.

Overflowing

I very frequently encounter an Overflowing quality at this position when the person is affected by deep emotional problems causing anxiety and worry; more often than not, these problems are due to relationship difficulties. It is important to stress that the pulse quality may be 'Overflowing' at this position only in relation to the rest of the pulse and, when it is so, it 'stands out' and attracts our attention; thus, if all the other pulse positions are quite weak and the pulse on the Heart position is much stronger and more superficial, we may classify this as being 'Overflowing' although the same quality in a person with strong pulses would be normal. It is essential that a relatively Overflowing quality on this position when the rest of the positions are very weak is not interpreted as being normal: when that particular position stands out and is out of tune with the rest of the pulse, it usually indicates where the main problem lies.

The Overflowing quality on the Heart position also indicates that, as a consequence of deep emotional stress, Qi rebels upwards towards the chest and face

and the patient would experience a feeling of heat in the face, a sense of constriction of the throat and a feeling of energy rising to the head.

Short

A Short quality on the Heart position also indicates emotional problems usually deriving from sadness and grief. The Short pulse lacks a 'wave', that is, it does not flow smoothly with a wave-like movement towards the wrist; Dr Shen calls this pulse 'Sad pulse' as it is nearly always due to this emotion. I frequently see this pulse in people who are sad from being lonely and who crave love and affection; this pulse is also seen in people who tend to hide their emotions.

If both Heart and Lung positions feel Short, this can be due to two causes: either it is due to sadness as above, or to an accident to the chest. To differentiate these two conditions one must refer to the other aspects of diagnosis; for example, in a case of sadness, the eyes might lack spirit (*shen*), the tongue might be Red on the tip or have a Heart crack and the complexion might be pale.

Weak

A Weak position on the Heart pulse often indicates a functional weakness of the heart and circulation rather than emotional problems, although the two conditions may of course occur simultaneously. Thus, a Weak pulse on the left Front position often indicates Heart-Qi, Heart-Yang or Heart-Blood deficiency and the patient would suffer from cold hands, tiredness, slight breathlessness, slight depression and palpitations. If the Heart position is very Weak while the other pulses are not Weak and there is a Heart crack on the tongue, these signs indicate a constitutional weakness of the Heart.

Floating

A pulse that is Floating in one position only is not so floating as the Floating pulse seen in external invasions of Wind. When the pulse is Floating only in one position (that is not the Lung position), it does not indicate an exterior invasion of Wind but a pathology of that particular organ. In mild invasions of external Wind, the pulse may be Floating only on the Lung position.

A Floating quality on the Heart pulse often indicates a problem with the heart itself. For example, a Floating-Hollow quality felt on the lateral and medial side of the pulse position may indicate high blood pressure. A Floating-Weak-Hollow quality indicates that

the heart is dilated; this occurs often in people who jog for long distances every day. A Floating-Tight-Hollow quality may indicate hardening of the arteries.

Slippery

A Slippery quality on the Heart position, especially on its medial and lateral sides, often indicates heart disease; in such a case, the pulse on the heart position is often Deep, Fine and Slippery.

Hollow

If the whole pulse is Hollow this of course indicates loss of blood, but the significance is different if only the Heart position is Hollow. In such a case, it usually denotes that the heart is permanently dilated or enlarged, often from excessive jogging. If the pulse feels Hollow and Overflowing with strength on the distal or proximal side of the Heart position, this may indicate arteriosclerosis, stroke or high blood pressure.

Choppy

A Choppy quality on the Heart position indicates Heart-Blood deficiency often deriving from emotional problems such as sadness. If both the Heart and Liver positions are Choppy, this indicates general deficiency of Blood which may derive from other than emotional causes (such as overwork or childbirth).

Wiry

A Wiry quality on the Heart position usually indicates stagnation in the chest. If the pulse is Wiry and strong,

it indicates stagnation of Qi in the chest with the patient most probably suffering from chest pain. If it is Wiry but Fine and Rapid, this may indicate that the heart has been affected by shock. If both the Heart and Lung positions are Wiry with strength, this may indicate stagnation of Qi in the chest, probably due to a previous accident or blow to the chest.

Box 50.38 summarizes the left Front pulse position.

Left Middle position (Liver)

The structure of the left Middle position is illustrated in Figure 50.3.

The left Middle position corresponds to the Liver and Gall-Bladder and there is little disagreement on this by various authors.

Floating

A Floating quality on this position is quite common and it usually indicates Liver-Yang rising or Liver-Qi rebelling horizontally. Of course, this assumes that the pulse is Floating only in this position and not Floating in general and that there are not symptoms and signs of an exterior invasion of Wind.

If the pulse feels Floating and Wiry on the Liver position, this indicates Liver-Yang rising; if it is Floating but Weak and slightly Hollow, it indicates stagnation of Liver-Qi in the epigastrium and hypochondrium.

Deep

If the pulse on the Liver position is Deep and Slippery, this indicates Phlegm affecting the Liver and Gall-Bladder. If it is Deep, Wiry and Slippery, it indicates Gall-Bladder disease. If it is Deep and Weak, it indicates Liver-Blood deficiency.

Slippery

A Slippery quality on the Liver pulse indicates poor liver function due to affliction from Phlegm. If the pulse is Slippery on the proximal side of the pulse

---

BOX 50.38 LEFT-FRONT POSITION (HEART)

- Overflowing: Deep emotional problems (anxiety, worry), Qi rebelling upwards
- Short: sadness or grief, accident to chest
- Weak: functional weakness of the heart and circulation, Heart-Qi, Heart-Yang or Heart-Blood deficiency
- Floating: possibly a heart problem, high blood pressure (Floating-Hollow on lateral and medial side), heart dilated (Floating-Weak-Hollow), hardening of arteries (Floating-Tight-Hollow)
- Slippery: heart disease (Slippery on medial and lateral sides)
- Hollow: heart dilated, usually from excessive jogging, (Hollow-Overflowing) hardening of arteries, stroke, high blood pressure
- Choppy: Heart-Blood deficiency usually from sadness, general Blood deficiency
- Wiry: stagnation of Qi in the chest, shock (Wiry-Fine-Rapid), accident to the chest (both Heart and Lung positions Wiry)

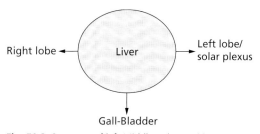

Right lobe ← Liver → Left lobe/ solar plexus

Gall-Bladder

Fig. 50.3 Structure of left Middle pulse position

position, this indicates Dampness in the Gall-Bladder. If it is Slippery and Wiry on the proximal side, it may indicate the presence of gall-bladder stones (in which case there may also be small blood spots on the sclera of the eyes).

Overflowing

An Overflowing quality on the Liver position indicates Liver-Yang rising or Liver-Fire blazing.

Wiry

A Wiry quality on the Liver position is very common as this quality is indicative of Liver disharmonies. If it is Wiry but also 'stagnant', (i.e. without a wave but strong), this indicates repressed anger.

If both left and right Middle positions are Wiry it indicates rebellious Liver-Qi invading the Stomach.

Box 50.39 summarizes the left Middle pulse position.

BOX 50.39 LEFT MIDDLE POSITION (LIVER)

- Floating: Liver-Yang rising or Liver-Qi rebelling horizontally, stagnation of Liver-Qi (Floating-Weak and slightly Hollow)
- Deep: Phlegm in Liver and Gall-Bladder, Gall-Bladder disease (Deep-Wiry-Slippery), Liver-Blood deficiency (Deep-Weak)
- Slippery: Liver affected by Phlegm, Dampness in the Gall-Bladder (Slippery on the proximal side), gall-bladder stones (Slippery-Wiry on the proximal side)
- Overflowing: Liver-Yang rising or Liver-Fire blazing
- Wiry: Liver disharmony, repressed anger (Wiry-Stagnant), Liver-Qi invading the Stomach (both Middle positions Wiry)

Left Rear position (Kidney)

The structure of the left Rear position is illustrated in Figure 50.4. The left Rear position reflects the state of the Kidneys, Large Intestine, Bladder and Uterus.

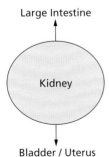

Large Intestine

Kidney

Bladder / Uterus

Fig. 50.4 Structure of left Rear pulse position

Floating

A Floating quality with strength usually relates to Large Intestine problems, whereas a Floating quality without strength usually reflects Kidney problems.

A Floating, Fine, Wiry and Rapid quality on the left Rear position indicates stagnation in the Large Intestines with Damp-Heat. A Floating, Weak quality indicates weak Kidneys. In a woman, a Floating-Wiry quality here indicates Blood-Heat in the Uterus. A Floating-Rapid quality on the left Kidney position in a pregnant woman indicates the danger of miscarriage.

Deep

A Deep quality here usually indicates Kidney deficiency and especially Kidney-Yang deficiency; it is an extremely common quality at the Kidney position, especially after the age of 40, and is more often met in women. Two factors should be taken into account when judging whether this position is Deep or not: first, it is normal for this position to be deeper than the Front and Middle ones, and secondly, it is normal for this position to be somewhat deeper in winter.

A Deep, Fine and Weak quality on the left Kidney position indicates a severe deficiency of the Kidneys; if, in addition, it is also Slow, this indicates a severe deficiency of Kidney-Yang.

If the pulse is Deep, Full and Slippery on the distal side, this indicates Dampness in the Large Intestine. If it is Deep, Weak and Slippery in the same position, it indicates weak Large Intestine-Qi and diarrhoea.

Slippery

A Slippery quality on the Kidney position usually indicates retention of Dampness in the Kidneys and Bladder. According to Dr Shen, a Slippery pulse in this position in men may indicate the tendency to have frequent nocturnal emissions.

If the pulse is Slippery, Deep and Full on the distal side (Large Intestine), this indicates Dampness in the Large Intestine and possibly diarrhoea; if it is Slippery, Deep and Weak, it indicates weak Large Intestine-Qi and possibly diarrhoea.

If the pulse is Slippery on the proximal side (Uterus), this indicates pregnancy if the Heart pulse is strong and amenorrhoea if the Heart pulse is weak.

Weak

A Weak quality on the left Kidney position is extremely common in both men and women, especially after 40, and it indicates a Kidney deficiency. In men it may be

due to excessive sexual activity, whereas in women it may be due to having had too many children too close together, to menorrhagia, or to hysterectomy; in both men and women it is often due to overwork.

If the left Kidney pulse is Weak and Intermittent this indicates a deficiency of the Kidneys and the Original Qi; it may be due to excessive sexual activity (or indeed any level of sexual activity) before puberty.

Fine

A Fine pulse on the Kidney position indicates deficiency of the Original Qi and Essence; in men, this may be due to excessive sexual activity (including masturbation).

If this pulse is Fine, Hidden and Wiry, it indicates inflammation in the Large Intestine.

Overflowing

An Overflowing quality here is usually related to the Intestines rather than the Kidneys: it indicates Heat in the Large Intestine. If it is Overflowing on both left and right Kidney positions, this may indicate prostatic hypertrophy.

Hollow

A Hollow quality on the Kidney position is usually seen in diabetes when the patient has been on insulin for many years.

Box 50.40 summarizes the left Rear pulse position.

Right Front position (Lungs)

The structure of the right Front position is illustrated in Figure 50.5.

The right Front position reflects the state of the Lungs. It should be remembered that the Lung pulse is naturally quite soft and this should be taken into account when identifying a particular pathological quality especially the full-type ones: in other words, a Tight or Wiry or Slippery quality on the Lung pulse is less obvious than in other positions. Thus, a quality that might be considered 'Slippery' or 'Tight' on the Lung pulse may be normal for other pulse positions.

When feeling the Lung pulse, we should also check a position distal and medial to it which Dr Shen calls the 'special' Lung pulse (Fig. 50.6). In normal conditions, there is no pulse in this position. If the 'special' Lung pulse is present while the Lung pulse itself is Weak, this indicates that the patient had a lung disease as a child, or that the parents had a lung disease, possibly TB of the lungs, and that these factors have adversely affected the patient's lungs. If a 'special' Lung pulse can be felt but the Lung pulse itself is normal, this indicates either that the patient has suffered a lung disease during childhood (e.g. whooping cough, pneumonia) or that the parents had suffered from a lung disease (e.g. TB of the lungs). If the 'special' Lung pulse is soft and the Lung pulse itself normal, this indicates a past problem in the lung. If the 'special' Lung pulse is Floating, this indicates a present problem in the lungs, such as asthma or TB. If the 'special' Lung pulse is Slippery and the Lung pulse itself normal, this indicates retention of old Phlegm in the lungs. If the

---

BOX 50.40 LEFT REAR POSITION (LARGE INTESTINE AND KIDNEY)

- Floating: Large Intestine pattern (with strength), Kidney pattern (without strength), Damp-Heat in the Large Intestine (Floating-Fine-Wiry-Rapid), weak Kidneys (Floating-Weak), Blood-Heat affecting Uterus (Floating-Wiry), danger of miscarriage (Floating-Rapid)
- Deep: Kidney-Yang deficiency, severe Kidney deficiency (Deep-Fine-Weak), severe Kidney-Yang deficiency (Deep-Fine-Weak-Slow), Dampness in the Large Intestine (Deep-Full-Slippery on distal side), weak Large Intestine Qi (Deep-Weak-Slippery on distal side)
- Slippery: Dampness in Kidneys and Bladder, Dampness in Large Intestine (Slippery-Deep-Full on distal side), Weak Large Intestine-Qi (Slippery-Deep-Weak), amenorrhoea (Slippery on proximal side and Weak Heart pulse), pregnancy (Slippery on proximal side and strong Heart pulse)
- Weak: Kidney deficiency, deficiency of the Original Qi (Weak and Intermittent)
- Fine: deficiency of the Original Qi and Essence, inflammation of the Large Intestine (Fine-Hidden-Wiry)
- Overflowing: Heat in the Large Intestine, prostatic hypertrophy (Overflowing on both left and right Rear positions)
- Hollow: diabetes after long-tem insulin administration

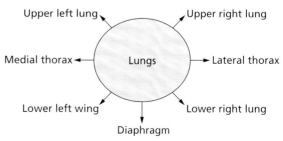

Fig. 50.5 Structure of right Front pulse position

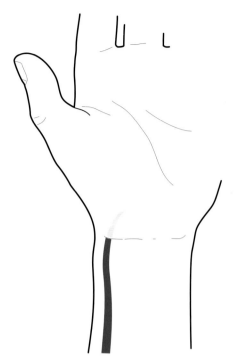

Fig. 50.6 'Special' Lung pulse (distal and medial location)

'special' Lung pulse is Slippery and Weak and the Lung pulse itself also Weak, it may indicate TB of the lungs.

Floating

A Floating quality on the Lung position is very commonly seen in invasions of external Wind; if the pathogenic factor is particularly strong, the pulse will be Floating in all positions. A Floating-Tight quality on this position indicates invasion of Wind-Cold with prevalence of Cold, a Floating-Slow quality indicates invasion of Wind-Cold with prevalence of Wind, and a Floating-Rapid quality indicates invasion of Wind-Heat.

If the pulse in this position is Floating but Weak, this indicates a previous invasion of Wind with retention of a residual pathogenic factor in the Interior. If it is Floating, Hollow and soft, it indicates stagnation of Qi in the Lungs from emotional problems.

Slippery

A Slippery quality on the Lung position indicates retention of Phlegm in the Lungs.

Overflowing

An Overflowing quality on the Lung position indicates Lung-Heat. In the absence of Heat signs, a relatively

Overflowing quality in this position indicates emotional problems deriving from grief or worry.

Hollow

A Hollow quality with strength indicates that there might be bleeding in the lungs; if it is also Rapid, this indicates a forthcoming bleeding in the lungs.

Box 50.41 summarizes the right Front pulse position.

BOX 50.41 RIGHT FRONT POSITION (LUNG)

- Floating: invasion of external Wind, invasion of Wind-Cold with prevalence of Cold (Floating-Tight), invasion of Wind-Cold with prevalence of Wind (Floating-Slow), invasion of Wind-Heat (Floating-Rapid), residual pathogenic factor (Floating-Weak), stagnation of Qi in the Lungs from emotional problems (Floating-Hollow and soft)
- Slippery: Phlegm in the Lungs
- Overflowing: Lung-Heat, emotional problems from grief or worry
- Hollow: bleeding in the lungs

Right Middle position (Stomach and Spleen)

The structure of the right Middle position is illustrated in Figure 50.7.

As explained in the introduction to pulse diagnosis, the terms 'external' and 'internal' describing the different location of Yang and Yin organs on the pulse can be interpreted in three ways: they can mean superficial and deep, lateral and medial, or distal and proximal. In the case of the right Middle position, the most widely used interpretations are the first two, that is, the Stomach is felt on the surface or lateral side, and the Spleen at the deep level or medial side. However, in the case of Stomach and Spleen, more than any other Yin–Yang organ systems, the relationship between the

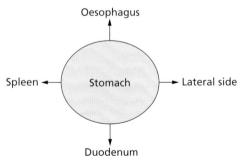

Fig. 50.7 Structure of right Middle pulse position

two is extremely close so that the pulse position needs to be taken as a whole indicating the state of the Earth Element; the differentiation between Stomach and Spleen should be seen not mechanically but dynamically according to clinical manifestations. As a rough rule of thumb, full-type qualities on this position reflect a Stomach pathology whereas empty-type ones reflect a Spleen pathology.

Floating

A Floating quality on this position is very common and it always reflects a Stomach pathology. It usually indicates Stomach-Heat or Qi stagnation in the Stomach: when the Stomach pulse is Floating, the patient experiences a pronounced feeling of distension in the epigastrium.

If the pulse is slightly Floating but empty at the deep level, it indicates Stomach-Yin deficiency; this quality is also frequently seen in practice.

Wiry

A Wiry quality on the right Middle position indicates stagnation of Qi in the Stomach, usually from dietary irregularities such as eating too much, eating in a hurry, eating under stress, etc. If Wiry on the distal position, this may indicate hiatus hernia. If both Middle positions are Wiry, this indicates that rebellious Liver-Qi is invading the Stomach.

Weak

A Weak quality on this position is extremely common and it usually indicates a Spleen deficiency. If the pulse feels very Weak on the Stomach position but slightly Wiry on its proximal side (when rolling the finger very slightly proximally) this may indicate a prolapse of the Stomach. A Stomach prolapse may cause considerable digestive problems even when it is minimal and the pulse reflects this accurately: the patient experiences a poor digestion, feels sleepy after eating, suffers a feeling of heaviness of the epigastrium and is very tired in general.

If the pulse is Weak, relatively Floating and Hollow, this indicates Stomach-Yin deficiency with slight Qi stagnation; the patient experiences excessive stomach acidity and pronounced epigastric distension.

If the pulse is Weak, and very slightly Wiry, and the Lung pulse is Weak, it may indicate a stomach ulcer.

If both right and left Middle positions are Weak, Deep and Slow, this indicates a deficiency of Stomach and Spleen

Fine

A Fine quality on the right Middle position is common, and indicates a deficiency of both Spleen and Stomach. If it is Fine, Deep and very slightly Wiry, this may indicate a stomach ulcer; if it is Fine, Deep, Slippery and Rapid, it indicates Damp-Heat in the Stomach and Spleen.

Slippery

A Slippery quality on this position indicates Dampness or Phlegm: Dampness may affect both Spleen and Stomach, whereas Phlegm usually affects only the Stomach. If the pulse is Slippery and Full, this usually indicates Phlegm in the Stomach; if it is Slippery but Weak and relatively soft, it indicates chronic Dampness in the Spleen.

Soggy

A Soggy quality on this position is common and it indicates chronic Dampness in the Spleen: with Spleen-Qi deficiency; it is frequently seen in postviral fatigue syndrome.

Hollow

A Hollow quality on the right Middle position indicates bleeding in the stomach; if the pulse is Hollow and Rapid, it may indicate a forthcoming stomach haemorrhage.

BOX 50.42 RIGHT MIDDLE POSITION (STOMACH AND SPLEEN)

- Floating: Stomach-Heat, Qi stagnation in the Stomach, Stomach-Yin deficiency (Floating but Empty at the deep level)
- Wiry: Qi stagnation in the Stomach, eating too fast, possibly hiatus hernia (Wiry on distal position), rebellious Liver-Qi invading the Stomach (both Middle positions Wiry)
- Weak: Spleen-Qi deficiency, prolapse of the Stomach (Weak on the main position and slightly Wiry on the proximal side), Stomach-Yin deficiency (Weak-Floating-Hollow), stomach ulcer (Weak and slightly Wiry, with Weak Lung pulse), deficiency of Stomach and Spleen (Weak-Deep-Slow on both Middle positions)
- Fine: deficiency of Stomach and Spleen, stomach ulcer (Fine-Deep and very slightly Wiry), Damp-Heat in Stomach and Spleen (Fine-Deep-Slippery-Rapid)
- Slippery: Dampness or Phlegm in the Stomach (Slippery-Full) or Dampness in Spleen (Slippery-Weak)
- Soggy: chronic Dampness in the Spleen with Spleen-Qi deficiency
- Hollow: bleeding in the stomach with forthcoming stomach haemorrhage (Hollow-Rapid)

Box 50.42 summarizes the right Middle pulse position.

Right Rear position (Small Intestine and Kidneys)

The structure of the right Rear position is illustrated in Figure 50.8. This position reflects the state of the Kidneys, Small Intestine and Lower Burner.

Floating

A Floating quality on the right Rear position usually reflects a pathology of the Small Intestine (i.e. Heat in the Small Intestine).

Weak

A Weak quality on the right Rear position usually reflects a deficiency of the Kidneys. If the pulse is Deep and Weak it usually indicates a deficiency of Kidney-Yang.

Slippery

A Slippery quality on the right Rear position usually reflects a pathology of the Small Intestine (i.e. Dampness). If it is Slippery and Wiry it indicates Damp-Heat in the Small Intestine with Qi stagnation; this pulse quality on both rear positions is frequently seen in ulcerative colitis. If the pulse is Slippery but Deep and slightly Weak, this indicates retention of Dampness in the Small Intestine and Kidneys.

Wiry

A Wiry quality on the right Rear position usually reflects a pathology of the Small Intestine and particularly indicates Qi stagnation. If the pulse in this position is Wiry, Long and Rapid it indicates Damp-Heat and Qi stagnation in the Small Intestine; this pulse picture is frequently seen in ulcerative colitis. If the

pulse is Wiry but Fine and Rapid, this indicates Damp-Heat in the Small Intestine occurring against a background of Kidney deficiency.

Box 50.43 summarizes the right Rear pulse position.

> ### BOX 50.43 RIGHT REAR POSITION (SMALL INTESTINE AND KIDNEYS)
>
> - Floating: Heat in the Small Intestine
> - Weak: Kidney deficiency, Kidney-Yang deficiency (Weak and Deep)
> - Slippery: Dampness in the Small-Intestine, Damp-Heat with Qi stagnation in the Small Intestine (Slippery-Wiry), ulcerative colitis (Slippery-Wiry on both rear positions, retention of Dampness in the Small Intestine and Kidneys (Slippery-Deep-Weak)
> - Wiry: stagnation of Qi in the Small Intestine, Damp-Heat with Qi stagnation in the Small Intestine (Wiry-Long-Rapid), Damp-Heat in the Small Intestine with Kidney deficiency (Wiry-Fine-Rapid)

PULSE QUALITIES INDICATING DANGEROUS CONDITIONS

Traditionally, there are 10 pulse qualities that indicate dangerous conditions and a poor prognosis. These dangerous qualities are:

> - Boiling cauldron pulse
> - Circling fish pulse
> - Swimming shrimp pulse
> - Leaking roof pulse
> - Pecking bird pulse
> - Untying rope pulse
> - Bouncing stone pulse
> - Upturned knife pulse
> - Spinning bean pulse
> - Sesame seed hasty pulse.

Boiling cauldron pulse

This pulse is in the skin, floating and extremely rapid so that it cannot be counted. It feels like water boiling furiously in a cauldron; it is without root.

This pulse indicates extreme Heat in the three Yang and complete drying up of Yin.

Circling fish pulse

This pulse is in the skin, it is like a fish with the head still and the tail waving and shaking; it is sometimes there and sometimes not. It is also extremely rapid.

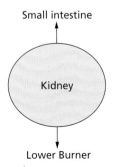

Fig. **50.8** Structure of right Rear pulse position

This pulse indicates extreme Cold in the three Yin and Collapse of Yang.

Swimming shrimp pulse

This pulse is in the skin but its shape is somewhat hidden; sometimes it comes, sometimes it does not; it jumps and darts like a shrimp.

This pulse indicates collapse of both Yin and Yang.

Leaking roof pulse

This pulse is in between the muscles and sinews, it is like water dripping, one drop at a time, at long, uneven intervals, each drop splashing without strength.

This pulse indicates collapse of Qi of the Stomach and Spleen.

Pecking bird pulse

This pulse is in between the muscles and sinews, it is rapid and irregular, stopping and starting. It is like a bird pecking at food three then five times in a row, stopping and starting at irregular intervals.

This pulse indicates exhaustion of Spleen-Qi and of Food-Qi (*Gu Qi*).

Untying rope pulse

This pulse is in between the muscles and sinews; it is rapid and chaotic beating at irregular intervals.

This pulse indicates collapse of Kidney-Qi.

Bouncing stone pulse

This pulse is in between the muscles and sinews and is like a finger tapping hard on a stone at irregular intervals.

This pulse denotes exhaustion of Kidney-Water.

Upturned knife pulse

This pulse is like the blade of a knife upside down; it is thin but hard and tense. On the superficial level it is thin, hard and tense and at the deep level it is large, hard and tense.

This pulse indicates exhaustion of Liver- and Kidney-Yin.

Spinning bean pulse

This pulse feels as it is were spinning, it is short and moving and feels like Coix seeds (Yi Yi Ren *Semen Coicis lachryma jobi*). It feels also like rolling pearls.

This pulse indicates exhastion of all the Internal Organs.

Sesame seed hasty pulse

This pulse is rapid and stops at irregular intervals (like the Hasty pulse); it is small and shaped like a sesame seed.

This pulse indicates exhaustion of Qi and Blood.

A common characteristic of most of the danger pulse qualities is the irregularity of the beat; they therefore indicate a pathology of the heart in a Western sense. Many of them are also rapid indicating not necessarily Heat but a complete collapse of Qi and Blood, which makes the pulse rapid.

THE INFLUENCE OF DRUGS ON THE PULSE

I list below some drugs and their effect on the pulse. This list is not comprehensive but is limited only to the effects I have observed in clinical practice. It should be remembered that drugs will not always have the effects listed below as different people react in different ways to the same drug. For example, it is common for antibiotics to cause a partial peeling of the tongue but, in some patients, they tend to make the coating thick.

Tranquillizers and hypnotics

Tranquillizers (anxiolytics) and hypnotics (sleeping pills) have a definite influence on the pulse. In my experience, they cause what I call the 'Stagnant' pulse quality (see above).

The tranquillizers cause a pulse that feels reluctant to come, as if being suppressed, and seems unlikely to last; it does not flow smoothly and does not have a 'wave'. It is somewhat Wiry but it does not have the strength or wave of a truly Wiry pulse.

Antidepressants
Tricyclic antidepressants

Tricyclic antidepressants tend to cause the pulse to lose its 'root', that is, it becomes slightly empty at the deep level and very slightly Floating.

Selective serotonin reuptake inhibitors (SSRI)

SSRI antidepressants tend to cause Qi stagnation in the digestive system and affect the Stomach and Spleen. The Stomach and Spleen pulse position tends to become somewhat Slippery or Wiry, or both.

Monoamine oxidase inhibitors (MAOI)

These antidepressants tend to affect the Liver and often cause Liver-Yang rising. They tend to make the pulse Wiry.

Beta blockers

Beta blockers are probably the drugs with the clearest effect on the pulse. They make the pulse slow and this should definitely be taken into account, lest we conclude wrongly that the patient suffers from a Cold syndrome. They also tend to make the pulse Deep and somewhat Weak. In my experience, this type of drug makes pulse reading very difficult and I almost tend to discount the pulse altogether when a patient is on beta blockers.

ACE inhibitors

ACE inhibitors affects the Kidneys and make the pulse Deep and Weak on both Rear positions.

Warfarin

Warfarin tends to make the pulse relatively Over-flowing and slightly Empty at the middle level.

Diuretics

Diuretics tend to make the pulse slightly Empty at the deep level. They may also affect the Kidneys

and make the pulse very Weak on both Rear positions.

H₂-Receptor antagonists

These drugs tend to affect the Stomach and Spleen and may make the right Middle position slightly Floating-Empty.

Insulin

Long-term use of insulin makes the pulse slightly Slippery but Hollow.

Box 50.44 summarizes the effects of drugs on the pulse.

BOX 50.44 EFFECTS OF DRUGS ON THE PULSE

- Tranquillizers and hypnotics: Stagnant pulse
- Tricyclic antidepressants: Empty at deep level and slightly Floating
- Selective serotonin reuptake inhibitors: Slippery or Wiry on right Middle position
- Monoamine oxidase inhibitors: Wiry
- Beta blockers: Slow
- ACE inhibitors: Deep and Weak on both Rear positions
- Warfarin: Overflowing and slightly Empty at middle level
- Diuretics: Empty at the deep level or very Weak on both Rear positions
- H₂-receptor antagonists: Floating-Empty on right Middle position
- Insulin: Slippery and Hollow

NOTES

1. Nanjing College of Traditional Chinese Medicine 1979 A Revised Explanation of the Classic of Difficulties (*Nan Jing Jiao Shi* 难经校释), People's Health Publishing House, Beijing, p. 47. First published c. AD100.
2. Shang Han Lun Research Group of the Nanjing College of Traditional Chinese Medicine 1980 An Explanation of the Discussion of Cold-induced Diseases (*Shang Han Lun Shi* 伤寒论校释), Shanghai Science Publishing House, Shanghai, p. 8. 'The Discussion of Cold-induced Diseases' was written by Zhang Zhong Jing in c. 220BC.
3. Nanjing College of Traditional Chinese Medicine 1979 A Revised Explanation of the Classic of Difficulties (*Nan Jing Jiao Shi* 难经校释), People's Health Publishing House, Beijing, p. 19. First published c. AD 100.
4. The Lilium Syndrome is described in Chapter 3 of the 'Synopsis of Prescriptions from the Golden Cabinet'. The syndrome is described as follows: '*The patient wants to eat but is reluctant to swallow food and unwilling to speak. He prefers to lie in bed yet cannot lie quietly due to restlessness. He may want to walk about but soon becomes tired. Now and then he may enjoy eating certain foods but at other times he cannot even tolerate the smell of food. He may feel either too cold or too hot but without fever or aversion to cold. He also has a bitter taste in the mouth and the urine is dark. No drugs appear to be effective to cure this syndrome; after taking the medicine there may be vomiting and diarrhoea. The disease haunts the patient and although his appearance is normal, he is actually suffering. His pulse is Rapid.*' This apparently strange syndrome does occur in practice and is seen in patients who are depressed.
5. 1979 The Yellow Emperor's Classic of Internal Medicine – Simple Questions (*Huang Di Nei Jing Su Wen* 黄帝内经素问), People's Health Publishing House, Beijing, p. 98. First published c. 100BC.
6. Cited in Liu Guan Jun 1981 Pulse Diagnosis (*Mai Zhen* 脉诊), Shanghai Science Publishing House, Shanghai, p. 90.
7. Simple Questions, p. 98.
8. Ibid., p. 118.
9. Ibid., p. 107.
10. Ibid., p. 116.
11. Ibid., p. 98.
12. 1981 Spiritual Axis (*Ling Shu Jing* 灵枢经), People's Health Publishing House, Beijing, p. 17. First published c. 100BC.

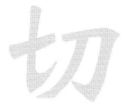

Chapter **51**

PALPATION OF PARTS OF THE BODY

Chapter contents

INTRODUCTION   *509*

PALPATION OF THE CHEST AND ABDOMEN   *510*
    Palpation of the chest   *512*
    Palpation of the abdomen   *513*

PALPATION OF THE SKIN   *516*
    Body skin   *516*
    Forearm diagnosis   *517*
    Palpation of temples in children   *518*

PALPATION OF HANDS AND FEET   *519*
    Temperature   *519*
    Palpation and comparison of dorsum and palm   *520*
    Palpation of feet and hands in children   *520*
    Palpation of the nails   *520*

PALPATION OF ACUPUNCTURE POINTS   *520*
    Front Collecting (*Mu*) points   *521*
    Back Transporting (*Bei Shu*) points   *522*
    Source (*Yuan*) points   *522*

INTRODUCTION

Palpation is used to detect the temperature, moisture and texture of the skin, the consistency of the deeper tissues and the presence of masses. Palpation is carried out on the skin, hands and feet, chest, abdomen and acupuncture points and channels.

There are three different palpation techniques:

- touching
- stroking
- pressing

Touching   This consists simply in touching the skin of the patient lightly. This is done to detect the temperature and moisture of the skin and to check whether the patient is sweating. Detecting whether the patient is sweating is important in exterior invasions of Wind to differentiate between an Attack of Wind and an Attack of Cold within the Greater-Yang pattern of invasion of Wind-Cold. The temperature of the skin of the forehead is also important in exterior invasions of Wind because it reflects the intensity of the 'fever' (or heat emission as defined in Chapter 43).

Stroking   This consists in stroking the skin and deeper tissues of the patient and it is usually carried out on the chest, abdomen and limbs. Stroking serves to determine the presence of tenderness or swelling and it is used to distinguish Full from Empty conditions.

Pressing   This consists in pressing relatively hard to still deeper levels usually of the abdomen. It serves to determine the presence of pain or masses and is used to establish the Full or Empty condition of the Internal Organs.

These three techniques correspond to three different degrees of pressures reflecting the state of different energetic layers. Thus, *touching* reveals the state of the skin, *stroking* that of the flesh and muscles and *pressing* that of the sinews and bones and of the Internal Organs.

PALPATION OF THE CHEST AND ABDOMEN

Palpation of the chest and abdomen is an important part of diagnosing by palpation because it reveals the state of the Internal Organs. Chapter 35 of the 'Spiritual Axis' says: *'The internal organs reside inside the chest and abdominal cavity like precious objects in a chest,*

each with its own specific location.'[1] The 'Simple Questions' in Chapter 22 says: *'When the Heart is diseased there is pain in the centre of the chest and hypochondrial fullness and pain . . . When the Kidneys are diseased there is swelling of the abdomen.'*[2]

The chest and abdominal areas influenced by the various Internal Organs are illustrated in Figure 51.1.

Temperature

When palpating the abdomen one should first of all feel the temperature of different areas: if the abdomen feels cold on palpation this indicates either Cold or Yang deficiency; if it feels hot on palpation this indicates Heat. If the pulse picture indicates Heat but the abdomen is not hot on palpation, this indicates exter-

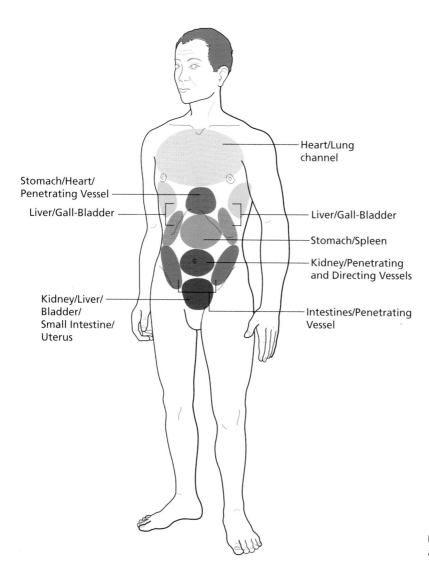

Stomach/Heart/Penetrating Vessel

Liver/Gall-Bladder

Heart/Lung channel

Liver/Gall-Bladder

Stomach/Spleen

Kidney/Penetrating and Directing Vessels

Kidney/Liver/Bladder/Small Intestine/Uterus

Intestines/Penetrating Vessel

Fig. 51.1 Areas of the chest and abdomen and the Internal Organs

nal Heat. In children, a hot sensation of the abdomen on palpation often indicates retention of food.

Texture

Next, one should check the texture of the abdomen, that is, whether it feels soft or hard. The normal abdomen should feel relatively soft on a superficial palpation but firm with a deeper pressure. If the abdomen feels very soft and flaccid on palpation, this indicates a deficiency condition of the Spleen and Stomach if it is the epigastrium, or the Spleen and Kidneys if the lower abdomen; the latter sign is common in women who have had several children.

If the abdomen feels hard on palpation, this indicates a Full condition, which is usually Qi stagnation, Blood stasis, Dampness or retention of food; each of these conditions presents with different subjective symptoms, which are distension, pain and fullness respectively.

Palpation of the abdomen is quite important in invasions of Wind, especially in children, because if the abdomen feels soft the pathogenic factor is usually still on the Exterior, whereas if it feels hard the pathogenic factor has penetrated to the Interior.

Box 51.1 summarizes the significance of different textures on palpation.

> ### BOX 51.1 TEXTURE OF THE ABDOMEN
>
> - Soft and flaccid epigastrium: Stomach and Spleen deficiency
> - Soft and flaccid lower abdomen: Spleen and Kidney deficiency
> - Hard: Full condition
>   —stagnation (with feeling of distension)
>   —Dampness (with feeling of fullness)
>   —Blood stasis (with pain)
>   —retention of food (with feeling of fullness)
> - Soft during invasions of Wind in children: pathogenic factor still on the Exterior
> - Hard during invasions of Wind in children: pathogenic factor in the Interior

Distension versus fullness

One can distinguish distension from fullness on palpation. Besides being subjective symptoms, distension and fullness are also objective signs. The distended abdomen feels hard but elastic, like a drum, whereas fullness of the abdomen manifests with a hardness of the abdomen but without distension on palpation.

Tenderness

The abdomen should then be palpated to check for tenderness and pain. If a light palpation elicits tenderness or pain, this indicates a Full condition, which may be Qi stagnation, Blood stasis, Dampness, retention of food, Heat or Cold. If the pressure of palpation relieves the pain, this indicates a deficient condition of the Spleen and Stomach if it is in the epigastrium, or of the Spleen, Kidneys and Liver if in the lower abdomen. If the abdomen feels tender only under deep pressure, this usually indicates Blood stasis. If superficial pressure of the abdomen relieves a pain but deeper pressure elicits a discomfort, this indicates a combined condition of Deficiency and Excess (e.g. stagnation of Liver-Qi with Spleen-Qi deficiency).

Box 51.2 summarizes the significance of tenderness on palpation.

> ### BOX 51.2 TENDERNESS ON PALPATION
>
> - Tenderness on light palpation: Full condition (Qi stagnation, Blood stasis, Dampness, Retention of Food, Heat or Cold)
> - Tenderness relieved by palpation: Stomach and Spleen deficiency (epigastrium) or Liver and Kidney deficiency (lower abdomen)
> - Tender on deep pressure: Blood stasis
> - Tenderness relieved by superficial pressure and elicited by deeper pressure: combined Deficiency and Excess

Lumps

Abdominal masses are called *Ji Ju*. *Ji* indicates actual abdominal masses which are fixed and immovable; if there is an associated pain, its location is fixed. These masses are due to stasis of Blood and I call them 'Blood masses'. *Ju* indicates abdominal masses which come and go, do not have a fixed location and are movable. If there is an associated pain, it too comes and goes and changes location. Such masses are due to stagnation of Qi and I call them 'Qi masses'.

Actual abdominal lumps therefore pertain to the category of abdominal masses and specifically *Ji* masses (i.e. Blood masses).

Another name for abdominal masses was *Zheng Jia*, *Zheng* being equivalent to *Ji* (i.e. acute, fixed masses) and *Jia* being equivalent to *Ju* (i.e. non-substantial masses from stagnation of Qi). The term *Zheng Jia* normally referred to abdominal masses occurring only in women, but although these masses are more frequent in women they do occur in men as well.

When palpating the abdomen one should feel for lumps. Lumps that come and go and are associated with distension indicate Qi stagnation, whereas lumps that are fixed and painful indicate Blood stasis. Soft and movable abdominal lumps may indicate Phlegm. Lumps in the left-lower abdominal region may simply indicate faeces in the colon.

Palpable lumps in the lower abdomen may be due to Qi stagnation, Blood stasis, Damp-Phlegm or Damp-Heat.

Abdominal lumps, if due to Qi stagnation, normally feel soft and come and go with emotional moods; if due to Blood stasis they feel hard on palpation and are usually associated with pain; if from Damp-Heat they may also be painful and, when palpated, very tender; if from Damp-Phlegm, they feel softer than lumps from Blood stasis or Damp-Heat. A typical example of an abdominal lump from Blood stasis is a myoma, whereas an example of that from Damp-Phlegm or Damp-Heat is an ovarian cyst.

Box 51.3 summarizes the types of abdominal masses.

BOX 51.3 TWO TYPES OF ABDOMINAL MASSES

- Qi (*Ju* or *Jia*): relatively soft masses that come and go
- Blood (*Ji* or *Zheng*): hard, fixed masses

Palpation of the chest

Palpation of the chest includes palpation of the following areas:

- apical pulse
- chest
- area under xyphoid process
- breast.

Apical pulse

The apical pulse can be palpated in the fifth intercostal space; from a Western, anatomical point of view, it is the palpation of the left ventricle of the heart, whereas in ancient Chinese medicine it was called the pulsation of *Xu Li*, which relates to the Great Connecting channel of the Stomach and reflects the state of the Gathering Qi (*Zong Qi*). For a description of the ancient interpretation of this pulsation, see Chapter 13 in Part 1, 'Diagnosis by Observation'.

The pulsation of the apical pulse reflects the state of the Gathering Qi and, under normal conditions, it

should be felt clearly but not be hard and it should be relatively slow; this indicates a normal state of the Gathering Qi. If the pulsation of the apical pulse is feeble and without strength, this indicates a deficiency of the Gathering Qi and therefore of Lungs and Heart. If the pulsation feels too strong and hard, this indicates an Excess condition of the Lungs or Heart, or both. However, in some cases, when the left ventricle is enlarged, the apical pulse may feel 'large' but empty and this indicates Heart-Qi deficiency.

If the apical pulse stops and starts, this may indicate that the patient has suffered a severe shock; the same sign may also be seen in alcoholism.

The pulsation of the apical pulse should also be compared with that of the radial pulse and the two should be similar to each other (e.g. if the apical pulse feels feeble, the radial pulse should also feel Weak, Empty or Choppy). A discrepancy between the apical and the radial pulse is a poor prognostic sign and it often indicates heart disease.

The apical pulse may become affected by short-term influences such as shock, fright or a severe outburst of anger in which case it becomes very rapid.

Box 51.4 summarizes findings on palpation of the apical pulse.

BOX 51.4 APICAL PULSE

- Clearly felt, not hard, relatively slow: normal
- Feeble and without strength: deficiency of the Gathering Qi (*Zong Qi*)
- Strong and hard: Excess condition of the Lungs and/or Heart
- Large but empty: Heart-Qi deficiency
- Stopping and starting: severe shock or alcoholism
- Discrepancy between apical and radial pulse: poor prognosis
- Rapid: shock, fright or outburst of anger

Chest

The centre of the chest corresponds to the Heart and the rest of it to the Lungs. Palpation of the chest reveals the state of the Heart, Lungs and Pericardium and generally speaking, tenderness on palpation indicates a Full condition of one of these organs. For example, if the chest feels very tender even on light palpation in the centre, in the area of Ren-17 Shanzhong, this may indicate Heart-Blood stasis.

If the chest is tender on palpation in the areas around the centre, it usually indicates an Excess condition of the Lungs and often retention of Phlegm in the

Lungs. By contrast, if palpation of the chest relieves discomfort, it indicates Deficiency of the Heart or Lungs. If superficial palpation of the chest relieves a pain but the patient feels discomfort with a deeper pressure, it indicates a combined condition of Deficiency and Excess.

Box 51.5 summarizes findings on palpation of the chest.

BOX 51.5 CHEST

- Tender with light palpation of Ren-17: Heart-Blood stasis
- Tender around the centre: Excess condition of the Lungs
- Tenderness relieved by palpation: Deficiency condition of Heart or Lungs
- Tenderness relieved by light palpation but elicited by deeper palpation: combined Deficiency and Excess

---

Area under xyphoid process

The area under the xyphoid process reflects the state of the Stomach, Heart and Penetrating Vessel. This area readily reflects patterns deriving from emotional problems. For example, if the area feels relatively hard and knotted, this indicates Heart-Qi stagnation from emotional problems such as sadness and grief. If the area is soft but painful, it indicates Stomach-Heat combined with Stomach-Qi deficiency. The Penetrating Vessel also affects this area and a knotted and full feeling in this area occurs often in the pattern of rebellious Qi of the Penetrating Vessel, but only when it is associated with other abdominal, chest and throat symptoms.

Box 51.6 summarizes findings on palpation of the area under the xyphoid process.

BOX 51.6 AREA UNDER THE XYPHOID PROCESS

- Hard and knotted: stagnation of Heart-Qi
- Soft on palpation and painful: Stomach-Heat with Stomach-Qi deficiency
- Hard and full: rebellious Qi of the Penetrating Vessel

Breast

Palpation of the breasts in women is carried out when there are breast lumps. Breast lumps may be malignant or benign. The purpose of palpation in Chinese medicine is never to replace the Western diagnosis – we should never rely on palpation to distinguish benign from malignant lumps – but to identify the patterns causing them. The palpation of lumps should take into consideration their hardness, their edges and their mobility:

- relatively soft: Phlegm
- relatively hard: Blood stasis
- distinct edges: Phlegm
- indistinct edges: Toxic Heat
- mobile on palpation: Phlegm
- immovable on palpation: Blood stasis or Toxic Heat.

Small, movable lumps with distinct edges that change size according to the menstrual cycle normally indicate fibrocystic disease of the breast, which is usually due to a combination of Phlegm and Qi stagnation. A single, relatively hard, movable lump with distinct edges which may be also slightly painful usually indicates a fibroadenoma, which from the Chinese point of view is due to a combination of Phlegm and Blood stasis. A single, hard, immovable lump with indistinct margins, without pain, may indicate carcinoma of the breast which, in Chinese medicine, is usually due to a combination of Phlegm, Qi stagnation and Blood stasis occurring against a background of disharmony of the Penetrating and Directing Vessels.

Box 51.7 summarizes the causes of the most common breast lumps.

BOX 51.7 COMMON CAUSES OF BREAST LUMPS

- Fibrocystic disease (Qi stagnation and Phlegm): small, multiple, movable lumps with distinct edges, changing size according to the menstrual cycle
- Fibroadenoma (Phlegm and Blood stasis): single, relatively hard, movable lump with distinct edges, possibly painful
- Carcinoma of the breast (Blood stasis and Phlegm): single, hard, immovable, painless lump with indistinct margins

---

Palpation of the abdomen

The palpation areas of the abdomen are as follows (Fig. 51.2):

- hypochondrium
- epigastrium
- umbilical area
- lateral-lower abdomen
- central-lower abdomen.

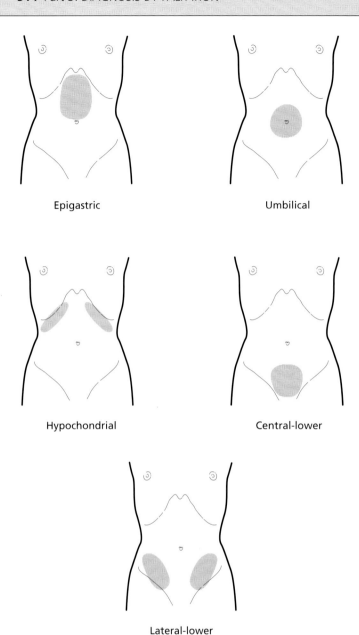

Epigastric

Umbilical

Hypochondrial

Central-lower

Lateral-lower

Fig. 51.2 Abdominal areas

Hypochondrium

The hypochondrium includes the lateral side of the rib cage and also the area immediately below it. It reflects the state of the Liver and Gall-Bladder. If the hypochondrium is distinctly tender on palpation, this indicates stagnation of Liver-Qi, Liver-Blood stasis or Damp-Heat in the Liver and Gall-Bladder. If palpation of the hypochondrium relieves the patient's discomfort, this may indicate Liver-Blood deficiency.

Box 51.8 summarizes findings on palpation of the hypochondrium.

BOX 51.8 HYPOCHONDRIUM

- Tender on palpation: Liver-Qi stagnation, Liver-Blood stasis, Damp-Heat in Liver and Gall-Bladder
- Discomfort relieved by palpation: Liver-Blood deficiency

Epigastrium

The epigastric area is the area contained between the xyphoid process, the costal margins and the umbilicus. Palpation of the epigastrium reveals primarily the condition of the Stomach and Spleen. The normal epigastrium should feel elastic but neither hard nor too soft. The area immediately below the xyphoid process reflects the condition of both the Stomach and the Heart and should feel relatively softer than the rest of the epigastrium; if this area feels hard on palpation, it often indicates stagnation of Qi or Blood of the Heart, which is usually due to emotional problems.

If the epigastrium feels hard on palpation, this indicates an Excess condition of the Stomach, which may be stagnation of Qi, Blood stasis, Dampness or retention of food. If the epigastrium feels distended like a drum, this indicates Qi stagnation. If the patient has a subjective sensation of fullness but the epigastrium is soft on palpation, this indicates a condition of mixed Deficiency and Excess, which is often characterized by Stomach-Heat and Spleen-Qi deficiency. If palpation of the epigastrium relieves the patient's discomfort, this indicates a Deficiency condition of the Stomach.

Box 51.9 summarizes findings on palpation of the epigastrium.

BOX 51.9 EPIGASTRIUM

- Elastic, neither hard nor soft: healthy state of Stomach and Spleen
- Hardness in the area below the xyphoid process: stagnation of Qi or Blood of the Heart, usually due to emotional problems
- Hard: Excess condition of the Stomach (Qi stagnation, Blood stasis, Dampness or retention of Food)
- Distended like a drum: Qi stagnation
- Soft on palpation with subjective sensation of Fullness: Stomach-Heat and Spleen-Qi deficiency

---

Umbilical region

The umbilical region reflects the state of the Kidneys and of the Penetrating and Directing Vessels. It should feel elastic but not hard. If it feels hard and full on palpation, this indicates either stagnation of Qi or Blood stasis in the Penetrating Vessel. If it is painful on palpation, this indicates Blood stasis in the Penetrating Vessel. If it feels very soft on palpation, this indicates a Kidney deficiency and a deficiency of the Penetrating and Directing Vessels.

Box 51.10 summarizes findings on palpation of the unbilical region.

BOX 51.10 UMBILICAL REGION

- Hard and full: stagnation of Qi or Blood stasis in Penetrating Vessel
- Pain: Blood stasis in the Penetrating Vessel
- Soft: Kidney deficiency and deficiency of Penetrating and Directing Vessels

---

Umbilical pulse

Palpation of the abdomen should always include palpation of the pulse around the umbilicus by using three fingers and the thumb simultaneously, that is the middle finger above the umbilicus, the index and ring finger to the right and left respectively and the thumb below the umbilicus. From the Chinese point of view this is the pulsation of the Original Qi, which should be strong and regular. If this pulse pulsates more than five times per breathing cycle, it indicates Heat in the Penetrating and Directing Vessels. If this pulse feels faint, and there is a feeling of heat on palpation, it indicates Yin deficiency in the Penetrating Vessel. If this pulse is slower than two pulsations per breathing cycle it indicates a severe deficiency of the Original Qi. If the pulsation around the umbilicus is slow and it feels cold on palpation, it indicates a deficiency of the Fire of the Gate of Life.

Box 51.11 summarizes findings on palpation of the umbilical pulse.

BOX 51.11 UMBILICAL PULSE

- Strong and regular umbilical pulse: healthy Original Qi
- Umbilical pulse which beats more than five times per breathing cycle: Heat in the Penetrating and Directing Vessels
- Faint umbilical pulse with a feeling of heat on palpation: Yin deficiency in the Penetrating Vessel
- Umbilical pulse slower than two pulsations per breathing cycle: severe deficiency of the Original Qi
- Slow umbilical pulse with a feeling of cold on palpation: deficiency of the Fire of the Gate of Life

---

Lateral-lower abdomen

The lateral-lower abdominal areas are called *Shao Fu* and they reflect the state of the Intestines and of the Penetrating Vessel. If hard on palpation, they indicate either Dampness in the Intestines or Blood stasis

in the Penetrating Vessel. If painful on palpation, they indicate Blood stasis in the Penetrating Vessel. A feeling of mass in the lateral lower abdomen also indicates Blood stasis in the Intestines or in the Penetrating Vessel.

Box 51.12 summarizes findings on palpation of the lateral-lower area.

BOX 51.12 LATERAL-LOWER ABDOMEN

- Hard: Dampness in Intestines or Blood stasis in Penetrating Vessel
- Pain: Blood stasis in Penetrating Vessel
- Feeling of mass: Blood stasis in the Intestines or Penetrating Vessel

---

Central-lower abdomen

The central-lower abdominal area is called *Xiao Fu* and it reflects the state of the Small Intestine, Kidneys, Bladder, Uterus and Liver. If this area feels hard on palpation, it may indicate Dampness in the Intestines or Bladder. If it is painful on palpation, it may indicate Qi stagnation or Blood stasis in the Intestines or Bladder.

Box 51.13 summarizes findings on palpation of the central-lower area.

BOX 51.13 CENTRAL-LOWER ABDOMEN

- Hard: Dampness in the Small Intestine or Bladder
- Pain: Qi stagnation of Blood stasis in Small Intestine or Bladder

---

PALPATION OF THE SKIN

Palpation of the skin includes palpation of the body skin and palpation of the forearm. Palpation of the skin includes the following areas:

- body skin
- forearm diagnosis
- palpation of temples in children.

Body skin

Palpation of the body skin is aimed at assessing its temperature, moistness and texture.

Temperature

The temperature of the skin reflects conditions of Heat or Yang deficiency. If the skin feels hot on palpation it usually indicates a condition of Heat, whereas if it feels Cold this indicates Yang deficiency or Cold. Sometimes the pulse is Rapid but the abdomen does not feel hot; this indicates external Heat. A hot abdomen in children indicates retention of food.

Box 51.14 summarizes findings of heat and cold on palpation.

BOX 51.14 TEMPERATURE

- Cold: Cold or Yang deficiency
- Hot: Heat
- Pulse Rapid but abdomen not hot: external Heat
- Hot abdomen in children: retention of food

Energetic layers

A hot feeling of the skin on palpation may be related more specifically to the five energetic layers of skin, muscles, blood vessels, sinews and bones according to the amount of pressure exerted. These five energetic layers reflect the state of the Lungs, Spleen, Heart, Liver and Kidneys and they may be grouped into three, (i.e. skin, muscles and blood vessels, and sinews and bones), corresponding to three different pressures of palpation.

!

There are three energetic layers of palpation:
- skin
- muscles and blood vessels
- sinews and bones.

Skin   The skin energetic layer is felt by palpating very lightly; if it feels hot on palpation and the feeling of heat subsides after several minutes, this indicates exterior Heat from invasion of Wind or Empty-Heat from Yin deficiency affecting the Lungs.

Muscles and blood vessels   The muscles and blood vessels energetic layer is felt by palpating the skin with a slightly harder pressure; if it feels hot at this level, this indicates interior Heat affecting the Heart or Spleen.

Sinews and bones   The sinews and bones energetic layer is felt by palpating the skin with a still harder pressure; if it feels hot at this level, this indicates Empty-Heat from Yin deficiency usually affecting the Liver and Kidneys.

Box 51.15 summarizes findings on palpation of the energetic layers.

Moisture

Palpation of the skin should take into consideration the moisture of the skin: the normal skin should be slightly moist and elastic. If the skin is too moist from sweat, this indicates either Yang deficiency or Heat, whereas if moist and greasy, it indicates Dampness or Phlegm. If the skin feels dry on palpation, this indicates Blood deficiency, Yin deficiency or severe Blood stasis. If the skin feels rough on palpation, this indicates severe Blood deficiency, often as an underlying condition of Painful Obstruction Syndrome (*Bi*).

Texture

If the skin feels rough and very dry and scaly, this indicates severe deficiency and Dryness of Blood together with a deficiency of the Spleen. If the skin feels swollen on palpation and the exerting of pressure with the thumb leaves it dented, this indicates oedema from Yang deficiency; if the skin feels swollen but the exerting of pressure with the thumb does not leave it dented, this indicates Qi stagnation or Blood stasis.

Forehead

Palpating the forehead to feel its temperature was, in ancient China, a method of ascertaining whether or not the patient was suffering from a 'fever'. An objective sensation of heat on palpation of the forehead is called *fa re*, which literally means 'emission of heat' and which is often translated as 'fever'; however, this is not entirely correct as the patient may or may not have a fever. Whenever 'fever' is mentioned in this context, it is intended as an objective feeling of heat of the forehead on palpation. An objective sensation of heat on palpation of the forehead together with a subjective feeling of aversion to cold indicates invasion of external Wind; such a sensation together with a subjective feeling of heat indicates internal Heat.

The temperature of the forehead should be compared with that of the palms: if the forehead is hotter than the palms, this generally indicates exterior Heat, while if the palms are hotter than the forehead, this generally indicates interior Heat.

Box 51.16 summarizes the findings on palpation of skin.

Forearm diagnosis

Diagnosis by palpating the palmar surface of the forearm between the elbow and the wrist crease was described in Chapter 74 of the 'Spiritual Axis', which says: '*The rapid or slow, large or small and slippery or rough condition of the skin of the forearm, as well as the firmness of the muscles, reflects the location of the disease.*'[3] This quotation refers to palpation of the palmar surface of the forearm. 'Rapid or slow' refers to how the hand glides over the patient's skin, that is 'rapid' means that the patient's skin is smooth and the practitioner's hand glides easily and 'slow' means that the patient's skin is rough and the practitioner's hand does not glide easily. 'Large or small' refers to the size of the muscles of this part of the arm and 'slippery or rough' refers to the texture of the skin of the forearm.

The same chapter of the 'Spiritual Axis' says:

When the skin of the forearm is slippery and moist, it indicates invasion of Wind; if it is rough, it indicates Wind Painful Obstruction Syndrome; if it is like fish scales, it indicates Phlegm-Fluids; if it feels hot and the pulse is Full, it indicates a Heat disease; if the skin is cold and the pulse is small, it indicates diarrhoea and deficiency of Qi; if the skin is extremely hot and then becomes cold, it indicates combined Heat and Cold; if the skin feels cold but becomes gradually hotter on palpation, it also indicates combined Heat and Cold.[4]

In other words, the texture of the skin of the inner surface of the forearm reflects invasions of external Wind if it feels slightly moist, Blood deficiency if it feels dry, Wind Painful Obstruction syndrome if it feels rough and severe Spleen deficiency with Phlegm if it

feels rough and coarse like fish scales. In addition to this, the temperature of the skin of the inner forearm reflects conditions of Heat (particularly of the Intestines) if it feels hot or conditions of Cold (particularly of the Intestines) if it feels cold.

The same chapter of the 'Spiritual Axis' describes the correspondences between the areas of the forearm and the Internal Organs; these are summarized in Box 51.17.

BOX 51.17 PALPATION OF THE FOREARM (Chapter 74 of the 'Spiritual Axis')

- Hot elbow: Heat above the waist
- Hot hand: Heat below the waist
- Hot inner flexure of the elbow: Heat in the chest
- Hot lateral side of the elbow: Heat in the upper back
- Hot inner aspect of the arm: Heat in the abdomen
- Hot 3–4 cun below the lateral side of the elbow: worms in the Intestines
- Hot palm: Heat in the abdomen
- Cold palm: Cold in the abdomen
- Bluish blood vessels on thenar eminence: Cold in the Stomach

---

The 'Detailed Discussion of the Essence of Pulse Diagnosis' (*Mai Yao Jing Wei Lun*) developed the above topography of the forearm from Chapter 74 of the 'Spiritual Axis' into a detailed map of correspondence between areas of the inner forearm and parts of the body (Fig. 51.3).[5]

Besides palpation, the skin of the inner aspect of the forearm should be observed for slackness, tightness, moistness, dryness, protrusion and shrinking. If the inner aspect of the forearm looks slack and loose, it indicates Heat; if it is tight, this indicates Cold. If the forearm is moist this indicates Wind invasion; if it is dry it indicates Blood or Yin deficiency. If the forearm skin seems to be protruding and sticking out this indicates a Full condition; if it looks shrinking and withered it indicates an Empty condition.

Palpation of temples in children

In babies under 6 months, palpation of the temples is used for diagnosis. The area to palpate is that between the end of the eyebrow and the temple hairline (Fig. 51.4).

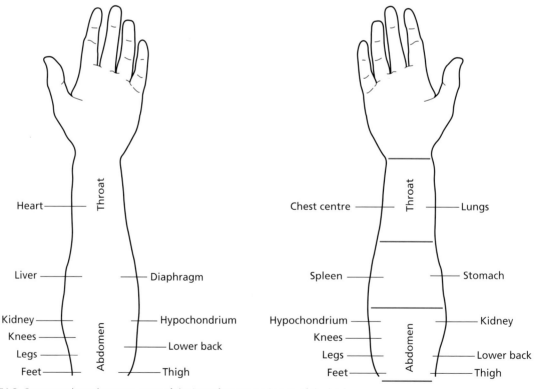

Fig. 51.3 Correspondence between areas of the inner forearm and parts of the body

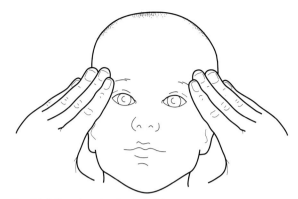

Fig. 51.4 Temple palpation in babies

This area is palpated by gently resting the index, middle and ring fingers between the end of the eyebrow and the temporal hairline with the ring finger nearest the end of the eyebrow. The right hand should be used to feel the left side of the child's temple while the left hand should be used to feel the right side. If this area feels hot under all three fingers, this indicates an external invasion of Wind; if it feels cold under all three fingers, this indicates an external invasion of Wind-Cold or Accumulation Disorder from stagnation in the digestive system. If it feels hot under the index and middle fingers, this indicates Heat above and Cold below. If it feels hot under the middle and ring fingers, this indicates Heat from fright. If it feels hot under the index finger only, this indicates Accumulation Disorder, stagnation of Qi in the chest or breast-feeding problems. Of course, a hot feeling in this area also corresponds to the objective feeling of heat called *fa re*, which may or may not correspond to an actual fever.

Finally, the temperature of this area of the baby's forehead should be compared with that of the palms. If the palms are hotter than the temples, this indicates Empty-Heat; if the temples are hotter than the palms, this indicates Full Heat.

BOX 51.18 TEMPLE PALPATION IN BABIES

- Hot under three fingers: external invasion of Wind-Heat
- Cold under three fingers: external invasion of Wind-Cold or Accumulation Disorder
- Hot under index and middle fingers: Heat above, Cold below
- Hot under middle and ring fingers: Heat from fright
- Hot under the index finger only: Accumulation Disorder, stagnation of Qi in the chest or breast-feeding problems
- Temples hotter than palms: Full Heat
- Palms hotter than temples: Empty Heat

Box 51.18 summarizes findings on temple palpation in babies.

PALPATION OF HANDS AND FEET

Temperature

Palpation of the hands and feet, particularly in regard to their temperature, is important to diagnose conditions of Heat and Cold. The most common cause of cold hands and cold feet is Yang deficiency. Lung- or Heart-Yang deficiency, or both, will cause coldness of the hands only. Kidney-Yang deficiency will cause coldness of the feet; if associated with Spleen-Yang deficiency, the hands may be cold as well. Stomach-Yang deficiency may cause coldness of both hands and feet. With Spleen- and Kidney-Yang deficiency a particular feature is that not only the hands and feet but the whole limbs are cold.

In women, cold hands and feet may also be caused by Blood deficiency. Heart-Blood deficiency may cause cold hands, whereas Liver-Blood deficiency may cause cold feet.

Stagnation of Liver-Qi may cause coldness of the hands and feet but particularly of the fingers and toes. In this case, the cold feeling is due not to a Yang deficiency but to Qi that is stagnant being unable to reach the extremities.

> ! In cold hands and feet from Liver-Qi stagnation, it is the fingers and toes particularly that are cold.

There are other less common causes of cold hands and feet. One is Phlegm in the Interior, which may obstruct the circulation of Qi to the limbs and cause cold hands; this may happen also in the case of Phlegm-Heat giving rise to contradictory hot and cold symptoms. Another less common situation of cold hands and feet is when there is a very pronounced and intense Heat in the Interior obstructing the circulation of Qi so that it cannot warm the hands and feet; this condition will also give rise to contradictory hot and cold symptoms. An example of this situation is the condition of Heat in the Pericardium at the Nutritive-Qi level within the Four Levels, which is characterized by symptoms and signs of intense Heat (i.e. dark-Red tongue without coating, fever at night, mental restlessness, etc.) but cold hands.

Box 51.19 summarizes the causes of cold hands and feet.

BOX 51.19 COLD HANDS AND FEET

Common causes
- Cold hands: Lung/Heart-Yang deficiency
- Cold feet: Kidney-Yang deficiency
- Cold of whole limbs: Spleen- and Kidney-Yang deficiency
- Cold hands and feet: Stomach-Yang deficiency, Kidney- with Spleen-Yang deficiency
- Cold hands and feet in women: Blood deficiency
- Cold hands in women: Heart-Blood deficiency
- Cold feet in women: Liver-Blood deficiency
- Cold fingers and toes: Liver-Qi stagnation

Less common cause
- Cold hands and feet: Phlegm or Interior Heat obstructing circulation of Qi
- Contradictory hot and cold symptoms: Phlegm-Heat or intense interior Heat

---

Palpation and comparison of dorsum and palm

When palpating the hands to feel their temperature, we should distinguish between the dorsum and the palm of the hand: a hot dorsum reflects more conditions of Full-Heat, whereas a hot palm reflects more conditions of Empty-Heat, though not exclusively so.

!

Hot dorsum of the hand indicates Full-Heat; a hot palm usually indicates Empty-Heat.

In the context of exterior invasions of Wind, palpation of the dorsum of the hands is important because it confirms the exterior nature of the condition. In fact, in exterior invasions of Wind (whether Wind-Cold or Wind-Heat) there is the characteristic contradiction between the patient's subjective sensation of cold ('aversion to cold') or even shivering and the objective hot feeling of the dorsum of the hands on palpation. The Chinese term *fa re*, which is often translated as 'fever' in the context of exterior invasions of Wind, actually refers precisely to this (i.e. the *objective* hot feeling of the dorsum of the hands and forehead on palpation); the patient may or may not have an actual fever.

Therefore, the comparison between the temperature of the dorsum and the palms of the hands has two interpretations: on the one hand, it helps to distinguish Full- from Empty-Heat; on the other, in the context of acute diseases it confirms their exterior nature.

Chapter 74 of the 'Spiritual Axis' relates the temperature of the palm of the hand to the condition of the Intestines: if the palm is hot, this indicates Heat in the Intestines, whereas if cold it indicates Cold in the Intestines.[6]

Palpation of feet and hands in children

In children, conditions of Heat are normally reflected on the soles of the feet, which become hot, whereas conditions of Cold are normally reflected on the dorsum of the foot and on the leg, which become cold. Also in children, cold tips of the fingers may indicate shock or fright, whereas if the middle section of the fingers is hot this indicates an external invasion of Wind.

Palpation of the nails

Palpation of the hands should include pressing of the nails. When a fingernail is pressed, a white discoloration appears. Under normal conditions, the nail should resume its normal pinky colour as soon as the pressure is released. If the resumption of the normal pinky colour occurs slowly, this indicates either Blood deficiency or Blood stasis.

PALPATION OF ACUPUNCTURE POINTS

Palpation of acupuncture points is aimed primarily at checking for tenderness. If a point is very tender on even superficial pressure, this indicates a Full condition of that channel or local stagnation. If pressure on the point relieves a particular pain, this indicates an Empty condition of that channel. If pressure of the point initially relieves a particular pain but then causes a discomfort, this indicates a condition of mixed Deficiency and Excess.

Any acupuncture point may be used diagnostically, and indeed the *Ah Shi* points may be used as well. However, some points have a particular diagnostic significance; these are the Front Collecting (*Mu*) points, the Back Transporting (*Shu*) points and the Source (*Yuan*) points.

Front Collecting (*Mu*) points

With a single exception, the Front Collecting points are all located on the chest and abdomen. The Chinese character *Mu* literally means to 'raise, collect, enlist, recruit'. In this context, it has the meaning of collecting, that is, these are the points where the Qi of the relevant organs collects or gathers. These points are frequently used in palpation diagnosis because they easily become tender on palpation or even spontaneously when the relevant organ is diseased. They are used diagnostically particularly, but not exclusively, in acute conditions. For example, the point LU-1 Zhongfu will be tender in acute lung diseases, such as bronchitis; however, the same point may also be tender in chronic asthma.

The Front-Collecting points are listed in Box 51.20.

BOX 51.20 FRONT COLLECTING POINTS

- Lungs: LU-1 Zhongfu
- Large Intestine: ST-25 Tianshu
- Stomach: Ren-12 Zhongwan
- Spleen: Liv-13 Zhangmen
- Heart: Ren-14 Juque
- Small Intestine: Ren-4 Guanyuan
- Bladder: Ren-3 Zhongji
- Kidneys: GB-25 Jingmen
- Pericardium: Ren-17 Shanzhong
- Triple Burner: Ren-5 Shimen
- Gall-Bladder: GB-24 Riyue
- Liver: LIV-14 Qimen

LU-1 Zhongfu This point is particularly useful to diagnose conditions of Emptiness or Fullness of the Lung in interior diseases, such as acute or chronic bronchitis, asthma and emphysema. LU-2 Yunmen is also frequently tender on palpation in the same conditions.

ST-25 Tianshu This point is a very important point in abdominal diagnosis because it readily reflects Full or Empty conditions not only of the Large Intestine, of which it is the Front Collecting point, but also of the Small Intestine. ST-25 is also often the centre of stagnation of Qi or Blood stasis in the Intestines, in which case the abdomen feels distended on palpation. This point is also one where Dampness in the Intestines frequently accumulates, in which case it will feel hard on palpation.

Ren-12 Zhongwan This point is an extremely important point which should always be palpated because it reflects Full or Empty conditions of the Stomach. A distended feeling on palpation indicates stagnation of Qi, a hard feeling on palpation indicates Dampness or retention of food, whereas if the point feels very soft on palpation and the hand sinks down easily this indicates a condition of deficiency of the Stomach. When palpating Ren-12, other associated points should be palpated because they all reflect the state of the Stomach; these points are ST-20 Chengman, KI-17 Shangqu and ST-21 Liangmen.

LIV-13 Zhangmen This point reflects Full and Empty conditions of the Spleen and one can frequently feel a feeling of distension on palpation of this point, which indicates stagnation of Qi in the Spleen. When palpating LIV-13, other associated points indicating the state of the Spleen should also be palpated and especially KI-18 Shiguan, Ren-9 Shuifen and ST-21 Liangmen.

Ren-14 Juque This point is very important to palpate because it readily reflects Full and Empty conditions of the Heart, especially when caused by emotional problems. The consistency and feeling of the area around this point should be compared and contrasted with that of the lower abdomen around Ren-6 Qihai: the area around Ren-14 should feel relatively soft compared with the area around Ren-6, which should not be hard but should be harder than Ren-14. When the area around this point feels distended or hard, it usually indicates stagnation of Qi affecting not only the Heart but often the Lungs and Stomach as well, and generally caused by emotional problems. If the area around Ren-14 feels too soft and the hand sinks easily this indicates a deficiency condition of the Heart. When palpating Ren-14, we should also always palpate Ren-15 Jiuwei because, although it is not the Front Collecting point of the Heart, it very much functions as one and palpation of this point therefore has the same diagnostic significance as that of Ren-14.

Ren-4 Guanyuan This point indicates Full or Empty conditions of the Small Intestine but in my experience this is a secondary aspect of its palpation. I feel that the condition of the Small Intestine is also reflected by palpation of other points such as ST-25 Tianshu, ST-27 Daju, ST-28 Shuidao and ST-29 Guilai. By contrast, palpation of Ren-4 Guanyuan is important to show Full or Empty conditions of the Uterus and of the Penetrating and Directing Vessels. If this point feels distended on palpation this indicates stagnation of Qi in the Uterus, if it feels hard on palpation it indicates retention of Dampness in the Uterus, and if it feels hard with a sensation of a mass it indicates Blood stasis

in the Uterus. If this point feels very soft and the hand sinks easily, it indicates a condition of deficiency of the Uterus and of the Penetrating and Directing Vessels (this finding is common in multiparous women).

Ren-3 Zhongji This point readily reflects Full or Empty conditions of the Bladder on palpation. However, palpation of this point also reflects the condition of the Liver channel, especially in urinary conditions. For example, if this point feels distended on palpation, it indicates stagnation of Qi, not only in the Bladder, but also in the Liver channel, usually causing urinary problems; if this point feels hard on palpation it indicates retention of Dampness in the Bladder or in the Liver channel, or both.

GB-25 Jingmen This point reflects diseases of the Kidney organ; if it is tender on palpation, this may indicate the presence of a kidney infection.

Ren-17 Shanzhong This point indicates Full and Empty conditions of the Pericardium according to the same general principles, depending on whether it feels hard or soft on palpation. However, to determine conditions of the Heart and Pericardium, palpation of Ren-14 Juque and Ren-15 Jiuwei is more important.

Ren-5 Shimen This point reflects the condition of the Lower Burner and particularly Small Intestine, Bladder, Uterus and Kidneys. Hardness here indicates a Full condition of one of these organs, while a softness indicates a deficiency of one of these organs but also of the Original Qi (*Yuan Qi*).

GB-24 Riyue This point indicates the state of the Gall-Bladder. A hardness at this point indicates Dampness in the Gall-Bladder while a softness indicates Gall-Bladder Qi deficiency.

LIV-14 Qimen This point reflects the condition of the Liver. A hardness at this point and tenderness on palpation indicate a Full condition of the Liver (Qi stagnation, Blood stasis, Dampness). A softness on palpation indicates Liver-Blood deficiency.

Back Transporting (*Bei Shu*) points

The Back Transporting points are all located on the Bladder channel on the back and may also be used diagnostically. The same principles that apply to Front Collecting points apply to these points, that is, if they are tender on palpation this indicates a Full condition of the relevant organ, whereas if palpation relieves a particular pain it indicates an Empty condition of that organ. A particular diagnostic significance of the palpation of these points is that they reflect specifically a condition of the relevant Internal Organ as opposed to its channel. For example, tenderness on BL-18 Ganshu may indicate a Full condition of the Liver.

The Back Transporting points are listed in Box 51.21.

BOX 51.21 BACK TRANSPORTING POINTS

- Lungs: BL-13 Feishu
- Pericardium: BL-14 Jueyinshu
- Heart: BL-15 Xinshu
- Liver: BL-18 Ganshu
- Gall-Bladder: BL-19 Danshu
- Spleen: BL-20 Pishu
- Stomach: BL-21 Weishu
- Triple Burner: BL-22 Sanjiaoshu
- Kidneys: BL-23 Shenshu
- Large Intestine: BL-25 Dachangshu
- Small Intestine: BL-27 Xiaochangshu
- Bladder: BL-28 Pangguangshu

Source (*Yuan*) points

The diagnostic use of the Source points is described in Chapter 1 of the 'Spiritual Axis', which says: '*If the 5 Yin organs are diseased, abnormal reactions will appear at the 12 Source points. If we know the correspondence of Source points to the relevant Yin organ, we can diagnose when a Yin organ is diseased.*'[7] This statement clearly indicates that the Source points have a relationship with the Original Qi and that changes on the skin over the Source points or tenderness on palpation indicate abnormalities in the relevant Yin organ. It should be noted that Chapter 1 of the 'Spiritual Axis' lists Source points only for the Yin organs (Box 51.22).

BOX 51.22 SOURCE POINTS FOR THE YIN ORGANS

- Lungs: LU-9 Taiyuan
- Heart: PE-7 Daling
- Spleen: SP-3 Taibai
- Liver: LIV-3 Taichong
- Kidneys: KI-3 Taixi

This makes a total of 10 points (each point being bilateral); the other two source points listed in that chapter are Ren-15 Jiuwei for Fat tissues, and Ren-6 Qihai for the Membranes.

NOTES

1. 1981 Spiritual Axis (*Ling Shu Jing* 灵枢经), People's Health Publishing House, Beijing, p. 75. First published c. 100BC.
2. 1979 The Yellow Emperor's Classic of Internal Medicine – Simple Questions (*Huang Di Nei Jing Su Wen* 黄帝内经素问), People's Health Publishing House, Beijing, p. 146. First published c. 100BC.
3. Spiritual Axis, p. 133.
4. Ibid., p. 133.
5. Cited in Deng Tie Tao, Practical Chinese Diagnosis (*Shi Yong Zhong Yi Zhen Duan Xue* 实用中医诊断学), Shanghai Science Publishing House, Shanghai, 1988, p. 167.
6. Spiritual Axis, p. 133.
7. Ibid., p. 3.

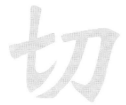

Chapter **52**

PALPATION OF CHANNELS

Chapter contents

INTRODUCTION   *525*

CONNECTING CHANNELS   *525*

MUSCLE CHANNELS   *527*

PALPATION OF THE CHANNELS IN PAINFUL OBSTRUCTION
   SYNDROME (*BI*)   *527*

PALPATION OF CHANNELS   *528*
   Lung channel   *528*
   Large Intestine channel   *528*
   Stomach channel   *529*
   Spleen channel   *530*
   Heart channel   *531*
   Small Intestine channel   *532*
   Bladder channel   *533*
   Kidney channel   *533*
   Pericardium channel   *534*
   Triple Burner channel   *535*
   Gall-Bladder channel   *536*
   Liver channel   *536*

INTRODUCTION

Besides palpating specific points with a particular diagnostic significance (as described in the previous chapter), palpation diagnosis must include also palpation of the channels. Before discussing the palpation of channels proper, we must discuss the energetic significance of the secondary channels, and in particular the Connecting (*Luo*) channels and the Muscle (*Jing Jin*) channels: these are the two secondary channels that are mostly involved in palpation. The other secondary channels, the Divergent (*Jing Bie*) channels, are not involved in palpation because they lie at a deep level, deeper than the Main channels.

CONNECTING CHANNELS

The Connecting channels are called *Luo Mai*: *Luo* implies the meaning of 'network'. (The Main channels are called *Jing Mai*, and *Jing* implies the meaning of 'line', 'route', 'way'.) Chapter 17 of the 'Spiritual Axis' confirms that the Connecting channels are 'horizontal' or 'crosswise': '*The Main channels are in the Interior, their branches are horizontal [or crosswise] forming the Luo channels*'.[1]

The Connecting channels are more superficial than the Main channels and they run in all directions, horizontally rather than vertically. In particular, they fill the space between skin and muscles (i.e. the *Cou Li* space). The components of each channel system correspond to different energetic layers pertaining to that channel. For example, if we take the Lung channel, the most superficial part of it is the skin overlying the channel pathway; below that, there is the *space between skin and muscles* or *Li* space, that is, the space between the skin and muscles where the Superficial Connecting

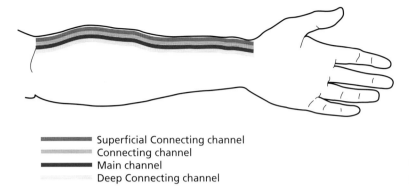

Superficial Connecting channel
Connecting channel
Main channel
Deep Connecting channel

Fig. 52.1 Energetic layers of a channel (Lung)

channels course; below that, the Connecting channel proper fills the space between the muscles and sinews: below that, there is the Lung Main channel and below that, the Lung Deep Connecting channel (Fig. 52.1). It is important to visualize the Connecting channels not as lines but as spaces filled by channels.

Thus, the Connecting channels occupy the space between the Main channels and the skin; however, within this space, there are also degrees of depth. On the superficial layers just below the skin there are smaller Connecting channels called Minute and Superficial Connecting channels.

The main branches of the Connecting channels are called *Bie*, that is, 'divergent' (same word as that used for Divergent channels). The Minute Connecting channels are called *Sun*, whereas the Superficial ones are called are called *Fu*.

Chapter 17 of the 'Spiritual Axis' says: *'The Main channels are in the Interior, their branches are horizontal [or crosswise] forming the Luo channels: branching out from these are the Minute Luo'*.[2] Chapter 10 of the same book says: *'The more superficial branches of the channels which can be seen are the Luo channels'*.[3] Chapter 58 of the 'Simple Questions' states: *'The Minute Luo [Sun Luo] communicate with the 365 points'*.[4]

However, the Connecting channels have also a deeper layer beyond the Main channels: these can be called the Deep Connecting channels and they are connected to the blood vessels and Blood in general.

The 12 Main channels are situated between the Yang and Yin Connecting channels. It is through the Yin and Yang Connecting channels that Nutritive and Defensive Qi and Qi and Blood of the main channels spread in all directions, permeate and irrigate the Internal Organs. It is also through the Connecting channels that the essence of the Internal Organs is transported to the Main channels and, through them, to the whole body.

The Connecting channels cannot penetrate the big joints of the body (as do the Main channels) and they are therefore restricted to the spaces in between the deep pathway of the Main channels and the surface of the body. The Connecting channels also fill the spaces and 'cavities' of the body, which are all part of the Triple Burner. This means that most of the stagnation in the body actually occurs in the Connecting channels because they are 'constricted' in these spaces (as they cannot course through the large joints) and because they form like a net which easily 'catches' pathogenic factors or in which Qi or Blood, or both, become stagnant. Chapter 10 of the 'Spiritual Axis' says:

The Luo channels cannot course through the large joints; in order to [enter and] exit they must move by alternate routes. They then enter and come together again under the skin and therefore they can be seen from the outside. To needle the Luo channel one must needle above the accumulation where Blood is concentrated. Even if there is no blood accumulation, one must prick to cause bleeding quickly to drain the pathogenic factors out: if this is not done, Bi syndrome may develop.[5]

Palpation

Palpation of the limbs involves essentially palpation of the Connecting channels and especially the Superficial Connecting channels and the Connecting channels proper. Generally speaking, the more distal the point, the more it reflects the state of the Connecting channels, whereas the more proximal the point, the more it reflects the state of the Main channels. For example, palpation of the forearm from LU-10 to LU-3 and slightly beyond reflects the state of the Lung Connecting channel portion; palpation in the area of

LU-2 and LU-1 reflects more the state of the Lung Main channel (and the organ itself).

Palpation should include the following techniques.

Touching

Touching the skin reveals its temperature and moisture and reflects the state of the Superficial Connecting channels. A hot sensation indicates Heat of the Superficial Connecting channel; a cold sensation indicates Cold of that particular channel. Dryness of the skin indicates lack of Body Fluids in the Superficial Connecting channels (related to Lungs and Spleen), whereas excessive sweating indicates a weak state of the space between skin and muscles (related to Lung-Qi deficiency).

Stroking

Stroking the skin reveals the texture and firmness of the skin and flesh and reflects the state of the Connecting channels. A flaccid feel indicates a weakness of the Connecting channel of the particular channel palpated; a hardness indicates stagnation there.

Pressing

Pressing the muscles reveals the firmness of the muscles and sinews and possible lumps or masses. Stiffness and hardness of the layers below the flesh of the limb indicate a Full condition of the Connecting channels (stagnation of Qi or Blood, or both). Flaccidity indicates a condition of Emptiness of the Connecting channel.

MUSCLE CHANNELS

The Muscle channels are called *Jing Jin*, which could be translated as 'channel-like muscles' or 'muscles of the channels'. They are discussed in Chapter 13 of the 'Spiritual Axis'.

Characteristics

The Muscle channels have the following characteristics:

- they are on the surface of the body
- they do not connect with the Internal Organs
- they all originate at the extremities
- they broadly follow the course of the Main channel (with exceptions, e.g. the Bladder Muscle channel)
- they follow the contours of the major muscles overlying the Main channels.

Functions

- They protect the body from trauma.
- They sustain the body in its erect position.
- They maintain the integrity of the body by connecting the '100 bones'.
- They govern the movement of joints.
- They allow movement of the body.
- They contribute to the integration of the surface of the body with the Interior.
- They contribute to the integration and connection within the Yang and within the Yin channels (i.e. the connections between Greater-Yang, Bright-Yang and Lesser-Yang channels and those between Greater-Yin, Lesser-Yin and Terminal-Yin channels).

Palpation

Palpation of the Muscle channels is done relatively firmly and it reveals the consistency of the muscles. A hard and stiff feel on palpation indicates either stagnation of Qi or Cold in the Muscle channels, whereas a flaccid feel indicates a deficiency of Qi or Blood, or both, in the Muscle channels.

The pathology of Muscle channels is essentially related only to invasion of external pathogenic factors or trauma.

PALPATION OF THE CHANNELS IN PAINFUL OBSTRUCTION SYNDROME (BI)

Palpation of points along the channel is essential in the treatment of Painful Obstruction Syndrome; this consists in the palpation not only of actual acupuncture points but also of Ah Shi points. Therefore, in order to find the Ah Shi points, the whole channel needs to be palpated.

The choice of points in the treatment of Painful Obstruction Syndrome is based primarily on one or more distal points of the affected channel (which are usually needled with reducing or even method) and on several local points according to tenderness on palpation. Palpating the Ah Shi points serves two purposes: in diagnosis, it allows us to identify the affected channel precisely; in treatment, it allows us to treat the reactive points (because their tenderness indicates the points of local stagnation).

Identifying the affected channel through palpation is absolutely essential for the choice of both distal and local points. For example, in shoulder problems, one must clearly identify the channel involved, which may be Small Intestine, Triple Burner, Large Intestine or Lung channel.

PALPATION OF CHANNELS

Each channel has specific areas that have a particular diagnostic significance on palpation. The following is a discussion of these areas for each channel.

For each channel, two aspects of palpation are discussed, that is palpation of a blood vessel overlying the channel and palpation of the skin overlying the channel. For palpation of the skin, three aspects are discussed, that is, temperature, texture and tenderness.

Lung channel

Apart from the palpation of points along the channels, the palpation of the Front position of the radial artery on the right side itself is a form of palpation of the Lung channel.

Palpation of blood vessel

The axillary artery can be palpated along the channel in the region extending from LU-1 Zhongfu to LU-4 Xiabai. If this feels superficial on palpation, it indicates an external invasion of Wind in the Lung-Defensive-Qi portion; if it feels deep this indicates an internal Lung problem. If it is rapid, this indicates Lung-Heat; if it is slow, this denotes Damp-Phlegm or Cold-Phlegm in the Lungs. If the artery pulsation feels empty this indicates Lung-Qi deficiency; if it feels full, this denotes a Full condition of the Lung such as Phlegm in the Lungs.

Palpation of skin
Temperature

Besides feeling the pulsation of the axillary artery, one should palpate the skin overlying the Lung channel, again in the area extending from LU-1 Zhongfu to LU-4 Xiabai. If the skin feels hot, this indicates Lung-Heat, whereas if it feels cold, this indicates Cold-Phlegm in the Lungs.

Texture

If the skin feels flaccid, it denotes Lung-Qi deficiency. If it feels rough and stiff, this indicates a Full condition of the Lungs.

Tenderness

Tenderness on palpation indicates stagnation of Qi and Blood in the Lung channel. If the tenderness is elicited with a light pressure this indicates stagnation in the superficial layers at the level of the Lung Connecting channel energetic layer; if it is elicited with a deep pressure this indicates stagnation at the deep energetic layers of the channel, that is, the sinew and bone energetic layers.

Box 52.1 summarizes the findings on palpation of the Lung channel.

BOX 52.1 PALPATION OF LUNG CHANNEL

Palpation of blood vessel: Axillary artery from LU-1 Zhongfu to LU-4 Xiabai
- Superficial: external invasion of Wind in the Lungs' Defensive-Qi portion
- Deep: internal Lung problem
- Rapid: Lung-Heat
- Slow: Damp-Phlegm or Cold-Phlegm in the Lungs
- Empty: Lung-Qi deficiency
- Full: Full condition of the Lung

Palpation of skin
Temperature
- Hot: Lung-Heat
- Cold: Cold-Phlegm in the Lungs
Texture
- Flaccid: Lung-Qi deficiency
- Rough and stiff: Full condition of the Lungs
Tenderness
- Tenderness with a light pressure: stagnation in the superficial layers of the Lung Connecting channel
- Tenderness with a deep pressure: stagnation at the deep energetic layers of the channel, i.e. sinew and bone energetic layers

---

Large Intestine channel

The diagnostic area for palpation on the Large Intestine channel is the area from LI-4 Hegu to LI-5 Yangxi and especially the latter where the radial artery can be felt.

Palpation of blood vessel

If the pulsation in the area of LI-5 Yangxi is superficial and large, this indicates conditions such as facial paralysis, tooth abscess or external Wind-Heat; if it is deep it may indicate an intestinal pathology such as abdominal pain, constipation or diarrhoea. If it is rapid this denotes a Heat condition of the Large Intestine and if it is slow a Cold condition. If the pulsation feels empty this denotes an Empty condition of the Large Intestine,

and if it feels full a Full condition with stagnation and abdominal pain.

Palpation of skin
Temperature

If the skin in the area of LI-4 Hegu and LI-5 Yangxi feels hot, this indicates a Heat condition of the channel often causing a tooth abscess or tonsillitis. If it feels cold, this denotes a Cold condition.

Texture

If the skin in the same area feels flaccid, this indicates an Empty condition of the Large Intestine with symptoms such as chronic diarrhoea. If the skin feels rough and hard it denotes a Full condition of the Large Intestine with symptoms such as Damp-Heat diarrhoea.

Tenderness

If the area between LI-4 Hegu and LI-5 Yangxi is tender on a light palpation, this indicates a stagnation in the Superficial Connecting channels (with symptoms such as facial tingling). If it is tender on deep pressure, it indicates a stagnation in the Connecting

---

BOX 52.2 LARGE INTESTINE CHANNEL PALPATION

Palpation of blood vessel: from LI-4 Hegu to LI-5 Yangxi
- Superficial and large: facial paralysis, tooth abscess or external Wind-Heat
- Deep: intestinal pathology
- Rapid: Heat
- Slow: Cold
- Empty: Empty condition
- Full: Full condition with stagnation and abdominal pain

Palpation of skin
Temperature
- Hot: Heat condition (teeth, tonsils)
- Cold: Cold condition
Texture
- Flaccid: Empty (diarrhoea)
- Rough and hard: Full (Damp-Heat diarrhoea)
Tenderness
- Tender on a light palpation: stagnation in the Superficial Connecting channels
- Tender on deep pressure: stagnation in the Connecting channels proper and Deep Connecting channels
- Spontaneous tenderness that is alleviated by palpation: Empty condition of the channel
- Tenderness aggravated by palpation: Full condition of the channel

---

channels proper, and possibly also the Deep Connecting channels, with symptoms such as chronic tendinitis of the shoulder or elbow with long-standing stagnation. If there is a spontaneous tenderness that is alleviated by palpation, this indicates an Empty condition of the channel, whereas if the tenderness is aggravated by palpation it denotes a Full condition of the channel.

Box 52.2 summarizes the findings on palpation of the Large Intestine channel

Stomach channel
Palpation of blood vessel

The two areas with diagnostic significance are ST-42 Chongyang and ST-9 Renying.

ST-42 Chongyang

The dorsal artery can be felt at this point. If the pulsation feels superficial, this indicates problems of the Stomach channel such as headache or sore throat; if it feels deep, it denotes problems of the Stomach organ with symptoms such as epigastric pain. If the pulsation is rapid, this indicates Heat in the Stomach channel with symptoms such as thirst and problems of the teeth or gums from Heat; if it feels slow, it indicates Cold in the Stomach channel. If the pulsation feels empty, this denotes an Empty condition of the Stomach with symptoms such as a dull epigastric pain; if it is full, it indicates a Full condition of the Stomach with symptoms such as epigastric pain from stagnation.

ST-9 Renying

The carotid artery can be felt at this point. This point is a Window of Heaven point regulating the flow of Qi to and from the head. If the carotid pulse feels full and rapid, this indicates a Full condition with excess of Yang in the head; if it feels empty, this indicates an Empty condition with a deficiency of Qi or Blood, or both, in the head.

Palpation of skin

The area around ST-42 Chongyang is palpated.

Temperature

If the skin feels hot on palpation this indicates a condition of Heat of the Stomach channel, which may be causing gum or breast problems (in women); if the skin feels cold, it indicates a Cold condition of the Stomach with symptoms such as dull epigastric pain.

Texture

If the skin in the area of ST-42 Chongyang feels flaccid, this indicates an Empty condition of the Stomach with symptoms such as dull epigastric pain, if it feels rough and hard, it denotes a Full condition of the Stomach, which may be causing a sharp epigastric pain or a breast pathology (in women).

Tenderness

If the area is tender on light palpation, this indicates a stagnation in the Superficial Connecting channels with symptoms such as facial paralysis; if it is tender

---

BOX 52.3 STOMACH CHANNEL PALPATION

Palpation of blood vessel: ST-42 Chongyang and ST-9 Renying

ST-42 Chongyang
- Superficial: Stomach channel problems (headache, sore throat)
- Deep: problems of the Stomach organ (epigastric pain)
- Rapid: Heat in the Stomach channel (thirst, problems in gums and mouth)
- Slow: Cold in the Stomach channel
- Empty: Empty condition of the Stomach (dull epigastric pain)
- Full: Full condition of the Stomach (dull pain from stagnation)

ST-9 Renying
- Full and rapid: Full condition with excess of Yang in the head
- Empty: Empty condition with a deficiency of Qi/Blood in the head

Palpation of skin: around ST-42 Chongyang

Temperature
- Hot: Heat of the Stomach channel (problems with gums or breast in women)
- Cold: Cold condition of the Stomach (epigastrium)

Texture
- Flaccid: Empty condition of the Stomach (pain in epigastrium)
- Rough and hard: Full condition of the Stomach (could be sharp epigastric pain or breast pathology in women)

Tenderness
- Tender on light palpation: stagnation in the Superficial Connecting channels, with facial paralysis
- Tender on deep pressure: stagnation of Qi/Blood in the Connecting channels proper and Main channels with symptoms such as chronic Painful Obstruction Syndrome along the Stomach channel
- Tenderness that is alleviated by pressure: Empty condition of the channel
- Tenderness aggravated by pressure: Full condition of the channel

---

on deep pressure it indicates stagnation of Qi or Blood, or both, in the Connecting channels proper and Main channels, with symptoms such as chronic Painful Obstruction Syndrome along the Stomach channel.

If there is tenderness that is alleviated by pressure, this indicates an Empty condition of the channel; if it is aggravated by pressure it indicates a Full condition of the channel.

Box 52.3 summarizes the findings on palpation of the stomach channel.

Spleen channel

The diagnostic area for palpation on the Spleen channel is the area from SP-11 Jimen to SP-12 Chongmen where the femoral artery can felt.

Palpation of blood vessel

If the pulsation in the area of SP-11 Jimen to SP-12 Chongmen is superficial and large, this indicates skin conditions such as erysipelas; if it is deep it may indicate an intestinal pathology such as abdominal pain or fullness. If it is rapid, this denotes a Heat condition of the Spleen channel, and if it is slow a Cold condition of the organ with symptoms such a diarrhoea from Cold. If the pulsation feels empty, this denotes an Empty condition of the Spleen with symptoms such as lassitude, weakness and loose stools; if it feels full, this denotes a Full condition with stagnation and abdominal pain.

Palpation of skin
Temperature

If the skin in the area of SP-11 Jinmen and SP-12 Chongmen feels hot, this indicates a Heat condition of the channel often causing erysipelas; if it feels cold, it denotes a Cold condition with symptoms such as cold limbs.

Texture

If the skin in the same area feels flaccid, this indicates an Empty condition of the Spleen with symptoms such as chronic diarrhoea; if the skin feels rough and hard it denotes a Full condition of the Spleen with symptoms such as Damp-Heat diarrhoea.

Tenderness

If the area between SP-11 Jinmen and SP-12 Chongmen is tender on a light palpation, this indicates a stagnation in the Superficial Connecting channels; if it is

tender on deep pressure, it indicates a stagnation in the Connecting channels proper and possibly also Deep Connecting channels with symptoms such as chronic groin pain. If there is a spontaneous tenderness that is alleviated by palpation, this indicates an Empty condition of the channel, whereas if the tenderness is aggravated by palpation it denotes a Full condition of the channel.

BOX 52.4 SPLEEN CHANNEL PALPATION

Palpation of blood vessel: from SP-11 Jimen to SP-12 Chongmen
- Superficial and large: skin rashes
- Deep: intestinal pathology
- Rapid: Heat in Spleen channel
- Slow: Cold condition (diarrhoea)
- Empty: Empty condition (loose stools, weakness, tiredness)
- Full: stagnation in Intestines

Palpation of skin
Temperature
- Hot: Heat in channel
- Cold: Cold (limbs)
Texture
- Flaccid: Empty condition (diarrhoea)
- Rough and hard: Full condition (Damp-Heat diarrhoea)
Tenderness
- Tender on light palpation: stagnation in Superficial Connecting channels
- Tender on deep pressure: stagnation in Connecting channel proper and Deep Connecting channel
- Spontaneous tenderness alleviated by pressure: Empty condition of channel
- Spontaneous tenderness aggravated by pressure: Full condition of channel

---

Box 52.4 summarizes the findings on palpation of the Spleen channel.

Heart channel

The diagnostic areas for palpation on the Heart channel are HE-7 Shenmen, where the ulnar artery can be felt, and HE-1 Jiquan, where the axillary artery can be felt.

Palpation of blood vessel

If the pulsation in the area of HE-7 Shenmen and HE-1 Jiquan is superficial and large, this indicates conditions such as red eyes from Heart-Heat or erysipelas; if it is deep it may indicate a condition with palpitations and chest pain. If it is rapid, this denotes a Heat condition of the Heart channel with symptoms such as tongue ulcers, whereas if it is slow it denotes a Cold condition such as Chest Painful Obstruction Syndrome. If the pulsation feels empty, it denotes an Empty condition of the Heart with symptoms such as anxiety and poor memory, and if it feels full a Full condition with symptoms such as mental restlessness.

Palpation of skin
Temperature

If the skin in the area of HE-7 Shenmen and HE-1 Jiquan feels hot, this indicates a Heat condition of the channel often causing red eyes, hot palms or erysipelas; if it feels cold it denotes a Cold condition often causing chest pain.

Texture

If the skin in the same area feels flaccid, this indicates an Empty condition of the Heart channel with symptoms such as contraction of the little finger; if the skin feels rough and hard it denotes a Full condition of the Heart channel such as Heart-Heat causing tongue ulcers.

BOX 52.5 HEART CHANNEL PALPATION

Palpation of blood vessel: From HE-7 Shenmen to HE-1 Jiquan
- Superficial and large: Heart-Heat (e.g. red eyes)
- Deep: palpitations and chest pain
- Rapid: Heat in Heart channel (e.g. tongue ulcers)
- Slow: Chest Painful Obstruction Syndrome
- Empty: Empty condition (e.g. anxiety, poor memory)
- Full: Full condition (e.g. mental restlessness)

Palpation of skin
Temperature
- Hot: Heat (e.g. red eyes)
- Cold: Cold (e.g. chest pain)
Texture
- Flaccid: Empty condition of channel (e.g. contraction in little finger)
- Rough and hard: Full condition of channel (e.g. tongue ulcers)
Tenderness
- Tenderness on light palpation: stagnation in Superficial Connecting channel
- Tenderness on deep pressure: stagnation in Connecting channel proper and Deep Connecting channel
- Spontaneous tenderness alleviated by pressure: Empty condition of the channel
- Spontaneous tenderness aggravated by pressure: Full condition of the channel

---

Tenderness

If the areas of HE-7 Shenmen and HE-1 Jiquan are tender on a light palpation, this indicates a stagnation in the Superficial Connecting channels, whereas if it is tender on deep pressure it indicates a stagnation in the Connecting channels proper and possibly also Deep Connecting channels with symptoms such as chronic Chest Painful Obstruction Syndrome. If there is a spontaneous tenderness that is alleviated by palpation, this indicates an Empty condition of the channel; if the tenderness is aggravated by palpation it denotes a Full condition of the channel.

Box 52.5 summarizes findings on palpation of the Heart channel.

Small intestine channel

The diagnostic area for palpation on the Small Intestine channel is the area around SI-16 Tianchuang where the cervical artery can be felt.

Palpation of blood vessel

If the pulsation in the area of SI-16 Tianchuang is superficial and large, this indicates conditions such as headache from invasion of external Wind; if it is deep it may indicate a urinary pathology such as urinary retention. If it is rapid, this denotes a Heat condition of the Small Intestine with symptoms such as burning on urination; if it is slow, it indicates a Cold condition with symptoms such as pale-frequent urination. If the pulsation feels empty, this denotes an Empty condition of the Small Intestine with urinary symptoms, and if it feels full a Full condition with stagnation and abdominal pain or urinary retention.

Palpation of skin
Temperature

If the skin in the area of SI-16 Tianchuang feels hot, this indicates a Heat condition of the channel often causing tonsillitis or ear infections; if it feels cold it denotes a Cold condition of the Small Intestine with borborygmi and diarrhoea.

Texture

If the skin in the same area feels flaccid, this indicates an Empty condition of the Small Intestine with symptoms such as frequent-pale urination. If the skin feels

rough and hard it denotes a Full condition of the Small Intestine, often with symptoms such as stiff and painful neck.

Tenderness

If the area around SI-16 Tianchuang is tender on a light palpation, this indicates a stagnation in the Superficial Connecting channels (with symptoms such as numbness of the neck muscles), while if it is tender on deep pressure it indicates a stagnation in the Connecting channels proper and possibly also Deep Connecting channels with symptoms such as chronic tendinitis of the shoulder or stiff neck with long-standing stagnation. If there is a spontaneous tenderness that is alleviated by palpation it indicates an Empty condition of the channel, while if the tenderness is aggravated by palpation it denotes a Full condition of the channel.

BOX 52.6 SMALL INTESTINE CHANNEL PALPATION

Palpation of blood vessel: area around SI-16 Tianchuang
- Superficial and large: external Wind
- Deep: urinary pathology
- Rapid: Heat with urinary symptoms
- Slow: Cold with urinary symptoms
- Empty: Empty condition with urinary symptoms
- Full: Full condition with abdominal pain and urinary retention

Palpation of skin
Temperature
- Hot: Heat in channel (e.g. tonsillitis, ear infection)
- Cold: Cold in organ (e.g. diarrhoea)
Texture
- Flaccid: Empty condition with urinary symptoms
- Rough and hard: Full condition of channel (e.g. neck numbness)
Tenderness
- Tenderness on light palpation: stagnation in Superficial Connecting channel (e.g. numb neck muscles)
- Tenderness on deep pressure: stagnation in Connecting channel proper and Deep Connecting channel (e.g. shoulder and neck stiffness)
- Spontaneous tenderness alleviated by pressure: Empty condition of channel
- Spontaneous tenderness aggravated by pressure: Full condition of channel

---

Box 52.6 summarizes findings on palpation of the Small Intestine channel.

Bladder channel

The diagnostic area for palpation on the Bladder channel is the area around BL-40 Weizhong where the popliteal artery can be felt.

Palpation of blood vessel

If the pulsation in the area of BL-40 Weizhong is superficial and large, this indicates conditions such as headache and neck ache from invasion of external Wind; if it is deep it may indicate a urinary pathology such as scanty urination with oedema. If it is rapid, this denotes a Heat condition of the Bladder with symptoms such as burning on urination, and if it is slow, it denotes a Cold condition with symptoms such as frequent-pale urination. If the pulsation feels empty, this denotes an Empty condition of the Bladder with symptoms such as urinary incontinence or enuresis, and if it feels full, it denotes a Full condition with symptoms such as urinary retention.

Palpation of skin
Temperature

If the skin in the area of BL-40 Weizhong feels hot, this indicates a Heat condition of channel, which may cause skin eruptions along the channel. If it feels cold it denotes a Cold condition with symptoms such as cold and weak legs.

Texture

If the skin in the same area feels flaccid, this indicates an Empty condition of the Bladder with symptoms such as backache from Deficiency and weak legs; if the skin feels rough and hard it denotes a Full condition of the Bladder with symptoms such as urinary retention.

Tenderness

If the area around BL-40 Weizhong is tender on a light palpation, this indicates a stagnation in the Superficial Connecting channels (with symptoms such as scalp tingling), while if it is tender on deep pressure it indicates a stagnation in the Connecting channels proper and possibly also the Deep Connecting channels with symptoms such as chronic backache from long-standing stagnation. If there is a spontaneous tenderness that is alleviated by palpation, this indicates an Empty condition of the channel, whereas if the tenderness is aggravated by palpation it denotes a Full condition of the channel.

BOX 52.7 BLADDER CHANNEL PALPATION

Palpation of blood vessel: area around BL-40 Weizhong
- Superficial and large: external Wind
- Deep: urinary pathology
- Rapid: Heat (e.g. burning on urination)
- Slow: Cold (e.g. frequent urination)
- Empty: Empty condition of organ
- Full: Full condition of organ

Palpation of skin
Temperature
- Hot: Heat condition of channel
- Cold: Cold condition of channel (e.g. cold and weak legs)

Texture
- Flaccid: Empty condition (e.g. weak legs, backache)
- Rough and hard: Full condition (e.g. urinary retention)

Tenderness
- Tenderness on light palpation: stagnation in Superficial Connecting channel
- Tenderness on deep pressure: stagnation in Connecting channel proper and Deep Connecting channel
- Spontaneous tenderness alleviated by pressure: Empty condition of channel
- Spontaneous tenderness aggravated by pressure: Full condition of channel

---

Box 52.7 summarizes the findings on palpation of the Bladder channel.

Kidney channel

The diagnostic area for palpation on the Kidney channel is the area around KI-3 Taixi where the posterior tibial artery can be felt.

Palpation of blood vessel

If the pulsation in the area of KI-3 Taixi is superficial and large, this indicates conditions such as headache and neck ache from invasion of external Wind; if it is deep it may indicate a urinary pathology such as scanty urination with oedema or gynaecological problems. If it is rapid, this denotes a Heat condition of the Kidneys with symptoms such as burning on urination, and if slow a Cold condition with symptoms such as frequent-pale urination. If the pulsation feels empty, this denotes an Empty condition of the Kidneys with symptoms such as urinary incontinence or enuresis, and if it feels full a Full condition with symptoms such as urinary retention.

Palpation of skin

Temperature

If the skin in the area of KI-3 Taixi feels hot, this indicates a Heat condition of the channel which may cause skin eruptions along the channel; if it feels cold it denotes a Cold condition with symptoms such as feeling cold, backache and frequent-pale urination.

Texture

If the skin in the same area feels flaccid, this indicates an Empty condition of the Kidney with symptoms such as backache from Deficiency and weak legs; if the skin feels rough and hard it denotes a Full condition of the Kidney with symptoms such as urinary retention.

Tenderness

If the area around KI-3 Taixi is tender on a light palpation, this indicates a stagnation in the Superficial Connecting channels (with symptoms such as scalp tingling), whereas if tender on deep pressure, it indicates a stagnation in the Connecting channels proper, and possibly also the Deep Connecting channels, with symptoms such as chronic backache from long-standing stagnation. If there is a spontaneous tenderness that is alleviated by palpation, this indicates an Empty condition of the channel, whereas if the tenderness is aggravated by palpation it denotes a Full condition of the channel.

Box 52.8 summarizes findings on palpation of the Kidney channel.

Pericardium channel

The diagnostic area for palpation on the Pericardium channel is the area around PE-8 Laogong where the common palmar digital artery can be felt.

Palpation of blood vessel

If the pulsation in the area of PE-8 Laogong is superficial and large, this indicates conditions such as fullness of the chest; if it is deep it may indicate chest pain from stagnation. If it is rapid, this denotes a Heat condition of the Pericardium with symptoms such as mental restlessness and hot chest, whereas if slow a Cold condition with symptoms such as chest pain from Yang deficiency. If the pulsation feels empty, this denotes an Empty condition of the Pericardium, with symptoms such as palpitations, insomnia and an empty feeling of the chest, and if it feels full a Full condition, with symptoms such as mental restlessness and manic behaviour.

Palpation of skin

Temperature

If the skin in the area of PE-8 Laogong feels hot, this indicates a Heat condition of channel, which may cause hot palms; if it feels cold it denotes a Cold condition, with symptoms such as feeling of cold and dull chest ache.

Texture

If the skin in the same area feels flaccid, this indicates an Empty condition of the Pericardium, with symptoms such as an empty feeling of the chest; if it feels rough and hard it denotes a Full condition of the Pericardium, with symptoms such as chest pain.

Tenderness

If the area around PE-8 Laogong is tender on a light palpation, this indicates a stagnation in the Superficial Connecting channels (with symptoms such as scalp tingling) whereas if tender on deep pressure, it indicates a stagnation in the Connecting channels proper, and possibly also Deep Connecting channels, with symptoms such as chest pain from long-standing stagnation. If there is a spontaneous tenderness that is

---

BOX 52.8 KIDNEY CHANNEL PALPATION

Palpation of blood vessel: area around KI-3 Taixi
- Superficial and large: external Wind
- Deep: urinary or gynaecological condition
- Rapid: Heat (urinary)
- Slow: Cold (urinary)
- Empty: Empty condition (urinary)
- Full: Full condition (urinary)

Palpation of skin
Temperature
- Hot: Heat condition of channel
- Cold: Cold condition of channel
Texture
- Flaccid: Empty condition (back)
- Rough and hard: Full condition (urinary)
Tenderness
- Tenderness on light palpation: stagnation in Superficial Connecting channel
- Tenderness on deep pressure: stagnation in Connecting channel proper and Deep Connecting channel
- Spontaneous tenderness alleviated by pressure: Empty condition of channel
- Spontaneous tenderness aggravated by pressure: Full condition of channel

alleviated by palpation, this indicates an Empty condition of the channel, whereas if the tenderness is aggravated by palpation it denotes a Full condition of the channel.

BOX 52.9 PERICARDIUM CHANNEL PALPATION

Palpation of blood vessel: area around PE-8 Laogong
- Superficial and large: fullness of the chest
- Deep: chest pain from stagnation
- Rapid: Heat condition of Pericardium (e.g. mental restlessness)
- Slow: chest pain from Yang deficiency
- Empty: Empty condition (e.g. insomnia)
- Full: Full condition (e.g. mental restlessness, mania)

Palpation of skin
Temperature
- Hot: Heat condition of channel (e.g. hot palms)
- Cold: Cold condition (e.g. dull chest ache)
Texture
- Flaccid: Empty condition (e.g. empty feeling in chest)
- Rough and hard: Full condition (e.g. chest pain)
Tenderness
- Tenderness on light palpation: stagnation in Superficial Connecting channel
- Tenderness on deep pressure: stagnation in Connecting channel proper and Deep Connecting channel
- Spontaneous tenderness alleviated by pressure: Empty condition of channel
- Spontaneous tenderness aggravated by pressure: Full condition of channel

---

Box 52.9 summarizes findings on palpation of the Pericardium channel.

Triple Burner channel

The diagnostic area for palpation on the Triple Burner channel is the area around TB-22 Heliao where the superficial temporal artery can be felt.

Palpation of blood vessel

If the pulsation in the area of TB-22 Heliao is superficial and large, this indicates conditions such as headache and neck ache from invasion of external Wind; if it is deep it may indicate a urinary pathology. If it is rapid, this denotes a Heat condition of the Triple Burner with symptoms such as earache, and if it is slow a Cold condition, with symptoms such as frequent-pale urination. If the pulsation feels empty, this denotes an Empty condition of the Triple Burner, with symptoms such as urinary incontinence or enuresis,

and if it feels full a Full condition, with symptoms such as fullness of the chest.

Palpation of skin
Temperature

If the skin in the area of TB-22 Heliao feels hot, this indicates a Heat condition of channel, which may cause ear infections; if it feels cold it denotes a Cold condition, with symptoms such as cold and weak legs or a urinary pathology.

Texture

If the skin in the same area feels flaccid, this indicates an Empty condition of the Triple Burner, with symptoms such as weak arms; if the skin feels rough and hard it denotes a Full condition of the Triple Burner, with symptoms such as red skin eruptions along the channel.

Tenderness

If the area around TB-22 Heliao is tender on a light palpation, this indicates a stagnation in the Superficial Connecting channels (with symptoms such as face tingling), while if tender on deep pressure it indicates a stagnation in the Connecting channels proper, and

---

BOX 52.10 TRIPLE BURNER CHANNEL PALPATION

Palpation of blood vessel: area around TB-22 Heliao
- Superficial and large: external Wind
- Deep: urinary pathology
- Rapid: Heat (e.g. earache)
- Slow: Cold (e.g. frequent urination)
- Empty: Empty condition (e.g. urinary incontinence)
- Full: Full condition (e.g. chest fullness)

Palpation of skin
Temperature
- Hot: Heat condition of channel
- Cold: Cold condition of channel
Texture
- Flaccid: Empty condition (e.g. weak arms)
- Rough and hard: Full condition (e.g. eruptions along channel)
Tenderness
- Tenderness on light palpation: stagnation in the Superficial Connecting channel
- Tenderness on deep pressure: stagnation in the Connecting channel proper and Deep Connecting channel
- Spontaneous tenderness alleviated by pressure: Empty condition of the channel
- Spontaneous tenderness aggravated by pressure: Full condition of the channel

---

possibly also Deep Connecting channels, with symptoms such as chronic tendinitis of the shoulder from long-standing stagnation. If there is spontaneous tenderness that is alleviated by palpation, this indicates an Empty condition of the channel, while if the tenderness is aggravated by palpation it denotes a Full condition of the channel.

Box 52.10 Summarizes findings on palpation of the Triple Burner channel.

Gall-Bladder channel

The diagnostic area for palpation on the Gall-Bladder channel is the area around GB-2 Tinghui where the superficial temporal artery can be felt.

Palpation of blood vessel

If the pulsation in the area of GB-2 Tinghui is superficial and large, this indicates conditions such as headache and neck ache from invasion of external Wind; if it is deep it may indicate a Gall-Bladder pathology, with symptoms such as hypochondrial pain. If it is rapid, this denotes a Heat condition of the Gall-Bladder, with symptoms such as earache or red eyes, and if slow a Cold condition, with symptoms such as headache or watering eyes. If the pulsation feels empty, this denotes an Empty condition of the Gall-Bladder, with symptoms such as chronic leucorrhoea, and if it feels full a Full condition, with symptoms such as earache.

Palpation of skin
Temperature

If the skin in the area of GB-2 Tinghui feels hot, this indicates a Heat condition of channel, which may cause ear infections; if it feels cold it denotes a Cold condition, with symptoms such as cold and weak legs.

Texture

If the skin in the same area feels flaccid, this indicates an Empty condition of the Gall-Bladder, with symptoms such as backache from Deficiency and weak legs; if the skin feels rough and hard it denotes a Full condition of the Gall-Bladder, with symptoms such as hypochondrial pain.

Tenderness

If the area around GB-2 Tinghui is tender on a light palpation, this indicates a stagnation in the Superficial Connecting channels (with symptoms such as face and ear tingling), while if tender on deep pressure it indicates a stagnation in the Connecting channels proper, and possibly also the Deep Connecting channels, with symptoms such as chronic hip or knee pain from long-standing stagnation. If there is a spontaneous tenderness that is alleviated by palpation, this indicates an Empty condition of the channel, whereas if aggravated by palpation it denotes a Full condition of the channel.

BOX 52.11 GALL-BLADDER CHANNEL PALPATION

Palpation of blood vessel: area around GB-2 Tinghui
- Superficial and large: external Wind
- Deep: hypochondrial pain
- Rapid: Heat (e.g. earache, red eyes)
- Slow: Cold (e.g. headache, watery eyes)
- Empty: Empty condition (e.g. vaginal discharge)
- Full: Full condition (e.g. earache)

Palpation of skin
Temperature
- Hot: Heat (e.g. ear infection)
- Cold: Cold (e.g. cold/weak legs)
Texture
- Flaccid: Empty condition (e.g. backache, weak legs)
- Rough and hard: Full condition (e.g. hypochondrial pain)
Tenderness
- Tenderness on light palpation: stagnation in the Superficial Connecting channel
- Tenderness on deep pressure: stagnation in the Connecting channel proper and Deep Connecting channel
- Spontaneous tenderness alleviated by pressure: Empty condition of the channel
- Spontaneous tenderness aggravated by pressure: Full condition of the channel

---

Box 52.11 summarizes findings on palpation of the Gall-Bladder channel.

Liver channel

The diagnostic area for palpation on the Liver channel is the area around LIV-3 Taichong (where the dorsal metatarsal artery can be felt), LIV-9 Yinbao and LIV-10 Wuli (where the femoral artery can be felt).

Palpation of blood vessel

If the pulsation in the area of LIV-3 Taichong, LIV-9 Yinbao and LIV-10 Wuli is superficial and large, this indicates conditions such as headache and painful eyes; if it is deep it may indicate a Liver pathology such as Liver-Qi stagnation, with symptoms of abdominal pain. If it is

rapid, this denotes a Heat condition of the Liver, with symptoms such as headache, red eyes and epistaxis; if slow it denotes a Cold condition, with symptoms such as headache or watering eyes. If the pulsation feels empty, this denotes an Empty condition of the Liver such as Liver-Blood deficiency, with symptoms such as blurred vision and scanty periods; if it feels full, it denotes a Full condition such as Liver-Qi stagnation, with symptoms such as hypogastric distension and urinary problems.

Palpation of skin
Temperature

If the skin in the area of LIV-3 Taichong, LIV-9 Yinbao and LIV-10 Wuli feels hot, this indicates a Heat con-

---

BOX 52.12 LIVER CHANNEL PATHOLOGY

Palpation of blood vessel: from LIV-3 Taichong to LIV-10 Wuli
- Superficial and large: pain in head and eyes
- Deep: Liver-Qi stagnation
- Rapid: Liver-Heat (e.g. headache, red eyes)
- Slow: headache with watery eyes
- Empty: Liver-Blood deficiency
- Full: Liver-Qi stagnation (e.g. urinary problems)

Palpation of skin
Temperature
- Hot: Heat in channel (e.g. inflammation of genitalia)
- Cold: Cold in channel (e.g. cold genitalia)
Texture
- Flaccid: Empty condition (e.g. numb/weak legs)
- Rough and hard: Full condition (e.g. hypochondrial pain)
Tenderness
- Tenderness on light palpation: stagnation in the Superficial Connecting channel
- Tenderness on deep pressure: stagnation in the Connecting channel proper and Deep Connecting channel
- Spontaneous tenderness alleviated by pressure: Empty condition of the channel
- Spontaneous tenderness aggravated by pressure: Full condition of the channel

---

dition of channel, which may cause erysipelas or inflammation of the external genitalia; if it feels cold it denotes a Cold condition, with symptoms such as cold hypogastrium and external genitalia.

Texture

If the skin in the same area feels flaccid, this indicates an Empty condition of the Liver, with symptoms such as numbness and weakness of the legs; if it feels rough and hard it denotes a Full condition of the Liver, with symptoms such as hypochondrial pain.

Tenderness

If the area around LIV-3 Taichong, LIV-9 Yinbao and LIV-10 Wuli is tender on light palpation, this indicates a stagnation in the Superficial Connecting channels (with symptoms such as genital itching), whereas if tender on deep pressure, it indicates a stagnation in the Connecting channels proper, and possibly also Deep Connecting channels, with symptoms such as hypogastric pain and urinary symptoms. If there is a spontaneous tenderness that is alleviated by palpation, this indicates an Empty condition of the channel; if the tenderness is aggravated by palpation it denotes a Full condition of the channel.

Box 52.12 summarizes the findings on palpations of the Liver channel.

NOTES

1. 1981 Spiritual Axis (*Ling Shu Jing* 灵枢经), People's Health Publishing House, Beijing, p. 50. First published c. 100BC.
2. Ibid., p. 50.
3. Ibid., p. 37.
4. 1979 The Yellow Emperor's Classic of Internal Medicine – Simple Questions (*Huang Di Nei Jing Su Wen* 黄帝内经素问), People's Health Publishing House, Beijing, p. 301. First published c. 100 BC.
5. Spiritual Axis, p. 37.

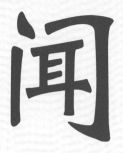

PART 4

DIAGNOSIS BY HEARING AND SMELLING

Part contents

53 Diagnosis by hearing *541*
54 Diagnosis by smelling *549*

INTRODUCTION

Diagnosis by hearing and smelling is called *Wen* in Chinese and, interestingly, this character can mean both 'to hear' and 'to smell'. Diagnosis by these means has been an integral part of Chinese medicine since early times. Chapter 5 of the 'Simple Questions' mentions hearing in the context of diagnosis in general: '*A good diagnostician will observe the patient's complexion and feel his pulse to distinguish Yin from Yang; he will examine whether the complexion is clear or turbid to identify the location of the disease; he will listen to the patient's panting and breathing and the patient's voice to diagnose the affliction.*'[1]

In ancient times the Yin organs were correlated with the five musical notes (the scale of Chinese music has five rather than seven notes) and the five sounds. These were:

- the Liver has the note *jue* and the sound of shouting
- the Heart has the note *zhi* and the sound of laughing
- the Spleen has the note *gong* and the sound of singing
- the Lungs have the note *shang* and the sound of weeping
- the Kidneys have the note *yu* and the sound of groaning.

The 'Classic of Difficulties' mentions the sounds and smells in several passages. Chapter 34 lists the colours, sounds, smells, tastes and fluids of each Yin organ. The sounds and smells of each Yin organ in this classic are listed as follows.[2]

Organ	Sound	Smell
Liver	Shouting	Foul
Heart	Talking	Scorched
Spleen	Singing	Fragrant
Lungs	Weeping	Rotten
Kidneys	Groaning	Putrid

Chapter 49 of the 'Classic of Difficulties' says: *'The Heart controls the sense of smell. When this enters the Heart itself the smell is scorched, when it enters the Spleen it is fragrant, when it enters the Liver it is foul, when it enters the Kidneys it is putrid, when it enters the Lungs it is rotten.'*[3] It is interesting that this passage relates the sense of smell to the Heart.

The same chapter of the 'Classic of Difficulties' discusses the sounds related to the Yin organs: *'The Lungs control the voice [or sound]. When this enters the Liver the sound is shouting, when it enters the Heart it is talking, when it enters the Spleen it is singing, when it enters the Kidneys it is groaning, and when it enters the Lung itself it is weeping.'*[4] Chapter 61 of the same classic says: *'By hearing the five sounds we can diagnose the disease.'*[5]

Chapter 17 of the 'Simple Questions' has an interesting description of the voice of a patient suffering from Dampness: *'When the Centre [i.e. Middle Burner] suffers from fullness, the rising Qi will cause fear and the voice [of the patient] sounds as if it were coming from the inside of a room [i.e. between walls] and this is due to Dampness in the Centre.'*[6] The same passage then describes the clinical significance of a weak voice and of incoherent speech: *'When the voice is feeble and interrupted Qi is depleted. If a person cannot look after his personal hygiene [literally the clothes and bedding are messy] and the speech is incoherent, it means that the Mind is chaotic.'*[7]

NOTES

1. 1979 The Yellow Emperor's Classic of Internal Medicine – Simple Questions (*Huang Di Nei Jing Su Wen* 黄帝内经素问), People's Health Publishing House, Beijing, p. 46. First published c. 100BC.
2. Nanjing College of Traditional Chinese Medicine 1979 A Revised Explanation of the Classic of Difficulties (*Nan Jing Jiao Shi* 难经校释), People's Health Publishing House, Beijing, p. 85. First published c. AD100.
3. Ibid., p. 113.
4. Ibid., p. 114.
5. Ibid., p. 135.
6. Simple Questions, pp. 99–100.
7. Ibid., p. 100.

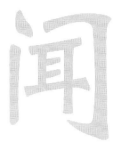

Chapter **53**

DIAGNOSIS BY HEARING

Chapter contents

INTRODUCTION   *541*

VOICE   *541*
  Normal voice   *542*
  The voice and the Five Elements   *542*
  Strength and quality of the voice   *543*

SPEECH   *544*

CRYING IN BABIES   *544*

BREATHING AND SIGHING   *544*
  Breathing   *544*
  Pathological breathing sounds   *545*
  Sighing   *545*

COUGHING AND SNEEZING   *545*
  Coughing   *545*
  Sneezing   *546*

HICCUP   *546*

BELCHING   *546*

VOMITING   *547*

INTRODUCTION

We may start using 'hearing' as an aid to diagnosis as soon as patients begin to speak, or even when they telephone to make an appointment. The sound of the voice gives us an immediate indication of the state of patients' Qi and, in particular, of their Lung-Qi, which is directly reflected in the voice. The voice also reflects the state of the Mind and Spirit: a quiet voice without force and with a sad tone indicates that the Mind and Spirit are affected.

VOICE

The sound of the voice is produced by the combined function of many parts of the body which are influenced by various Internal Organs in Chinese medicine (indicated in brackets). They are: the lungs themselves (Lungs), larynx (Lungs), epiglottis (Kidneys), tongue (Heart), teeth (Kidneys), lips (Spleen) and nose (Lungs). For this reason, the voice can reflect the state of Qi in general because several organs are involved in its production and, particularly, the Lungs, Heart, Spleen and Kidneys.

> **!**
>
> The voice is produced by the following organs:
> - lungs (Lungs)
> - larynx (Lungs)
> - epiglottis (Kidneys)
> - tongue (Heart)
> - teeth (Kidneys)
> - lips (Spleen)
> - nose (Lungs).

The voice is an important diagnostic element and one that is used as soon as the patient comes in and greets us. This gives us the very first impression of the person's Qi in general, a strong voice reflecting a strong Qi (and possibly pathogenic factors) and a weak voice indicating Qi deficiency.

The voice is an important reflection of the state of the Mind and Spirit as well because talking in general is controlled by the Heart. Our voice of course reflects very closely our mental–emotional state and we can easily detect sadness, fear or anger in someone's voice.

The voice is a direct manifestation of Lung-Qi and it readily reflects the state of the Lung-Qi; the Lungs influence the tone and strength of the voice.

The Heart influences the speech itself in two ways. First, the Heart has a profound influence on the tone and texture of the voice because it controls the tongue, which is a crucial organ in the production of speech. Secondly, the Heart houses the Mind and Spirit, and the tone and strength of the voice are very much affected by the speaker's mental–emotional state.

The Spleen controls the lips, which are also a crucial factor in the production of speech, and, obviously, this influences the strength and tone of the voice. First, if Spleen-Qi is deficient, the lips may lack strength and the speech may be unclear. Secondly, although the tone and strength of the voice reflect primarily the state of Lung-Qi, they also reflect the state of Qi in general and therefore of the Spleen, which is the root of Postnatal Qi.

The Kidneys influence the pitch and the quality of the voice because the Original Qi emerging from between the Kidneys reaches the root of the tongue allowing the larynx to emit sounds.

When listening to the voice, one should assess the overall strength, tone, pitch and quality of the voice itself and the manner of speech, that is, whether it is rapid, slow, confused, slurred, etc. The manner of speech is discussed in the next section, under the heading 'Speech'.

Normal voice

The normal voice should be harmonious, relatively soft, rounded, clear and of the right strength (not too loud or too weak). The normal voice is often compared with the sound emitted by a bell and the Lungs are compared with the bell itself. Therefore, when the bell is intact its ringing sound is clear. In a similar way, when Lung-Qi is good and the Lungs are unobstructed by Phlegm, the voice is clear, its tone is melodious and

its pitch is not too high and not too low. When assessing whether the quality, pitch and tone of the voice are normal, however, one should be aware that there is no universal standard because the voice should be related to the sex, age and body build of the patient. Therefore what is too weak a voice for a well-built man might be normal for a small-built old lady.

Allowance should be made also for the emotional state of the patient as this will easily affect the voice. For example, the 'Golden Mirror of Medicine' (*Yi Zong Jin Jian*) says: '*When the Heart is affected by excess joy, the voice becomes scattered; when the Heart is affected by anger, the voice becomes indignant and stern; when the Heart is affected by grief, the voice becomes sad and hoarse . . . when the Heart is affected by love the voice is warm and harmonious. When the Heart is happy, the voice is slow and relaxed.*'[1]

The voice and the Five Elements

From a Five-Element perspective, there are five tones of voice: shouting for Wood, laughing for Fire, singing for Earth, weeping for Metal and groaning for Water. These tones of voice can be interpreted in two ways: under physiological conditions, these tones are normal for those types, that is, it is normal for a Wood type to have a relatively loud, 'shouting' voice; under pathological conditions, the tone of voice may deviate from its standard by excess or deficiency, that is, a Wood type may have a voice that is either 'too shouting' or not strong enough.

A shouting voice is loud and is emitted in short, sharp bursts as if that person were reproaching someone. A person with a laughing voice will often have short bursts of laughter within their speech and the voice itself may have an edge of laughter. A singing tone of voice has a relatively high pitch, is melodious and has a flow of high and low tones like a song. A weeping voice is somewhat hesitant, with a relatively low pitch and a sad tone; in some cases it may sound almost as if the person were about to burst into tears. A groaning voice sounds guttural, has a low pitch and is somewhat croaky.

Box 53.1 lists the correspondences between the Five Elements and voice tones.

BOX 53.1 FIVE-ELEMENT VOICES

- Shouting: Wood
- Laughing: Fire
- Singing: Earth
- Weeping: Metal
- Groaning: Water

Strength and quality of the voice

A strong, loud voice generally indicates a Full condition, whereas a weak, low and quiet voice indicates an Empty condition.

When considering the quality of the voice we should include the following various sounds:

- nasal voice
- hoarse voice
- snoring
- groaning
- crying out
- stuttering.

Nasal voice

Symptoms and Signs, Chapter 83

Apart from the strength of the voice, one should also assess its clarity. As mentioned above, the normal voice should sound as clear as a bell. If the voice sounds muffled, this indicates that the passages of the Lungs are obstructed. This obstruction may be caused by external Wind, Phlegm or Dampness.

In Deficiency, if the voice sounds muffled but weak this indicates a deficiency of Qi and Blood or a deficiency of Lung-Qi, which is usually combined with retention of Dampness or Phlegm in the nasal passages.

Hoarse voice

Symptoms and Signs, Chapter 83

A hoarse voice in acute conditions always indicates an invasion of Wind-Heat with Dryness in the Lung Defensive-Qi system. If we compare the Lungs to a metal instrument or a bell, in this case the voice becomes hoarse because the bell is 'full' (i.e. the Lungs are obstructed by Wind); in ancient times this was called '*Jin* full not ringing', *Jin* being an ancient, metal percussion instrument.

A sudden hoarse voice may also be due to stagnation of Liver- or Lung-Qi affecting the throat from emotional problems.

A hoarse voice in chronic conditions is due to a deficiency of Yin of the Lungs and Kidneys; in this case, the voice becomes hoarse because the bell is cracked and, in ancient times, this was called '*Jin* broken and not ringing'. If the voice becomes hoarse suddenly in the course of a serious, chronic disease (such as cancer), this indicates a collapse of Yin or Yang and it is a bad prognostic sign.

A chronic hoarse voice with a swelling of the pharynx may be due to Phlegm and Blood stasis obstructing the throat.

A hoarse voice during pregnancy is due to a pathology of the Connecting channel which links the Uterus to the Kidneys. As the Kidney channel reaches the root of the tongue, a disturbance of the Connecting channel connecting the Kidneys to the Uterus during pregnancy prevents Kidney-Qi from rising to the tongue and it affects the voice. This condition is mentioned in Chapter 47 of the 'Simple Questions'.[2] It normally improves by itself and does not require treatment; in fact, the 'Simple Questions' says that this problem does not require treatment because '*it will be resolved in the tenth month*', that is, when the woman gives birth.

A coarse, deep, raucous voice with sudden onset indicates an invasion of Wind; a nasal voice indicates an invasion of Wind-Cold or Wind-Dampness.

A difficulty in producing sound with breathlessness and a rattling sound in the throat like the sound of a saw indicates retention of Phlegm in the Lungs.

Snoring

Symptoms and Signs, Chapters 81 and 83

Snoring is generally due to Phlegm or Dampness obstructing the nasal passages, but we should distinguish loud snoring, reflecting a purely Full condition of Dampness or Phlegm, from weak snoring, reflecting a condition of Dampness or Phlegm against a background of Qi deficiency.

Groaning

Symptoms and Signs, Chapter 83

Groaning generally indicates pain, but we still need to differentiate loud groaning, reflecting a Full condition causing the pain, from weak and feeble groaning, reflecting a mixed Full and Empty condition as the cause of the pain. Groaning from pain is usually due to Dampness or Qi stagnation.

Crying out

Symptoms and Signs, Chapter 83

Crying out indicates severe pain, usually always of a Full nature; it is usually due to Blood stasis, Damp-Heat or Toxic Heat.

Stuttering

Symptoms and Signs, Chapter 83

Stuttering may be due to Heart-Blood deficiency or Heart-Fire.

Box 53.2 summarizes patterns underlying voice strengths and qualities.

BOX 53.2 VOICE

- Loud voice: Full condition
- Weak voice: Empty condition
- Muffled voice in acute conditions: invasion of Wind
- Muffled voice in chronic conditions: deficiency of Qi and Blood
- Nasal voice: invasion of Wind-Cold or Wind-Dampness, Phlegm
- Hoarse voice in acute conditions: invasion of Wind-Heat or Qi stagnation
- Hoarse voice in chronic conditions: Yin deficiency (of Lungs and/or Kidneys)
- Hoarse voice in chronic conditions with swelling of the pharynx: Phlegm and Blood stasis
- Sudden hoarse voice in chronic disease: collapse of Yin or Yang
- Hoarse voice during pregnancy: Kidney channel pathology
- Coarse, deep, raucous voice with sudden onset: invasion of Wind
- Difficulty in emitting sound with breathlessness and throat rattling: Phlegm in the Lungs
- Snoring: Phlegm or Dampness obstructing the nasal passages
- Weak snoring: Dampness or Phlegm with Qi deficiency
- Groaning: pain from Dampness or Qi stagnation
- Crying out: severe pain of a Full nature from Blood stasis, Damp-Heat or Toxic Heat
- Stuttering: Heart-Blood deficiency or Heart-Fire.

Delirious speech occurs in high fevers and it indicates Heat invading the Pericardium during a febrile disease. Speaking with a very feeble voice, with the speech frequently interrupted and with great difficulty in starting speaking again after stopping, indicates a severe depletion of Qi and is called *Duo Qi*, which literally means 'Robbing of Qi'.

Talking in one's sleep may be due to Full conditions such as Heart-Fire, Gall-Bladder Heat or Stomach-Heat or to Empty conditions such as Heart-Blood deficiency: in the former case, the talking in one's sleep is agitated and loud while in the latter it is weak.

Box 53.3 summarizes patterns underlying various speech symptoms and signs.

BOX 53.3 SPEECH

- Dislike of speaking: Qi deficiency (Lungs/Spleen)
- Speaking too much: Full condition
- Slurred speech: Phlegm, Wind-stroke
- Incoherent, incessant speech: Phlegm-Fire
- Muttering to oneself: Phlegm obstructing the Mind's orifices
- Hesitation in speech with difficulty in finding words: Dampness or Phlegm
- Speaking and laughing a lot: manic behaviour (*Kuang*)
- Delirious speech: Heat in the Pericardium in febrile diseases
- Very feeble, interrupted speech: severe depletion of Qi
- Talking in one's sleep: Heart-Fire, Gall-Bladder Heat, Stomach-Heat, Heart-Blood deficiency

---

SPEECH

Symptoms and Signs, Chapter 83

Dislike of speaking generally indicates Qi deficiency of the Lungs or Spleen, or both, whereas speaking a lot generally indicates a Full condition and especially Heat of the Heart.

Slurred speech indicates retention of Phlegm and is frequently seen in patients after Wind-stroke. Incoherent, incessant speech indicates Phlegm-Fire obstructing the Mind's orifices. Muttering to oneself with a low voice indicates Phlegm obstructing the Mind's orifices.

Hesitation in speech with difficulty in finding words usually indicates Dampness or Phlegm obstructing the brain; this symptom is frequently seen in postviral fatigue syndrome. Speaking and laughing a lot together with abnormal activity at night-time may indicate the manic phase (*Kuang*) of bipolar disorder.

CRYING IN BABIES

Symptoms and Signs, Chapter 90

Listening to a baby's cry forms part of the diagnosis by hearing. If the baby cries with a high pitch and moves its head from side to side, this indicates Accumulation Disorder. If the baby cries with a low sound and intermittently, this indicates Spleen deficiency. If the baby cries with a long, continuous but soft sound, this indicates a Deficient condition and possibly swollen tonsils.

BREATHING AND SIGHING

Breathing

The sound of breathing reflects the condition of the Lungs and of the Kidneys. The general principle is the same as for the voice sound; that is, breathing with a weak, low sound indicates a deficiency of the Lungs or

Kidneys, or both, whereas loud breathing indicates a Full condition. A shallow breathing sound indicates deficiency of Yang, whereas breathing with a loud sound often indicates Lung-Heat.

Apart from these general principles, pathological breathing sounds may be classified as breathlessness, wheezing, shortness of breath, rebellious Qi and weakness of Qi.

Pathological breathing sounds

Symptoms and Signs, Chapter 63

Breathlessness (Chuan)   This is characterized by difficulty in breathing and shortness of breath with raising of the shoulders; it is a feature of patients suffering from asthma or other obstructive pulmonary diseases. Such breathlessness can be of a Full or an Empty type. In the Full type, the breathing is irregular, loud and coarse, whereas in the Empty type the breathing sound is lower and the voice weak.

Breathlessness of the Full type is usually due to retention of Phlegm in the Lungs, whereas that of the Empty type is due to Phlegm in the Lungs combined with a deficiency of the Lungs, Spleen or Kidneys.

Symptoms and Signs, Chapter 63

Wheezing (Xiao)   This is characterized by a whistling sound emitted on breathing, often on exhalation; this is often a symptom of asthma. Wheezing indicates retention of Phlegm in the Lungs. Phlegm is the traditional explanation for wheezing in Chinese medicine but, in my experience, in young people suffering from allergic asthma there is little or no Phlegm and wheezing is caused by Wind in the Lungs. For a more complete explanation of this concept see Chapter 5 of 'The Practice of Chinese Medicine'.[3]

Shortness of breath (Duan Qi)   This is characterized by short, irregular and rapid breaths but without the pronounced struggling for breath and raising of shoulders seen in breathlessness. Shortness of breath indicates retention of Phlegm in the Lungs combined with Lung deficiency.

Weak breathing (Qi Shao)   This is characterized by weak, low and short breathing sounds, which indicate a deficiency of Qi of the Lungs or Kidneys, or both.

Rebellious-Qi breathing (Shang Qi)   This is characterized by rapid, short breaths, a cough and a sensation of oppression of the throat and of energy rising; this is accompanied by a feeling of anxiety and it is worse lying down. Rebellious Qi may be due to the rising of the Qi of the Penetrating Vessel or to Liver-Fire insulting the Lungs.

> **BOX 53.4 THE FIVE PATHOLOGICAL BREATHING SOUNDS**
> ___
> - Breathlessness (*Chuan*): Phlegm in the Lungs
> - Wheezing (*Xiao*): Phlegm or Wind in the Lungs
> - Shortness of breath (*Duan Qi*): Phlegm in the Lungs with Lung-Qi deficiency
> - Weakness of Qi (*Qi Shao*): Qi deficiency (Lungs/Kidneys)
> - Rebellious Qi (*Shang Qi*): Rebellious Qi of the Penetrating Vessel or Liver-Fire insulting the Lungs

Box 53.4 summarizes the patterns underlying abnormal breathing sounds.

Sighing

Sighing generally indicates Qi stagnation of the Liver or Lungs, which derives from emotional problems such as repressed anger or frustration if the Liver is involved, or worry and sadness if the Lungs are involved. Sighing with a weak sound may also be due to deficiency of the Spleen and Heart deriving from sadness, grief or pensiveness.

COUGHING AND SNEEZING

Coughing

Symptoms and Signs, Chapter 63

The same general principles apply to the sound of coughing, that is, a cough with a loud sound indicates a Full condition, whereas a cough with a weak sound indicates an Empty condition. Apart from this, a cough which is loud and 'rich' and which sounds 'loose' indicates Damp-Phlegm in the Lungs. A barking cough which sounds loud indicates Phlegm-Heat in the Lungs. A persistent, loud, dry cough with the occasional expectoration of sputum in acute conditions indicates residual Dryness and Phlegm in the Lungs after an invasion of Wind-Heat. A persistent, weak, dry cough with the occasional expectoration of sputum in chronic conditions indicates Dry-Phlegm in the Lungs. A persistent, dry, weak cough with a low sound indicates Lung-Yin deficiency.

In children, a barking, loud cough coming in violent bouts with a characteristic whooping sound and often ending with vomiting indicates whooping cough.

Box 53.5 summarizes the patterns underlying coughing.

BOX 53.5 COUGH

- Loud sound: Full condition
- Weak sound: Empty condition
- Loud, rich, loose sound: Damp-Phlegm in the Lungs
- Barking cough with loud sound: Phlegm-Heat in the Lungs
- Persistent, dry, loud cough with occasional expectoration of scanty sputum in acute conditions: residual Dryness and Phlegm in the Lungs after an invasion of Wind-Heat
- Persistent, dry, weak cough with occasional expectoration of scanty sputum in chronic conditions: Dry-Phlegm in the Lungs
- Persistent, dry, weak cough with low sound: Lung-Yin deficiency
- Barking, loud cough in violent bouts in children: whooping cough

---

Sneezing

Interrogation, Chapter 35; Symptoms and Signs, Chapter 58

Sneezing is usually due to an impairment of the Lung's diffusing of Qi. The normal sneezing that occurs as a reaction to airborne particles entering the nose is an expression of a good state of Yang-Qi. Chapter 28 of the 'Spiritual Axis' attributes this normal sneezing to the Heart: '*When Yang-Qi is harmonized, it fills the Heart, exits at the nose and causes sneezing.*'[4] Chapter 23 of the 'Simple Questions' relates sneezing also to the Kidneys; it says: '*The Heart controls belching, the Lungs control coughing, the Liver controls the flow of speech, the Spleen controls swallowing and the Kidneys control sneezing.*'[5]

Sneezing with a loud sound indicates a Full condition, which is usually due to invasion of external Wind, whereas sneezing with a weak sound indicates an Empty condition of the Lungs as, for example, in allergic rhinitis. Acute sneezing is due to invasion of Wind; if this is accompanied by profuse nasal discharge this indicates invasion of Wind-Cold. According to

---

BOX 53.6 SNEEZING

- Loud sound: Full condition
- Weak sound: Empty condition
- Acute sneezing: invasion of Wind
- Weak chronic sneezing: chronic retention of Wind in the nose (allergic rhinitis)
- Sneezing with profuse nasal discharge: invasion of Wind-Cold

---

some doctors, if, after an invasion of Wind, the pathogenic factor penetrates the Interior and the patient suddenly starts sneezing again, this indicates that the body's Qi is recovering.

Box 53.6 summarizes the patterns underlying sneezing.

HICCUP

Symptoms and Signs, Chapter 69

Hiccup with a loud, high-pitched sound indicates a Full condition and often Heat; this type of hiccup may be due to Stomach-Qi rebelling upwards, Stomach-Heat or Liver-Qi invading the Stomach. Infrequent hiccup with a deep but strong sound may be due to Cold in the Stomach. Infrequent, weak hiccup with a low sound indicates Stomach deficiency. Frequent but weak hiccup indicates Stomach-Yin deficiency.

Box 53.7 summarizes the patterns underlying hiccup.

BOX 53.7 HICCUP

- Loud, high-pitched sound: Stomach-Qi rebelling upwards, Stomach-Heat, Liver-Qi invading the Somach
- Deep and strong sound: Cold in the Stomach
- Weak with low sound: Stomach deficiency
- Weak and frequent: Stomach-Yin deficiency

BELCHING

Interrogation, Chapter 30; Symptoms and Signs, Chapter 69

Belching with a loud and long sound indicates a Full condition, which may be retention of food, Stomach-Heat or Liver-Qi invading the Stomach. Belching with a short and low sound indicates a deficient condition, which may be Stomach-Qi deficiency or Stomach deficient and cold.

Box 53.8 summarizes the patterns underlying belching.

BOX 53.8 BELCHING

- Loud and long: retention of food, Stomach-Heat, Liver-Qi invading the Stomach
- Short and low: Stomach-Qi deficiency, Stomach deficient and cold

VOMITING

Interrogation, Chapter 30; Symptoms and Signs, Chapter 69

Vomiting with a loud sound indicates a Full condition, which may be retention of food, Stomach-Heat, Liver- and Stomach-Heat or Full-Cold in the Stomach. Vomiting with a weak sound indicates Deficiency, which may be Stomach-Qi deficiency, Stomach deficient and cold or Stomach-Yin deficiency. Bouts of vomiting depending on the emotional state usually indicate rebellious Liver-Qi invading the Stomach.

Box 53.9 summarizes the patterns underlying vomiting.

BOX 53.9 VOMITING

- Loud sound: retention of food, Stomach-Heat, Liver- and Stomach-Heat, Full-Cold in the stomach
- Weak sound: Stomach-Qi deficiency, Stomach deficient and cold, Stomach-Yin deficiency
- Bouts of vomiting depending on emotional state: Liver-Qi rebellious invading the Stomach

---

NOTES

1. Wu Qian 1977 Golden Mirror of Medicine (*Yi Zong Jin Jian* 医宗金鉴), People's Health Publishing House, Beijing, Vol. 2, p. 877. First published in 1742.
2. 1979 The Yellow Emperor's Classic of Internal Medicine – Simple Questions (*Huang Di Nei Jing Su Wen* 黄帝内经素问), People's Health Publishing House, Beijing, p. 259. First published c. 100BC.
3. Maciocia G. 2000 The Practice of Chinese Medicine. Churchill Livingstone, Edinburgh.
4. 1981 Spiritual Axis (*Ling Shu Jing* 灵枢经), People's Health Publishing House, Beijing, p. 67. First published c. 100BC.
5. Simple Questions, p. 150.

Chapter **54**

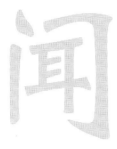

DIAGNOSIS BY SMELLING

Chapter contents

INTRODUCTION *549*

BODY ODOUR *549*

ODOUR OF BODILY SECRETIONS *550*
   Breath *550*
   Sweat *550*
   Sputum *550*
   Urine and stools *550*
   Vaginal discharge and lochia *551*
   Intestinal gas *551*

INTRODUCTION

Diagnosis by smelling is not a major part of the diagnostic process. It is used mostly to confirm our diagnosis and is seldom a clinching factor. The Five-Element smells mentioned below are useful mostly to correlate to the patient's Element type and to indicate accordance with or discordance from it. For example, a rancid smell in a Wood Element is a pathological exaggeration of a constitutional Wood smell and therefore is less serious than another smell would be.

There are two quite distinct aspects to diagnosis by smelling: the first is the odour of the patient's body itself, which can give us an idea not only of the prevailing pattern of disharmony but also of the patient's constitutional type; the second is the odour of certain bodily secretions, which is used only to identify the prevailing pattern of disharmony.

Assuming the patient is not wearing perfume or strong after-shave (I normally ask my patients not to use perfume or after-shave when they come for their first consultation), diagnosis by smelling is carried out as the interrogation progresses. In some cases, the body odour is quite clear, even overwhelming. If there is no particular odour emanating from the body at the start of the interrogation, in most cases it will become apparent when the patient is lying down, undressed, for acupuncture.

BODY ODOUR

From a Five-Element perspective, the five body odours are: rancid for Wood, scorched for Fire, fragrant or sweetish for Earth, rotten for Metal and putrid for Water. From this point of view, these body odours

reflect a disharmony in the relevant Element, which may be a Deficiency or an Excess. In a few cases, these body odours are very apparent as soon as the patient comes in, but in most cases these odours are detected only when the patient undresses and especially on the back.

Sometimes, the Five-Element body odour emanates after the needles have been in for about 20 minutes. In my experience, the two most common Five-Element body odours are the putrid and rancid ones; the putrid odour is relatively common in the elderly (presumably caused by a decline of Kidney-Qi).

The body odour can be used diagnostically in two ways. In the absence of patterns of disharmony accounting for a particular odour, the body odour reflects the patient's constitutional Element type in the same way as do the body shape and facial structures. Thus, a slightly rancid odour will emanate from a Wood type, a slightly scorched one from a Fire type, etc. In addition to the constitutional body odour, patients' body odour reflects the patterns they are suffering from and these may not necessarily accord with their Element type. For example, a Wood type may emanate a slightly scorched smell, indicating the presence of a Heart pattern. Indeed, if the body odour contradicts the constitutional Element type, this is a bad sign. In other words, it is worse for a Wood type to have a scorched odour (for example) than a rancid one.

Box 54.1 summarizes the correspondences between the Five Elements and body odours.

BOX 54.1 FIVE-ELEMENT ODOURS

- Rancid: Wood
- Scorched: Fire
- Fragrant/sweetish: Earth
- Rotten: Metal
- Putrid: Water

ODOUR OF BODILY SECRETIONS

Diagnosis by smelling is based also on detecting the smell of bodily secretions. Obviously it is impractical for a practitioner to be able to smell a patient's urine or vaginal discharge. However, I usually ask patients if they have noticed a strong smell; most people are very aware if any of their bodily secretions are particularly smelly.

Bodily secretions include:

- breath
- sweat
- sputum
- urine and stools
- vaginal discharge and lochia
- intestinal gas.

Breath

The odour emanating from the mouth is closely related to the condition of the digestive system. Generally speaking, a strong, unpleasant breath indicates Stomach-Heat or retention of food. A sour-smelling breath indicates retention of food, or in children Accumulation Disorder. A foul and somewhat pungent breath indicates Damp-Heat in the Stomach and Spleen. A rotten-smelling breath may indicate Damp-Heat in the Large Intestine, which may be due to ulcerative colitis.

Box 54.2 summarizes the patterns underlying breath smells.

BOX 54.2 BREATH SMELLS

- Strong, foul: Stomach-Heat or Retention of Food
- Sour: Retention of Food, Accumulation Disorder (in children)
- Foul, pungent: Damp-Heat in Stomach and Spleen
- Rotten: Damp-Heat in Large Intestine

Sweat

The smell of sweat is often related to Dampness because the fluids forming sweat come from the space between the skin and muscles where Dampness often accumulates. Any strong-smelling sweat often indicates Damp-Heat. Putrid-smelling sweat may indicate a disease of the lungs, liver or kidneys.

Sputum

A strong-smelling sputum, often smelling rotten, indicates Heat in the Lungs and usually Phlegm-Heat or Toxic Heat. A fishy-smelling sputum may also indicate Lung-Heat. Sputum without smell indicates Cold.

Urine and stools

Foul-smelling stools always indicate Heat or Damp-Heat in the Intestines, whereas an irregularity of the

bowel movement and an absence of smell indicates usually a Cold condition.

As for urine, strong-smelling urine indicates Damp-Heat in the Bladder; absence of smell indicates Cold.

Vaginal discharge and lochia

A strong-smelling, leathery smell of vaginal discharge indicates Damp-Heat; a fishy smell indicates Damp-Cold.

Strong-smelling lochia after childbirth may indicate Damp-Heat or Toxic Heat in the Uterus.

Intestinal gas

A strong, foul-smelling intestinal gas indicates Damp-Heat in the Large Intestine. If the gas smells rancid and rotten like rotten eggs, this indicates Toxic Heat in the Large Intestines.

The release of gas without smell usually indicates Spleen-Qi deficiency.

证
候

PART 5

SYMPTOMS AND SIGNS

Part contents

SECTION 1
SYMPTOMS AND SIGNS OF PARTS OF THE BODY
55 Head, hair and face   *559*
56 Face colour   *575*
57 Ears   *581*
58 Nose   *589*
59 Throat   *601*
60 Mouth, tongue, teeth, gums, lips, palate and philtrum   *609*
61 Eyes   *627*
62 Neck, shoulders and upper back   *653*
63 Chest   *659*
64 Limbs   *671*
65 Arms   *679*
66 Legs   *693*
67 Lower back   *703*
68 Body   *709*
69 Digestive system and taste   *717*
70 Thirst and drink   *731*
71 Abdomen   *735*
72 Defecation   *747*
73 Urination   *753*
74 Anus   *761*
75 Men's sexual and genital symptoms   *765*
76 Sweating   *775*
77 Skin signs   *781*
78 Emotional symptoms   *791*
79 Mental and emotional symptoms   *797*
80 Mental difficulties   *803*
81 Sleep problems   *807*
82 Feeling of cold, feeling of heat, fever   *813*
83 Voice, speech and sounds   *819*

SECTION 2
GYNAECOLOGICAL SYMPTOMS AND SIGNS
84 Menstrual symptoms   *825*
85 Problems at period time   *831*
86 Problems during pregnancy   *837*
87 Problems after childbirth   *843*
88 Breast signs   *849*
89 Miscellaneous gynaecological symptoms   *855*

SECTION 3
PAEDIATRIC SYMPTOMS AND SIGNS
90 Children's problems   *863*

INTRODUCTION

Whereas Part 1 on Observation lists the signs, which can be observed, and Part 2 on Interrogation discusses symptoms that are elicited on interrogation, Part 5 lists both symptoms and signs, according to area of the body, without distinction between what is seen on observation and what is elicited from asking the patient. The separation between observation and interrogation is made purely for didactic purposes and does not correspond to clinical reality where what is seen on observation and what is elicited on interrogation occurs simultaneously and may be integrated automatically. For example, the separation between bloodshot eyes (observation) and eye pain (interrogation) is artificial and unrealistic.

Moreover, the combination of both symptoms and signs for each area corresponds also to how we normally proceed with the patient. For example, when patients come in with their clinical manifestations mainly concentrated in one area of the body, we would naturally investigate that area by asking about symptoms and observing any outward sign without distinction between interrogation and observation; if a patient complains of blurred vision, for instance, we would immediately and automatically observe the eyes to see whether they are dry or bloodshot.

To clarify the links between Part 5, on Symptoms and Signs, Part 1, on Observation, and Part 2, on Interrogation, I have indicated them in each of these Parts (e.g. 'Dizziness' found in Chapter 55 of Part 5 is also found in Chapter 34 of Part 2).

The symptoms and signs listed in Part 5 are mostly described in terms taken from Chinese books, but with the following adaptations:

1. I have integrated into the listed symptoms and signs some symptoms (e.g. constant picking) and signs (e.g. blushing) which I felt are common in the West but which are missing from the Chinese texts.
2. For many symptoms and signs I have introduced new patterns which I have not found in the Chinese source texts.
3. I have eliminated certain symptoms and signs or patterns that are seen only in China and added some that are typical of Western patients.
4. Within each pattern I have added symptoms and signs specific to the symptom or sign discussed.

Part 5 is divided into three sections, arranged by body area, as follows:

Section 1: Symptoms and signs of parts of the body
Section 2: Gynaecological symptoms and signs
Section 3: Paediatric symptoms and signs.

For each symptom or sign I list the most common patterns that cause it. I would like to draw the reader's attention to the following points:

- The symptoms/signs are arranged, as much as possible, in order of frequency within each chapter, or (in longer chapters) within each chapter section.
- The patterns pertaining to each symptom/sign are arranged generally in the order of Excess and then Deficiency patterns; within each of these groups, they appear in order of frequency.
- There are more symptoms and signs in Part 5 than there are in Part 1 on Observation and Part 2 on Interrogation, but all the symptoms and signs in these two Parts are found in the present Part 5.
- The patterns pertaining to each symptom/sign in Part 5 do not necessarily correspond exactly to those in the Appendixes for various reasons:
  —Whenever possible, the pattern has been changed to make it more specific to the symptom/sign in which it appears (e.g. the Liver-Blood deficiency pattern for blurred vision will contain more eye or face symptoms).
  —The patterns have also been changed by listing the symptoms and signs that are more closely related to the presenting symptom.
  —There are certain patterns that are peculiar to the symptom/sign discussed and which do not occur in other cases (e.g. Fetus-Toxin Heat in the children's section). This reflects also the fact that, in clinical practice, conditions do not always neatly fall into the standard patterns.
  —The list of all possible manifestations in each pattern has usually been shortened in Part 5 compared with the patterns in the Appendixes.
- Whenever appropriate, I have indicated, with small figures, the kind of patient in whom that particular pattern occurs more frequently. If the symbol for a man or woman is combined with the symbol for the elderly, this means that that pattern is more common in an elderly man or woman respectively. Of course, these symbols should not be interpreted too rigidly; that is, if there is the symbol of a woman against a particular pattern, that simply means that the pattern is more frequent in women and *not* that that pattern cannot occur in men. The symbolic figures are as follows:
  —a man, indicating that that pattern is more common in men
  —a woman, indicating that that pattern is more common in women
  —a child, indicating that that pattern is more common in children
  —an old person, indicating that that pattern is more common in the elderly (man or woman)
  —a pregnant woman, indicating that that pattern is more common in pregnant women or women after childbirth

The main Chinese source texts used for Part 5 are:

1. Zhang Zhu Sheng 1995 Great Treatise of Diagnosis by Observation in Chinese Medicine (*Zhong Hua Yi Xue Wang Shen Da Quan*), Shanxi Science Publishing House, Taiyuan.

2. Zhao Jin Duo 1985 Identification of Patterns and Diagnosis in Chinese Medicine (*Zhong Yi Zheng Zhuang Jian Bie Zhen Duan Xue*), People's Health Publishing House, Beijing.

3. Zhu Wen Feng 1999 Diagnosis in Chinese Medicine (*Zhong Yi Zhen Duan Xue*), People's Health Publishing House, Beijing.

4. Zhao Jin Duo 1991 Differential Diagnosis and Patterns in Chinese Medicine (*Zhong Yi Zheng Hou Jian Bie Zhen Duan Xue*), People's Health Publishing House, Beijing.

For ease of consultation, there are two lists of the Symptoms and Signs (see Index of symptoms and signs, p. xlix): the first arranged according to body area and the second alphabetically irrespective of body area.

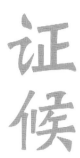

SECTION 1

SYMPTOMS AND SIGNS OF PARTS OF THE BODY

Section contents

55 Head and face 559
56 Face colour 575
57 Ears 581
58 Nose 589
59 Throat 601
60 Mouth, tongue, teeth, gums, lips, palate and philtrum 609
61 Eyes 627
62 Neck, shoulders and upper back 653
63 Chest 659
64 Limbs 671
65 Arms 679
66 Legs 693
67 Lower back 703
68 Body 709
69 Digestive system and taste 717
70 Thirst and drink 731
71 Abdomen 735
72 Defecation 747
73 Urination 753
74 Anus 761
75 Men's sexual and genital symptoms 765
76 Sweating 775
77 Skin signs 781
78 Emotional symptoms 791
79 Mental and emotional symptoms 797
80 Mental difficulties 803
81 Sleep problems 807
82 Feeling of cold, feeling of heat, fever 813
83 Voice, speech and sounds 819

INTRODUCTION

This first section of Part 5 deals with general symptoms and signs of the whole body. Part 5 lists both symptoms and signs, by area of the body, without distinction between what is seen on observation and what is elicited from asking the patient. The separation between observation and interrogation does not correspond to clinical reality where what is seen on observation and what is elicited on interrogation occurs simultaneously and may be integrated automatically. For example, the separation between bloodshot eyes (observation) and eye pain (interrogation) is artificial and unrealistic. The collection of both symptoms (elicited by interrogation) and signs (elicited by observation) for each part of the body corresponds to clinical reality. To give another example, if a patient complains of joint ache (interrogation), the first thing we would naturally do is to look at the joint to see whether it is swollen (observation) and we would also palpate the joint (palpation); thus, in this example, observation, interrogation and palpation all converge into one.

Moreover, the combination of both symptoms and signs for each area corresponds to how we normally proceed with the patient. For example, if a patient's clinical manifestations are mainly concentrated in one area of the body, we would naturally investigate that area by asking about symptoms and observing any outward sign without distinction between interrogation and observation; if the patient complains of blurred vision, for instance, we would immediately and automatically observe the eyes to see if they are dry or bloodshot.

To clarify the links between Part 5, on Symptoms and Signs, Part 1, on Observation, and Part 2, on Interrogation, I have indicated them in each of these parts (e.g. 'Dizziness' found in Chapter 55 of Part 5 is also found in Chapter 34 of Part 2).

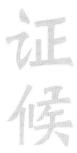

Chapter **55**

HEAD, HAIR AND FACE

Chapter contents

HEAD *559*
  Dizziness *559*
  Fainting *560*
  Feeling of heaviness of the head *561*
  Headache *561*
  Feeling of distension of the head *562*
  Feeling of muzziness (fuzziness) of the head *563*
  Feeling of cold of the head *563*
  Feeling of heat of the head *563*
  Numbness of the head *563*
  Drooping head *563*
  Leaning of the head to one side *564*
  Tremor of the head *564*
  Brain noise *564*
  Swelling of the whole head *564*
  Ulcers in the mastoid region *564*
  Head tilted backwards *565*

HAIR AND SCALP *565*
  Premature greying of the hair *565*
  Hair falling out *565*
  Alopecia *566*
  Dry and brittle hair *566*
  Greasy hair *566*
  Dandruff *567*
  Itchy scalp *567*
  Dry scalp *568*
  Redness and pain of the scalp *568*
  Boils on the scalp *568*
  Erosion of the scalp *568*
  Ulcers on the scalp *568*

FACE *569*
  Acne *569*
  Feeling of heat of the face *569*
  Facial pain *571*
  Numbness of the face *572*
  Oedema of the face *572*
  Tic *572*
  Deviation of eye and mouth *573*
  Facial paralysis *573*

Papular/macular eruptions *573*
Swelling and redness of the face *573*
Swelling, redness and pain of the cheeks *573*
Ulcers below the zygomatic arch *574*
Lines on the face *574*

HEAD

Dizziness

Interrogation, Chapter 34

The dizziness from a Full condition is always more severe than that from an Empty condition.

Liver-Blood deficiency

Mild dizziness, blurred vision, floaters, numbness/tingling of limbs, scanty menstruation, dull-pale complexion, Pale tongue, Choppy or Fine pulse.

Kidney deficiency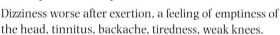

Dizziness worse after exertion, a feeling of emptiness of the head, tinnitus, backache, tiredness, weak knees.

Other symptoms and signs depend on whether there is a Kidney-Yin or Kidney-Yang deficiency.

Liver-Yang rising

Dizziness with headache, headache, dizziness, tinnitus, irritability, propensity to outbursts of anger, Wiry pulse.

Phlegm obstructing the head

Dizziness, a feeling of heaviness and muzziness of the head, a feeling of oppression of the chest, dizziness, blurred vision, somnolence, nausea, sputum in the throat, muzziness of the head, Swollen tongue with sticky coating, Slippery pulse.

Liver-Fire

Dizziness, headache, red face, tinnitus, irritability, propensity to outbursts of anger, thirst, bitter taste, constipation, dark urine, Red tongue with redder sides and dry yellow coating, Wiry-Rapid pulse.

Liver-Wind

Severe dizziness, vertigo, tremors, tinnitus, headache, numbness of limbs, tics, Stiff, Deviated or Moving tongue, Wiry pulse.

This is the most severe type of dizziness.

Qi and Blood deficiency of the Spleen and Heart

Mild, postural dizziness, palpitations, insomnia, dream-disturbed sleep, poor memory, anxiety, tendency to be easily startled, dull-pale complexion, pale lips, tiredness, weak muscles, loose stools, poor appetite, scanty periods, Pale and Thin tongue, Choppy or Fine pulse.

Stomach- and Spleen-Qi deficiency

Mild dizziness, poor appetite, slight abdominal distension after eating, tiredness, lassitude, pale complexion, weakness of the limbs, loose stools, an uncomfortable feeling in the epigastrium, lack of sense of taste, Pale tongue, Empty pulse.

> **Clinical note**
>
> - In women, Liver-Blood deficiency is the most common cause of dizziness. A Kidney deficiency is also common.
> - In the elderly, look for Phlegm as a cause of dizziness.
> - When it is clearly due to emotional problems, dizziness is often due to Liver-Yang rising.

Fainting

Interrogation, Chapter 34

Liver-Qi stagnation with Liver-Qi rebelling upwards to cloud the orifices

Fainting, mouth closed and hands clenched, coarse breathing, cold hands and feet, Wiry-Deep pulse.

Blood-Heat with Liver-Fire blazing upwards to cloud the orifices

Sudden fainting, unconsciousness, clenched teeth, closed mouth, clenched fists, red face, red lips, blood-shot eyes, Red tongue with yellow coating, Wiry-Overflowing-Rapid pulse.

Phlegm clouding the orifices

Sudden fainting with unconsciousness or episodes of fainting without complete loss of consciousness, sputum in the throat, a feeling of oppression of the chest, nausea, vomiting, coarse breathing, Swollen tongue with sticky coating, Slippery pulse.

Retention of food

Episodes of fainting after overeating, breathlessness, epigastric fullness and distension, foul breath, sour regurgitation, thick sticky tongue coating, Slippery pulse.

Heart-Blood deficiency

Short, transient episodes of fainting, often without complete loss of consciousness, dull-pale complexion, palpitations, anxiety, insomnia, cold hands, pale lips, Pale tongue, Choppy pulse.

Heart-Yin deficiency

Short, transient episodes of fainting, often without complete loss of consciousness, dull-pale complexion with floating-red cheekbones, palpitations, anxiety, insomnia, dry throat at night, tongue without coating, Floating-Empty pulse.

Liver-Blood deficiency

Short, transient episodes of fainting, often without complete loss of consciousness, in women often coinciding with the period, dull-pale face, pale lips, cold hands, dizziness, blurred vision, sweating, weak breathing, Pale tongue, Choppy or Fine pulse.

Liver-Yin deficiency

Short, transient episodes of fainting, often without complete loss of consciousness, in women often coinciding with the period, dull-pale face with red cheekbones, dizziness, blurred vision, sweating, weak breathing, dry hair, tongue without coating, Floating-Empty pulse.

Kidney-Yang deficiency and deficiency of the Original Qi

Short, transient episodes of fainting, often without loss of consciousness, open mouth, relaxed hands, weak breathing, pale complexion, sweating, cold limbs, Pale tongue, Deep-Weak pulse.

Feeling of heaviness of the head

Interrogation, Chapter 34

A feeling of heaviness of the head is always caused by Dampness or Phlegm obstructing the head.

Damp-Phlegm

A feeling of heaviness and muzziness of the head and body, dizziness, blurred vision, somnolence, a feeling of oppression of the chest, nausea, Swollen tongue with sticky coating, Slippery pulse.

Dampness

A feeling of heaviness of the head and body that is worse in the afternoon, a feeling of heaviness of the head and body, a sticky taste, epigastric fullness, a feeling of oppression of the chest, excessive vaginal discharge, sticky tongue coating, Slippery or Soggy pulse.

Other symptoms and signs depend on whether there is Damp-Heat or Cold-Dampness.

Headache

Interrogation, Chapter 34

Liver-Yang rising

Distending headache, which can be on the side of the head on the Gall-Bladder channel, on the temples or behind the eyes, dizziness, tinnitus, irritability, propensity to outbursts of anger, Wiry pulse.

This is probably the most common type of headache. Liver-Yang rising may arise from deficiency of Liver-Blood or Liver-Yin, or both, or from Kidney-Yin deficiency and the clinical manifestations will vary accordingly.

Wind-Phlegm

Pulling headache with a feeling of heaviness of the head, severe dizziness, blurred vision, tremors, numbness/tingling of the limbs, tinnitus, nausea, sputum in the throat, a feeling of oppression of the chest, Stiff or Deviated and Swollen tongue, Wiry-Slippery pulse.

Dampness obstructing the head

Headache with a feeling of heaviness of the head, head feeling as if wrapped in cotton wool, a sticky taste, a feeling of heaviness of the head and body, epigastric fullness, a feeling of oppression of the chest, excessive vaginal discharge, sticky tongue coating, Slippery or Soggy pulse.

Turbid Phlegm obstructing the head

Dull headache with a feeling of heaviness and muzziness of the head, poor memory and concentration, dizziness, blurred vision, sputum in the throat, a feeling of oppression of the chest, nausea, Swollen tongue with sticky coating, Slippery pulse.

Liver-Fire

Distending headache, which can be on the side of the head on the Gall-Bladder channel, on the temples or behind the eyes, red and bloodshot eyes, red face, dizziness, tinnitus, irritability, propensity to outbursts of anger, thirst, bitter taste, constipation, dark urine, Red tongue with redder sides and dry yellow coating, Wiry-Rapid pulse.

Liver-Wind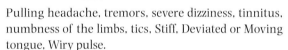

Pulling headache, tremors, severe dizziness, tinnitus, numbness of the limbs, tics, Stiff, Deviated or Moving tongue, Wiry pulse.

Liver-Qi stagnation

Distending headache on the temples or forehead, or both, hypochondrial or epigastric distension, irritability, moodiness, a feeling of a lump in the throat, premenstrual tension, Wiry pulse.

Blood stasis

Stabbing headache fixed in a small area, purple lips, dark complexion, Purple tongue.

Stomach-Heat

Severe headache on the forehead, burning epigastric pain, thirst, sour regurgitation, nausea, excessive hunger, foul breath, a feeling of heat, Red tongue with a yellow coating, Overflowing-Rapid pulse.

Qi deficiency

Dull headache on the forehead that is aggravated by overwork and alleviated by rest and by lying down, uncomfortable feeling in the epigastrium, no appetite, lack of sense of taste, loose stools, tiredness especially in the morning, weak limbs, Pale tongue, Empty pulse.

This is generally due to Stomach-Qi deficiency.

Blood deficiency

Dull headache on the forehead or the vertex, dizziness, blurred vision, poor memory, Pale and Thin tongue, Choppy or Fine pulse.

Other symptoms and signs depend on whether the Liver or Heart is affected.

Kidney deficiency

Dull headache with a feeling of emptiness of the head, aggravated by overexertion, dizziness, lower backache, weak knees, tinnitus.

The other clinical manifestations depend on whether there is a Kidney-Yin or Kidney-Yang deficiency.

Retention of food

Headache on the forehead that is worse after eating, fullness, pain and distension of the epigastrium which are relieved by vomiting, nausea, vomiting of sour fluids, foul breath, sour regurgitation, belching, insomnia, loose stools or constipation, poor appetite, thick tongue coating, Full-Slippery pulse.

This type of headache is usually seen only in children.

Invasion of Wind-Cold

Occipital headache, stiff neck, aversion to cold, fever, cough, itchy throat, slight breathlessness, stuffed or runny nose with clear watery discharge, sneezing, body aches, thin white tongue coating, Floating-Tight pulse.

Invasion of Wind-Heat

Headache of the whole head, aversion to cold, fever, cough, sore throat, stuffed or runny nose with yellow discharge, headache, body aches, slight sweating, slight thirst, swollen tonsils, tongue slightly Red on the sides in the chest area or on front part, Floating-Rapid pulse.

Invasion of Wind-Dampness

Frontal headache, feeling of heaviness of the head, aversion to cold, fever, epigastric fullness, body aches, tongue with thin, sticky white coating, Floating-Slippery pulse.

Apart from the above pattern identification according to Internal Organs, it is also important, especially from an acupuncturist's perspective, to differentiate headaches according to the channel involved.

Greater-Yang channels

Occipital headache radiating to the back of the neck and top of the back.

Bright-Yang channels

Headache on the forehead.

Lesser-Yang channels

Headaches on the temples, the sides of the head and neck along the Gall-Bladder channel and Triple Burner channel.

Greater-Yin channels

Frontal headache.

Lesser-Yin channels

Headache felt inside the head or on the occiput, dull in character.

Terminal-Yin channels

Headache on the vertex.

Clinical note

- In my experience, the combination of Liver-Yang rising and Phlegm is the most common cause of chronic headaches.
- In women, Liver-Yang rising (causing chronic headaches) usually arises from Liver-Blood deficiency

---

Feeling of distension of the head

Interrogation, Chapter 34

Liver-Yang rising

A feeling of distension of the head, headache, dizziness, tinnitus, irritability, propensity to outbursts of anger, Wiry pulse.

Liver-Fire

A feeling of distension of the head, eye ache, bloodshot eyes, headaches, red face, dizziness, tinnitus, irritability, propensity to outbursts of anger, thirst, bitter taste, constipation, dark urine, Red tongue with redder sides and dry yellow coating, Wiry-Rapid pulse.

Invasion of Wind-Heat

An acute feeling of distension of the head, aversion to cold, fever, cough, sore throat, stuffed or runny nose with yellow discharge, headache, body aches, slight sweating, slight thirst, swollen tonsils, tongue slightly Red on the sides in the chest area or on front part, Floating-Rapid pulse.

Feeling of muzziness (fuzziness) of the head

Interrogation, Chapter 34

Dampness

Muzziness of the head, a feeling of heaviness of the head, chronic sinusitis, stuffed nose, sticky nasal discharge, dull frontal headache as if the head were wrapped in cotton wool, epigastric fullness, a sticky taste, a feeling of oppression of the chest, excessive vaginal discharge, sticky tongue coating, Slippery or Soggy pulse.

Phlegm

Severe muzziness of the head, dizziness, a feeling of heaviness of the head, blurred vision, excessive production of ear wax, stuffed nose, dull frontal headache, sputum in the throat, a feeling of oppression of the chest, Swollen tongue with sticky coating, Slippery pulse.

> ## Clinical note
>
> - Phlegm is by far the most common cause of a feeling of muzziness (fuzziness) of the head.

Feeling of cold of the head

Interrogation, Chapter 34

This includes an actual feeling of cold of the head but also a propensity to wearing a hat and a strong dislike of wind.

Governing Vessel empty and cold

A feeling of cold of the head and back, cold limbs, a feeling of cold, sore back, cold feet, dizziness, tinnitus, weak knees, pale complexion, pulse Floating but Weak on all three positions on the left.

Cold in the Liver channel

A feeling of cold of the head, vertical headache, bluish complexion, cold hands and feet, Deep-Tight pulse.

Feeling of heat of the head

Interrogation, Chapter 34

Liver-Fire

A feeling of heat of the head, red face, red and bloodshot eyes, eye ache, headaches, red face, dizziness, tin-

nitus, irritability, propensity to outbursts of anger, thirst, bitter taste, constipation, dark urine, Red tongue with redder sides and dry yellow coating, Wiry-Rapid pulse.

Kidney-Yin deficiency with Empty-Heat

A feeling of heat of the head especially in the evening, dizziness, tinnitus, hardness of hearing, night sweating, dry mouth at night, five-palm heat, a feeling of heat in the evening, malar flush, thirst with a desire to drink in small sips, lower backache, dark scanty urine, insomnia, Red tongue without coating, Floating-Empty and Rapid pulse.

Numbness of the head

Interrogation, Chapter 34

Liver-Blood deficiency

Numbness of the skin of the head, especially on the vertex, dull headache, dizziness, blurred vision, floaters, numbness/tingling of limbs, scanty menstruation, dull-pale complexion, Pale tongue, Choppy or Fine pulse.

Damp-Phlegm

Numbness of the skin of the head, especially on the forehead, a feeling of heaviness and muzziness of the head, a feeling of oppression of the chest, dizziness, blurred vision, somnolence, nausea, sputum in the throat, muzziness of the head, Swollen tongue with sticky coating, Slippery pulse.

Liver-Wind

Unilateral numbness of the head, tremors, severe dizziness, tinnitus, headache, numbness of limbs, tics, Stiff, Deviated or Moving tongue, Wiry pulse.

Drooping head
Stomach- and Spleen-Qi deficiency

Head drooping, poor appetite, tiredness, slight abdominal distension, pale complexion, loose stools, Pale tongue, Empty pulse.

Emptiness of the Sea of Marrow

Head drooping, dizziness, tinnitus, deafness, sore back, poor memory, weak knees, difficulty in walking. This is

usually, but not always, accompanied by Kidney-Yin deficiency.

Leaning of the head to one side

Observation, Chapter 5

Spleen-Qi sinking

Leaning of the head to one side, poor appetite, slight abdominal distension after eating, tiredness, lassitude, pale complexion, weakness of the limbs, loose stools, depression, tendency to obesity, a bearing-down sensation in the abdomen, prolapse of stomach, uterus, anus or bladder, frequency and urgency of urination, Pale tongue, Weak pulse.

Emptiness of the Sea of Marrow

Leaning of the head to one side, dizziness, tinnitus, deafness, sore back, poor memory, weak knees, difficulty in walking. This is usually, but not always, accompanied by Kidney-Yin deficiency.

Tremor of the head

Observation, Chapters 4 and 5

Liver-Wind

Tremor of the head, vertigo, tremors, severe dizziness, tinnitus, headache, numbness of limbs, tics, Stiff, Deviated or Moving tongue, Wiry pulse.

Empty-Wind from Blood deficiency

Slight tremor of the head, slight tremor of the hand, facial tic, dizziness, poor memory, blurred vision, Pale and Thin tongue, Choppy or Fine and slightly Wiry pulse.

Empty-Wind from Yin deficiency

Slight tremor of the head, slight tremor of the hand, dizziness, tinnitus, night sweating, tongue without coating, Floating-Empty or Fine and slightly Wiry pulse.

Brain noise

Interrogation, Chapter 34

'Brain noise' is similar to the sound of tinnitus in the ears but it is experienced in the centre of the head. The Chinese name for it is *nao ting*, which means 'brain tinnitus', its old name was *lei tou feng*, which means 'thunder head wind'.

Emptiness of the Sea of Marrow

Brain noise like tinnitus, dizziness, tinnitus, brain noise, poor memory, deafness, a feeling of emptiness of the head, blurred vision.

Deficiency of Qi and Blood of the Spleen and Heart

Brain noise like tinnitus, poor memory, dizziness, insomnia, palpitations, poor appetite, loose stools, Pale tongue, Weak or Choppy pulse.

Phlegm-Heat rising

Brain noise like tinnitus, a feeling of heaviness and muzziness of the head, headache, dizziness, blurred vision, nausea, a feeling of oppression of the chest, Red-Swollen tongue with sticky yellow coating, Slippery pulse.

Liver-Qi stagnation

Brain noise like tinnitus, tense neck muscles, hypochondrial or epigastric distension, irritability, moodiness, a feeling of a lump in the throat, premenstrual tension, Wiry pulse.

Stagnant Liver-Qi impairs the ascending and descending of Qi, clear Qi cannot rise, and turbid Qi cannot descend so that turbidity accumulates in the head.

Swelling of the whole head

Observation, Chapter 5

'Big Head Warm Disease' (invasion of Toxic Heat in the head)

Swelling of the head and face, swollen glands, swelling of the parotid gland, swollen tonsils, aversion to cold, fever, cough, sore throat, stuffed or runny nose with yellow discharge, headache, body aches, slight sweating, slight thirst, tongue slightly Red on the sides in the chest area or on front part, Floating-Rapid pulse.

Ulcers in the mastoid region

Observation, Chapter 5

Damp-Heat in the Gall-Bladder channel

Ulcers in the mastoid region, hypochondrial pain, fullness and distension, nausea, vomiting, inability to digest fats, yellow complexion and eyes, dizziness, tin-

nitus, irritability, a feeling of heaviness, unilateral or bilateral thick, sticky yellow coating, Slippery-Rapid pulse.

Liver-Fire

Ulcers in the mastoid region, headache, red face, dizziness, tinnitus, irritability, propensity to outbursts of anger, thirst, bitter taste, constipation, dark urine, Red tongue with redder sides and dry yellow coating, Wiry-Rapid pulse.

Head tilted backwards

Observation, Chapter 5

Internal Wind in acute febrile diseases

Head tilted backwards, with eyes rolled up, opisthotonos, fever at night, convulsions, macular rash, Red tongue without coating, Fine and Wiry pulse.

HAIR AND SCALP

Premature greying of the hair

Observation, Chapter 5

Liver-Blood deficiency

Premature greying of the hair especially on the vertex, dizziness, blurred vision, floaters, numbness/tingling of limbs, scanty menstruation, dull-pale complexion, Pale tongue, Choppy or Fine pulse.

Liver and Kidney deficiency

Premature greying of the hair over the whole head, balding, dizziness, tinnitus, blurred vision, backache, decreased libido. Other clinical manifestations depend on whether there is Kidney-Yin or Kidney-Yang deficiency.

Kidney-Yin deficiency with Empty-Heat

Premature greying of the hair, balding, dizziness, tinnitus, hardness of hearing, night sweating, dry mouth at night, five-palm heat, a feeling of heat in the evening, malar flush, thirst with a desire to drink in small sips, lower backache, dark scanty urine, insomnia, Red tongue without coating, Floating-Empty and Rapid pulse.

Kidney-Essence deficiency

Premature greying of the hair, poor bone development in children, softening of the bones in adults, deafness,

weakness of the knees and legs, poor memory, loose teeth, falling hair or premature greying of the hair, weakness from sexual activity, lower backache, infertility, sterility, dizziness, tinnitus, normal-coloured tongue and Floating-Empty or Leather pulse if Kidney-Essence deficiency occurs against a background of Kidney-Yin deficiency, or Pale tongue and Deep-Weak pulse if against a background of Kidney-Yang deficiency.

Deficiency of Qi and Blood

Premature greying of the hair, poor appetite, loose stools, weak voice, tiredness, blurred vision, dizziness, numbness/tingling of limbs, palpitations, dull-pale complexion, Pale tongue, Weak or Choppy pulse.

Liver- and Heart-Fire

Hair turning white suddenly after a shock or a very intense emotional upset such as anger, headaches, bloodshot eyes, dizziness, tinnitus, irritability, red face, thirst, bitter taste, palpitations, agitation, insomnia, dream-disturbed sleep, a feeling of heat, Red tongue with redder sides and tip and dry yellow coating, Wiry-Overflowing-Rapid pulse.

Liver-Qi stagnation

Premature greying of the hair in patches which may appear in a relatively short time, hypochondrial or epigastric distension, irritability, moodiness, a feeling of a lump in the throat, premenstrual tension, Wiry pulse.

This pattern is due to worry, pensiveness or anger causing Qi stagnation, which turns into Heat, which, in turn, damages Yin.

Hair falling out

Observation, Chapter 5

This refers to hair falling out gradually and uniformly (as opposed to in clumps).

Liver-Blood deficiency

Gradual loss of hair, dull headache, dizziness, blurred vision, floaters, numbness or tingling of limbs, scanty menstruation, dull-pale complexion, Pale tongue, Choppy or Fine pulse.

Kidney deficiency

Gradual loss of hair, which may improve during pregnancy, dizziness, tinnitus, backache, tiredness.

Other symptoms and signs, including pulse and tongue, depend on whether there is a deficiency of Kidney-Yin, Kidney-Yang or Kidney-Essence.

Blood-Heat from Liver-Fire

Gradual loss of hair especially on the vertex, red face, bloodshot eyes, headache, red face, dizziness, tinnitus, irritability, propensity to outbursts of anger, thirst, bitter taste, constipation, dark urine, Red tongue with redder sides and dry yellow coating, Wiry-Rapid pulse.

Alopecia

Observation, Chapter 5

Alopecia refers to the loss of hair falling out in clumps.

Empty Liver-Wind from Blood deficiency

Sudden loss of hair in clumps, slight tremor of the head or hand, or both, facial tic, dizziness, blurred vision, unilateral numbness/tingling of a limb, Pale and Thin tongue, Choppy or Fine and slightly Wiry pulse.

Full Liver-Wind

Sudden loss of hair in clumps, tremors, severe dizziness, tinnitus, headache, numbness of limbs, tics, Stiff, Deviated or Moving tongue, Wiry pulse.

Blood Heat from Liver-Fire

Hair falling out in clumps, dry hair, headache, red face, dizziness, tinnitus, irritability, propensity to outbursts of anger, thirst, bitter taste, constipation, dark urine, Red tongue with redder sides and dry yellow coating, Wiry-Rapid pulse.

Liver-Blood stasis

Hair falling out in clumps, hypochondrial/abdominal pain, painful periods, dark and clotted menstrual blood, masses in the abdomen, purple nails and lips, purple or dark complexion, Purple tongue, Wiry or Firm pulse.

> **Clinical note**
> - Remember: as a rule of thumb, if the hair falls gradually it is due to a deficiency (of Liver-Blood or Kidneys), whereas if it falls out in clumps it is due to a Fullness (often internal Wind).

Dry and brittle hair

Observation, Chapter 5

Liver-Blood deficiency

Dry hair without lustre, dizziness, blurred vision, floaters, numbness/tingling of limbs, scanty menstruation, dull-pale complexion, Pale tongue, Choppy or Fine pulse.

Kidney-Yin deficiency

Dry hair without lustre, dizziness, tinnitus, hardness of hearing, poor memory, hardness of hearing, night sweating, vertigo, dry mouth and throat at night, lower backache, ache in bones, nocturnal emissions, constipation, dark scanty urine, infertility, premature ejaculation, tiredness, lassitude, depression, slight anxiety, normal-coloured tongue without coating, Floating-Empty pulse.

Deficiency of Qi and Blood

Thin and brittle hair, poor appetite, loose stools, weak voice, tiredness, blurred vision, dizziness, numbness/tingling of limbs, palpitations, dull-pale complexion, Pale tongue, Weak or Choppy pulse.

Stomach- and Spleen-Qi deficiency

Thin and brittle hair, poor appetite, slight abdominal distension after eating, tiredness, lassitude, pale complexion, weakness of the limbs, loose stools, an uncomfortable feeling in the epigastrium, lack of taste sensation, Pale tongue, Empty pulse.

Loss of Blood

Dry and lifeless hair without lustre, dry skin, pale complexion, menorrhagia, Pale and dry tongue, Hollow pulse.

> **Clinical note**
> - In women patients, I always observe the hair early on during the consultation to check the state of Liver-Blood.

Greasy hair

Observation, Chapter 5

Dampness

Greasy hair, a feeling of heaviness of the head and body, epigastric fullness, a sticky taste, a feeling of

oppression of the chest, excessive vaginal discharge, sticky tongue coating, Slippery or Soggy pulse.

Damp-Heat

Greasy hair, epigastric fullness, a sticky taste, thirst with no desire to drink, a feeling of heaviness of the head and body, a feeling of heat, sticky yellow tongue coating, Slippery-Rapid pulse.

Phlegm

Greasy hair, a feeling of oppression of the chest, sputum in the throat, Swollen tongue with sticky coating, Slippery pulse.

Dandruff

Observation, Chapter 5

Liver-Blood deficient and dry

Dandruff, dry hair, dry skin, dry eyes, dizziness, blurred vision, floaters, numbness/tingling of limbs, dull-pale complexion, Pale tongue, Choppy or Fine pulse.

Liver-Blood deficiency with Liver-Wind

Dandruff, dry hair, dry skin, slight tremor of the head or hand or both facial tic, dizziness, blurred vision, unilateral numbness/tingling of a limb, Pale and Thin tongue, Choppy or Fine and slightly Wiry pulse.

Liver-Fire

Dandruff, a feeling of heat of the head, headache, red face, dizziness, tinnitus, irritability, propensity to outbursts of anger, thirst, bitter taste, constipation, dark urine, Red tongue with redder sides and dry yellow coating, Wiry-Rapid pulse.

Damp-Heat in the Liver

Dandruff, greasy hair, yellow eyes, excessive ear wax production, fullness of the hypochondrium, abdomen or hypogastrium, bitter taste, nausea, a feeling of heaviness of the body, excessive vaginal discharge and itching, mid-cycle bleeding/pain, genital papular or vesicular skin rashes and itching, urinary difficulty, burning on urination with dark urine, Red tongue with redder sides and sticky yellow coating, Slippery-Wiry-Rapid pulse.

Toxic Heat

Dandruff, scalp skin infections, boils on the head, a feeling of heat of the head, red eyes, thirst, Red tongue

with red points and thick, dry yellow coating, Slippery-Overflowing-Rapid pulse.

Invasion of Wind-Heat with Dryness

Dandruff with acute onset, dry cough, aversion to cold, fever, dry throat, tickly throat, dry nose, discomfort of the chest, thin, dry white coating, Floating pulse.

Itchy scalp

Interrogation, Chapter 34

Liver-Blood deficiency

Itchy scalp, dandruff, dry scalp and hair, dizziness, blurred vision, floaters, numbness/tingling of limbs, scanty menstruation, dull-pale complexion, Pale tongue, Choppy or Fine pulse.

Liver-Blood deficiency with Liver-Wind

Itchy scalp, dandruff, dry scalp and hair, dry skin, slight tremor of the head or hand or both, facial tic, dizziness, blurred vision, unilateral numbness/tingling of a limb, Pale and Thin tongue, Choppy or Fine and slightly Wiry pulse.

Liver-Yin deficiency

Itchy scalp, dry scalp and hair, dizziness, numbness/tingling of the limbs, blurred vision, floaters in the eyes, dry eyes, scanty menstruation, dull-pale complexion but with red cheekbones, withered and brittle nails, night sweating, normal-coloured tongue without coating, Fine or Floating-Empty pulse.

Liver-Fire

Itchy scalp, feeling of heat of the head, dry scalp, headache, red face, dizziness, tinnitus, irritability, propensity to outbursts of anger, thirst, bitter taste, constipation, dark urine, Red tongue with redder sides and dry yellow coating, Wiry-Rapid pulse.

Damp-Heat in the Liver channel

Itchy scalp, skin eruptions on the scalp, psoriasis of scalp, fullness of the hypochondrium, abdomen or hypogastrium, bitter taste, nausea, feeling of heaviness of the body, yellow vaginal discharge, vaginal itching, mid-cycle bleeding/pain, genital papular or vesicular shin rashes and itching, urinary difficulty, burning on urination, dark urine, Red tongue with redder sides and sticky yellow coating, Slippery-Wiry-Rapid pulse.

Dry scalp

Observation, Chapter 5

Liver-Yin deficiency

Dry scalp, dry hair, dandruff, blurred vision, floaters, dry eyes, dizziness, numbness/tingling of the limbs, scanty menstruation, withered and brittle nails, normal colour tongue without coating, Fine or Floating-Empty pulse.

Kidney-Yin deficiency

Dry scalp, dry hair, dandruff, blurred vision, floaters, dry eyes, dizziness, tinnitus, poor memory, hardness of hearing, night sweating, dry mouth and throat at night, lower backache, dry stools, dark scanty urine, normal-coloured tongue without coating, Floating-Empty pulse.

Redness and pain of the scalp

Observation, Chapter 5

Invasion of Wind-Heat

Acute redness and pain of the scalp, aversion to cold, fever, cough, sore throat, stuffed or runny nose with yellow discharge, headache, body aches, slight sweating, slight thirst, swollen tonsils, tongue slightly Red on the sides in the chest area or on front part, Floating-Rapid pulse.

Liver-Fire

Redness and pain of the scalp, headache, red face, dizziness, tinnitus, irritability, propensity to outbursts of anger, thirst, bitter taste, constipation, dark urine, Red tongue with redder sides and dry yellow coating, Wiry-Rapid pulse.

Boils on the scalp

Observation, Chapter 5

Liver-Fire

Chronic boils on the scalp, headache, red face, dizziness, tinnitus, irritability, propensity to outbursts of anger, thirst, bitter taste, constipation, dark urine, Red tongue with redder sides and dry yellow coating, Wiry-Rapid pulse.

Damp-Heat in the Liver channel

Chronic boils on the scalp, fullness of the hypochondrium, abdomen or hypogastrium, bitter taste, poor appetite, nausea, feeling of heaviness of the body, yellow vaginal discharge, vaginal itching, urinary difficulty, burning on urination, dark urine, Red tongue with redder sides and a sticky yellow coating, Slippery-Wiry-Rapid pulse.

Toxic Heat in the head

Acute boils on the scalp, redness, pain and swelling of the scalp, headache, swollen glands, red and swollen tonsils, aversion to cold, fever, thirst, tongue that is Red on the front with red points and a thick, sticky yellow coating, Slippery-Overflowing-Rapid pulse.

Erosion of the scalp

Observation, Chapter 5

Damp-Heat in the Liver channel

Erosion of the scalp with itching and oozing of fluid, fullness of the hypochondrium, abdomen or hypogastrium, bitter taste, poor appetite, nausea, a feeling of heaviness of the body, yellow vaginal discharge, urinary difficulty, burning on urination, dark urine, Red tongue with redder sides and a sticky yellow coating, Slippery-Wiry-Rapid pulse.

Ulcers on the scalp

Observation, Chapter 5

Liver-Fire

Chronic ulcers on the scalp, headache, red face, dizziness, tinnitus, irritability, propensity to outbursts of anger, thirst, bitter taste, constipation, dark urine, Red tongue with redder sides and dry yellow coating, Wiry-Rapid pulse.

Damp-Heat in the Liver channel

Chronic ulcers on the scalp, fullness of the hypochondrium, abdomen or hypogastrium, bitter taste, poor appetite, nausea, a feeling of heaviness of the body, yellow vaginal discharge, vaginal itching, urinary difficulty, burning on urination, dark urine, Red tongue with redder sides and a sticky yellow coating, Slippery-Wiry-Rapid pulse.

Heat in the Governing Vessel

Ulcers on the crown of the head, a feeling of heat in the head, redness of the scalp, headache, insomnia, dark scanty urine, Red tongue with yellow coating, Floating-Rapid pulse on all three positions on the left.

FACE

Acne

Observation, Chapter 5; Symptoms and Signs, Chapter 77

Damp-Heat in the skin

Facial acne with red, papular eruptions, greasy skin, puffy face, sticky yellow tongue coating, Slippery-Rapid pulse.

This is the most common pattern causing acne in young people.

Toxic Heat in the skin

Facial acne with large, red, pustular eruptions that are painful, a feeling of heat, red face, red eyes, Red tongue with red points and thick, sticky yellow coating, Slippery-Overflowing-Rapid pulse.

Toxic Heat with Blood stasis in the skin

Facial acne with large, dark red or purple, pustular eruptions that are painful, a feeling of heat, dark face, red eyes, Reddish-Purple tongue with red points and thick, sticky yellow coating, Slippery-Overflowing-Wiry-Rapid pulse.

Spleen-Qi deficiency with Dampness

Chronic, facial acne with pale-red, papular or vesicular eruptions which take a long time to come to a head, greasy skin, dull-pale complexion, Pale tongue with sticky coating, Soggy pulse.

Heat in the Stomach and Lungs

Facial acne with small, red, papular eruptions, on the face, chest and upper back, dry skin, blackheads, red face, a feeling of heat, Red tongue with dry yellow coating, Overflowing-Rapid pulse.

Damp-Phlegm in the skin

Facial acne with large, pale, vesicular eruptions, greasy skin, puffy face, greasy hair, Swollen tongue with sticky coating, Slippery pulse.

Damp-Phlegm with Blood stasis in the skin

Facial acne with large, dark, purple, papular eruptions, dark complexion, puffy face, dry skin if Blood stasis predominates, or greasy skin if Damp-Phlegm predominates, Purple and Swollen tongue, Slippery-Wiry pulse.

Disharmony of Penetrating and Directing Vessels

Facial acne that starts with puberty, especially on the chin, greasy skin, papular eruptions which are aggravated before the period in girls.

Rather than being a separate pattern causing acne, a disharmony of the Penetrating and Directing Vessels is the condition underlying the development of acne at puberty time and one that continues to be an underlying condition when the acne persists for several years, especially in women.

> **Clinical note**
>
> - When treating acne, I always harmonize the Directing and Penetrating Vessels, irrespective of the pattern, in order to balance the hormone levels.

Feeling of heat of the face

Interrogation, Chapter 35

A feeling of heat of the face includes menopausal hot flushes.

Liver-Yang rising

A feeling of heat of the face, red face, headache, dizziness, tinnitus, irritability, propensity to outbursts of anger, Wiry pulse.

Liver-Fire

A feeling of heat of the face and head, worse when anxious or upset, red face, red eyes, headache, red face, dizziness, tinnitus, irritability, propensity to outbursts of anger, thirst, bitter taste, constipation, dark urine, Red tongue with redder sides and dry yellow coating, Wiry-Rapid pulse.

Heart-Fire

A feeling of heat of the face, palpitations, thirst, mouth and tongue ulcers, mental restlessness, a feeling of agitation, insomnia, dream-disturbed sleep, a feeling of

heat, red face, bitter taste, Red tongue with redder tip and yellow coating, Overflowing-Rapid pulse.

Heart-Yin deficiency with Empty-Heat

A feeling of heat of the face in the afternoon and evening, malar flush, palpitations, insomnia, dream-disturbed sleep, poor memory, anxiety, tendency to be easily startled, mental restlessness, uneasiness, 'feeling hot and bothered', dry mouth and throat, thirst with a desire to sip fluids, a feeling of heat in the evening, malar flush, night sweating, five-palm heat, Red tongue, redder on the tip, no coating, Floating-Empty and Rapid pulse.

Kidney-Yin deficiency with Empty-Heat

A feeling of heat of the face in the afternoon or evening, dizziness, tinnitus, hardness of hearing, night sweating, dry mouth at night, five-palm heat, a feeling of heat in the evening, malar flush, thirst with a desire to drink in small sips, lower backache, dark scanty urine, insomnia, Red tongue without coating, Floating-Empty and Rapid pulse.

Lung-Heat

A feeling of heat of the face, redness of the right cheek, cough, slight breathlessness, feeling of heat, chest ache, flaring of nostrils, thirst, red face, Red tongue with yellow coating, Overflowing-Rapid pulse.

Lung-Yin deficiency with Empty-Heat

A feeling of heat of the face in the afternoon and evening, malar flush, dry cough or with scanty, sticky sputum which could be blood-tinged, dry mouth and throat at night, weak/hoarse voice, night sweating, tiredness, malar flush, a feeling of heat or a low-grade fever in the evening, five-palm heat, thin body or thin chest, insomnia, anxiety, Red tongue without coating, Floating-Empty and Rapid pulse.

Stomach-Heat

A feeling of heat of the face, worse after eating, burning epigastric pain, thirst, sour regurgitation, nausea, excessive hunger, foul breath, a feeling of heat, Red tongue with a yellow coating, Overflowing-Rapid pulse.

Stomach-Yin deficiency with Empty-Heat

A feeling of heat of the face in the afternoon and evening, dull or burning epigastric pain, feeling of heat in the afternoon, dry mouth and throat especially in the afternoon, thirst with desire to drink in small sips, dry stools, slight feeling of fullness after eating, night sweating, five-palm heat, bleeding gums, Red tongue (or Red centre only) without coating in the centre, Floating-Empty and Rapid pulse.

Damp-Heat in the Spleen

A feeling of heat of the face, sticky taste, thirst with no desire to drink, a feeling of fullness of the epigastrium, epigastric or abdominal pain, poor appetite, a feeling of heaviness of the body, nausea, vomiting, loose stools with offensive odour, a feeling of heat, scanty dark urine, headache with a feeling of heaviness of the head, dull-yellow complexion, bitter taste, Red tongue with sticky yellow coating, Slippery-Rapid pulse.

Spleen-Heat

A feeling of heat of the face, red and dry lips, red tip of the nose, burning epigastric/abdominal pain, excessive hunger, mouth ulcers, thirst, dry stools, a feeling of heat, scanty dark urine, yellow complexion, Red tongue with dry yellow coating, Overflowing-Rapid pulse.

Spleen-Yin deficiency with Empty-Heat

A feeling of heat of the face in the afternoon and evening, poor appetite, poor digestion, retching, gnawing hunger, loss of taste, slight epigastric pain, dry mouth and lips, dry stools, thin body, sallow complexion with red tip of the nose, night sweating, malar flush, a feeling of heat in the evening, Red tongue without coating and transversal cracks on the sides, Floating-Empty and Rapid pulse.

Yin Fire

A feeling of heat of the face but cold limbs, slightly red face or pale face with a floating red colour on the cheeks, intermittent sore throat, dry mouth, dry lips, mouth ulcers, exhaustion, poor appetite, poor digestion, weak limbs, Pale tongue, Weak or Overflowing-Empty pulse.

Yin Fire is a pathological Minister Fire that arises when the Original Qi (*Yuan Qi*) becomes depleted from overwork. Since the Minister Fire and the Original Qi reside in the same place, the pathological Minister Fire 'robs' the Original Qi and rises to the head. This pattern is treated by tonifying the Original Qi and lightly clearing Heat; the representative prescription is Bu Zhong Yi Qi Tang *Tonifying the Centre and Benefiting Qi Decoction.*

Clinical note

- In women, a feeling of heat of the face by no means always indicates Heat. In women, a feeling of heat of the face contradicting other symptoms and signs is very common. In particular, it may be due to:
  —a simultaneous deficiency of Kidney-Yin and Kidney-Yang
  —Empty-Heat from Blood deficiency
  —Yin Fire.

Facial pain

Interrogation, Chapter 35

Facial pain such as in trigeminal neuralgia is often due to invasion of Wind in the channels of the face. This is an invasion of Wind purely in the channels of the face and it is not accompanied by the symptoms of invasion of Wind in the Lung Defensive-Qi system (as in common cold and influenza). The pattern of Wind in the channels causing facial pain may be associated with any of the other patterns listed; for example, the association of invasion of Wind in the channels of the face with Yin deficiency is a common cause of facial pain, especially in the elderly.

Invasion of Wind-Cold in the channels

Facial pain in repeated bouts, spastic, unbearable pain, face becoming ashen-pale during a bout of pain, aggravated by exposure to cold and alleviated by heat, Pale tongue, Tight pulse.

Invasion of Wind-Heat in the channels

Facial pain with a burning sensation in repeated bouts, stabbing, unbearable pain, pain in nose and lips, touching the face may suddenly provoke the pain, the pain is more often along the central axis of the face rather than on the right and left sides, face becomes red during a bout of pain, sweating, pain alleviated by exposure to cold and aggravated by exposure to heat, a feeling of heat, thirst, yellow tongue coating, Rapid pulse.

Liver-Fire

Burning facial pain that comes and goes according to emotional moods, pain aggravated by exposure to heat, red face, bloodshot eyes, headache, dizziness, tinnitus, irritability, propensity to outbursts of anger, thirst, bitter taste, constipation, dark urine, Red tongue with redder sides and dry yellow coating, Wiry-Rapid pulse.

Damp-Heat

Severe pain in the cheeks and forehead accompanied by a sticky yellow or greenish nasal discharge, epigastric fullness, a sticky taste, thirst with no desire to drink, a feeling of heaviness of the head and body, a feeling of heat, sticky yellow tongue coating, Slippery-Rapid pulse.

Deficiency of Qi and Blood

Chronic, dull facial pain that is aggravated by overexertion and alleviated by rest, pale face, poor appetite, loose stools, weak voice, tiredness, blurred vision, dizziness, numbness/tingling of limbs, palpitations, dull-pale complexion, Pale tongue, Weak or Choppy pulse.

Blood stasis

Stabbing facial pain, dark complexion, headache, purple lips, dark rings under the eyes, Purple tongue, Wiry or Choppy pulse.

This is Blood stasis affecting the channels of the face, which may occur against a background of Heart- or Liver-Blood deficiency.

Yin deficiency with Empty-Heat

Facial pain, malar flush, dry mouth with no desire to drink, a feeling of heat in the evening, night sweating, Red tongue without coating, Floating-Empty and Rapid pulse.

Other symptoms and signs depend on the organ involved.

Yin deficiency with Empty-Heat and internal Wind

Facial pain aggravated by exposure to wind, malar flush, dry mouth with no desire to drink, a feeling of heat in the evening, night sweating, vertigo, facial tics, tremor, Stiff, Red tongue without coating, Floating-Empty, Rapid and slightly Wiry pulse.

Phlegm-Heat

Facial pain, a feeling of heaviness and muzziness of the head, a feeling of heat, red face, swelling of the face, dark rings under the eyes, greasy skin, a feeling of oppression of the chest, sputum in the throat, expectoration of yellow sputum, dizziness, nausea, Red and Swollen tongue with sticky yellow coating, Slippery-Rapid pulse.

Yin deficiency with Phlegm-Heat

Facial pain, malar flush, dry mouth with no desire to drink, a feeling of heat in the evening, night sweating,

a feeling of heat, red face, a feeling of heaviness and muzziness of the head, swelling of the face, greasy skin, dizziness, nausea, a feeling of oppression of the chest, sputum in the throat, Red, Swollen tongue with coating, Floating-Empty or Fine and slightly Slippery pulse.

> ### Clinical note
> - In the elderly with facial pain (often trigeminal neuralgia), Yin deficiency is nearly always the background for an invasion of Wind.

Numbness of the face

Interrogation, Chapter 35

Blood deficiency

Mild numbness of the face, dull-pale complexion, dull headache, blurred vision, dizziness, Pale tongue, Choppy or Fine pulse.

Other symptoms and signs depend on the organs involved (which may be the Liver or Heart).

Liver-Wind

Unilateral numbness of the face, tremors, severe dizziness, tinnitus, headache, numbness of limbs, tics, Stiff, Deviated or Moving tongue, Wiry pulse.

Stomach-Fire

Numbness of the face, bleeding gums, burning epigastric pain, intense thirst with desire to drink cold liquids, mental restlessness, dry mouth, mouth ulcers, dry stools, sour regurgitation, foul breath, nausea, vomiting soon after eating, a feeling of heat, sour regurgitation, tongue Red with a thick, dry, dark-yellow coating, Deep-Full-Rapid pulse.

Wind-Phlegm

Numbness of the face, deviation of the mouth, slurred speech, severe dizziness, blurred vision, tremors, numbness/tingling of the limbs, tinnitus, nausea, sputum in the throat, a feeling of oppression of the chest, Stiff or Deviated and Swollen tongue, Wiry-Slippery pulse.

Invasion of Wind

Numbness of the face with a sudden onset and short duration, deviation of eye and mouth, Floating pulse.

Oedema of the face

Observation, Chapter 5

Lung-Qi deficiency

Oedema of the face and hands, slight shortness of breath, slight cough, weak voice, spontaneous daytime sweating, dislike of speaking, bright-white complexion, tendency to catch colds, tiredness, dislike of cold, Pale tongue, Empty pulse.

Spleen-Yang deficiency

Oedema of the face, abdomen and legs, poor appetite, slight abdominal distension after eating, tiredness, lassitude, pale complexion, weakness of the limbs, loose stools, slight depression, tendency to obesity, a feeling of cold, cold limbs, oedema, Pale and wet tongue, Deep-Weak pulse.

Wind-Water invading the Lungs

Oedema of the face and hands with sudden onset, bright-shiny complexion, scanty and pale urination, aversion to wind, fever, cough, slight breathlessness, sticky white tongue coating, Floating-Slippery pulse.

Tic

Observation, Chapter 4

'Tic' indicates an involuntary, recurrent twitching of facial muscles, usually involving the eyes or mouth, or both.

Liver-Wind

Severe eye tic, tremors, severe dizziness, tinnitus, headache, numbness of limbs, Stiff, Deviated or Moving tongue, Wiry pulse.

Liver-Blood deficiency leading to Liver-Wind

Occasional facial tic, slight tremor of the head/hand, dizziness, blurred vision, unilateral numbness/tingling of a limb, Pale and Thin tongue, Choppy or Fine and slightly Wiry pulse.

Liver-Wind and Phlegm

Facial tic, severe dizziness, blurred vision, tremors, numbness/tingling of the limbs, tinnitus, nausea, sputum in the throat, a feeling of oppression of the chest, Stiff or Deviated and Swollen tongue, Wiry-Slippery pulse.

This condition is more common in old people.

Liver-Qi stagnation

Eye tic, hypochondrial or epigastric distension, irritability, moodiness, a feeling of a lump in the throat, premenstrual tension, Wiry pulse.

External invasion of Wind-Cold in the channels of the face

Short-lasting tic with sudden onset, stiff neck, occipital headache, Floating-Tight pulse.

Deviation of eye and mouth

Observation, Chapters 4 and 5

Liver-Wind

Deviation of eye and mouth, tremors, severe dizziness, tinnitus, headache, numbness of limbs, tics, Stiff, Deviated or Moving tongue, Wiry pulse.

This corresponds to Wind-stroke.

Liver-Wind and Phlegm

Deviation of eye and mouth, hypertension, tremors, severe dizziness, tinnitus, headache, numbness of limbs, tics, a feeling of oppression of the chest, expectoration of sputum, Deviated or Stiff and Swollen tongue with a sticky coating, Wiry-Slippery pulse.

This condition is more common in old people.

External invasion of Wind-Cold in the channels of the face

Sudden deviation of mouth and eye, incomplete closure of the eye, inability to raise the eyebrow. This corresponds to facial paralysis (Bell's palsy) and it is due to an invasion of Wind-Cold, not in the Lung's Defensive-Qi portion (as in the common cold and influenza), but in the channels of the face.

Liver-Qi stagnation

Intermittent deviation of eye and mouth depending on emotional moods, hypochondrial or epigastric distension, irritability, moodiness, a feeling of a lump in the throat, premenstrual tension, Wiry pulse.

Deficiency of Qi and Blood

Slight deviation of eye and mouth, poor appetite, loose stools, weak voice, tiredness, blurred vision, dizziness, numbness/tingling of limbs, palpitations, dull-pale complexion, Pale tongue, Weak or Choppy pulse.

Toxic Heat in the channels of the face

Deviation of mouth only, thirst, bitter taste, swelling and pain of the face, toothache, headache, red eyes, Red tongue with red points with thick, sticky, yellow coating, Overflowing-Slippery-Rapid pulse.

Facial paralysis

Observation, Chapter 4

External invasion of Wind-Cold in the channels of the face

Facial paralysis with a sudden onset, incomplete closure of the eye, inability to raise eyebrow.

This corresponds to facial paralysis (Bell's palsy) and it is due to an invasion of Wind-Cold, not in the Lung's Defensive-Qi portion (as in the common cold and influenza), but in the channels of the face.

Papular/macular eruptions

Observation, Chapter 5

Lung-Heat

Papular eruptions on the face and nose, cough, slight breathlessness, a feeling of heat, chest ache, flaring of nostrils, thirst, red face, Red tongue with yellow coating, Overflowing-Rapid pulse.

Blood-Heat

Macular eruptions on the face, red face, a feeling of heat of the head, thirst, insomnia, agitation, heavy periods, Red tongue, Overflowing-Rapid pulse.

Swelling and redness of the face

Observation, Chapter 5

Invasion of Toxic Heat

Acute swelling and redness of the face, swollen tonsils, swollen glands, swelling of the parotid gland, aversion to cold, fever, headache, tongue Red in the front with red points and thick, sticky yellow coating, Overflowing-Slippery-Rapid pulse.

Swelling, redness and pain of the cheeks

Observation, Chapter 5

Toxic Heat in the face

Swelling, redness and pain of the cheeks, thirst, bitter taste, toothache, headache, red eyes, Red tongue with

red points with thick, sticky yellow coating, Overflowing-Slippery-Rapid pulse.

Ulcers below the zygomatic arch

Observation, Chapter 5

Toxic Heat in the Stomach

Ulcers below the zygomatic arch, swelling and redness of the cheeks, red and swollen tonsils, burning epigastric pain, thirst, sour regurgitation, nausea, excessive hunger, foul breath, a feeling of heat, Red tongue with a thick, sticky yellow coating and red points, Overflowing-Slippery-Rapid pulse.

Lines on the face

Observation, Chapter 5

Blood deficiency

Lines on the face, dry skin of the face, dry scalp and hair, dry eyes, floaters, blurred vision, numbness/tingling of the limbs, scanty menstruation, Pale and Thin tongue, Fine or Choppy pulse.

Heat with Dryness

Lines on the face, dry skin of the face, dry scalp and hair, red face, dry mouth, dry eyes, thirst, a feeling of heat, Red tongue with yellow coating, Overflowing-Rapid pulse.

Other symptoms and signs depend on the organ involved.

证
候

Chapter **56**

FACE COLOUR

Chapter contents

WHITE/PALE   *575*

YELLOW   *576*

RED   *577*

BLUISH/GREENISH   *577*

PURPLE   *578*

DARK   *578*

SALLOW   *578*

BLUSHING   *579*

WHITE/PALE

Observation, Chapter 3

Qi deficiency

Slightly pale face, tiredness, poor appetite, loose stools, weak voice, slight shortness of breath, Empty pulse.

Other symptoms and signs depend on the organ involved, which may be especially the Lungs, Spleen or Heart.

Yang deficiency

Bright-pale complexion, tiredness, poor appetite, loose stools, weak voice, slight shortness of breath, spontaneous sweating, cold limbs, Pale tongue, Weak pulse.

Yang deficiency of any organ, but especially the Stomach, Spleen, Kidneys, Lungs and Heart, may cause a bright-pale complexion.

Blood deficiency

Dull-pale complexion, blurred vision, poor memory, dizziness, scanty periods, Pale tongue, Choppy or Fine pulse.

Blood deficiency of the Heart, Spleen or Liver may cause a dull-pale complexion.

Full-Cold

Greyish-pale complexion, abdominal pain, epigastric pain cold limbs, pain alleviated by exposure to heat and by drinking warm drinks, and aggravated by exposure to cold and by drinking cold drinks, thick white tongue coating, Tight pulse.

This is Full-Internal-Cold, which may affect the Stomach, Spleen, Liver channel and Intestines.

Collapse of Yang

Greyish-pale complexion, sweating on the forehead like oil beads, chilliness, cold limbs, weak breathing,

absence of thirst, profuse pale urination or incontinence of urine, loose stools, incontinence of faeces, mental confusion or unconsciousness, Pale-Short and wet tongue, Deep-Minute pulse.

Invasion of Wind-Cold

Greyish-pale complexion, aversion to cold, fever, cough, itchy throat, slight breathlessness, stuffed or runny nose with clear watery discharge, sneezing, occipital headache, body aches, thin white tongue coating, Floating-Tight pulse.

Heat stagnating in the Interior (True Heat–False Cold)

Greyish-pale complexion, dark face, bright eyes with lustre, red dry lips, irritability, strong body, noisy breathing, loud voice, thirst with a desire to drink cold fluids, scanty-dark urine, constipation, burning sensation in the anus, hot chest, cold limbs, aversion to heat, mental restlessness, thirst, dark urine, dry stools, Red tongue with yellow coating, Deep-Full-Rapid pulse.

> ### Clinical note
>
> - Do not be surprised if, in women, a pale face has some redness on the cheeks. This may be due to:
> —simultaneous Kidney-Yin and Kidney-Yang deficiency
> —Empty-Heat from Blood deficiency
> —Yin Fire.

YELLOW

Observation, Chapter 3

Dampness

Yellow complexion (which may be bright if Dampness is combined with Heat), a feeling of heaviness of the head and body, epigastric fullness, a sticky taste, a feeling of oppression of the chest, excessive vaginal discharge, sticky tongue coating, Slippery or Soggy pulse.

Chronic Spleen-Qi deficiency

Dull yellow, greyish-yellow complexion, poor appetite, slight abdominal distension after eating, tiredness, weakness of the limbs, loose stools, Pale tongue, Empty pulse.

Chronic Damp-Heat

Ash-like yellow complexion, a feeling of fullness and pain of the epigastrium and lower abdomen, poor appetite, a feeling of heaviness, thirst without a desire to drink, nausea, loose stools with offensive odour, a feeling of heat, sticky taste, Red tongue with sticky-yellow coating, Slippery-Rapid pulse.

Liver-Blood deficiency

Dull-yellow or greyish-yellow complexion, dizziness, blurred vision, floaters, numbness/tingling of limbs, scanty menstruation, Pale tongue, Choppy or Fine pulse.

Spleen-Qi deficiency with stagnation of Liver-Qi

Greyish yellow complexion, poor appetite, slight abdominal distension after eating, tiredness, weakness of the limbs, loose stools, hypochondrial or epigastric distension, irritability, moodiness, a feeling of a lump in the throat, premenstrual tension, pulse Weak on the right and Wiry on the left.

Damp-Heat with Blood stasis

Bluish yellow complexion, a feeling of fullness and pain of the epigastrium and lower abdomen, poor appetite, a feeling of heaviness, thirst without a desire to drink, nausea, loose stools with offensive odour, a feeling of heat, sticky taste, purple lips and nails, Reddish-purple tongue with sticky yellow coating, Slippery-Rapid pulse.

Stomach-Heat

Dry yellow complexion, burning epigastric pain, thirst, sour regurgitation, nausea, excessive hunger, foul breath, a feeling of heat, Red tongue with a yellow coating, Overflowing-Rapid pulse.

Stomach Empty-Heat

Thin, dry, yellow complexion, malar flush, poor appetite, poor digestion, retching, loss of taste, slight epigastric pain, dry mouth and lips, dry stools, thin body, a feeling of heat in the evening, Red tongue without coating, Floating-Empty and Rapid pulse.

Spleen-Heat

Dry yellow complexion, burning epigastric/abdominal pain, excessive hunger, red tip of the nose, dry lips, mouth ulcers, thirst, dry stools, a feeling of heat, scanty dark urine, Red tongue with dry yellow coating, Overflowing-Rapid pulse.

Blood stasis

Very dull and sallow yellow complexion, mental restlessness, abdominal pain, Purple tongue, Firm pulse.

Other symptoms and signs depend on the organ involved.

Invasion of Wind-Heat

Floating, reddish-yellow complexion, aversion to cold, fever, cough, sore throat, stuffed or runny nose with yellow discharge, headache, body aches, slight sweating, slight thirst, swollen tonsils, tongue slightly Red on the sides in the chest area or on front part, Floating-Rapid pulse.

Invasion of Wind-Dampness

Floating yellow complexion, aversion to cold, fever, nausea, a feeling of heaviness, headache, body aches, slight sweating, Floating-Slippery pulse.

RED

Observation, Chapter 3

Full-Heat

Bright-red face, a feeling of heat, thirst, mental restlessness, Red tongue with yellow coating, Overflowing-Rapid pulse.

Heat of any organ, but especially the Heart, Lungs, Liver and Stomach, may cause a red face.

Yin deficiency with Empty-Heat

Malar flush, a feeling of heat in the evening, night sweating, mental restlessness, five-palm heat, Red tongue without coating, Rapid and Floating-Empty pulse.

This may be Empty-Heat of any organ but especially of the Stomach, Heart, Lungs, Kidneys, Spleen and Liver.

Liver-Yang rising

Slightly red face, headache, dizziness, tinnitus, irritability, propensity to outbursts of anger, Wiry pulse.

Damp-Heat

Red face, swollen face, greasy skin, epigastric fullness, sticky taste, thirst with no desire to drink, a feeling of heaviness of the head and body, a feeling of heat, sticky yellow tongue coating, Slippery-Rapid pulse.

Blood deficiency with Empty-Heat

Floating red colour on cheekbones, dull-pale complexion, blurred vision, dizziness, scanty periods, amenorrhoea, insomnia, Pale tongue, Choppy or Fine pulse.

Empty-Heat deriving from Blood deficiency is usually seen only in women and, although it may cause the cheekbones to become red, it is not usually associated with other Heat symptoms such as thirst or feeling of heat.

Yin Fire

Slightly red face or pale face with a floating red colour on the cheeks, intermittent and recurrent feeling of heat in the face but cold limbs, intermittent sore throat, dry mouth, dry lips, mouth ulcers, exhaustion, poor appetite, poor digestion, weak limbs, Pale tongue, Weak or Overflowing-Empty pulse.

Yin Fire is a pathological Minister Fire that arises when the Original Qi (*Yuan Qi*) becomes depleted from overwork. Since the Minister Fire and the Original Qi reside in the same place, the pathological Minister Fire 'robs' the Original Qi and rises to the head. This pattern is treated by tonifying the Original Qi and lightly clearing Heat; the representative prescription is Bu Zhong Yi Qi Tang *Tonifying the Centre and Benefiting Qi Decoction*.

Invasion of Wind-Heat

Red face, aversion to cold, fever, cough, sore throat, stuffed or runny nose with yellow discharge, headache, body aches, slight sweating, slight thirst, swollen tonsils, tongue slightly Red on the sides in the chest area or on front part, Floating-Rapid pulse.

Deficient Yang floating

Malar flush, feeling of heat, desire to remove clothes, thirst with a desire to drink warm liquids, slight shortness of breath, cold sweating, cold limbs, pale urine, pale lips, Pale tongue, Weak pulse.

This condition is quite rare and is due to the Yang being so weak that the little Yang there is floats upwards.

BLUISH/GREENISH

Observation, Chapter 3

'Bluish/greenish' is a translation of the Chinese word *qing*, which, unfortunately, may mean both 'green' and 'blue', leading to difficulties in translating this term.

Full-Cold

Bright-bluish face, abdominal pain, epigastric pain, facial pain, pain alleviated by exposure to heat and aggravated by exposure to cold, cold limbs, white tongue coating, Tight pulse.

Heart- and Kidney-Yang deficiency

Dull-bluish face, ashen face, greenish lips, palpitations, shortness of breath, discomfort of the chest, cold limbs, oedema, backache, dizziness, tinnitus, pale abundant urination, Pale and wet tongue, Deep-Weak pulse.

Chronic pain

Dull-greenish face, abdominal pain, epigastric pain, facial pain, painful periods.

A chronic pain from any origin or organ may cause the face to become dull greenish.

Lung- and Kidney-Yang deficiency

Dull-greenish-purplish face, breathlessness that is worse on exertion, weak voice, cold limbs, sweating, pale frequent urination, backache, dizziness, tinnitus, Pale tongue, Deep-Weak pulse.

Liver-Qi stagnation

Very slightly greenish complexion especially around the mouth, hypochondrial or epigastric distension, irritability, moodiness, a feeling of a lump in the throat, premenstrual tension, Wiry pulse.

Liver-Wind

Greenish face, tremors, severe dizziness, tinnitus, headache, numbness of the limbs, tics, Stiff, Deviated or Moving tongue, Wiry pulse.

PURPLE

Observation, Chapter 3

Blood stasis from Cold

Bluish-purple face, chest pain, palpitations, abdominal pain, Bluish-Purple tongue, Tight pulse.

Other manifestation depend on the organ involved, which may be the Heart, Liver, Lungs or Intestines.

Blood stasis from Heat

Reddish-purple face, a feeling of heat, chest pain, abdominal pain, Reddish-Purple tongue, Wiry pulse.

This is usually due to Liver-Blood stasis associated with Blood-Heat.

DARK

Observation, Chapter 3

A 'dark' complexion is a mixture of a greyish-purplish colour, usually without 'spirit', that is, dull in appearance; in extreme cases, it can be very dark, almost black.

Severe Kidney-Yang deficiency

Dark complexion, backache, dizziness, tinnitus, feeling cold, weak knees, bright-white complexion, tiredness, depression, exhaustion, abundant clear urination, Pale and wet tongue, Deep-Weak pulse.

Severe Blood stasis

Dark complexion, purple nails, dry skin, purple lips, abdominal or chest pain, painful periods, Purple tongue, Choppy pulse.

Kidney-Essence deficiency

Dark complexion, backache, dizziness, tinnitus, weak knees, poor memory, loose teeth, premature greying of hair, infertility, sterility, Leather pulse.

SALLOW

Observation, Chapter 3

A 'sallow' complexion indicates a pale-yellowish colour of the skin that is dull and without lustre.

Spleen-Qi deficiency with Dampness

Sallow complexion, poor appetite, slight abdominal distension after eating, tiredness, lassitude, weakness of the limbs, loose stools, slight depression, tendency to obesity, abdominal fullness, a feeling of heaviness, a sticky taste, poor digestion, undigested food in the stools, nausea, dull frontal headache, excessive vaginal discharge, Pale tongue with sticky coating, Soggy pulse.

Chronic Spleen-Qi deficiency

Sallow complexion, poor appetite, slight abdominal distension after eating, tiredness, lassitude, pale complexion, weakness of the limbs, loose stools, slight depression, tendency to obesity, Pale tongue, Empty pulse.

Blood deficiency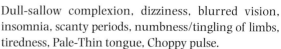

Dull-sallow complexion, dizziness, blurred vision, insomnia, scanty periods, numbness/tingling of limbs, tiredness, Pale-Thin tongue, Choppy pulse.

Other symptoms and signs depend on the organ involved, which may be the Liver, Heart or Spleen.

Blood stasis

Very dull-sallow complexion, mental restlessness, abdominal pain, Purple tongue, Firm pulse.

Other symptoms and signs depend on the organ involved.

BLUSHING

Heart-Heat

Blushing easily when excited or anxious, palpitations, a feeling of heat, anxiety, insomnia, tongue with Red tip, Overflowing-Rapid pulse.

Heart-Yin deficiency with Empty-Heat

Blushing easily when excited or anxious, palpitations, insomnia, dream-disturbed sleep, poor memory, anxiety, tendency to be easily startled, mental restlessness, uneasiness, 'feeling hot and bothered', dry mouth and throat, thirst with a desire to sip fluids, a feeling of heat in the evening, malar flush, night sweating, five-palm heat, Red tongue, redder on the tip, no coating, Floating-Empty and Rapid pulse.

Liver-Yang rising

Blushing easily when upset, headache, dizziness, tinnitus, irritability, propensity to outbursts of anger, Wiry pulse.

Liver-Fire

Blushing easily after drinking alcohol, headache, red face, dizziness, tinnitus, irritability, propensity to outbursts of anger, thirst, bitter taste, constipation, dark urine, Red tongue with redder sides and dry yellow coating, Wiry-Rapid pulse.

Lung-Yin deficiency with Empty-Heat

Blushing easily when worried, dry cough or with scanty, sticky sputum, which could be blood tinged, dry mouth and throat at night, weak/hoarse voice, night sweating, tiredness, malar flush, a feeling of heat or a low-grade fever in the evening, five-palm heat, thin body or thin chest, insomnia, anxiety, Red tongue without coating, Floating-Empty and Rapid pulse.

证候

Chapter **57**

EARS

Chapter contents

TINNITUS/DEAFNESS **581**

ITCHY EARS **582**

EARACHE **582**

BLEEDING FROM THE EARS **583**

DISCHARGE FROM THE EARS **583**

EXCESSIVE WAX PRODUCTION **583**

ABNORMAL SIZE **584**
Swollen ears **584**
Contracted ears **584**

DRY AND CONTRACTED HELIX **584**

SORES ON THE EAR **584**

WARTS ON THE EAR **585**

ABNORMAL HELIX COLOUR **585**
Yellow **585**
Pale **585**
Bluish-greenish (*Qing*) **585**
Dark **585**
Red **586**

RED BACK OF THE EAR **586**

DISTENDED BLOOD VESSELS ON THE EAR **586**

SWELLING AND REDNESS OF THE CONCHA **586**

TINNITUS/DEAFNESS

Interrogation, Chapter 42

Kidney deficiency

Tinnitus/deafness with gradual onset, tinnitus with low rushing sound, dizziness, backache, tiredness.

Other symptoms and signs, including tongue and pulse, depend on whether there is Kidney-Yin or Kidney-Yang deficiency.

Liver-Yang rising

Tinnitus/deafness, tinnitus with a high-pitched sound, headaches, dizziness, irritability, propensity to outbursts of anger, red face, Wiry pulse.

Liver-Fire

Tinnitus/deafness with sudden onset, tinnitus with high-pitched sound, red face, bloodshot eyes, headache, dizziness, tinnitus, irritability, propensity to outbursts of anger, thirst, bitter taste, constipation, dark urine, Red tongue with redder sides and dry yellow coating, Wiry-Rapid pulse.

Phlegm-Fire affecting the Liver channel

Tinnitus/deafness with sudden onset, tinnitus with high-pitched sound, thirst, bitter taste, red face, a feeling of oppression of the chest, sputum in the throat, catarrh, Red tongue with redder sides, or Swollen with a sticky yellow coating, Wiry-Slippery-Rapid pulse.

Heart- and Kidney-Yin deficiency

Tinnitus/deafness with gradual onset, tinnitus with low-pitched sound, dizziness, insomnia, anxiety, palpitations, night sweating, tongue without coating, Floating-Empty pulse.

Heart-Blood deficiency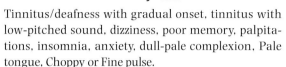

Tinnitus/deafness with gradual onset, tinnitus with low-pitched sound, dizziness, poor memory, palpitations, insomnia, anxiety, dull-pale complexion, Pale tongue, Choppy or Fine pulse.

Heart- and Lung-Qi deficiency (deficiency of Gathering-Qi)

Tinnitus/deafness with gradual onset, tinnitus with low-pitched sound, tiredness, palpitations, depression, shortness of breath, Pale tongue, pulse Weak on both Front positions.

Liver-Blood deficiency

Tinnitus/deafness with gradual onset, tinnitus with low-pitched sound, dizziness, blurred vision, insomnia, poor memory, Pale tongue, Choppy or Fine pulse.

Invasion of Wind-Heat (in the Lesser-Yang channels)

Sudden Tinnitus/deafness, tinnitus with high-pitched sound, headache, stiff neck, sore throat, burning eyes, slight sweating, fever, aversion to cold, tongue Red in the front or sides, Floating-Rapid pulse.

> **Clinical note**
>
> • In my experience, tinnitus from a Deficiency is easier to treat than one from a Fullness.

ITCHY EARS

Interrogation, Chapter 42

Damp-Heat in the Gall-Bladder

Itchy ears, earache, dizziness, tinnitus, headache, sticky taste, hypochondrial pain, fullness and distension, nausea, vomiting, inability to digest fats, yellow complexion and eyes, irritability, a feeling of heaviness, unilateral or bilateral thick, sticky yellow coating, Slippery-Rapid pulse.

Invasion of Wind-Heat

Itchy ears with sudden onset, aversion to cold, fever, sore throat, headache, body aches, slight sweating, tongue with Red sides/front, Floating-Rapid pulse.

Blood deficiency with internal Wind

Itchy ears, dryness of the skin around the ears, crusts on the ear, blurred vision, dizziness, giddiness, numbness, Pale and Stiff tongue, Choppy or Fine and slightly Wiry pulse.

Kidney-Yin deficiency with Empty-Heat

Itchy ears, dizziness, tinnitus, night-sweating, dry mouth with a desire to drink in small sips, backache, poor memory, dark scanty urine, five-palm heat, malar flush, a feeling of heat in the evening, Red tongue without coating, Floating-Empty and Rapid pulse.

EARACHE

Interrogation, Chapter 42

Invasion of Wind-Heat

Earache with acute onset, aversion to cold, fever, sore throat, headache, body aches, slight sweating, tongue with Red sides/front, Floating-Rapid pulse.

Damp-Heat in the Gall-Bladder

Earache, yellow discharge from the ear, dizziness, tinnitus, hypochondrial pain, fullness and distension, nausea, vomiting, inability to digest fats, yellow complexion and eyes, irritability, a feeling of heaviness, unilateral or bilateral thick, sticky yellow coating, Slippery-Rapid pulse.

Liver-Fire

Earache with sudden onset, worse with pressure, headaches, dizziness, red face, bloodshot eyes, thirst, bitter taste, tinnitus, irritability, propensity to outbursts of anger, constipation, dark urine, Red tongue with redder sides and dry yellow coating, Wiry-Rapid pulse.

Stagnation of Qi and stasis of Blood

Severe earache, headache, tinnitus, Purple tongue, Wiry pulse.

> **Clinical note**
>
> • Chronic earache in children is always due to residual pathogenic factor (usually Damp-Heat) after repeated upper respiratory or ear infections treated with antibiotics.

BLEEDING FROM THE EARS

Damp-Heat in the Gall-Bladder

Bleeding from the ears, earache, yellow discharge from the ear, dizziness, tinnitus, headache, hypochondrial pain, fullness and distension, nausea, vomiting, inability to digest fats, yellow complexion and eyes, irritability, a feeling of heaviness, unilateral or bilateral thick, sticky yellow coating, Slippery-Rapid pulse.

Liver-Fire

Sudden bleeding from the ear, red face, bloodshot eyes, thirst, bitter taste, headaches, dizziness, tinnitus, irritability, propensity to outbursts of anger, constipation, dark urine, Red tongue with redder sides and dry yellow coating, Wiry-Rapid pulse.

Kidney-Yin deficiency with Empty-Heat

Bleeding from the ear that comes and goes, scanty amount, ear not swollen or red, dizziness, tinnitus, night sweating, dry mouth with a desire to drink in small sips, backache, poor memory, dark scanty urine, five-palm heat, malar flush, a feeling of heat in the evening, Red tongue without coating, Floating-Empty and Rapid pulse.

Spleen-Qi deficiency

Occasional, slight bleeding from the ear, poor appetite, tiredness, slight abdominal distension, pale complexion, loose stools, Pale tongue, Empty pulse.

DISCHARGE FROM THE EARS

Observation, Chapter 9

Invasion of Wind-Heat

Yellow discharge from the ear, earache, aversion to cold, fever, sore throat, headache, body aches, slight sweating, tongue with Red sides/front, Floating-Rapid pulse.

Damp-Heat in the Gall-Bladder

Sticky, thick yellow discharge from the ear, earache, tinnitus, dizziness, headache, hypochondrial pain, fullness and distension, nausea, vomiting, inability to digest fats, yellow complexion and eyes, irritability, a feeling of heaviness, unilateral or bilateral thick, sticky yellow coating, Slippery-Rapid pulse.

Kidney-Yin deficiency with Empty-Heat

Thin discharge from the ear that comes and goes, dizziness, tinnitus, night sweating, dry mouth with a desire to drink in small sips, backache, poor memory, dark scanty urine, five-palm heat, malar flush, a feeling of heat in the evening, Red tongue without coating, Floating-Empty and Rapid pulse.

Toxic Heat in the Liver and Gall-Bladder

Foul-smelling yellow discharge from the ear, severe earache, irritability, headache, a feeling of heat, fever, bitter taste, sticky taste, Red tongue with redder sides and red points with sticky yellow coating, Overflowing-Slippery-Rapid pulse.

Spleen-Qi deficiency with Dampness

Slight discharge from the ear without pain, tiredness, loose stools, a feeling of heaviness, a feeling of fullness, Pale tongue with white sticky coating, Soft pulse.

EXCESSIVE WAX PRODUCTION

Observation, Chapter 9

Phlegm

Excessive wax production, dizziness, a feeling of muzziness of the head, a feeling of oppression of the chest, a feeling of heaviness, sputum in the throat, Swollen tongue with sticky coating, Slippery pulse.

Other symptoms and signs depend on the organ involved.

Damp-Heat in the Gall-Bladder

Excessive wax production, discharge of bright-yellow wax, earache, headache, hypochondrial pain, fullness and distension, nausea, vomiting, inability to digest fats, yellow complexion and eyes, dizziness, tinnitus, irritability, a feeling of heaviness, unilateral or bilateral thick, sticky yellow coating, Slippery-Rapid pulse.

Spleen- and Kidney-Yang deficiency

Excessive wax production, discharge of dull-yellow wax, dizziness, tinnitus, tiredness, poor appetite, loose stools, backache, a feeling of cold, Pale tongue, Weak pulse.

Kidney-Yin deficiency with Empty-Heat

Excessive ear wax production, dizziness, tinnitus, night sweating, dry mouth with a desire to drink in small sips, backache, poor memory, scanty dark urine, five-palm heat, malar flush, a feeling of heat in the evening, Red tongue without coating, Floating-Empty and Rapid pulse.

Toxic Heat with stagnation of Qi and stasis of Blood

Excessive wax production, earache, occasional discharge of dull wax, bleeding from the ear, discharge from the ear, Red tongue with red points and sticky yellow coating, Slippery-Wiry-Rapid pulse.

ABNORMAL SIZE

Swollen ears

Observation, Chapter 9

Damp-Heat in the Gall-Bladder

Swollen and red ears, earache, ear discharge, a sticky taste, hypochondrial pain, fullness and distension, nausea, vomiting, inability to digest fats, yellow complexion and eyes, dizziness, tinnitus, irritability, a feeling of heaviness, unilateral or bilateral thick, sticky yellow coating, Slippery-Rapid pulse.

Heat in the Gall-Bladder

Swollen and red ears, earache, thirst, bitter taste, irritability, headache, unilateral yellow tongue coating, Wiry-Rapid pulse.

Invasion of Wind-Water in the Lungs

Swollen ears with acute onset, oedema of the face and hands, aversion to cold, fever, headache, white tongue coating, Floating-Slippery pulse.

Contracted ears

Observation, Chapter 9

Kidney-Yin deficiency

Contracted and dry ears, dizziness, tinnitus, night sweating, dry mouth with a desire to drink in small sips, backache, poor memory, scanty dark urine, tongue without coating, Floating-Empty pulse.

Aftermath of acute Heat in febrile diseases

Contracted, dry ears, dry mouth, exhaustion, dry skin, dry tongue, Fine pulse.

Severe Blood stasis in the abdomen with abdominal masses

Contracted, dry, dull and dark ears, dry mouth, dry skin, abdominal pain, loss of weight, Purple tongue, Wiry or Choppy pulse.

DRY AND CONTRACTED HELIX

Observation, Chapter 9

Blood stasis

Dry, contracted and dark helix, abdominal pain, chest pain, Purple tongue, Wiry or Choppy pulse.

Other symptoms and signs depend on the organs involved, which may be the Liver, Heart, Stomach or Intestines.

Blood stasis with Damp-Heat

Dry and contracted helix, abdominal pain, mucus in the stools, loose stools, Purple tongue with sticky yellow coating, Wiry-Slippery pulse.

Kidney-Yin deficiency

Dry, dark and contracted helix, tinnitus, dizziness, night sweating, dry mouth with desire to sip water, backache, poor memory, dark scanty urine, tongue without coating, Floating-Empty pulse.

SORES ON THE EAR

Observation, Chapter 9

Heat in the Liver and Gall-Bladder

Sores on the ear, red face, headache, irritability, bitter taste, dizziness, hypochondrial pain, Red tongue with yellow coating, Wiry-Rapid pulse.

Invasion of Wind-Heat in the Lesser-Yang channels

Sores on the ear, earache, alternating chills and fever, irritability, headache, tongue with Red sides and possibly unilateral white coating, Floating-Rapid and Wiry pulse.

WARTS ON THE EAR

Observation, Chapter 9

Heat in the Liver and Gall-Bladder

Warts on the ear, red face, headache, irritability, dizziness, bitter taste, hypochondrial pain, Red tongue with yellow coating, Wiry-Rapid pulse.

Stomach-Fire

Warts on the ear, burning epigastric pain, intense thirst with a desire to drink cold liquids, mental restlessness, bleeding gums, dry stools, sour regurgitation, foul breath, a feeling of heat, tongue Red with a thick, dry, dark-yellow coating, Deep-Full-Rapid pulse.

ABNORMAL HELIX COLOUR

Yellow

Observation, Chapter 9

Damp-Heat in the Gall-Bladder

Yellow helix, bitter and sticky taste, earache, hypochondrial pain, fullness and distension, nausea, vomiting, inability to digest fats, yellow complexion and eyes, dizziness, tinnitus, irritability, a feeling of heaviness, unilateral or bilateral thick, sticky yellow coating, Slippery-Rapid pulse.

Blood stasis deriving from Heat (Liver and Gall-Bladder)

Dull, dark-yellow helix, earache, hypochondrial pain, thirst, dry mouth, headache, irritability, Reddish-purple tongue with unilateral yellow coating, Wiry-Rapid pulse.

Pale

Observation, Chapter 9

Yang deficiency

Pale helix, feeling cold, tiredness, cold limbs, loose stools, Pale and wet tongue, Deep-Weak pulse.
  Other symptoms and signs depend on the organ involved.

Blood deficiency

Pale, dry helix, dry skin, blurred vision, dizziness, numbness of the limbs, scanty periods, Pale tongue, Choppy or Fine pulse.

Bluish-greenish (*Qing*)

Observation, Chapter 9

Blood stasis from Heat

Greenish, dry helix, abdominal pain, chest pain, Reddish-Purple tongue, Wiry or Choppy pulse.
  Other symptoms and signs depend on the organ involved.

Blood stasis from Cold

Bluish, wet helix, abdominal pain, chest pain, Bluish-Purple tongue, Wiry or Choppy pulse.
  Other symptoms and signs depend on the organ involved.

Internal Wind in children

Greenish helix, tremor, convulsions, fever, opisthotonos, Stiff tongue, Wiry pulse.

Dark

Observation, Chapter 9

Blood stasis

Dark and dry helix, dry mouth, dark complexion, dry skin, abdominal pain, chest pain, Purple tongue, Wiry or Choppy pulse.

Blood stasis from Cold

Dark, moist helix, abdominal pain, chest pain, Bluish-Purple tongue, Wiry or Choppy pulse.

Chronic Heat

Dark and dry helix, red face, thirst, dry skin, dry mouth, dry stools, Red tongue with yellow coating, Overflowing-Rapid pulse.
  Other symptoms and signs depend on the organ involved.

Red

Observation, Chapter 9

Lung-Heat

Red helix, flaring of nostrils, thirst, red face, cough, slight breathlessness, a feeling of heat, chest ache, Red tongue with yellow coating, Overflowing-Rapid pulse.

Heart-Fire

Red helix, red face, bitter taste, thirst, palpitations, agitation, insomnia, dream-disturbed sleep, a feeling of heat, Red tongue with redder tip and yellow coating, Overflowing-Rapid pulse.

Heat in the Lesser-Yang channels

Red helix, bitter taste, hypochondrial discomfort, dry throat, alternation of cold and hot feeling with predominance of the latter, irritability, tongue with unilateral yellow coating, Wiry-Rapid pulse.

Damp-Heat in the Liver and Gall-Bladder.

Red and swollen helix, bitter and sticky taste, burning on urination, excessive vaginal discharge, irritability, a feeling of oppression of the chest, nausea, vomiting, dark urine, tongue with Red sides and sticky-yellow tongue coating, Wiry-Slippery-Rapid pulse.

Kidney-Yin deficiency with Empty-Heat 🧍

Red and dry helix, tinnitus, malar flush, dry mouth with a desire to sip water, dizziness, night sweating, backache, poor memory, dark scanty urine, five-palm heat, a feeling of heat in the evening, Red tongue without coating, Floating-Empty and Rapid pulse.

RED BACK OF THE EAR

Observation, Chapter 9

Invasion of Wind-Heat (especially in children) ⚛

Red back of the ear, aversion to cold, fever, sore throat, headache, body aches, slight sweating, tongue with Red sides/front, Floating-Rapid pulse.

Measles ⚛

Red back of the ear, papular rash, fever, thirst, sweating, Red tongue with yellow coating, Overflowing-Rapid pulse.

DISTENDED BLOOD VESSELS ON THE EAR

Observation, Chapter 9

Lung deficiency with Phlegm-Heat

Distended, red blood vessels on the ear, cough, breathlessness, expectoration of sticky sputum, weak voice, tiredness, a feeling of oppression of the chest, Pale and Swollen tongue with sticky coating, pulse Slippery in general but Weak on the right Front position.

Blood stasis

Distended, purple blood vessels on the ear, dark complexion, headache, abdominal pain, chest pain, Purple tongue, Wiry or Choppy pulse. Other symptoms and signs depend on the organ involved.

Damp-Heat in the Gall-Bladder

Distended, red blood vessels on the ear, earache, dizziness, tinnitus, hypochondrial pain, fullness and distension, nausea, vomiting, inability to digest fats, yellow complexion and eyes, irritability, a feeling of heaviness, unilateral or bilateral thick, sticky yellow coating, Slippery-Rapid pulse.

Heart-Heat

Distended, red blood vessels on the ear, especially on the lobe, palpitations, feeling of heat, anxiety, insomnia, Red tip of the tongue, Overflowing-Rapid pulse.

SWELLING AND REDNESS OF THE CONCHA

Observation, Chapter 9

Damp-Heat in the Gall-Bladder

Swelling and redness of the concha, earache, ear discharge, itchy ear, headache, hypochondrial pain, fullness and distension, nausea, vomiting, inability to digest fats, yellow complexion and eyes, dizziness, tinnitus, irritability, a feeling of heaviness, unilateral or bilateral thick, sticky yellow coating, Slippery-Rapid pulse.

Kidney-Yin deficiency with Empty-Heat 🧍

Redness and slight swelling of the concha, earache, dizziness, tinnitus, night sweating, dry mouth with a

desire to drink in small sips, backache, poor memory, scanty dark urine, five-palm heat, malar flush, a feeling of heat in the evening, Red tongue without coating, Floating-Empty and Rapid pulse.

Toxic Heat

Swelling and redness of the concha, earache, discharge from the ear, swollen neck glands, headache, thirst, Red tongue with red points and thick, sticky yellow coating, Overflowing-Slippery-Rapid pulse.

Chapter **58**

NOSE

Chapter contents

ABNORMAL COLOUR　*589*
　Pale　*589*
　Yellow　*589*
　Red　*590*
　Bluish-greenish　*590*
　Reddish-purple　*591*
　Dark　*591*

SNEEZING　*591*

BLOCKED NOSE　*591*

RUNNY NOSE　*592*

ITCHY NOSE　*593*

DRY NOSTRILS　*593*

NOSEBLEED　*594*

NOSE ACHE　*595*

NOSE PAIN　*595*

SWOLLEN NOSE　*596*

BAD SMELL　*597*

LOSS OF SENSE OF SMELL　*597*

POLYPS　*598*

FLAPPING ALAE NASI (THE OUTSIDE OF THE NOSTRILS)　*598*

ULCERS ON THE NOSE　*598*

PAPULES ON THE NOSE　*598*

ABNORMAL COLOUR

Pale

Observation, Chapter 7

Stomach- and Spleen-Yang deficiency with Empty-Cold

Pale tip of the nose, discomfort or dull pain in the epigastrium, better after eating and better with pressure or massage, no appetite, preference for warm drinks and foods, vomiting of clear fluid, absence of thirst, cold and weak limbs, tiredness, pale complexion, loose stools, a feeling of cold, cold limbs, Pale and wet tongue, Deep-Weak-Slow pulse.

Liver-Blood deficiency

Pale bridge of the nose, dull-pale face, dizziness, blurred vision, floaters, numbness/tingling of limbs, scanty menstruation, Pale tongue, Choppy or Fine pulse.

Phlegm-Fluids

Pale and swollen tip of the nose, swollen face, greasy skin, abdominal fullness and distension, nausea, vomiting or watery fluids, dry mouth without a desire to drink, shortness of breath, dizziness, a feeling of oppression of the chest, swelling of the limbs, expectoration of thin watery sputum, inability to lie down, Swollen tongue with sticky coating, Deep-Wiry or Deep-Slippery pulse.

Yellow

Observation, Chapter 7

Damp-Heat in the Spleen

Bright-yellow nose if Heat predominates, dull-yellow nose if Dampness predominates, greasy skin, fullness of the epigastrium, epigastric or abdominal pain, sticky

taste, thirst with no desire to drink, poor appetite, a feeling of heaviness of the body, thirst, nausea, vomiting, loose stools with offensive odour, a feeling of heat, scanty dark urine, headache with a feeling of heaviness of the head, dull-yellow complexion, bitter taste, Red tongue with sticky yellow coating, Slippery-Rapid pulse.

Chronic Spleen-Qi deficiency with retention of Dampness

Dull-yellow tip of the nose, dull-pale face, poor appetite, slight abdominal distension after eating, tiredness, lassitude, pale or sallow complexion, weakness of the limbs, loose stools, slight depression, tendency to obesity, abdominal fullness, a feeling of heaviness, a sticky taste, poor digestion, undigested food in the stools, nausea, dull frontal headache, excessive vaginal discharge, Pale tongue with sticky coating, Soggy pulse.

Liver-Blood stasis

Dull, dark-yellow bridge of the nose, dark complexion, hypochondrial pain, abdominal pain, painful periods, dark and clotted menstrual blood, masses in the abdomen, purple nails and lips, Purple tongue, Wiry or Firm pulse.

Spleen-Heat

Bright-yellow and dry tip of the nose, burning epigastric/abdominal pain, excessive hunger, red tip of the nose, dry lips, mouth ulcers, thirst, dry stools, a feeling of heat, scanty dark urine, yellow complexion, Red tongue with dry yellow coating, Overflowing-Rapid pulse.

Phlegm-Fluids

Dull-yellow and swollen tip of the nose, abdominal fullness and distension, nausea, vomiting of watery fluids, dry mouth without a desire to drink, shortness of breath, dizziness, a feeling of oppression of the chest, swelling of the limbs, expectoration of thin watery sputum, inability to lie down, Swollen tongue with sticky coating, Deep-Wiry or Deep-Slippery pulse.

Red

Observation, Chapter 7

Lung-Heat

Red bridge of the nose in its upper part, flaring of nostrils, red face, cough, slight breathlessness, a feeling of heat, chest ache, flaring of nostrils, thirst, red face, Red tongue with yellow coating, Overflowing-Rapid pulse.

Liver-Fire

Red bridge of the nose in its central part, red face, headache, dizziness, tinnitus, irritability, propensity to outbursts of anger, thirst, bitter taste, constipation, dark urine, Red tongue with redder sides and dry yellow coating, Wiry-Rapid pulse.

Spleen-Heat

Red and dry tip of the nose, thirst, dry lips, dry mouth, burning epigastric/abdominal abdominal pain, excessive hunger, red tip of the nose, mouth ulcers, dry stools, a feeling of heat, scanty dark urine, yellow complexion, Red tongue with dry yellow coating, Overflowing-Rapid pulse.

Invasion of Wind-Heat

Red bridge of the nose with acute onset, aversion to cold, fever, cough, sore throat, stuffed or runny nose with yellow discharge, headache, body aches, slight sweating, slight thirst, swollen tonsils, tongue slightly Red on the sides in the chest area or on front part, Floating-Rapid pulse.

Bluish-greenish

Observation, Chapter 7

Liver-Blood stasis

Greenish bridge of the nose, dark complexion, headache, hypochondrial/abdominal pain, painful periods, dark and clotted menstrual blood, masses in the abdomen, purple nails and lips, Purple tongue, Wiry or Firm pulse.

Internal Cold

Bluish bridge of the nose, greyish-pale face, abdominal pain, cold limbs, a feeling of cold, diarrhoea, Pale and wet tongue, Deep-Tight-Slow pulse.

Phlegm-Fluids

Bluish and swollen tip of the nose, swollen face, abdominal fullness and distension, nausea, vomiting of watery fluids, dry mouth without a desire to drink, shortness of breath, dizziness, a feeling of oppression of the chest, swelling of the limbs, expectoration of thin watery sputum, inability to lie down, Swollen tongue with sticky coating, Deep-Wiry or Deep-Slippery pulse.

Reddish-purple

Observation, Chapter 7

Liver-Blood stasis

Reddish-purple bridge of the nose, dark complexion, hypochondrial/abdominal pain, painful periods, dark and clotted menstrual blood, masses in the abdomen, purple nails and lips, Purple tongue, Wiry or Firm pulse.

Heart-Blood stasis

Reddish-purple colour on the bridge between the eyes, palpitations, stabbing or pricking chest pain which may radiate to the inner aspect of the left arm or to the shoulder, a feeling of oppression or constriction of the chest, cyanosis of lips and nails, cold hands, tongue entirely Purple or Purple only on the sides in the chest areas, Choppy or Wiry pulse.

Blood stasis in the Stomach

Dark reddish-purple alae nasi, bleeding gums, stabbing epigastric pain, vomiting of blood, tongue Purple in the centre, Wiry or Choppy pulse.

Dark

Observation, Chapter 7

Liver-Fire

Dark bridge of the nose, red face, thirst, bitter taste, headaches, dizziness, tinnitus, irritability, propensity to outbursts of anger, constipation, dark urine, Red tongue with redder sides and dry yellow coating, Wiry-Rapid pulse.

Exhaustion (Xu Lao)

Dark, bluish-purple bridge of the nose, extreme exhaustion, weight loss, Red tongue without coating, Fine-Rapid pulse.

Other symptoms and signs depend on the organ involved.

SNEEZING

Interrogation, Chapter 35

Invasion of Wind

Acute sneezing, aversion to cold, fever, body aches, occipital headache, Floating pulse.

Other manifestations depend on whether it is Wind-Cold or Wind-Heat.

Lung-Qi deficiency

Chronic sneezing, allergy to house-dust mites or pollen, itchy nose, tiredness, slight shortness of breath, slight cough, weak voice, spontaneous daytime sweating, dislike of speaking, bright-white complexion, tendency to catch colds, tiredness, dislike of cold, Pale tongue, Empty pulse.

Kidney-Yang deficiency

Chronic sneezing, allergy to house-dust mites or pollen, worse after sex, lower backache, cold knees, sensation of cold in the lower back, feeling cold, weak legs, bright-white complexion, weak knees, tiredness, lassitude, abundant clear or scanty clear urination, urination at night, apathy, oedema of lower legs, infertility in women, loose stools, depression, impotence, premature ejaculation, low sperm count, cold and thin sperm, decreased libido, Pale and wet tongue, Deep-Weak pulse.

Clinical note

- Remember that sneezing is due not only to the lack of diffusing of Lung-Qi but also to a deficiency of the Kidney's Defensive-Qi system. The Governing Vessel is also involved as it runs through the nose.

BLOCKED NOSE

Interrogation, Chapter 35

Invasion of Wind

Acute blocked nose, aversion to cold, fever, occipital headache, stiff neck, Floating pulse.

Other symptoms and signs depend on whether it is Wind-Cold or Wind-Heat.

Lung- and Spleen-Qi deficiency

Chronic blocked nose, pale nose, poor appetite, slight abdominal distension after eating, tiredness, pale complexion, weakness of the limbs, loose stools, slight shortness of breath, weak voice, slight cough, spontaneous daytime sweating, tendency to catch colds, Pale tongue, Empty pulse.

Lung-Heat

Blocked nose, dry nose, red nose, cough, slight breathlessness, a feeling of heat, chest ache, flaring of the

nostrils, thirst, red face, Red tongue with yellow coating, Overflowing-Rapid pulse.

Damp-Heat in the Stomach and Spleen

Blocked nose, facial pain, sinusitis, dull headache, a feeling of fullness and pain of the epigastrium and lower abdomen, poor appetite, a feeling of heaviness, thirst without a desire to drink, nausea, loose stools with offensive odour, a feeling of heat, dull-yellow complexion, sticky taste, Red tongue with sticky yellow coating, Slippery-Rapid pulse.

Heat in the Gall-Bladder

Blocked nose, red and swollen membranes, sticky yellow nasal discharge, dry throat, bitter taste, red face and ears, dizziness, tinnitus, irritability, hypochondrial fullness, unilateral or bilateral yellow tongue coating, Wiry-Rapid pulse.

Damp-Heat in the Liver and Gall-Bladder

Blocked nose with occasional yellow discharge, sinusitis, bitter taste, fullness/pain pain of the hypochondrium, abdomen or epigastrium, bitter taste, poor appetite, nausea, a feeling of heaviness of the body, yellow vaginal discharge, vaginal itching, mid-cycle bleeding/pain, burning on urination, dark urine, yellow complexion and eyes, vomiting, Red tongue with redder sides and unilateral or bilateral sticky yellow coating, Wiry-Slippery-Rapid pulse.

Lung- and Kidney-Yang deficiency

Blocked nose, cough, shortness of breath, backache, dizziness, tinnitus, a feeling of cold, cold limbs, abundant pale urination, Pale tongue, Weak pulse.

Stagnation of Qi and stasis of Blood

Blocked nose, purple and swollen nose bridge with an uneven surface, headache, chest pain, Purple tongue.

Clinical note

- Sinusitis is the most common cause of blocked nose. In children, this is nearly always due to residual pathogenic factor (Damp-Heat) from repeated upper respiratory infections treated with antibiotics.

RUNNY NOSE

Observation, Chapter 20; Interrogation, Chapter 35

Invasion of Wind-Cold

Runny nose with profuse white watery discharge, itchy throat, acute onset, aversion to cold, fever, cough, slight breathlessness, stuffed or runny nose with clear watery discharge, sneezing, occipital headache, body aches, thin white tongue coating, Floating-Tight pulse.

Invasion of Wind-Heat

Runny nose with yellow discharge, acute onset, red nostrils, aversion to cold, fever, cough, sore throat, stuffed or runny nose with yellow discharge, headache, body aches, slight sweating, slight thirst, swollen tonsils, tongue slightly Red on the sides in the chest area or on front part, Floating-Rapid pulse.

Damp-Heat in the Stomach and Spleen

Runny nose with sticky yellow, foul-smelling discharge, facial pain, a feeling of heaviness of the head, sticky taste, a feeling of fullness and pain of the epigastrium and lower abdomen, poor appetite, thirst without a desire to drink, nausea, loose stools with offensive odour, a feeling of heat, dull-yellow complexion, Red tongue with sticky yellow coating, Slippery-Rapid pulse.

Lung-Qi deficiency with Empty-Cold

Chronic runny nose with white watery discharge, sneezing, slight shortness of breath, slight cough, weak voice, spontaneous daytime sweating, dislike of speaking, bright-white complexion, tendency to catch cold, tiredness, dislike of cold, a feeling of cold, cold limbs, Pale tongue, Weak pulse.

This may correspond to allergic rhinitis in Western medicine.

Kidney-Yang deficiency

Lower backache, cold knees, a feeling of cold, bright-white complexion, weak knees, tiredness, lassitude, abundant clear urination, urination at night, impotence, decreased libido, Pale and wet tongue, Deep-Weak pulse.

This may also correspond to allergic rhinitis in Western medicine.

Toxic Heat in the Lungs and Stomach

Runny nose with yellow, red and swollen nose, bloody discharge, breathlessness, foul breath, cough, headache, swollen and red face, epigastric pain, thirst,

tongue Red with red points and thick, sticky, dry, dark-yellow coating, Overflowing-Slippery-Rapid pulse.

> ## Clinical note
>
> - Remember: a white watery-runny nasal discharge indicates allergic rhinitis, whereas a sticky thick discharge indicates sinusitis.

ITCHY NOSE

Interrogation, Chapter 35

Invasion of Wind

Itchy nose, sneezing, nasal discharge, itchy throat, aversion to cold, fever, cough, slight breathlessness, stuffed or runny nose with clear watery discharge, sneezing, occipital headache, body aches, thin white tongue coating, Floating pulse.

Dry-Heat in the Lungs

Itchy and dry nose, dry throat, dry cough, slight breathlessness, a feeling of heat, chest ache, flaring of nostrils, thirst, dry mouth and throat, red face, Red tongue with dry yellow coating, Overflowing-Rapid pulse.

Toxic Heat in the Lungs

Itchy nose, painful and swollen nostrils, mental restlessness, red nose, skin spots (papules), headache, cough, slight breathlessness, a feeling of heat, chest ache, flaring of nostrils, thirst, red face, Red tongue with red points in the front and a sticky yellow coating, Overflowing-Rapid-Slippery pulse.

Damp-Heat in the Spleen channel

Itchy nose with a sticky yellow discharge, painful and red tip of the nose, facial pain, a feeling of heaviness of the head, fullness of the epigastrium, epigastric or abdominal pain, sticky taste, thirst with no desire to drink, poor appetite, thirst, nausea, vomiting, loose stools with offensive odour, a feeling of heat, scanty dark urine, headache with a feeling of heaviness of the head, dull-yellow complexion, bitter taste, Red tongue with sticky yellow coating, Slippery-Rapid pulse.

Lung-Qi deficiency

Chronic itchy nose, white watery nasal discharge, sneezing, slight shortness of breath, slight cough, weak voice, spontaneous daytime sweating, dislike of speaking, bright-white complexion, tendency to catch colds, tiredness, dislike of cold, Pale tongue, Empty pulse.

Lung-Qi and Kidney-Yang deficiency (Governing Vessel deficient)

Chronic itchy nose, white watery nasal discharge, sneezing, allergic rhinitis, allergic asthma, history of childhood eczema, abundant pale urination, lower backache, Pale and wet tongue, Deep-Weak pulse.

This is often seen in atopic individuals suffering from allergic rhinitis and it corresponds to what I call a deficiency of the Defensive-Qi systems of the Lungs and Kidneys.

Nose Childhood Nutritional Impairment ⌗

Itchy nose, scabs or ulcers on the nose, a watery yellow nasal discharge, dry skin, hot hands and feet, itchy nostrils, a tendency for the child to pick the nose.

DRY NOSTRILS

Observation, Chapter 7; Interrogation, Chapter 35

Dryness injuring the Lungs

Dry nostrils, dry throat, dry cough, blocked nose, itchy nose, dry tongue, pulse Fine on the right Front position.

Lung-Heat

Dry and red nostrils, itchy nose, flaring of nostrils, epistaxis, red face, cough, slight breathlessness, a feeling of heat, chest ache, flaring of nostrils, thirst, Red tongue with yellow coating, Overflowing-Rapid pulse.

Stomach-Heat

Dry and red nostrils, epistaxis, crusts around the nostrils, burning epigastric pain, thirst, sour regurgitation, nausea, excessive hunger, foul breath, a feeling of heat, Red tongue with a yellow coating, Overflowing-Rapid pulse.

Lung-Yin deficiency with Empty-Heat ⌀

Dry nostrils, itchy nose, dry cough or with scanty, sticky sputum which could be blood tinged, dry mouth and throat at night, weak/hoarse voice, night sweating, tiredness, malar flush, a feeling of heat or a low-grade fever in the evening, five-palm heat, thin body or thin chest, insomnia, anxiety, Red tongue without coating, Floating-Empty and Rapid pulse.

Stomach-Yin deficiency with Empty-Heat

Dry nostrils, dry mouth and throat especially in the afternoon, dull or burning epigastric pain, a feeling of heat in the afternoon, dry mouth and throat especially in the afternoon, thirst with a desire to drink in small sips, dry stools, a slight feeling of fullness after eating, night sweating, five-palm heat, bleeding gums, Red tongue (or Red centre only) without coating in the centre, Floating-Empty and Rapid pulse.

Lung- and Spleen-Qi deficiency

Dry and itchy nostrils, dry crusts on the nostrils, poor appetite, slight abdominal distension after eating, tiredness, lassitude, pale complexion, weakness of the limbs, loose stools, slight depression, tendency to obesity, slight shortness of breath, slight cough, weak voice, spontaneous daytime sweating, dislike of speaking, tendency to catch colds, dislike of cold, Pale tongue, Empty pulse, especially on the right side.

Blood stasis

Dry nostrils, dry nose bridge, thirst without a desire to swallow, headache, dark rings under the eyes, Purple tongue.

Invasion of Wind-Heat

Dry nostrils, acute onset, aversion to cold, fever, cough, sore throat, stuffed or runny nose with yellow discharge, headache, body aches, slight sweating, slight thirst, swollen tonsils, tongue slightly Red on the sides in the chest area or on front part, Floating-Rapid pulse.

Invasion of Wind-Dryness

Dry nostrils, acute onset, dry cough, dry throat, aversion to cold, fever, dry throat, tickly throat, dry nose, discomfort of the chest, thin, dry white tongue coating, Floating pulse.

Toxic Heat in the Lungs

Dry nostrils, swollen and red nose, flaring of the nostrils, cough with expectoration of bloody sputum, fever, chest pain, mental restlessness, cough, breathlessness, a feeling of heat, thirst, red face, Red tongue with red points in the front and thick, sticky, dry, dark-yellow coating, Overflowing-Slippery-Rapid pulse.

NOSEBLEED

Observation, Chapter 7

Liver-Fire insulting the Lungs

Nosebleed often induced by emotional stress, bloodshot eyes, breathlessness, asthma, a feeling of fullness and distension of the chest and hypochondrium, cough with a yellow or blood-tinged sputum, headache, dizziness, red face, thirst, bitter taste, scanty dark urine, constipation, Red tongue with redder sides and dry yellow coating, Wiry pulse.

Acute Lung-Heat

Nosebleed, flapping of the alae nasi, flaring of nostrils, red face, cough, slight breathlessness, a feeling of heat, chest ache, thirst, Red tongue with yellow coating, Overflowing-Rapid pulse.

Spleen-Qi deficiency

Chronic nosebleed with pale blood, often induced by overwork, poor appetite, slight abdominal distension after eating, tiredness, lassitude, pale complexion, weakness of the limbs, loose stools, slight depression, tendency to obesity, Pale tongue, Empty pulse.

Stomach-Fire

Nosebleed with dark-red blood, red nose, bleeding gums, burning epigastric pain, intense thirst with a desire to drink cold liquids, mental restlessness, dry mouth, mouth ulcers, bleeding gums, dry stools, sour regurgitation, foul breath, nausea, vomiting soon after eating, a feeling of heat, sour regurgitation, tongue Red with a thick, dry dark-yellow coating, Deep-Full-Rapid pulse.

Kidney-Yin deficiency with Empty-Heat

Chronic nosebleed with scanty bleeding, dizziness, tinnitus, vertigo, poor memory, hardness of hearing, night sweating, dry mouth at night, five-palm heat, a feeling of heat in the evening, malar flush, menopausal hot flushes, thirst with desire to sip fluids, lower backache, ache in bones, nocturnal emissions with dreams, constipation, scanty dark urine, infertility, premature ejaculation, tiredness, depression, anxiety, insomnia, excessive menstrual bleeding, Red tongue without coating, Floating-Empty and Rapid pulse.

Liver-Blood stasis

Nosebleed with dark blood, which may be associated with the period in women, dark bridge of the nose, headache, hypochondrial/abdominal pain, painful periods, dark and clotted menstrual blood, masses in the abdomen, purple nails and lips, purple or dark complexion, Purple tongue, Wiry or Firm pulse.

Invasion of Wind-Heat

Nosebleed, aversion to cold, fever, cough, sore throat, stuffed or runny nose with yellow discharge, headache, body aches, slight sweating, slight thirst, swollen tonsils, tongue slightly Red on the sides in the chest area or on front part, Floating-Rapid pulse.

Residual Dry-Heat in the Lungs

Slight nosebleed, dry cough, a feeling of heat, dry throat, chest pain, tongue Red in the front and dry, Overflowing-Empty and Rapid pulse.

Collapse of both Yin and Yang

Profuse unstoppable nosebleed, bleeding gums, macules, blood in the urine, profuse sweating like oily beads, ashen-grey face, mouth open, cold limbs, hands open, incontinence of urine, unconsciousness, weak breathing, Pale-Short tongue, Scattered-Minute pulse.

> **Clinical note**
>
> - The Xi-Cleft points are good to stop bleeding. In the case of the nose, LU-6 Kongzui is applicable.

NOSE ACHE

Interrogation, Chapter 35

Invasion of Wind-Heat

Nose ache, runny nose, aversion to cold, fever, cough, sore throat, stuffed or runny nose with yellow discharge, headache, body aches, slight sweating, slight thirst, swollen tonsils, tongue slightly Red on the sides in the chest area or on front part, Floating-Rapid pulse.

Phlegm-Heat in the Lungs

Nose ache, sticky yellow nasal discharge, red nose, barking cough with profuse, sticky yellow or green sputum, shortness of breath, wheezing, a feeling of oppression of the chest, a feeling of heat, thirst, insomnia, agitation, Red and Swollen tongue with a sticky yellow coating, Slippery-Rapid pulse.

Lung- and Spleen-Qi deficiency

Nose ache, watery nasal discharge, decreased sense of smell, sneezing, poor appetite, slight abdominal distension after eating, tiredness, lassitude, pale complexion, weakness of the limbs, loose stools, slight depression, tendency to obesity, slight shortness of breath, slight cough, weak voice, spontaneous daytime sweating, dislike of speaking, tendency to catch colds, dislike of cold, Pale tongue, Empty pulse, especially on the right side.

NOSE PAIN

Interrogation, Chapter 35

Invasion of Wind

Nose pain, runny nose, sneezing, aversion to cold, fever, headache, stiff neck, Floating pulse. Other symptoms and signs depend on whether it is Wind-Cold or Wind-Heat.

Lung- and Stomach-Heat

Nose pain, blocked nose, red nose, nose bleed, cough, slight breathlessness, a feeling of heat, chest ache, flaring of the nostrils, thirst, red face, burning epigastric pain, sour regurgitation, nausea, excessive hunger, foul breath, Red tongue with a yellow coating, Overflowing-Rapid pulse.

Stomach channel Damp-Heat

Nose pain, sticky yellow nasal discharge, facial pain, redness of the nose and forehead, blocked nose, sticky yellow tongue coating.

Lung-Yin deficiency with Empty-Heat

Nose pain, dryness and a feeling of heat of the nose, scabs on the nose, red nose, malar flush, dry cough or with scanty, sticky sputum which could be blood tinged, dry mouth and throat at night, weak/hoarse voice, night sweating, tiredness, a feeling of heat or a low-grade fever in the evening, five-palm heat, thin body or thin chest, insomnia, anxiety, Red tongue without coating, Floating-Empty and Rapid pulse.

Liver-Blood stasis

Severe nose pain, nosebleed with dark blood, which may be associated with the period in women, dark nose

bridge, headache, hypochondrial/abdominal pain, painful periods, dark and clotted menstrual blood, masses in the abdomen, purple nails and lips, purple or dark complexion, Purple tongue, Wiry or Firm pulse.

Carcinoma of the nose

Nose pain extending to the head, nosebleed with a swelling of the nasal mucosa.

SWOLLEN NOSE

Observation, Chapter 7

Damp-Heat in the Stomach and Spleen

Swollen nose, especially the tip, red nose, sticky yellow nasal discharge, itchy nose, spots on the nose, a feeling of heaviness especially of the head, a feeling of fullness and pain of the epigastrium and lower abdomen, poor appetite, thirst without a desire to drink, nausea, loose stools with offensive odour, a feeling of heat, dull-yellow complexion, sticky taste, Red tongue with sticky yellow coating, Slippery-Rapid pulse.

Lung-Heat

Swollen and red nose, especially in its upper part, flaring of the nostrils, cough, slight breathlessness, a feeling of heat, chest ache, thirst, red face, Red tongue with yellow coating, Overflowing-Rapid pulse.

Liver-Fire

Swollen and red bridge of the nose, headache, red face, dizziness, tinnitus, irritability, propensity to outbursts of anger, thirst, bitter taste, constipation, dark urine, Red tongue with redder sides and dry yellow coating, Wiry-Rapid pulse.

Heart-Fire

Swollen and red bridge of the nose, especially in the area between the eyes, red face, bitter taste, palpitations, thirst, mouth and tongue ulcers, mental restlessness, a feeling of agitation, insomnia, dream-disturbed sleep, a feeling of heat, Red tongue with redder tip and yellow coating, Overflowing and Rapid pulse.

Heart-Yin deficiency with Empty-Heat

Swollen bridge of the nose, especially its upper part, palpitations, insomnia, dream-disturbed sleep, poor memory, anxiety, tendency to be easily startled, mental restlessness, uneasiness, 'feeling hot and bothered', dry mouth and throat, thirst with a desire to sip fluids, a feeling of heat in the evening, malar flush, night sweating, five-palm heat, Red tongue, redder on the tip, no coating, Floating-Empty and Rapid pulse.

Kidney-Yin deficiency with Empty-Heat

Swollen nose, dizziness, tinnitus, vertigo, poor memory, hardness of hearing, night sweating, dry mouth at night, five-palm heat, a feeling of heat in the evening, malar flush, menopausal hot flushes, thirst with a desire to sip fluids, lower backache, ache in bones, nocturnal emissions with dreams, constipation, scanty dark urine, infertility, premature ejaculation, tiredness, depression, anxiety, insomnia, excessive menstrual bleeding, Red tongue without coating, Floating-Empty and Rapid pulse.

Damp-Phlegm in the Lungs

Swollen nose, especially on the tip and alae nasi (outside of the nostrils), greasy skin, chronic cough coming in bouts with profuse white sticky sputum that is easy to expectorate, white pasty complexion, a feeling of oppression in the chest, shortness of breath, dislike of lying down, wheezing, nausea, Swollen tongue with a sticky white coating, Slippery pulse.

Toxic Heat in the Lungs

Swelling of the nose, spots (red papules) on the nose, whole nose feels hard to touch, pain in the nose, purulent spots on the head appearing 3 to 5 days after the swelling of the nose, flaring of the nostrils, fever, headache, cough, slight breathlessness, a feeling of heat, chest ache, thirst, red face, Red tongue with red points and thick, sticky yellow coating, Overflowing-Slippery-Rapid pulse.

Toxic Heat at Nutritive-Qi or Blood level

Swollen nose, painful nose, top of the nose feels hard to touch, tip of the nose oozing pus, red and swollen nose, dark macules, red cheeks, lips and eyes, fever at night, mental confusion, thirst at night, tremor of the limbs, Deep-Red tongue without coating, Floating-Empty-Rapid pulse.

Heat Childhood Nutritional Impairment ⚅

Swelling of the nose, spots on the nose, nose pain, itching of the nose, crusts on the nose, epistaxis, poor appetite, headache, loose stools, thin body, Red tongue with yellow coating, Rapid pulse.

Worms in children

Swollen and itchy nose in children, white vesicles on the face, sallow complexion, emaciation, small white spots inside the lips, purple spots inside the eyelids, loss of appetite or a desire to eat strange objects (such as wax, leaves, raw rice), abdominal pain, itchy anus.

BAD SMELL

'Bad smell' refers to the subjective sensation of a bad smell in the nose when breathing in.

Phlegm-Heat in the Lungs

Bad smell in the nose, blocked nose, yellow nasal discharge, facial pain, swollen face, barking cough with profuse, sticky yellow or green sputum, shortness of breath, wheezing, a feeling of oppression of the chest, a feeling of heat, thirst, insomnia, agitation, Red and Swollen tongue with a sticky yellow coating, Slippery-Rapid pulse.

Lung-Qi deficiency with Damp-Heat

Bad smell in the nose, blocked nose, yellow nasal discharge, sinusitis, facial pain, dull frontal headache, a feeling of heaviness of the head, epigastric fullness, sticky taste, tiredness, slight shortness of breath, slight cough, weak voice, spontaneous daytime sweating, dislike of speaking, bright-white complexion, tendency to catch colds, tiredness, dislike of cold, Pale tongue with sticky yellow coating, Soggy pulse.

Damp-Heat in the Gall-Bladder and Liver

Bad smell in the nose, sticky yellow nasal discharge, facial pain, fullness/pain of the hypochondrium, abdomen or epigastrium, bitter taste, poor appetite, nausea, feeling of heaviness of the body, yellow vaginal discharge, vaginal itching, mid-cycle bleeding/pain, burning on urination, dark urine, yellow complexion and eyes, vomiting, Red tongue with redder sides and unilateral or bilateral sticky yellow coating, Wiry-Slippery-Rapid pulse.

Spleen-Qi deficiency with Damp-Heat

Bad smell in the nose, slight nasal discharge, crusts on the nostrils, dull frontal headache, poor appetite, slight abdominal distension after eating, tiredness, lassitude, pale or sallow complexion, weakness of the limbs, loose stools, abdominal fullness, a feeling of heaviness, a sticky taste, poor digestion, thirst without a desire to drink, undigested food in the stools, nausea, excessive vaginal discharge, Pale tongue with sticky yellow coating, Soggy pulse.

LOSS OF SENSE OF SMELL

Interrogation, Chapter 35

Invasion of Wind-Heat

Sudden loss of sense of smell, aversion to cold, fever, sore throat, headache, body aches, slight sweating, tongue with Red sides/front, Floating-Rapid pulse.

Lung- and Spleen-Qi deficiency

Gradual loss of sense of smell, runny nose with white watery discharge, tiredness, weak voice, tendency to catch colds, poor appetite, loose stools, Pale tongue, Weak pulse.

Deficiency of Qi and Blood

Gradual loss of sense of smell, pale nose, tiredness, poor appetite, loose stools, palpitations, dizziness, Pale tongue, Weak or Choppy pulse.

Damp-Heat in the Gall-Bladder

Loss of sense of smell, blocked nose, yellow nasal discharge, headache, hypochondrial pain, fullness and distension, nausea, vomiting, inability to digest fats, yellow complexion and eyes, dizziness, tinnitus, irritability, a feeling of heaviness, unilateral or bilateral thick, sticky yellow coating, Slippery-Rapid pulse.

Damp-Heat in the Stomach and Spleen

Loss of sense of smell, yellow nasal discharge, facial pain, headache, a feeling of heaviness especially of the head, a feeling of fullness and pain of the epigastrium and lower abdomen, poor appetite, thirst without a desire to drink, a feeling of heat, dull-yellow complexion, sticky taste, Red tongue with sticky yellow coating, Slippery-Rapid pulse.

Cold-Dampness in the Stomach and Spleen

Loss of sense of smell, white nasal discharge, facial pain, headache, a feeling of heaviness of the head, abdominal fullness, loose stools, tongue with sticky white coating, Slippery pulse.

Blood stasis in the Lungs

Gradual loss of sense of smell, blocked nose, pain in the nose, headache, chest pain, cough, Purple tongue, Wiry pulse.

POLYPS

Damp-Heat in the Stomach and Spleen

Polyps, sinusitis, facial pain, swollen nose, sticky taste, loss of sense of smell, a feeling of heaviness especially of the head, a feeling of fullness and pain of the epigastrium and lower abdomen, poor appetite, thirst without a desire to drink, nausea, loose stools with offensive odour, a feeling of heat, dull-yellow complexion, sticky taste, Red tongue with sticky yellow coating, Slippery-Rapid pulse.

Cold-Dampness in the Stomach and Spleen

Polyps, loss of sense of smell, white nasal discharge, facial pain, headache, a feeling of heaviness of the head, abdominal fullness, loose stools, tongue with sticky white coating, Slippery pulse.

Phlegm in the Lungs

Polyps, cough with expectoration of sticky sputum, a feeling of oppression of the chest, a feeling of heaviness, Swollen tongue with sticky coating, Slippery pulse.

FLAPPING ALAE NASI (THE OUTSIDE OF THE NOSTRILS)

Observation, Chapter 7

Acute Lung-Heat

Flapping alae nasi, flaring of the nostrils, red face, cough, slight breathlessness, a feeling of heat, chest ache, thirst, red face, Red tongue with yellow coating, Overflowing-Rapid pulse.

Lung-Yin deficiency with Empty-Heat

Slightly flapping alae nasi, dry nose, dry cough or with scanty, sticky sputum which could be blood tinged, dry mouth and throat at night, weak/hoarse hoarse voice, night sweating, tiredness, malar flush, a feeling of heat or a low-grade fever in the evening, five-palm heat, thin body or thin chest, insomnia, anxiety, Red tongue without coating, Floating-Empty and Rapid pulse.

Invasion of Wind-Heat

Flapping alae nasi, aversion to cold, fever, cough, sore throat, stuffed or runny nose with yellow discharge, headache, body aches, slight sweating, slight thirst, swollen tonsils, tongue slightly Red on the sides in the chest area or on front part, Floating-Rapid pulse.

ULCERS ON THE NOSE

Observation, Chapter 7

Lung-Heat

Ulcers on the nose, red nose, dry nose, cough, slight breathlessness, a feeling of heat, chest ache, flaring of the nostrils, thirst, red face, Red tongue with yellow coating, Overflowing-Rapid pulse.

Damp-Heat in the Stomach and Spleen

Ulcers on the nose, swelling of the nose, sticky taste, a feeling of fullness and pain of the epigastrium and lower abdomen, poor appetite, a feeling of heaviness, thirst without a desire to drink, nausea, loose stools with offensive odour, a feeling of heat, dull-yellow complexion, sticky taste, Red tongue with sticky yellow coating, Slippery-Rapid pulse.

Liver-Fire

Ulcers on the bridge of the nose, red bridge of the nose, headache, red face, dizziness, tinnitus, irritability, propensity to outbursts of anger, thirst, bitter taste, constipation, dark urine, Red tongue with redder sides and dry yellow coating, Wiry-Rapid pulse.

Toxic Heat in the Liver

Ulcers on the bridge of the nose, nose pain, red and swollen nose, fever, red face, macular eruptions, agitation, headache, dizziness, tinnitus, irritability, propensity to outbursts of anger, thirst, bitter taste, constipation, dark urine, Red tongue with red points, thick, sticky, dry dark-yellow coating, Overflowing-Slippery-Rapid pulse.

PAPULES ON THE NOSE

Observation, Chapter 7

Stomach-Heat

Papules on the nose, burning epigastric pain, thirst, sour regurgitation, nausea, excessive hunger, foul

breath, a feeling of heat, Red tongue with a yellow coating, Overflowing-Rapid pulse.

Lung-Heat

Papules on the nose, cough, slight breathlessness, a feeling of heat, chest ache, flaring of nostrils, thirst, red face, Red tongue with yellow coating, Overflowing-Rapid pulse.

Blood-Heat in the Lungs

Dark papules on the nose, cough, coughing of blood, slight breathlessness, a feeling of heat, chest ache, flaring of nostrils, thirst, red face, Red tongue without coating, Overflowing-Rapid pulse.

Chapter **59**

THROAT

Chapter contents

SORE THROAT   *601*

REDNESS OF THE PHARYNX   *602*

REDNESS AND SWELLING OF THE PHARYNX   *602*

REDNESS AND EROSION OF THE PHARYNX   *602*

SWOLLEN TONSILS   *603*

PHLEGM IN THE THROAT   *603*

GOITRE (SWELLING OF THE SIDES OF THE NECK)   *604*

ITCHY THROAT   *605*

DRY THROAT   *605*

HOARSE VOICE OR LOSS OF VOICE   *606*

WHITE PURULENT SPOTS IN THE THROAT   *606*

FEELING OF OBSTRUCTION OF THE THROAT   *607*

REDNESS ON THE THROAT   *607*

SORE THROAT

Interrogation, Chapter 36

Invasion of Wind-Heat

Acute sore throat, itchy throat, shivers, fever, slight sweating, headache, tongue Red on the sides or front, thin white coating, Floating-Rapid pulse.

Lung- and Kidney-Yin deficiency with Empty-Heat

Chronic sore throat, dry and red throat, dry cough, dizziness, tinnitus, night sweating, five-palm heat, dry throat at night, Red tongue without coating, Floating-Empty and Rapid pulse.

Damp-Heat in the Stomach

Chronic sore throat, swollen throat with purulent spots, a feeling of fullness and pain of the epigastrium, a feeling of heaviness, facial pain, stuffed nose or thick sticky nasal discharge, thirst without a desire to drink, nausea, a feeling of heat, dull-yellow complexion, a sticky taste, Red tongue with sticky yellow coating, Slippery-Rapid pulse.

Stomach-Fire

Sore throat with severe pain, swollen and red throat, intense thirst with a desire to drink cold liquids, burning epigastric pain, mental restlessness, dry mouth, mouth ulcers, bleeding gums, dry stools, sour regurgitation, foul breath, nausea, vomiting soon after eating, a feeling of heat, sour regurgitation, tongue Red with a thick, dry dark-yellow coating, Deep-Full-Rapid pulse.

Deficiency of Qi and Yin

Chronic sore throat, slight pain, often aggravated by exertion, shortness of breath, tiredness, weak voice, dry cough, Pale tongue, Weak pulse.

Qi stagnation

Chronic 'sore throat' that comes and goes according to the emotional state, a feeling of a lump in the throat with a feeling of difficulty in swallowing, irritability, sighing, moodiness, depression, sadness, Wiry pulse.

Other symptoms and signs depend on the organ involved, which may be the Liver or the Lungs.

> ### Clinical note
>
> - Apart from Qi stagnation, the throat area can suffer only from Heat (Full or Empty) conditions.
> - **Remember**: Qi stagnation in the throat does not always derive from the Liver but it may derive also from the Lungs, Heart and Stomach.

REDNESS OF THE PHARYNX

Observation, Chapter 10

Invasion of Wind-Heat

Redness of the pharynx, sore throat, aversion to cold, fever, cough, sore throat, stuffed or runny nose with yellow discharge, headache, body aches, slight sweating, slight thirst, swollen tonsils, tongue slightly Red on the sides in the chest area or on front part, Floating-Rapid pulse.

Stomach-Heat

Redness of the pharynx, thirst, foul breath, burning epigastric pain, thirst, sour regurgitation, nausea, excessive hunger, foul breath, a feeling of heat, Red tongue with a yellow coating, Overflowing-Rapid pulse.

Lung-Yin deficiency with Empty-Heat

Pale-red pharynx, dry cough or with scanty, sticky sputum, dry mouth and throat at night, night sweating, tiredness, malar flush, a feeling of heat or a low-grade fever in the evening, five-palm heat, thin body, Red tongue without coating, Floating-Empty and Rapid pulse.

Kidney-Yin deficiency with Empty-Heat

Pale-red pharynx, dry mouth with desire to sip water, dizziness, tinnitus, hardness of hearing, night sweating, dry mouth at night, five-palm heat, a feeling of heat in the evening, malar flush, thirst with a desire to drink in small sips, lower backache, dark scanty urine, insomnia, Red tongue without coating, Floating-Empty and Rapid pulse.

REDNESS AND SWELLING OF THE PHARYNX

Observation, Chapter 10

Invasion of Wind-Heat

Red and swollen throat with sudden onset, sore throat, swollen tonsils, aversion to cold, fever, cough, sore throat, stuffed or runny nose with yellow discharge, headache, body aches, slight sweating, slight thirst, swollen tonsils, tongue slightly Red on the sides in the chest area or on front part, Floating-Rapid pulse.

Heat in the Lungs and Stomach

Red and swollen throat with sudden onset, sore throat, a feeling of obstruction in the throat, Cough, slight breathlessness, a feeling of heat, chest ache, flaring of nostrils, thirst, red face, burning epigastric pain, sour regurgitation, nausea, excessive hunger, foul breath, Red tongue with a yellow coating, Overflowing-Rapid pulse.

Toxic Heat

Red and swollen throat with purulent spots, swollen tonsils with yellow purulent spots, sore throat, fever, thirst, headache, Red tongue with red points and thick, sticky yellow coating, Overflowing-Rapid-Slippery pulse.

Lung- and Kidney-Yin deficiency with Empty-Heat

Chronic slightly swollen throat, red throat, dry throat at night with desire to drink in small sips, dry cough which is worse in the evening, thin body, breathlessness on exertion, lower backache, night sweating, dizziness, tinnitus, hardness of hearing, scanty urination, a feeling of heat in the evening, five-palm heat, malar flush, thirst with a desire to drink in small sips, Red tongue without coating, Floating-Empty and Rapid pulse.

REDNESS AND EROSION OF THE PHARYNX

Observation, Chapter 10

Toxic Heat

Redness, erosion, swelling and severe pain of the pharynx, swollen tonsils with yellow purulent spots, sore throat, fever, thirst, headache, Red tongue with red points and thick, sticky yellow coating, Overflowing-Rapid-Slippery pulse.

Heat in the Stomach and Intestines

Erosion, swelling and a yellowish-red colour of the pharynx, burning epigastric pain, thirst, sour regurgitation, nausea, excessive hunger, foul breath, a feeling of heat, Red tongue with a yellow coating, Overflowing-Rapid pulse.

Yin deficiency with Empty-Heat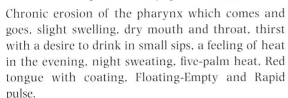

Chronic erosion of the pharynx which comes and goes, slight swelling, dry mouth and throat, thirst with a desire to drink in small sips, a feeling of heat in the evening, night sweating, five-palm heat, Red tongue with coating, Floating-Empty and Rapid pulse.

Other symptoms and signs depend on the organ affected, which may be Stomach, Lungs or Kidneys.

Severe Yin deficiency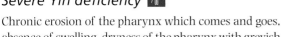

Chronic erosion of the pharynx which comes and goes, absence of swelling, dryness of the pharynx with greyish ulcers, dry throat, thirst with a desire to drink in small sips, night sweating, a feeling of heat in the evening, tongue dry without coating, Floating-Empty pulse.

Other symptoms and signs depend on the organ involved, which may be Lungs or Kidneys.

Blood stasis with Phlegm-Heat

Chronic erosion of the pharynx with ulcers with raised, hard edges, dark, dull colour of the pharynx, sore throat, mental restlessness, abdominal pain, a feeling of oppression of the chest, sputum in the throat, a feeling of heat, thirst with no desire to drink, Reddish-Purple and Swollen tongue with sticky yellow coating, Wiry-Slippery pulse.

SWOLLEN TONSILS

Observation, Chapter 10

Invasion of Wind-Heat with Toxic Heat

Acute swelling and redness of the tonsils, in severe cases oozing pus, severe sore throat, aversion to cold, fever, cough, stuffed or runny nose with yellow discharge, headache, body aches, slight sweating, slight thirst, swollen tonsils, tongue slightly Red on the sides in the chest area or on front part, Floating-Rapid pulse.

Toxic Heat in the throat at the Qi level

Acute redness and swelling of the tonsils, which ooze pus, severe sore throat, difficulty in swallowing, high fever, thirst, mental restlessness, a feeling of heat, dark Red tongue with red points and thick, dark-yellow coating, Overflowing-Slippery-Rapid pulse.

Toxic Heat in the Stomach and Intestines

Chronic redness and swelling of the tonsils, thirst, foul breath, burning epigastric pain, thirst, sour regurgitation, nausea, excessive hunger, foul breath, a feeling of heat, constipation, Red tongue with a yellow coating, Overflowing-Rapid pulse.

Stomach- and Lung-Yin deficiency with Empty-Heat

Chronic swelling and redness of the tonsils, which come and go, dry cough or with scanty, sticky sputum, dry mouth and throat especially in the afternoon, thirst with a desire to drink in small sips, dull or burning epigastric pain, a feeling of heat in the afternoon, night sweating, five-palm heat, bleeding gums, tiredness, malar flush, thin body, Red tongue without coating, Floating-Empty and Rapid pulse.

> **Clinical note**
>
> - In my experience, a chronic swelling of the tonsils in children denotes a residual pathogenic factor, usually Dampness.
> - Heat in the Stomach and Large Intestine may also cause a chronic swelling of the tonsils in children.

PHLEGM IN THE THROAT

Phlegm with Lung-Qi stagnation

Phlegm in the throat, a feeling of a lump in the throat, a feeling of oppression or distension of the chest, slight breathlessness, difficulty in swallowing, sighing, sadness, irritability, depression, sputum in the throat, tongue slightly Swollen on the sides in the chest areas, Slippery pulse that is also very slightly Tight on the right Front position.

Phlegm obstructing the clear orifices

Phlegm in the throat, difficulty in speech, rattling sound in the throat, a feeling of oppression of the

chest, dull headache as if the head were full of cotton wool, dizziness, blurred vision, expectoration of phlegm, nausea, vomiting, Swollen tongue with sticky tongue coating, Slippery pulse.

Phlegm-Heat in the Lungs

Phlegm in the throat, a rattling sound in the throat, barking cough with profuse, sticky yellow or green sputum, shortness of breath, wheezing, a feeling of oppression of the chest, a feeling of heat, thirst, insomnia, agitation, Red and Swollen tongue with a sticky yellow coating, Slippery-Rapid pulse.

Phlegm-Heat and Wind

Phlegm in the throat, a feeling of oppression of the chest, a feeling of heat, thirst with no desire to drink, headache, breathlessness, a rattling sound in the throat, expectoration of yellow sputum, dizziness, giddiness, numbness/tingling of the limbs, Red, Swollen and Stiff tongue with sticky yellow coating, Slippery-Wiry-Rapid pulse.

Spleen- and Kidney-Yang deficiency

Scanty phlegm in the throat, weak rattling sound in the throat, expectoration of white watery phlegm, lower backache, cold and weak knees, a feeling of cold, bright-white complexion, impotence, decreased libido, tiredness, lassitude, abundant clear urination, urination at night, loose stools, poor appetite, slight abdominal distension, a desire to lie down, early-morning diarrhoea, Pale and wet tongue, Deep-Weak pulse.

> ### Clinical note
>
> - When I suspect Phlegm, I always ask patients whether they experience some phlegm in the throat, even if only in the morning. If they reply affirmatively, I take this as a sign of Phlegm, even in the absence of other symptoms.

GOITRE (*swelling of the sides of the neck*)

Observation, Chapter 10; Interrogation, Chapter 36

Qi stagnation and Phlegm

Relatively soft and large goitre with indistinct margins, normal skin colour, not painful, a feeling of oppression of the chest, a feeling of a lump in the throat, sighing, sputum in the throat, hypochondrial distension, irritability, Swollen tongue, Wiry pulse.

Liver-Qi stagnation, Spleen-Qi deficiency and Phlegm

Large, soft goitre, depression, irritability, a feeling of a lump in the throat, difficulty in swallowing, a feeling of oppression or distension of the chest and hypochondrium, moodiness, premenstrual tension, nausea, vomiting of watery fluids, tiredness, poor appetite, a feeling of heaviness, weak limbs, loose stools, dull-pale complexion, cold limbs, Pale, and Swollen tongue with sticky coating, Soggy or Weak and slightly Slippery or Wiry pulse.

Liver-Fire blazing with Phlegm-Heat

Small- or medium-sized goitre that is relatively soft and slippery under the finger, headache, exophthalmos (bulging eyeballs), red face, dizziness, tinnitus, irritability, propensity to outbursts of anger, thirst, bitter taste, constipation, dark urine, barking cough with profuse, sticky yellow or green sputum, shortness of breath, wheezing, a feeling of oppression of the chest, a feeling of heat, insomnia, agitation, Swollen and Red tongue with redder sides and tip, Wiry-Slippery-Rapid pulse.

Phlegm and Blood stasis

Relatively hard goitre with distinct margins, nodules on the thyroid, dark skin colour, painful, a feeling of oppression of the chest, headache, insomnia, anxiety, chest or abdominal pain, sputum in the throat, Purple and Swollen tongue with sticky coating, Wiry-Slippery pulse.

Heart- and Liver-Yin deficiency with Phlegm

Chronic goitre that may be large or small and relatively soft with slow onset, tremor of hands, palpitations, insomnia, dream-disturbed sleep, anxiety, dry mouth and throat, night sweating, dizziness, numbness or tingling of the limbs, blurred vision, floaters in eyes, dry eyes, scanty menstruation, dull-pale complexion but with red cheekbones, withered and brittle nails, dry skin and hair, normal-coloured Swollen tongue without coating, Fine or Floating-Empty pulse.

> ### Clinical note
>
> - Goitre is by definition due to Phlegm.

ITCHY THROAT

Interrogation, Chapter 36

Invasion of Wind

Itchy throat with sudden onset, aversion to cold, stiff neck, fever, headache, Floating pulse.

Other symptoms and signs depend on whether it is Wind-Cold or Wind-Heat.

Lung-Yin deficiency

Chronic itchy throat, dry cough, weak voice, dry throat with a desire to sip water, hoarse voice, night sweating, tiredness, tongue without coating in the front, Floating-Empty pulse.

Lung Dryness

Itchy throat, dry cough, dry skin, dry throat, dry mouth, thirst, hoarse voice, dry tongue, Fine pulse.

Dryness invading the Lungs

Itchy throat with sudden onset, dry cough, aversion to cold, fever, dry nose, dry and sore throat, tongue Red in the front with dry, thin white coating, Floating pulse.

DRY THROAT

Interrogation, Chapter 36

Lung-Yin deficiency

Chronic dry throat, hoarse voice, dry cough, weak voice, dry throat with desire to sip water, night sweating, tiredness, tongue without coating in the front, Floating-Empty pulse.

Kidney-Yin deficiency

Chronic dry throat, dry throat at night with a desire to drink in small sips, dizziness, tinnitus, hardness of hearing, poor memory, night sweating, vertigo, lower backache, ache in bones, nocturnal emissions, constipation, scanty dark urine, infertility, premature ejaculation, tiredness, lassitude, depression, slight anxiety, normal-coloured tongue without coating, Floating-Empty pulse.

Stomach-Yin deficiency

Chronic dryness of the throat, no appetite or slight hunger but no desire to eat, constipation (dry stools), dull or slightly burning epigastric pain, dry mouth especially in the afternoon, thirst but no desire to drink, or a desire to drink in small sips, a slight feeling of fullness after eating, normal-coloured tongue without coating in the centre, Floating-Empty pulse.

Liver-Yin deficiency

Chronic dryness of the throat, dizziness, numbness/tingling of the limbs, insomnia, blurred vision, floaters in the eyes, dry eyes, diminished night vision, scanty menstruation or amenorrhoea, dull-pale complexion without lustre but with red cheekbones, muscular weakness, cramps, withered and brittle nails, very dry skin and hair, night sweating, depression, a feeling of aimlessness, normal-coloured tongue without coating, Fine or Floating-Empty pulse.

Invasion of Wind-Heat

Dry throat with sudden onset, itchy throat, sore throat, aversion to cold, fever, cough, stuffed or runny nose with yellow discharge, headache, body aches, slight sweating, slight thirst, swollen tonsils, tongue slightly Red on the sides in the chest area or on front part, Floating-Rapid pulse.

Heat in the Stomach and Spleen

Dry throat, swollen throat, burning epigastric pain, thirst, sour regurgitation, nausea, foul breath, a feeling of heat, excessive hunger, red tip of the nose, dry lips, mouth ulcers, dry stools, scanty dark urine, yellow complexion, Red tongue with dry yellow coating, Overflowing-Rapid pulse.

Heat in the Liver and Gall-Bladder

Dry throat, bitter taste, thirst, blurred vision, hypochondrial pain, nausea, headache, red eyes, Red tongue with redder sides and dry yellow coating, Wiry-Rapid pulse.

Lesser-Yang pattern (Six Stages)

Dry throat, bitter taste, hypochondriac fullness and pain, alternation of chills and feeling of heat with predominance of the former, irritability, unilateral white tongue coating, Wiry pulse.

Gall-Bladder-Heat pattern (Qi level of Four levels)

Dryness of the throat, thirst, bitter taste, hypochondrial pain, alternation of chills and feeling of heat with predominance of the latter, irritability, unilateral yellow tongue coating, Wiry-Rapid pulse.

Wind-Dryness-Heat invading the Lungs

Dry throat with sudden onset, sore throat, itchy throat, aversion to cold, fever, dry cough, stuffed or runny nose with yellow discharge, headache, body aches, slight sweating, slight thirst, swollen tonsils, dry nose, tongue slightly Red on the sides in the chest area or on front part, Floating-Rapid pulse.

HOARSE VOICE OR LOSS OF VOICE

Interrogation, Chapter 36; Hearing, Chapter 53

Lung- and Kidney-Yin deficiency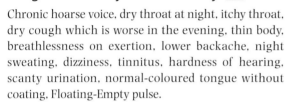

Chronic hoarse voice, dry throat at night, itchy throat, dry cough which is worse in the evening, thin body, breathlessness on exertion, lower backache, night sweating, dizziness, tinnitus, hardness of hearing, scanty urination, normal-coloured tongue without coating, Floating-Empty pulse.

Lung-Yin deficiency

Chronic hoarse voice, cough which is dry or with scanty sticky sputum, weak voice, dry mouth and throat, tickly throat, tiredness, dislike of speaking, thin body or thin chest, night sweating, normal-coloured tongue without coating (or with rootless coating) in the front part, Floating-Empty pulse.

Invasion of Wind-Heat and Dryness

Hoarse voice with sudden onset, dry throat with sudden onset, sore throat, itchy throat, aversion to cold, fever, dry cough, stuffed or runny nose with yellow discharge, headache, body aches, slight sweating, slight thirst, swollen tonsils, dry nose, tongue slightly Red on the sides in the chest area or on front part, Floating-Rapid pulse.

Lung-Heat

Hoarse voice, sore throat, a feeling of blockage of the throat, cough, slight breathlessness, a feeling of heat, chest ache, flaring of nostrils, thirst, red face, Red tongue with yellow coating, Overflowing-Rapid pulse.

Blood stasis and Phlegm

Chronic hoarse voice, sore throat, a feeling of obstruction of the throat, thickening of the vocal chords, nodules on the vocal chords, swelling of the throat, headache, chest pain, a feeling of oppression of the chest, sputum in the throat, Purple tongue, Wiry pulse.

WHITE PURULENT SPOTS IN THE THROAT

Epidemic Toxic Heat on the Exterior

White purulent spots in the throat, small and with distinct margins, sore and swollen throat, swollen tonsils, fever, aversion to cold, headache, body aches, thin white tongue coating, Floating-Rapid pulse.

Epidemic Toxic Heat in the Interior

White purulent spots in the throat, large spots which may ooze blood, red, swollen and sore throat, high fever, profuse sweating, red face, thirst, mental restlessness, a feeling of heat, Red tongue with yellow coating, Overflowing-Rapid pulse.

Turbid Phlegm in the throat

Chronic white purulent spots in the throat, dull-pasty complexion, mental restlessness, a feeling of oppression of the chest, wheezing, expectoration of sputum, barking voice, hoarse voice, Swollen tongue with white coating, Slippery pulse.

Lung- and Kidney-Yin deficiency

White purulent spots in the throat, dry throat, dry cough which is worse in the evening, dry throat and mouth, thin body, breathlessness on exertion, lower backache, night sweating, dizziness, tinnitus, hardness of hearing, scanty urination, normal-coloured tongue without coating, Floating-Empty pulse.

Lung- and Kidney-Yin deficiency with Empty-Heat

White purulent spots in the throat, dry throat at night, dry cough which is worse in the evening, thin body, breathlessness on exertion, lower backache, night sweating, dizziness, tinnitus, hardness of hearing, scanty urination, a feeling of heat in the evening, five-palm heat, malar flush, thirst with a desire to drink in small sips, Red tongue without coating, Floating-Empty and Rapid pulse.

Heat in the Lungs and Stomach

White purulent spots in the throat, swollen throat, painful throat, swollen tonsils, cough, slight breathlessness, a feeling of heat, chest ache, flaring of nostrils, thirst, red face, burning epigastric pain, thirst, sour regurgitation, nausea, excessive hunger,

foul breath, Red tongue with a yellow coating, Overflowing-Rapid pulse.

Kidney-Yang deficiency

White purulent spots in the throat, lower backache, cold knees, a sensation of cold in the lower back, a feeling of cold, weak legs, bright-white complexion, weak knees, tiredness, lassitude, abundant clear or scanty clear urination, urination at night, apathy, oedema of lower legs, infertility in women, loose stools, depression, impotence, premature ejaculation, low sperm count, cold and thin sperm, decreased libido, Pale and wet tongue, Deep-Weak pulse.

FEELING OF OBSTRUCTION OF THE THROAT

Interrogation, Chapter 36

Liver-Qi stagnation

A feeling of lump in the throat that comes and goes according to the emotional state, hypochondrial or epigastric distension, irritability, moodiness, a feeling of lump in the throat, premenstrual tension, Wiry pulse.

Lung- and Stomach-Qi stagnation

A feeling of lump in the throat that comes and goes according to the emotional state, sadness, worry, grief, depression, a slight feeling of tightness, oppression or distension of the chest, slight breathlessness, difficulty in swallowing, sighing, irritability, epigastric pain and distension, belching, nausea, vomiting, hiccup, tongue slightly Red on the sides in the chest areas, pulse slightly Wiry on the right.

Qi stagnation and Phlegm

A feeling of lump in the throat, phlegm in the throat that needs frequent clearing, expectoration of scanty sputum, a feeling of oppression of the chest, irritability, Swollen tongue with sticky coating, Slippery-Wiry pulse.

Lung-Yin deficiency

A feeling of lump in the throat, dry throat at night, tickly throat, cough which is dry or with scanty sticky sputum, weak/hoarse voice, tiredness, dislike of speaking, thin body or thin chest, night sweating, normal-coloured tongue without coating (or with rootless coating) in the front part, Floating-Empty pulse.

Kidney-Yin deficiency

A slight feeling of lump in the throat, dry throat at night, dizziness, tinnitus, hardness of hearing, poor memory, night sweating, vertigo, lower backache, ache in bones, nocturnal emissions, constipation, scanty dark urine, infertility, premature ejaculation, tiredness, lassitude, depression, slight anxiety, normal-coloured tongue without coating, Floating-Empty pulse.

Clinical note

- In my experience, a feeling of obstruction in the throat strongly indicates emotional stress with Qi stagnation.
- Note that this is not always related to the Liver and may be related also to Lungs or Heart.
- Ban Xia Hou Po Tang is for stagnation of Lung-Qi in the throat from worry or grief.

REDNESS ON THE THROAT

Observation, Chapter 10

By 'redness on the throat' is meant not a redness inside the throat (pharynx) but a redness on the skin overlying the throat.

Heart-Fire

Redness on the throat that gets worse when patient talks, thirst, bitter taste, palpitations, anxiety, red face, Red tongue with redder tip and yellow coating, Overflowing-Rapid pulse.

Heart-Yin deficiency with Empty-Heat

'Floating' redness on the throat, dry mouth and throat, palpitations, insomnia, dream-disturbed sleep, poor memory, anxiety, mental restlessness, a feeling of heat in the evening, malar flush, night sweating, five-palm heat, Red tongue with redder tip and without coating, Floating-Empty and Rapid pulse.

Lung-Heat

Redness on the throat, dry throat, thirst, cough, slight breathlessness, a feeling of heat, chest ache, flaring of the nostrils, red face, Red tongue with yellow coating, Overflowing-Rapid pulse.

Lung-Yin deficiency with Empty-Heat

'Floating' redness on the throat, malar flush, dry cough or with scanty, sticky sputum, dry mouth and throat at night, night sweating, tiredness, a feeling of

heat or a low-grade fever in the evening, five-palm heat, thin body, Red tongue without coating, Floating-Empty and Rapid pulse.

Liver-Yang rising

'Floating' redness on the throat, headache, dizziness, tinnitus, irritability, red face, Wiry pulse.

Liver-Fire

Redness on the throat, thirst, bitter taste, red face, irritability, propensity to outbursts of anger, headache, constipation, dark urine, Red tongue with redder sides and dry-yellow coating, Wiry-Rapid pulse.

Clinical note

- I have noticed that a redness on the throat appearing as the patient talks, indicates severe anxiety with Heat or Empty-Heat.

Chapter **60**

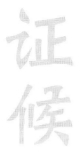

MOUTH, TONGUE, TEETH, GUMS, LIPS, PALATE AND PHILTRUM

Chapter contents

MOUTH   *609*
   Mouth ulcers   *609*
   Cold sores   *610*
   Cracked corners of the mouth   *611*
   Itching around the mouth   *611*
   Dribbling from the corners of the mouth   *612*
   Trembling mouth   *612*
   Mouth open   *612*
   Deviation of the mouth   *613*

TONGUE   *613*
   Itchy tongue   *613*
   Painful tongue   *613*
   Numbness of the tongue   *614*
   Tongue ulcers   *614*

TEETH   *615*
   Toothache   *615*
   Tooth cavities   *616*
   Loose teeth   *616*
   Grinding teeth   *616*
   Plaque   *617*
   Dry and white teeth   *617*
   Dry and dull teeth   *617*
   Yellow and dry teeth   *618*
   Grey teeth   *618*
   Upper teeth moist and lower teeth dry   *618*

GUMS   *618*
   Inflamed gums   *618*
   Bleeding gums   *619*
   Receding gums   *619*
   Gums oozing pus   *620*
   Pale gums   *620*
   Red gums   *620*
   Purple gums   *620*

LIPS   *621*
   Pale lips   *621*
   Red lips   *621*

Purple lips   *621*
Bluish-greenish lips   *622*
Yellow lips   *622*
Dry or cracked lips   *622*
Trembling lips   *623*
Peeled lips   *623*
Swollen lips   *623*
Inverted lips   *624*
Drooping lips   *624*
Abnormal lip colour in pregnancy   *624*

PALATE   *624*
Pale palate   *624*
Dull-pale palate   *624*
Yellow palate   *625*
Red palate   *625*
Purple palate   *625*

PHILTRUM   *625*
Flat philtrum   *625*
Stiff-looking philtrum   *625*
Pale philtrum   *625*
Red philtrum   *626*
Bluish-greenish philtrum   *626*
Dark philtrum   *626*

MOUTH

Mouth ulcers

Observation, Chapter 8; Interrogation, Chapter 35

Stomach-Heat

Ulcers with a red rim on the gums or inside cheeks, bleeding gums, thirst, foul breath, burning epigastric pain, sour regurgitation, nausea, excessive hunger, a feeling of heat, Red tongue with a yellow coating, Overflowing-Rapid pulse.

Heart-Fire

Tongue ulcers, thirst, bitter taste, palpitations, mental restlessness, a feeling of agitation, insomnia, dream-disturbed sleep, a feeling of heat, red face, Red tongue with redder tip and yellow coating, Overflowing and Rapid pulse.

Yin deficiency with Empty-Heat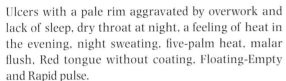

Ulcers with a pale rim aggravated by overwork and lack of sleep, dry throat at night, a feeling of heat in the evening, night sweating, five-palm heat, malar flush, Red tongue without coating, Floating-Empty and Rapid pulse.

Other symptoms and signs depend on the organ involved.

Stomach- and Spleen-Qi deficiency with Yin Fire

Pale ulcers on the gums or inside cheeks, slightly red face or pale face with a floating red colour on the cheeks, an intermittent and recurrent feeling of heat in the face but cold limbs, intermittent sore throat, dry mouth, dry lips, exhaustion, poor appetite, poor digestion, weak limbs, Pale tongue, Weak or Overflowing-Empty pulse.

These ulcers are due to Yin Fire as described by Li Dong Yuan in his 'Discussion on Stomach and Spleen' (see Chapter 55).

Liver-Fire

Ulcers inside the cheeks, very painful and red in colour, thirst, bitter taste, headache, red face, dizziness, tinnitus, irritability, propensity to outbursts of anger, constipation, dark urine, Red tongue with redder sides and dry yellow coating, Wiry-Rapid pulse.

Toxic Heat

Ulcers inside the cheeks, red and festering, oozing sticky yellow pus, fever, thirst, Red tongue with red points and thick, sticky yellow coating, Overflowing-Slippery-Rapid pulse.

Invasion of Wind-Heat with Phlegm

Ulcers inside the cheeks, red and swollen, oozing thin yellow pus, aversion to cold, fever, cough, sore throat, stuffed or runny nose with yellow discharge, headache, body aches, slight sweating, slight thirst, swollen tonsils, nausea, vomiting, a feeling of oppression of the chest, tongue slightly Red on the sides in the chest area or on front part, Floating-Rapid pulse.

Invasion of Wind-Cold with Kidney deficiency

Ulcers inside the cheeks, white rim around them, swollen, aversion to cold, fever, cough, itchy throat, slight breathlessness, stuffed or runny nose with clear watery discharge, sneezing, occipital headache, body aches, thin white tongue coating, lower backache, dizziness, tinnitus, Pale tongue, Floating-Tight pulse.

> **Clinical note**
>
> - **Remember**: for mouth ulcers on gums and inside cheeks in women treat the Directing Vessel irrespective of the pattern causing them.
> - If they are on the tongue, treat the Heart channel and especially HE-5 Tongli.

Cold sores

Observation, Chapter 8; Interrogation, Chapter 35

Invasion of Wind-Heat

Cold sores at the corner of the mouth or on the edge of the upper lip, aversion to cold, fever, cough, sore throat, stuffed or runny nose with yellow discharge, headache, body aches, slight sweating, slight thirst, swollen tonsils, tongue slightly Red on the sides in the chest area or on front part, Floating-Rapid pulse.

Stomach Damp-Heat

Cold sores at the corner of the mouth or on the edge of the lower lip, a sticky taste, thirst with no desire to drink, facial pain, stuffed nose or thick sticky nasal discharge, a feeling of fullness and pain of the epigastrium, a feeling of heaviness, nausea, a feeling of heat, dull-yellow complexion, Red tongue with sticky yellow coating, Slippery-Rapid pulse.

Stomach-Heat

Cold sores at the corner of the mouth or on the edge of the lower lip, foul breath, thirst, burning epigastric pain, sour regurgitation, nausea, excessive hunger, a feeling of heat, Red tongue with a yellow coating, Overflowing-Rapid pulse.

Stomach-Yin deficiency with Empty-Heat

Cold sores at the corner of the mouth or on the edge of the lower lip, dry mouth in the evening, dull or burning epigastric pain, a feeling of heat in the afternoon, thirst with a desire to drink in small sips, dry stools, a slight feeling of fullness after eating, night

sweating, five-palm heat, bleeding gums, Red tongue (or Red centre only) without coating in the centre, Floating-Empty and Rapid pulse.

Heat in the Large Intestine

Cold sores on the upper lip, constipation with dry stools, a burning sensation in the mouth, dry tongue, burning and swelling in the anus, scanty dark urine, thick yellow (or brown or black) dry tongue coating, Full-Rapid pulse (often Wiry on both Rear positions).

Damp-Heat in the Large Intestine

Cold sores on the upper lip, abdominal pain that is not relieved by a bowel movement, diarrhoea, mucus and blood in stools, offensive odour of stools, burning in the anus, scanty dark urine, fever, sweating which does not decrease the fever, a feeling of heat, thirst without a desire to drink, a feeling of heaviness of the body and limbs, a feeling of oppression of the chest and epigastrium, Red tongue with sticky yellow coating, Slippery-Rapid pulse or pulse that is Slippery and Wiry on both the Rear positions.

Clinical note

- I use LI-4 Hegu contralaterally for the corners of the mouth, that is, on the left for cold sore on the right and vice versa.

Cracked corners of the mouth

Observation, Chapter 8

Stomach-Heat

Cracked corners of the mouth, thirst, burning epigastric pain, sour regurgitation, nausea, excessive hunger, foul breath, a feeling of heat, Red tongue with a yellow coating, Overflowing-Rapid pulse.

Stomach-Yin deficiency

Cracked corners of the mouth, dry mouth with desire to sip water, no appetite or slight hunger but no desire to eat, constipation (dry stools), dull or slightly burning epigastric pain, dry mouth and throat especially in the afternoon, a slight feeling of fullness after eating, normal-coloured tongue without coating, or without coating in the centre, Floating-Empty pulse.

Stomach-Yin deficiency with Empty-Heat

Cracked corners of the mouth, dry mouth and throat especially in the afternoon, thirst with a desire to drink in small sips, bleeding gums, dull or burning epigastric pain, a feeling of heat in the afternoon, dry stools, a slight feeling of fullness after eating, night sweating, five-palm heat, bleeding gums, Red tongue (or Red centre only) without coating in the centre, Floating-Empty and Rapid pulse.

Itching around the mouth
Stomach-Heat

Intense itching around mouth and especially at the corners and below the mouth, cold sores, foul breath, burning epigastric pain, thirst, sour regurgitation, nausea, excessive hunger, foul breath, a feeling of heat, Red tongue with a yellow coating, Overflowing-Rapid pulse.

Liver-Blood deficiency with Empty-Wind 👤

Slight itching around the mouth, dryness around the mouth, greenish colour around the mouth, trembling mouth, facial tic, slight flapping of the eyelid, blurred vision, floaters, unilateral numbness/tingling of a limb, Pale and Thin tongue, Choppy or Fine and slightly Wiry pulse.

Damp-Heat in Stomach and Spleen

Itching around mouth, wet rash around mouth, cold sores, sticky taste, thirst with no desire to drink, a feeling of fullness and pain of the epigastrium and lower abdomen, poor appetite, a feeling of heaviness, thirst without a desire to drink, nausea, loose stools with offensive odour, a feeling of heat, dull-yellow complexion, sticky taste, Red tongue with sticky yellow coating, Slippery-Rapid pulse.

Disharmony of Penetrating and Directing Vessels 👤

Itching around mouth at period time or during the menopausal time, lower backache, dizziness, tinnitus, irregular periods.

Other symptoms and signs depend on whether there is a deficiency of Kidney-Yin or Kidney-Yang.

Clinical note

- The area around the mouth is controlled by the Liver channel and the Penetrating and Directing Vessels.

Dribbling from the corners of the mouth

Observation, Chapter 8

Spleen-Qi deficiency

Dribbling from the corners of the mouth, poor appetite, tiredness, slight abdominal distension, pale complexion, loose stools, Pale tongue, Empty pulse.

Lung-Qi deficiency with Empty-Cold

Dribbling from the corners of the mouth, chronic runny nose with watery white discharge, sneezing, slight shortness of breath, slight cough, weak voice, spontaneous daytime sweating, dislike of speaking, bright-white complexion, tendency to catch cold, tiredness, dislike of cold, a feeling of cold, cold limbs, Pale tongue, Weak pulse.

Stomach- and Spleen-Heat

Dribbling from the corners of the mouth, painful tongue, mouth ulcers, dry mouth and lips, burning epigastric/abdominal pain, thirst, sour regurgitation, nausea, excessive hunger, foul breath, a feeling of heat, excessive hunger, red tip of the nose, dry stools, scanty dark urine, yellow complexion, Red tongue with dry yellow coating, Overflowing-Rapid pulse.

This dribbling is due to Stomach-Heat flaring upwards causing the fluids in the mouth to evaporate.

Wind-Phlegm

Dribbling from the corners of the mouth, severe dizziness, blurred vision, tremors, numbness or tingling of the limbs, tinnitus, nausea, sputum in the throat, a feeling of oppression of the chest, Stiff or Deviated and Swollen tongue, Wiry-Slippery pulse.

Invasion of external Wind

Dribbling from the corners of the mouth, numbness of the face, deviation of eye and mouth, inability to shut eyelid completely, watery eyes.

This is not an invasion of external Wind in the Lung's Defensive-Qi system (as when one catches a cold) but an invasion of external Wind attacking the channels of the face causing facial paralysis (Bell's palsy).

Trembling mouth
Liver-Blood and Liver-Yin deficiency with internal Wind

Slightly trembling mouth, dizziness, numbness/tingling of the limbs, blurred vision, floaters in the eyes, dry eyes, scanty menstruation, dull-pale complexion but with red cheek bones, withered and brittle nails, dry skin and hair, night sweating.

The tongue and pulse presentation depends on whether Blood or Yin deficiency predominates.

Qi stagnation and Phlegm

Trembling mouth, dribbling from the corners of the mouth, epigastric or abdominal distension, a feeling of muzziness of the head, sputum in the throat, a feeling of oppression of the chest, irritability, a feeling of a lump in the throat, Wiry-Slippery pulse.

Stomach-Heat

Trembling mouth, thirst, foul breath, burning epigastric pain, sour regurgitation, nausea, excessive hunger, a feeling of heat, Red tongue with a yellow coating, Overflowing-Rapid pulse.

Liver-Wind

Trembling mouth, tremors, severe dizziness, tinnitus, headache, numbness of limbs, tics, Stiff, Deviated or Moving tongue, Wiry pulse.

Mouth open

Observation, Chapter 8

Lung-Qi deficiency with Phlegm

Mouth open, chronic cough which is worse on exertion, scanty phlegm that is difficult to expectorate or dilute watery phlegm, spontaneous sweating, a feeling of cold, shortness of breath, a feeling of oppression of the chest, weak voice, tongue Pale and slightly Swollen in the front, pulse Empty on the right Front position and slightly Slippery.

Heart-Fire

Mouth open, tongue ulcers, red face, palpitations, thirst, mental restlessness, feeling agitated, insomnia, dream-disturbed sleep, a feeling of heat, bitter taste, Red tongue with redder tip and yellow coating, Overflowing-Rapid pulse.

Heart-Qi deficiency

Mouth open, palpitations, mental dullness, palpitations, shortness of breath on exertion, pale face, tiredness, slight depression, spontaneous sweating, Pale tongue, Empty pulse.

Deviation of the mouth

Observation, Chapter 8

Liver-Wind

Deviation of mouth, tremors, severe dizziness, tinnitus, headache, numbness of the limbs, tics, Stiff, Deviated or Moving tongue, Wiry pulse.

Liver-Wind and Phlegm

Deviation of mouth, severe dizziness, blurred vision, tremors, numbness/tingling of the limbs, tinnitus, nausea, sputum in the throat, a feeling of oppression of the chest, Stiff or Deviated and Swollen tongue, Wiry-Slippery pulse.

Invasion of Wind-Cold in the channels of the face

Sudden deviation of mouth, numbness of the face.
    This is due to an invasion of Wind-Cold, not in the Lungs Defensive-Qi portion (as in the common cold and influenza) but in the channels of the face.

Liver-Qi stagnation

Intermittent deviation of mouth depending on emotional moods, hypochondrial or epigastric distension, irritability, moodiness, a feeling of a lump in the throat, premenstrual tension, Wiry pulse.

Deficiency of Qi and Blood

Slight deviation of mouth, poor appetite, loose stools, weak voice, tiredness, blurred vision, dizziness, numbness/tingling of limbs, palpitations, dull-pale complexion, Pale tongue, Weak or Choppy pulse.

Toxic Heat in the channels of the face

Deviation of mouth, thirst, bitter taste, swelling and pain of the face, toothache, headache, red eyes, swollen face, Red tongue with red points with thick, sticky yellow coating, Overflowing-Slippery-Rapid pulse.

TONGUE

The tongue signs discussed in this chapter deal only with a few unusual tongue signs; tongue diagnosis itself is discussed in full in Chapters 23–27.

Itchy tongue

Interrogation, Chapter 35

Heart-Fire

Itchy tip or front of the tongue, burning sensation of the tongue, palpitations, thirst, mouth and tongue ulcers, mental restlessness, a feeling of agitation, insomnia, dream-disturbed sleep, a feeling of heat, red face, bitter taste, Red tongue with redder tip and yellow coating, Overflowing-Rapid pulse.

Heart-Yin deficiency with Empty-Heat

Slight itching of the tongue especially in the evening, dry mouth and throat, palpitations, insomnia, dream-disturbed sleep, poor memory, anxiety, tendency to be easily startled, mental restlessness, uneasiness, 'feeling hot and bothered', thirst with a desire to sip fluids, a feeling of heat in the evening, malar flush, night sweating, five-palm heat, Red tongue redder on the tip with no coating, Floating-Empty and Rapid pulse.

Heart- and Kidney-Yin deficiency

Itchy tongue, palpitations, insomnia, dream-disturbed sleep, anxiety, poor memory, dizziness, tinnitus, hardness of hearing, lower backache, night sweating, scanty dark urine, normal-coloured tongue without coating, Floating-Empty pulse.

Invasion of Wind-Heat

Itchy tongue with acute onset, aversion to cold, fever, cough, sore throat, stuffed or runny nose with yellow discharge, headache, body aches, slight sweating, slight thirst, swollen tonsils, tongue slightly Red on the sides in the chest area or on front part, Floating-Rapid pulse.

Painful tongue

Interrogation, Chapter 35

Heart-Fire

Painful tongue especially on the tip, tongue ulcers, palpitations, thirst, mouth and tongue ulcers, mental restlessness, a feeling of agitation, insomnia, dream-disturbed sleep, a feeling of heat, red face, bitter taste, Red tongue with redder tip and yellow coating, Overflowing-Rapid pulse.

Heart-Yin deficiency with Empty-Heat

Slight pain of the tongue especially in the evening, dry mouth and throat, palpitations, insomnia, dream-

disturbed sleep, poor memory, anxiety, tendency to be easily startled, mental restlessness, uneasiness, 'feeling hot and bothered', dry mouth and throat, thirst with a desire to sip fluids, a feeling of heat in the evening, malar flush, night sweating, five-palm heat, Red tongue redder on the tip with no coating, Floating-Empty and Rapid pulse.

Stomach-Fire

Painful tongue, bleeding gums, foul breath, intense thirst with a desire to drink cold liquids, burning epigastric pain, mental restlessness, dry mouth, mouth ulcers, dry stools, sour regurgitation, nausea, vomiting soon after eating, a feeling of heat, sour regurgitation, Red tongue with a thick, dry dark-yellow coating, Deep-Full-Rapid pulse.

Stomach-Yin deficiency with Empty-Heat

Slightly painful tongue, dull or burning epigastric pain, a feeling of heat in the afternoon, dry mouth and throat especially in the afternoon, thirst with desire to drink in small sips, dry stools, a slight feeling of fullness after eating, night sweating, five-palm heat, bleeding gums, Red tongue (or Red centre only) without coating in the centre, Floating-Empty and Rapid pulse.

Liver-Fire

Painful tongue, thirst, bitter taste, headache, red face, dizziness, tinnitus, irritability, propensity to outbursts of anger, constipation, dark urine, Red tongue with redder sides and dry yellow coating, Wiry-Rapid pulse.

Phlegm-Fire harassing the Heart

Painful tongue, thirst, bitter taste, sputum in throat, palpitations, mental restlessness, red face, a feeling of oppression of the chest, expectoration of phlegm, sputum in the throat, insomnia, dream-disturbed sleep, agitation, mental confusion, incoherent speech, rash behaviour, uncontrolled laughter or crying, shouting, depression, manic behaviour, Red tongue with redder swollen tip and Heart crack with a sticky, dry yellow coating inside it, Slippery-Rapid or Slippery-Overflowing-Rapid pulse.

Numbness of the tongue

Interrogation, Chapter 35

Heart-Blood deficiency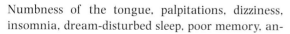

Numbness of the tongue, palpitations, dizziness, insomnia, dream-disturbed sleep, poor memory, an-

xiety, tendency to be easily startled, dull-pale complexion, pale lips, Pale and Thin tongue, Choppy or Fine pulse.

Phlegm obstructing the Heart

Numbness of the tongue, swollen tongue, dizziness, a feeling of oppression of the chest, sputum in the throat, numbness/tingling of the limbs, sticky tongue coating, Slippery pulse.

Liver-Wind

Numbness of the tongue, tremors, severe dizziness, tinnitus, headache, tics, convulsions, rigidity of the neck, tremor of limbs, stiff neck, opisthotonos, in severe cases coma, Stiff, Moving or Deviated tongue, Wiry pulse.

Liver Wind-Phlegm

Numbness of the tongue, deviated tongue, severe dizziness, blurred vision, tremors, numbness or tingling of the limbs, tinnitus, nausea, sputum in the throat, a feeling of oppression of the chest, Stiff or Deviated and Swollen tongue, Wiry-Slippery pulse.

Spleen-Qi deficiency

Numbness of the tongue, poor appetite, tiredness, slight abdominal distension, pale complexion, loose stools, Pale tongue, Empty pulse.

Chronic Blood stasis

Numbness of the tongue, dark complexion, headache, chest pain, mental restlessness, abdominal pain, dark nails, Purple tongue, Wiry pulse.

Tongue ulcers

Observation, Chapter 8; Interrogation, Chapter 35

Heart-Fire

Painful tongue ulcers with raised, red rim, bitter taste, thirst, palpitations, mouth and tongue ulcers, mental restlessness, a feeling of agitation, insomnia, dream-disturbed sleep, a feeling of heat, red face, Red tongue with redder tip and yellow coating, Overflowing-Rapid pulse.

Heart-Yin deficiency with Empty-Heat

Tongue ulcers with white rims, dry mouth and throat, palpitations, insomnia, dream-disturbed sleep, poor memory, anxiety, tendency to be easily startled, mental restlessness, uneasiness, 'feeling hot and bothered', thirst with a desire to sip fluids, a feeling of heat in the

evening, malar flush, night sweating, five-palm heat, Red tongue redder on the tip with no coating, Floating-Empty and Rapid pulse.

Full-Heat in the Small Intestine

Tongue ulcers with red rims, dry stools, dark urine, painful urination, blood in the urine, abdominal pain, dry yellow tongue coating, Overflowing-Rapid pulse.

Clinical note

- I use HE-5 Tongli as a point to reach the tongue (in addition to other points for the relevant pattern).

TEETH

Toothache

Interrogation, Chapter 35

Toothache obviously excludes causes such as abscesses or root canal problems.

Stomach-Fire

Toothache especially on the lower teeth, mouth ulcers, foul breath, intense thirst with a desire to drink cold liquids, bleeding gums, burning epigastric pain, mental restlessness, dry mouth, dry stools, sour regurgitation, nausea, vomiting soon after eating, a feeling of heat, sour regurgitation, Red tongue with a thick, dry, dark-yellow coating, Deep-Full-Rapid pulse.

Damp-Heat in the Stomach

Toothache, swollen gums, sticky taste, thirst with no desire to drink, a feeling of fullness and pain of the epigastrium, a feeling of heaviness, facial pain, stuffed nose or thick sticky nasal discharge, nausea, a feeling of heat, dull-yellow complexion, Red tongue with sticky yellow coating, Slippery-Rapid pulse.

Stomach-Yin deficiency with Empty-Heat

Toothache, mouth ulcers, dry mouth or thirst with a desire to drink in small sips, dull or burning epigastric pain, a feeling of heat in the afternoon, dry mouth and throat especially in the afternoon, dry stools, a slight feeling of fullness after eating, night sweating, five-palm heat, bleeding gums, Red tongue (or Red centre only) without coating in the centre, Floating-Empty and Rapid pulse.

Stomach- and Spleen-Qi deficiency

Dull toothache that comes and goes, weak gums, poor appetite, slight abdominal distension after eating, tiredness, lassitude, pale complexion, weakness of the limbs, loose stools, an uncomfortable feeling in the epigastrium, lack of sense of taste, Pale tongue, Empty pulse.

Heat in Large Intestine

Severe toothache, especially of the upper teeth, mouth ulcers, bleeding gums, constipation with dry stools, burning sensation in the mouth, dry tongue, burning and swelling in the anus, scanty dark urine, thick yellow (or brown or black) dry tongue coating, Full-Rapid pulse.

Damp-Heat in Large Intestine

Toothache, especially of upper teeth, thirst with no desire to drink, mouth ulcers, a sticky taste, abdominal pain that is not relieved by a bowel movement, diarrhoea, mucus and blood in stools, offensive odour of stools, burning in the anus, scanty dark urine, fever, sweating which does not decrease the fever, a feeling of heat, a feeling of heaviness of the body and limbs, Red tongue with sticky yellow coating, Slippery-Rapid pulse.

Heat in the Spleen and Heart

Toothache, bleeding gums, red lips, palpitations, thirst, mouth and tongue ulcers, mental restlessness, a feeling of agitation, insomnia, dream-disturbed sleep, a feeling of heat, red face, bitter taste, burning epigastric/abdominal pain, excessive hunger, red tip of the nose, dry lips, dry stools, Red tongue with dry yellow coating, Overflowing-Rapid pulse.

Invasion of external Wind

Toothache, aversion to cold, fever, stiff neck, occipital headache, sneezing.

Other symptoms and signs, including tongue and pulse, depend on whether the pattern is Wind-Cold or Wind-Heat.

'Wind-Cold in the Brain'

Severe toothache extending to the brain after an invasion of external Wind that has not been cleared, Purple tongue.

Tooth cavities

Observation, Chapter 8

Damp-Heat in the Stomach and Spleen

Tooth cavities, especially of lower teeth, bleeding gums, red lips, thirst with no desire to drink, sticky taste, a feeling of fullness and pain of the epigastrium and lower abdomen, poor appetite, a feeling of heaviness, nausea, loose stools with offensive odour, a feeling of heat, dull-yellow complexion, Red tongue with sticky yellow coating, Slippery-Rapid pulse.

Stomach- and Spleen-Qi deficiency

Tooth cavities, loose teeth, poor appetite, slight abdominal distension after eating, tiredness, lassitude, pale complexion, weakness of the limbs, loose stools, uncomfortable feeling in the epigastrium, lack of sense of taste, Pale tongue, Empty pulse.

Damp-Heat in the Large Intestine

Tooth cavities, especially of upper teeth, thirst with no desire to drink, mouth ulcers, abdominal pain that is not relieved by a bowel movement, diarrhoea, mucus and blood in stools, offensive odour of stools, burning in the anus, scanty dark urine, fever, sweating which does not decrease the fever, a feeling of heat, feeling of heaviness of the body and limbs, Red tongue with sticky yellow coating, Slippery-Rapid pulse.

Kidney deficiency

Tooth cavities, loose teeth, lower backache, dizziness, tinnitus, weak knees.

Other symptoms and signs, including pulse and tongue, depend on whether there is a Kidney-Yin or Kidney-Yang deficiency.

Loose teeth

Observation, Chapter 8

Stomach-Heat

Loose teeth, toothache, mouth ulcers, thirst, foul breath, burning epigastric pain, sour regurgitation, nausea, excessive hunger, a feeling of heat, Red tongue with a yellow coating, Overflowing-Rapid pulse.

Kidney deficiency

Loose teeth, lower backache, dizziness, tinnitus, tiredness, pulse Weak on both Rear positions.

Other symptoms and signs depends on whether there is a Kidney-Yang or Kidney-Yin deficiency.

Spleen-Yin deficiency with Empty-Heat

Loose teeth, toothache, red cheeks, poor appetite, poor digestion, retching, gnawing hunger, loss of sense of taste, slight epigastric pain, dry mouth and lips, dry stools, thin body, sallow complexion with red tip of the nose, night sweating, a feeling of heat in the evening, Red tongue without coating and transversal cracks on the sides, Floating-Empty and Rapid pulse.

Kidney-Yin deficiency with Empty-Heat

Loose teeth, dizziness, tinnitus, vertigo, poor memory, hardness of hearing, night sweating, dry mouth at night, five-palm heat, a feeling of heat in the evening, malar flush, menopausal hot flushes, thirst with a desire to sip fluids, lower backache, ache in bones, nocturnal emissions with dreams, constipation, scanty dark urine, infertility, premature ejaculation, tiredness, depression, anxiety, insomnia, excessive menstrual bleeding, Red tongue without coating, Floating-Empty and Rapid pulse.

Grinding teeth

Liver-Qi invading the Spleen

Grinding teeth when tense, irritability, abdominal distension and pain, alternation of constipation and diarrhoea, stools sometimes dry and bitty (small pieces) and sometimes loose, flatulence, tiredness, tongue normal coloured or slightly Red on the sides, pulse Wiry on the left and Weak on the right.

Stomach- and Heart-Fire

Grinding teeth, bleeding gums, burning epigastric pain, intense thirst with desire to drink cold liquids, mental restlessness, dry mouth, mouth ulcers, bleeding gums, dry stools, sour regurgitation, foul breath, nausea, vomiting soon after eating, a feeling of heat, sour regurgitation, palpitations, insomnia, dream-disturbed sleep, red face, bitter taste, tongue Red with a thick, dry, dark-yellow coating, Deep-Full-Rapid pulse.

Retention of food

Grinding of teeth in children, fullness, pain and distension of the epigastrium which are relieved by vomiting, nausea, vomiting of sour fluids, foul breath, sour regurgitation, belching, insomnia, loose stools or

constipation, poor appetite, thick tongue coating, Full-Slippery pulse.

Deficiency of Qi and Blood

Weakly grinding teeth, poor appetite, loose stools, weak voice, tiredness, blurred vision, dizziness, numbness/tingling of limbs, palpitations, dull-pale complexion, Pale tongue, Weak or Choppy pulse.

Internal Empty-Wind

Grinding teeth, dizziness, headache, tics, fine tremors, tiredness, blurred vision, poor memory, Fine and slightly Wiry pulse.

The tongue may be Pale or Red without coating depending on whether there is an underlying Blood or Yin deficiency.

Invasion of External Wind

Grinding teeth, shivering, aversion to cold, fever, stiff neck, occipital headache, body aches, Floating pulse.

Plaque

Observation, Chapter 8

Stomach-Heat

Plaque, teeth yellow at the junction with the gums, thirst, foul breath, burning epigastric pain, sour regurgitation, nausea, excessive hunger, a feeling of heat, Red tongue with a yellow coating, Overflowing-Rapid pulse.

Heat in the Stomach and Kidneys

Plaque, teeth yellow at the junction with the gums, burning epigastric pain, thirst, sour regurgitation, nausea, excessive hunger, foul breath, a feeling of heat, dark urine, painful urination, backache, Red tongue with yellow coating, Overflowing-Rapid pulse.

Kidney-Yin deficiency

Plaque, teeth dull yellow at the junction with the gums, dizziness, tinnitus, hardness of hearing, poor memory, night sweating, vertigo, dry mouth and throat at night, lower backache, ache in the bones, nocturnal emissions, constipation, dark scanty urine, infertility, premature ejaculation, tiredness, lassitude, depression, slight anxiety, normal-coloured tongue without coating, Floating-Empty pulse.

Dry and white teeth

Observation, Chapter 8

Acute interior Heat following an invasion of Wind-Heat

White, dry teeth, a feeling of heat, fever, thirst, sweating, Red tongue with yellow coating, Overflowing-Rapid pulse.

Stomach-Heat

White, dry teeth, thirst, foul breath, burning epigastric pain, sour regurgitation, nausea, excessive hunger, a feeling of heat, Red tongue with a yellow coating, Overflowing-Rapid pulse.

Dry and dull teeth

Observation, Chapter 8

Kidney-Yin deficiency

Dry, dull teeth which look like dry bones, dizziness, tinnitus, hardness of hearing, poor memory, night sweating, vertigo, dry mouth and throat at night, lower backache, ache in the bones, nocturnal emissions, constipation, dark scanty urine, infertility, premature ejaculation, tiredness, lassitude, depression, slight anxiety, normal-coloured tongue without coating, Floating-Empty pulse.

Kidney-Yin deficiency with Empty-Heat

Very dry, dull teeth which look like dry bones, dizziness, tinnitus, vertigo, poor memory, hardness of hearing, night sweating, dry mouth at night, five-palm heat, a feeling of heat in the evening, malar flush, menopausal hot flushes, thirst with desire to sip fluids, lower backache, ache in the bones, nocturnal emissions with dreams, constipation, dark scanty urine, infertility, premature ejaculation, tiredness, depression, anxiety, insomnia, excessive menstrual bleeding, Red tongue without coating, Floating-Empty and Rapid pulse.

Liver-Blood deficiency

Dry, dull teeth, dizziness, blurred vision, floaters, numbness/tingling of limbs, scanty menstruation, dull-pale complexion, Pale tongue, Choppy or Fine pulse.

Yellow and dry teeth

Observation, Chapter 8

Damp-Heat in the Stomach and Spleen with predominance of Heat

Yellow and dry teeth, dull-yellow complexion, a feeling of fullness and pain of the epigastrium and lower abdomen, poor appetite, a feeling of heaviness, thirst without desire to drink, nausea, loose stools with offensive odour, a feeling of heat, dull-yellow complexion, sticky taste, Red tongue with sticky yellow coating, Slippery-Rapid pulse.

Kidney-Yin deficiency

Dull-yellow and dry teeth, dizziness, tinnitus, hardness of hearing, poor memory, night sweating, vertigo, dry mouth and throat at night, lower backache, ache in the bones, nocturnal emissions, constipation, dark scanty urine, infertility, premature ejaculation, tiredness, lassitude, depression, slight anxiety, normal-coloured tongue without coating, Floating-Empty pulse.

Accumulation of Cold in the abdomen with false Yang above

Yellow and dry teeth, abdominal pain, a feeling of cold, cold feet, Pale tongue, Tight-Slow pulse.

Grey teeth

Observation, Chapter 8

Kidney-Yin deficiency with Empty-Heat

Grey and dry teeth, dizziness, tinnitus, vertigo, poor memory, hardness of hearing, night sweating, dry mouth at night, five-palm heat, a feeling of heat in the evening, malar flush, menopausal hot flushes, thirst with a desire to sip fluids, lower backache, ache in the bones, nocturnal emissions with dreams, constipation, dark scanty urine, infertility, premature ejaculation, tiredness, depression, anxiety, insomnia, excessive menstrual bleeding, Red tongue without coating, Floating-Empty and Rapid pulse.

Upper teeth moist and lower teeth dry

Observation, Chapter 8

Kidney- and Heart-Yin deficiency with Heart Empty-Heat (Kidneys and Heart not harmonized)

Upper teeth moist and lower teeth dry, dry mouth with a desire to sip water, palpitations, mental restlessness, insomnia, dream-disturbed sleep, anxiety, poor memory, dizziness, tinnitus, hardness of hearing, lower backache, nocturnal emissions with dreams, a feeling of heat in the evening, night sweating, five-palm heat, scanty dark urine, dry stools, Red tongue with redder tip and a Heart crack, Floating-Empty and Rapid pulse or a pulse that is Deep and Weak on both Rear positions and Overflowing on both Front positions.

GUMS

Inflamed gums

Observation, Chapter 8; Interrogation, Chapter 35

Stomach-Heat

Inflamed gums, foul breath, mouth ulcers especially on the lower gum, thirst, burning epigastric pain, sour regurgitation, nausea, excessive hunger, a feeling of heat, Red tongue with a yellow coating, Overflowing-Rapid pulse.

Stomach-Yin deficiency with Empty-Heat

Inflamed gums, especially lower gum, bleeding gums, mouth ulcers with a white rim, dry mouth and throat especially in the afternoon, thirst with a desire to drink in small sips, dull or burning epigastric pain, a feeling of heat in the afternoon, dry stools, a slight feeling of fullness after eating, night sweating, five-palm heat, Red tongue (or Red centre only) without coating in the centre, Floating-Empty and Rapid pulse.

Invasion of Wind-Heat

Inflamed gums, aversion to cold, fever, cough, sore throat, stuffed or runny nose with yellow discharge, headache, body aches, slight sweating, slight thirst, swollen tonsils, tongue slightly Red on the sides in the chest area or on front part, Floating-Rapid pulse.

Purple Leg and Teeth Nutritional Impairment Pattern

Swollen, inflamed and bleeding gums, cracked lips, painful legs, swelling of the legs in patches like clouds and discoloured like unripe aubergine seeds, hardness of the flesh, difficulty in walking.

There are actually two manifestations of this pattern, one with Damp-Cold and the other with Toxic Heat. If there is Damp-Cold there will also be a feeling of heaviness, cold limbs, oedema and ache in the joints. If there is Toxic Heat, there will be a bitter taste, dry mouth, thirst, foul breath, Red tongue with red points and thick, sticky, dry yellow coating and an Overflowing-Slippery-Rapid pulse.

'Walking Crow' Teeth Nutritional Impairment Pattern

In the beginning hard, red nodules on the gum, after 1 or 2 days the gums become inflamed and then greyish-black, bleeding gums that are neither painful nor itchy, foul breath, Red tongue with sticky yellow coating.

This pattern is more common in children.

Bleeding gums

Observation, Chapter 8: Interrogation, Chapter 35

Deficient Spleen-Qi not holding Blood

Bleeding gums, poor appetite, slight abdominal distension after eating, tiredness, lassitude, pale complexion, weakness of the limbs, loose stools, slight depression, tendency to obesity, Pale tongue, Empty pulse.

Stomach-Fire

Bleeding and painful gums, foul breath, intense thirst with a desire to drink cold liquids, burning epigastric pain, mental restlessness, dry mouth, mouth ulcers, bleeding gums, dry stools, sour regurgitation, nausea, vomiting soon after eating, a feeling of heat, sour regurgitation, Red tongue with a thick, dry, dark-yellow coating, Deep-Full-Rapid pulse.

Stomach-Yin deficiency with Empty Heat

Bleeding gums, dry mouth and throat especially in the afternoon, thirst with a desire to drink in small sips, dull or burning epigastric pain, a feeling of heat in the afternoon, constipation (dry stools), a feeling of hunger but no desire to eat, a slight feeling of fullness after eating, night sweating, five-palm heat, bleeding gums, Red tongue (or Red centre only) without coating in the centre, Floating-Empty and Rapid pulse.

Kidney-Yin deficiency with Empty-Heat

Bleeding gums, dizziness, tinnitus, vertigo, poor memory, deafness, night sweating, dry mouth at night, five-palm heat, a feeling of heat in the evening, malar flush, menopausal hot flushes, thirst with a desire to sip fluids, lower backache, ache in bones, nocturnal emissions with dreams, constipation, scanty dark urine, infertility, premature ejaculation, tiredness, depression, anxiety, insomnia, excessive menstrual bleeding, Red tongue without coating, Floating-Empty and Rapid pulse.

Receding gums

Observation, Chapter 8: Interrogation, Chapter 35

Deficiency of Qi and Blood

Receding gums, pale lips, pale gums, poor appetite, loose stools, weak voice, tiredness, blurred vision, dizziness, numbness/tingling of limbs, palpitations, dull-pale complexion, Pale tongue, Weak or Choppy pulse.

Stomach-Fire

Receding gums, red gums, mouth ulcers, bleeding gums, foul breath, burning epigastric pain, intense thirst with a desire to drink cold liquids, mental restlessness, bleeding gums, dry stools, dry mouth, mouth ulcers, nausea, vomiting soon after eating, sour regurgitation, a feeling of heat, tongue Red with a thick, dry, dark-yellow coating, Deep-Full-Rapid pulse.

Kidney-Yin deficiency with Empty-Heat

Receding gums, bleeding gums, dizziness, tinnitus, vertigo, poor memory, deafness, night sweating, dry mouth at night, five-palm heat, a feeling of heat in the evening, malar flush, menopausal hot flushes, thirst with desire to sip fluids, lower backache, ache in bones, nocturnal emissions with dreams, constipation, scanty dark urine, infertility, premature ejaculation, tiredness, depression, anxiety, insomnia, excessive menstrual bleeding, Red tongue without coating, Floating-Empty and Rapid pulse.

Clinical note

- Remember that, apart from the Stomach, the Kidneys also influence the gums. 'Loose teeth' is a sign associated with a Kidney deficiency in Chinese medicine, but teeth also become loose from gum disease.

Gums oozing pus

Observation, Chapter 8

Stomach-Fire

Gums oozing pus, tooth abscess, red and swollen gums, bleeding gums, toothache, foul breath, burning epigastric pain, intense thirst with a desire to drink cold liquids, mental restlessness, dry stools, dry mouth, mouth ulcers, nausea, vomiting soon after eating, sour regurgitation, a feeling of heat, Red tongue with a thick, dry, dark-yellow coating, Deep-Full-Rapid pulse.

Invasion of Wind-Heat with Toxic Heat

Gums oozing pus, swollen glands, bleeding gums, aversion to cold, sore throat, fever, tonsillitis, tonsils oozing pus, headache, tongue red on the sides with red points and a yellow coating, Floating-Rapid pulse.

Severe deficiency of Qi and Blood with Toxic Heat

Chronic, recurrent bouts of gums oozing pus, ulcers on the gums which are slow to heal, poor appetite, loose stools, weak voice, tiredness, blurred vision, dizziness, numbness/tingling of limbs, palpitations, dull-pale complexion, Pale tongue, Weak or Choppy pulse.

Pale gums

Observation, Chapter 8

Spleen-Qi deficiency

Pale gums, pale lips, poor appetite, tiredness, slight abdominal distension, pale complexion, loose stools, Pale tongue, Empty pulse.

Blood deficiency

Dull-pale gums, tiredness, dizziness, blurred vision, scanty periods, Pale tongue, Choppy or Weak pulse.

Spleen-Yang deficiency with Empty-Cold

Bright-pale gums, poor appetite, slight abdominal distension after eating, tiredness, lassitude, pale complexion, weakness of the limbs, loose stools, slight depression, tendency to obesity, a feeling of cold, cold limbs, oedema. Pale and wet tongue, Deep-Weak pulse.

Red gums

Observation, Chapter 8

Stomach-Heat

Bright-red gums, swollen gums, bleeding gums, thirst, foul breath, burning epigastric pain, sour regurgitation, nausea, excessive hunger, a feeling of heat, Red tongue with a yellow coating, Overflowing-Rapid pulse.

Stomach-Yin deficiency with Empty-Heat

Red gums, bleeding gums, a feeling of heat in the afternoon, dry mouth and throat especially in the afternoon, thirst with a desire to drink in small sips, dull or burning epigastric pain, a feeling of heat in the afternoon, constipation (dry stools), feeling of hunger but no desire to eat, a slight feeling of fullness after eating, night sweating, five-palm heat, Red tongue (or Red centre only) without coating in the centre, Floating-Empty and Rapid pulse.

Spleen-Heat

Red gums, dry and red lips, burning epigastric/abdominal pain, excessive hunger, red tip of the nose, mouth ulcers, thirst, dry stools, a feeling of heat, scanty dark urine, yellow complexion, Red tongue with dry yellow coating, Overflowing-Rapid pulse.

Spleen Empty-Heat

Pale-red gums, poor appetite, poor digestion, retching, gnawing hunger, loss of taste, slight epigastric pain, dry mouth and lips, dry stools, thin body, sallow complexion with red tip of the nose, night sweating, a feeling of heat in the evening, malar flush, Red tongue without coating and transversal cracks on the sides, Floating-Empty and Rapid pulse.

Purple gums

Observation, Chapter 8

Blood stasis in the Stomach

Purple gums, bleeding gums, toothache, purple lips, severe, stabbing epigastric pain that may be worse at night, dislike of pressure, nausea, vomiting, possibly vomiting of blood, vomiting of food looking like coffee grounds, Purple tongue, Wiry pulse.

Heat at the Blood level in febrile diseases

Purple gums, bleeding gums, dark macular rash. mental confusion, fever at night, high fever, irritability, vomiting of blood, epistaxis, blood in stools, blood in urine, Dark-Red tongue without coating, Fine-Wiry-Rapid pulse.

LIPS

Pale lips

Observation, Chapter 8

Deficiency of Qi and Blood of the Spleen

Pale lips, dull-pale complexion, poor appetite, slight abdominal distension after eating, tiredness, lassitude, weakness of the limbs, loose stools, thin body, scanty periods or amenorrhoea, insomnia, joint ache, Pale tongue, Weak or Choppy pulse.

Liver-Blood deficiency

Pale lips, dull-pale complexion, dizziness, blurred vision, floaters, numbness/tingling of limbs, scanty menstruation, Pale tongue, Choppy or Fine pulse.

Spleen-Yang deficiency with Empty-Cold

Pale and slightly bluish lips or bright-white lips, pale complexion, poor appetite, slight abdominal distension after eating, abdominal pain, tiredness, lassitude, weakness of the limbs, loose stools, a feeling of cold, cold limbs, Pale and wet tongue, Deep-Weak-Slow pulse.

Red lips

Observation, Chapter 8

Full-Heat

Red and swollen lips, thirst, dry stools, a feeling of heat, Red tongue with yellow coating, Overflowing-Rapid pulse.

Heat in the Heart, Lungs, Stomach, Liver, Kidneys and Spleen may all cause red lips and other symptoms and signs depend on the organ involved.

Yin deficiency with Empty-Heat

Red, cracked and dry lips, dry mouth, thirst with a desire to drink in small sips, feeling of heat in the evening, night sweating, five-palm heat, Red tongue without coating, Floating-Empty and Rapid pulse.

Empty-Heat in the Heart, Lungs, Stomach, Liver, Kidneys and Spleen may all cause red lips and other symptoms and signs depend on the organ involved.

Invasion of Wind-Heat

Red lips (especially in children), aversion to cold, fever, sore throat, headache, body aches, slight sweating, tongue with Red sides or front or both, Floating-Rapid pulse.

Acute Heat at the Qi level in febrile diseases (Heat)

Red and swollen lips, fever, a feeling of heat, throwing off of the bedclothes, thirst, profuse sweating, Red tongue with yellow coating, Overflowing-Rapid pulse.

Acute Heat at the Qi level in febrile diseases (Fire)

Red, swollen, dry and cracked lips, fever, a feeling of heat, thirst, dry mouth, dry stools, dark urine, mental restlessness, Red tongue with dry, dark-yellow or brown coating, Deep-Full-Rapid pulse.

Purple lips

Observation, Chapter 8

Blood stasis

Purple lips, dark complexion, headache, chest, hypochondrial or abdominal pain, palpitations, Purple tongue, Wiry pulse.

Other symptoms and signs depend on the organ involved, which may be the Liver or the Heart.

Severe Spleen-Yang deficiency with Empty-Cold

Purple lips, pale complexion, poor appetite, slight abdominal distension after eating, abdominal pain, tiredness, lassitude, weakness of the limbs, loose stools, a feeling of cold, cold limbs. Pale and wet tongue, Deep-Weak-Slow pulse.

Severe Kidney-Yang deficiency with Empty-Cold

Purple lips, lower backache, cold knees, a feeling of cold, bright-white complexion, weak knees, tiredness, lassitude, abundant clear urination, urination at night, impotence, decreased libido, Pale and wet tongue, Deep-Weak pulse.

This is a severe deficiency of Kidney-Yang with internal Empty-Cold that leads to some Blood stasis; for this reason the complexion is dark rather than pale, as it should be in Yang deficiency.

Internal Full-Cold

Bluish-purple lips, bright-white complexion, a feeling of cold, cold limbs, abdominal pain, bright-pale complexion, thick white tongue coating, Deep-Full-Tight-Slow pulse.

Other symptoms and signs depend on the organ involved.

Turbid Phlegm in the Lungs

Bluish-purple lips, sticky taste, breathlessness, expectoration of phlegm, wheezing, inability to lie down, a feeling of oppression of the chest, sticky, dirty tongue coating, Slippery pulse.

Heat at the Nutritive-Qi or Blood level in acute febrile diseases

Reddish-purple lips, fever at night, mental restlessness and confusion, macular rash, bleeding, Red tongue without coating, Fine-Rapid pulse.

Bluish-greenish lips

Observation, Chapter 8

Internal Cold

Bluish lips, bluish-white complexion, a feeling of cold, cold limbs, abdominal pain.

Other symptoms, including tongue and pulse, depend on whether it is Full- or Empty-Cold and also on the organ involved.

Stagnation of Qi and stasis of Blood

Greenish lips, greenish complexion, abdominal distension and pain, irritability, chest pain, Purple tongue, Wiry or Choppy pulse.

Qi and Blood stagnation of the Heart, Lungs, Stomach or Liver may cause greenish lips and other symptoms and signs depend on the organ involved.

Yellow lips

Observation, Chapter 8

Damp-Heat in the Stomach and Spleen

Bright-yellow lips, sticky taste, dull-yellow complexion, a feeling of fullness and pain of the epigastrium and lower abdomen, poor appetite, a feeling of heaviness, thirst without desire to drink, nausea, loose stools with offensive odour, a feeling of heat, dull-yellow complexion, Red tongue with sticky yellow coating, Slippery-Rapid pulse.

Cold-Dampness in the Stomach and Spleen

Dull-yellow lips, dull-yellowish complexion, sticky taste, abdominal pain, a feeling of cold in the abdomen, cold limbs, a feeling of fullness and heaviness, Pale tongue with sticky white coating, Slippery-Slow pulse.

Full-Heat with Blood stasis

Dark-yellow lips, a feeling of heat, thirst, abdominal pain, headache, chest pain, Reddish-Purple tongue, Wiry or Choppy and Rapid pulse.

Other symptoms and signs depend on the organ involved.

Dry or cracked lips

Observation, Chapter 8

Stomach- and Spleen-Yin deficiency

Dry lips, dry mouth, no appetite or slight hunger but no desire to eat, constipation (dry stools), dull or slightly burning epigastric pain, dry mouth and throat especially in the afternoon, thirst but with no desire to drink, or a desire to drink in small sips, a slight feeling of fullness after eating, normal-coloured tongue without coating in the centre, Floating-Empty pulse.

Full-Heat

Cracked, red and swollen lips, thirst, dry stools, a feeling of heat, Red tongue with yellow coating, Overflowing-Rapid pulse.

Heat of the Lungs, Stomach, Spleen and Large Intestine may cause cracked lips and other symptoms and signs depend on which organ is involved.

Yin deficiency with Empty-Heat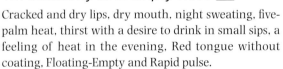

Cracked and dry lips, dry mouth, night sweating, five-palm heat, thirst with a desire to drink in small sips, a feeling of heat in the evening, Red tongue without coating, Floating-Empty and Rapid pulse.

Empty-Heat of the Lungs, Stomach, Spleen and Large Intestine may cause cracked lips and other symptoms and signs depend on which organ is involved.

Liver-Blood deficiency

Slightly cracked and dry lips, dizziness, blurred vision, floaters, numbness/tingling of limbs, scanty menstruation, dull-pale complexion, Pale tongue, Choppy or Fine pulse.

Blood stasis

Cracked, dry and purple lips, dry mouth with desire to drink without swallowing, headache, chest pain, abdominal pain, Purple tongue, Wiry or Choppy pulse.

Blood stasis of the Heart, Lungs, Stomach or Liver may cause cracked lips and other symptoms and signs depend on the organ involved. As there is an interchange between Blood and Body Fluids, severe, long-standing Blood stasis impairs the metabolism of Body Fluids and causes Dryness.

> ### Clinical note
>
> - In women, dry lips is often a sign 'clinching' the diagnosis of Spleen-Yin deficiency.

Trembling lips

Observation, Chapter 8

Spleen-Qi deficiency

Slow, trembling lips, pale lips, pale complexion, poor appetite, tiredness, slight abdominal distension, loose stools, Pale tongue, Empty pulse.

Blood deficiency with Empty-Wind

Trembling and dry lips, itching around the mouth, dry skin, slight tremor of the head or hand or both, facial tic, dizziness, blurred vision, unilateral numbness/tingling of a limb, Pale and Thin tongue, Choppy or Fine and slightly Wiry pulse.

Stomach-Fire

Fast, trembling lips, red lips, bleeding gums, intense thirst with a desire to drink cold liquids, foul breath, dry mouth, mouth ulcers, burning epigastric pain, mental restlessness, bleeding gums, dry stools, sour regurgitation, nausea, vomiting soon after eating, a feeling of heat, sour regurgitation, tongue Red with a thick, dry dark-yellow coating, Deep-Full-Rapid pulse.

Peeled lips

Observation, Chapter 8

Spleen-Heat

Peeled, fresh red, cracked and swollen lips, dry lips, mouth ulcers, thirst, burning epigastric/abdominal pain, excessive hunger, red tip of the nose, dry stools, a feeling of heat, scanty dark urine, yellow complexion, Red tongue with dry yellow coating, Overflowing-Rapid pulse.

Spleen-Yin deficiency with Empty-Heat

Peeled, dry, cracked lips, poor appetite, poor digestion, retching, gnawing hunger, loss of taste, slight epigastric pain, dry stools, thin body, sallow complexion with red tip of the nose, night sweating, a feeling of heat in the evening, malar flush, Red tongue without coating and transversal cracks on the sides, Floating-Empty and Rapid pulse.

Swollen lips

Observation, Chapter 8

Toxic Heat affecting Stomach and Spleen

Swollen, dark lips, thirst, feeling of heat, mental restlessness, pustular rashes, swelling, pain, headache, Red tongue with red points and thick, sticky yellow coating, Overflowing-Slippery-Rapid pulse.

Damp-Heat in the Stomach and Spleen

Swollen and bright red lips, a feeling of fullness and pain of the epigastrium and lower abdomen, poor appetite, a feeling of heaviness, thirst without a desire to drink, nausea, loose stools with offensive odour, a feeling of heat, dull-yellow complexion, sticky taste, Red tongue with sticky yellow coating, Slippery-Rapid pulse.

Wind-Heat in the skin

Swollen and bright-red lips with acute onset, urticarial rash, swelling of the throat, itching, red eyes.

This corresponds to an allergic reaction to foods or a bee sting.

Inverted lips

Observation, Chapter 8

Severe Yang deficiency

Inverted lips, cold limbs, sweating, feeling cold, lassitude, backache, dizziness, tinnitus, loose stools, Pale and wet tongue, Deep-Weak or Scattered pulse.

Other symptoms and signs depend on the organ involved.

Severe Yin deficiency

Inverted lips, a feeling of heat, dry skin, dry mouth, dry nails, dizziness, tinnitus, night sweating, tongue without coating, Fine or Minute pulse.

Other symptoms and signs depend on the organ involved.

Drooping lips

Observation, Chapter 8

Spleen-Qi deficient and sinking

Drooping lips, a feeling of bearing down in the abdomen, prolapse, poor appetite, slight abdominal distension after eating, tiredness, lassitude, pale complexion, weakness of the limbs, loose stools, Pale tongue, Empty pulse.

Spleen- and Kidney-Yang deficiency

Drooping lips, lower backache, cold and weak knees, a feeling of cold, bright-white complexion, impotence, decreased libido, tiredness, lassitude, abundant clear urination, urination at night, loose stools, poor appetite, slight abdominal distension, a desire to lie down, early-morning diarrhoea, Pale and wet tongue, Deep-Weak pulse.

Abnormal lip colour in pregnancy

Observation, Chapter 8

Blood deficiency

Pale lips in pregnancy, dizziness, blurred vision, floaters, numbness/tingling of limbs, dull-pale complexion, palpitations, Pale tongue, Choppy or Fine pulse.

Severe Blood deficiency

White-coloured lips, dryness of the corners of the mouth, exhaustion, palpitations, dizziness, blurred vision, floaters, numbness/tingling of limbs, dull-pale complexion, dry skin, tongue Pale and dry or Pale and without coating, Choppy or Fine pulse.

Blood stasis from Cold

Bluish lips in pregnancy, abdominal pain that is alleviated by the application of heat, chest pain, headache, cold limbs, Bluish-purple tongue, Tight pulse.

PALATE

Pale palate

Observation, Chapter 8

Stomach- and Spleen-Qi deficiency

Pale palate that looks like the skin of milk, poor appetite, slight abdominal distension after eating, tiredness, lassitude, pale complexion, weakness of the limbs, loose stools, an uncomfortable feeling in the epigastrium, lack of sense of taste, Pale tongue, Empty pulse.

Stomach- and Spleen-Yang deficiency

Pale palate that looks almost white, poor appetite, slight abdominal distension after eating, tiredness, pale complexion, weakness of the limbs, loose stools, uncomfortable feeling of the epigastrium, lack of taste sensation, a feeling of cold, cold limbs, Pale and wet tongue, Weak-Deep pulse.

Dull-pale palate

Observation, Chapter 8

Spleen- and Liver-Blood deficiency

Dull-pale palate, poor appetite, slight abdominal distension after eating, tiredness, dull-pale complexion, weakness of the limbs, loose stools, thin body, scanty periods or amenorrhoea, insomnia, dizziness, numbness of limbs, blurred vision, 'floaters' in eyes, pale lips, cramps, withered and brittle nails, dry hair and skin, Pale and dry tongue, Choppy or Fine pulse.

Deficiency of Qi and Blood

Dull-pale palate, poor appetite, loose stools, weak voice, tiredness, blurred vision, dizziness, numbness/tingling of limbs, palpitations, dull-pale complexion, Pale tongue, Weak or Choppy pulse.

Yellow palate

Observation, Chapter 8

Chronic Stomach- and Spleen-Qi deficiency

Dull-yellow palate, poor appetite, slight abdominal distension after eating, tiredness, pale complexion, weakness of the limbs, loose stools, uncomfortable feeling of the epigastrium, lack of sense of taste, Pale tongue, Empty pulse.

Dampness in the Stomach and Spleen

Bright-yellow palate, a feeling of fullness and pain of the epigastrium and lower abdomen, poor appetite, a feeling of heaviness, thirst without a desire to drink, nausea, loose stools with offensive odour, a feeling of heat, dull-yellow complexion, sticky taste, Red tongue with sticky yellow coating, Slippery-Rapid pulse.

Red palate

Observation, Chapter 8

Full-Heat

Red palate, thirst, mouth ulcers, a feeling of heat, mental restlessness, Red tongue with yellow coating, Overflowing-Rapid pulse.

Other symptoms and signs depend on the organ involved.

Purple palate

Observation, Chapter 8

Blood stasis

Purple palate, abdominal pain, chest pain, headache, mental restlessness, Purple tongue, Wiry or Choppy pulse.

Other symptoms and signs depend on the organ involved (usually the Liver, Lungs, Stomach or Heart).

PHILTRUM

Flat philtrum

Observation, Chapter 8

Kidney deficiency

Flat philtrum, lower backache, dizziness, tinnitus, tiredness.

Other symptoms and signs, including pulse and tongue, depend on whether there is a Kidney-Yang or Kidney-Yin deficiency.

Damp-Heat in the Stomach and Spleen

Flat philtrum, a feeling of fullness and pain of the epigastrium and lower abdomen, poor appetite, a feeling of heaviness, thirst without a desire to drink, nausea, loose stools with offensive odour, a feeling of heat, dull-yellow complexion, sticky taste, Red tongue with sticky yellow coating, Slippery-Rapid pulse.

> ### Clinical note
>
> - According to the ancient Chinese art of face reading, a flat philtrum in women may indicate infertility.

Stiff-looking philtrum

Observation, Chapter 8

Blood stasis

Stiff-looking philtrum, dark lips, abdominal pain, chest pain, headache, Purple tongue, Wiry or Choppy pulse.

Pale philtrum

Observation, Chapter 8

Qi deficiency

Pale philtrum, tiredness, poor appetite, loose stools, weak voice, Pale tongue, Empty pulse.

Other symptoms and signs depend on the organ involved.

Full-Cold

Bright-pale philtrum, greyish-pale complexion, abdominal pain, epigastric pain, cold limbs, pain alleviated by exposure to heat and by drinking warm drinks and aggravated by exposure to cold and by drinking cold drinks, thick white tongue coating, Tight pulse.

Other symptoms and signs depend on the organ involved.

Empty-Cold

Pale philtrum, greyish-pale complexion, dull abdominal pain, dull epigastric pain, cold limbs, pain alleviated by exposure to heat and by drinking warm drinks, and aggravated by exposure to cold and by drinking cold drinks, a feeling of cold, tiredness, Pale tongue with thin white tongue coating, Deep-Weak pulse.

Other symptoms and signs depend on the organ involved.

Red philtrum

Observation, Chapter 8

Heat in the Blood

Red philtrum, skin rashes, a feeling of heat, thirst, bleeding, mental restlessness, Red tongue, Overflowing-Rapid pulse.

Invasion of Wind-Heat

Red philtrum, aversion to cold, fever, sore throat, headache, body aches, slight sweating, tongue with Red sides/front, Floating-Rapid pulse.

Damp-Heat in the Intestines

Red philtrum with skin spots oozing fluid, abdominal pain that is not relieved by a bowel movement, diarrhoea, mucus and blood in stools, offensive odour of stools, burning in the anus, scanty dark urine, fever, sweating which does not decrease the fever, a feeling of heat, thirst without a desire to drink, a feeling of heaviness of the body and limbs, Red tongue with sticky yellow coating, Slippery-Rapid pulse.

Bluish-greenish philtrum

Observation, Chapter 8

Internal Cold

Bluish philtrum, a feeling of cold, abdominal pain, cold limbs, Pale tongue, Deep pulse.

Other symptoms and signs depend on whether there is Full- or Empty-Cold.

Liver-Qi stagnation

Greenish philtrum, hypochondrial or epigastric distension, irritability, moodiness, a feeling of a lump in the throat, premenstrual tension, Wiry pulse.

Dark philtrum

Observation, Chapter 8

Heat in the Blood

Dark philtrum, skin rashes, a feeling of heat, thirst, bleeding, mental restlessness, Red tongue, Overflowing-Rapid pulse.

Damp-Heat in the Lower Burner

Dark philtrum, yellow, itchy vaginal discharge, lower abdominal pain, dark/cloudy urine, tongue with sticky yellow coating on the root, Slippery-Rapid pulse.

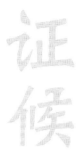

Chapter **61**

EYES

Chapter contents

VISION   *628*
  Blurred vision and floaters   *628*
  Strabismus   *628*
  Myopia   *629*
  Hyperopia   *629*
  Decreased night vision   *630*
  Decreased visual acuity   *630*
  Sudden blindness   *630*

ITCHY EYES   *631*

DRY EYES   *631*

HOT AND PAINFUL EYES   *632*

STREAMING EYES   *633*

DISCHARGE FROM THE EYES   *634*

EYE COLOUR   *634*
  Yellow (sclera)   *634*
  Red (sclera)   *635*
  Bluish-greenish (sclera)   *635*
  Dark (sclera)   *636*
  Pale corners   *636*
  Red corners   *636*

EYELIDS   *637*
  Stye   *637*
  Red eyelids   *637*
  Dark eyelids   *638*
  Green eyelids   *638*
  Pale eyelids   *638*
  Swollen eyelids   *638*
  Boil on the eyelid   *639*
  Pain of the eyelids   *639*
  Flapping eyelids   *639*
  Drooping eyelids   *640*
  Loss of control of the eyelids   *640*
  Nodules within the eyelids   *640*
  Small red grains inside the eyelids   *641*
  Redness inside the lower lids   *641*

GLAUCOMA   *641*

FEELING OF DISTENSION OF THE EYES   *641*

EYEBALL   *642*
  Protruding eyeball   *642*
  Sunken eyeball   *643*
  Scaly eyeballs   *643*
  Quivering eyeball   *644*
  Eyeball turning up   *644*

ECCHYMOSIS UNDER CONJUNCTIVA   *644*

RED VEINS/MEMBRANE   *645*
  Red veins in the eyes   *645*
  Drooping red membrane   *645*
  Red membrane in the corner of the eye   *646*

CORNEA   *646*
  Corneal opacity   *646*
  Scarring after corneal opacity   *647*

WHITE SPECKS   *647*

PUPILS   *647*
  Red ring around the pupil   *647*
  White membrane on the pupil in children   *648*
  Yellow fluid between pupil and iris   *648*
  Bleeding between pupil and iris   *649*
  Dilated pupils   *649*
  Contracted pupils   *649*

STARING, FIXED EYES   *650*

CLOSED EYES   *650*

OPEN EYES   *650*

INVERTED EYELASHES   *650*

CATARACT   *651*

VISION

Blurred vision and floaters

Interrogation, Chapter 42

There are three Chinese terms which may be translated as 'blurred vision'. The first is *mu xuan* (*mu* meaning 'eye'), in which the term *xuan* suggests also dizziness; the second is *mu hun*, in which the term *hun* suggests 'faint feeling'; the third is *mu hua*, in which the term *hua* means 'flower' and the two terms together indicate that the patient sees objects that look like flowers or butterfly wings (i.e. floaters). This third term could therefore be translated more specifically as 'seeing floaters'. Therefore, the Chinese term for blurred vision also implies the symptom of dizziness and there is a certain overlap between these two terms and symptoms. In fact, the term for 'dizziness' is *xuan yun*, *xuan* being the same character as in *mu xuan* meaning blurred vision.

Liver-Blood deficiency

Blurred vision or floaters or both, dizziness, numbness/tingling of the limbs, scanty menstruation, dull-pale complexion, Pale tongue, Choppy or Fine pulse.

Liver-Yin deficiency

Blurred vision or floaters or both, dry eyes, diminished night vision, dizziness, dry hair, numbness/tingling of the limbs, insomnia, scanty menstruation or amenorrhoea, dull-pale complexion without lustre but with red cheekbones, cramps, withered and brittle nails, night sweating, normal-coloured tongue without coating, Fine or Floating-Empty pulse.

Kidney-Yin deficiency

Blurred vision or floaters or both, dry eyes, dizziness, tinnitus, hardness of hearing, poor memory, night sweating, vertigo, dry mouth and throat at night, lower backache, constipation, scanty dark urine, tiredness, normal-coloured tongue without coating, Floating-Empty pulse.

Turbid Phlegm in the head

Blurred vision or floaters or both, dull headache with a feeling of heaviness and muzziness of the head, poor memory and concentration, dizziness, sputum in the throat, a feeling of oppression of the chest, nausea, Swollen tongue with sticky coating, Slippery pulse.

Liver-Yang rising

Blurred vision or floaters or both, often occurring during a headache attack, headache, dizziness, tinnitus, irritability, propensity to outbursts of anger, Wiry pulse.

Heart-Blood deficiency

Blurred vision or floaters or both, palpitations, dizziness, insomnia, dream-disturbed sleep, poor memory, anxiety, tendency to be easily startled, dull-pale complexion, pale lips, Pale and Thin tongue, Choppy or Fine pulse.

Liver-Fire

Blurred vision, bloodshot eyes, painful eyes, headache, red face, dizziness, tinnitus, irritability, propensity to outbursts of anger, thirst, bitter taste, constipation, dark urine, Red tongue with redder sides and dry yellow coating, Wiry-Rapid pulse.

Heat in the Gall-Bladder

Blurred vision, dizziness, tinnitus, bitter taste, dry throat, irritability, red face and ears, hypochondrial fullness, unilateral or bilateral yellow tongue coating, Wiry-Rapid pulse.

Deficiency of Minister Fire (Kidney-Yang deficiency)

Blurred vision or floaters or both, watery eyes, lower backache, cold knees, sensation of cold in the lower back, a feeling of cold, weak legs, bright-white complexion, weak knees, tiredness, lassitude, abundant clear or scanty clear urination, urination at night, infertility in women, impotence, premature ejaculation, decreased libido, Pale and wet tongue, Deep-Weak pulse.

Spleen-Qi deficiency

Blurred vision or floaters or both, tired eyes, poor appetite, slight abdominal distension after eating, tiredness, lassitude, pale complexion, weakness of the limbs, loose stools, slight depression, tendency to obesity, Pale tongue, Empty pulse.

Strabismus

Observation, Chapter 6

Kidney-Essence deficiency

Strabismus from childhood, short-sightedness, weak constitution as a child, poor bone development in children, softening of bones in adults, deafness, weakness

of the knees and legs, poor memory, loose teeth, falling hair or premature greying of the hair, lower backache, dizziness, tinnitus, normal-coloured tongue and Floating-Empty or Leather pulse if Kidney-Essence deficiency occurs against a background of Kidney-Yin deficiency, or Pale tongue and Deep-Weak pulse if against a background of Kidney-Yang deficiency.

Liver-Wind

Strabismus, headaches, vertigo, tremors, tinnitus, tics, convulsions, rigidity of the neck, tremor of the limbs, stiff neck, opisthotonos, in severe cases coma, Stiff, Moving or Deviated tongue, Wiry pulse.

Liver-Yang rising

Strabismus, headache, dizziness, tinnitus, irritability, propensity to outbursts of anger, Wiry pulse.

Severe, chronic deficiency of Qi and Blood of the Liver

Strabismus, extreme exhaustion, dizziness, blurred vision, floaters, numbness/tingling of limbs, scanty menstruation, dull-pale complexion, dry skin and hair, Pale tongue, Choppy or Fine pulse.

Internal Cold

Strabismus, greyish-pale complexion, abdominal pain, epigastric pain, cold limbs, pain alleviated by exposure to heat and by drinking warm drinks and aggravated by exposure to cold and by drinking cold drinks, thick white tongue coating, Tight pulse.

Liver-Blood stasis

Strabismus, hypochondrial/abdominal pain, painful periods, dark and clotted menstrual blood, masses in the abdomen, purple nails and lips, purple or dark complexion, Purple tongue, Wiry or Firm pulse.

Toxic Heat

Strabismus, fever, a feeling of agitation, mental restlessness, red skin rashes, Red tongue with red points and thick, sticky, dry dark-yellow coating, Overflowing-Rapid pulse.

Phlegm obstructing Lungs and Spleen

Strabismus, blurred vision, chronic cough coming in bouts with profuse sticky white sputum which is easy to expectorate, pasty-white complexion, a feeling of oppression in the chest and epigastrium, shortness of breath, dislike of lying down, wheezing, nausea,

Swollen tongue with a sticky white coating, Slippery pulse.

Myopia
Liver-Blood deficiency

Myopia, blurred vision, floaters, dizziness, numbness/tingling of the limbs, scanty menstruation, dull-pale complexion, Pale tongue, Choppy or Fine pulse.

Liver- and Kidney-Yin deficiency

Myopia from childhood, blurred vision, floaters, weak child, nocturnal enuresis, pulse Weak on both Rear positions.

This is a congenital Kidney and Liver deficiency in children causing myopia; due to their young age, there are not many symptoms. The myopia itself, the weakness of the child, possibly nocturnal enuresis and a Weak pulse on the Kidney positions are enough to diagnose this pattern.

Hyperopia

'Hyperopia' is the opposite of myopia; that is, the vision is better for far objects than for near.

Kidney-Essence deficiency

Hyperopia, poor bone development in children, softening of the bones in adults, deafness, weakness of the knees and legs, poor memory, loose teeth, falling hair or premature greying of the hair, weakness from sexual activity, lower backache, infertility, sterility, dizziness, tinnitus, normal-coloured tongue and Floating-Empty or Leather pulse if Kidney-Essence deficiency occurs against a background of Kidney-Yin deficiency, or Pale tongue and Deep-Weak pulse if against a background of Kidney-Yang deficiency.

Kidney-Yin deficiency with Empty-Heat

Hyperopia, red and dry eyes, blurred vision, dizziness, tinnitus, hardness of hearing, night sweating, dry mouth at night, five-palm heat, a feeling of heat in the evening, malar flush, thirst with a desire to drink in small sips, lower backache, scanty dark urine, insomnia, Red tongue without coating, Floating-Empty and Rapid pulse.

Deficiency of Qi and Blood

Hyperopia, blurred vision, poor appetite, loose stools, weak voice, tiredness, dizziness, numbness/tingling of

limbs, palpitations, dull-pale complexion, Pale tongue, Weak or Choppy pulse.

Decreased night vision
Liver-Blood deficiency

Decreased night vision, blurred vision, floaters, dizziness, numbness/tingling of limbs, scanty menstruation, dull-pale complexion, Pale tongue, Choppy or Fine pulse.

Liver- and Kidney-Yin deficiency

Decreased night vision, blurred vision, floaters, dry eyes, dizziness, tinnitus, hardness of hearing, lower backache, dull occipital or vertical headache, insomnia, numbness/tingling of limbs, dry throat, dry hair and skin, brittle nails, night sweating, dry stools, scanty menstruation or amenorrhoea, normal-coloured without coating, Floating-Empty pulse.

Spleen-Qi deficiency

Decreased night vision, poor appetite, slight abdominal distension after eating, tiredness, pale complexion, weakness of the limbs, loose stools, Pale tongue, Empty pulse.

Spleen- and Kidney-Yang deficiency

Decreased night vision, lower backache, cold knees, a sensation of cold in the back, a feeling of cold, weak legs, bright-white complexion, weak knees, impotence, tiredness, abundant clear or scanty clear urination, urination at night, loose stools, poor appetite, slight abdominal distension, a desire to lie down, early-morning diarrhoea, chronic diarrhoea, Pale and wet tongue, Deep-Weak pulse.

Deficiency of Qi and Blood

Decreased night vision, blurred vision, poor appetite, loose stools, weak voice, tiredness, dizziness, numbness/tingling of limbs, palpitations, dull-pale complexion, Pale tongue, Weak or Choppy pulse.

Decreased visual acuity
Liver-Blood deficiency

Decreased visual acuity, dizziness, blurred vision, floaters, numbness/tingling of limbs, scanty menstruation, dull-pale complexion, Pale tongue, Choppy or Fine pulse.

Liver-Yin deficiency

Decreased visual acuity, blurred vision, floaters, dry eyes, dizziness, numbness/tingling of the limbs, scanty menstruation, dull-pale complexion but with red cheekbones, withered and brittle nails, dry skin and hair, night sweating, normal-coloured tongue without coating, Fine or Floating-Empty pulse.

Kidney-Yin deficiency

Decreased visual acuity, dry eyes, floaters, dizziness, tinnitus, hardness of hearing, poor memory, night sweating, dry mouth and throat at night, lower backache, constipation, scanty dark urine, tiredness, normal-coloured tongue without coating, Floating-Empty pulse.

Turbid Phlegm obstructing the head's orifices

Decreased visual acuity, blurred vision, floaters, dizziness, dull headache with a feeling of heaviness and muzziness of the head, poor memory and concentration, sputum in the throat, a feeling of oppression of the chest, nausea, Swollen tongue with sticky coating, Slippery pulse.

Heart-Blood deficiency

Decreased visual acuity, blurred vision, palpitations, dizziness, insomnia, dream-disturbed sleep, poor memory, anxiety, tendency to be easily startled, dull-pale complexion, pale lips, Pale and Thin tongue, Choppy or Fine pulse.

Sudden blindness
Liver-Fire

Sudden unilateral blindness, bloodshot eyes, headaches, dizziness, tinnitus, irritability, propensity to outbursts of anger, red face, thirst, bitter taste, constipation, dark urine, Red tongue with redder sides and dry yellow coating, Wiry-Rapid pulse.

Liver-Blood stasis

Sudden unilateral blindness, pain in the eyes, hypochondrial/abdominal pain, painful periods, dark and clotted menstrual blood, masses in abdomen, purple nails and lips, purple or dark complexion, Purple tongue, Wiry or Firm pulse.

Phlegm-Heat in the Liver

Sudden blindness, red face and eyes, irritability, propensity to outbursts of anger, tinnitus/deafness (with sudden onset), temporal headache, dizziness, thirst, bitter taste, dream-disturbed sleep, constipation with dry stools, dark-yellow urine, epistaxis, haematemesis, haemoptysis, a feeling of oppression of the chest, rattling sound in the throat, a feeling of muzziness of the head, expectoration of sputum, hypertension, Red and Swollen tongue with redder sides and with sticky yellow coating, Wiry-Slippery-Rapid pulse.

Phlegm-Heat in the Heart

Sudden blindness, red face, red eyes, palpitations, mental restlessness, thirst, red face, a feeling of oppression of the chest, dark urine, expectoration of phlegm, rattling sound in the throat, bitter taste, insomnia, dream-disturbed sleep, a feeling of agitation, mental confusion, incoherent speech, rash behaviour, tendency to hit or scold people, uncontrolled laughter or crying, shouting, muttering to oneself, depression, manic behaviour, Red tongue with redder-swollen tip and Heart crack with a sticky yellow coating inside it, Slippery-Rapid or Slippery-Overflowing-Rapid pulse.

Liver-Wind

Sudden unilateral blindness, tremors, severe dizziness, tinnitus, headache, numbness of limbs, tics, Stiff, Deviated or Moving tongue, Wiry pulse.

Heat at the Blood level (within the Four Levels)

Sudden blindness, high fever at night, macular skin eruptions, mental confusion, coma, bleeding, Dark-Red and dry tongue without coating, Fine-Rapid pulse.

ITCHY EYES

Interrogation, Chapter 42

Liver-Blood deficiency

Slightly itchy eyes, blurred vision, floaters, dizziness, numbness/tingling of limbs, dull-pale complexion, scanty menstruation, Pale tongue, Choppy or Fine pulse.

Liver-Yin deficiency

Itchy eyes, floaters, dry eyes, blurred vision, dizziness, numbness/tingling of the limbs, scanty menstruation,

dull-pale complexion but with red cheekbones, withered and brittle nails, dry skin and hair, night sweating, normal-coloured tongue without coating, Fine or Floating-Empty pulse.

Liver-Fire

Severely itchy eyes, bloodshot eyes, painful eyes, headache, red face, dizziness, tinnitus, irritability, propensity to outbursts of anger, thirst, bitter taste, constipation, dark urine, Red tongue with redder sides and dry yellow coating, Wiry-Rapid pulse.

Heart-Fire

Itchy eyes, red eyes, burning sensation in the eyes, redness in the inner canthus of the eyes, palpitations, thirst, mouth and tongue ulcers, mental restlessness, a feeling of agitation, insomnia, dream-disturbed sleep, feeling of heat, red face, bitter taste, Red tongue with redder tip and yellow coating, Overflowing-Rapid pulse.

Liver-Wind

Itchy eyes, dry eyes, blurred vision, tremors, severe dizziness, tinnitus, headache, numbness of the limbs, tics, Stiff, Deviated or Moving tongue, Wiry pulse.

Damp-Heat in the Gall-Bladder

Itchy eyes, discharge from the eyes, yellow complexion and eyes, blurred vision, a heavy feeling in the eyelids, dizziness, hypochondrial pain, fullness and distension, nausea, vomiting, inability to digest fats, tinnitus, irritability, a feeling of heaviness, unilateral or bilateral thick, sticky yellow coating, Slippery-Rapid pulse.

Invasion of Wind-Heat

Itchy eyes with sudden onset, unbearable itching, aversion to cold, fever, cough, sore throat, stuffed or runny nose with yellow discharge, headache, body aches, slight sweating, slight thirst, swollen tonsils, tongue slightly Red on the sides in the chest area or on front part, Floating-Rapid pulse.

DRY EYES

Interrogation, Chapter 42

Liver-Yin deficiency

Dry eyes, blurred vision, floaters, dizziness, numbness/tingling of the limbs, scanty menstruation, dull-pale

complexion but with red cheekbones, withered and brittle nails, dry skin and hair, night sweating, normal-coloured tongue without coating, Fine or Floating-Empty pulse.

Kidney-Yin deficiency

Dry eyes, blurred vision, floaters, dizziness, tinnitus, hardness of hearing, poor memory, night sweating, vertigo, dry mouth and throat at night, lower back-ache, constipation, scanty dark urine, tiredness, lassitude, normal-coloured tongue without coating, Floating-Empty pulse.

Liver-Fire

Dry and red eyes with burning sensation, bloodshot eyes, painful eyes, headache, red face, dizziness, tinnitus, irritability, propensity to outbursts of anger, thirst, bitter taste, constipation, dark urine, Red tongue with redder sides and dry yellow coating, Wiry-Rapid pulse.

Heart-Yin deficiency

Dry eyes, palpitations, insomnia, dream-disturbed sleep, poor memory, anxiety, tendency to be easily startled, mental restlessness, uneasiness, 'feeling hot and bothered', dry mouth and throat, night sweating, normal-coloured tongue without coating or with rootless coating, Floating-Empty pulse, especially on the left Front position.

Severe Liver-Blood deficiency

Dry eyes, blurred vision, floaters, dizziness, numbness/tingling of limbs, scanty menstruation, dull-pale complexion, Pale and Thin tongue with very Pale or orangey sides, Choppy or Fine pulse.

Lung- and Kidney-Yin deficiency

Dry eyes, blurred vision, floaters, dry cough which is worse in the evening, dry throat and mouth, thin body, breathlessness on exertion, lower backache, night sweating, dizziness, tinnitus, hardness of hearing, scanty urination, normal-coloured tongue without coating, Floating-Empty pulse.

HOT AND PAINFUL EYES

Interrogation, Chapter 42

Liver-Fire

Hot and painful eyes, bloodshot eyes, headaches, dizziness, tinnitus, irritability, propensity to outbursts of anger, red face, thirst, bitter taste, constipation, dark urine, Red tongue with redder sides and dry yellow coating, Wiry-Rapid pulse.

Liver-Yang rising

Hot and painful eyes, a feeling of distension of the eyes, headache, dizziness, tinnitus, irritability, propensity to outbursts of anger, Wiry pulse.

Heart-Fire

Hot and painful eyes, red eyes, redness of the inner canthus of the eyes, burning sensation in the eyes, palpitations, thirst, mouth and tongue ulcers, mental restlessness, a feeling of agitation, insomnia, dream-disturbed sleep, a feeling of heat, red face, bitter taste, Red tongue with redder tip and yellow coating, Overflowing-Rapid pulse.

Liver-Wind

Painful eyes (not necessarily hot), tremors, severe dizziness, tinnitus, headache, numbness of limbs, tics, Stiff, Deviated or Moving tongue, Wiry pulse.

Damp-Heat in the head

Hot and painful eyes, sticky eyelids, heaviness of the eyelids, sticky taste, facial pain, sticky yellow nasal discharge, a feeling of heaviness of the head, thirst without desire to drink, a feeling of heat, dull-yellow complexion, sticky yellow tongue coating, Slippery-Rapid pulse.

Phlegm-Heat

Hot and painful eyes, sticky eyelids, blurred vision, a feeling of heaviness and muzziness of the head, a feeling of heat, red face, greasy skin, a feeling of oppression of the chest, sputum in the throat, expectoration of yellow sputum, dizziness, nausea, Red and Swollen tongue with sticky yellow coating, Slippery-Rapid pulse.

Blood stasis in the head

Painful eyes (not necessarily hot), dark rings under the eyes, headache, dark complexion, bulging eyes, mental agitation, Purple tongue, Wiry pulse.

Liver-Blood deficiency

Dull ache in the eyes (not necessarily hot), blurred vision, floaters, dizziness, numbness/tingling of limbs, scanty menstruation, dull-pale complexion, Pale tongue, Choppy or Fine pulse.

Heart-Blood deficiency

Dull ache in the eyes (not necessarily hot), dull headache, palpitations, dizziness, insomnia, dream-disturbed sleep, poor memory, anxiety, tendency to be easily startled, dull-pale complexion, pale lips, Pale and Thin tongue, Choppy or Fine pulse.

Kidney deficiency

Dull ache in the eyes (not necessarily hot), dull occipital headache, blurred vision, floaters, dizziness, tinnitus, lower backache, poor memory.

Other manifestations, including tongue and pulse, depend on whether there is Kidney-Yang or Kidney-Yin deficiency.

Deficiency of Qi and Yin

Slightly hot and painful eyes, mild pain, a desire to shut the eyes, dry eyes, slightly red eyes, dizziness, tiredness, dry throat, loose stools, poor appetite, Pale tongue or normal-coloured tongue without coating, Weak or Floating-Empty pulse.

Invasion of Wind-Heat

Hot and painful eyes with sudden onset, red eyes, aversion to cold, fever, cough, sore throat, stuffed or runny nose with yellow discharge, headache, body aches, slight sweating, slight thirst, swollen tonsils, tongue slightly Red on the sides in the chest area or on front part, Floating-Rapid pulse.

STREAMING EYES

Observation, Chapter 6; Interrogation, Chapter 42

There are traditionally two types of streaming eyes: one is called *liu lei*, which indicates runny and streaming eyes and is described here; the other is called *yan chi*, which indicates a thick discharge from the eye and is described under 'Discharge from the eyes'.

Liver-Blood deficiency

Streaming eyes, floaters, blurred vision, dizziness, numbness/tingling of limbs, scanty menstruation, dull-pale complexion, Pale tongue, Choppy or Fine pulse.

This is called 'cold streaming'.

Kidney-Yang deficiency

Streaming eyes, lower backache, cold knees, a feeling of cold, bright-white complexion, weak knees, tired-ness, abundant clear urination, urination at night, Pale and wet tongue, Deep-Weak pulse.

This is called 'cold streaming'.

Liver-Blood deficiency with Liver-Heat

Streaming eyes, itchy eyes, dizziness, blurred vision, floaters, numbness/tingling of the limbs, scanty menstruation, dull pale face with 'floating' red colour on the cheeks, thirst, irritability, headache, tongue Pale but also slightly Red on the sides, pulse Choppy or Fine and slightly Rapid.

Liver-Fire

Streaming eyes, bloodshot eyes, headaches, dizziness, tinnitus, irritability, propensity to outbursts of anger, red face, thirst, bitter taste, constipation, dark urine, Red tongue with redder sides and dry yellow coating, Wiry-Rapid pulse.

Kidney- and Liver-Yin deficiency with Empty-Heat

Streaming eyes, itchy eyes, red and dry eyes, dizziness, tinnitus, hardness of hearing, dull occipital or vertical headache, insomnia, numbness/tingling of the limbs, malar flush, lower backache, dry throat, dry hair and skin, brittle nails, dry vagina, night sweating, dry stools, scanty menstruation or amenorrhoea, five-palm heat, a feeling of heat in the evening, Red tongue without coating, Floating-Empty and Rapid pulse.

Heart-Fire

Streaming eyes, red, red inner canthus of the eyes, painful eyes, palpitations, thirst, mouth and tongue ulcers, mental restlessness, a feeling of agitation, insomnia, dream-disturbed sleep, a feeling of heat, red face, bitter taste, Red tongue with redder tip and yellow coating, Overflowing-Rapid pulse.

Damp-Phlegm in the Spleen and Lungs

Streaming eyes, swollen eyelids, sticky eyelids, chronic cough coming in bouts with profuse sticky white sputum which is easy to expectorate, pasty-white complexion, a feeling of oppression in the chest, shortness of breath, a dislike of lying down, wheezing, nausea, abdominal fullness, tendency to obesity, Swollen tongue with a sticky white coating, Slippery pulse.

Empty-Cold in the Liver channel

Streaming eyes, fullness and distension of the hypogastrium with pain which refers downwards to the

scrotum and testis and upwards to the hypochondrium, alleviation of the pain by warmth, straining of the testis or contraction of the scrotum, vertical headache, a feeling of cold, cold hands and feet, vomiting of clear watery fluid or dry vomiting, Pale and wet tongue with a white coating, Deep-Wiry-Fine-Slow pulse.

Invasion of Wind-Heat

Streaming eyes with sudden onset, itchy eyes, pain in the eye, aversion to cold, fever, cough, sore throat, stuffed or runny nose with yellow discharge, headache, body aches, slight sweating, slight thirst, swollen tonsils, tongue slightly Red on the sides in the chest area or on front part, Floating-Rapid pulse.

This is called 'hot streaming'.

Invasion of Wind-Cold

Streaming eyes with sudden onset, itchy eyes, aversion to cold, fever, cough, itchy throat, slight breathlessness, stuffed or runny nose with clear watery discharge, sneezing, occipital headache, body aches, thin white tongue coating, Floating-Tight pulse.

DISCHARGE FROM THE EYES

Observation Chapter 6; Interrogation, Chapter 42

'Discharge from the eyes' is a translation of the Chinese term *yan chi*, which indicates a thick discharge from the eyes as opposed to a watery one, which is called *liu lei*.

Liver-Fire

Yellow discharge from the eyes, bloodshot eyes, painful eyes, headache, red face, dizziness, tinnitus, irritability, propensity to outbursts of anger, thirst, bitter taste, constipation, dark urine, Red tongue with redder sides and dry yellow coating, Wiry-Rapid pulse.

Heart-Fire

Yellow discharge from the eyes, red, painful eyes, palpitations, thirst, agitation, insomnia, dream-disturbed sleep, a feeling of heat, red face, bitter taste, Red tongue with redder tip and yellow coating, Overflowing-Rapid pulse.

Yin deficiency with Empty-Heat

Yellow, thin discharge from the eyes, dry and red eyes, a feeling of heat in the evening, dry mouth at night, night sweating, five-palm heat, Red tongue without coating, Floating-Empty and Rapid pulse.

Other symptoms and signs depend on the organ involved, which may be the Liver, Heart, Kidneys or Lungs.

Deficiency of Qi and Blood

Chronic light watery discharge from the eyes that is aggravated by overexertion, poor appetite, loose stools, weak voice, tiredness, blurred vision, dizziness, numbness/tingling of the limbs, palpitations, dull-pale complexion, Pale tongue, Weak or Choppy pulse.

Invasion of Wind-Heat

Yellow discharge from the eyes, itchy and red eyes, aversion to cold, fever, cough, sore throat, stuffed or runny nose with yellow discharge, headache, body aches, slight sweating, slight thirst, swollen tonsils, tongue slightly Red on the sides in the chest area or on front part, Floating-Rapid pulse.

Toxic Heat (measles)

Thick, yellow discharge from the eyes, fever, thirst, restlessness, red eyes, Red tongue with red points and thick, dark-yellow coating, Overflowing-Rapid pulse.

This corresponds to the Qi level of measles.

EYE COLOUR

Yellow (sclera)

Observation, Chapter 6

Damp-Heat with predominance of Heat

Bright-yellow sclera like tangerine peel, thirst, dry mouth, a feeling of heat, bitter taste, epigastric fullness, a sticky taste, a feeling of heaviness of the head and body, Red tongue with sticky yellow tongue coating, Slippery-Rapid pulse.

Damp-Heat with predominance of Dampness

Dull-yellow sclera, thirst without desire to drink, epigastric fullness, a sticky taste, abdominal fullness, a feeling of heaviness of the head and body, sticky yellow tongue coating, Slippery-Rapid pulse.

Cold-Dampness

Dull, dark-yellow sclera, epigastric fullness, a sticky taste, abdominal fullness, a feeling of heaviness of the head and body, cold limbs, loose stools, sticky white tongue coating, Slippery-Slow pulse.

Toxic Heat

Deep-yellow sclera, bloodshot eyes, fever, a feeling of heat, agitation, red skin rashes, boils, headache, Red tongue with red points and thick, sticky, dark-yellow coating, Overflowing-Slippery-Rapid pulse.

Liver-Blood deficiency

Light-yellow sclera, dizziness, blurred vision, floaters, numbness/tingling of the limbs, scanty menstruation, dull-pale complexion, Pale tongue, Choppy or Fine pulse.

Blood stasis

Dark, dull-yellow or brown sclera, dark rings under the eyes, headache, abdominal pain, agitation, Purple tongue, Wiry or Choppy pulse.

Other symptoms and signs depend on the organ involved, which could be the Heart or Liver.

Red (sclera)

Observation, Chapter 6

Liver-Fire

Red eyes, burning eyes, painful eyes, headache, red face, dizziness, tinnitus, irritability, propensity to outbursts of anger, thirst, bitter taste, constipation, dark urine, Red tongue with redder sides and dry yellow coating, Wiry-Rapid pulse.

Heart-Fire

Red eyes, painful eyes, palpitations, thirst, mouth and tongue ulcers, mental restlessness, feeling agitated, insomnia, dream-disturbed sleep, a feeling of heat, red face, bitter taste, Red tongue with redder tip and yellow coating, Overflowing-Rapid pulse.

Liver- and Kidney-Yin deficiency with Empty-Heat

Red eyes, blurred vision, dry eyes, dizziness, tinnitus, dull occipital or vertical headache, insomnia, numbness/tingling of the limbs, malar flush, dry eyes, blurred vision, lower backache, dry throat, dry hair and skin, brittle nails, dry vagina, night sweating, dry stools, scanty menstruation, five-palm heat, a feeling of heat in the evening, Red tongue without coating, Floating-Empty and Rapid pulse.

Invasion of Wind-Heat

Red eyes with sudden onset, itchy eyes, aversion to cold, fever, cough, sore throat, stuffed or runny nose with yellow discharge, headache, body aches, slight sweating, slight thirst, swollen tonsils, tongue slightly Red on the sides in the chest area or on front part, Floating-Rapid pulse.

Lung-Heat or Phlegm-Heat

Red eyes, flaring of nostrils, red face, fever, cough with profuse yellow sputum, a feeling of muzziness of the head, a feeling of oppression of the chest, breathlessness, thirst, a feeling of heat, chest ache, tongue with sticky yellow tongue coating, Overflowing-Rapid or Slippery-Rapid pulse.

Damp-Heat in the Bladder

Red eyes, especially the inner corner, headache from occiput to top of head and eyes, a feeling of heat, burning on urination, difficult urination, scanty dark urine, sticky yellow tongue coating on the root, Slippery-Rapid pulse.

Bluish-greenish (sclera)

Observation, Chapter 6

'Bluish-greenish' is a translation of the Chinese colour *qing*, which in certain pathologies (such as Cold) refers to a bluish colour and in others (such as Liver patterns) to a greenish colour.

Liver-Wind

Greenish sclera, headaches, tremors, severe dizziness, tinnitus, headache, numbness of the limbs, tics, Stiff, Deviated or Moving tongue, Wiry pulse.

Internal Cold

Bluish sclera, a feeling of cold, cold limbs, abdominal pain, chronic pain, abundant pale urine, Pale tongue, Tight-Slow pulse.

Other symptoms and signs depend on the organ involved and on whether it is Full- or Empty-Cold.

Kidney-Yin deficiency

Bluish sclera, dizziness, tinnitus, hardness of hearing, poor memory, night sweating, dry mouth and throat at night, lower backache, constipation, scanty dark urine, tiredness, normal-coloured tongue without coating, Floating-Empty pulse.

Dark (sclera)

Observation, Chapter 6

Phlegm

Dark, brownish sclera, a feeling of muzziness of the head, a feeling of oppression of the chest, a feeling of heaviness, sputum in the throat, dizziness, nausea, Swollen tongue with sticky coating, Slippery pulse.

Liver- and Kidney-Yin deficiency

Dark sclera, dry eyes, dizziness, tinnitus, hardness of hearing, lower backache, dull occipital or vertical headache, insomnia, numbness/tingling of the limbs, dry eyes, blurred vision, dry throat, dry hair and skin, brittle nails, dry vagina, night sweating, dry stools, nocturnal emissions, scanty menstruation or amenorrhoea, delayed cycle, infertility, normal-coloured tongue without coating, Floating-Empty pulse.

Severe Full-Heat

Dark sclera, a feeling of heat, thirst, a feeling of agitation, mental restlessness, Red tongue with yellow coating, Overflowing-Rapid pulse.

Other symptoms and signs depend on the organ involved.

Pale corners

Observation, Chapter 6

Blood deficiency

Pale corners, blurred vision, floaters, dizziness, numbness, Pale tongue, Choppy or Fine pulse.

Other symptoms depend on the organ involved, which may be the Liver or Heart.

Yang deficiency

Pale corners, a feeling of cold, cold limbs, tiredness, Pale and wet tongue, Deep-Weak pulse.

Other symptoms and signs depend on the organ involved, which may be the Spleen or Kidneys.

Red corners

Observation, Chapter 6

Heat of the Liver, Heart or Lungs may manifest with a redness in the corners of the eyes and this may not necessarily coincide with the areas described by the Five Wheels (see Chapter 6, p. 78).

Liver-Fire

Redness of either corner of the eye, pain in the eyes, headaches, dizziness, tinnitus, irritability, propensity to outbursts of anger, red face, thirst, bitter taste, constipation, dark urine, Red tongue with redder sides and dry yellow coating, Wiry-Rapid pulse.

Heart-Fire

Red inner corner, pain in the eyes, palpitations, thirst, mouth and tongue ulcers, mental restlessness, a feeling of agitation, insomnia, dream-disturbed sleep, a feeling of heat, red face, bitter taste, Red tongue with redder tip and yellow coating, Overflowing-Rapid pulse.

Lung-Heat

Red inner corner, red face, cough, slight breathlessness, a feeling of heat, chest ache, flaring of the nostrils, thirst, red face, Red tongue with yellow coating, Overflowing-Rapid pulse.

Liver-Yin deficiency with Empty-Heat

Slight redness of either corner, blurred vision, floaters in the eyes, dry eyes, diminished night vision, dizziness, numbness/tingling of the limbs, insomnia, scanty menstruation or heavy menstrual bleeding (if Empty-Heat is severe), red cheekbones, cramps, withered and brittle nails, very dry hair and skin, anxiety, a feeling of heat in the evening, night sweating, five-palm heat, thirst with a desire to drink in small sips, Red tongue without coating, Floating-Empty Rapid pulse.

Heart-Yin deficiency with Empty-Heat

Slight redness of the inner corner, malar flush, palpitations, insomnia, dream-disturbed sleep, poor memory, anxiety, mental restlessness, dry mouth and throat, a feeling of heat in the evening, night sweating, five-palm heat, Red tongue with redder tip and without coating, Floating-Empty and Rapid pulse.

Lung-Yin deficiency with Empty-Heat

Slight redness of the inner corner, dry cough or with scanty, sticky sputum which could be blood tinged, dry mouth and throat at night, weak/hoarse voice, night sweating, tiredness, malar flush, a feeling of heat or a low-grade fever in the evening, five-palm heat, thin body or thin chest, insomnia, anxiety, Red tongue without coating, Floating-Empty and Rapid tongue.

Kidney-Yin deficiency with Empty-Heat

Slight redness of the inner corner, dry eyes, dizziness, tinnitus, hardness of hearing, night sweating, dry mouth at night, five-palm heat, a feeling of heat in the evening, malar flush, thirst with a desire to drink in small sips, lower backache, scanty dark urine, insomnia, Red tongue without coating, Floating-Empty and Rapid pulse.

Damp-Heat

Red corners, yellow, sticky discharge from the eyes, red and swollen eyelids, epigastric fullness, a sticky taste, thirst with no desire to drink, a feeling of heaviness of the head and body, a feeling of heat, sticky yellow tongue coating, Slippery-Rapid pulse.

Invasion of Wind-Heat

Red corners with sudden onset, itchy eyes, aversion to cold, fever, cough, sore throat, stuffed or runny nose with yellow discharge, headache, body aches, slight sweating, slight thirst, swollen tonsils, tongue slightly red on the sides in the chest area or on front part, Floating-Rapid pulse.

EYELIDS

Stye

Heat in Lungs and Spleen

Stye on the upper eyelid, red eyes, tears flowing from the eyes, swollen and hard eyelids, pain in the eye, cough, slight breathlessness, a feeling of heat, chest ache, flaring of the nostrils, thirst, red face, burning epigastric/abdominal pain, excessive hunger, red tip of the nose, dry lips, mouth ulcers, dry stools, scanty dark urine, Red tongue with dry yellow coating, Overflowing-Rapid pulse.

Heat in Lungs and Stomach

Stye on the lower eyelid, red eyes, tears flowing from the eyes, swollen and hard eyelids, pain in the eye, cough, slight breathlessness, a feeling of heat, chest ache, flaring of nostrils, thirst, red face, burning epigastric pain, thirst, sour regurgitation, nausea, excessive hunger, foul breath, Red tongue with yellow coating, Overflowing-Rapid pulse.

Spleen-Qi deficiency with Dampness

Chronic styes on the upper eyelid that come and go and are aggravated by overexertion, swollen and soft eyelids, poor appetite, slight abdominal distension after eating, tiredness, pale or sallow complexion, weakness of the limbs, loose stools, abdominal fullness, a feeling of heaviness, a sticky taste, poor digestion, undigested food in the stools, nausea, dull frontal headache, excessive vaginal discharge, Pale tongue with sticky coating, Soggy pulse.

Damp-Heat in the Stomach and Spleen

Stye, red and swollen eyelids, a feeling of fullness and pain of the epigastrium and lower abdomen, poor appetite, a feeling of heaviness, thirst without a desire to drink, nausea, loose stools with offensive odour, a feeling of heat, dull-yellow complexion, sticky taste, Red tongue with sticky yellow coating, Slippery-Rapid pulse.

Red eyelids

Observation, Chapter 6

Damp-Heat in the Stomach and Spleen

Red eyelids, discharge from the eye, swollen eyelids, painful and itchy eyes, a feeling of heaviness of the head, dull headache, a feeling of fullness and pain of the epigastrium and lower abdomen, poor appetite, thirst without a desire to drink, nausea, loose stools with offensive odour, a feeling of heat, dull-yellow complexion, sticky taste, Red tongue with sticky yellow coating, Slippery-Rapid pulse.

Spleen-Heat

Redness and heat of the upper eyelids, red and dry lips, burning epigastric/abdominal pain, excessive hunger, red tip of the nose, dry lips, mouth ulcers, thirst, dry stools, a feeling of heat, scanty dark urine, yellow complexion, Red tongue with dry yellow coating, Overflowing-Rapid pulse.

Stomach-Heat

Redness and heat of the lower eyelids, burning epigastric pain, thirst, sour regurgitation, nausea, excessive hunger, foul breath, a feeling of heat, Red tongue with a yellow coating, Overflowing-Rapid pulse.

Invasion of Wind-Heat

Red eyelids with sudden onset, red eyes, aversion to cold, fever, cough, sore throat, stuffed or runny nose

with yellow discharge, headache, body aches, slight sweating, slight thirst, swollen tonsils, tongue slightly Red on the sides in the chest area or on front part, Floating-Rapid pulse.

Dark eyelids
Kidney deficiency

Dark eyelids, lower backache, dizziness, tinnitus, Weak pulse.

Other symptoms and signs depend on whether there is Kidney-Yin or Kidney-Yang deficiency.

Cold-Phlegm

Greyish, dull eyelids like soot, cough with expectoration of watery white sputum, feeling cold, cold hands and feet, nausea, vomiting, a feeling of oppression of the chest and epigastrium, dull-white complexion, pale urine, Pale and Swollen tongue with wet white coating, Slippery-Slow pulse.

Phlegm-Heat

Dark, red and swollen eyelids, a feeling of heaviness and muzziness of the head, a feeling of heat, red face, greasy skin, a feeling of oppression of the chest, sputum in the throat, expectoration of yellow sputum, dizziness, nausea, Red and Swollen tongue with sticky yellow coating, Slippery-Rapid pulse.

Wind-Phlegm

Dark eyelids, a dull-yellow complexion, severe dizziness, blurred vision, tremors, numbness/tingling of the limbs, tinnitus, nausea, sputum in the throat, a feeling of oppression of the chest, Stiff or Deviated and Swollen tongue, Wiry-Slippery pulse.

Green eyelids
Stomach-Cold

Green eyelids, severe pain in the epigastrium, a feeling of cold, cold limbs, preference for warmth, vomiting of clear fluids (which may alleviate the pain), nausea, aggravation by swallowing cold fluids, which are quickly vomited, preference for warm liquids, thick white tongue coating, Deep-Tight-Slow pulse.

Pale eyelids
Blood deficiency

Pale eyelids, pale inside the eyelids, dull-pale complexion, dry hair, dizziness, blurred vision, floaters, numbness/

tingling of limbs, scanty menstruation, Pale tongue, Choppy or Fine pulse.

Yang deficiency

Pale eyelids, paleness inside the eyelids, a feeling of cold, cold limbs, loose stools, abundant clear urination, tiredness, Pale and wet tongue, Deep-Weak pulse.

Other symptoms and signs depend on the organ involved.

Retention of food

Pale colour inside the eyelids surrounded by yellow, fullness, pain and distension of the epigastrium, which are relieved by vomiting, nausea, vomiting of sour fluids, foul breath, sour regurgitation, belching, insomnia, loose stools or constipation, poor appetite, thick tongue coating, Full-Slippery pulse.

Swollen eyelids

Observation, Chapter 6

Invasion of Wind-Heat

Swollen, red and itchy eyelids, aversion to cold, fever, cough, sore throat, stuffed or runny nose with yellow discharge, headache, body aches, slight sweating, slight thirst, swollen tonsils, tongue slightly Red on the sides in the chest area or on front part, Floating-Rapid pulse.

Spleen-Yin deficiency with Empty-Heat

Swollen and dry eyelids, poor appetite, poor digestion, retching, gnawing hunger, loss of taste, slight epigastric pain, dry mouth and lips, dry stools, thin body, sallow complexion with red tip of the nose, night sweating, a feeling of heat in the evening, malar flush, Red tongue without coating and transversal cracks on the sides, Floating-Empty and Rapid pulse.

Spleen-Heat

Swollen and red eyelids, red and dry lips, burning epigastric/abdominal pain, excessive hunger, red tip of the nose, mouth ulcers, thirst, dry stools, a feeling of heat, scanty dark urine, yellow complexion, Red tongue with dry yellow coating, Overflowing-Rapid pulse.

Water overflowing

Gradual swelling of the eyelids, pale eyelids, oedema of the face and hands, cold hands and feet, scanty urination, pale complexion, a feeling of cold, loose stools, Pale and wet tongue, Deep-Weak pulse.

Cold-Phlegm

Gradual swelling of the eyelids, pale eyelids, cough with expectoration of white watery sputum, a feeling of cold, cold hands and feet, nausea, vomiting, a feeling of oppression of the chest and epigastrium, dull-white complexion, pale urine, Pale and Swollen tongue with wet white coating, Slippery-Slow pulse.

Boil on the eyelid
Toxic Heat in the Stomach

Boil on the lower eyelid, red eyes, painful eyes, swollen eyelids, burning epigastric pain, intense thirst with a desire to drink cold liquids, mental restlessness, dry mouth, mouth ulcers, bleeding gums, dry stools, sour regurgitation, foul breath, nausea, vomiting soon after eating, a feeling of heat, sour regurgitation, tongue Red with a thick, dry, dark-yellow coating, Deep-Full-Slippery-Rapid pulse.

Deficiency of Qi and Yin

Chronic boil on the eyelid that comes and goes, shaped like a small bean, pale in colour, dry eyes, dull pain of the eye, tiredness, shortness of breath, weak/hoarse voice, spontaneous daytime sweating, night sweating, dry mouth and throat at night, loose stools, tongue Pale or normal-coloured without coating, Empty or Floating-Empty pulse.

Spleen-Qi deficiency

Chronic boils on the upper eyelid that come and go and may move from eye to eye, aggravated by overexertion, poor appetite, slight abdominal distension after eating, tiredness, pale complexion, weakness of the limbs, loose stools, Pale tongue, Empty pulse.

Spleen-Qi deficiency with Damp-Heat

Chronic boils on the upper eyelid that come and go, greasy skin, sinus problems, facial ache, headache with a feeling of heaviness of the head, sticky taste, a feeling of fullness of the epigastrium/abdomen, epigastric/abdominal pain, poor appetite, a sticky taste, a feeling of heaviness of the body, thirst without a desire to drink, nausea, vomiting, loose stools, dull-yellow complexion like tangerine peel, Pale tongue with sticky yellow coating, Soggy-Rapid pulse.

Invasion of Wind-Heat

Boil of the eyelid with sudden onset, red and itchy eyes, aversion to cold, fever, cough, sore throat, stuffed or runny nose with yellow discharge, headache, body aches, slight sweating, slight thirst, swollen tonsils, tongue slightly Red on the sides in the chest area or on front part, Floating-Rapid pulse.

Pain of the eyelids
Heat in Lungs and Spleen

Pain of the upper eyelid, red eyes, tears flowing from the eyes, swollen and hard eyelids, pain in the eye, headache, cough, slight breathlessness, a feeling of heat, chest ache, flaring of nostrils, thirst, red face, burning epigastric/abdominal pain, excessive hunger, red tip of the nose, dry lips, mouth ulcers, dry stools, scanty dark urine, yellow complexion, Red tongue with dry yellow coating, Overflowing-Rapid pulse.

Heat in Lungs and Stomach

Pain of the lower eyelid, red eyes, tears flowing from the eyes, swollen and hard eyelids, pain in the eye, cough, slight breathlessness, a feeling of heat, chest ache, flaring of the nostrils, thirst, red face, burning epigastric pain, sour regurgitation, nausea, excessive hunger, foul breath, Red tongue with a yellow coating, Overflowing-Rapid pulse.

Flapping eyelids
Blood deficiency with internal Wind

Flapping eyelids, facial tic, slight tremor of the head or hand or both, dizziness, blurred vision, unilateral numbness/tingling of a limb, Pale and Thin tongue, Choppy or Fine and slightly Wiry pulse.

Stomach- and Spleen-Qi deficiency

Slightly flapping eyelids, a feeling of tiredness of the eyelids, a desire to shut the eyes, poor appetite, slight abdominal distension after eating, tiredness, lassitude, pale complexion, weakness of the limbs, loose stools, an uncomfortable feeling in the epigastrium, lack of sense of taste, Pale tongue, Empty pulse.

Invasion of Wind-Cold

Flapping of the eyelids with sudden onset, itchy eyes, aversion to cold, fever, occipital headache, stiff neck, sneezing, body aches, tongue with thin white coating, Floating-Tight pulse.

Drooping eyelids

Stomach- and Spleen-Qi deficient and sinking

Drooping eyelids, aggravated by overexertion and alleviated by rest, depression, poor appetite, slight abdominal distension after eating, tiredness, pale complexion, weakness of the limbs, loose stools, a bearing-down feeling, prolapse of uterus, an uncomfortable feeling in the epigastrium, lack of sense of taste, Pale tongue, Empty pulse.

Deficiency of Qi and Blood

Drooping eyelids, blurred vision, poor appetite, loose stools, weak voice, tiredness, dizziness, numbness/tingling of limbs, palpitations, dull-pale complexion, Pale tongue, Weak or Choppy pulse.

Liver and Kidney deficiency

Drooping eyelids, dry eyes, blurred vision, floaters, dizziness, tinnitus, lower backache.

Other symptoms depend on whether there is Yin or Yang deficiency.

Stagnation of Qi and stasis of Blood

Drooping eyelids, irritability, headache, chest pain, abdominal distension, Purple tongue, Wiry pulse.

Stomach-Heat

Drooping eyelids, red and swollen eyelids, burning epigastric pain, thirst, sour regurgitation, nausea, excessive hunger, foul breath, a feeling of heat, Red tongue with a yellow coating, Overflowing-Rapid pulse.

Invasion of Wind

Drooping of the eyelids, aversion to cold, fever, occipital headache, stiff neck, Floating pulse.

Other symptoms and signs depend on whether it is Wind-Cold or Wind-Heat.

Loss of control of the eyelids

'Loss of control of the eyelid' indicates a condition in which the patient cannot open the eyes, the eyelids tremble, and there is loss of voluntary control of the eyelids; this condition is more common in children.

Liver-Blood deficiency

Loss of control of both eyelids, uncomfortable sensation of the eyes, blurred vision, floaters, dizziness, numbness/tingling of limbs, scanty menstruation, dull-pale complexion, Pale tongue, Choppy or Fine pulse.

Liver-Qi invading the Spleen

Loss of control of both eyelids, trembling eyelids, greenish complexion, irritability, abdominal distension and pain, alternation of constipation and diarrhoea, stools sometimes dry and bitty (small pieces) and sometimes loose, flatulence, tiredness, tongue normal coloured or slightly Red on the sides, pulse Wiry on the left and Weak on the right.

Wind-Heat affecting the Liver channel

Loss of control of both eyelids, eyelids trembling upwards and downwards and from side to side as if blown by the wind, fever, aversion to cold, tongue Red in the front and with a thin white coating, Floating-Rapid pulse.

Childhood Nutritional Impairment

Loss of control of both eyelids, trembling eyelids, streaming eyes, uncomfortable sensation of the eyes, red sclera, worse in the afternoon, abdominal distension, diarrhoea, thin body, sticky tongue coating, Weak pulse.

Nodules within the eyelids

In Western medicine, nodules within the eyelids correspond to external hordeolum or meibomian cyst. External hordeolum (stye) is a small abscess caused by an acute staphylococcal infection of a lash follicle. A meibomian cyst is a chronic lipogranulomatous inflammation secondary to retention of sebum caused by obstruction of a duct of a meibomian gland.

Damp-Phlegm obstructing the Spleen

Nodules within the eyelids, shaped like grains of rice or small beans, discharge from the eyes, neither painful nor itchy, eyelids not red, nodules movable, a feeling of oppression of the chest and epigastrium, somnolence, nausea, sputum in the throat, muzziness of the head, Swollen tongue with sticky coating, Slippery pulse.

Phlegm-Heat obstructing the Spleen

Nodules within the eyelids, shaped like grains of rice or small beans, yellow discharge from the eyes, painful eyelids, red eyelids, nodules movable, a feeling of oppression of the chest and epigastrium, somnolence,

nausea, sputum in the throat, muzziness of the head, thirst without a desire to drink, a feeling of heat, Red and Swollen tongue with sticky yellow coating, Slippery-Rapid pulse.

Small red grains inside the eyelids

'Small red grains inside the eyelids' corresponds to vernal keratoconjunctivitis in Western medicine. This is an allergic disorder which is common in atopic patients but occurs also in non-atopic patients; it manifests with intense itching, lachrymation, photophobia, burning and a sensation of a foreign body in the eye.

Damp-Heat in the Spleen

Small red grains inside the eyelids, yellow discharge from the eyes, itchy eyes, a feeling of heaviness of the head, fullness of the epigastrium, epigastric or abdominal pain, sticky taste, thirst with no desire to drink, poor appetite, a feeling of heaviness of the body, thirst, nausea, vomiting, loose stools with offensive odour, a feeling of heat, scanty dark urine, headache with a feeling of heaviness of the head, dull-yellow complexion, bitter taste, Red tongue with sticky yellow coating, Slippery-Rapid pulse.

Wind-Heat affecting the Spleen channel

Small red grains inside the eyelids with sudden onset, red eyes, sore throat, itchy throat, itchy eyes, aversion to cold, fever, headache, tongue Red in the front or sides, Floating-Rapid pulse.

Redness inside the lower lids
Full-Heat

Redness inside the lower lids, thirst, mental restlessness, a feeling of heat, Red tongue with dry yellow coating, Overflowing-Rapid pulse.

Other symptoms and signs depend on the organ involved.

Yin deficiency with Empty-Heat

Thin, red line inside the lower lids, thirst with a desire to drink in small sips, mental restlessness, a feeling of heat in the evening, dry throat at night, night sweating, Red tongue without coating, Floating-Empty and Rapid pulse.

GLAUCOMA

Stagnant Liver-Qi turned into Heat rebelling upwards

Glaucoma, eye pain, red eyes, red face, hypochondrial or epigastric distension, a slight feeling of oppression of the chest, irritability, premenstrual tension, premenstrual breast distension, a feeling of lump in the throat, a feeling of heat, red face, thirst, propensity to outbursts of anger, heavy periods, tongue Red on the sides, Wiry pulse especially on the left side and slightly Rapid.

Liver-Fire

Glaucoma, red eyes, eye pain, headache, red face, dizziness, tinnitus, irritability, propensity to outbursts of anger, thirst, bitter taste, constipation, dark urine, Red tongue with redder sides and dry yellow coating, Wiry-Rapid pulse.

Kidney-Yin deficiency with Empty-Heat

Glaucoma, dry eyes, dizziness, tinnitus, hardness of hearing, night sweating, dry mouth at night, five-palm heat, a feeling of heat in the evening, malar flush, thirst with a desire to drink in small sips, lower backache, scanty dark urine, insomnia, Red tongue without coating, Floating-Empty and Rapid pulse.

Empty-Cold in the Liver channel

Glaucoma, eye pain, fullness and distension of the hypogastrium with pain which refers downwards to the scrotum and testis and upwards to the hypochondrium, and is alleviated by warmth, vertical headache, a feeling of cold, cold hands and feet, vomiting of clear watery fluid or dry vomiting, Pale tongue with a wet and white coating, Deep-Tight-Slow.

FEELING OF DISTENSION OF THE EYES

Interrogation, Chapter 42

Liver-Fire

Pronounced feeling of distension of the eye, pain in the eye, bloodshot eyes, dry eyes, headache, red face, dizziness, tinnitus, irritability, propensity to outbursts of anger, thirst, bitter taste, constipation, dark urine, Red tongue with redder sides and dry yellow coating, Wiry-Rapid pulse.

Liver-Yang rising

Feeling of distension of the eye, headache, dizziness, tinnitus, irritability, propensity to outbursts of anger, Wiry pulse.

Liver-Wind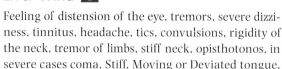

Feeling of distension of the eye, tremors, severe dizziness, tinnitus, headache, tics, convulsions, rigidity of the neck, tremor of limbs, stiff neck, opisthotonos, in severe cases coma, Stiff, Moving or Deviated tongue, Wiry pulse.

Phlegm obstructing the Lungs and Spleen

Feeling of distension of the eye, enlarged pupil, chronic cough coming in bouts with profuse sticky white sputum which is easy to expectorate, pasty-white complexion, a feeling of oppression in the chest and epigastrium, shortness of breath, wheezing, nausea, epigastric fullness, Swollen tongue with a sticky white coating, Slippery pulse.

Liver- and Kidney-Yin deficiency with Empty-Heat

Slight feeling of distension of the eye, blurred vision, dry eyes, a feeling of heat in the eyes, dizziness, tinnitus, hardness of hearing, dull occipital or vertical headache, insomnia, numbness/tingling of the limbs, malar flush, lower backache, dry throat, dry hair and skin, brittle nails, dry vagina, night sweating, dry stools, scanty menstruation or amenorrhoea, five-palm heat, a feeling of heat in the evening, Red tongue without coating, Floating-Empty and Rapid pulse.

Liver-Qi stagnation

A feeling of distension of the eyes when tense, frontal headache, hypochondrial or epigastric distension, irritability, moodiness, a feeling of a lump in the throat, premenstrual tension, Wiry pulse.

Damp-Heat in Liver and Gall-Bladder

Feeling of distension of the eyes, swollen red eyelids, fullness/pain of the hypochondrium, abdomen or epigastrium, bitter taste, poor appetite, nausea, a feeling of heaviness of the body, yellow vaginal discharge, vaginal itching, mid-cycle bleeding/pain, burning on urination, dark urine, yellow complexion and eyes, vomiting, Red tongue with redder sides and unilateral or bilateral sticky yellow coating, Wiry-Slippery-Rapid pulse.

EYEBALL

Protruding eyeball

Observation, Chapter 6

In Western medicine, protruding eyeball is called proptosis and in 80% of cases it is due to a thyroid ophthalmopathy; it may also be due to a tumour in the orbit of the eye.

Liver-Fire

Protruding eyeball, pain in the eye, bloodshot eyes, headache, red face, dizziness, tinnitus, irritability, propensity to outbursts of anger, thirst, bitter taste, constipation, dark urine, Red tongue with redder sides and dry yellow coating, Wiry-Rapid pulse.

Heart-Fire

Protruding eyeball, pain in the eye, palpitations, thirst, mouth and tongue ulcers, mental restlessness, a feeling of agitation, insomnia, dream-disturbed sleep, a feeling of heat, red face, bitter taste, Red tongue with redder tip and yellow coating, Overflowing-Rapid pulse.

Liver-Qi stagnation and Phlegm

Protruding eyeball, pain in the eye, a feeling of distension of the eye, hypochondrial or epigastric distension, irritability, moodiness, a feeling of a lump in the throat, premenstrual tension, a feeling of oppression of the chest, sputum in the throat, Swollen tongue, Wiry-Slippery pulse.

Liver-Wind

Protruding eyeball, tremors, severe dizziness, tinnitus, headache, tics, convulsions, rigidity of the neck, tremor of the limbs, stiff neck, opisthotonos, in severe cases coma, Stiff, Moving or Deviated tongue, Wiry pulse.

Liver-Wind with Phlegm-Heat

Protruding eyeball, dark sclera, tremors, severe dizziness, tinnitus, headache, tics, convulsions, rigidity of the neck, tremor of the limbs, stiff neck, opisthotonos, in severe cases coma, feeling of oppression of the chest, sputum in the throat, a feeling of heat, a feeling of heaviness, Red and Swollen tongue which may also be Stiff, Moving or Deviated, Wiry-Slippery-Rapid pulse.

Liver-Qi stagnation

Protruding eyeball, an uncomfortable sensation of the eye, a feeling of distension of the eye, hypochondrial or epigastric distension, irritability, moodiness, a feeling of a lump in the throat, premenstrual tension, Wiry pulse.

Liver-Qi stagnation and Liver-Blood stasis

Protruding eyeball, pain in the eye, hypochondrial or epigastric distension, irritability, moodiness, a feeling of a lump in the throat, premenstrual tension, painful periods, Purple tongue, Wiry or Firm pulse.

Damp-Heat in Liver and Gall-Bladder

Protruding eyeball, eye ache, earache, headache, fullness/pain of the hypochondrium, abdomen or epigastrium, bitter taste, poor appetite, nausea, a feeling of heaviness of the body, yellow vaginal discharge, vaginal itching, mid-cycle bleeding/pain, burning on urination, dark urine, yellow complexion and eyes, vomiting, Red tongue with redder sides and unilateral or bilateral sticky yellow coating, Wiry-Slippery-Rapid pulse.

Toxic Heat

Protruding and painful eyeball, red sclera, gum in the eye, a feeling of heat, agitation, fever, Red tongue with red points and thick, sticky, dry dark-yellow coating, Overflowing-Slippery-Rapid pulse.

Deficiency of Kidney-Yin and Kidney-Yang

Slightly protruding eyeball, dizziness, floaters, tinnitus, night sweating, lower backache, cold limbs, loose stools.

Other symptoms and signs, including tongue and pulse, depend on whether there is a predominance of Kidney-Yin or Kidney-Yang deficiency.

Deficiency of Qi and Blood

Slightly protruding eyeball, blurred vision, poor appetite, loose stools, weak voice, tiredness, dizziness, numbness/tingling of the limbs, palpitations, dull-pale complexion, Pale tongue, Weak or Choppy pulse.

Rebellious Lung-Qi (Lung-Qi not descending)

Protruding eyeball, chronic cough or asthma, a feeling of oppression of the chest.

Invasion of Wind-Heat

Protruding eyeball with sudden onset, pain in the eye, itchy eyes, aversion to cold, fever, cough, sore throat, stuffed or runny nose with yellow discharge, headache, body aches, slight sweating, slight thirst, swollen tonsils, tongue slightly Red on the sides in the chest area or on front part, Floating-Rapid pulse.

Sunken eyeball

Observation, Chapter 6

Severe, chronic, Lung- and Spleen-Qi deficiency

Sunken eyeballs, drooping eyelids, shortness of breath, slight cough, weak voice, spontaneous daytime sweating, dislike of speaking, dull-white complexion, tendency to catch colds, tiredness, dislike of cold, poor appetite, slight abdominal distension after eating, weakness of the limbs, loose stools, Pale tongue, Empty pulse.

Spleen-Qi deficiency following food poisoning

Sunken eyeballs following profuse vomiting and diarrhoea, poor appetite, loose stools, Empty pulse.

Collapse of Yin or Yang

Sunken eyeballs with sudden onset, drooping eyelids, Deep-Scattered pulse.

Other symptoms and signs depend on whether there is collapse of Yin or of Yang.

Scaly eyeballs

In Western medicine, 'scaly eyeballs' corresponds to blepharoconjunctivitis, which is characterized by burning, itching, mild photophobia, dilated blood vessels and brittle fibrinous scales.

Lung-Heat

Scaly eyeballs, burning eyes, red eyes, desire to keep eyes shut, streaming eyes, cough, slight breathlessness, a feeling of heat, chest ache, flaring of the nostrils, thirst, red face, Red tongue with yellow coating, Overflowing-Rapid pulse.

Heart-Yin deficiency with Empty-Heat

Scaly eyeballs, burning eyes, red eyes, palpitations, insomnia, dream-disturbed sleep, poor memory,

anxiety, tendency to be easily startled, mental restlessness, uneasiness, 'feeling hot and bothered', dry mouth and throat, thirst with a desire to sip fluids, a feeling of heat in the evening, malar flush, night sweating, five-palm heat, Red tongue, redder on the tip, no coating, Floating-Empty and Rapid pulse.

Invasion of Wind-Heat

Scaly eyeballs with sudden onset, itchy eyes, burning eyes, aversion to cold, fever, cough, sore throat, stuffed or runny nose with yellow discharge, headache, body aches, slight sweating, slight thirst, swollen tonsils, tongue slightly Red on the sides in the chest area or on front part, Floating-Rapid pulse.

Quivering eyeball

This is called nystagmus in Western medicine.

Internal Wind (acute stage of Wind-stroke)

Quivering eyeballs, open eyes, unconsciousness, clenched fists, urinary retention, Red tongue, Rapid pulse.

Empty-Wind from Blood deficiency

Quivering eyeballs, slight tremor of the head or hand or both, facial tic, dizziness, blurred vision, unilateral numbness/tingling of a limb, Pale and Thin tongue, Choppy or Fine and slightly Wiry pulse.

Kidney-Essence deficiency

Quivering eyeballs, poor bone development in children, softening of the bones in adults, deafness, weakness of knees and legs, poor memory, loose teeth, falling hair or premature greying of the hair, weakness of sexual activity, lower backache, infertility, sterility, dizziness, tinnitus, normal-coloured tongue and Floating-Empty or Leather pulse if Kidney-Essence deficiency occurs against a background of Kidney-Yin deficiency, and Pale tongue and Deep-Weak pulse if against a background of Kidney-Yang deficiency.

Liver-Qi invading the Spleen

Quivering eyeballs, irritability, abdominal distension and pain, alternation of constipation and diarrhoea, stools sometimes dry and bitty and sometimes loose, flatulence, tiredness, poor appetite, normal-coloured tongue (or slightly Red on the sides in severe cases of Liver-Qi stagnation), pulse Wiry on the left and Weak on the right.

Eyeball turning up

The eyeball turning up is seen in acute conditions of internal Wind; it is also seen in chronic conditions, in which case the eyeball turns upwards slightly so that the white sclera can be seen under the eye.

Heat generating Wind (Blood level of the Four Levels)

Eyeballs turning up, eyes open, coma, tremor, macular rash, Red tongue without coating, Fine-Rapid pulse.

Stagnant Blood generating Wind

Eyeballs turning up, open eyes, open mouth, dribbling from the corners of the mouth, dark complexion, headache, dark rings under eyes, chest pain, Purple and Deviated tongue, Wiry pulse.

Internal Wind

Eyeballs turning up, tremors, severe dizziness, tinnitus, headache, numbness of limbs, tics, Stiff, Deviated or Moving tongue, Wiry pulse.

Kidney deficiency

Eyeballs slightly turning up, lower backache, dizziness, tinnitus, exhaustion.

Other symptoms and signs depend on whether there is a Kidney-Yang or Kidney-Yin deficiency.

ECCHYMOSIS UNDER CONJUNCTIVA

In Western medicine, ecchymosis under conjunctiva corresponds to a subconjunctival haemorrhage, which may manifest with excessive lachrymation, gritty sensation, retrobulbar discomfort and photophobia.

Liver-Fire

Large ecchymosis under conjunctiva, red and painful eyes, headache, red face, dizziness, tinnitus, irritability, propensity to outbursts of anger, thirst, bitter taste, constipation, dark urine, Red tongue with redder sides and dry yellow coating, Wiry-Rapid pulse.

Kidney-Yin deficiency with Empty-Heat

Small ecchymosis under conjunctiva, dizziness, tinnitus, poor memory, hardness of hearing, night sweat-

ing, dry mouth at night, five-palm heat, a feeling of heat in the evening, malar flush, thirst with a desire to sip fluids, lower backache, constipation, scanty dark urine, tiredness, anxiety, insomnia, Red tongue without coating, Floating-Empty and Rapid pulse.

Invasion of Wind-Heat

Ecchymosis under conjunctiva with sudden onset, burning and red eyes, aversion to cold, fever, cough, sore throat, stuffed or runny nose with yellow discharge, headache, body aches, slight sweating, slight thirst, swollen tonsils, tongue slightly Red on the sides in the chest area or on front part, Floating-Rapid pulse.

Dry-Heat invading the Lungs

Ecchymosis under conjunctiva, headache, red and burning eyes, dry eyes, dry throat, dry cough, Red tongue with dry coating, Fine pulse.

Liver Phlegm-Fire

Ecchymosis under conjunctiva, eye ache, protruding eyeball, red face, red eyes, palpitations, mental restlessness, thirst, red face, a feeling of oppression of the chest, dark urine, expectoration of phlegm, rattling sound in the throat, bitter taste, insomnia, dream-disturbed sleep, agitation, mental confusion, incoherent speech, rash behaviour, tendency to hit or scold people, uncontrolled laughter or crying, shouting, muttering to oneself, depression, manic behaviour, Red tongue with redder-swollen tip, Heart crack with a sticky yellow coating inside it, Slippery-Rapid or Slippery-Overflowing-Rapid pulse.

RED VEINS/MEMBRANE

Red veins in the eyes

'Red veins in the eyes' indicates visible veins on the sclera running horizontally from the corners of the eyes. In Western medicine this corresponds to an engorgement of the subconjunctival vessels.

Liver-Fire

Large red veins in the eyes, running horizontally from the outer corner, headaches, dizziness, tinnitus, irritability, propensity to outbursts of anger, red face, thirst, bitter taste, constipation, dark urine, Red tongue with redder sides and dry yellow coating, Wiry-Rapid pulse.

Liver-Yin deficiency with Empty-Heat

Small red veins in the eyes running horizontally from the outer corner, blurred vision, dry eyes, diminished night vision, red eyes, floaters, dizziness, numbness/tingling of the limbs, insomnia, scanty menstruation or heavy menstrual bleeding (if Empty-Heat is severe), red cheekbones, cramps, withered and brittle nails, very dry hair and skin, anxiety, a feeling of heat in the evening, night sweating, five-palm heat, thirst with a desire to drink in small sips, Red tongue without coating, Floating-Empty Rapid pulse.

Heart-Fire

Red veins in the eyes, running horizontally from the inner corner, red painful eyes, palpitations, thirst, mouth and tongue ulcers, mental restlessness, a feeling of agitation, insomnia, dream-disturbed sleep, a feeling of heat, red face, bitter taste, Red tongue with redder tip and yellow coating, Overflowing-Rapid pulse.

Heart-Yin deficiency with Empty-Heat

Red veins in the eyes running horizontally from the inner corner, palpitations, insomnia, dream-disturbed sleep, poor memory, anxiety, mental restlessness, dry mouth and throat, a feeling of heat in the evening, malar flush, night sweating, five-palm heat, Red tongue with redder tip and without coating, Floating-Empty and Rapid pulse.

Kidney-Essence deficiency

Thin, red veins in the eyes, dry eyes, poor bone development in children, softening of bones in adults, deafness, weakness of the knees and legs, poor memory, loose teeth, falling hair or premature greying of the hair, weakness from sexual activity, lower backache, infertility, sterility, dizziness, tinnitus, normal-coloured tongue and Floating-Empty or Leather pulse if Kidney-Essence deficiency occurs against a background of Kidney-Yin deficiency, or Pale tongue and Deep-Weak pulse if against a background of Kidney-Yang deficiency.

Drooping red membrane

'Drooping red membrane' indicates a condition in which fine streaks of blood on the upper border of the pupil gradually grow into a red membrane, which spreads downward covering the pupil. In Western

medicine, this corresponds to trachoma; the pathogen of this disease is carried by flies and it is usually seen only in developing countries.

Liver-Fire

Fine blood streaks becoming a membrane, often shaped like a half-moon, covering the pupil, headache, red face, dizziness, tinnitus, irritability, propensity to outbursts of anger, thirst, bitter taste, constipation, dark urine, Red tongue with redder sides and dry yellow coating, Wiry-Rapid pulse.

Heat in the Lungs and Spleen

Small ulcers inside the upper eyelid which give rise to streaks of blood from the upper border of the pupil, painful and itchy eyes, cough, slight breathlessness, a feeling of heat, chest ache, flaring of the nostrils, thirst, red face, burning epigastric/abdominal pain, excessive hunger, red tip of the nose, dry lips, mouth ulcers, dry stools, scanty dark urine, Red tongue with dry yellow coating, Overflowing-Rapid pulse.

Wind-Heat affecting the Liver and Lung channels

Red eyes, fine streaks of blood over the eye, thickening of the eyelid, pain in the eye, sticky discharge in the eye, streaming eyes, a feeling of heat, slight thirst, yellow tongue coating, Wiry-Rapid pulse.

Red membrane in the corner of the eye

Observation, Chapter 6

'Red membrane in the corner of the eye' indicates a condition in which a large red membrane, shaped like the wing of a fly, extends horizontally from the corner of the eyes towards the pupil, eventually covering the pupil. In Western medicine, this corresponds to pterygium, which consists in overgrowth of the cornea by the conjunctiva; this disease is usually seen only in hot and dry climates.

Liver-Fire

Membrane in the corner of the eye that looks like butter, later becoming dark red, pain in the eyes, dry eyes, headache, red face, dizziness, tinnitus, irritability, propensity to outbursts of anger, thirst, bitter taste, constipation, dark urine, Red tongue with redder sides and dry yellow coating, Wiry-Rapid pulse.

Heart-Fire

Red membrane in the corners of the eye, rather thick, pain in the eye, palpitations, thirst, mouth and tongue ulcers, mental restlessness, a feeling of agitation, insomnia, dream-disturbed sleep, a feeling of heat, red face, bitter taste, Red tongue with redder tip and yellow coating, Overflowing-Rapid pulse.

Heart-Yin deficiency with Empty-Heat

Red membrane in the corners of the eyes running horizontally from the inner corner, palpitations, insomnia, dream-disturbed sleep, poor memory, anxiety, mental restlessness, dry mouth and throat, a feeling of heat in the evening, malar flush, night sweating, five-palm heat, Red tongue with redder tip and without coating, Floating-Empty and Rapid pulse.

Heat in the Lung channel

Red membrane in the corner of the eye extending horizontally towards the pupil, pain in the eye, cough, slight breathlessness, a feeling of heat, chest ache, flaring of the nostrils, thirst, red face, Red tongue with yellow coating, Overflowing-Rapid pulse.

Heat in the Stomach and Spleen

Red membrane in the corner of the eye with a small head, constipation, burning epigastric pain, thirst, sour regurgitation, nausea, excessive hunger, foul breath, a feeling of heat, abdominal pain, red tip of the nose, dry lips, mouth ulcers, dry stools, scanty dark urine, Red tongue with dry yellow coating, Overflowing-Rapid pulse.

Kidney-Yin deficiency with Empty-Heat

Pale red membrane in the corner of the eye, varying in thickness, dizziness, tinnitus, night sweating, dry mouth with a desire to drink in small sips, backache, poor memory, scanty dark urine, five-palm heat, malar flush, a feeling of heat in the evening, Red tongue without coating, Floating-Empty and Rapid pulse.

CORNEA

Corneal opacity

In Western medicine, corneal opacity may be caused by trauma, bacterial or viral infections or systemic diseases such as rheumatoid arthritis or lupus erythematosus.

Kidney-Yin deficiency

Corneal opacity over the pupil, red in colour, no pain or streaming of the eye, dizziness, tinnitus, hardness of hearing, poor memory, night sweating, dry mouth and throat at night, lower backache, constipation, scanty dark urine, tiredness, normal-coloured tongue without coating, Floating-Empty pulse.

Deficiency of Qi and Blood

Corneal opacity over the pupil, red in colour, streaming eyes, blurred vision, poor appetite, loose stools, weak voice, tiredness, dizziness, numbness/tingling of the limbs, palpitations, dull-pale complexion, Pale tongue, Weak or Choppy pulse.

Wind-Heat affecting the Liver channel

Corneal opacity over the pupil, bright white in colour, oozing of fluid, pain in the eye, streaming eyes, itchy eyes, headache, yellow tongue coating, Wiry-Rapid pulse.

Toxic Heat

Corneal opacity over the pupil, grey or yellow in colour, fine granular nebulas in pupil, greyish-white or yellowish in colour with indistinct borders, sinking in the centre, which may cover the whole pupil, nebulas which may be densely or sparsely distributed, or extend sharply like tree branches, or mat together into patches so as to be covered by a yellow membrane that looks like fat, pain in the eye, eyes streaming with a thick fluid, a feeling of heat, thirst, Red tongue with red point and thick, sticky yellow coating, Deep-Rapid-Slippery pulse.

Scarring after corneal opacity
Kidney-Yin deficiency

Scarring after corneal opacity, dry eyes, dizziness, tinnitus, hardness of hearing, poor memory, night sweating, dry mouth and throat at night, lower backache, constipation, scanty dark urine, tiredness, normal-coloured tongue without coating, Floating-Empty pulse.

Stomach-Yin deficiency

Scarring after corneal opacity, pale red sclera, dry eyes, no appetite or slight hunger but no desire to eat, constipation (dry stools), dull or slightly burning epigastric pain, dry mouth and throat especially in the afternoon, thirst but no desire to drink, or a desire to drink in small sips, a slight feeling of fullness after eating, normal-coloured tongue without coating or without coating in the centre, Floating-Empty pulse.

Stagnation of Qi and stasis of Blood

Scarring after corneal opacity, red or dark yellow sclera, looking like an agate (a precious stone with multicoloured stripes), abdominal distension and pain, headache, Purple tongue, Wiry pulse.

WHITE SPECKS

Observation, Chapter 6

White specks may occur on the sclera or pupil and may be bright or dull white.

Phlegm obstructing the Lungs

Dull-white specks on the sclera/pupil, a feeling of oppression in the chest, a feeling of heaviness, dizziness, nausea, phlegm in the throat, cough with expectoration of sticky sputum, Swollen tongue with sticky coating, Slippery pulse.

Liver- and Kidney-Yin deficiency

Dull-white specks on the sclera, dry eyes, blurred vision, dizziness, tinnitus, hardness of hearing, lower backache, dull occipital or vertical headache, insomnia, numbness/tingling of limbs, dry throat, dry hair and skin, brittle nails, night sweating, dry stools, scanty menstruation or amenorrhoea, normal-coloured tongue without coating, Floating-Empty pulse.

Yang deficiency with internal Cold

Bright-white specks on the sclera, a feeling of cold, cold limbs, abdominal pain, loose stools, tiredness, Pale and wet tongue, Deep-Weak-Slow pulse.

Other symptoms and signs depend on the organ involved.

PUPILS

Red ring around the pupil

In Western medicine, 'red ring around the pupil' corresponds to anterior uveitis or iritis, the main symptoms of which are photophobia, pain, redness, decreased vision and lachrymation.

Liver-Fire

Red ring around the pupil, contracted pupil, pain in the eye aggravated by heat and alleviated by the application of cold, streaming eye, headache, red face, dizziness, tinnitus, irritability, propensity to outbursts of anger, thirst, bitter taste, constipation, dark urine, Red tongue with redder sides and dry yellow coating, Wiry-Rapid pulse.

Heat in the Stomach and Spleen

Red ring around the pupil with yellow fluid flowing upwards, pain in the eye aggravated by heat and alleviated by the application of cold, streaming eyes, burning epigastric/abdominal pain, excessive hunger, red tip of the nose, dry lips, mouth ulcers, thirst, dry stools, a feeling of heat, scanty dark urine, foul breath, Red tongue with dry yellow coating, Overflowing-Rapid pulse.

Qi deficiency with Internal Wind

Pale-red ring around the pupil, eye not painful, chronic condition, eyelashes falling out, fine tremor of the hand, facial tic, tiredness, poor appetite, loose stools, weak voice, shortness of breath, Pale tongue, Weak pulse.

White membrane on the pupil in children

'White membrane on the pupil in children' is called *gan yi* in Chinese, which means Childhood Nutritional Impairment Nebula; it consists of a white membrane covering the pupil, often starting with the symptom of decreased vision at night. As its name implies, it occurs in children suffering from nutritional impairment. A nebula is a translucent, greyish corneal haze, scarring or opacity.

Spleen-Qi deficiency with Dampness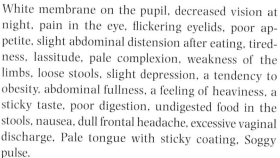

White membrane on the pupil, decreased vision at night, pain in the eye, flickering eyelids, poor appetite, slight abdominal distension after eating, tiredness, lassitude, pale complexion, weakness of the limbs, loose stools, slight depression, a tendency to obesity, abdominal fullness, a feeling of heaviness, a sticky taste, poor digestion, undigested food in the stools, nausea, dull frontal headache, excessive vaginal discharge, Pale tongue with sticky coating, Soggy pulse.

Spleen-Qi deficiency

White membrane on the pupil, frequent blinking, oozing of fluid, poor appetite, tiredness, slight abdominal distension, pale complexion, loose stools, Pale tongue, Empty pulse.

Retention of food

White membrane on the pupil, decreased vision at night, pain in the eye, thin body, fullness, pain and distension of the epigastrium, which are relieved by vomiting, nausea, vomiting of sour fluids, foul breath, sour regurgitation, belching, insomnia, loose stools or constipation, poor appetite, thick tongue coating, Full-Slippery pulse.

Spleen- and Kidney-Yang deficiency

Greyish membrane on the pupil, decreased vision at night, uncomfortable sensation in the eye, dull in colour, corneal erosion, lower backache, cold and weak knees, a feeling of cold, bright-white complexion, impotence, decreased libido, tiredness, lassitude, abundant clear urination, urination at night, loose stools, poor appetite, slight abdominal distension, a desire to lie down, early-morning diarrhoea, Pale and wet tongue, Deep-Weak pulse.

Yellow fluid between pupil and iris

In Western medicine, yellow fluid between the pupil and iris corresponds to hypopyon, which is a sterile pus formation in the anterior chamber, that is, between the back of the cornea and iris. Diseases such as pneumococcal keratitis or pseudomonas keratitis could show this phenomenon.

Heat in the Stomach and Spleen

Yellow fluid between the pupil and the iris streaming upwards, shaped like a crescent, pain in the eye with acute onset, photophobia, streaming eyes, sticky discharge from the eyes, burning epigastric/abdominal pain, excessive hunger, red tip of the nose, dry lips, mouth ulcers, thirst, dry stools, a feeling of heat, scanty dark urine, foul breath, Red tongue with dry yellow coating, Overflowing-Rapid pulse.

Stomach and Spleen deficient and cold

Yellow fluid between the pupil and the iris streaming upwards, uncomfortable sensation of the eye, chronic

condition, discomfort or dull pain in the epigastrium, better after eating and better with pressure or massage, no appetite, preference for warm drinks and foods, vomiting of clear fluid, no thirst, cold and weak limbs, tiredness, pale complexion, slight abdominal distension after eating, loose stools, feeling of cold, Pale and wet tongue, Deep-Weak pulse.

Damp-Heat in Stomach and Spleen

Yellow fluid between the pupil and iris streaming upwards, eye ache, sticky discharge from the eyes, greasy skin, sinus problems, sticky taste, thirst with no desire to drink, a feeling of fullness of the epigastrium, epigastric or abdominal pain, poor appetite, a feeling of heaviness of the body, nausea, vomiting, loose stools with offensive odour, a feeling of heat, scanty dark urine, headache with a feeling of heaviness of the head, dull-yellow complexion, bitter taste, Red tongue with sticky yellow coating, Slippery-Rapid pulse.

Bleeding between pupil and iris
Liver-Fire

Bleeding between pupil and iris, headaches, dizziness, tinnitus, irritability, propensity to outbursts of anger, red face, thirst, bitter taste, constipation, dark urine, Red tongue with redder sides and dry yellow coating, Wiry-Rapid pulse.

Liver- and Kidney-Yin deficiency and Blood deficiency

Bleeding between pupil and iris, uncomfortable sensation of the eyes, streaming eyes, red eyes, blurred vision, dry eyes, dizziness, tinnitus, lower backache, dull occipital or vertical headache, insomnia, numbness/tingling of limbs, dry throat, dry hair and skin, brittle nails, night sweating, dry stools, scanty menstruation or amenorrhoea, normal coloured without coating, Floating-Empty pulse.

Deficient Spleen-Qi not holding Blood

Bleeding between pupil and iris, tiredness, poor appetite, loose stools, pale complexion, Pale tongue, Weak pulse.

Dilated pupils
Kidney-Yang deficiency

Dilated pupils, lower backache, cold knees, a feeling of cold, bright-white complexion, weak knees, tiredness,

lassitude, abundant clear urination, urination at night, impotence, decreased libido, Pale and wet tongue, Deep-Weak pulse.

Deficiency of Qi and Yin

Dilated pupil, uncomfortable sensation of the eye, floaters, blurred vision, tiredness, shortness of breath, weak/hoarse voice, spontaneous daytime sweating, night sweating, dry mouth and throat at night, loose stools, tongue Pale or normal coloured without coating, Empty or Floating-Empty pulse.

Kidney-Yin deficiency with Empty-Heat

Dilated pupil, floaters, dizziness, tinnitus, night sweating, dry mouth with a desire to drink in small sips, backache, poor memory, scanty dark urine, five-palm heat, malar flush, a feeling of heat in the evening, Red tongue without coating, Floating-Empty and Rapid pulse.

Liver-Wind with Phlegm

Dilated pupil, severe dizziness, blurred vision, tremors, numbness/tingling of the limbs, tinnitus, nausea, sputum in the throat, a feeling of oppression of the chest, Stiff or Deviated and Swollen tongue, Wiry-Slippery pulse.

Collapse of Yang

Dilated pupils, profuse sweating, cyanosis of the lips, open eyes, open mouth, open fists, incontinence, Pale and Short tongue, Minute or Scattered pulse.

Contracted pupils
Liver-Fire

Contracted pupils, bloodshot eyes, pain in the eyes, headaches, dizziness, tinnitus, irritability, propensity to outbursts of anger, red face, thirst, bitter taste, constipation, dark urine, Red tongue with redder sides and dry yellow coating, Wiry-Rapid pulse.

Liver-Wind

Contracted pupils, tremors, severe dizziness, tinnitus, headache, numbness of the limbs, tics, Stiff, Deviated or Moving tongue, Wiry pulse.

Liver-Blood stasis in the Connecting channels of the Brain (Eye System)

Contracted pupils, pain in the eyes, headache, dark complexion, Purple tongue, Wiry pulse.

Toxic Heat at the Blood level

Contracted pupils, mental confusion, tremor, macular rash, fever at night, Red tongue with red points and no coating, Fine-Rapid pulse.

Damp-Heat in the Stomach and Spleen

Contracted pupils, sticky taste, thirst with no desire to drink, a feeling of fullness of the epigastrium, epigastric or abdominal pain, poor appetite, a feeling of heaviness of the body, nausea, vomiting, loose stools with offensive odour, a feeling of heat, scanty dark urine, headache with a feeling of heaviness of the head, dull-yellow complexion, bitter taste, Red tongue with sticky yellow coating, Slippery-Rapid pulse.

Invasion of Wind-Heat

Contracted pupils with sudden onset, aversion to cold, fever, cough, sore throat, stuffed or runny nose with yellow discharge, headache, body aches, slight sweating, slight thirst, swollen tonsils, tongue slightly Red on the sides in the chest area or on front part, Floating-Rapid pulse.

STARING, FIXED EYES

Observation, Chapter 6

Heart-Fire

Staring, fixed eyes, pain in the eyes, palpitations, thirst, agitation, insomnia, dream-disturbed sleep, a feeling of heat, red face, bitter taste, Red tongue with redder tip and yellow coating, Overflowing-Rapid pulse.

Phlegm-Heat in the Heart

Staring, fixed eyes, protruding eyeballs, a feeling of muzziness of the head, palpitations, anxiety, insomnia, thirst, a feeling of heat, a feeling of oppression of the chest, manic behaviour, Red-Swollen tongue with redder tip, Overflowing-Slippery-Rapid pulse.

CLOSED EYES

'Closed eyes' refers to the inability of the patient to keep the eyes open.

Excess of Yin

Closed eyes, cold limbs, open palms, Pale tongue, Deep-Full-Slow pulse.

Heat in febrile disease (Blood level)

Closed eyes, fever at night, macular rash, Red tongue without coating, Fine-Rapid pulse.

Wind-stroke (acute stage)

Closed eyes, unconsciousness, open palms, incontinence of urine, cold limbs, Pale and Short tongue, Deep-Full-Slow pulse.

OPEN EYES

'Open eyes' refers to the inability of the patient to keep the eyes shut.

Wind-stroke (acute stage)

Open eyes, unconsciousness, closed palms, urinary retention, hot limbs, Red tongue, Rapid pulse.

Stomach- and Spleen-Qi deficiency

Open eyes, poor appetite, slight abdominal distension after eating, tiredness, pale complexion, weakness of the limbs, loose stools, an uncomfortable feeling in the epigastrium, lack of sense of taste, Pale tongue, Empty pulse.

INVERTED EYELASHES

Lung- and Spleen-Qi deficiency

Inverted eyelashes, no pain, itchy eyes, aggravated by overexertion, tiredness, weak voice, shortness of breath, loose stools, poor appetite, Pale tongue, Empty pulse.

Damp-Heat in Stomach and Spleen

Inverted eyelashes, red and swollen eyelids, sticky taste, thirst with no desire to drink, a feeling of fullness of the epigastrium, epigastric or abdominal pain, poor appetite, a feeling of heaviness of the body, nausea, vomiting, loose stools with offensive odour, a feeling of heat, scanty dark urine, headache with a feeling of heaviness of the head, dull-yellow complexion, bitter taste, Red tongue with sticky yellow coating, Slippery-Rapid pulse.

Empty-Cold in the Bladder

Inverted eyelashes, a feeling of cold, cold legs, frequent, pale and abundant urination, Pale and wet tongue, Deep-Weak pulse.

Invasion of Wind-Heat

Inverted eyelashes, red and itchy eyes, tears flowing from the eyes, aversion to cold, fever, cough, sore throat, stuffed or runny nose with yellow discharge, headache, body aches, slight sweating, slight thirst, swollen tonsils, tongue slightly Red on the sides in the chest area or on front part, Floating-Rapid pulse.

CATARACT

Stomach- and Spleen-Qi deficiency

Cataract, poor appetite, tiredness, slight abdominal distension, pale complexion, loose stools, discomfort in the epigastrium, Pale tongue, Empty pulse.

Liver- and Kidney-Yin deficiency

Cataract, tiredness, dry eyes, blurred vision, floaters, dizziness, tinnitus, lower backache, dull occipital or vertical headache, insomnia, numbness/tingling of the limbs, dry throat, dry hair and skin, brittle nails, night sweating, dry stools, scanty menstruation or amenorrhoea, normal coloured without coating, Floating-Empty pulse.

Heart- and Kidney-Yin deficiency

Cataract, dry eyes, Dizziness, tinnitus, poor memory, night sweating, dry mouth and throat at night, lower backache, scanty dark urine, tiredness, slight anxiety, palpitations, insomnia, normal-coloured tongue without coating, Floating-Empty pulse.

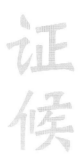

Chapter **62**

NECK, SHOULDERS AND UPPER BACK

Chapter contents

NECK AND SHOULDERS   *653*
  Stiff neck   *653*
  Rigidity of the neck   *654*
  Neck pain   *654*
  Soft neck   *654*
  Deviated neck   *654*
  Wide neck   *655*
  Thin neck   *655*
  Swollen neck glands   *655*
  Pulsation of the carotid artery   *655*
  Shoulder ache   *656*
  Frozen shoulder   *656*

UPPER BACK   *656*
  Upper backache   *656*
  Cold upper back   *656*
  Hot upper back   *656*
  Stiffness of the back as if wearing a tight belt   *657*

NECK AND SHOULDERS

Stiff neck

Interrogation, Chapter 36

Wind-Damp Painful Obstruction Syndrome

Stiff neck, body aches, a feeling of heaviness of the body.

Liver-Qi stagnation

Stiff neck when tense, tense upper back muscles, hypochondrial or epigastric distension, irritability, moodiness, a feeling of a lump in the throat, premenstrual tension, Wiry pulse.

Liver-Yang rising

Stiff neck, tense upper back muscles, headache, dizziness, tinnitus, irritability, propensity to outbursts of anger, Wiry pulse.

Kidney deficiency

Slightly stiff neck, dizziness, tinnitus, lower backache.
  Other symptoms depend on whether there is a Kidney-Yin or Kidney-Yang deficiency.

Invasion of Wind-Cold

Stiff neck with acute onset, aversion to cold, fever, occipital headache, stiff neck, sneezing, body aches, tongue with thin white coating, Floating-Tight pulse.

Liver-Wind

Stiff neck, headaches, tremors, severe dizziness, tinnitus, headache, numbness of the limbs, tics, Stiff, Deviated or Moving tongue, Wiry pulse.

Rigidity of the neck

Observation, Chapter 10

Cold Painful Obstruction Syndrome

Rigidity of the neck with acute onset which may continue for months, neck ache that is aggravated by exposure to cold and damp weather and ameliorated by the application of heat.

Liver-Qi stagnation

Rigidity of the neck which is aggravated by emotional upsets, hypochondrial or epigastric distension, irritability, moodiness, a feeling of a lump in the throat, premenstrual tension, Wiry pulse.

Liver-Yang rising

Rigidity of the neck, headache, dizziness, tinnitus, irritability, propensity to outbursts of anger, Wiry pulse.

Liver-Wind

Rigidity of the neck, stiff neck, tremors, severe dizziness, tinnitus, headache, tics, tremor of limbs, Stiff, Moving or Deviated tongue, Wiry pulse.

Neck pain

Interrogation, Chapter 36

Wind-Damp Painful Obstruction Syndrome

Neck pain, stiff neck, body aches, a feeling of heaviness of the body.

Liver-Qi stagnation

Chronic neck ache, tense upper back muscles, hypochondrial or epigastric distension, irritability, moodiness, a feeling of a lump in the throat, premenstrual tension, Wiry pulse.

Liver-Yang rising

Chronic neck ache, tense upper back muscles, headache, dizziness, tinnitus, irritability, propensity to outbursts of anger, Wiry pulse.

Invasion of Wind

Neck pain, stiff neck, aversion to cold, fever, occipital headache, body aches, Floating pulse.

Other symptoms and signs depend on whether it is Wind-Cold or Wind-Heat.

Liver-Wind

Neck pain, stiff neck, tremors, severe dizziness, tinnitus, headache, numbness of the limbs, tics, Stiff, Deviated or Moving tongue, Wiry pulse.

Soft neck

Observation, Chapter 10

'Soft neck' refers not only to a feeling of softness of the neck on palpation but also to a subjective feeling of softness and weakness of the neck, as if the patient found it difficult to keep the head up.

Severe deficiency of Qi and Blood

Soft neck, exhaustion, poor appetite, loose stools, weak voice, tiredness, blurred vision, dizziness, numbness/tingling of limbs, palpitations, dull-pale complexion, Pale tongue, Weak or Choppy pulse.

Kidney-Yang deficiency

Soft neck, lower backache, dizziness, tinnitus, a feeling of cold, weak knees, bright-white complexion, tiredness, abundant clear urination, Pale and wet tongue, Deep-Weak pulse.

Deviated neck

Observation, Chapter 10

'Deviated neck' indicates the leaning of the neck to one side.

Kidney-Essence deficiency

Deviated neck, poor constitution, poor bone development in children, softening of the bones in adults, deafness, weakness of the knees and legs, poor memory, loose teeth, falling hair or premature greying of the hair, weakness from sexual activity, lower backache, infertility, sterility, dizziness, tinnitus, normal-coloured tongue and Floating-Empty or Leather pulse if Kidney-Essence deficiency occurs against a background of Kidney-Yin deficiency, or Pale tongue and Deep-Weak pulse if against a background of Kidney-Yang deficiency.

Liver-Qi stagnation

Deviated neck, stiff neck, headache, dizziness, tinnitus, irritability, propensity to outbursts of anger, Wiry pulse.

Wide neck

Observation, Chapter 10

Qi stagnation with Phlegm

Wide neck, a feeling of a lump in the throat, irritability, phlegm in the throat, a feeling of oppression of the chest, abdominal distension, Swollen tongue with sticky coating, Wiry-Slippery pulse.

Phlegm with Blood stasis

Wide neck, a feeling of a lump in the throat, a feeling of oppression of the chest, a feeling of heaviness, dizziness, abdominal pain, chest pain, Purple and Swollen tongue, Wiry-Slippery pulse.

Liver-Fire

Wide neck, headaches, dizziness, tinnitus, irritability, propensity to outbursts of anger, red face, thirst, bitter taste, constipation, dark urine, Red tongue with redder sides and dry yellow coating, Wiry-Rapid pulse.

Thin neck

Observation, Chapter 10

Severe deficiency of Qi and Blood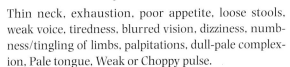

Thin neck, exhaustion, poor appetite, loose stools, weak voice, tiredness, blurred vision, dizziness, numbness/tingling of limbs, palpitations, dull-pale complexion, Pale tongue, Weak or Choppy pulse.

Chronic Yin deficiency

Thin neck, dizziness, tinnitus, night sweating, dry throat, tongue without coating, Floating-Empty pulse.

Other symptoms and signs depend on the organ involved.

Swollen neck glands

Observation, Chapter 10

Invasion of Wind-Heat with Toxic Heat

Swollen neck glands with acute onset, swollen tonsils, sore throat, aversion to cold, fever, cough, sore throat, stuffed or runny nose with yellow discharge, headache, body aches, slight sweating, slight thirst, tongue slightly Red on the sides in the chest area or on front part, Floating-Rapid pulse.

Toxic Heat with Qi and Yin deficiency

Chronic swelling of neck glands which comes and goes, sore throat that comes and goes, tiredness, breathlessness, weak voice, dry throat, loose stools, night sweating, tongue without coating in the centre, Empty or Floating-Empty pulse.

Residual Damp-Heat with Qi deficiency

Chronic swelling of neck glands which comes and goes, aggravated by periods of overwork and alleviated by periods of rest, chronic sore throat that comes and goes, a feeling of heaviness, muscle ache, tiredness, poor appetite, loose stools, Pale tongue with sticky yellow coating, Soggy pulse.

This condition is very common in postviral fatigue syndrome.

Toxic Heat with Blood stasis

Chronic, swollen neck glands, dark colour on the neck, dark complexion, chest pain, headache, abdominal pain, Purple tongue, Wiry-Rapid or Choppy-Rapid pulse.

Pulsation of the carotid artery

Observation, Chapter 10

'Pulsation of the carotid artery' indicates an excessive pulsation of this artery which is clearly visible.

Kidney- and Heart-Yang deficiency with Water overflowing to the Heart

Pulsation of the carotid artery, oedema especially of the legs and ankles, a cold feeling in legs and back, fullness and distension of abdomen, soreness of the lower back, a feeling of cold, scanty clear urination, palpitations, breathlessness, vomiting of watery, frothy white fluid, cold hands, Pale and Swollen tongue with a wet white coating, Deep-Wiry or Deep-Fine-Slippery pulse.

Chronic Phlegm in the Lungs

Pulsation of the carotid artery, sputum in the throat, wheezing, breathlessness, inability to lie down, a feeling of oppression of the chest, cough with expectoration of profuse sputum, Swollen tongue with sticky coating, Slippery pulse.

Shoulder ache
Damp-Cold
Ache in the shoulder region that may extend to the scapula region, a feeling of heaviness, numbness, coldness on palpation.

Wind-Cold
Acute pain in the shoulder joint that is aggravated by exposure to cold and application of heat, a feeling of cold.

Stagnation of Qi and stasis of Blood
Pain in the shoulder joint, rigidity of the shoulder, a feeling of distension, Purple tongue.

Frozen shoulder
Cold
Severe pain in the shoulder joint that is aggravated by exposure to cold and alleviated by application of heat, inability to abduct the arm, a feeling of cold.

Damp-Cold
Severe pain in the shoulder joint that is aggravated by exposure to cold and dampness and alleviated by the application of heat, inability to abduct the arm, a feeling of heaviness and numbness of the arm, feeling of cold.

Blood stasis
Severe pain in the shoulder joint that is worse at night, rigidity of the shoulder joint, Purple tongue.

UPPER BACK

Upper backache
Interrogation, Chapter 37

Invasion of Wind-Cold
Upper backache, stiffness of the neck and top of the shoulders, aversion to cold, fever, occipital headache, stiff neck, sneezing, body aches, tongue with thin white coating, Floating-Tight pulse.

Stagnation of Qi and stasis of Blood
Upper backache that may be worse at night, rigidity of the neck, pain relieved by exercise and aggravated by rest, tense muscles, headache, abdominal distension and pain, Purple tongue, Wiry pulse.

Damp-Cold
Severe pain in the upper back that is aggravated by exposure to cold and dampness and alleviated by the application of heat, a feeling of heaviness and numbness of the upper back, a feeling of cold.

Liver-Yang rising
Pain and stiffness of the upper back, stiff neck, tense muscles, headache, dizziness, tinnitus, irritability, propensity to outbursts of anger, Wiry pulse.

Liver-Qi stagnation
Pain and stiffness of the upper back, stiff neck, tense muscles, hypochondrial or epigastric distension, irritability, moodiness, a feeling of lump in the throat, premenstrual tension, Wiry pulse.

Cold upper back
Interrogation, Chapter 37

Invasion of Wind-Cold
A feeling of cold of the upper back, stiff neck and shoulders, aversion to cold, fever, occipital headache, stiff neck, sneezing, body aches, tongue with thin white coating, Floating-Tight pulse.

Yang deficiency
A feeling of cold of the upper back or in general, cold limbs, tiredness, depression, Pale tongue, Deep-Weak pulse.

Hot upper back
Lung-Heat
A feeling of heat of the upper back or in general, cough, slight breathlessness, chest ache, flaring of the nostrils, thirst, red face, Red tongue with yellow coating, Overflowing-Rapid pulse.

Lung-Yin deficiency
A feeling of heat in the upper back that is worse at night, dry cough, weak voice, dry throat with a desire to drink in small sips, hoarse voice, night sweating, tiredness, tongue without coating in the front, Floating-Empty pulse.

Stiffness of the back as if wearing a tight belt
Girdle Vessel pathology

A feeling of stiffness of the back and waist as if wearing a belt which is too tight, backache radiating horizontally to the front or abdominal pain radiating towards the back, a feeling as if sitting in cold water, a feeling of heaviness of the abdomen as if wearing a heavy money-belt (ancient texts describe this symptom as 'feeling as if wearing a belt with 3000 coins').

Damp-Heat in the Liver channel

A feeling of stiffness of the back and waist as if wearing a belt which is too tight, a pricking feeling of the skin around the waist, inability to breathe deeply, fullness of the hypochondrium, abdomen or hypogastrium, bitter taste, poor appetite, nausea, a feeling of heaviness of the body, yellow vaginal discharge, mid-cycle bleeding/pain, pain, urinary difficulty, burning on urination, dark urine, Red tongue with redder sides and a sticky-yellow coating, Slippery-Wiry-Rapid pulse.

Chapter **63**

CHEST

Chapter contents

COUGH   *659*
  Acute cough   *659*
  Chronic cough   *660*
  Coughing blood   *660*

BREATHLESSNESS   *661*

WHEEZING   *662*

PAIN   *663*
  Chest pain   *663*
  Pain in the ribs   *664*

FEELINGS IN THE CHEST AND HEART   *664*
  Feeling of oppression of the chest   *664*
  Feeling of distension of the chest   *664*
  Feeling of heat of the chest   *665*
  Heart feeling vexed   *665*
  Feeling of stuffiness under the heart   *666*

PALPITATIONS   *666*
  Palpitations under the heart   *666*

DISPLACED HEARTBEAT   *667*
  Heartbeat displaced downwards   *667*
  Heartbeat displaced upwards   *667*
  Heartbeat displaced to the left   *668*
  Heartbeat displaced to the right   *668*
  Heartbeat below the xyphoid process   *668*

ABNORMAL CHEST SHAPE   *668*
  Protruding chest   *668*
  Sunken chest   *668*
  Protruding sternum   *669*
  Chest sunken on one side   *669*
  Chest protruding on one side   *669*

GYNAECOMASTIA   *669*

YAWNING   *670*

SIGHING   *670*

COUGH

Acute cough

Observation, Chapter 20; Hearing and Smelling, Chapter 53

Invasion of Wind-Cold

Acute cough with expectoration of white sputum, aversion to cold, fever, itchy throat, slight breathlessness, stuffed or runny nose with clear watery discharge, sneezing, occipital headache, body aches, thin white tongue coating, Floating-Tight pulse.

Invasion of Wind-Heat

Acute cough with expectoration of yellow sputum, aversion to cold, fever, sore throat, stuffed or runny nose with yellow discharge, headache, body aches, slight sweating, slight thirst, swollen tonsils, tongue slightly Red on the sides in the chest area or on front part, Floating-Rapid pulse.

Invasion of Wind-Dryness

Acute, dry cough, aversion to cold, fever, dry throat, tickly throat, dry nose, discomfort of the chest, thin, dry white tongue coating, Floating pulse.

Phlegm-Heat in the Lungs

Acute, barking cough following an invasion of external Wind with profuse, sticky yellow or green sputum, shortness of breath, wheezing, a feeling of oppression of the chest, a feeling of heat, thirst, insomnia, agitation, Red and Swollen tongue with a sticky yellow coating, Slippery-Rapid pulse.

Lung-Heat

Acute, barking cough following an invasion of external Wind, expectoration of scanty yellow sputum,

slight breathlessness, a feeling of heat, chest ache, flaring of the nostrils, thirst, red face, Red tongue with yellow coating, Overflowing-Rapid pulse.

Residual dryness and Phlegm in the Lungs

Acute, dry cough after an invasion of Wind-Heat, difficult expectoration of scanty sputum after repeated bouts of dry coughing, persistent tickling sensation in the throat, dry throat, dry mouth, Swollen and dry tongue, Slippery pulse.

Residual dryness in the Lungs

Acute, dry cough after an invasion of Wind-Heat, repeated bouts of dry coughing, persistent tickling sensation in the throat, dry throat, dry mouth, dry tongue.

> ### Clinical note
>
> - In my experience, coughs following acute upper respiratory infections are due either to Phlegm-Heat or to Dryness with Phlegm. For the former I use Qing Qi Hua Tan Tang *Clearing Heat-Resolving Phlegm Decoction*, and for the latter Qing Zao Jiu Fei Tang *Clearing Dryness and Rescuing the Lungs Decoction*.

Chronic cough

Hearing and Smelling, Chapter 53

Damp-Phlegm in the Lungs

Chronic cough with easy expectoration of profuse white sputum, rattling sound in the throat, pasty-white complexion, a feeling of oppression in the chest, shortness of breath, a dislike of lying down, wheezing, nausea, Swollen tongue with a sticky white coating, Slippery pulse.

Phlegm-Dryness in the Lungs

Chronic, dry cough with a weak sound and occasional, difficult expectoration of scanty sputum, shortness of breath, a feeling of oppression of the chest, dry throat, wheezing, pasty dry complexion, Swollen tongue with a dry sticky coating, Fine-Slippery pulse.

Lung-Yin deficiency

Chronic cough that is dry or with difficult expectoration of scanty sputum, weak/hoarse voice, dry mouth and throat, tickly throat, tiredness, dislike of speaking, thin body or thin chest, night sweating, normal-coloured tongue without coating (or with rootless coating) in the front part, Floating-Empty pulse.

Lung-Yin deficiency with Empty-Heat

Chronic cough that is dry or with difficult expectoration of scanty sputum, which may be blood tinged, dry mouth and throat at night, tickly throat, tiredness, dislike of speaking, thin body or thin chest, night sweating, malar flush, a feeling of heat or a low-grade fever in the evening, five-palm heat, thin body, Red tongue without coating, Floating-Empty and Rapid pulse.

Lung-Dryness

Chronic, dry cough, dry skin, dry throat, dry mouth, thirst, hoarse voice, dry tongue, Floating-Empty pulse.

Lung-Qi deficiency

Chronic, slight cough with a weak sound, slight shortness of breath, weak voice, spontaneous daytime sweating, dislike of speaking, bright-white complexion, tendency to catch colds, tiredness, dislike of cold, Pale tongue, Empty pulse.

Cold-Phlegm in the Lungs

Chronic cough with expectoration of watery white sputum, aggravated by exposure to cold, a feeling of cold, cold hands, phlegm in the throat, dizziness, a feeling of oppression of the chest, a feeling of cold of the chest, Swollen and wet tongue with a sticky white coating, Slippery-Slow pulse.

Liver-Fire insulting the Lungs

Chronic, barking cough with a yellow or blood-tinged sputum, breathlessness, asthma, a feeling of fullness and distension of the chest and hypochondrium, headache, dizziness, red face, thirst, bitter taste, bloodshot eyes, scanty dark urine, constipation, Red tongue with redder sides and dry yellow coating, Wiry pulse.

Phlegm-Fluids in the Lungs

Chronic cough with expectoration of watery, frothy white sputum, breathlessness, splashing sound in the chest, vomiting of watery, frothy white sputum, feeling of cold, cough which may be elicited by a scare, Pale tongue with thick, sticky white coating, Fine-Slippery or Weak-Floating pulse.

Coughing blood
Lung-Heat

Cough with blood-tinged sputum, slight breathlessness, a feeling of heat, chest ache, flaring of nostrils,

thirst, red face, Red tongue with yellow coating, Overflowing-Rapid pulse.

Phlegm-Heat in the Lungs

Barking cough with expectoration of blood-tinged sputum, shortness of breath, wheezing, a feeling of oppression of the chest, a feeling of heat, thirst, insomnia, agitation, Red and Swollen tongue with a sticky yellow coating, Slippery-Rapid pulse.

Lung-Yin deficiency with Empty-Heat

Dry cough with difficult expectoration of scanty, blood-tinged sputum, dry mouth and throat at night, night sweating, tiredness, malar flush, a feeling of heat or a low-grade fever in the evening, five-palm heat, thin body, Red tongue without coating, Floating-Empty and Rapid pulse.

Invasion of Wind-Heat

Cough with blood-tinged sputum, aversion to cold, fever, sore throat, stuffed or runny nose with yellow discharge, headache, body aches, slight sweating, slight thirst, swollen tonsils, tongue slightly Red on the sides in the chest area or on front part, Floating-Rapid pulse.

Lung- and Spleen-Qi deficiency

Slight cough with expectoration of scanty, blood-tinged sputum, fresh-red blood, tiredness, loose stools, poor appetite, slight abdominal distension, weak voice, slight shortness of breath, spontaneous sweating, dislike of speaking, Pale tongue, Empty pulse.

Lung-Heat at the Blood level (Four Levels)

Coughing of blood, fever at night, macular skin eruptions, mental confusion, night sweating, five-palm heat, dry throat, Red tongue with red points and without coating, Fine-Rapid pulse.

BREATHLESSNESS

Hearing and Smelling, Chapter 53

The symptom of breathlessness comprises four slightly different symptoms. These are:

> • breathlessness (*Chuan*): severe difficulty in breathing with shortness of breath and raising of the shoulders

> • shortness of breath (*Duan Qi*): short, irregular, rapid breaths without pronounced struggling for breath and raising of shoulders seen in breathlessness
> • weak breathing (*Qi Shao*): weak, low, short breathing sounds
> • rebellious-Qi breathing (*Shang Qi*): rapid short breaths, cough, a sensation of oppression of the throat and feeling of energy rising accompanied by a feeling of anxiety.

Lung-Qi deficiency

Shortness of breath or weak breathing, slight cough, weak voice, spontaneous daytime sweating, dislike of speaking, bright-white complexion, tendency to catch colds, tiredness, dislike of cold, Pale tongue, Empty pulse.

Lung-Yin deficiency

Shortness of breath or weak breathing with difficulty in exhaling, cough which is dry or with scanty sticky sputum, weak/hoarse voice, dry mouth and throat, tickly throat, tiredness, dislike of speaking, thin body or thin chest, night sweating, normal-coloured tongue without coating (or with rootless coating) in the front part, Floating-Empty pulse.

Kidneys not receiving Qi

Shortness of breath or weak breathing with difficulty in inhaling, rapid and weak breathing, chronic cough/asthma, spontaneous sweating, cold limbs, cold limbs after sweating, swelling of the face, thin body, mental listlessness, clear urination during asthma attack, soreness of the back, dizziness, tinnitus, Pale tongue, Deep-Weak-Tight pulse.

Lung-Qi stagnation

Shortness of breath, a feeling of a lump in the throat, difficulty in swallowing, a feeling of oppression or distension of the chest, slight breathlessness, sighing, sadness, worry, irritability, depression, tongue slightly Red on the sides in the chest areas, pulse very slightly Tight on the right Front position.

Phlegm-Heat in the Lungs

Acute breathlessness, barking cough with expectoration of blood-tinged sputum, shortness of breath, wheezing, a feeling of oppression of the chest, a feeling of heat, thirst, insomnia, agitation, Red and Swollen

tongue with a sticky yellow coating, Slippery-Rapid pulse.

Damp-Phlegm in the Lungs

Breathlessness, wheezing, chronic cough coming in bouts with profuse sticky white sputum which is easy to expectorate, pasty-white complexion, a feeling of oppression in the chest, dislike of lying down, wheezing, nausea, Swollen tongue with a sticky white coating, Slippery pulse.

Lung-Heat

Acute breathlessness, cough with expectoration of scanty yellow sputum, a feeling of heat, chest ache, flaring of nostrils, thirst, red face, Red tongue with yellow coating, Overflowing-Rapid pulse.

Cold-Phlegm in the Lungs

Breathlessness, chronic cough with expectoration of watery white sputum, aggravated by exposure to cold, a feeling of cold generally or in the chest, cold hands, phlegm in the throat, dizziness, a feeling of oppression of the chest, Swollen and wet tongue with a sticky white coating, Slippery-Slow pulse.

Kidney-Yang deficiency with Phlegm

Shortness of breath with difficulty in inhaling, cough with expectoration of watery white sputum, a feeling of cold, cold feet, lower backache, dizziness, tinnitus, frequent pale urination, Pale, Swollen and wet tongue, Weak and slightly Slippery pulse.

Kidney-Yang deficiency with Water overflowing to the Lungs

Severe breathlessness, oedema especially of the legs and ankles, a feeling of cold in legs and back, fullness and distension of abdomen, soreness of lower back, a feeling of cold, scanty clear urination, expectoration of thin, watery frothy sputum, cough, Pale and Swollen tongue with a wet white coating, Deep-Weak-Slow pulse.

Phlegm in the Lungs with Lung-Qi deficiency

Shortness of breath, chronic cough which is worse on exertion, scanty phlegm that is difficult to expectorate or dilute watery phlegm, spontaneous sweating, a feeling of cold, a feeling of oppression of the chest, weak voice, tongue Pale and slightly Swollen in the front, pulse Empty on the right Front position and slightly Slippery.

Lung-Qi and Kidney-Yang deficiency

Slight shortness of breath, weak breathing, low, short breathing sounds, lower backache, cold knees, a feeling of cold, bright-white complexion, weak knees, tiredness, lassitude, abundant clear urination, urination at night, slight cough, weak voice, spontaneous daytime sweating, dislike of speaking, bright-white complexion, tendency to catch colds, tiredness, dislike of cold, Pale tongue, Deep-Weak pulse.

Rebellious Qi of the Penetrating Vessel 👩 👨

Slight shortness of breath, rapid, short breaths, cough, a feeling of tightness of the chest, palpitations, anxiety, epigastric and abdominal fullness, painful periods, Firm pulse.

Liver-Fire insulting the Lungs 👨

Shortness of breath, rapid, short breaths, chronic, barking cough with a yellow or blood-tinged sputum, asthma, a feeling of fullness and distension of the chest and hypochondrium, headache, dizziness, red face, thirst, bitter taste, bloodshot eyes, scanty dark urine, constipation, Red tongue with redder sides and dry yellow coating, Wiry pulse.

WHEEZING

Hearing and Smelling, Chapter 53

Cold-Phlegm in the Lungs

Wheezing, cough with expectoration of watery white sputum, a feeling of cold, cold hands and feet, nausea, vomiting, a feeling of oppression of the chest and epigastrium, dull-white complexion, pale urine, Pale and Swollen tongue with wet white coating, Slippery-Slow pulse.

Phlegm-Heat in the Lungs

Noisy wheezing, feeling of heaviness and muzziness of the head, a feeling of heat, red face, greasy skin, a feeling of oppression of the chest, sputum in the throat, expectoration of yellow sputum, dizziness, nausea, Red and Swollen tongue with sticky yellow coating, Slippery-Rapid pulse.

Damp-Phlegm in the Lungs

Wheezing, chronic cough with expectoration of profuse, sticky white sputum which is easy to expecto-

rate, a feeling of oppression of the chest, dizziness, blurred vision, somnolence, nausea, sputum in the throat, muzziness of the head, Swollen tongue with sticky coating, Slippery pulse.

Lung-Yang deficiency with Phlegm

Slight wheezing, expectoration of watery white sputum, breathlessness, rattling sound in the throat, cold limbs, worse on exercise, pale face, sweating, feeling of cold, tendency to catch colds, Pale and wet tongue, Deep-Weak and slightly Slippery pulse.

Lung-Yin deficiency with Phlegm

Slight wheezing, expectoration of scanty sputum, breathlessness, a feeling of oppression of the chest, dry cough, weak voice, dry throat with desire to sip water, hoarse voice, night sweating, tiredness, tongue without coating in the front, Floating-Empty pulse.

Lung-Qi deficiency with Phlegm

Chronic wheezing, shortness of breath, slight cough, weak voice, spontaneous daytime sweating, dislike of speaking, pale complexion, tendency to catch colds, a feeling of oppression of the chest, sputum in the throat, Pale and Swollen tongue, Soggy pulse.

Spleen-Qi deficiency with Phlegm

Slight, chronic wheezing, sputum in the throat, a feeling of oppression of the chest, poor appetite, tiredness, slight abdominal distension, pale complexion, loose stools, Pale and Swollen tongue, Soggy pulse.

Kidney-Yang deficiency with Phlegm

Chronic wheezing, lower backache, cold knees, a feeling of cold, bright-white complexion, weak knees, tiredness, lassitude, abundant clear urination, urination at night, impotence, decreased libido, Pale and wet tongue, Deep-Weak pulse.

PAIN

Chest pain

Interrogation, Chapter 38

Heart-Blood stasis

Stabbing or pricking chest pain which may radiate to the inner aspect of the left arm or to the shoulder, palpitations, a feeling of oppression or constriction of the chest, cyanosis of lips and nails, cold hands, tongue entirely Purple or Purple only on the sides in the chest areas, Choppy or Wiry pulse.

Heart-Yang deficiency

A feeling of discomfort or very slight pain of the chest, palpitations, shortness of breath on exertion, tiredness, slight depression, spontaneous sweating, a feeling of cold, cold hands, bright-pale face, slightly dark lips, Pale tongue, Deep-Weak pulse.

Heart-Yang deficiency with Phlegm

Dull chest pain, a feeling of oppression or tightness of the chest, palpitations, shortness of breath on exertion, tiredness, slight depression, spontaneous sweating, a feeling of cold, cold hands, bright-pale face, slightly dark lips, Pale and Swollen tongue, Deep-Weak-Slippery pulse.

Phlegm-Heat in the Lungs

Chest pain, a feeling of oppression of the chest, shortness of breath, a feeling of heaviness and muzziness of the head, a feeling of heat, red face, greasy skin, sputum in the throat, expectoration of yellow sputum, dizziness, nausea, Red and Swollen tongue with sticky yellow coating, Slippery-Rapid pulse.

Liver-Qi stagnation

Dull chest and hypochondrial distension and pain, irritability, moodiness, a feeling of a lump in the throat, premenstrual tension, Wiry pulse.

Rebellious Qi in the Penetrating Vessel

Dull chest pain, a feeling of tightness of the chest, palpitations, anxiety, a feeling of a lump in the throat, abdominal and umbilical fullness, epigastric fullness, irregular periods, painful periods, a feeling of energy rising in the abdomen to the chest, a feeling of heat in the face, nausea, Firm pulse.

Lung-Qi stagnation

Slight chest pain, a feeling of a lump in the throat, difficulty in swallowing, a feeling of oppression or distension of the chest, slight breathlessness, sighing, sadness, irritability, depression, tongue slightly Red on the sides in the chest areas, pulse very slightly Tight on the right Front position.

Damp-Heat in the Liver and Gall-Bladder channels

Chest pain extending to the hypochondrium, a feeling of oppression and heaviness of the chest, bitter taste, poor appetite, nausea, a feeling of heaviness of the body, yellow vaginal discharge, vaginal itching, mid-cycle bleeding/pain, burning on urination, dark urine, yellow complexion and eyes, vomiting, Red tongue with redder sides and unilateral or bilateral sticky yellow coating, Wiry-Slippery-Rapid pulse.

Pain in the ribs

Interrogation, Chapter 38

'Pain in the ribs' refers to pain on the lateral aspect of the rib cage above the hypochondrial area.

Liver-Qi stagnation

Pain in the ribs with a feeling of distension, hypochondrial or epigastric distension, irritability, moodiness, a feeling of a lump in the throat, premenstrual tension, Wiry pulse.

Liver-Blood stasis

Severe pain in the ribs, hypochondrial pain, abdominal pain, painful periods, irregular periods, dark and clotted menstrual blood, masses in the abdomen, purple nails and lips, purple or dark complexion, dry skin, Purple tongue, Wiry or Firm pulse.

Damp-Heat in the Liver and Gall-Bladder

Pain in the ribs, a feeling of oppression and heaviness in the ribs, bitter and sticky taste, burning on urination, excessive vaginal discharge, irritability, a feeling of oppression of the chest, nausea, vomiting, dark urine, tongue with Red sides and sticky yellow tongue coating, Wiry-Slippery-Rapid pulse.

FEELINGS IN THE CHEST AND HEART

Feeling of oppression of the chest

Interrogation, Chapter 38

Please note that this particular feeling is sometimes described as a 'feeling of tightness' of the chest by many patients.

Phlegm in the Lungs

A feeling of oppression of the chest, breathlessness, sputum in the throat, a feeling of heaviness, Swollen tongue with sticky coating, Slippery pulse.

Other symptoms and signs depend on whether there is Cold-Phlegm, Damp-Phlegm or Phlegm-Heat.

Lung-Qi stagnation

A feeling of oppression of the chest, slight chest pain, a feeling of tightness of the chest, a feeling of a lump in the throat, difficulty in swallowing, slight breathlessness, sighing, sadness, irritability, depression, tongue slightly Red on the sides in the chest areas, pulse very slightly Tight on the right Front position.

Liver-Qi stagnation

A feeling of oppression and distension of the chest and hypochondrium, epigastric distension, irritability, moodiness, a feeling of a lump in the throat, premenstrual tension, Wiry pulse.

Rebellious Qi in the Penetrating Vessel

A feeling of oppression of the chest, dull chest pain, a feeling of tightness of the chest, a feeling of heat in the face, a feeling of a lump in the throat, palpitations, anxiety, nausea, slight breathlessness, epigastric fullness or stuffiness, umbilical and abdominal fullness, irregular/painful periods, a feeling of energy rising in the abdomen to the chest, Firm pulse.

Heart-Yang deficiency with Phlegm

A feeling of oppression or tightness of the chest, slight chest pain or discomfort, palpitations, shortness of breath on exertion, tiredness, slight depression, spontaneous sweating, a feeling of cold, cold hands, bright-pale face, slightly dark lips, Pale tongue, Deep-Weak pulse.

> ### Clinical note
>
> - 'A feeling of oppression of the chest' is the translation of the Chinese term '*men*', which nearly always indicates that emotional problems are at the root of this symptom. P-6 Neiguan and ST-40 Fenglong used unilaterally and crossed over is a good combination for this symptom.

Feeling of distension of the chest
Liver-Qi stagnation

Feeling of distension of the chest and hypochondrium, epigastric distension, irritability, moodiness, a feeling of a lump in the throat, premenstrual tension, Wiry pulse.

Lung-Qi stagnation

Feeling of distension, oppression or tightness of the chest, a feeling of a lump in the throat, difficulty in swallowing, slight breathlessness, sighing, sadness, irritability, depression, tongue slightly Red on the sides in the chest areas, pulse very slightly Tight on the right Front position.

Feeling of heat of the chest

Interrogation, Chapter 38

Lung-Heat

A feeling of heat of the chest, cough, slight breathlessness, a feeling of heat, chest ache, flaring of nostrils, thirst, red face, Red tongue with yellow coating, Overflowing-Rapid pulse.

Lung-Yin deficiency with Empty-Heat

A feeling of heat in the chest in the afternoon or evening, dry cough or with scanty, sticky sputum, dry mouth and throat at night, night sweating, tiredness, malar flush, a feeling of heat or a low-grade fever in the evening, five-palm heat, thin body, Red tongue without coating, Floating-Empty and Rapid pulse.

Heart-Fire

A feeling of heat of the chest, palpitations, thirst, mouth and tongue ulcers, mental restlessness, a feeling of agitation, insomnia, dream-disturbed sleep, a feeling of heat, red face, bitter taste, Red tongue with redder tip and yellow coating, Overflowing-Rapid pulse.

Heart-Yin deficiency with Empty-Heat

A feeling of heat of the chest that is worse in the evening, palpitations, insomnia, dream-disturbed sleep, poor memory, anxiety, mental restlessness, dry mouth and throat, malar flush, night sweating, five-palm heat, Red tongue with redder tip and without coating, Floating-Empty and Rapid pulse.

Residual Heat in the diaphragm

A feeling of heat in the chest, thirst, dry throat, irritability, restlessness, a feeling of fullness and stuffiness of the diaphragm and epigastrium, which feels soft on pressure, nausea, slight shortness of breath, tongue Red in the front, Deep-Rapid pulse.

This is residual Heat following an invasion of Wind-Heat, which later progressed to the Qi level.

Heart feeling vexed

The term 'Heart feeling vexed' (called *Xin Zhong Ao Nong*) includes a feeling of anxiety and mental restlessness with heat, a slight feeling of oppression and uneasiness of the chest and a feeling of constriction between the heart and the diaphragm.

Heart-Fire

Heart feeling vexed, a feeling of tightness of the chest, palpitations, thirst, mouth and tongue ulcers, mental restlessness, feeling of agitation, insomnia, dream-disturbed sleep, a feeling of heat, red face, bitter taste, Red tongue with redder tip and yellow coating, Overflowing-Rapid pulse.

Heart-Yin deficiency with Empty-Heat

Heart feeling vexed, a slight feeling of emptiness of the chest, anxiety, mental restlessness, palpitations, insomnia, dream-disturbed sleep, poor memory, dry mouth and throat, a feeling of heat in the evening, malar flush, night sweating, five-palm heat, Red tongue with redder tip and without coating, Floating-Empty and Rapid pulse.

Qi and Yin deficiency of the Heart

Heart feeling vexed, a slight feeling of tightness of the chest, slight anxiety, palpitations, sweating, slight shortness of breath, dry throat, dry mouth, insomnia, tongue without coating, Weak pulse.

Phlegm-Heat in the Heart

Heart feeling vexed, palpitations, mental restlessness, thirst, red face, a feeling of oppression of the chest, expectoration of phlegm, sputum in the throat, bitter taste, insomnia, dream-disturbed sleep, a feeling of agitation, mental confusion, incoherent speech, rash behaviour, uncontrolled laughter or crying, shouting, depression, manic behaviour, Red tongue with redder swollen tip, and Heart crack with a sticky, dry yellow coating inside it, Slippery-Rapid or Slippery-Overflowing-Rapid pulse.

Residual Heat in the diaphragm

Heart feeling vexed, a feeling of heat in the chest, thirst, dry throat, irritability, restlessness, a feeling of fullness and stuffiness of the diaphragm and epigastrium, which feels soft on pressure, nausea, slight shortness of breath, tongue Red in the front, Deep-Rapid pulse.

This is residual Heat following an invasion of Wind-Heat, which later progressed to the Qi level.

Feeling of stuffiness under the heart

'A feeling of stuffiness' indicates a subjective feeling of fullness or oppression of a certain area of the body, which, however, feels soft on palpation. It is a translation of the Chinese term *pi*.

Heat

A feeling of stuffiness under the heart, a feeling of heat, palpitations, thirst, nausea, dark urine, Red tongue with yellow tongue coating, Overflowing-Rapid pulse.

Other symptoms and signs depend on the organ involved, which may be the Heart or Lungs.

Cold

A feeling of stuffiness under the heart, a feeling of cold, cold limbs, white tongue coating, Tight pulse.

Other symptoms and signs depend on the organ involved, which may be the Lungs or Stomach.

Phlegm

A feeling of stuffiness under the heart, sputum in the throat, a feeling of oppression of the chest, nausea, vomiting, dizziness, blurred vision, Swollen tongue with sticky coating, Slippery pulse.

Other symptoms and signs depend on the organ involved, which may be the Lungs, Heart or Stomach, and on the type of Phlegm.

Rebellious Qi in the Penetrating Vessel

A feeling of stuffiness under the heart, palpitations under the heart, feeling of heat in the face, a feeling of a lump in the throat, anxiety, a feeling of tightness of the chest, nausea, slight breathlessness, epigastric fullness or stuffiness, umbilical and abdominal fullness, irregular/painful periods, a feeling of energy rising in the abdomen to the chest, Firm pulse.

Phlegm-Fluids

A feeling of stuffiness under the heart, abdominal fullness and distension, nausea, vomiting of watery fluids, dry mouth without a desire to drink, shortness of breath, dizziness, a feeling of oppression of the chest, swelling of the limbs, expectoration of thin watery sputum, inability to lie down, Swollen tongue with sticky coating, Deep-Wiry or Deep-Slippery pulse.

PALPITATIONS

Interrogation, Chapter 38

'Palpitations' indicates a subjective sensation of the patient who is aware of the heart beating and may have the impression that it is fast or irregular. This is a subjective sensation and the pulse may in fact be neither rapid nor irregular. 'Palpitations' should therefore not be confused or identified with the Western symptom of tachycardia, which refers to the objective rapidity of the pulse, nor to arrhythmia.

Palpitations is a symptom that may appear in any Heart pattern (to avoid repetition, please refer to the Heart patterns in Chapter 91). Below are listed three more conditions that may cause palpitations.

Shock affecting the Heart

Palpitations after a shock, anxiety, agitation, restless sleep, Moving pulse.

Kidney-Yang deficiency with Water overflowing to the Heart

Palpitations, oedema especially of the legs and ankles, a feeling of cold generally or in legs and back, fullness and distension of abdomen, soreness of the lower back, scanty clear urination, breathlessness, cold hands, Pale and Swollen tongue with a wet white coating, Deep-Weak-Slow pulse.

Rebellious-Qi in the Penetrating Vessel affecting the Heart

Severe palpitations, anxiety, feeling of energy rising from the abdomen to the chest, a feeling of heat in the face, a feeling of a lump in the throat, a feeling of tightness of the chest, nausea, slight breathlessness, epigastric fullness or stuffiness, umbilical and abdominal fullness, irregular/painful periods, Firm pulse.

Palpitations under the heart

'Palpitations under the heart' indicates a feeling of pulsation in the epigastrium or the area between the heart and epigastrium. Western patients may express this symptom in different ways, such as 'a feeling of pulsation in the stomach', 'butterflies in the stomach', 'a jumping feeling in the stomach' and 'a feeling of anxiety in the stomach'.

Heart-Yang deficiency

Slight palpitations under the heart, a desire to press or massage the area between the heart and the stomach, shortness of breath on exertion, tiredness, slight depression, spontaneous sweating, a slight feeling of discomfort or stuffiness in the heart region, a feeling of cold, cold hands, bright-pale face, slightly dark lips, Pale tongue, Deep-Weak pulse.

Heart-Yin deficiency with Empty-Heat

Slight palpitations under the heart, insomnia, dream-disturbed sleep, poor memory, anxiety, mental restlessness, dry mouth and throat, a feeling of heat in the evening, malar flush, night sweating, five-palm heat, Red tongue with redder tip and without coating, Floating-Empty and Rapid pulse.

Phlegm-Fire harassing the Heart

Severe palpitations under the heart, a feeling of oppression of the chest, mental restlessness, thirst, red face, dark urine, expectoration of phlegm, rattling sound in the throat, bitter taste, insomnia, dream-disturbed sleep, a feeling of agitation, mental confusion, incoherent speech, rash behaviour, tendency to hit or scold people, uncontrolled laughter or crying, shouting, muttering to oneself, depression, manic behaviour, Red tongue with redder swollen tip, Heart crack with a sticky yellow coating inside it, Slippery-Rapid or Slippery-Overflowing-Rapid pulse.

Rebellious Qi in the Penetrating Vessel

Palpitations under the heart, a feeling of heat in the face, a feeling of a lump in the throat, anxiety, a feeling of tightness of the chest, nausea, slight breathlessness, epigastric fullness or stuffiness, umbilical and abdominal fullness, irregular/painful periods, a feeling of energy rising in the abdomen to the chest, Firm pulse.

Kidney-Yang deficiency with Water overflowing to the Heart

Slight palpitations under the heart, oedema especially of the legs and ankles, a feeling of cold in the legs and back, fullness and distension of the abdomen, soreness of the lower back, a feeling of cold, scanty clear urination, palpitations, breathlessness, cold hands, Pale and Swollen tongue with a wet white coating, Deep-Weak-Slow pulse.

DISPLACED HEARTBEAT

Heartbeat displaced downwards

Observation, Chapter 13

Heart-Qi deficiency with Heart-Blood stasis

Heartbeat displaced downwards, exhaustion, palpitations, shortness of breath on exertion, pale face, tiredness, slight depression, spontaneous sweating, chest pain, purple lips, Bluish-Purple tongue, Choppy pulse.

Liver- and Kidney-Yin deficiency

Heartbeat displaced downwards, palpitations, dizziness, tinnitus, hardness of hearing, lower backache, dull occipital or vertical headache, insomnia, numbness/tingling of limbs, dry eyes, blurred vision, dry throat, dry hair and skin, brittle nails, dry vagina, night sweating, dry stools, nocturnal emissions, scanty menstruation or amenorrhoea, delayed cycle, infertility, normal-coloured tongue without coating, Floating-Empty pulse.

Phlegm-Fluids obstructing the Heart

Heartbeat displaced downwards, palpitations, abdominal fullness and distension, nausea, vomiting of watery fluids, dry mouth without a desire to drink, shortness of breath, dizziness, a feeling of oppression of the chest, swelling of the limbs, expectoration of thin watery sputum, inability to lie down, Swollen tongue with sticky coating, Deep-Wiry or Deep-Slippery pulse.

Toxic Heat invading the Heart

Heartbeat displaced downwards, palpitations, a feeling of oppression of the chest, breathlessness, mental restlessness, fever, Red tongue with red points and thick, sticky yellow coating, Overflowing-Slippery-Rapid pulse.

Heartbeat displaced upwards

Observation, Chapter 13

Kidney- and Heart-Yang deficiency with Water overflowing

Heartbeat displaced upwards, oedema especially of the legs and ankles, a feeling of cold generally or in legs and back, fullness and distension of the abdomen, soreness of the lower back, scanty clear urination, palpitations, breathlessness, cold hands, Pale and Swollen

tongue with a wet white coating, Deep-Weak-Slow pulse.

Heartbeat displaced to the left

Observation, Chapter 13

Phlegm-Fluids in the chest and hypochondrium

Heartbeat displaced to the left, hypochondrial pain which is worse on coughing and breathing, a feeling of distension and pulling of the hypochondrium, shortness of breath, cough with expectoration of watery white sputum, breathlessness, oedema, dizziness, hypochondrial pain, Swollen tongue with sticky coating, Deep-Slippery-Wiry pulse.

Liver-Blood stasis with Water overflowing

Heartbeat displaced to the left, hypochondrial pain, abdominal pain, painful periods, dark and clotted menstrual blood, masses in the abdomen, purple nails and lips, purple or dark complexion, oedema of the abdomen, Purple and Swollen tongue, Wiry or Firm pulse.

Heartbeat displaced to the right

Observation, Chapter 13

Heart-Qi deficiency with Heart-Blood stasis

Heartbeat displaced to the right, exhaustion, palpitations, shortness of breath on exertion, pale face, spontaneous sweating, stabbing or pricking chest pain which may radiate to the inner aspect of the left arm or to the shoulder, a feeling of oppression or constriction of the chest, cyanosis of lips and nails, cold hands, tongue entirely Purple or Purple only on the sides in the chest areas, Choppy pulse.

Phlegm-Fluids in the chest and hypochondrium

Heartbeat displaced to the right, hypochondrial pain which is worse on coughing and breathing, a feeling of distension and pulling of the hypochondrium, shortness of breath, cough with expectoration of watery white sputum, breathlessness, oedema, dizziness, hypochondrial pain, Swollen tongue with sticky coating, Deep-Slippery-Wiry pulse.

Heartbeat below the xyphoid process

Observation, Chapter 13

Heart-Blood stasis

Heartbeat below the xyphoid process, palpitations, stabbing or pricking chest pain which may radiate to the inner aspect of the left arm or to the shoulder, a feeling of oppression or constriction of the chest, cyanosis of lips and nails, cold hands, tongue entirely Purple or Purple only on the sides in the chest areas, Choppy or Wiry pulse.

Heart-Qi deficiency

Heartbeat below the xyphoid process, palpitations, shortness of breath on exertion, pale face, tiredness, slight depression, spontaneous sweating, Pale tongue, Empty pulse.

ABNORMAL CHEST SHAPE

Protruding chest

Observation, Chapter 16

Chronic Phlegm in the Lungs

Protruding chest, a feeling of oppression of the chest, cough with expectoration of profuse sputum, breathlessness, sputum in the throat, wheezing, Swollen tongue with sticky coating, Slippery pulse.

Severe Liver-Qi stagnation

Protruding chest, hypochondrial or epigastric distension, irritability, moodiness, a feeling of a lump in the throat, premenstrual tension, Wiry pulse.

Liver-Blood stasis

Protruding chest, chest pain, hypochondrial pain, abdominal pain, painful periods, dark and clotted menstrual blood, masses in the abdomen, purple nails and lips, purple or dark complexion, Purple tongue, Wiry or Firm pulse.

Sunken chest

Observation, Chapter 16

Lung-Qi deficiency

Sunken chest, slight shortness of breath, slight cough, weak voice, spontaneous daytime sweating, dislike of speaking, bright-white complexion, tendency to catch

colds, tiredness, dislike of cold, Pale tongue, Empty pulse.

Lung-Yin deficiency

Sunken chest, dry cough, weak voice, dry throat with desire to sip water, hoarse voice, night sweating, tiredness, tongue without coating in the front, Floating-Empty pulse.

Kidney-Yang deficiency

Sunken chest, lower backache, cold knees, a feeling of cold, bright-white complexion, weak knees, tiredness, lassitude, abundant clear urination, urination at night, impotence, decreased libido, Pale and wet tongue, Deep-Weak pulse.

Lung- and Kidney-Yin deficiency

Sunken chest, dry cough which is worse in the evening, dry throat and mouth, thin body, breathlessness on exertion, lower backache, night sweating, dizziness, tinnitus, hardness of hearing, scanty urination, normal-coloured tongue without coating, Floating-Empty pulse.

Protruding sternum

Observation, Chapter 16

Constitutional deficiency of Lungs and Kidneys

Protruding sternum, poor constitution, tendency to catch colds, lower backache, a history of repeated chest infections during childhood.

Other symptoms and signs depend on whether there is Yin or Yang deficiency.

Phlegm in the Lungs

Protruding sternum, a feeling of oppression of the chest, cough with expectoration of profuse sputum, sputum in the throat, breathlessness, wheezing, Swollen tongue with sticky coating, Slippery pulse.

Chest sunken on one side

Observation, Chapter 16

Lung-Yin deficiency

Chest sunken on one side, dry cough, weak voice, dry throat with desire to sip water, hoarse voice, night sweating, tiredness, tongue without coating in the front, Floating-Empty pulse.

Phlegm-Fluids in the Lungs

Chest sunken on one side, abdominal fullness and distension, nausea, vomiting of watery fluids, dry mouth without a desire to drink, shortness of breath, dizziness, a feeling of oppression of the chest, swelling of the limbs, expectoration of thin watery sputum, inability to lie down, Swollen tongue with sticky coating, Deep-Wiry or Deep-Slippery pulse.

Phlegm-Fluids in the Lungs with Blood stasis

Chest sunken on one side, abdominal fullness and distension, nausea, vomiting of watery fluids, dry mouth without a desire to drink, shortness of breath, dizziness, a feeling of oppression of the chest, swelling of the limbs, expectoration of thin watery sputum, inability to lie down, Swollen tongue with sticky coating, purple lips, chest pain, Purple and Swollen tongue with sticky coating, Slippery or Wiry pulse.

Chest protruding on one side

Observation, Chapter 16

Phlegm-Fluids in the Lungs

Chest protruding on one side, abdominal fullness and distension, nausea, vomiting of watery fluids, dry mouth without a desire to drink, shortness of breath, dizziness, a feeling of oppression of the chest, swelling of the limbs, expectoration of thin watery sputum, inability to lie down, Swollen tongue with sticky coating, Deep-Wiry or Deep-Slippery pulse.

Severe Liver-Qi stagnation

Chest protruding on one side, hypochondrial or epigastric distension, irritability, moodiness, a feeling of a lump in the throat, premenstrual tension, Wiry pulse.

Heart-Qi deficiency with Blood stasis

Chest protruding on one side, palpitations, shortness of breath on exertion, pale face, tiredness, spontaneous sweating, chest pain, purple lips, cold hands, tongue Purple on the sides towards the front, Choppy pulse.

GYNAECOMASTIA

Observation, Chapter 16

Gynaecomastia is a swelling of the breasts in males.

Liver-Blood stasis

Gynaecomastia, hypochondrial pain, abdominal pain, vomiting of blood, epistaxis, infertility, masses in the abdomen, purple nails and lips, purple or dark complexion, dry skin (only in severe cases), purple petechiae, Purple tongue, Wiry or Firm pulse.

Damp-Heat in the Penetrating Vessel

Gynaecomastia, abdominal fullness and pain, pain in the testicles, turbid urine, tongue with sticky yellow coating, Slippery-Rapid pulse.

YAWNING

Yawning is considered a symptom only if it occurs very frequently; yawning when one is sleepy and tired is normal.

Liver-Qi stagnation

Frequent yawning, hypochondrial or epigastric distension, irritability, moodiness, a feeling of a lump in the throat, premenstrual tension, Wiry pulse.

Lung-Qi stagnation

Frequent yawning, a feeling of a lump in the throat, difficulty in swallowing, a feeling of oppression or distension of the chest, slight breathlessness, sighing, sadness, irritability, depression, tongue slightly Red on the sides in the chest areas, pulse very slightly Tight on the right Front position.

Stagnation of Qi and stasis of Blood

Frequent yawning, a feeling of tightness of the chest, chest pain, abdominal distension, palpitations, agitation, Purple tongue, Wiry pulse.

Spleen- and Kidney-Yang deficiency

Frequent yawning, lower backache, cold and weak knees, a feeling of cold, bright-white complexion, impotence, decreased libido, tiredness, lassitude, abundant clear urination, urination at night, loose stools, poor appetite, slight abdominal distension, a desire to lie down, early-morning diarrhoea, Pale and wet tongue, Deep-Weak pulse.

SIGHING

Liver-Qi stagnation

Bouts of sighing preceded by emotional problems, long sighs, hypochondrial or epigastric distension, irritability, moodiness, a feeling of a lump in the throat, premenstrual tension, Wiry pulse.

Lung-Qi stagnation

Short sighs, a feeling of a lump in the throat, difficulty in swallowing, a feeling of oppression or distension of the chest, slight breathlessness, sighing, sadness, irritability, depression, tongue slightly Red on the sides in the chest areas, pulse very slightly Tight on the right Front position.

Spleen- and Heart-Qi deficiency

Short sighs, poor appetite, slight abdominal distension after eating, tiredness, pale complexion, weakness of the limbs, loose stools, palpitations, shortness of breath on exertion, spontaneous sweating, Pale tongue, Empty pulse.

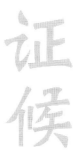

Chapter **64**

LIMBS

Chapter contents

MUSCLE ACHE IN THE LIMBS   *671*

PAIN IN THE LIMBS   *672*

HANDS AND FEET   *672*
Cold hands and feet   *672*
Hot hands and feet   *672*

ABNORMAL FEELINGS IN THE LIMBS   *673*
Numbness/tingling of the limbs   *673*
Feeling of heaviness of the limbs   *673*
Feeling of distension of the limbs   *674*

WEAKNESS AND ATROPHY   *674*
Weakness of the limbs   *674*
Atrophy of the limbs   *674*
Flaccidity of the limbs   *675*

LIMB SWELLING   *675*
Oedema of the limbs   *675*
Swelling of the joints of the limbs   *676*

LIMB MOVEMENT   *676*
Rigidity of the limbs   *676*
Paralysis of the limbs   *676*
Contraction of the limbs   *677*
Tremor or spasticity of the limbs   *678*
Convulsions of the limbs   *678*

MUSCLE ACHE IN THE LIMBS

Interrogation, Chapter 39

Dampness in the muscles

Muscle ache, a feeling of heaviness of the limbs, a feeling of heaviness in general, lassitude, sleepiness, epigastric fullness, sticky tongue coating, Slippery pulse.

Other symptoms and signs depend on whether the Dampness is associated with Cold or Heat.

Phlegm-Heat in the muscles

Muscle ache, a feeling of heaviness of the limbs, numbness/tingling of the limbs, sputum in the throat, a feeling of oppression of the chest, thirst without a desire to drink, Swollen tongue with sticky yellow coating, Slippery-Rapid pulse.

Liver-Qi stagnation

Distending muscle ache, hypochondrial or epigastric distension, irritability, moodiness, a feeling of a lump in the throat, premenstrual tension, Wiry pulse.

Liver-Blood deficiency

Dull muscle ache which is aggravated by physical exertion, dizziness, blurred vision, floaters, numbness/tingling of limbs, scanty menstruation, dull-pale complexion, Pale tongue, Choppy or Fine pulse.

> ## Clinical note
> - Dampness is by far the most common cause of muscle ache. This is a common symptom in postviral fatigue syndrome.

PAIN IN THE LIMBS

Interrogation, Chapter 39

Wind

Wandering pain in the joints that may come and go, especially in the upper part of the body.

This pattern is Wind Painful Obstruction Syndrome and, in acute cases, the pulse is Floating.

Cold

Pain in the joints that is aggravated by exposure to cold and alleviated by application of heat, usually in one joint only, cold limbs.

This is Cold Painful Obstruction Syndrome and, in acute cases, the pulse is Tight.

Dampness

Pain in the joints with swelling, a feeling of heaviness, numbness of the limbs.

This is Damp Painful Obstruction Syndrome and, in acute cases, the pulse is Slippery.

Damp-Heat

Pain in the joints with swelling and redness, hot to touch, a feeling of heaviness and numbness of the limbs, Red tongue with sticky yellow coating, Slippery-Rapid pulse.

Qi and Blood deficiency

Chronic, dull ache in the joints that is aggravated when tired and alleviated by rest, poor appetite, loose stools, weak voice, tiredness, blurred vision, dizziness, numbness/tingling of limbs, palpitations, dull-pale complexion, Pale tongue, Weak or Choppy pulse.

Liver and Kidney deficiency

Dull ache in the joints especially in the lower part of the body, weak knees, dizziness, lower backache, tinnitus.

Other clinical manifestations, including tongue and pulse, depend on whether there is Yin or Yang deficiency.

HANDS AND FEET

Cold hands and feet

Interrogation, Chapter 39

Yang deficiency

Coldness of hands and feet, the cold feeling extending to arms and legs, feeling of cold in general, bright-pale complexion, Pale tongue, Deep-Weak pulse.

These are the symptoms of a general Yang deficiency and other manifestations depend on the organ involved, which may be the Heart, Lungs, Spleen or Kidneys.

Blood deficiency

Coldness of hands and feet, numbness/tingling of the limbs, blurred vision, dizziness, insomnia, Pale tongue, Choppy or Fine pulse.

This pattern is much more common in women and it may be due to either Liver-Blood or Heart-Blood deficiency.

Qi stagnation

Coldness of hands and feet, especially of the fingers and toes, hypochondrial or epigastric distension, irritability, moodiness, a feeling of a lump in the throat, premenstrual tension, Wiry pulse.

Phlegm

Coldness of hands and feet, a feeling of heaviness of the limbs, numbness/tingling of the limbs, a feeling of oppression of the chest, Swollen tongue, Slippery pulse.

Heat stagnating in the Interior (True Heat–False Cold)

Coldness of hands and feet, dark face, bright eyes with lustre, dry red lips, irritability, strong body, breathing noisy, loud voice, thirst with a desire to drink cold fluids, scanty dark urine, constipation, a burning sensation in the anus, coldness of the limbs, hot chest, a feeling of heat of the face, red face, mental restlessness, thirst, Red tongue, Rapid pulse.

This pattern is quite rare and the cold hands and feet are due to Heat stagnating in the Interior and preventing Qi from reaching the extremities.

> ### Clinical note
>
> - Cold hands and feet are a reliable indication of Yang deficiency or Cold. In women, do not be surprised if this symptom is accompanied by a feeling of heat of the face.

Hot hands and feet

Interrogation, Chapter 39

Damp-Heat

Heat in hands and feet, sweating of hands and feet, swollen, red and hot joints of the hands and feet, a

feeling of heaviness and numbness of the limbs, Red tongue with sticky yellow coating, Slippery-Rapid pulse.

Heart- and Kidney-Yin deficiency with Empty-Heat

Heat in hands and feet, or in palms and soles, palpitations, mental restlessness, insomnia, dream-disturbed sleep, anxiety, poor memory, dizziness, tinnitus, hardness of hearing, lower backache, a feeling of heat in the evening, night sweating, five-palm heat, scanty dark urine, dry stools, Red tongue with redder tip and a Heart crack, Floating-Empty and Rapid pulse.

Stomach-Heat

Heat in hands and feet, burning epigastric pain, thirst, sour regurgitation, nausea, excessive hunger, foul breath, a feeling of heat, Red tongue with a yellow coating, Overflowing-Rapid pulse.

Stomach-Yin deficiency with Empty-Heat

Heat in hands and feet worse in the afternoon, dull or burning epigastric pain, a feeling of heat in the afternoon, dry stools, dry mouth and throat especially in the afternoon, thirst with a desire to drink in small sips, a feeling of hunger but no desire to eat, night sweating, five-palm heat, bleeding gums, Red tongue without coating in the centre, Floating-Empty and Rapid pulse.

ABNORMAL FEELINGS IN THE LIMBS

Numbness/tingling of the limbs

Interrogation, Chapter 39

Liver-Blood deficiency

Tingling and weakness of the limbs, dizziness, blurred vision, floaters, numbness/tingling of limbs, scanty menstruation, dull-pale complexion, Pale tongue, Choppy or Fine pulse.

Phlegm in the limbs

Numbness of the limbs, a feeling of heaviness of the limbs, tendency to obesity, Swollen tongue, Slippery pulse.

Wind-Phlegm

Numbness of the limbs, especially the upper limbs and often unilateral, a feeling of heaviness of the limbs, tremor, dizziness, headache, Swollen and Stiff tongue, Wiry-Slippery pulse.

Liver-Wind

Numbness of the limbs, especially the upper limbs and often unilateral, tremors, severe dizziness, tinnitus, headache, numbness of the limbs, tics, Stiff, Deviated or Moving tongue, Wiry pulse.

Dampness

Numbness of the limbs, especially the legs, pain in the joints with swelling, muscle ache, a feeling of heaviness, sticky tongue coating, Slippery pulse.

Damp-Heat

Numbness of the limbs, especially the lower limbs, ache, redness, heat and swelling of the joints, muscle ache, Red tongue with sticky yellow coating, Slippery-Rapid pulse.

Qi stagnation and Blood stasis

Numbness/tingling of the limbs, stiffness and pain of the limbs, dark complexion, Purple tongue.

Invasion of Wind-Cold

Numbness/tingling of the limbs, aversion to cold, fever, occipital headache, stiff neck, sneezing, body aches, tongue with thin white coating, Floating-Tight pulse.

> **Clinical note**
> - Numbness is more indicative of Phlegm or Wind, whereas tingling is more indicative of a deficiency of Blood.

Feeling of heaviness of the limbs

Interrogation, Chapter 39

Dampness

A feeling of heaviness of the limbs, especially the legs, numbness, swelling of the legs, a feeling of heaviness in general, epigastric fullness, sticky tongue coating, Slippery pulse.

Damp-Heat

A feeling of heaviness of the limbs, especially the legs, swelling of the legs, hot feet, muscle ache, numbness, epigastric fullness, sticky yellow coating, Slippery-Rapid pulse.

Spleen-Qi deficiency with Dampness

A slight feeling of heaviness of the limbs, especially of the legs, weakness of the limbs, poor appetite, slight abdominal distension after eating, tiredness, lassitude,

pale complexion, loose stools, abdominal fullness, a sticky taste, poor digestion, undigested food in the stools, nausea, dull frontal headache, Pale tongue with sticky coating, Soggy pulse.

Kidney-Yang deficiency with Dampness

A slight feeling of heaviness of the limbs, especially the legs, weak and cold knees, lower backache, a feeling of cold, bright-white complexion, tiredness, lassitude, abundant clear urination, urination at night, impotence, decreased libido, excessive vaginal discharge, Pale and wet tongue with a sticky coating, Deep-Weak and slightly Slippery pulse.

Stomach- and Spleen-Qi deficiency with Dampness

A slight feeling of heaviness of the limbs, weakness of the limbs, poor appetite, slight abdominal distension after eating, tiredness, lassitude, pale complexion, loose stools, abdominal fullness, sticky taste, uncomfortable sensation in the epigastrium, Pale tongue with sticky coating, Soggy pulse.

Phlegm in the limbs

A feeling of heaviness of the limbs, numbness of the limbs, sputum in the throat, a feeling of oppression of the chest, Swollen tongue with sticky coating, Slippery pulse.

> **Clinical note**
>
> - A feeling of heaviness of the limbs is a very reliable symptom of Dampness in the lower part of the body.

Feeling of distension of the limbs

Interrogation, Chapter 39

Qi stagnation with Dampness

A feeling of distension or heaviness of the limbs, swelling of the skin, sticky tongue coating, Wiry-Slippery pulse.

Blood stasis from Qi deficiency

A feeling of distension of the limbs, aggravated by overexertion, pain in the limbs, purple colour of the lower legs, tiredness, poor appetite, loose stools, weak voice, shortness of breath, Wiry or Choppy pulse.

Wind-Phlegm

A feeling of distension or heaviness of the limbs, numbness/tingling of the limbs, severe dizziness, blurred vision, tremors, tinnitus, nausea, sputum in the throat, a feeling of oppression of the chest, Stiff or Deviated and Swollen tongue, Wiry-Slippery pulse.

WEAKNESS AND ATROPHY

Weakness of the limbs

Interrogation, Chapter 39

Stomach-Qi deficiency

Weakness of the four limbs, especially of the legs, an uncomfortable feeling in the epigastrium, no appetite, lack of sense of taste, loose stools, tiredness especially in the morning, Pale tongue, Empty pulse.

Deficiency of Qi and Blood

Weakness of all limbs, poor appetite, loose stools, weak voice, tiredness, blurred vision, dizziness, numbness/tingling of limbs, palpitations, dull-pale complexion, Pale tongue, Weak or Choppy pulse.

Kidney-Yang deficiency

Weakness of the limbs, especially the legs, weak knees, lower backache, cold knees, a feeling of cold, bright-white complexion, tiredness, lassitude, abundant clear urination, urination at night, impotence, decreased libido, Pale and wet tongue, Deep-Weak pulse.

Atrophy of the limbs

Observation, Chapter 18

Stomach- and Spleen-Qi deficiency

Atrophy or thinning of the muscles of the four limbs, weakness of the limbs, muscular weakness, gait like a duck, feet turning in or out, poor appetite, slight abdominal distension after eating, tiredness, lassitude, pale complexion, loose stools, an uncomfortable feeling in the epigastrium, lack of sense of taste, Pale tongue, Empty pulse.

In children this corresponds to the sequelae stage of poliomyelitis.

Liver- and Kidney-Yin deficiency

Atrophy or thinning of the muscles, especially of the legs, weak knees, staggering gait, dizziness, tinnitus, hardness of hearing, lower backache, dull occipital or vertical headache, insomnia, numbness/tingling of limbs, dry eyes, blurred vision, dry throat, dry hair and

skin, brittle nails, night sweating, dry stools, scanty menstruation or amenorrhoea, normal-coloured tongue without coating, Floating-Empty pulse.

This pattern is more common in the elderly.

Spleen- and Kidney-Yang deficiency

Atrophy or thinning of the muscles, muscular weakness, cold limbs, cold knees, weak legs, feeling of cold generally or in the back, oedema of the lower legs, lower backache, bright-white complexion, weak knees, decreased libido, tiredness, lassitude, abundant clear or scanty clear urination, urination at night, loose stools, poor appetite, slight abdominal distension, early-morning diarrhoea, chronic diarrhoea, Pale and wet tongue, Deep-Weak pulse.

Deficiency of Qi and Blood

Atrophy or thinning of the muscles, poor appetite, loose stools, weak voice, tiredness, blurred vision, dizziness, numbness/tingling of limbs, palpitations, dull-pale complexion, Pale tongue, Weak or Choppy pulse.

Kidney-Essence deficiency

Atrophy or thinning of the muscles, late development in children, hands unable to grasp, inability to put feet down, slow mental development.

This pattern occurs only in children or babies and is often associated with the Five Retardations (slow development in children involving standing, walking, teeth development, hair development and speech) and the Five Flaccidities (late closure of the fontanelles, flaccidity of mouth, hands, feet and muscles).

Flaccidity of the limbs

Observation, Chapter 18

Stomach- and Spleen-Qi deficiency

Flaccidity of the four limbs, cold and weak limbs, poor appetite, slight abdominal distension after eating, tiredness, lassitude, pale complexion, weakness of the limbs, loose stools, uncomfortable feeling in the epigastrium, lack of sense of taste, Pale tongue, Empty pulse.

Damp-Heat in the Stomach and Spleen

Flaccidity of the four limbs, a feeling of fullness and pain of the epigastrium and lower abdomen, poor appetite, a feeling of heaviness, thirst without a desire to drink, nausea, loose stools with offensive odour, a feeling of heat, dull-yellow complexion, sticky taste,

Red tongue with sticky yellow coating, Slippery-Rapid pulse.

Kidney-Yin deficiency

Flaccidity of the four limbs, dizziness, tinnitus, hardness of hearing, poor memory, night sweating, dry mouth and throat at night, lower backache, constipation, scanty dark urine, tiredness, normal-coloured tongue without coating, Floating-Empty pulse.

Qi deficiency with Blood stasis

Flaccidity of the four limbs in children, pain in the limbs especially at night, listlessness, poor appetite, tendency to catch colds, weak voice, shortness of breath, loose stools, Bluish-Purple tongue, Weak or Choppy pulse.

Heat at the Nutritive-Qi level

Flaccidity of the four limbs with acute onset, fever at night, mental confusion, delirium, Red tongue without coating, Fine-Rapid pulse.

LIMB SWELLING

Oedema of the limbs

Observation, Chapters 18 and 19; Interrogation, Chapter 39; Symptoms and Signs, Chapters 65, 66, 68

Spleen-Yang deficiency

Pitting oedema of the limbs and abdomen, feeling of cold generally or in limbs, poor appetite, slight abdominal distension after eating, tiredness, lassitude, pale complexion, weakness of the limbs, loose stools, slight depression, tendency to obesity, Pale and wet tongue, Deep-Weak pulse.

Kidney-Yang deficiency

Pitting oedema of the ankles and legs, weak knees, lower backache, a feeling of cold generally or in the knees, bright-white complexion, weak knees, tiredness, lassitude, abundant clear urination, urination at night, impotence, decreased libido, Pale and wet tongue, Deep-Weak pulse.

Lung-Qi deficiency

Pitting oedema of the hands and face, slight shortness of breath, slight cough, weak voice, spontaneous daytime sweating, dislike of speaking, bright-white complexion, tendency to catch colds, tiredness, dislike of cold, Pale tongue, Empty pulse.

Damp-Heat

Swelling of the legs and ankles, aching, swelling, redness and heat of the joints, hot limbs, sticky yellow tongue coating, Slippery-Rapid pulse.

Other symptoms and signs depend on the organ involved.

Qi stagnation

Non-pitting oedema of the limbs, with the skin spring-ings back on pressing the swollen area, a feeling of distension of the limbs.

Cold-Dampness

Swelling of the legs and ankles, a feeling of heaviness of the limbs, cold limbs, ache in the joints, a feeling of cold, sticky white tongue coating, Slippery-Slow pulse.

Qi deficiency and Blood stasis

Oedema of the limbs, cold hands and feet, numbness of the limbs, muscular weakness, purple colour of hands or feet or both, tiredness, poor appetite, loose stools, weak voice, Bluish-Purple tongue, Choppy pulse.

Wind-Water invading the Lungs

Sudden swelling of the eyes, face and hands gradually spreading to the whole body, bright-shiny complexion, scanty and pale urination, aversion to wind, fever, cough, slight breathlessness, sticky white tongue coating, Floating-Slippery pulse.

This is an acute type of oedema and this pattern is a type of external Wind-Cold.

Swelling of the joints of the limbs

Observation, Chapter 18

Damp Painful Obstruction (Bi) Syndrome

Swelling and pain of the joints, a feeling of heaviness of the limbs and the body.

In the case of Damp-Heat, in addition to the above symptoms, the joints would be also red and hot to the touch.

Phlegm in the joints

Long-term, chronic swelling and deformities of joints, osteophytes, a feeling of heaviness of the limbs and body, sputum in the throat, a feeling of oppression of the chest, Swollen tongue with sticky coating, Slippery pulse.

LIMB MOVEMENT

Rigidity of the limbs

Observation, Chapter 18

Wind in the joints

Stiffness of the limbs, difficulty in extending the limbs, pain in the joints.

This pattern corresponds to Wandering Painful Obstruction Syndrome.

Qi stagnation and Blood stasis

Rigidity of the limbs, pain in the muscles and joints, inability to bend arms, abdominal distension, irritability, Purple tongue, Wiry pulse.

Liver-Yang rising

Rigidity of the upper limbs, tense upper back muscles, headache, dizziness, tinnitus, irritability, propensity to outbursts of anger, Wiry pulse.

Liver- and Kidney-Yin deficiency

Rigidity of the lower limbs, thin limbs, weak knees, numbness/tingling of the limbs, dizziness, tinnitus, hardness of hearing, lower backache, dull occipital or vertical headache, insomnia, dry eyes, blurred vision, dry throat in the evening, dry hair and skin, brittle nails, night sweating, dry stools, scanty menstruation or amenorrhoea, normal-coloured tongue without coating, Floating-Empty pulse.

Liver-Wind

Rigidity of the upper limbs, tremors, severe dizziness, tinnitus, headache, numbness of limbs, tics, Stiff, Deviated or Moving tongue, Wiry pulse.

Wind-Phlegm

Rigidity of the limbs, numbness or tingling of limbs, severe dizziness, blurred vision, tremors, tinnitus, nausea, sputum in the throat, a feeling of oppression of the chest, Stiff or Deviated and Swollen tongue, Wiry-Slippery pulse.

Paralysis of the limbs

Observation, Chapter 18

Stomach- and Spleen-Qi deficiency

Paralysis of the four limbs, weak and cold limbs, poor appetite, slight abdominal distension after eating,

tiredness, lassitude, pale complexion, loose stools, an uncomfortable feeling in the epigastrium, lack of sense of taste, Pale tongue, Empty pulse.

Deficiency of Qi and Blood

Paralysis of the four limbs, weak limbs, poor appetite, loose stools, weak voice, tiredness, blurred vision, dizziness, numbness/tingling of limbs, palpitations, dull-pale complexion, Pale tongue, Weak or Choppy pulse.

Liver- and Kidney-Yin deficiency

Paralysis of the four limbs, dizziness, tinnitus, weak knees, hardness of hearing, lower backache, dull occipital or vertical headache, insomnia, numbness/tingling of the limbs, dry eyes, blurred vision, dry throat in the evening, dry hair and skin, brittle nails, night sweating, dry stools, scanty menstruation or amenorrhoea, normal-coloured tongue without coating, Floating-Empty pulse.

Liver- and Kidney-Yin deficiency with internal Wind

Tremor or spasms of limbs, weak limbs, weak knees, numbness/tingling of the limbs, lower backache, dizziness, tinnitus, hardness of hearing, dull occipital or vertical headache, insomnia, dry eyes, blurred vision, dry throat in the evening, dry hair and skin, brittle nails, night sweating, dry stools, scanty menstruation or amenorrhoea, normal-coloured Deviated or Moving tongue without coating, Floating-Empty and slightly Wiry pulse.

Retention of Dampness in the muscles

Paralysis of the four limbs, a feeling of heaviness of the body on limbs, swelling of the limbs and joints, epigastric fullness, sticky taste, sticky tongue coating, Slippery pulse.

Liver-Blood stasis

Paralysis of the four limbs, pain in the limbs which may be worse at night, hypochondrial/abdominal pain, painful periods, dark and clotted menstrual blood, masses in the abdomen, purple nails and lips, purple or dark complexion, Purple tongue, Wiry or Firm pulse.

Wind and Phlegm in the channels

Hemiplegia, numbness/tingling of the limbs (usually unilateral), sputum in the throat, feeling of oppression of the chest, Swollen and Deviated tongue, Slippery and Wiry pulse.

This corresponds to the sequelae stage of Wind-stroke.

Contraction of the limbs

Observation, Chapter 18

Liver-Blood deficiency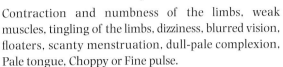

Contraction and numbness of the limbs, weak muscles, tingling of the limbs, dizziness, blurred vision, floaters, scanty menstruation, dull-pale complexion, Pale tongue, Choppy or Fine pulse.

Liver- and Kidney-Yin deficiency

Contraction of the lower limbs, thin limbs, weak knees, dizziness, tinnitus, hardness of hearing, lower backache, dull occipital or vertical headache, insomnia, numbness/tingling of the limbs, dry eyes, blurred vision, dry throat in the evening, dry hair and skin, brittle nails, night sweating, dry stools, scanty menstruation or amenorrhoea, normal-coloured tongue without coating, Floating-Empty pulse.

Cold-Dampness

Contraction and swelling of the limbs, a feeling of cold generally or in the limbs, ache in the joints, a feeling of heaviness of the limbs, sticky white tongue coating, Slippery-Slow pulse.

Internal Wind

Contraction of the upper limbs, tremors, severe dizziness, tinnitus, headache, numbness of the limbs, tics, Stiff, Deviated or Moving tongue, Wiry pulse.

Invasion of Wind-Cold

Contraction of the upper limbs, aversion to cold, fever, cough, itchy throat, slight breathlessness, stuffed or runny nose with clear watery discharge, sneezing, occipital headache, body aches, thin white tongue coating, Floating-Tight pulse.

Phlegm

Contraction of the limbs, a feeling of heaviness of the limbs, numbness/tingling of the limbs, a feeling of oppression of the chest, sputum in the throat, Swollen tongue, Slippery pulse.

Blood stasis

Contraction of the limbs, pain of the limbs, hypochondrial pain, abdominal pain, painful periods, dark complexion, Purple tongue, Wiry pulse.

Tremor or spasticity of the limbs

Observation, Chapters 4 and 18; Interrogation, Chapter 39; Symptoms and Signs, Chapter 66

Liver-Wind

Pronounced tremor of the limbs, severe dizziness, tinnitus, headache, numbness of the limbs, tics, Stiff, Deviated or Moving tongue, Wiry pulse.

Wind-Phlegm 👤

Tremor of the limbs, severe dizziness, blurred vision, numbness/tingling of the limbs, tinnitus, nausea, sputum in the throat, a feeling of oppression of the chest, Stiff or Deviated and Swollen tongue, Wiry-Slippery pulse.

Liver-Blood or -Yin deficiency leading to Empty-Wind 👤

Mild tremor of the limbs, slight tremor of the head or hand or both, facial tic, dizziness, blurred vision, numbness/tingling of a limb, dry eyes.

The tongue and pulse presentation depends on whether there is Liver-Blood or Liver-Yin deficiency.

Heat generating Wind

Tremor of the limbs, convulsions, twitching of limbs, high fever, fainting, rigidity of neck, opisthotonos, macular rash, eyeballs turning up, clenching of teeth, Dark-Red tongue without coating, Wiry-Rapid pulse.

This is an acute pattern occurring during a febrile disease and it corresponds to the Blood level within the identification of patterns according to the Four Levels.

Convulsions of the limbs

Observation, Chapter 18

Liver-Yang rising generating Liver-Wind

Convulsions of the four limbs, tremors, severe dizziness, tinnitus, headache, numbness of the limbs, tics, irritability, propensity to outbursts of anger, Stiff, Deviated or Moving tongue, Wiry pulse.

Liver-Blood deficiency generating Liver-Wind

Slight convulsions or twitching of the four limbs, numbness/tingling of the limbs, dizziness, blurred vision, floaters, facial tics, dull-pale complexion, Pale and Stiff tongue, Choppy or Fine and slightly Wiry pulse.

Liver-Wind and Phlegm

Convulsions of the four limbs, facial tic, tremors, numbness/tingling of the limbs, severe dizziness, blurred vision, tinnitus, nausea, sputum in the throat, a feeling of oppression of the chest, Stiff or Deviated and Swollen tongue, Wiry-Slippery pulse.

Liver- and Kidney-Yin deficiency and Liver-Blood deficiency giving rise to Liver-Wind

Slight convulsions of the four limbs, dizziness, tinnitus, weak knees, hardness of hearing, lower backache, dull occipital or vertical headache, insomnia, numbness/tingling of the limbs, dry eyes, blurred vision, floaters, dry throat in the evening, dry hair and skin, brittle nails, night sweating, dry stools, scanty menstruation or amenorrhoea, dull-pale complexion with red cheekbones, normal-coloured or Pale tongue without coating, Choppy, Fine or Floating-Empty pulse.

This pattern usually occurs during pregnancy or after childbirth.

Heat victorious stirring Wind (Blood level)

Convulsions of the four limbs with acute onset, tremor or twitching of the limbs, high fever, fainting, neck rigidity, opisthotonos, macular rash, turning up of the eyeballs, clenching of the teeth, Dark-Red tongue without coating, Wiry-Rapid pulse.

Yin deficiency generating Empty-Wind (Blood level)

Slight convulsions or twitching of the four limbs with acute onset, low-grade fever, tremor of the limbs, loss of weight, malar flush, listlessness, Dark-Red tongue without coating and Dry, Fine-Rapid pulse.

Chapter **65**

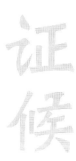

ARMS

Chapter contents

PAIN IN THE ELBOW   679

HANDS   680
  Cold hands   680
  Hot hands   680
  Pale hands   681
  Red dorsum of the hands   681
  Red palms   681
  Sweaty palms   681
  Pain in the hands   682
  Itchy hands   683
  Numbness/tingling of the hands   683
  Tremor of the hands   684
  Oedema of the hands   684
  Deformed knuckles   684
  Tinea (ringworm)   684
  Dry, cracked and peeling palms   684
  Venules on the thenar eminence   685
  Atrophy of the thenar eminence   685
  Atrophy of the muscles of the dorsum of the
    hands   685

FINGERS   686
  Swollen fingers   686
  Contraction of the fingers   686
  Spoon-shaped fingers   687
  Thin, pointed fingers   687
  Cracked fingers   687
  Thickened fingers   688
  Shrivelled and wrinkled fingers   688

NAILS   688
  Ridged nails   688
  Thickening of the nails   688
  Coarse and thick nails   688
  Cracked nails   688
  Nails falling off   689
  Indented nails   689
  Thin and brittle nails   689
  Withered and brittle nails   689
  Withered and thickened nails   690

Curling nails   690
Flaking nails   690
Twisted nails   691
Nails with white spots   691
Pale-white nails   691
Dull-white nails   691
Red nails   691
Yellow nails   691
Bluish-greenish nails   691
Dark nails   692
Purple nails   692
Small or absent lunulae   692
Large lunulae   692

PAIN IN THE ELBOW

Interrogation, Chapter 39

Invasion of Cold

Unilateral, severe pain in the elbow that is aggravated by exposure to cold and alleviated by the application of heat.

Invasion of Cold-Dampness

Unilateral pain in the elbow that is aggravated by exposure to cold and dampness and alleviated by the application of heat, swelling of the joint, a feeling of heaviness and numbness of the affected arm.

Stagnation of Qi and stasis of Blood

Unilateral pain in the elbow that is aggravated by rest and slightly ameliorated by movement. This is usually due to repetitive strain injury.

Damp-Heat

Pain in the elbow with swelling, redness and heat of the joint, a feeling of heaviness and numbness of the affected arm.

HANDS

Cold hands

Interrogation, Chapter 39

Heart-Yang deficiency

Cold hands, sweaty hands, palpitations, shortness of breath on exertion, tiredness, spontaneous sweating, a slight feeling of discomfort or stuffiness in the heart region, a feeling of cold, bright-pale face, slightly dark lips, Pale tongue, Deep-Weak pulse.

Lung-Yang deficiency

Cold hands, sweaty hands, slight shortness of breath, slight cough with profuse watery sputum, weak voice, spontaneous daytime sweating, dislike of speaking, bright-white complexion, tendency to catch colds, tiredness, dislike of cold, a feeling of cold generally or of the upper back, absence of thirst, Pale and slightly wet tongue, Weak pulse.

Heart-Blood deficiency

Cold hands, palpitations, dizziness, insomnia, dream-disturbed sleep, poor memory, anxiety, tendency to be easily startled, dull-pale complexion, pale lips, Pale and Thin tongue, Choppy or Fine pulse.

Spleen-Yang deficiency

Cold hands and often cold feet, poor appetite, slight abdominal distension after eating, tiredness, lassitude, pale complexion, weakness of the limbs, loose stools, a feeling of cold, oedema, Pale and wet tongue, Deep-Weak pulse.

Liver-Qi stagnation

Cold hands, especially fingers, hypochondrial or epigastric distension, irritability, moodiness, a feeling of a lump in the throat, premenstrual tension, Wiry pulse.

Phlegm in the channels

Cold hands, numbness or tingling of the limbs, a feeling of heaviness, or of oppression of the chest, sputum in the throat, Swollen tongue with sticky coating, Slippery pulse.

Clinical note

- Cold hands are a reliable symptom of Yang deficiency.

Hot hands

Interrogation, Chapter 39

Heart-Fire

Hot hands, especially the dorsum, palpitations, thirst, mouth and tongue ulcers, mental restlessness, a feeling of agitation, insomnia, dream-disturbed sleep, a feeling of heat, red face, bitter taste, Red tongue with redder tip and yellow coating, Overflowing-Rapid pulse.

Lung-Heat

Hot hands, especially the dorsum, cough, slight breathlessness, a feeling of heat, chest ache, flaring of the nostrils, thirst, red face, Red tongue with yellow coating, Overflowing-Rapid pulse.

Stomach-Heat

Hot hands, especially the dorsum, burning epigastric pain, thirst, sour regurgitation, nausea, excessive hunger, foul breath, a feeling of heat, Red tongue with a yellow coating, Overflowing-Rapid pulse.

Heart-Yin deficiency with Empty-Heat

Hot palms, five-palm heat, palpitations, insomnia, dream-disturbed sleep, poor memory, anxiety, tendency to be easily startled, mental restlessness, uneasiness, 'feeling hot and bothered', dry mouth and throat, thirst with a desire to sip fluids, a feeling of heat in the evening, malar flush, night sweating, Red tongue with redder tip and no coating, Floating-Empty and Rapid pulse.

Lung-Yin deficiency with Empty-Heat

Hot palms, five-palm heat, dry cough or with scanty, sticky sputum which could be blood tinged, dry mouth and throat at night, weak/hoarse voice, night sweating, tiredness, malar flush, a feeling of heat or a low-grade fever in the evening, thin body or chest, insomnia, anxiety, Red tongue without coating, Floating-Empty and Rapid pulse.

Stomach-Yin deficiency with Empty-Heat

Hot palms, five-palm heat, dull or burning epigastric pain, a feeling of heat in the afternoon, constipation (dry stools), dry mouth and throat especially in the afternoon, thirst with a desire to drink in small sips, a feeling of hunger but no desire to eat, a slight feeling of fullness after eating, night sweating, five-palm heat,

bleeding gums, Red tongue (or Red centre only) without coating in the centre, Floating-Empty and Rapid pulse.

Stomach Damp-Heat

Hot hands (dorsum), swelling and redness of the joints, pain in the hands, a feeling of fullness and pain of the epigastrium, a feeling of heaviness, facial pain, stuffed nose or thick sticky nasal discharge, thirst without a desire to drink, nausea, a feeling of heat, dull-yellow complexion, a sticky taste, Red tongue with sticky yellow coating, Slippery-Rapid pulse.

Invasion of Wind

Dorsum of the hands hot to touch, aversion to cold, chills, fever, stiff neck, occipital headache, Floating pulse.

Other symptoms and signs depend on whether it is Wind-Cold or Wind-Heat.

Pale hands

Observation, Chapter 14

Heart-Yang deficiency

Pale hands, cold hands, palpitations, shortness of breath on exertion, tiredness, spontaneous sweating, a slight feeling of discomfort or stuffiness in the heart region, a feeling of cold, bright-pale face, slightly dark lips, Pale tongue, Deep-Weak pulse.

Lung-Yang deficiency

Pale hands, cold hands, slight shortness of breath, slight cough with profuse watery sputum, weak voice, spontaneous daytime sweating, dislike of speaking, bright-white complexion, tendency to catch colds, tiredness, dislike of cold, a feeling of cold generally or of the upper back, absence of thirst, Pale and slightly wet tongue, Weak pulse.

Liver-Blood deficiency

Pale hands, dizziness, blurred vision, floaters, numbness/tingling of the limbs, scanty menstruation, dull-pale complexion, Pale tongue, Choppy or Fine pulse.

Heart-Blood deficiency

Pale hands, palpitations, dizziness, insomnia, dream-disturbed sleep, poor memory, anxiety, tendency to be easily startled, dull-pale complexion, pale lips, Pale and Thin tongue, Choppy or Fine pulse.

Red dorsum of the hands

Observation, Chapter 14

Full-Heat

Red dorsum of the hands, hot hands, a feeling of heat, thirst, red face.

Other symptoms and signs depend on which organ is involved, which may be the Heart, Lungs or Stomach.

Red palms

Observation, Chapter 14

Empty-Heat

Red palms of the hands, hot hands, becoming hotter in the afternoon and evening, a feeling of heat in the afternoon or evening, thirst with a desire to drink in small sips.

Other symptoms and signs depend on which organ is involved, which may be the Heart, Lungs or Stomach.

Sweaty palms

Observation, Chapter 14

Lung-Qi deficiency

Sweaty palms, slight shortness of breath, slight cough, weak voice, spontaneous daytime sweating, dislike of speaking, bright-white complexion, tendency to catch colds, tiredness, dislike of cold, Pale tongue, Empty pulse.

Lung-Yang deficiency

Sweaty palms, pale hands, cold hands, slight shortness of breath, slight cough with profuse watery sputum, weak voice, spontaneous daytime sweating, dislike of speaking, bright-white complexion, tendency to catch colds, tiredness, dislike of cold, a feeling of cold generally or of the upper back, absence of thirst, Pale and slightly wet tongue, Weak pulse.

Lung-Yin deficiency

Sweaty palms which are worse in the afternoon, hot palms, cough which is dry or with scanty sticky sputum, weak/hoarse voice, dry mouth and throat, tickly throat, tiredness, dislike of speaking, thin body or thin chest, night sweating, normal-coloured tongue without coating (or with rootless coating) in the front part, Floating-Empty pulse.

Heart-Qi deficiency

Sweaty palms when nervous, palpitations, shortness of breath on exertion, pale face, tiredness, slight depression, spontaneous sweating, Pale tongue, Empty pulse.

Heart-Yang deficiency

Sweaty palms with cold sweat when nervous, cold hands, palpitations, shortness of breath on exertion, tiredness, spontaneous sweating, a slight feeling of discomfort or stuffiness in the heart region, a feeling of cold, bright-pale face, slightly dark lips, Pale tongue, Deep-Weak pulse.

Heart-Yin deficiency

Sweaty palms which are worse in the evening or when nervous, palpitations, insomnia, dream-disturbed sleep, poor memory, anxiety, tendency to be easily startled, mental restlessness, uneasiness, 'feeling hot and bothered', dry mouth and throat, night sweating, normal-coloured tongue without coating or with rootless coating, Floating-Empty pulse, especially on the left Front position.

Lung-Heat

Sweaty palms, hot hands, cough, slight breathlessness, a feeling of heat, chest ache, flaring of the nostrils, thirst, red face, Red tongue with yellow coating, Overflowing-Rapid pulse.

Heart-Fire

Sweaty palms and hot hands, especially when anxious, palpitations, thirst, mouth and tongue ulcers, mental restlessness, a feeling of agitation, insomnia, dream-disturbed sleep, a feeling of heat, red face, bitter taste, Red tongue with redder tip and yellow coating, Overflowing-Rapid pulse.

Pain in the hands

Interrogation, Chapter 39

Wind

Wandering pain in the hands, fingers and other joints.

Cold

Pain in the hands that is aggravated by exposure to cold and alleviated by application of heat, contraction of fingers, a feeling of cold, cold hands.

Dampness

Ache and swelling of the hand or fingers or both, numbness of the hands.

Damp-Heat in the channels

Pain, swelling and redness of the hands, numbness/tingling of the hands, a feeling of heaviness of the arms, muscle ache.

Liver-Qi stagnation

Pain in the hands (often in feet as well), hypochondrial or epigastric distension, irritability, moodiness, a feeling of a lump in the throat, premenstrual tension, Wiry pulse.

Stagnation of Qi and stasis of Blood

Pain in the hands that is worse at night, rigidity of the fingers, hypochondrial or epigastric distension, irritability, moodiness, a feeling of a lump in the throat, premenstrual tension, abdominal pain, chest pain, Purple tongue, Wiry pulse.

Blood deficiency

Dull ache of the hands, cold hands, dizziness, blurred vision, scanty periods, Pale tongue, Choppy or Fine pulse.

Other symptoms and signs depend on the organ affected, which may be Heart, Liver or Spleen. This pattern is more common in women.

Heart-Yang deficiency

Dull ache in the hands, cold hands, palpitations, shortness of breath on exertion, tiredness, spontaneous sweating, a slight feeling of discomfort or stuffiness in the heart region, a feeling of cold, bright-pale face, slightly dark lips, Pale tongue, Deep-Weak pulse.

Lung-Yang deficiency

Dull ache in the hands, cold hands, slight shortness of breath, slight cough with profuse watery sputum, weak voice, spontaneous daytime sweating, dislike of speaking, bright-white complexion, tendency to catch colds, tiredness, dislike of cold, a feeling of cold generally or of the upper back, absence of thirst, Pale and slightly wet tongue, Weak pulse.

Stomach-Yang deficiency

Dull ache in the hands, cold hands (and often feet), discomfort or dull pain in the epigastrium, better after

eating and with pressure or massage, no appetite, preference for warm drinks and foods, vomiting of clear fluid, absence of thirst, cold and weak limbs, tiredness, pale complexion, Pale and wet tongue, Deep-Weak pulse.

Heart-Yin deficiency

Dull ache in the hands that is worse in the evening, hot palms, palpitations, insomnia, dream-disturbed sleep, poor memory, anxiety, a tendency to be easily startled, mental restlessness, uneasiness, 'feeling hot and bothered', dry mouth and throat, night sweating, normal-coloured tongue without coating or with rootless coating, Floating-Empty pulse, especially on the left Front position.

Lung-Yin deficiency

Dull ache in the hands that is worse in the evening, hot palms, dry cough, weak voice, dry throat with a desire to sip water, hoarse voice, night sweating, tiredness, tongue without coating in the front, Floating-Empty pulse.

Itchy hands

Interrogation, Chapter 39

Dampness

Itchy hands, swollen fingers with small white vesicles, fungal infections, sticky tongue coating, Slippery pulse.

Damp-Heat

Itchy hands, swollen and red fingers, small yellow vesicles, fungal infections, sticky yellow tongue coating, Slippery-Rapid pulse.

Invasion of Wind

Itchy hands with acute onset, itching spreading up the arms and towards the face, red rash on hands.

Blood deficiency leading to Wind in the skin

Itchy hands, pale and cold hands, tingling of the hands, Pale tongue, Choppy or Fine pulse.

Numbness/tingling of the hands

Interrogation, Chapter 39

Liver-Blood deficiency

Numbness/tingling of the hands and limbs, more tingling than numbness, dizziness, blurred vision, floaters, numbness or tingling of limbs, scanty menstruation, dull-pale complexion, Pale tongue, Choppy or Fine pulse.

Phlegm

Numbness/tingling of the hands and limbs, more numbness than tingling, dizziness, feeling of heaviness of the body, sputum in the throat, a feeling of oppression of the chest, Swollen tongue, Slippery pulse.

Wind-Phlegm

Unilateral numbness of a hand and especially the first three fingers, severe dizziness, blurred vision, tremors, tinnitus, nausea, sputum in the throat, a feeling of oppression of the chest, Stiff or Deviated and Swollen tongue, Wiry-Slippery pulse.

Liver-Wind

Unilateral numbness of a hand and especially the first three fingers, tremors, severe dizziness, tinnitus, headache, numbness of limbs, tics, Stiff, Deviated or Moving tongue, Wiry pulse.

Dampness

Numbness/tingling of the hands, swelling of the fingers, muscle ache, a feeling of heaviness of the limbs, sticky tongue coating, Slippery pulse.

Damp-Heat

Numbness/tingling of the hands, hot and swollen fingers, redness of the hands and fingers, ache in the wrist, muscle ache, a feeling of heaviness of the limbs, sticky yellow tongue coating, Slippery-Rapid pulse.

Stagnation of Qi and stasis of Blood

Numbness/tingling of the hands, hypochondrial or epigastric distension, irritability, moodiness, a feeling of a lump in the throat, premenstrual tension, abdominal pain, chest pain, painful periods, dark complexion, Purple tongue, Wiry pulse.

Invasion of external Wind

Numbness/tingling of the hands with acute onset, aversion to cold, fever, stiff neck, occipital headache, Floating pulse.

Other symptoms and signs depend on whether it is Wind-Cold or Wind-Heat.

Tremor of the hands

Observation, Chapter 14

Liver-Wind

Tremor of the hands, unilateral numbness/tingling of a hand, severe dizziness, tinnitus, headache, tics, Stiff, Deviated or Moving tongue, Wiry pulse.

Liver-Wind with Phlegm

Tremor of the hands, swollen hands, unilateral numbness/tingling of a hand, severe dizziness, blurred vision, tinnitus, nausea, sputum in the throat, a feeling of oppression of the chest, Stiff or Deviated and Swollen tongue, Wiry-Slippery pulse.

Liver-Blood or Liver-Yin deficiency leading to Wind

Mild tremor of the hands, numbness/tingling of the hands or limbs, dizziness, blurred vision, floaters, scanty menstruation, dull-pale complexion, dry eyes, night sweating, Pale or normal-coloured tongue, Choppy or Fine pulse.

Heat generating Wind

Tremor of hands, convulsions, twitching of limbs, high fever, fainting, rigidity of neck, opisthotonos, macular rash, eyeballs turning up, clenching of teeth, Dark-Red tongue without coating, Wiry-Rapid pulse.

Oedema of the hands

Observation, Chapter 18; Interrogation, Chapter 39; Symptoms and Signs, Chapters 64, 68

Lung-Yang deficiency

Oedema of the hands with slight pitting, cold hands, slight shortness of breath, slight cough, weak voice, spontaneous daytime sweating, dislike of speaking, bright-white complexion, tendency to catch colds, tiredness, a feeling of cold, Pale and wet tongue, Deep-Weak pulse.

Spleen-Yang deficiency

Pitting oedema of the hands, cold limbs, weakness of the limbs, poor appetite, slight abdominal distension after eating, tiredness, lassitude, pale complexion, loose stools, a feeling of cold, Pale and wet tongue, Deep-Weak pulse.

Liver-Qi stagnation

Non-pitting oedema of the hands, cold fingers and toes, hypochondrial or epigastric distension, irritability, moodiness, a feeling of a lump in the throat, premenstrual tension, Wiry pulse.

Deformed knuckles

Observation, Chapter 14

Chronic Painful Obstruction Syndrome with Phlegm

Deformed knuckles, pain in the fingers, numbness/tingling of the hands. If Phlegm is combined with Heat, the fingers will be red and hot to the touch.

Chronic Painful Obstruction Syndrome with Phlegm and Blood stasis

Deformed knuckles, severe pain in the fingers, dark complexion, rigidity of the finger joints.

Chronic Painful Obstruction Syndrome with Phlegm and Qi/Yin deficiency

Deformed knuckles, dull ache in the fingers, shiny skin, atrophy of muscles of the dorsum of the hand, tiredness, loose stools, poor appetite, dry skin, night sweating.

The pulse and tongue depend on whether deficiency of Qi or Yin predominates.

Tinea (ringworm)

Observation, Chapter 14

External invasion of Wind-Heat

Tinea of the hands, dry skin, itchy skin.

External invasion of Damp-Heat

Tinea of the hands, itchy skin, swollen hands, vesicles.

Toxic Heat in the skin

Tinea of the hands, intensely red rash with red papules that spreads quickly, unbearable itching, Red tongue with red points and thick, sticky yellow coating, Overflowing-Slippery-Rapid pulse.

Dry, cracked and peeling palms

Observation, Chapter 14

Blood deficiency

Dry, cracked and peeling palms, dry and brittle nails, dry skin, dizziness, tiredness, Pale tongue, Choppy or Fine pulse.

Other symptoms and signs depend on whether there is Liver-Blood or Heart-Blood deficiency.

Blood deficiency with Wind

Dry, cracked and peeling palms, severe itching, dry and brittle nails, dry skin, slight tremor of the head or hand or both, facial tic, dizziness, blurred vision, unilateral numbness/tingling of a limb, Pale and Thin tongue, Choppy or Fine and slightly Wiry pulse.

Venules on the thenar eminence

Observation, Chapter 14

Cold in the Stomach

Bluish or bluish-purple venules on the thenar eminence, pain in the epigastrium, a feeling of cold, cold limbs, preference for warmth, vomiting of clear fluids (which may alleviate the pain), nausea, feeling worse after swallowing cold fluids which are quickly vomited, preference for warm liquids, tongue with thick white coating, Deep-Tight-Slow pulse.

Stomach deficient and cold

Short, bluish venules on the thenar eminence, discomfort or dull pain in the epigastrium, better after eating and better with pressure or massage, no appetite, preference for warm drinks and foods, vomiting of clear fluid, no thirst, cold and weak limbs, tiredness, pale complexion, Pale and wet tongue, Deep-Weak-Slow pulse.

Full-Heat

Reddish venules on the thenar eminence, hot hands, red hands, thirst, a feeling of heat, red face.

Other symptoms and signs depend on which organ is involved, which may be the Stomach or Lungs.

Empty-Heat

Reddish venules on the thenar eminence, worse in the afternoon and evening, malar flush, a feeling of heat in the evening, night sweating, five-palm heat.

Other symptoms and signs depend on which organ is involved, which may be the Stomach or Lungs.

Blood stasis in the Stomach

Reddish-purple venules on the thenar eminence, severe, stabbing epigastric pain that may be worse at night, dislike of pressure, nausea, vomiting, possibly of blood, vomiting of food looking like coffee grounds, Purple tongue, Wiry pulse.

Damp-Heat in the Stomach

Yellowish-red venules on the thenar eminence, a feeling of fullness and pain of the epigastrium, a feeling of heaviness, facial pain, stuffed nose or thick sticky nasal discharge, thirst without a desire to drink, nausea, a feeling of heat, dull-yellow complexion, a sticky taste, Red tongue with sticky yellow coating, Slippery-Rapid pulse.

Atrophy of the thenar eminence

Observation, Chapter 14

Liver-Blood deficiency

Atrophy of the thenar eminence, dizziness, blurred vision, floaters, numbness or tingling of limbs, scanty menstruation, dull-pale complexion, Pale tongue, Choppy or Fine pulse.

Kidney-Yin deficiency

Atrophy of the thenar eminence, dizziness, tinnitus, hardness of hearing, poor memory, night sweating, dry mouth and throat at night, lower backache, constipation, scanty dark urine, tiredness, normal-coloured tongue without coating, Floating-Empty pulse.

Stomach- and Spleen-Qi deficiency

Atrophy of the thenar eminence, poor appetite, slight abdominal distension after eating, tiredness, lassitude, pale complexion, weakness of the limbs, loose stools, an uncomfortable feeling in the epigastrium, lack of sense of taste, Pale tongue, Empty pulse.

Atrophy of the muscles of the dorsum of the hands

Observation, Chapter 14

Liver-Blood deficiency

Atrophy of the muscles of the dorsum of the hands, dizziness, blurred vision, floaters, numbness/tingling of the limbs, scanty menstruation, dull-pale complexion, Pale tongue, Choppy or Fine pulse.

Kidney-Yin deficiency

Atrophy of the muscles of the dorsum of the hand, dizziness, tinnitus, hardness of hearing, poor memory, night sweating, dry mouth and throat at night, lower backache, constipation, scanty dark urine, tiredness, normal-coloured tongue without coating, Floating-Empty pulse.

Stomach- and Spleen-Qi deficiency

Atrophy of the muscles of the dorsum of the hand, poor appetite, slight abdominal distension after eating, tiredness, lassitude, pale complexion, weakness of the limbs, loose stools, uncomfortable feeling in the epigastrium, lack of sense of taste, Pale tongue, Empty pulse.

FINGERS

Swollen fingers

Observation, Chapter 14

Cold-Dampness Painful Obstruction Syndrome

Swelling and pain of the fingers, which is aggravated by exposure to cold and damp weather and alleviated by the application of heat or by exposure to dry weather, cold hands.

Damp-Heat Painful Obstruction Syndrome

Swelling, heat and pain of the fingers, which is aggravated by exposure to damp weather and alleviated in dry weather.

Wind-Dampness Painful Obstruction Syndrome

Swelling and pain of the fingers, which is aggravated by damp weather, itching of the hands, vesicles on the skin of the hands.

Lung- and Spleen-Yang deficiency

Swelling of the fingers and hands, cold and pale hands, poor appetite, slight abdominal distension after eating, tiredness, lassitude, pale complexion, weakness of the limbs, loose stools, a feeling of cold, slight shortness of breath, slight cough with profuse watery sputum, weak voice, spontaneous daytime sweating, dislike of speaking, bright-white complexion, tendency to catch colds, tiredness, dislike of cold, a feeling of cold generally or of the upper back, absence of thirst, Pale and slightly wet tongue, Deep-Weak pulse.

Qi stagnation

Swelling of the fingers before the period in women, hypochondrial or epigastric distension, irritability, moodiness, a feeling of a lump in the throat, premenstrual tension, Wiry pulse.

Blood stasis

Swelling and severe pain of the fingers, contraction of the fingers, dark complexion, purple nails, Purple tongue, Wiry or Choppy pulse.

Other symptoms and signs depend on the organ involved, which, in this case, may be the Liver or Heart.

Liver- and Kidney-Yin deficiency with Blood-Heat

Swollen, red and hot fingers, aggravated by exposure to heat, numbness/tingling of limbs, dizziness, tinnitus, hardness of hearing, dull occipital or vertical headache, insomnia, malar flush, dry eyes, blurred vision, lower backache, dry throat, dry hair and skin, brittle nails, night sweating, dry stools, scanty menstruation or amenorrhoea, five-palm heat, a feeling of heat in the evening, Red tongue without coating, Floating-Empty and Rapid pulse.

Wind-Water invading the Lungs

Sudden swelling of fingers and face gradually spreading to the whole body, bright-shiny complexion, scanty and pale urination, aversion to wind, fever, cough, slight breathlessness, sticky white tongue coating, Floating-Slippery pulse.

Contraction of the fingers

Observation, Chapter 14

Liver-Blood deficiency

Contraction of the fingers, cold hands, tingling of limbs, dizziness, blurred vision, floaters, numbness/tingling of limbs, scanty menstruation, dull-pale complexion, Pale tongue, Choppy or Fine pulse.

Liver-Yin deficiency

Contraction of the fingers, thinning of muscles, hot palms, tingling of the limbs, dizziness, blurred vision, floaters in eyes, dry eyes, scanty menstruation, dull-pale complexion but with red cheekbones, withered and brittle nails, dry skin and hair, night sweating, normal-coloured tongue without coating, Fine or Floating-Empty pulse.

Blood stasis

Contraction of the fingers, pain in the hands that is worse at night, rigidity of the limbs, Purple tongue, Wiry or Choppy pulse.

Liver-Wind

Unilateral contraction of the fingers, unilateral numbness/tingling of a hand, tremors, severe dizziness, tinnitus, headache, tics, Stiff, Deviated or Moving tongue, Wiry pulse.

Wind-Phlegm

Unilateral contraction of the fingers, unilateral numbness of a hand, severe dizziness, blurred vision, tremors, numbness/tingling of the limbs, tinnitus, nausea, sputum in the throat, a feeling of oppression of the chest, Stiff or Deviated and Swollen tongue, Wiry-Slippery pulse.

Cold-Dampness

Contraction and swelling of the fingers, numbness, a feeling of heaviness, cold hands.

Liver-Qi stagnation

Contraction of the fingers that comes and goes according to emotional moods, hypochondrial/epigastric distension, irritability, moodiness, a feeling of a lump in the throat, premenstrual tension, Wiry pulse.

Invasion of external Wind-Cold

Contraction of the fingers with acute onset, aversion to cold, fever, occipital headache, stiff neck, Floating pulse.

Spoon-shaped fingers

Observation, Chapter 14

Cold-Phlegm in the Lungs

Spoon-shaped fingers, cough with expectoration of watery white sputum, a feeling of cold, cold hands and feet, nausea, vomiting, a feeling of oppression of the chest and epigastrium, dull-white complexion, pale urine, Pale and Swollen tongue with wet-white coating, Slippery-Slow pulse.

Phlegm-Heat in the Lungs

Spoon-shaped fingers, hot fingers, barking cough with profuse, sticky yellow or green sputum, shortness of breath, wheezing, a feeling of oppression of the chest, a feeling of heat, thirst, insomnia, agitation, Red and Swollen tongue with a sticky yellow coating, Slippery-Rapid pulse.

Lung and Kidney-Yin deficiency

Spoon-shaped fingers, dry cough which is worse in the evening, dry throat and mouth, thin body, breathlessness on exertion, lower backache, night sweating, dizziness, tinnitus, hardness of hearing, scanty urination, normal-coloured tongue without coating, Floating-Empty pulse.

Thin, pointed fingers

Observation, Chapter 14

Cold-Dampness in the Stomach

Thin, pointed fingers, pain and distension in the abdomen, a feeling of cold in the abdomen, worsened by ingestion of cold liquids, a feeling of fullness and pain in the epigastrium, a sticky taste, sticky white tongue coating, Slippery-Slow pulse.

Damp-Heat in the Stomach

Thin, pointed fingers, a feeling of fullness and pain of the epigastrium, a feeling of heaviness, facial pain, stuffed nose or thick sticky nasal discharge, thirst without a desire to drink, nausea, a feeling of heat, dull-yellow complexion, a sticky taste, Red tongue with sticky yellow coating, Slippery-Rapid pulse.

Stomach- and Spleen-Qi deficiency

Thin, pointed fingers, poor appetite, slight abdominal distension after eating, tiredness, lassitude, pale complexion, weakness of the limbs, loose stools, an uncomfortable feeling in the epigastrium, lack of sense of taste, Pale tongue, Empty pulse.

Cracked fingers

Observation, Chapter 14

Liver-Blood deficiency

Cracked fingers, dizziness, blurred vision, floaters, numbness/tingling of limbs, scanty menstruation, dull-pale complexion, Pale tongue, Choppy or Fine pulse.

Liver-Blood stasis

Cracked fingers, purplish hands, hypochondrial/abdominal pain, painful periods, dark and clotted menstrual blood, masses in abdomen, purple nails and lips, purple or dark complexion, Purple tongue, Wiry or Firm pulse.

Yang deficiency with Empty-Cold

Cracked fingers, cold and pale hands, a feeling of cold, a slight feeling of discomfort in the chest, Pale and wet tongue, Deep-Weak pulse.

Yang deficiency with Empty-Cold causing cracked fingers may be either of the Heart or of the Lungs.

Thickened fingers

Observation, Chapter 14

Deficiency of Qi and Blood

Thickened fingers, poor appetite, loose stools, weak voice, tiredness, blurred vision, dizziness, numbness/tingling of limbs, palpitations, dull-pale complexion, Pale tongue, Weak or Choppy pulse.

Shrivelled and wrinkled fingers

Observation, Chapter 14

Loss of Body Fluids

Shrivelled and wrinkled fingers, dry skin, pale complexion, dry stools.

This is a state of Dryness that may occur after a prolonged spell of vomiting, sweating or diarrhoea.

NAILS

Ridged nails

Observation, Chapter 15

Liver-Blood deficiency

Ridged nails, dizziness, blurred vision, floaters, numbness/tingling of limbs, scanty menstruation, dull-pale complexion, Pale tongue, Choppy or Fine pulse.

Liver-Yin deficiency

Ridged, withered and brittle nails, dry nails, dizziness, numbness/tingling of the limbs, insomnia, blurred vision, floaters in eyes, dry eyes, diminished night vision, scanty menstruation or amenorrhoea, dull-pale complexion without lustre but with red cheekbones, muscular weakness, cramps, very dry skin and hair, night sweating, depression, a feeling of aimlessness, normal-coloured tongue without coating, Fine or Floating-Empty pulse.

Thickening of the nails

Observation, Chapter 15

Liver-Fire

Thickening of the nails, headache, red face, dizziness, tinnitus, irritability, propensity to outbursts of anger, thirst, bitter taste, constipation, dark urine, Red tongue with redder sides and dry yellow coating, Wiry-Rapid pulse.

Liver-Blood stasis

Thickening of the nails, dark nails, hypochondrial/abdominal pain, painful periods, dark and clotted menstrual blood, masses in abdomen, purple lips, purple or dark complexion, Purple tongue, Wiry or Firm pulse.

Phlegm

Thickening of the nails, yellowish nails, swollen hands, a feeling of heaviness of the limbs, sputum in the throat, a feeling of oppression of the chest, Swollen tongue, Slippery pulse.

Coarse and thick nails

Observation, Chapter 15

Qi and Blood deficiency with dryness of Blood generating Wind

Coarse and thick nails, ridged nails, dizziness, blurred vision, floaters, numbness/tingling of limbs, dull-pale complexion, dry skin, Pale and dry tongue, Choppy or Fine pulse.

Cracked nails

Observation, Chapter 15

Qi and Blood deficiency with dryness of Blood

Cracked, coarse and thick nails, poor appetite, loose stools, weak voice, tiredness, blurred vision, dizziness, numbness/tingling of limbs, palpitations, dull-pale complexion, dry skin, Pale and dry tongue, Weak or Choppy pulse.

Yin deficiency

Cracked nails, night sweating, dry mouth with a desire to drink in small sips, dry throat in the evening, scanty dark urine, dry stools, normal-coloured tongue without coating, Floating-Empty pulse.

Liver-Blood stasis

Cracked and dark-purplish nails, hypochondrial/abdominal pain, painful periods, dark and clotted menstrual blood, masses in the abdomen, purple lips, purple or dark complexion, Purple tongue, Wiry or Firm pulse.

Nails falling off

Observation, Chapter 15

Toxic Heat in the Liver

Nails falling off, swollen, hot and painful nails, pus in the nails, a feeling of heat, mental restlessness, thirst, Red tongue with red points and thick, sticky yellow coating, Overflowing-Slippery-Rapid pulse.

Indented nails

Observation, Chapter 15

Liver-Blood deficient and dry

Indented nails, brittle nails, withered nails, dry skin, dizziness, blurred vision, floaters, numbness/tingling of limbs, dull-pale complexion, scanty menstruation, Pale and dry tongue, Choppy or Fine pulse.

This is often seen in chronic skin diseases such as eczema and psoriasis.

Deficiency of Qi and Blood

Indented nails, brittle nails, poor appetite, loose stools, weak voice, tiredness, blurred vision, dizziness, numbness/tingling of limbs, palpitations, dull-pale complexion, Pale tongue, Weak or Choppy pulse.

Heat injuring Body Fluids

Indented nails, dry nails, a feeling of heat, thirst, mental restlessness, dry skin, Red tongue with dry yellow coating, Overflowing-Rapid pulse.

Other symptoms and signs depend on the organ involved.

Thin and brittle nails

Observation, Chapter 15

Qi and Blood deficiency

Thin and brittle nails, dry nails, poor appetite, loose stools, weak voice, tiredness, blurred vision, dizziness, numbness/tingling of limbs, palpitations, dull-pale complexion, Pale tongue, Weak or Choppy pulse.

Liver-Yin deficiency

Thin and brittle nails, dry nails, dry skin, dry eyes, dizziness, numbness/tingling of the limbs, insomnia, blurred vision, floaters in eyes, scanty menstruation or amenorrhoea, dull-pale complexion without lustre but with red cheekbones, cramps, night sweating, normal-coloured tongue without coating, Fine or Floating-Empty pulse.

Liver-Blood stasis

Thin and brittle nails, dark nails, thick nails, dry skin, hypochondrial/abdominal pain, painful periods, dark and clotted menstrual blood, masses in the abdomen, purple nails and lips, purple or dark complexion, Purple tongue, Wiry or Firm pulse.

Phlegm in the joints

Thin and brittle nails, dry nails, swollen and painful joints, joint deformities.

Kidney-Essence deficiency

Thin and brittle nails, poor bone development in children, softening of bones in adults, deafness, weakness of knees and legs, poor memory, loose teeth, falling hair or premature greying of the hair, weakness of sexual activity, lower backache, infertility, sterility, dizziness, tinnitus, normal-coloured tongue and Floating-Empty or Leather pulse if Kidney-Essence deficiency occurs against a background of Kidney-Yin deficiency, or Pale tongue and Deep-Weak pulse if against a background of Kidney-Yang deficiency.

Withered and brittle nails

Observation, Chapter 15

Liver-Blood deficiency

Withered and brittle nails, dizziness, blurred vision, floaters, numbness/tingling of limbs, scanty menstruation, dull-pale complexion, Pale tongue, Choppy or Fine pulse.

Liver-Yin deficiency

Withered and brittle nails, dizziness, numbness/tingling of limbs, blurred vision, floaters, dry eyes, scanty menstruation, dry skin and hair, night sweating, normal-coloured tongue without coating, Fine or Floating-Empty pulse.

Liver-Blood stasis

Withered and brittle nails, purple nails and lips, hypochondrial/abdominal pain, painful periods, dark and clotted menstrual blood, masses in the abdomen, purple or dark complexion, Purple tongue, Wiry or Firm pulse.

Liver-Blood stasis may cause Dryness and withered and brittle nails only in severe and advanced cases.

Liver-Fire

Withered and brittle nails, headache, red face, dizziness, tinnitus, irritability, propensity to outbursts of anger, thirst, bitter taste, constipation, dark urine, Red tongue with redder sides and dry yellow coating, Wiry-Rapid pulse.

Kidney-Yin deficiency

Withered and brittle nails, dizziness, tinnitus, hardness of hearing, poor memory, night sweating, vertigo, dry mouth and throat at night, lower backache, ache in bones, constipation, scanty dark urine, tiredness, lassitude, normal-coloured tongue without coating, Floating-Empty pulse.

Phlegm

Withered and brittle nails, thickened and yellow nails, numbness of the limbs, sputum in the throat, a feeling of oppression of the chest, Swollen tongue with sticky coating, Slippery pulse.

Blood Dryness and Empty-Heat in acute febrile diseases

Withered and brittle nails with acute onset in the aftermath of an acute febrile disease with high temperature reaching the Blood level, Red tongue without coating, Fine-Rapid pulse.

Withered and thickened nails

Observation, Chapter 15

Severe Stomach- and Spleen-Qi deficiency

Withered and thickened nails, poor appetite, slight abdominal distension after eating, tiredness, lassitude, pale complexion, weakness of the limbs, loose stools, an uncomfortable feeling in the epigastrium, lack of sense of taste, Pale tongue, Empty pulse.

Liver-Blood deficient and dry

Withered and thickened nails, brittle nails, dry skin, dizziness, blurred vision, floaters, numbness/tingling of limbs, scanty menstruation, dull-pale complexion, Pale and dry tongue, Choppy or Fine pulse.

Liver-Yin deficiency

Withered and thickened but brittle nails, dry nails, dizziness, numbness/tingling of the limbs, insomnia, blurred vision, floaters in eyes, dry eyes, scanty menstruation or amenorrhoea, dull-pale complexion without lustre but with red cheekbones, cramps, dry skin and hair, night sweating, normal-coloured tongue without coating, Fine or Floating-Empty pulse.

Damp-Heat with Toxic Heat

Withered and thickened nails, nail infections, red nails, swollen junction of the nail and finger, swollen and painful fingers, a feeling of heat, sticky taste, thirst, mental restlessness, Red tongue with red points and thick, sticky yellow coating, Overflowing-Slippery-Rapid pulse.

Curling nails

Observation, Chapter 15

Qi and Blood deficiency with Blood stasis

Curling nails, purple nails, pain in the hands, poor appetite, loose stools, weak voice, tiredness, blurred vision, dizziness, numbness/tingling of the limbs, palpitations, dark complexion, Pale or Purple tongue, Weak or Choppy pulse.

Flaking nails

Observation, Chapter 15

Spleen and Kidney deficiency with Dampness

Flaking nails, lower backache, cold and weak knees, a feeling of cold, bright-white complexion, impotence, decreased libido, tiredness, lassitude, abundant clear urination, urination at night, loose stools, poor appetite, slight abdominal distension, a desire to lie down, early-morning diarrhoea, Pale and wet tongue, Deep-Weak pulse.

Twisted nails

Observation, Chapter 15

Liver-Blood deficiency

Twisted nails, ridged nails, dizziness, blurred vision, floaters, numbness/tingling of limbs, scanty menstruation, dull-pale complexion, Pale tongue, Choppy or Fine pulse.

Nails with white spots

Observation, Chapter 15

Qi deficiency

Nails with white spots, tiredness, loose stools, shortness of breath, weak voice, weak limbs, Pale tongue, Empty pulse.

This may be Qi deficiency of the Spleen, Heart, Lungs, Liver or Kidneys.

Pale-white nails

Observation, Chapter 15

Liver- and Spleen-Blood deficiency

Pale white nails, pale hands, cold hands, poor appetite, slight abdominal distension after eating, tiredness, lassitude, dull-pale complexion, weakness of the limbs, loose stools, thin body, scanty periods or amenorrhoea, insomnia, dizziness, numbness of the limbs, blurred vision, floaters, diminished night vision, pale lips, muscular weakness, cramps, withered and brittle nails, dry hair and skin, slight depression, a feeling of aimlessness, Pale tongue especially on the sides, Choppy or Fine pulse.

Dull-white nails

Observation, Chapter 15

Spleen- and Kidney-Yang deficiency

Dull-white nails, pale hands, cold hands, lower backache, cold knees, a feeling of cold generally or in the back, weak legs, bright-white complexion, weak knees, impotence, premature ejaculation, low sperm count, cold and thin sperm, decreased libido, tiredness, lassitude, abundant clear or scanty clear urination, urination at night, apathy, oedema of the lower legs, infertility in women, loose stools, depression, poor appetite, slight abdominal distension, a desire to lie down, early-morning or chronic diarrhoea, Pale and wet tongue, Deep-Weak pulse.

Loss of Body Fluids

Dull-white, dry nails after profuse sweating, vomiting or diarrhoea, dry skin.

Red nails

Observation, Chapter 15

Full-Heat

Red nails, red dorsum of the hands, hot hands, a feeling of heat, mental restlessness, thirst, Red tongue with dry yellow coating, Overflowing-Rapid pulse.

Other symptoms and signs depend on the organ involved.

Yellow nails

Observation, Chapter 15

Damp-Heat in the Stomach and Spleen

Yellow nails, swollen fingers, painful joints, a feeling of fullness and pain of the epigastrium and lower abdomen, poor appetite, a feeling of heaviness, thirst without a desire to drink, nausea, loose stools with offensive odour, a feeling of heat, dull-yellow complexion, sticky taste, Red tongue with sticky yellow coating, Slippery-Rapid pulse.

Damp-Heat in the Liver and Gall-Bladder

Yellow nails, swollen fingers, painful joints, fullness/pain of the hypochondrium, abdomen or epigastrium, bitter taste, poor appetite, nausea, a feeling of heaviness of the body, yellow vaginal discharge, vaginal itching, midcycle bleeding/pain, burning on urination, dark urine, yellow complexion and eyes, vomiting, Red tongue with redder sides and unilateral or bilateral sticky yellow coating, Wiry-Slippery-Rapid pulse.

Phlegm

Yellowish and thick nails, a feeling of heaviness of the limbs, swollen hands, sputum in the throat, a feeling of oppression of the chest, Swollen tongue with sticky coating, Slippery pulse.

Bluish-greenish nails

Observation, Chapter 15

Liver-Blood deficiency with internal Cold

Bluish nails, dry nails, pale and cold hands, dizziness, blurred vision, floaters, numbness/tingling of limbs,

scanty menstruation, dull-pale complexion, a feeling of cold, Pale tongue, Choppy or Fine pulse and Slow pulse.

Severe Spleen-Qi deficiency with internal Wind (children)

Greenish nails, thin fingers, poor appetite, thin body, retarded development, flaccid muscles, fine tremor of limbs, Pale tongue, Weak pulse.

Liver-Blood stasis

Dark, bluish-green nails, pain in the hands, rigidity of the fingers, hypochondrial/abdominal pain, painful periods, dark and clotted menstrual blood, masses in the abdomen, purple nails and lips, purple or dark complexion, Purple tongue, Wiry or Firm pulse.

Dark nails

Observation, Chapter 15

Kidney deficiency

Dark nails, lower backache, dizziness, tinnitus.

Other symptoms and signs depend on whether there is a deficiency of Kidney-Yin or Kidney-Yang.

Blood stasis

Dark nails, joint pain, dry nails, abdominal pain, dark complexion, Purple tongue, Wiry or Choppy pulse.

Purple nails

Observation, Chapter 15

Liver-Blood stasis

Purple nails, hypochondrial/abdominal pain, painful periods, dark and clotted menstrual blood, masses in the abdomen, purple lips, purple or dark complexion, Purple tongue, Wiry or Firm pulse.

Heat at the Blood level

Purple nails, fever at night, macular rash, bleeding, mental confusion, Red tongue without coating, Fine and Rapid pulse.

Small or absent lunulae

Observation, Chapter 15

Chronic Qi and Blood deficiency

Small or absent lunulae, ridged nails, poor appetite, loose stools, weak voice, tiredness, blurred vision, dizziness, numbness/tingling of limbs, palpitations, dull-pale complexion, Pale tongue, Weak or Choppy pulse.

Yang deficiency

Small or absent lunulae, a feeling of cold, cold limbs, loose stools, abundant pale urination, tiredness, Pale and wet tongue, Deep-Weak pulse.

Other symptoms and signs depend on the organ affected by Yang deficiency, which may be of the Stomach, Spleen, Heart, Kidneys or Lungs.

Internal Cold

Small or absent lunulae, a feeling of cold, cold limbs, abdominal pain which improves with the application of warmth, Pale tongue, Tight-Slow pulse.

Large lunulae

Observation, Chapter 15

Yin deficiency with Empty-Heat

Large lunulae, brittle nails, dry throat at night, a feeling of heat in the evening, night sweating, five-palm heat, malar flush, insomnia, anxiety, dry mouth with a desire to drink in small sips, Red tongue without coating, Floating-Empty and Rapid pulse.

Other symptoms and signs depend on the organ involved, which may be the Liver, Lungs, Heart, Stomach or Kidneys.

Chapter **66**

LEGS

Chapter contents

FEET *693*
  Oedema *693*
  Cold feet *694*

ATROPHY OF THE LEGS *694*

PARALYSIS OF THE LEGS *695*

GAIT *695*
  Festination *695*
  Unstable gait *695*
  Staggering gait *696*
  Stepping gait *696*
  Shuffling gait *696*

ARCHED LEGS *696*

PAIN *696*
  Pain in the thigh *696*
  Pain in the hip *697*
  Pain in the knee *697*
  Pain in the foot *697*
  Pain in the groin *698*
  Pain in the soles *698*

KNEES *698*
  Weak knees *698*
  Stiff knees *699*

WEAKNESS OF THE LEGS *699*

A FEELING OF HEAVINESS OF THE LEGS *699*

RESTLESS LEGS *700*

TREMOR OF THE LEGS *700*

CRAMPS IN THE CALVES *700*

LOWER LEG ULCERS *701*

TOE ULCERS *701*

BURNING SENSATION IN THE SOLES *701*

FEET

Oedema

Observation, Chapters 18 and 19; Interrogation, Chapter 39; Symptoms and Signs, Chapters 64 and 68

Spleen-Yang deficiency

Pitting oedema of legs and abdomen, cold limbs, poor appetite, slight abdominal distension after eating, tiredness, lassitude, pale complexion, weakness of the limbs, loose stools, a feeling of cold, Pale and wet tongue, Deep-Weak pulse.

Kidney-Yang deficiency

Pitting oedema of ankles and legs, weak knees, lower backache, cold knees, a feeling of cold, bright-white complexion, tiredness, lassitude, abundant clear urination, urination at night, impotence, decreased libido, Pale and wet tongue, Deep-Weak pulse.

Damp-Heat

Swelling of legs and ankles, ache, swelling, redness and heat of the joints, sticky yellow tongue coating, Slippery-Rapid pulse.

Other symptoms and signs depend on the location of the Damp-Heat.

Qi stagnation and stasis of Blood

Non-pitting oedema of the legs, in which the skin springs back on pressing the swollen area, a feeling of distension of the legs, purplish colour of the legs, hypochondrial/epigastric distension, irritability, moodiness, a feeling of a lump in the throat, premenstrual tension, hypochondrial pain, abdominal pain, painful periods, dark and clotted menstrual blood, masses in the abdomen, purple nails and lips, purple or dark complexion, Purple tongue, Wiry or Firm pulse.

Cold-Dampness

Swelling of legs and ankles, a feeling of heaviness of the limbs, puffy legs, ache in the joints, epigastric fullness, a feeling of heaviness of the head and body, a feeling of cold, cold limbs, sticky white tongue coating, Slippery-Slow pulse.

Qi deficiency and Blood stasis

Oedema of the limbs, cold hands and feet, pain in the legs, tiredness, poor appetite, loose stools, weak voice, slight shortness of breath, dark complexion, abdominal pain, Bluish-Purple tongue, Weak or Choppy pulse.

> ### Clinical note
>
> - Remember: if oedema is not pitting (i.e. leaves a dent when pressed with the finger), it is not 'true' oedema.

Cold feet

Interrogation, Chapter 39

Kidney-Yang deficiency

Cold feet, oedema of the feet, cold knees, lower backache, cold knees, feeling cold, bright-white complexion, weak knees, tiredness, lassitude, abundant clear urination, urination at night, impotence, decreased libido, Pale and wet tongue, Deep-Weak pulse.

Liver-Blood deficiency

Cold feet, numbness of the feet, dry feet, dizziness, blurred vision, floaters, numbness/tingling of limbs, scanty menstruation, dull-pale complexion, Pale tongue, Choppy or Fine pulse.

Spleen- and Kidney-Yang deficiency

Cold feet, oedema of the feet, cold and weak legs or knees, lower backache, a feeling of cold generally or in the back, or bright-white complexion, impotence, decreased libido, tiredness, abundant clear or scanty clear urination, urination at night, loose stools, poor appetite, slight abdominal distension, a desire to lie down, early-morning diarrhoea, Pale and wet tongue, Deep-Weak pulse.

Phlegm in the Lower Burner

Cold feet, a feeling of heaviness of the legs, numbness of the legs, abdominal pain, excessive vaginal discharge, Swollen tongue, Slippery pulse.

> ### Clinical note
>
> - Cold feet is often a reliable symptom of Kidney-Yang deficiency.

ATROPHY OF THE LEGS

Observation, Chapter 19

Stomach- and Spleen-Qi deficiency

Atrophy or thinning of the muscles of the legs, weakness of the limbs, muscular weakness, gait like a duck, feet turning in or out, poor appetite, slight abdominal distension after eating, tiredness, lassitude, pale complexion, loose stools, uncomfortable feeling in the epigastrium, lack of sense of taste, Pale tongue, Empty pulse.

In children this corresponds to the sequelae stage of poliomyelitis.

Liver- and Kidney-Yin deficiency

Atrophy or thinning of the leg muscles, weak knees, staggering gait, dizziness, tinnitus, weak knees, hardness of hearing, lower backache, dull occipital or vertical headache, insomnia, numbness/tingling of the limbs, dry eyes, blurred vision, dry throat in the evening, dry hair and skin, brittle nails, night sweating, dry stools, scanty menstruation or amenorrhoea, normal-coloured tongue without coating, Floating-Empty pulse.

This pattern is more common in the elderly.

Spleen- and Kidney-Yang deficiency

Atrophy or thinning of the leg muscles, cold and weak knees, oedema of the lower legs, muscular weakness, lower backache, feelings of cold generally or in the back, weak legs, bright-white complexion, decreased libido, tiredness, lassitude, abundant clear or scanty clear urination, urination at night, loose stools, poor appetite, slight abdominal distension, a desire to lie down, early-morning diarrhoea, Pale and wet tongue, Deep-Weak pulse.

Deficiency of Qi and Blood

Atrophy or thinning of the leg muscles, poor appetite, loose stools, weak voice, tiredness, blurred vision, dizziness, numbness/tingling of limbs, palpitations, dull-pale complexion, Pale tongue, Weak or Choppy pulse.

Kidney-Essence deficiency

Atrophy or thinning of the leg muscles, late physical/mental development in children, inability to grasp with the hands, inability to put feet down.

This pattern occurs only in children or babies and is often associated with the Five Retardations (slow development in children involving standing, walking, teeth development, hair development and speech) and the Five Flaccidities (late closure of the fontanelles, flaccidity of mouth, hands, feet and muscles).

PARALYSIS OF THE LEGS

Observation, Chapter 19

Stomach- and Spleen-Qi deficiency

Paralysis of the legs, weak and cold limbs, poor appetite, slight abdominal distension after eating, tiredness, lassitude, pale complexion, loose stools, an uncomfortable feeling in the epigastrium, lack of sense of taste, Pale tongue, Empty pulse.

Deficiency of Qi and Blood

Paralysis of the legs, weak limbs, poor appetite, loose stools, weak voice, tiredness, blurred vision, dizziness, numbness/tingling of limbs, palpitations, dull-pale complexion, Pale tongue, Weak or Choppy pulse.

Liver- and Kidney-Yin deficiency

Paralysis of the legs, dizziness, tinnitus, weak knees, hardness of hearing, lower backache, dull occipital or vertical headache, insomnia, numbness/tingling of the limbs, dry eyes, blurred vision, dry throat in the evening, dry hair and skin, brittle nails, night sweating, dry stools, scanty menstruation or amenorrhoea, normal-coloured tongue without coating, Floating-Empty pulse.

Retention of Dampness in the muscles

Paralysis of the legs, a feeling of heaviness of the body or limbs, swelling of the limbs, epigastric fullness, sticky taste, sticky tongue coating, Slippery pulse.

Liver-Blood stasis

Paralysis of the legs, pain in the limbs which may be worse at night, hypochondrial/abdominal pain, painful periods, dark and clotted menstrual blood, masses in the abdomen, purple nails and lips, purple or dark complexion, Purple tongue, Wiry or Firm pulse.

Wind and Phlegm in the channels

Paralysis of the leg on one side, numbness of the limbs, severe dizziness, blurred vision, tremors, numbness/tingling of the limbs, tinnitus, nausea, sputum in the throat, a feeling of oppression of the chest, Stiff or Deviated and Swollen tongue, Wiry-Slippery pulse.

This corresponds to the sequelae stage of Wind-stroke.

GAIT

Festination

Observation, Chapter 19

'Festination' refers to a particular gait whereby the patient lifts the feet up higher than necessary and then steps forward in a haste as if trying to avoid falling forwards.

Liver- and Kidney-Yin deficiency with internal Wind

Festination, tremors, severe dizziness, tinnitus, weak knees, hardness of hearing, lower backache, dull occipital or vertical headache, insomnia, numbness/tingling of the limbs, dry eyes, blurred vision, dry throat in the evening, dry hair and skin, brittle nails, night sweating, dry stools, scanty menstruation or amenorrhoea, tremors, tic, normal-coloured, Deviated or Moving tongue without coating, Floating-Empty and slightly Wiry pulse.

Qi and Blood deficiency with internal Wind

Festination, weak limbs, slight tremor of the limbs, tic, poor appetite, loose stools, weak voice, tiredness, blurred vision, dizziness, numbness/tingling of limbs, palpitations, dull-pale complexion, Pale and Deviated or Moving tongue, Weak or Choppy and slightly Wiry pulse.

Unstable gait

Observation, Chapter 19

Liver- and Kidney-Yin deficiency with internal Wind

Unstable gait, severe dizziness, tinnitus, weak knees, hardness of hearing, lower backache, dull occipital or vertical headache, insomnia, numbness/tingling of

the limbs, dry eyes, blurred vision, dry throat in the evening, dry hair and skin, brittle nails, night sweating, dry stools, scanty menstruation or amenorrhoea, tremors, tic, normal-coloured, Deviated or Moving tongue without coating, Floating-Empty and slightly Wiry pulse.

Qi and Blood deficiency with internal Wind 👤 👤

Unstable gait, weak limbs, slight tremor of the limbs, tic, poor appetite, loose stools, weak voice, tiredness, blurred vision, dizziness, numbness/tingling of limbs, palpitations, dull-pale complexion, Pale and Deviated or Moving tongue, Weak or Choppy and slightly Wiry pulse.

Staggering gait

Observation, Chapter 19

Liver- and Kidney-Yin deficiency

Staggering gait, dizziness, tinnitus, weak knees, hardness of hearing, lower backache, dull occipital or vertical headache, insomnia, numbness/tingling of the limbs, dry eyes, blurred vision, dry throat in the evening, dry hair and skin, brittle nails, night sweating, dry stools, scanty menstruation or amenorrhoea, normal-coloured tongue without coating, Floating-Empty pulse.

Phlegm and Blood stasis 👤

Staggering gait, pain in the legs which is worse at night, swollen legs, heaviness of the legs, Purple and Swollen tongue, Wiry-Slippery pulse.

Stepping gait

Observation, Chapter 19

Liver- and Kidney-Yin deficiency with internal Wind 👤

Stepping gait, severe dizziness, tinnitus, weak knees, hardness of hearing, lower backache, dull occipital or vertical headache, insomnia, numbness/tingling of the limbs, dry eyes, blurred vision, dry throat in the evening, dry hair and skin, brittle nails, night sweating, dry stools, scanty menstruation or amenorrhoea, tremors, tic, normal-coloured, Deviated or Moving tongue without coating, Floating-Empty and slightly Wiry pulse.

Qi and Blood deficiency with internal Wind 👤 👤

Stepping gait, weak limbs, slight tremor of the limbs, tic, poor appetite, loose stools, weak voice, tiredness, blurred vision, dizziness, numbness/tingling of limbs, palpitations, dull-pale complexion, Pale and Deviated or Moving tongue, Weak or Choppy and slightly Wiry pulse.

Shuffling gait

Observation, Chapter 19

Liver- and Kidney-Yin deficiency with Wind-Phlegm in the channels 👤

Shuffling gait, numbness/tingling of the limbs or legs, tremors, severe dizziness, tinnitus, weak knees, hardness of hearing, lower backache, dull occipital or vertical headache, insomnia, dry eyes, blurred vision, dry throat in the evening, dry hair and skin, brittle nails, night sweating, dry stools, scanty menstruation or amenorrhoea, tremors, tic, normal-coloured, Deviated or Moving and Swollen tongue without coating, Floating-Empty and slightly Wiry-Slippery pulse.

ARCHED LEGS

Observation, Chapter 19

Congenital deficiency of Stomach and Spleen 🔏

Arched legs in children, thinness and weakness in children, poor digestion, weakness of the legs, abdominal distension, poor appetite, loose stools, tiredness.

Congenital deficiency of Liver and Kidneys 🔏

Arched legs in children, thinness and weakness in children, weakness of the legs and knees, or back, nocturnal enuresis.

PAIN

Pain in the thigh

Interrogation, Chapter 39

Damp-Heat

Burning pain in the inner thigh that may extend to the external genitalia, a feeling of heaviness of the legs,

a feeling of heat, dull-yellow complexion, excessive vaginal discharge, vaginal redness or soreness and itching, sticky yellow tongue coating, Slippery-Rapid pulse.

Cold-Dampness

Ache in the inner thigh that is aggravated by exposure to cold and alleviated by application of heat, a feeling of heaviness of the legs, dull-pale complexion, cold limbs, excessive white vaginal discharge, sticky white tongue coating, Slippery-Slow pulse.

Qi deficiency and Blood stasis

Ache in the thigh that is worse at night, muscular weakness, weak limbs, tiredness, dark complexion, rigidity of the knees, Purple tongue, Wiry pulse.

Kidney-Yang deficiency

Chronic dull ache in the thigh, cold and weak knees, lower backache, a feeling of cold, bright-white complexion, tiredness, lassitude, abundant clear urination, urination at night, impotence, decreased libido, Pale and wet tongue, Deep-Weak pulse.

Stagnation of Qi and stasis of Blood in the descending branch of the Penetrating Vessel

Ache in the inner thigh, often in conjunction with the period in women, cold feet, a feeling of heat in the face, abdominal fullness and pain, irregular periods, visible venules on the inside of the legs, Firm pulse.

Pain in the hip

Interrogation, Chapter 39

Stagnation of Qi and stasis of Blood

Stabbing hip pain that is worse at night, marked rigidity of the joint, a feeling of distension of the legs, Purple tongue, Wiry pulse.

Invasion of Cold and Dampness

Unilateral, severe hip pain which is aggravated by exposure to cold and alleviated by application of heat, a feeling of heaviness of the legs, cold legs, rigidity.

Pain in the knee

Interrogation, Chapter 39

Invasion of Cold and Dampness

Unilateral severe pain in the knee that is aggravated by exposure to cold and alleviated by the application of heat, rigidity of the joint, swelling of the knee, a feeling of heaviness of the legs.

Invasion of Cold

Unilateral severe pain in the knee that is aggravated by exposure to cold and alleviated by the application of heat, better with exercise and worse with rest, rigidity of the joint.

Damp-Heat

Severe pain in the knee, with redness, swelling and heat.

Stagnation of Qi and stasis of Blood

Pain in the knee that does not react to weather conditions, pain aggravated by movement and ameliorated by rest, with no swelling. This is usually caused by repetitive strain injury or sprain.

Kidney deficiency

Chronic dull ache and weakness in both knees, of gradual onset, better with rest, worse with exercise, lower backache, dizziness, tinnitus.

Other symptoms and signs depend on whether there is a Kidney-Yin or Kidney-Yang deficiency.

Pain in the foot

Interrogation, Chapter 39

Dampness

Ache and swelling of the feet, cold feet, a feeling of heaviness of the legs.

Damp-Heat

Ache and swelling of the feet, hot, red and smelling feet, a feeling of heaviness of the legs.

Kidney deficiency

Dull ache in the feet, weak knees, lower backache, dizziness, tinnitus.

Other manifestations depend on whether there is Yin or Yang deficiency.

Deficiency of Qi and Blood

Dull ache in the feet, numbness of feet, poor appetite, loose stools, weak voice, tiredness, blurred vision, dizziness, numbness/tingling of limbs, palpitations, dull-pale complexion, Pale tongue, Weak or Choppy pulse.

Damp-Phlegm

Ache in the dorsum or ball of the foot, tingling of the feet, a feeling of heaviness of the legs, a tendency to obesity, Swollen tongue, Slippery pulse.

Pain in the groin
Dampness

Pain in the groin, a feeling of heaviness of the legs, swelling, sticky tongue coating, Slippery pulse.

Stagnation of Qi and stasis of Blood in the Liver channel

Severe pain in the groin that is alleviated by mild exercise, hypochondrial or epigastric distension, irritability, moodiness, a feeling of a lump in the throat, premenstrual tension, hypochondrial/abdominal pain, painful periods, dark and clotted menstrual blood, masses in the abdomen, purple nails and lips, purple or dark complexion, Purple tongue, Wiry or Firm pulse.

Girdle Vessel pathology (Damp-Heat)

Pain in the groin that radiates from the lower abdomen, a feeling of heaviness, abdominal fullness, excessive vaginal discharge, unilateral sticky yellow coating, Wiry pulse on both Middle positions.

Pain in the soles

Interrogation, Chapter 39

Stomach-Qi deficiency

Dull ache in the soles (ball of the foot) of slow onset, weak legs, an uncomfortable feeling in the epigastrium, no appetite, lack of sense of taste, loose stools, tiredness especially in the morning, weak limbs, Pale tongue, Empty pulse.

Stomach-Qi deficiency with Dampness

Dull ache in the soles (ball of the foot) of acute onset, swelling of the ball of the foot, a feeling of heaviness of the legs, weak legs, an uncomfortable feeling in the epigastrium, lack of appetite, lack of sense of taste, loose stools, tiredness especially in the morning, weak limbs, Pale tongue, Empty pulse.

Stomach-Heat

Burning pain in the ball of the foot, burning epigastric pain, thirst, sour regurgitation, nausea, excessive hunger, foul breath, a feeling of heat, Red tongue with a yellow coating, Overflowing-Rapid pulse.

Liver-Fire

Burning pain under the big toe, hot feet, headache, red face, dizziness, tinnitus, irritability, propensity to outbursts of anger, thirst, bitter taste, constipation, dark urine, Red tongue with redder sides and dry yellow coating, Wiry-Rapid pulse.

Dampness in the Spleen

Dull ache under the big toe, swelling of the foot, a feeling of heaviness of the legs, sweaty feet, a feeling of fullness in the epigastrium and abdomen, a sticky taste, sticky tongue coating, Slippery pulse.

Kidney-Yang deficiency

Dull ache in the soles, cold feet, cold and weak knees, lower backache, a feeling of cold, bright-white complexion, tiredness, lassitude, abundant clear urination, urination at night, impotence, decreased libido, Pale and wet tongue, Deep-Weak pulse.

Kidney-Yin deficiency

Dull ache in the soles in the evening or night, burning sensation in the soles, weak knees, dizziness, tinnitus, hardness of hearing, poor memory, night sweating, dry mouth and throat at night, lower backache, constipation, scanty dark urine, tiredness, normal-coloured tongue without coating, Floating-Empty pulse.

Kidney deficiency with Dampness

Dull ache in the soles with a slight puffiness, a feeling of heaviness and weakness of the legs, weak knees, lower backache, dizziness, tinnitus.

Other symptoms and signs depend on whether there is Kidney-Yin or Kidney-Yang deficiency.

KNEES

Weak knees

Interrogation, Chapter 39

Kidney-Yang deficiency

Weak and cold knees, lower backache, a feeling of cold, bright-white complexion, tiredness, lassitude, abundant clear urination, urination at night, impotence, decreased libido, Pale and wet tongue, Deep-Weak pulse.

Kidney- and Liver-Yin deficiency

Weak knees, dizziness, tinnitus, weak knees, hardness of hearing, lower backache, dull occipital or vertical headache, insomnia, numbness/tingling of the limbs, dry eyes, blurred vision, dry throat in the evening, dry hair and skin, brittle nails, night sweating, dry stools, scanty menstruation or amenorrhoea, normal-coloured tongue without coating, Floating-Empty pulse.

Stomach- and Spleen-Qi deficiency

Weak knees, poor appetite, slight abdominal distension after eating, tiredness, lassitude, pale complexion, weakness of the limbs, loose stools, an uncomfortable feeling in the epigastrium, lack of sense of taste, Pale tongue, Empty pulse.

Stiff knees

Cold-Dampness in the channels

Stiff and swollen knees, a cold feeling in the knees or legs, knee ache that is aggravated by exposure to cold and dampness and alleviated by the application of heat, a feeling of heaviness of the legs.

Cold in the channels

Stiff and painful knees, pain that is aggravated by exposure to cold and alleviated by the application of heat.

Dampness

Stiff knees, swollen knees, numbness of the legs, a feeling of heaviness of the legs, sticky tongue coating, Slippery pulse.

Damp-Heat

Stiff knees, swollen, red, painful and hot knees, numbness of the legs, a feeling of heaviness of the legs, sticky yellow tongue coating, Slippery-Rapid pulse.

Stagnation of Qi and stasis of Blood

Stiff knees, painful knees, ameliorated by mild exercise, stiff tendons, may be worse at night, Wiry pulse.

Kidney-Yang deficiency

Slight stiffness of the knees, lower backache, cold knees, a feeling of cold, bright-white complexion, weak knees, tiredness, lassitude, abundant clear urination, urination at night, impotence, decreased libido, Pale and wet tongue, Deep-Weak pulse.

WEAKNESS OF THE LEGS

Interrogation, Chapter 39

Stomach- and Spleen-Qi deficiency

Weakness of the limbs or legs, poor appetite, slight abdominal distension after eating, tiredness, lassitude, pale complexion, loose stools, an uncomfortable feeling in the epigastrium, lack of sense of taste, Pale tongue, Empty pulse.

Kidney-Yang deficiency

Weakness of the legs, cold feet and legs, oedema of the ankles, weak and cold knees, lower backache, a feeling of cold, bright-white complexion, tiredness, lassitude, abundant clear urination, urination at night, impotence, decreased libido, Pale and wet tongue, Deep-Weak pulse.

Kidney-Yin deficiency

Weakness of the legs, thin legs, unsteady walking, hot soles at night, dizziness, tinnitus, hardness of hearing, poor memory, night sweating, dry mouth and throat at night, lower backache, constipation, scanty dark urine, tiredness, normal-coloured tongue without coating, Floating-Empty pulse.

Liver- and Kidney-Yin deficiency

Weakness of the legs, thin legs, unsteady walking, hot soles at night, dizziness, tinnitus, weak knees, hardness of hearing, lower backache, dull occipital or vertical headache, insomnia, numbness/tingling of the limbs, dry eyes, blurred vision, dry throat in the evening, dry hair and skin, brittle nails, night sweating, dry stools, scanty menstruation or amenorrhoea, normal-coloured tongue without coating, Floating-Empty pulse.

A FEELING OF HEAVINESS OF THE LEGS

Interrogation, Chapter 39; Symptoms and Signs, Chapter 64

Dampness

A feeling of heaviness of the legs or in general, numbness, swelling of the legs, epigastric fullness, sticky tongue coating, Slippery pulse.

Damp-Heat

A feeling of heaviness of the legs, swelling of the legs, hot feet, muscle ache, numbness, epigastric fullness, sticky yellow coating, Slippery-Rapid pulse.

Spleen-Qi deficiency with Dampness

A slight feeling of heaviness of the legs, weakness of the limbs, poor appetite, slight abdominal distension after eating, tiredness, lassitude, pale complexion, loose stools, abdominal fullness, a feeling of heaviness, a sticky taste, poor digestion, undigested food in the stools, nausea, dull frontal headache, Pale tongue with sticky coating, Soggy pulse.

Kidney-Yang deficiency with Dampness

A slight feeling of heaviness of the legs, weak/cold knees, lower backache, feeling cold, bright-white complexion, tiredness, lassitude, abundant clear urination, urination at night, impotence, decreased libido, excessive vaginal discharge, Pale and wet tongue with a sticky coating, Deep-Weak and slightly Slippery pulse.

> ### Clinical note
>
> - A feeling of heaviness of the legs is a certain symptom of Dampness in the Lower Burner.

RESTLESS LEGS

Liver- and Kidney-Yin deficiency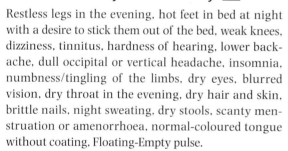

Restless legs in the evening, hot feet in bed at night with a desire to stick them out of the bed, weak knees, dizziness, tinnitus, hardness of hearing, lower backache, dull occipital or vertical headache, insomnia, numbness/tingling of the limbs, dry eyes, blurred vision, dry throat in the evening, dry hair and skin, brittle nails, night sweating, dry stools, scanty menstruation or amenorrhoea, normal-coloured tongue without coating, Floating-Empty pulse.

Stomach-Yin deficiency

Restless legs, weak legs, no appetite or slight hunger but no desire to eat, constipation (dry stools), dull or slightly burning epigastric pain, dry mouth and throat especially in the afternoon, thirst but no desire to drink, or a desire to drink in small sips, slight feeling of fullness after eating, normal-coloured tongue without coating or without coating in the centre, Floating-Empty pulse.

Liver-Blood deficiency

Restless legs, numbness/tingling of the legs, dizziness, blurred vision, floaters, scanty menstruation, dull-pale complexion, Pale tongue, Choppy or Fine pulse.

Deficiency of Blood in the Penetrating Vessel

Restless legs, anxiety, dizziness, scanty periods, irregular periods, abdominal and umbilical fullness, numbness/tingling of the legs and big toes, Pale tongue, Choppy or Fine pulse.

> ### Clinical note
>
> - I find ST-36 Zusanli, ST-37 Shangjuxu and ST-39 Xiajuxu in combination an effective treatment for restless legs.

TREMOR OF THE LEGS

Observation, Chapters 4 and 18; Symptoms and Signs, Chapter 64

Liver-Blood or Liver-Yin deficiency leading to Wind

Mild tremor of the legs, numbness/tingling of the limbs, dizziness, blurred vision, floaters, scanty menstruation, dry eyes, fine tremor of legs, tic, vertigo, Pale tongue with coating, or normal-coloured without coating, Choppy or Fine pulse.

Kidney-Yin deficiency with internal Wind

Mild tremor of the legs, vertigo, dizziness, tinnitus, hardness of hearing, poor memory, night sweating, vertigo, dry mouth and throat at night, lower backache, ache in bones, nocturnal emissions, constipation, scanty dark urine, infertility, premature ejaculation, tiredness, lassitude, depression, slight anxiety, normal-coloured tongue without coating, Floating-Empty pulse.

CRAMPS IN THE CALVES

Interrogation, Chapter 39

Liver-Blood deficiency

Cramps in the calves at night or during moderate exercise, numbness/tingling of legs, dizziness, blurred vision, floaters, scanty menstruation, dull-pale complexion, Pale tongue, Choppy or Fine pulse.

Liver-Blood deficiency with Empty-Wind

Severe cramps in the calves at night, numbness/tingling of the legs, dizziness, blurred vision, floaters,

scanty menstruation, dull-pale complexion, vertigo, tremors, Pale tongue, Fine and slightly Wiry pulse.

Wind-Phlegm

Severe cramps in the calves, numbness/tingling of the legs, a feeling of heaviness of the legs, severe dizziness, blurred vision, tremors, tinnitus, nausea, sputum in the throat, a feeling of oppression of the chest, Stiff or Deviated and Swollen tongue, Wiry-Slippery pulse.

Liver-Blood stasis

Severe cramps in the calves which are often worse at night, abdominal pain, Purple tongue, Wiry pulse.

> **Clinical note**
>
> - I find BL-57 Chengshan an effective point for cramps in the calves.

LOWER LEG ULCERS

Observation, Chapter 21

Damp-Heat

Ulcers on the lower legs, red, painful, swollen, oozing a sticky yellow fluid, itchy, hardness of the edges of the ulcer after oozing fluid, a feeling of heaviness, sticky yellow tongue coating, Slippery-Rapid pulse.

Spleen-Qi deficiency with Dampness

Ulcers on the lower leg, swollen, not painful, pale red, oozing a thin fluid, poor appetite, slight abdominal distension after eating, tiredness, pale complexion, weakness of the limbs, loose stools, abdominal fullness, a feeling of heaviness, a sticky taste, poor digestion, undigested food in the stools, nausea, dull frontal headache, Pale tongue with sticky coating, Soggy pulse.

Qi stagnation and Blood stasis

Ulcers on the lower legs, dark in colour, painful, hard, oozing a turbid fluid, pain in the legs, a feeling of distension of the legs, Purple tongue, Wiry pulse.

Liver- and Kidney-Yin deficiency

Ulcers on the lower leg, not painful, pale red, dizziness, tinnitus, weak knees, hardness of hearing, lower backache, dull occipital or vertical headache, insomnia, numbness/tingling of the limbs, dry eyes, blurred vision, dry throat in the evening, dry hair and skin, brittle nails, night sweating, dry stools, scanty menstruation or amenorrhoea, normal-coloured tongue without coating, Floating-Empty pulse.

TOE ULCERS

Observation, Chapter 21

Toxic Heat

Dark ulcers on the toes, oozing a dark fluid or blood and festering, a burning pain that is worse at night, insomnia, mental restlessness, thirst, Red tongue with red points and thick, sticky yellow coating, Overflowing-Slippery-Rapid pulse.

External Toxic Heat

Ulcers on the toes, especially the inner aspect of the big toe, dark nails, swelling on the side of the nail, pain, Floating pulse.

BURNING SENSATION IN THE SOLES

Interrogation, Chapter 39

Kidney-Yin deficiency with Empty-Heat

Burning sensation in the soles that is worse in the evening or at night, dizziness, tinnitus, hardness of hearing, night sweating, dry mouth at night, five-palm heat, a feeling of heat in the evening, malar flush, thirst with a desire to drink in small sips, lower backache, scanty dark urine, insomnia, Red tongue without coating, Floating-Empty and Rapid pulse.

Stomach-Heat

Burning sensation in the ball of the foot, burning epigastric pain, thirst, sour regurgitation, nausea, excessive hunger, foul breath, a feeling of heat, Red tongue with a yellow coating, Overflowing-Rapid pulse.

Liver-Fire

Burning sensation under the big toe, headache, red face, dizziness, tinnitus, irritability, propensity to outbursts of anger, thirst, bitter taste, constipation, dark urine, Red tongue with redder sides and dry yellow coating, Wiry-Rapid pulse.

Chapter **67**

LOWER BACK

Chapter contents

LOWER BACKACHE   703

SCIATICA   704

FEELING OF COLD AND HEAVINESS OF THE LOWER BACK   704

WEAKNESS OF THE LOWER BACK AND KNEES   704

STIFFNESS OF THE LOWER BACK   705

COCCYX PAIN   705

ATROPHY OF THE MUSCLES ALONG THE SPINE   705

RIGIDITY OF THE LOWER BACK   705

SKIN SIGNS   706
  Spots on the back   706
  Vesicles on the lower back   706
  Dryness and redness of the skin of the lower
    back   706
  Yellow colour of the lower back   706
  Skin marks on the lower back   706
  Boils on BL-23 Shenshu   706
  Ulcers on the buttocks   706
  Papules or pustules on the buttocks   707

SPINAL CURVATURE   707
  Scoliosis   707
  Lordosis   707
  Spine bent forward   707
  Kyphosis   708
  Flattening of lumbar spine   708
  List of spine   708

LOWER BACKACHE

Interrogation, Chapter 37

Kidney-Yang deficiency

Chronic lower backache, which may be unilateral, bilateral or on the midline and which may recur in bouts, a feeling of weakness and cold of the lower back, better with rest and worse with exercise, weak and cold knees, a feeling of cold, bright-white complexion, tiredness, lassitude, abundant clear urination, urination at night, impotence, decreased libido, Pale and wet tongue, Deep-Weak pulse.

Kidney-Yin deficiency

Chronic lower backache, which may be unilateral, bilateral or on the midline and which may recur in bouts, a feeling of weakness of the lower back, contraction of the muscles of the lower back, better with rest and worse with exercise, thin body, weak knees, dizziness, tinnitus, hardness of hearing, poor memory, night sweating, dry mouth and throat at night, constipation, scanty dark urine, tiredness, slight anxiety, normal-coloured tongue without coating, Floating-Empty pulse.

Sprain of the back

Acute, severe backache, which may be unilateral or on the midline, rigidity of the back with inability to bend forward, pain in the leg.

Cold-Dampness in the lower back

Acute or chronic backache that is worse in the morning and better as the day progresses, better with light exercise and worse with rest, feeling of heaviness, a feeling of cold.

Blood stasis in the back

Chronic, severe unilateral lower backache that improves with light exercise and worsens with rest, worse in the morning but also at night, rigidity of the back, pain centred in a small area, Purple tongue, Wiry pulse.

Invasion of Wind-Cold

Sudden backache on the midline extending from the occiput to the lower back, aversion to cold, fever, cough, itchy throat, slight breathlessness, stuffed or runny nose with clear watery discharge, sneezing, occipital headache, body aches, thin white tongue coating, Floating-Tight pulse.

Clinical note

- In chronic lower backache there is always a Kidney deficiency and I always use BL-23 Shenshu.

SCIATICA

Apart from identifying the pattern, the affected channel must be identified. The channels affected are the Bladder, Gall-Bladder or Stomach; often more than one channel is involved.

Cold-Dampness in the lower back and legs

Dull pain in the leg that is worse in the morning, numbness/tingling of the leg, a feeling of heaviness of the leg, pain aggravated by exposure to cold and dampness and ameliorated by the application of heat.

Damp-Heat in the lower back and legs

Severe pain in the leg that is worse in the afternoon or evening, numbness/tingling of the leg, a feeling of heaviness and heat of the leg.

Stagnation of Qi and stasis of Blood

Severe stabbing pain in the leg that is slightly better with movement and worse with rest or sitting and during the night, pain slightly ameliorated by the application of heat.

Kidney-Yang deficiency with Dampness

Dull ache in the leg that is better with rest and worse with overexertion, lower backache, cold and weak knees, a feeling of heaviness of the legs, a feeling of cold, bright-white complexion, tiredness, lassitude, abundant clear urination, urination at night, impotence, decreased libido, Pale and wet tongue with sticky coating, Deep-Weak and slightly Slippery pulse.

Clinical note

- In my experience, in sciatica if the pulse is Rapid and Slippery and the tongue is Red with a sticky yellow coating, it is more difficult to treat.

FEELING OF COLD AND HEAVINESS OF THE LOWER BACK

Kidney-Yang deficiency

A chronic feeling of cold and heaviness of the lower back, a desire to apply warmth to the lower back, worse for exposure to cold and dampness, weak and cold knees, a feeling as if sitting in cold water, cold feet, lower backache, a feeling of cold, bright-white complexion, tiredness, lassitude, abundant clear urination, urination at night, impotence, decreased libido, Pale and wet tongue, Deep-Weak pulse.

Cold-Dampness in the back

A feeling of cold and heaviness of the lower back, a feeling of heaviness in general, chronic backache, cold legs, sticky white tongue coating, Slippery-Slow pulse.

Invasion of Wind-Water

A sudden feeling of cold and heaviness of the lower back, oedema of the ankles, aversion to cold, Floating pulse.

WEAKNESS OF THE LOWER BACK AND KNEES

Kidney-Yang deficiency

Weak back and knees, lower backache, cold knees, better with rest and worse with exercise, a feeling of cold, cold feet, bright-white complexion, tiredness, lassitude, abundant clear urination, urination at night, impotence, decreased libido, Pale and wet tongue, Deep-Weak pulse.

Kidney-Yin deficiency

Weak back and knees, lower backache, a feeling of heat, hot feet in bed at night, dizziness, tinnitus, hardness of hearing, poor memory, night sweating, dry mouth and throat at night, lower backache, constipation, scanty dark urine, tiredness, normal-coloured tongue without coating, Floating-Empty pulse.

Cold-Dampness in the lower back

Weak back and knees, a feeling of heaviness and cold of the lower back, lower backache, swollen feet, worse with exposure to damp and cold and better with application of warmth.

Damp-Heat in the lower back

Weak back and knees, a feeling of heaviness and burning of the lower back, lower backache, swollen and hot feet, worse with exposure to damp and heat and better in dry weather.

STIFFNESS OF THE LOWER BACK

Stagnation of Qi and stasis of Blood

Severe stiffness of the lower back, inability or difficulty in bending forward or turning the waist, backache, stiffness alleviated by moderate exercise and aggravated by inactivity, Wiry pulse.

Cold-Dampness in the lower back

Stiffness of the lower back, a feeling of heaviness of the back, numbness/tingling of the legs, stiffness worse in the morning and better as the day progresses.

Kidney-Yang deficiency

Slight stiffness of the lower back, dull backache, weak and cold knees, lower backache, a feeling of cold, bright-white complexion, tiredness, lassitude, abundant clear urination, urination at night, impotence, decreased libido, Pale and wet tongue, Deep-Weak pulse.

COCCYX PAIN

Traumatic injury

Coccyx pain with history of traumatic injury, difficulty in walking, lying down or turning, pain aggravated by coughing and sneezing.

Kidney deficiency

Dull ache in the coccyx not related to movement numbness, with no history of traumatic injury, lower backache, dizziness, tinnitus, Weak pulse.

Other symptoms and signs depend on whether there is Kidney-Yin or Kidney-Yang deficiency.

Cold-Dampness in the Bladder channel

Coccyx pain, a feeling of heaviness of the legs, numbness/tingling of the legs, pain aggravated by exposure to cold or dampness and ameliorated by the application of heat.

Damp-Heat in the Bladder channel

Severe coccyx pain, a feeling of heaviness of the legs, numbness/tingling of the legs, a feeling of heat in the lower back.

ATROPHY OF THE MUSCLES ALONG THE SPINE

Observation, Chapter 11

Spleen-Qi deficiency

Atrophy of the muscles along the spine, weak muscles, poor appetite, slight abdominal distension after eating, tiredness, lassitude, pale complexion, weakness of the limbs, loose stools, slight depression, tendency to obesity, Pale tongue, Empty pulse.

RIGIDITY OF THE LOWER BACK

Observation, Chapter 11

Retention of Damp-Cold

Rigidity of the lower back, swelling of the muscles of the lower back, backache that is worse with rest and better with moderate activity, a feeling of cold of the back, a feeling of heaviness of the back.

Blood stasis

Rigidity of the lower back, backache that may be worse at night, stabbing pain of the lower back that is worse with rest and better with movement, Wiry pulse.

SKIN SIGNS

Spots on the back

Observation, Chapter 11

Wind-Heat with Toxic Heat

Red papules on the upper back with acute onset, aversion to cold, fever, tongue with red points and thick, sticky yellow coating, Floating-Overflowing-Rapid.

Damp-Heat

Red papules or pustules on the back, lower backache, a feeling of heaviness of the back, sticky yellow tongue coating, Slippery-Rapid pulse.

Other symptoms and signs depend on the organ involved, which may be the Stomach, Spleen or Liver.

Stagnant Liver-Qi turned into Heat

Red papules on the back which may be itchy and painful, hypochondrial or epigastric distension, a slight feeling of oppression of the chest, irritability, premenstrual tension, irregular periods, premenstrual breast distension, a feeling of a lump in the throat, a feeling of heat, red face, thirst, propensity to outbursts of anger, heavy periods, tongue Red on the sides, Wiry and slightly Rapid pulse.

Vesicles on the lower back

Observation, Chapter 11

Retention of Damp-Heat

Vesicles filled with clear fluid on the lower back which look like a string of pearls, backache, a feeling of heaviness of the back, sticky yellow tongue coating, Slippery-Rapid pulse.

Dryness and redness of the skin of the lower back

Observation, Chapter 11

Liver-Fire

Red and dry macular rash on the skin of the lower back that is itchy and hot, headache, red face, dizziness, tinnitus, irritability, propensity to outbursts of anger, thirst, bitter taste, constipation, dark urine, Red tongue with redder sides and dry yellow coating, Wiry-Rapid pulse.

Heart-Fire

Red and dry macular rash on the skin of the lower and upper back that is itchy and hot, dark urine, palpitations, thirst, mouth and tongue ulcers, mental restlessness, a feeling of agitation, insomnia, dream-disturbed sleep, a feeling of heat, red face, bitter taste, Red tongue with redder tip and yellow coating, Overflowing-Rapid pulse.

Yellow colour of the lower back

Observation, Chapter 11

Damp-Heat in the Spleen and Kidneys

Yellow colour of the lower back, small vesicles on the lower back, backache, a feeling of heaviness of the back, turbid urine, sticky yellow tongue coating, Slippery-Rapid pulse.

Skin marks on the lower back

Observation, Chapter 11

Girdle Vessel pathology with Kidney deficiency

A discoloration of the skin of the lower back like long skin marks often distributed like a belt, not itchy, not painful, lower backache, dizziness, tinnitus, a feeling of heaviness of the lower abdomen and back, urinary discomfort, excessive vaginal discomfort, a feeling of bearing down.

Boils on BL-23 Shenshu

Observation, Chapter 11

Phlegm with Kidney deficiency

Boils on BL-23 Shenshu, a feeling of heaviness of the back, swelling of the muscles of the back, lower backache that is alleviated by rest, weak knees, dizziness, tinnitus, a feeling of oppression of the chest, Swollen tongue, Weak pulse.

Ulcers on the buttocks
Toxic Heat

Unilateral ulcers on the buttock, red, swollen and painful in the centre with a red edge around, indistinct

margins, oozing a sticky yellow fluid and festering, thirst, a feeling of heat, Red tongue with red points and a thick, sticky yellow coating, Overflowing-Slippery-Rapid pulse.

External Toxic Heat

Ulcers on the buttocks, red, swollen and painful with sudden onset, Floating-Rapid pulse.

Papules or pustules on the buttocks

Observation, Chapter 11

Damp-Heat in the Bladder

Papules or pustules on buttocks, frequent and urgent urination, burning on urination, difficult urination, dark-yellow/turbid urine, thirst with no desire to drink, hypogastric fullness and pain, a feeling of heat, thick, sticky yellow coating on the tongue root with red spots, Slippery-Rapid pulse.

SPINAL CURVATURE

Scoliosis

Observation, Chapter 11

Kidney-Essence deficiency

Congenital scoliosis, lower backache, weakness of the knees and legs, poor bone development in children, softening of bones in adults, deafness, poor memory, loose teeth, falling hair or premature greying of the hair, weakness of sexual activity, infertility, sterility, dizziness, tinnitus, normal-coloured tongue and Floating-Empty or Leather pulse if Kidney-Essence deficiency occurs against a background of Kidney-Yin deficiency, or Pale tongue and Deep-Weak pulse if against a background of Kidney-Yang deficiency.

Kidney deficiency with Blood stasis

Scoliosis, severe lower backache, stiff back, dizziness, tinnitus.

Other symptoms and signs, including tongue and pulse, depend on whether there is Kidney-Yin or Kidney-Yang deficiency.

Retention of Wind-Dampness in the channels of the back

Scoliosis, backache that is aggravated by damp and cold weather, a feeling of heaviness in the back.

Lordosis

Observation, Chapter 11

Kidney-Essence deficiency

Congenital lordosis, lower backache, weak knees, poor bone development in children, softening of bones in adults, deafness, poor memory, loose teeth, falling hair or premature greying of the hair, weakness of sexual activity, infertility, sterility, dizziness, tinnitus, normal-coloured tongue and Floating-Empty or Leather pulse if Kidney-Essence deficiency occurs against a background of Kidney-Yin deficiency, or Pale tongue and Deep-Weak pulse if against a background of Kidney-Yang deficiency.

Deficiency of Liver- and Kidney-Yin

Lordosis, lower backache, weak knees, dizziness, tinnitus, hardness of hearing, dull occipital or vertical headache, insomnia, numbness/tingling of the limbs, dry eyes, blurred vision, dry throat in the evening, dry hair and skin, brittle nails, night sweating, dry stools, scanty menstruation or amenorrhoea, normal-coloured tongue without coating, Floating-Empty pulse.

Retention of Wind-Dampness in the channels of the back

Lordosis, backache that is aggravated by damp and cold weather, a feeling of heaviness in the back.

Deficiency of the Stomach and Spleen

Lordosis, weak limbs, poor appetite, slight abdominal distension after eating, tiredness, lassitude, pale complexion, weakness of the limbs, loose stools, an uncomfortable feeling in the epigastrium, lack of sense of taste, Pale tongue, Empty pulse.

Spine bent forward

Observation, Chapter 11

Kidney-Essence deficiency with weakness of the Governing Vessel

Spine bent forward, lower backache, weakness of the knees and legs, poor bone development in children, softening of bones in adults, deafness, poor memory, loose teeth, falling hair or premature greying of the hair, weakness of sexual activity, infertility, sterility, dizziness, tinnitus, normal-coloured tongue

and Floating-Empty or Leather pulse if Kidney-Essence deficiency occurs against a background of Kidney-Yin deficiency, or Pale tongue and Deep-Weak pulse if against a background of Kidney-Yang deficiency.

If a person is born with such deformity of the spine, the condition is constitutional and there may not be any other symptoms.

Kyphosis

Observation, Chapter 11

Kidney-Essence deficiency in the elderly

Kyphosis, softening of bones, deafness, weakness of knees and legs, poor memory, loose teeth, falling hair or premature greying of the hair, weakness of sexual activity, lower backache, infertility, sterility, dizziness, tinnitus, normal-coloured tongue and Floating-Empty or Leather pulse if Kidney-Essence deficiency occurs against a background of Kidney-Yin deficiency, or Pale tongue and Deep-Weak pulse if against a background of Kidney-Yang deficiency.

Liver- and Kidney-Yin deficiency

Kyphosis, lower backache, dizziness, tinnitus, weak knees, hardness of hearing, dull occipital or vertical headache, insomnia, numbness/tingling of the limbs, dry eyes, blurred vision, dry throat in the evening, dry hair and skin, brittle nails, night sweating, dry stools, scanty menstruation or amenorrhoea, normal-coloured tongue without coating, Floating-Empty pulse.

Deficiency of the Governing Vessel

Kyphosis, lower backache, dizziness, tinnitus, poor memory, weak sexual function.

Other symptoms and signs depend on whether there is a Kidney-Yin or Kidney-Yang deficiency.

Kidney-Essence deficiency in children

Congenital kyphosis, poor bone development, weakness of knees and legs, poor memory, loose teeth, lower backache, dizziness, tinnitus, normal-coloured tongue and Floating-Empty or Leather pulse if Kidney-Essence deficiency occurs against a background of Kidney-Yin deficiency, or Pale tongue and

Deep-Weak pulse if against a background of Kidney-Yang deficiency.

Flattening of lumbar spine

Observation, Chapter 11

Qi stagnation

Flattening of the lumbar spine, stiffness of the spinal muscles, backache that improves with gentle exercise, hypochondrial or epigastric distension, irritability, moodiness, a feeling of a lump in the throat, pre-menstrual tension, Wiry pulse.

Blood stasis

Flattening of the lumbar spine, stiffness of the spinal muscles, rigidity of the back, backache that improves with gentle exercise and is worse at night, Purple tongue, Wiry pulse.

Cold

Flattening of lumbar spine, backache that improves with the application of heat and is aggravated by exposure to cold and dampness, a feeling of cold, cold back and knees, Pale tongue, Tight-Slow pulse.

List of spine

Observation, Chapter 11

Qi stagnation

List of spine, stiffness of the spinal muscles, backache that improves with gentle exercise, hypochondrial or epigastric distension, irritability, moodiness, a feeling of a lump in the throat, premenstrual tension, Wiry pulse.

Blood stasis

List of spine, stiffness of the spinal muscles, rigidity of the back, backache that improves with gentle exercise and is worse at night, Purple tongue, Wiry pulse.

Cold

List of spine, backache that improves with the application of heat and is aggravated by exposure to cold and dampness, a feeling of cold, cold back and knees, Pale tongue, Tight-Slow pulse.

Chapter **68**

BODY

Chapter contents

BODY ACHES *709*

PAIN IN THE JOINTS *710*

LOSS OF FEELING *710*
  Paralysis *710*
  Hemiplegia *711*
  Numbness/tingling *712*
  Numbness of half the body *712*

ITCHING *713*

OEDEMA *713*

WEIGHT CHANGE *713*
  Obesity *713*
  Loss of weight *714*

JAUNDICE *714*

TWITCHING OF MUSCLES *714*

OPISTHOTONOS *715*

BODY ACHES

Interrogation, Chapter 37

Body aches include aches in the muscles or joints, or both.

Wind

Ache in the joints, aversion to cold, fever, occipital headache, Floating pulse.

This is a pain that occurs in acute invasions of Wind.

Dampness

Ache in the muscles and joints, a feeling of heaviness, headache with a feeling as if the head were wrapped in cotton wool, sticky tongue coating, Soggy or Slippery pulse.

This is probably the most common type of joint and muscle ache, and can be either acute of chronic. It is seen in Fixed Painful Obstruction Syndrome and in postviral fatigue syndrome.

Qi stagnation

Ache in the joints (especially of the upper part of the body) which is better with exercise, a feeling of distension of the limbs, Wiry pulse.

Blood stasis

Severe stabbing pain in the joints which is better with exercise, Purple tongue, Wiry pulse.

This pattern is more likely to occur in the elderly but it is also relatively frequent in women suffering from Blood stasis. For example, it may occur after childbirth if there is stasis of Blood.

Blood deficiency

Dull ache in all the muscles which is worse after exercise, frequently after childbirth, tingling of the limbs, Pale tongue, Choppy or Fine pulse.

Stomach-Heat

Pain in all the muscles, skin hot to the touch, Red tongue with a yellow coating, Overflowing-Rapid pulse.

PAIN IN THE JOINTS

Interrogation, Chapter 37

Invasion of Wind in the joints

Pain moving from joint to joint, in acute cases a Floating pulse.

Invasion of Dampness in the joints

Fixed pain, swelling of the joints, a feeling of heaviness and tingling of the joints.

Invasion of Cold in the joints

Fixed, severe pain, usually in one joint, aggravated by exposure to cold and alleviated by application of heat.

Damp-Heat in the joints

Fixed pain, swollen, hot and red joints.

Stagnation of Qi and stasis of Blood

Pain and rigidity of the joints, stiff limbs, pain ameliorated by moderate exercise and aggravated by inactivity, Wiry pulse.

Liver-Blood deficiency

Dull joint ache, worse with exercise or after the period, Pale tongue, Choppy or Fine pulse.

Kidney deficiency

Dull joint ache especially of the lower limbs that is worse with exercise, lower backache, weak knees, weak legs.

LOSS OF FEELING

Paralysis

Observation, Chapter 4

This refers to bilateral paralysis of the arms/legs and of the body itself.

Stomach- and Spleen-Qi deficiency

Paralysis, poor appetite, slight abdominal distension after eating, tiredness, lassitude, pale complexion, weakness of the limbs, loose stools, an uncomfortable feeling in the epigastrium, lack of sense of taste, Pale tongue, Empty pulse.

In neurological problems such as multiple sclerosis, this pattern corresponds to the middle stage.

Liver- and Kidney-Yin deficiency

Long-term paralysis of slow onset, weak limbs, weak knees, dizziness, tinnitus, hardness of hearing, lower backache, dull occipital or vertical headache, insomnia, numbness/tingling of the limbs, dry eyes, blurred vision, dry throat in the evening, dry hair and skin, brittle nails, night sweating, dry stools, scanty menstruation or amenorrhoea, normal-coloured tongue without coating, Floating-Empty pulse.

In neurological problems such as multiple sclerosis, this pattern corresponds to the late stage.

Liver- and Kidney-Yin deficiency with internal Wind

Long-term paralysis of slow onset, tremor/spasms of limbs, weak limbs, weak knees, numbness/tingling of the limbs, lower backache, dizziness, tinnitus, hardness of hearing, dull occipital or vertical headache, insomnia, dry eyes, blurred vision, dry throat in the evening, dry hair and skin, brittle nails, night sweating, dry stools, scanty menstruation or amenorrhoea, normal-coloured Deviated or Moving tongue without coating, Floating-Empty and slightly Wiry pulse.

In neurological problems such as multiple sclerosis, this pattern corresponds to the final stage.

Kidney-Yang deficiency

Paralysis, lower backache, cold and weak knees, a feeling of cold, bright-white complexion, tiredness, lassitude, abundant clear urination, urination at night, impotence, decreased libido, Pale and wet tongue, Deep-Weak pulse.

Qi and Blood deficiency

Paralysis of the four limbs and body, weak limbs, poor appetite, loose stools, weak voice, tiredness, blurred vision, dizziness, numbness/tingling of limbs, palpitations, dull-pale complexion, Pale tongue, Weak or Choppy pulse.

Liver-Blood stasis

Paralysis, stabbing pain in the joints, hypochondrial or abdominal pain, painful periods, dark and clotted menstrual blood, masses in the abdomen, purple nails and

lips, purple or dark complexion, Purple tongue, Wiry or Firm pulse.

Cold-Dampness

Paralysis, a feeling of heaviness of the limbs, numbness, oedema of the limbs, epigastric fullness, a feeling of heaviness of the head and body, a feeling of cold, cold limbs, sticky white tongue coating, Slippery-Slow pulse.

In neurological problems such as multiple sclerosis, this corresponds to the initial stage.

Damp-Heat

Paralysis of the lower limbs, hot limbs, a feeling of heaviness of the limbs, numbness of the limbs, epigastric fullness, a sticky taste, thirst with no desire to drink, a feeling of heaviness of the head and body, a feeling of heat, sticky yellow tongue coating, Slippery-Rapid pulse.

Liver-Qi stagnation and Liver-Blood deficiency

Paralysis, numbness/tingling of limbs, hypochondrial or epigastric distension, irritability, moodiness, a feeling of a lump in the throat, premenstrual tension, dizziness, blurred vision, floaters, scanty menstruation, dull-pale complexion, Pale tongue, Choppy or Fine and slightly Wiry pulse.

Stomach and Spleen Fluids injured

Paralysis with sudden onset after a febrile disease, weak limbs, inability to grasp with hands, dry skin and mouth.

This pattern corresponds to the aftermath of a febrile disease such as polio.

Hemiplegia

Observation, Chapter 4

This refers to unilateral paralysis of the arm/leg. The first six patterns correspond to different types of Wind-stroke.

Wind in the channels

Hemiplegia, deviation of eye and mouth, aphasia.

Liver-Wind

Hemiplegia, tremors, numbness of limbs, severe dizziness, tinnitus, headache, Stiff, Deviated or Moving tongue, Wiry pulse.

Wind-Phlegm

Hemiplegia, numbness or tingling of the limbs, severe dizziness, blurred vision, tinnitus, nausea, sputum in the throat, a feeling of oppression of the chest, Stiff or Deviated and Swollen tongue, Wiry-Slippery pulse.

Phlegm-Fire

Hemiplegia, numbness of the limbs, sudden unconsciousness, mental confusion, deviation of eye and mouth, contraction of the hands, clenched teeth, red eyes and face, rattling sound in the throat, a feeling of oppression of the chest, expectoration of sticky yellow sputum, Red and Swollen tongue with a sticky yellow coating, Slippery-Rapid pulse.

Damp-Phlegm

Hemiplegia, numbness of the limbs, sudden unconsciousness, mental confusion, phlegm in the throat, clenched teeth, a feeling of oppression of the chest, expectoration of profuse, sticky sputum, pasty-white complexion, cold limbs, Swollen tongue with a sticky white coating, Slippery pulse.

Qi deficiency and Blood stasis

Hemiplegia, dull skin colour, oedema, rigidity of the tendons, contraction of the upper limbs, lower limbs relaxed and stretched, stretching of the upper limbs or bending of the lower limbs causes pain, tiredness, poor appetite, loose stools, weak voice, slight shortness of breath, pale complexion, Bluish-Purple tongue, Weak or Choppy pulse.

This corresponds to the sequelae stage of Wind-stroke.

Liver and Kidney deficiency

Hemiplegia, lower backache, soft limbs, dizziness, tinnitus, poor memory, blurred vision, mental confusion.

This pattern may be associated with a Yin and or Yang deficiency and the tongue may be Red or Pale respectively. This pattern also corresponds to the sequelae stage of Wind-stroke.

Collapse of Yang

Hemiplegia, sudden unconsciousness, mental confusion, eyes shut, mouth and hands open, urinary incontinence, weak breathing, cold limbs, bright-white complexion, sweating on the forehead, Pale and Short tongue, Hidden or Scattered pulse.

This corresponds to an acute stage of Wind-stroke.

Collapse of Yin

Hemiplegia, sudden unconsciousness, deviation of eye and mouth, eyes shut, mouth and hands open, cold limbs but red face, weak breathing, Red tongue without coating, Minute pulse.

This corresponds to an acute stage of Wind-stroke.

Numbness/tingling

Interrogation, Chapter 37

'Numbness' includes numbness itself or a tingling sensation, or both together. Numbness is more common in Phlegm and Wind, whereas tingling is more common in deficiency patterns such as Liver-Blood deficiency. However, this is only a broad rule.

Liver-Blood deficiency

Tingling of limbs, dizziness, blurred vision, floaters, scanty menstruation, dull-pale complexion, Pale tongue, Choppy or Fine pulse.

This is a very common cause of numbness/tingling and it occurs more frequently in women.

Phlegm in the channels

Numbness, a feeling of heaviness, a feeling of oppression of the chest, phlegm in the throat, Swollen tongue with a sticky coating, Slippery pulse.

Dampness in the channels

Numbness/tingling, swollen joints, a feeling of heaviness of the body and limbs, sticky tongue coating, Slippery pulse.

Other symptoms and signs depend on whether the Dampness is associated with Cold or Heat.

Internal Wind

Unilateral numbness of a limb, tremors, severe dizziness, tinnitus, headache, numbness of the limbs, tics, Stiff, Deviated or Moving tongue, Wiry pulse.

Wind-Phlegm

Unilateral numbness of a limb, tingling, tremors, severe dizziness, blurred vision, tinnitus, nausea, sputum in the throat, a feeling of oppression of the chest, Stiff or Deviated and Swollen tongue, Wiry-Slippery pulse.

Stagnation of Qi and stasis of Blood

Numbness/tingling of limbs, joint pain that is ameliorated by moderate exercise and aggravated by inactiv-ity, tiredness, poor appetite, loose stools, weak voice, slight shortness of breath, pale complexion, Bluish-Purple tongue, Weak or Choppy pulse.

Numbness of half the body

Numbness of half the body usually occurs in the limbs.

Liver-Blood deficiency

Numbness of half the body, numbness/tingling of the limbs, dizziness, blurred vision, floaters, scanty menstruation, dull-pale complexion, Pale tongue, Choppy or Fine pulse.

This numbness often occurs on the left side and more frequently in women.

Damp-Phlegm

Numbness of half the body, chronic cough with expectoration of profuse, sticky white sputum which is easy to expectorate, a feeling of oppression of the chest, dizziness, blurred vision, somnolence, nausea, sputum in the throat, muzziness of the head, Swollen tongue with sticky coating, Slippery pulse.

Liver-Wind

Numbness of half the body and a hand, tremors, severe dizziness, tinnitus, headache, tics, Stiff, Deviated or Moving tongue, Wiry pulse.

This pattern is more likely to occur in old people. In the elderly, numbness of half the body may herald Wind-stroke.

Deficiency of Central Qi

Numbness of half the body, soft and weak limbs, Poor appetite, slight abdominal distension after eating, tiredness, lassitude, pale complexion, weakness of the limbs, loose stools, an uncomfortable feeling in the epigastrium, lack of sense of taste, Pale tongue, Empty pulse.

This pattern is due to a deficiency of Stomach and Spleen and the numbness often occurs on the right side.

Dampness

Numbness of half the body, a feeling of heaviness of the limbs, swelling of the limbs/joints, muscle ache, sticky tongue coating, Slippery pulse.

Other symptoms and signs depend on whether the Dampness is associated with Cold or Heat.

ITCHING

Interrogation, Chapter 37

Wind in the skin

Intense itching in the whole body or moving from place to place, more in the upper body, an unbearable desire to scratch, dry skin.

Dampness in the skin

Localized itching often in the lower part of the body, vesicles on the skin, oozing a fluid.

Damp-Heat in the skin

Localized itching, yellow vesicles oozing a yellow fluid, red papules or pustules, oozing blood on scratching, more in the lower part of the body.

Blood-Heat

Generalized itching, red rash, red papules, feeling of agitation, thirst.

Blood deficiency

Mild generalized itching, dry skin, scaly skin (with white scales), dry hair, possibly pale wheals.

Toxic Heat

Localized or generalized intense itching, pustules oozing pus and blood, festering skin, fever.

This kind of itching is seen in chronic eczema when the skin becomes infected.

Clinical note

- To treat itching with acupuncture, apart from using points that expel Wind (TB-6 Zhigou and GB-31 Fengshi), I use points on the Heart channel.

OEDEMA

Spleen-Yang deficiency

Chronic pitting oedema of the abdomen or limbs, slow onset, poor appetite, slight abdominal distension after eating, tiredness, lassitude, pale complexion, weakness of the limbs, loose stools, a feeling of cold, cold limbs, oedema, Pale and wet tongue, Deep-Weak pulse.

Kidney-Yang deficiency

Pitting oedema of the whole body starting from the legs, worse on the ankles, lower backache, cold knees, a feeling of cold, bright-white complexion, weak knees, tiredness, lassitude, abundant clear urination, urination at night, impotence, decreased libido, Pale and wet tongue, Deep-Weak pulse.

This is probably the most common cause of chronic oedema and it is nearly always associated with Spleen-Yang deficiency.

Deficiency of Qi and Blood

Oedema starting on the face and limbs, poor appetite, loose stools, weak voice, tiredness, blurred vision, dizziness, numbness/tingling of limbs, palpitations, dull-pale complexion, Pale tongue, Weak or Choppy pulse.

Dampness

Oedema of the limbs and abdomen, slow onset, tiredness, a feeling of heaviness of the body and limbs, a feeling of fullness of the epigastrium, ache in the muscles, sticky tongue coating, Slippery pulse.

Wind-Water invading the Lungs

Sudden swelling of eyes, face and hands gradually spreading to the whole body, bright-shiny complexion, scanty and pale urination, aversion to wind, fever, cough, slight breathlessness, sticky white tongue coating, Floating-Slippery pulse.

This is an acute type of oedema and this pattern is a type of external Wind-Cold.

Qi stagnation

Non-pitting oedema of the body or limbs, irritability, a feeling of distension especially of the limbs, Wiry pulse.

Qi deficiency and Blood stasis

Oedema of the body or limbs, cold hands and feet, numbness of the limbs, muscular weakness, purple colour of hands/feet, tiredness, poor appetite, loose stools, weak voice, Bluish-Purple tongue, Choppy pulse.

WEIGHT CHANGE

Obesity

Observation, Chapter 1; Interrogation, Chapter 37

Obesity in Chinese medicine is always due to Dampness or Phlegm (deriving from Qi or Yang deficiency) retained in the space between the skin and muscles.

Damp-Phlegm with Qi deficiency

Obesity, chronic cough with expectoration of profuse, sticky white sputum which is easy to expectorate, a feeling of oppression of the chest, dizziness, blurred vision, somnolence, nausea, sputum in the throat, muzziness of the head, tiredness, poor appetite, loose stools, weak voice, slight shortness of breath, pale complexion, Pale and Swollen tongue with sticky coating, Soggy pulse.

Loss of weight

Observation, Chapter 1; Interrogation, Chapter 37

Yin deficiency

Loss of weight, night sweating, dry mouth with a desire to drink in small sips, dry throat in the evening, dark-scanty urine, dry stools, normal-coloured tongue without coating, Floating-Empty pulse.

This may be Yin deficiency of various organs such as Lungs, Stomach, Heart, Kidneys, Liver and Spleen.

Liver-Blood deficiency

Loss of weight, dizziness, blurred vision, floaters, numbness/tingling of limbs, scanty menstruation, dull-pale complexion, Pale tongue, Choppy or Fine pulse.

Stomach- and Spleen-Qi deficiency

Loss of weight, poor appetite, slight abdominal distension after eating, tiredness, lassitude, pale complexion, weakness of the limbs, loose stools, an uncomfortable feeling in the epigastrium, lack of sense of taste sensation, Pale tongue, Empty pulse.

Normally Stomach- and Spleen-Qi deficiency leads to obesity but it may also lead to weight loss because the Food Essences are not absorbed by the body.

Liver-Fire

Loss of weight, headache, red face, dizziness, tinnitus, irritability, propensity to outbursts of anger, thirst, bitter taste, constipation, dark urine, Red tongue with redder sides and dry yellow coating, Wiry-Rapid pulse.

Stomach-Heat

Loss of weight, burning epigastric pain, thirst, sour regurgitation, nausea, excessive hunger, foul breath, a feeling of heat, Red tongue with a yellow coating, Overflowing-Rapid pulse.

JAUNDICE

Observation, Chapter 3

Damp-Heat in the Gall-Bladder

Jaundice, yellow eyes, bright-yellow complexion, hypochondrial pain, fullness and distension, nausea, vomiting, inability to digest fats, yellow sclera, scanty dark-yellow urine, thirst without a desire to drink, bitter taste, irritability, headache, a feeling of heaviness of the body, a feeling of heat, thick, sticky yellow tongue coating, either bilateral in two strips or unilateral, Slippery-Wiry-Rapid pulse.

Cold-Dampness in the Gall-Bladder

Jaundice, dull-yellow eyes and skin, hypochondrial pain, fullness and distension, nausea, vomiting, an inability to digest fats, dull-yellow sclera, turbid urine, no thirst, sticky taste, dull headache, a feeling of heaviness of the body, a feeling of cold, thick, sticky white tongue coating, either bilateral in two strips or unilateral, Slippery-Wiry-Slow pulse.

Blood stasis

Jaundice, dull-yellow skin, dark complexion, a feeling of mass in the hypochondrium, hypochondrial or abdominal pain, lines on the skin like a spider's web, dark stools, Purple tongue, Wiry pulse.

Spleen-Qi deficiency and Blood deficiency

Jaundice, dull-yellow skin, poor appetite, slight abdominal distension after eating, tiredness, lassitude, pale complexion, weakness of the limbs, loose stools, dizziness, blurred vision, floaters, numbness/tingling of limbs, scanty menstruation, dull-pale complexion, Pale tongue, Choppy or Fine pulse.

This pattern is due Liver-Blood deficiency which leads to Liver-Qi stagnation and bile not flowing; this is a deficient type of jaundice.

TWITCHING OF MUSCLES

Observation, Chapter 4

Spleen- and Kidney-Yang deficiency

Twitching of muscles, lower backache, cold and weak knees, a feeling of cold, bright-white complexion, impotence, decreased libido, tiredness, lassitude, abun-

dant clear urination, urination at night, loose stools, poor appetite, slight abdominal distension, a desire to lie down, early-morning diarrhoea, Pale and wet tongue, Deep-Weak pulse.

Heart- or Lung-Yang deficiency with Water overflowing

Twitching of muscles, palpitations, dizziness, nausea, vomiting of watery, frothy white fluid, a feeling of cold, cold limbs, severe shortness of breath, a feeling of fullness and stuffiness of the chest and epigastrium, thirst with no desire to drink, urinary retention, Pale, Swollen and wet tongue, Deep-Wiry or Deep-Fine-Slippery pulse.

Deficiency of Qi and Blood

Twitching of muscles, poor appetite, loose stools, weak voice, tiredness, blurred vision, dizziness, numbness/tingling of limbs, palpitations, dull-pale complexion, Pale tongue, Weak or Choppy pulse.

OPISTHOTONOS

Observation, Chapter 4

Liver-Wind

Opisthotonos, tremors, severe dizziness, tinnitus, headache, numbness of limbs, tics, Stiff, Deviated or Moving tongue, Wiry pulse.

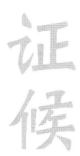
Chapter **69**

DIGESTIVE SYSTEM AND TASTE

Chapter contents

BELCHING 717

REGURGITATION 718
Sour regurgitation 718
Regurgitation of food 718

HICCUP 719

HUNGER AND EATING 719
Poor appetite 719
Excessive hunger 720
Aversion to food 721
Hunger with no desire to eat 721
Gnawing hunger 721
Craving for sweets/constant picking 722

SLEEPINESS AFTER EATING 722

NAUSEA, RETCHING AND VOMITING 723
Nausea 723
Vomiting 724
Retching 725
Vomiting of blood 725

DIFFICULTY IN SWALLOWING (DIAPHRAGM CHOKING) 726

TASTE 726
Bitter taste 726
Sweet taste 727
Salty taste 727
Sour taste 727
Sticky taste 728
Loss of taste 728
Foul breath 729

The symptoms of epigastric and abdominal pain are discussed in Chapter 71 (Abdomen).

BELCHING

Interrogation, Chapter 30; Hearing, Chapter 53

Liver-Qi invading the Stomach

Belching with loud sound, irritability, epigastric and hypochondrial distension and pain, a feeling of oppression of the epigastrium, sour regurgitation, hiccup, belching, nausea, vomiting, sighing, weak limbs, normal-coloured tongue (or slightly Red on the sides in severe cases of Liver-Qi stagnation), Pulse Wiry on the left and Weak on the right.

Stomach-Heat

Belching with loud sound, sour regurgitation, burning epigastric pain, thirst, nausea, excessive hunger, foul breath, a feeling of heat, Red tongue with a yellow coating, Overflowing-Rapid pulse.

Retention of food

Belching with loud sound, sour regurgitation, foul breath, nausea, fullness, pain and distension of the epigastrium which are relieved by vomiting, vomiting of sour fluids, insomnia, loose stools or constipation, poor appetite, thick tongue coating, Full-Slippery pulse.

Stomach- and Spleen-Qi deficiency

Belching with weak sound, slight nausea, vomiting of thin watery fluids, poor appetite, slight abdominal distension after eating, tiredness, lassitude, pale complexion, weakness of the limbs, loose stools, an uncomfortable feeling in the epigastrium, lack of sense of taste, Pale tongue, Empty pulse.

Stomach deficient and cold

Belching with weak sound, vomiting of clear fluid, discomfort or dull pain in the epigastrium, better after eating and with pressure or massage, lack of appetite, preference for warm drinks and foods, absence of thirst, cold and weak limbs, tiredness, pale complexion, Pale and wet tongue, Deep-Weak-Slow pulse.

Stomach-Yin deficiency

Belching with weak sound, no appetite or slight hunger but no desire to eat, constipation (dry stools), dull or slightly burning epigastric pain, dry mouth and throat especially in the afternoon, thirst but no desire to drink, or a desire to drink in small sips, slight feeling of fullness after eating, normal-coloured tongue without coating or without coating in the centre, Floating-Empty pulse.

REGURGITATION

Sour regurgitation

Interrogation, Chapter 30; Hearing, Chapter 53

Liver-Qi invading the Stomach

Sour regurgitation, a feeling of burning in the stomach coming in bouts, belching, irritability, epigastric/hypochondrial distension and pain, a feeling of oppression of the epigastrium, sour regurgitation, hiccup, belching, nausea, vomiting, sighing, weak limbs, normal-coloured tongue (or slightly red on the sides in severe cases of Liver-Qi stagnation), pulse Wiry on the left and Weak on the right.

Retention of food

Sour regurgitation, vomiting of sour fluids, belching, fullness, pain and distension of the epigastrium which are relieved by vomiting, nausea, foul breath, insomnia, loose stools or constipation, poor appetite, thick tongue coating, Full-Slippery pulse.

Damp-Heat in the Stomach

Sour regurgitation, nausea, a feeling of fullness and pain of the epigastrium, a feeling of heaviness, facial pain, stuffed nose or thick sticky nasal discharge, thirst without a desire to drink, a feeling of heat, dull-yellow complexion, a sticky taste, Red tongue with sticky yellow coating, Slippery-Rapid pulse.

Cold-Dampness in the Stomach

Sour regurgitation, epigastric fullness, a feeling of heaviness of the head and body, feeling cold, cold limbs, sticky white tongue coating, Slippery-Slow pulse.

Regurgitation of food

'Regurgitation of food', called *fan wei* in Chinese (meaning 'stomach reflux'), is characterized by food entering the stomach, not being digested and being regurgitated; this is different to vomiting. Regurgitation of food can take different forms: sometimes the food eaten in the morning may be regurgitated; sometimes the food eaten the previous evening may be regurgitated in the morning; sometimes the food may be regurgitated 1 or 2 hours after eating; sometimes there may be regurgitation only at night.

Cold in the Stomach

Regurgitation of thin watery fluids, nausea, hiccup, epigastric pain aggravated by cold liquids and alleviated by warm liquids, dribbling from the mouth, feeling worse after swallowing cold fluids (which are quickly vomited), severe pain in the epigastrium, a feeling of cold, cold limbs, preference for warmth and for warm liquids, thick white tongue coating, Deep-Tight-Slow pulse.

Stagnation of Qi and Phlegm in the Stomach

Regurgitation of food and phlegm, belching, nausea, vomiting, hiccup, epigastric pain and distension, a feeling of oppression of the chest, irritability, Swollen tongue, Slippery pulse.

Damp-Heat in the Stomach

Regurgitation of food, a feeling of fullness and pain of the epigastrium, a feeling of heaviness, thirst without desire to drink, nausea, a feeling of heat, dull-yellow complexion, sticky taste, Red tongue with sticky yellow coating, Slippery-Rapid pulse.

Stasis of Blood in the Stomach

Regurgitation of food and occasionally blood, nausea, vomiting, possibly vomiting of blood, vomiting of food looking like coffee grounds, severe, stabbing epigastric pain that may be worse at night, dislike of pressure, Purple tongue, Wiry pulse.

Retention of food

Regurgitation of food, sour regurgitation, sticky taste, nausea, fullness and pain of the epigastrium, restless sleep, thick sticky tongue coating, Slippery pulse.

Stomach-Yin deficiency with Blood dryness

Sour regurgitation, no appetite or slight hunger but no desire to eat, constipation (dry stools), dull or slightly burning epigastric pain, dry mouth and throat especially in the afternoon, thirst but no desire to drink, or a desire to drink in small sips, a slight feeling of fullness after eating, insomnia, dry skin, dull complexion, normal-coloured tongue without coating or without coating in the centre, Floating-Empty pulse.

Deficiency of Qi and Yin of the Stomach

Slight regurgitation of food, no appetite or slight hunger but no desire to eat, constipation (dry stools), dull or slightly burning epigastric pain, dry mouth and throat especially in the afternoon, thirst but no desire to drink, or a desire to drink in small sips, slight feeling of fullness after eating, loose stools, tiredness especially in the morning, weak limbs, Pale tongue without coating in the centre, Empty pulse or Floating-Empty pulse.

Deficiency of Minister Fire

Regurgitation of thin watery fluids, lower backache, cold knees, a feeling of cold, bright-white complexion, weak knees, tiredness, lassitude, abundant clear urination, urination at night, impotence, lack of libido, infertility, sterility, Pale and wet tongue, Deep-Weak pulse.

HICCUP

Hearing, Chapter 53

Cold in the Stomach

Forceful hiccup, nausea, feeling worse after swallowing cold fluids (which are quickly vomited), severe pain in the epigastrium, a feeling of cold, cold limbs, preference for warmth, vomiting of clear fluids (which may alleviate the pain), preference for warm liquids, thick white tongue coating, Deep-Tight-Slow pulse.

Stomach-Heat

Forceful hiccup, sour regurgitation, burning epigastric pain, thirst, nausea, excessive hunger, foul breath, a feeling of heat, Red tongue with a yellow coating, Overflowing-Rapid pulse.

Stomach-Qi deficiency

Weak, infrequent hiccup with low sound, an uncomfortable feeling in the epigastrium, no appetite, lack of sense of taste, loose stools, tiredness especially in the morning, weak limbs, Pale tongue, Empty pulse.

Stomach-Yin deficiency

Weak hiccup, no appetite or slight hunger but no desire to eat, constipation (dry stools), dull or slightly burning epigastric pain, dry mouth and throat especially in the afternoon, thirst but no desire to drink, or a desire to drink in small sips, slight feeling of fullness after eating, normal-coloured tongue without coating or without coating in the centre, Floating-Empty pulse.

Liver-Qi invading the Stomach

Pronounced hiccup, sour regurgitation, a feeling of burning in the stomach coming in bouts, belching, irritability, epigastric/hypochondrial distension and pain, a feeling of oppression of the epigastrium, sour regurgitation, hiccup, belching, nausea, vomiting, sighing, weak limbs, normal-coloured tongue (or slightly red on the sides in severe cases of Liver-Qi stagnation), Pulse Wiry on the left and Weak on the right.

Spleen- and Kidney-Yang deficiency

Incessant hiccup, lower backache, cold and weak knees, feeling cold, bright-white complexion, impotence, decreased libido, tiredness, lassitude, abundant clear urination, urination at night, loose stools, poor appetite, slight abdominal distension, a desire to lie down, early-morning diarrhoea, Pale and wet tongue, Deep-Weak pulse.

HUNGER AND EATING

Poor appetite

Interrogation, Chapter 30

Poor appetite is an important symptom in Chinese medicine frequently reported by Chinese patients; this is partially a culturally determined symptom given the history of frequent famines in China. Western patients seldom report this symptom spontaneously and we must therefore remember to ask always about appetite. In China, poor appetite is often a symptom of sadness and unhappiness; in contrast, Westerners tend to eat

more when they are unhappy or depressed.

Stomach- and Spleen-Qi deficiency

Poor appetite, slight abdominal distension after eating, tiredness, lassitude, pale complexion, weakness of the limbs, loose stools, an uncomfortable feeling in the epigastrium, lack of sense of taste, Pale tongue, Empty pulse.

Stomach and Spleen deficient and cold

Poor appetite, dull epigastric pain that is alleviated by warm liquids and aggravated by cold liquids, vomiting of thin watery fluids, slight abdominal distension after eating, tiredness, lassitude, pale complexion, weakness of the limbs, loose stools, an uncomfortable feeling in the epigastrium, lack of sense of taste, cold limbs, a feeling of cold, Pale and wet tongue, Deep-Weak pulse.

Spleen- and Kidney-Yang deficiency

Poor appetite, lower backache, cold and weak knees, a feeling of cold, bright-white complexion, impotence, decreased libido, tiredness, lassitude, abundant clear urination, urination at night, loose stools, slight abdominal distension, a desire to lie down, early-morning diarrhoea, Pale and wet tongue, Deep-Weak pulse.

Stomach-Yin deficiency

Poor appetite or slight hunger but no desire to eat, constipation (dry stools), dull or slightly burning epigastric pain, dry mouth and throat especially in the afternoon, thirst but no desire to drink, or a desire to drink in small sips, slight feeling of fullness after eating, normal-coloured tongue without coating or without coating in the centre, Floating-Empty pulse.

Cold-Dampness in the Stomach and Spleen

Poor appetite, epigastric fullness, a feeling of heaviness of the head and body, a feeling of cold, cold limbs, sticky-white tongue coating, Slippery-Slow pulse.

Damp-Heat in the Stomach and Spleen

Poor appetite, a feeling of fullness and pain of the epigastrium and lower abdomen, a feeling of heaviness, thirst without a desire to drink, nausea, loose stools with offensive odour, a feeling of heat, dull-yellow complexion, sticky taste, Red tongue with sticky yellow coating, Slippery-Rapid pulse.

Liver-Qi invading the Stomach

Poor appetite, irritability, epigastric/hypochondrial distension and pain, a feeling of oppression of the epigastrium, sour regurgitation, hiccup, belching, nausea, vomiting, sighing, weak limbs, normal-coloured tongue (or slightly Red on the sides in severe cases of Liver-Qi stagnation), Pulse Wiry on the left and Weak on the right.

Phlegm obstructing the Stomach

Poor appetite, nausea, vomiting, a feeling of oppression of the epigastrium, sputum in the throat, sticky taste, Swollen tongue with sticky coating, Slippery pulse.

Food poisoning

Poor appetite, vomiting, sour regurgitation, epigastric fullness and pain, thick tongue coating, Slippery pulse.

Excessive hunger

Interrogation, Chapter 30

Stomach-Heat

Excessive hunger, burning epigastric pain, thirst, sour regurgitation, nausea, foul breath, a feeling of heat, Red tongue with a yellow coating, Overflowing-Rapid pulse.

Stomach-Fire

Excessive hunger, bleeding gums, nausea, vomiting soon after eating, foul breath, intense thirst with a desire to drink cold liquids, burning epigastric pain, mental restlessness, mouth ulcers, dry stools, sour regurgitation, a feeling of heat, Red tongue with a thick, dry dark-yellow coating, Deep-Full-Rapid pulse.

Stomach-Yin deficiency with Empty-Heat

Excessive hunger but no desire to eat, dull or burning epigastric pain, a feeling of heat in the afternoon, constipation (dry stools), dry mouth and throat especially in the afternoon, thirst with a desire to drink in small sips, a slight feeling of fullness after eating, night sweating, five-palm heat, bleeding gums, Red tongue (or Red in centre only) without coating in the centre, Floating-Empty and Rapid pulse.

Aversion to food

Interrogation, Chapter 30

'Aversion to food' is different from 'poor appetite' as it implies not only no desire to eat, but also being disgusted at the sight and smell of food.

Food poisoning

Strong, acute aversion to food, nausea, especially at the smell of food, vomiting, diarrhoea with foul smell, sticky taste, epigastric pain, thick, sticky yellow tongue coating, Slippery pulse.

Retention of food

Chronic aversion to food, nausea, especially at the smell of food, sour regurgitation, sticky taste, fullness and pain of the epigastrium, restless sleep, thick sticky tongue coating, Slippery pulse.

Damp-Heat in the Liver, Gall-Bladder, Stomach and Spleen

Chronic aversion to food, nausea, especially at the smell of food, sticky taste, thirst, hypochondrial and epigastric fullness, irritability, a feeling of heaviness, sticky yellow tongue coating, Slippery-Wiry pulse.

Rebellious Qi in the Penetrating Vessel in pregnancy

Aversion to food during pregnancy, nausea, especially at the smell of food, a feeling of energy rising to the chest, restlessness, anxiety, a feeling of tightness of the chest, Firm pulse.

Hunger with no desire to eat

Interrogation, Chapter 30

Damp-Heat in the Stomach

Hunger with no desire to eat, a feeling of fullness of the epigastrium/abdomen, epigastric/abdominal pain, sticky taste, a feeling of heaviness of the body, thirst without a desire to drink, nausea, vomiting, loose stools with offensive odour, a feeling of heat, headache with a feeling of heaviness of the head, bitter taste, Red tongue with sticky yellow coating, Slippery-Rapid pulse.

'Stomach strong – Spleen weak'

Hunger with no desire to eat, thirst, burning epigastric pain, loose stools, tiredness.

This condition is characterized by the Full Stomach pattern (usually Heat), which causes the hunger, and an Empty Spleen pattern, which removes the desire to eat.

Gnawing hunger

'Gnawing hunger' is a translation of the Chinese term *cao za*, which literally means 'noisy', but the symptoms of this condition do not actually involve a gurgling noise. Chinese books usually explain that this condition is characterized by an uncomfortable sensation of the epigastrium that mimics pain but is not actually pain and mimics hunger but is not actually hunger; it also includes a vexed sensation felt in the epigastrium and a feeling of stuffiness of the epigastrium. This condition may also be accompanied by belching and sour regurgitation.

Liver-Qi invading the Stomach

Gnawing hunger, sour regurgitation, hiccup, belching, nausea, vomiting, irritability, epigastric and hypochondrial distension and pain, a feeling of oppression of the epigastrium, sighing, weak limbs, normal-coloured tongue (or slightly Red on the sides in severe cases of Liver-Qi stagnation), Pulse Wiry on the left and Weak on the right.

Stomach-Heat

Gnawing hunger, sour regurgitation, nausea, foul breath, burning epigastric pain, thirst, a feeling of heat, Red tongue with a yellow coating, Overflowing-Rapid pulse.

Cold in the Stomach

Gnawing hunger, nausea, vomiting of thin watery fluids, hiccup, epigastric pain aggravated cold liquids and alleviated by warm liquids, dribbling from the mouth, feeling worse after swallowing cold fluids (which are quickly vomited), severe pain in the epigastrium, a feeling of cold, cold limbs, preference for warmth and for warm liquids, thick white tongue coating, Deep-Tight-Slow pulse.

Food poisoning

Gnawing hunger, belching, nausea, vomiting, epigastric pain and fullness that is relieved by vomiting, thick tongue coating, Slippery pulse.

Case history 69.1

A 50-year-old woman complained of a 'bad' taste in her mouth (this was the first symptom she reported), a feeling of nausea, having either a poor appetite or being always hungry, and a feeling of fullness of the epigastrium for the past 20 years. When questioned further, she said 'I feel sick when I eat but also when I am hungry; I always want to eat in the late evening.' She also complained of abdominal distension and alternation of constipation and diarrhoea. She also felt tired, could not concentrate well and suffered from poor memory. Mentally, she felt depressed and often weepy. Her tongue was Purple and her pulse was Wiry.

This is a good example of a case of *cao za* (i.e. 'gnawing hunger' as described above) deriving from Liver-Qi stagnation. The characteristic symptom is that of 'feeling sick when she eats but also when she is hungry'; this corresponds to the description of this condition in Chinese books when they say that the condition *mimics hunger but is not hunger*.

Spleen-Yin deficiency

Slight gnawing hunger, poor appetite, poor digestion, retching, loss of taste, slight epigastric pain, dry mouth, dry lips, dry stools, thin body, sallow complexion with possibly a red tip of the nose, tongue with transverse cracks on the sides, Weak or Floating-Empty pulse.

Case history 69.1 illustrates a pattern causing gnawing hunger.

Craving for sweets/constant picking

Spleen-Qi deficiency

Craving for sweets when tired, constant picking, tendency to obesity, sweet taste, loss of taste, irregular appetite, poor appetite, slight abdominal distension after eating, tiredness, pale complexion, weakness of the limbs, loose stools, Pale tongue, Empty pulse.

Heart-Blood deficiency

Craving for sweets when upset, constant picking, irregular appetite, sadness, depression, loneliness, palpitations, dizziness, insomnia, dream-disturbed sleep, poor memory, anxiety, a tendency to be easily startled, dull-pale complexion, pale lips, Pale and Thin tongue, Choppy or Fine pulse.

Heart-Fire

Craving for sweets when worried, constant picking, hunger, irregular appetite, palpitations, thirst, mouth and tongue ulcers, mental restlessness, a feeling of agitation, insomnia, dream-disturbed sleep, a feeling of heat, red face, bitter taste, Red tongue with redder tip and yellow coating, Overflowing-Rapid pulse.

Liver-Qi invading the Spleen

Craving for sweets which is worse premenstrually, constant picking, irregular appetite, alternation of constipation and diarrhoea, epigastric/abdominal distension, irritability, moodiness, depression, tiredness, pulse Wiry on the left and Weak on the right.

Spleen- and Kidney-Yang deficiency

Craving for sweets when tired, constant picking, irregular appetite, lower backache, cold and weak knees, a feeling of cold, bright-white complexion, impotence, decreased libido, tiredness, lassitude, abundant clear urination, urination at night, loose stools, poor appetite, slight abdominal distension, a desire to lie down, early-morning diarrhoea, Pale and wet tongue, Deep-Weak pulse.

Spleen-Heat

Craving for sweets, constant picking, hunger, burning epigastric/abdominal pain, excessive hunger, red tip of the nose, dry lips, mouth ulcers, thirst, dry stools, a feeling of heat, scanty dark urine, yellow complexion, Red tongue with dry yellow coating, Overflowing-Rapid pulse.

SLEEPINESS AFTER EATING

Spleen-Qi deficiency

Sleepiness after eating, poor appetite, slight abdominal distension after eating, tiredness, lassitude, pale complexion, weakness of the limbs, loose stools, Pale tongue, Empty pulse.

Damp-Phlegm in the Spleen

Sleepiness after eating, a feeling of heaviness and muzziness of the head, a feeling of oppression or fullness of the chest and epigastrium, dizziness, blurred vision, somnolence, nausea, sputum in the throat, muzziness of the head, Swollen tongue with sticky coating, Slippery pulse.

Spleen-Qi deficiency with Dampness

Sleepiness after eating, poor appetite, slight abdominal distension after eating, tiredness, lassitude, pale complexion, weakness of the limbs, loose stools, abdominal fullness, a feeling of heaviness, a sticky taste, poor digestion, undigested food in the stools, nausea, dull frontal headache, excessive vaginal discharge, Pale tongue with sticky coating, Soggy pulse.

NAUSEA, RETCHING AND VOMITING

There are several Chinese terms referring to nausea and vomiting, expressing varying characteristics or degrees of severity. The Chinese term *e xin* means 'nausea', *ou* means vomiting with a sound, *tu* means vomiting without sound; *gan ou* indicates short retching with a low sound and *yue* indicates long retching with a loud sound (before the Ming dynasty this term indicated 'hiccup'). The two Chinese terms *ou* and *tu* are usually used together to indicate vomiting.

Nausea

Interrogation, Chapter 30

Liver-Qi invading the Stomach

Nausea, vomiting, belching, hiccup, irritability, epigastric and hypochondrial distension and pain, a feeling of oppression of the epigastrium, sour regurgitation, sighing, weak limbs, normal-coloured tongue (or slightly Red on the sides in severe cases of Liver-Qi stagnation), pulse Wiry on the left and Weak on the right.

Stomach-Qi deficiency

Very slight nausea especially in the morning, an uncomfortable feeling in the epigastrium, no appetite, lack of sense of taste, loose stools, tiredness especially in the morning, weak limbs, Pale tongue, Empty pulse.

Cold in the Stomach

Nausea, epigastric pain aggravated by cold liquids and alleviated by warm liquids, vomiting of thin watery fluid, dribbling from the mouth, hiccup, nausea, feeling worse after swallowing cold fluids (which are quickly vomited), severe pain in the epigastrium, a feeling of cold, cold limbs, preference for warmth, preference for warm liquids, thick white tongue coating, Deep-Tight-Slow pulse.

Stomach-Heat

Nausea, burning epigastric pain, thirst, sour regurgitation, excessive hunger, foul breath, a feeling of heat, Red tongue with a yellow coating, Overflowing-Rapid pulse.

Stomach-Yin deficiency

Slight nausea, no appetite or slight hunger but no desire to eat, constipation (dry stools), dull or slightly burning epigastric pain, dry mouth and throat especially in the afternoon, thirst but no desire to drink, or a desire to drink in small sips, a slight feeling of fullness after eating, normal-coloured tongue without coating or without coating in the centre, Floating-Empty pulse.

Phlegm obstructing the Stomach

Nausea, vomiting, poor appetite, a feeling of oppression of the epigastrium, sputum in the throat, sticky taste, Swollen tongue with sticky coating, Slippery pulse.

Cold-Dampness in the Stomach

Nausea, poor appetite, epigastric fullness, a feeling of heaviness of the head and body, a feeling of cold, cold limbs, sticky white tongue coating, Slippery-Slow pulse.

Food poisoning

Nausea aggravated by the smell of food, vomiting, epigastric fullness and pain alleviated by vomiting, thick tongue coating, Slippery pulse.

Heart-Qi stagnation

Nausea that is aggravated by emotional stress, palpitations, a feeling of oppression of the chest, depression, a slight feeling of a lump in the throat, slight shortness of breath, sighing, poor appetite, chest and epigastric distension, a dislike of lying down, weak and cold limbs, slightly purple lips, pale complexion,

tongue slightly Pale-Purple on the sides in the chest area, pulse Empty but very slightly Overflowing on the left Front position.

> **Clinical note**
>
> - Remember: nausea is not always due to Stomach-Qi not descending. It may also be due to Heart-Qi not descending (from emotional stress).

Vomiting

Interrogation, Chapter 30; Hearing, Chapter 53

Liver-Qi invading the Stomach

Vomiting with loud sound, nausea, belching, hiccup, irritability, epigastric and hypochondrial distension and pain, a feeling of oppression of the epigastrium, sour regurgitation, sighing, weak limbs, normal-coloured tongue (or slightly Red on the sides in severe cases of Liver-Qi stagnation), pulse Wiry on the left and Weak on the right.

Cold in the Stomach

Vomiting of thin watery fluids with low sound, dribbling from the mouth, hiccup, nausea, epigastric pain aggravated by cold liquids and alleviated by warm liquids, feeling worse after swallowing cold fluids which are quickly vomited, severe pain in the epigastrium, a feeling of cold, cold limbs, preference for warmth and for warm liquids, thick-white tongue coating, Deep-Tight-Slow pulse.

Stomach-Heat

Vomiting with loud sound soon after eating, belching, sour regurgitation, foul breath, nausea, burning epigastric pain, thirst, excessive hunger, a feeling of heat, Red tongue with a yellow coating, Overflowing-Rapid pulse.

Stomach-Qi deficiency

Vomiting with low sound, an uncomfortable feeling in the epigastrium, no appetite, lack of sense of taste, loose stools, tiredness especially in the morning weak limbs, Pale tongue, Empty pulse.

Stomach deficient and cold

Vomiting with low sound or vomiting of clear fluids, discomfort or dull pain in the epigastrium, better after eating and with pressure or massage, no appetite, preference for warm drinks and foods, no thirst, cold and weak limbs, tiredness, pale complexion, Pale and wet tongue, Deep-Weak-Slow pulse.

Stomach-Yin deficiency

Vomiting of thin fluids with low sound, no appetite or slight hunger but no desire to eat, constipation (dry stools), dull or slightly burning epigastric pain, dry mouth and throat especially in the afternoon, thirst but no desire to drink, or a desire to drink in small sips, a slight feeling of fullness after eating, normal-coloured tongue without coating or without coating in the centre, Floating-Empty pulse.

Heat in the Liver and Gall-Bladder

Vomiting of bitter fluids, headache, thirst, dizziness, tinnitus, bitter taste, dry throat, irritability, red face and ears, hypochondrial fullness, unilateral or bilateral yellow tongue coating, Wiry-Rapid pulse.

Stomach- and Liver-Fire

Vomiting, sour regurgitation, foul breath, nausea, burning epigastric pain, intense thirst with a desire to drink cold liquids, mental restlessness, dry mouth, mouth ulcers, bleeding gums, dry stools, a feeling of heat, headache, red face, dizziness, tinnitus, irritability, propensity to outbursts of anger, bitter taste, constipation, dark urine, Red tongue with redder sides and dry yellow coating, Wiry-Rapid pulse.

External Cold invading the Stomach

Sudden vomiting, epigastric pain aggravated by cold liquids and alleviated by warm liquids, vomiting of thin watery fluid, dribbling from the mouth, hiccup, nausea, feeling worse after swallowing cold fluids (which are quickly vomited), severe pain in the epigastrium, a feeling of cold, cold limbs, preference for warmth, preference for warm liquids, thick white tongue coating, Deep-Tight-Slow pulse.

Phlegm obstructing the Stomach

Vomiting, nausea, poor appetite, feeling of oppression of the epigastrium, sputum in the throat, sticky taste, Swollen tongue with sticky coating, Slippery pulse.

Cold-Dampness in the Stomach

Vomiting, nausea, poor appetite, epigastric fullness, a feeling of heaviness of the head and body, a feeling of

cold, cold limbs, sticky white tongue coating, Slippery-Slow pulse.

Retention of food

Vomiting of sour fluids, foul breath, sour regurgitation, belching, nausea, fullness, pain and distension of the epigastrium which are relieved by vomiting, insomnia, loose stools or constipation, poor appetite, thick tongue coating, Full-Slippery pulse.

Food poisoning

Vomiting, epigastric fullness and pain that is relieved by vomiting, sour regurgitation, belching, nausea at the smell of food, thick tongue coating, Slippery pulse.

Retching

Retching indicates the attempt and the sound of vomiting but without bringing up food. In Chinese it is called *gan ou*, indicating short retching with a low sound, or *yue*, indicating long retching with a loud sound.

Liver-Qi invading the Stomach

Retching with a loud sound coming in bouts according to the emotional state, irritability, epigastric and hypochondrial distension, pulse Wiry on both Middle positions.

Stomach-Heat

Retching with a loud sound, sour regurgitation, nausea, burning epigastric pain, thirst, excessive hunger, foul breath, a feeling of heat, Red tongue with a yellow coating, Overflowing-Rapid pulse.

Cold in the Stomach

Retching with a low sound, vomiting of thin watery fluids, hiccup, nausea, epigastric pain aggravated by cold liquids and alleviated by warm liquids, dribbling from the mouth, feeling worse after swallowing cold fluids (which are quickly vomited), severe pain in the epigastrium, a feeling of cold, cold limbs, preference for warmth and for warm liquids, thick white tongue coating, Deep-Tight-Slow pulse.

Retention of food

Retching with a loud sound, nausea, vomiting of sour fluids, sour regurgitation, foul breath, belching, fullness, pain and distension of the epigastrium which are relieved by vomiting, insomnia, loose stools or constipation, poor appetite, thick tongue coating, Full-Slippery pulse.

Spleen-Yin deficiency

Slight retching with a low sound, poor appetite, poor digestion, gnawing hunger, loss of sense of taste, slight epigastric pain, dry mouth, dry lips, dry stools, thin body, sallow complexion with possibly red tip of the nose, tongue with transverse cracks on the sides, Weak or Floating-Empty pulse.

Vomiting of blood
Stomach-Fire

Vomiting of food with bright-red or dark-red blood, sour regurgitation, foul breath, nausea, burning epigastric pain, intense thirst with a desire to drink cold liquids, mental restlessness, dry mouth, mouth ulcers, bleeding gums, dry stools, a feeling of heat, tongue Red with a thick, dry dark-yellow coating, Deep-Full-Rapid pulse.

Liver-Fire invading the Stomach

Vomiting of bright-red blood, headache, red face, dizziness, tinnitus, irritability, propensity to outbursts of anger, thirst, bitter taste, constipation, dark urine, epigastric and hypochondrial pain, insomnia, Red tongue with redder sides and yellow coating, Rapid-Wiry pulse.

Blood stasis in the Stomach

Vomiting of very dark blood which may look like coffee grounds, severe, stabbing epigastric pain that may be worse at night, dislike of pressure, Purple tongue, Wiry pulse.

Stomach-Yin deficiency with Empty-Heat

Vomiting of fresh red blood, feeling of hunger but no desire to eat, bleeding gums, dull or burning epigastric pain, feeling of heat in the afternoon, constipation (dry stools), dry mouth and throat especially in the afternoon, thirst with a desire to drink in small sips, night sweating, five-palm heat, Red tongue (or Red centre only) without coating in the centre, Floating-Empty and Rapid pulse.

Heart- and Spleen-Qi deficiency

Vomiting of bright red blood in small quantities, dull epigastric pain alleviated by pressure, poor appetite,

slight abdominal distension after eating, tiredness, pale complexion, weakness of the limbs, loose stools, palpitations, shortness of breath on exertion, spontaneous sweating, Pale tongue, Empty pulse.

Spleen- and Kidney-Yang deficiency

Vomiting of fresh red blood in small amounts, lingering chronic disease, lower backache, cold and weak knees, a feeling of cold, bright-white complexion, impotence, decreased libido, tiredness, lassitude, abundant clear urination, urination at night, loose stools, poor appetite, slight abdominal distension, a desire to lie down, early-morning diarrhoea, Pale and wet tongue, Deep-Weak pulse.

Difficulty in swallowing (diaphragm choking)

'Diaphragm choking' is a translation of the Chinese term *ye ge*: *ye* means 'choking' and *ge* literally means 'diaphragm' and, in this context, it indicates severe difficulty in swallowing. In fact, *ye* by itself indicates a mild degree of this condition while *ge* indicates a severe degree; one could also say that *ye* is the beginning stage of a condition later developing into *ge*. This condition is characterized by a difficulty in swallowing, a feeling of obstruction in the oesophagus and diaphragm and a feeling that the food cannot go down; it usually affects the elderly (especially men) and it is rare in young people.

The condition of 'diaphragm choking' (*ye ge*) should be differentiated from 'regurgitation of food' (*fan wei*): 'Diaphragm choking' is centred in the oesophagus and therefore above the neck of the stomach and it indicates that the food cannot enter the stomach, causing a difficulty in swallowing and a feeling of obstruction; 'regurgitation of food' is centred in the stomach itself and indicates that the food is regurgitated some hours after entering the stomach.

'Diaphragm choking' should also be differentiated from the 'Plum Stone Syndrome', which is characterized by a feeling of obstruction in the throat without any actual regurgitation of food.

'Diaphragm choking' often corresponds to the Western condition of hiatus hernia or, in more serious cases, to carcinoma of the oesophagus.

Stagnation of Qi and Phlegm

Difficulty in swallowing when tense, hypochondrial or epigastric distension, irritability, moodiness, a feeling of a lump in the throat, premenstrual tension, sputum in the throat, a feeling of oppression of the chest, Swollen tongue, Wiry pulse.

Blood stasis in the Stomach

Difficulty in swallowing, severe, stabbing epigastric pain that may be worse at night, dislike of pressure, nausea, vomiting, possibly of blood, vomiting of food looking like coffee grounds, Purple tongue, Wiry pulse.

Qi and Yang deficiency of the Stomach

Slight difficulty in swallowing, vomiting of thin watery fluids, discomfort or dull pain in the epigastrium, better after eating and with pressure or massage, lack of appetite, preference for warm drinks and foods, absence of thirst, cold and weak limbs, tiredness, pale complexion, Pale and wet tongue, Deep-Weak-Slow pulse.

Stomach-Yin deficiency

Slight difficulty in swallowing, no appetite or slight hunger but no desire to eat, thirst but no desire to drink, or a desire to drink in small sips, constipation (dry stools), dull or slightly burning epigastric pain, dry mouth and throat especially in the afternoon, slight feeling of fullness after eating, normal-coloured tongue without coating or without coating in the centre, Floating-Empty pulse.

Spleen- and Kidney-Yang deficiency

Chronic, slight difficulty in swallowing, lower backache, cold and weak knees, a feeling of cold, bright-white complexion, impotence, decreased libido, tiredness, lassitude, abundant clear urination, urination at night, loose stools, poor appetite, slight abdominal distension, a desire to lie down, early-morning diarrhoea, Pale and wet tongue, Deep-Weak pulse.

TASTE

Bitter taste

Interrogation, Chapter 30

A 'bitter' taste is a symptom that is very frequently reported by Chinese patients and, in Chinese culture, this symptom is very closely identified with emotional problems also because the word 'bitter' in Chinese is often used in that sense. In fact, when a Chinese patient complains of bitter taste, it almost always indicates emotional problems or serious life difficulties. In

the West there is no such correlation between this particular symptom and emotional problems.

Liver-Fire

Bitter taste throughout the day, headache, red face, dizziness, tinnitus, irritability, propensity to outbursts of anger, thirst, constipation, dark urine, Red tongue with redder sides and dry yellow coating, Wiry-Rapid pulse.

Heart-Fire

Bitter taste in the morning especially after a bad night's sleep, palpitations, thirst, mouth and tongue ulcers, mental restlessness, a feeling of agitation, insomnia, dream-disturbed sleep, a feeling of heat, red face, bitter taste, Red tongue with redder tip and yellow coating, Overflowing-Rapid pulse.

The difference between the bitter taste caused by Liver-Fire and that caused by Heart-Fire is that the former persists throughout the day, whereas the latter is experienced only in the morning after a bad night's sleep.

Damp-Heat in the Liver and Gall-Bladder

Bitter and sticky taste, fullness/pain of the hypochondrium, abdomen or epigastrium, poor appetite, nausea, a feeling of heaviness of the body, yellow vaginal discharge, vaginal itching, mid-cycle bleeding/pain, burning on urination, dark urine, yellow complexion and eyes, vomiting, Red tongue with redder sides and unilateral or bilateral sticky yellow coating, Wiry-Slippery-Rapid pulse.

Lesser-Yang pattern

Bitter taste, alternation of aversion to cold and a feeling of heat, headache, irritability, blurred vision, dry throat, hypochondrial pain, tongue with unilateral coating, Wiry pulse.

This is the Lesser-Yang pattern within the identification of patterns according to the Six Stages.

Sweet taste

Interrogation, Chapter 30

Deficiency of Qi/Yin of the Stomach and Spleen

Sweet taste, poor appetite, slight abdominal distension after eating, tiredness, lassitude, pale complexion, weakness of the limbs, loose stools, an uncomfortable feeling in the epigastrium, lack of taste sensation, dry mouth, night sweating.

The tongue and pulse presentation depends on whether Qi or Yin deficiency predominates.

Damp-Heat in the Spleen

Sweet or sticky taste, a feeling of fullness of the epigastrium/abdomen, epigastric/abdominal pain, poor appetite, a feeling of heaviness of the body, thirst without a desire to drink, nausea, vomiting, loose stools with an offensive odour, a feeling of heat, scanty dark urine, headache with a feeling of heaviness of the head, dull-yellow complexion, Red tongue with sticky yellow coating, Slippery-Rapid pulse.

Stomach- and Spleen-Heat

Sweet taste, burning epigastric pain, thirst, sour regurgitation, nausea, excessive hunger, foul breath, a feeling of heat, red tip of the nose, dry lips, mouth ulcers, dry stools, scanty dark urine, Red tongue with dry yellow coating, Overflowing-Rapid pulse.

Salty taste

Interrogation, Chapter 30

The salty taste is not very common in practice and very few patients will ever complain of this particular symptom.

Kidney-Yin deficiency

Salty taste, dry throat and mouth with a desire to drink in small sips, dizziness, tinnitus, hardness of hearing, poor memory, night sweating, dry mouth and throat at night, lower backache, constipation, scanty dark urine, tiredness, normal-coloured tongue without coating, Floating-Empty pulse.

Kidney-Yang deficiency

Salty taste, lower backache, cold knees, feeling cold, bright-white complexion, weak knees, tiredness, lassitude, abundant clear urination, urination at night, impotence, decreased libido, Pale and wet tongue, Deep-Weak pulse.

Sour taste

Interrogation, Chapter 30

Liver-Fire

A sour (or bitter) taste, headache, red face, dizziness, tinnitus, irritability, propensity to outbursts of anger, thirst, constipation, dark urine, Red tongue with

redder sides and dry yellow coating, Wiry-Rapid pulse.

Liver-Qi invading the Spleen

Sour taste, sour regurgitation, belching, epigastric fullness and distension, poor appetite, tiredness, alternation of constipation and diarrhoea, pulse Weak on the right and Wiry on the left.

Liver-Qi invading the Stomach

Sour taste, sour regurgitation, irritability, epigastric and hypochondrial distension and pain, a feeling of oppression of the epigastrium, sour regurgitation, hiccup, belching, nausea, vomiting, sighing, weak limbs, normal-coloured tongue (or slightly Red on the sides in severe cases of Liver-Qi stagnation), pulse Wiry on the left and Weak on the right.

Retention of food

Sour taste, foul breath, sour regurgitation, belching, fullness, pain and distension of the epigastrium which are relieved by vomiting, nausea, vomiting of sour fluids, insomnia, loose stools or constipation, poor appetite, thick tongue coating, Full-Slippery pulse.

Stomach-Heat

Sour taste, thirst, epigastric pain, sour regurgitation, nausea, excessive hunger, foul breath, a feeling of heat, Red tongue with a yellow coating, Overflowing-Rapid pulse.

Sticky taste

Interrogation, Chapter 30

Western patients often describe the sticky taste as a 'metallic' taste.

Cold-Dampness

Sticky taste, epigastric fullness, a feeling of heaviness of the head and body, a feeling of cold, cold limbs, sticky white tongue coating, Slippery-Slow pulse.

Damp-Heat

Sticky taste, thirst with no desire to drink, epigastric fullness, a feeling of heaviness of the head and body, a feeling of heat, sticky yellow tongue coating, Slippery-Rapid pulse.

Phlegm

Sticky taste, sputum in the throat, a feeling of oppression of the chest, Swollen tongue with sticky coating, Slippery pulse.

Phlegm-Heat in the Lungs

Sticky taste, thirst with no desire to drink, barking cough with profuse, sticky yellow or green sputum, shortness of breath, wheezing, a feeling of oppression of the chest, a feeling of heat, Red and Swollen tongue with a sticky yellow coating, Slippery-Rapid pulse.

Loss of taste

Interrogation, Chapter 30

Deficiency of Stomach- and Spleen-Qi

Gradual loss of sense of taste and possibly smell, poor appetite, slight abdominal distension after eating, tiredness, lassitude, pale complexion, weakness of the limbs, loose stools, an uncomfortable feeling in the epigastrium, Pale tongue, Empty pulse.

Dampness obstructing the Middle Burner

Loss of sense of taste, abdominal fullness and distension, poor appetite, no desire to drink, sleepiness after eating, thick sticky tongue coating, Slippery pulse.

Damp-Phlegm obstructing the Spleen

Loss of sense of taste, epigastric and abdominal fullness, a feeling of oppression of the chest, poor appetite, nausea, tiredness, feeling of heaviness, sputum in the throat, loose stools, sleepiness after eating, Swollen tongue with sticky coating, Slippery pulse.

Stomach- and Spleen-Qi deficiency with Cold in the Stomach

Loss of sense of taste, poor appetite, slight abdominal distension after eating, tiredness, lassitude, pale complexion, loose stools, discomfort or dull pain in the epigastrium, better after eating and with pressure or massage, preference for warm drinks and foods, vomiting of clear fluids, absence of thirst, cold and weak limbs, Pale and wet tongue, Deep-Weak-Slow pulse.

Foul breath

Stomach-Heat

Foul breath, thirst, sour regurgitation, nausea, excessive hunger, foul breath, burning epigastric pain, a feeling of heat, Red tongue with a yellow coating, Overflowing-Rapid pulse.

Phlegm-Heat in the Lungs

Foul breath, sticky taste, thirst with no desire to drink, barking cough with profuse, sticky yellow or green sputum, shortness of breath, wheezing, a feeling of oppression of the chest, a feeling of heat, insomnia, a feeling of agitation, Red and Swollen tongue with a sticky yellow coating, Slippery-Rapid pulse.

Retention of food

Foul breath, sour taste, belching, sour regurgitation, nausea, vomiting of sour fluids, fullness, pain and distension of the epigastrium which are relieved by vomiting, insomnia, loose stools or constipation, poor appetite, thick tongue coating, Full-Slippery pulse.

Chapter **70**

THIRST AND DRINK

Chapter contents

THIRST *731*

DRY MOUTH *732*

ABSENCE OF THIRST *733*

INCREASED SALIVATION *733*

THIRST

Interrogation, Chapter 32

Stomach-Heat

Thirst with a desire to drink cold fluids, foul breath, sour regurgitation, burning epigastric pain, nausea, excessive hunger, a feeling of heat, Red tongue with a yellow coating, Overflowing-Rapid pulse.

Liver-Fire

Thirst, bitter taste, red face, dizziness, tinnitus, headache, irritability, propensity to outbursts of anger, constipation, dark urine, Red tongue with redder sides and dry yellow coating, Wiry-Rapid pulse.

Heart-Fire

Thirst, mouth and tongue ulcers, palpitations, mental restlessness, a feeling of agitation, insomnia, dream-disturbed sleep, a feeling of heat, red face, bitter taste, Red tongue with redder tip and yellow coating, Overflowing-Rapid pulse.

Damp-Heat in Stomach and Spleen

Thirst with no desire to drink, sticky taste, a feeling of fullness and pain of the epigastrium and lower abdomen, poor appetite, a feeling of heaviness, nausea, loose stools with offensive odour, a feeling of heat, dull-yellow complexion, Red tongue with sticky yellow coating, Slippery-Rapid pulse.

Damp-Heat in Liver and Gall-Bladder

Thirst, bitter taste, fullness/pain of the hypochondrium, abdomen or epigastrium, poor appetite, nausea, a feeling of heaviness of the body, yellow vaginal discharge, vaginal itching, mid-cycle bleeding/pain, burning on urination, dark urine, yellow complexion

and eyes, vomiting, Red tongue with redder sides and unilateral or bilateral sticky yellow coating, Wiry-Slippery-Rapid pulse.

Phlegm-Heat in the Lungs

Thirst without desire to drink, barking cough with profuse, sticky yellow or green sputum, shortness of breath, wheezing, a feeling of oppression of the chest, a feeling of heat, insomnia, a feeling of agitation, Red and Swollen tongue with a sticky yellow coating, Slippery-Rapid pulse.

Heart-Yin deficiency with Empty-Heat

Thirst with desire to slip fluids that is more pronounced in the evening, dry mouth and throat, palpitations, insomnia, dream-disturbed sleep, poor memory, anxiety, propensity to be startled, mental restlessness, a feeling of heat in the evening, malar flush, night sweating, five-palm heat, Red tongue that is redder on the tip with no coating, Floating-Empty and Rapid pulse.

Stomach-Yin deficiency with Empty-Heat

Thirst with a desire to drink in small sips that is more pronounced in the evening, dry mouth and throat especially in the afternoon, dull or burning epigastric pain, a feeling of heat in the afternoon, constipation (dry stools), a feeling of hunger but no desire to eat, a slight feeling of fullness after eating, night sweating, five-palm heat, bleeding gums, Red tongue (or Red centre only) without coating in the centre, Floating-Empty and Rapid pulse.

Lung-Heat

Thirst with a desire to drink cold water, cough, slight breathlessness, a feeling of heat, chest ache, flaring of the nostrils, red face, Red tongue with yellow coating, Overflowing-Rapid pulse.

Lung-Yin deficiency with Empty-Heat

Slight thirst with a desire to drink in small sips that is more pronounced in the evening, dry mouth and throat at night, dry cough or with scanty, sticky sputum which could be blood tinged, weak/hoarse voice, night sweating, tiredness, malar flush, a feeling of heat or a low-grade fever in the evening, five-palm heat, thin body or thin chest, insomnia, anxiety, Red tongue without coating, Floating-Empty and Rapid tongue.

Heart-Yin deficiency

Slight thirst with a desire to drink in small sips, dry mouth and throat, palpitations, insomnia, dream-disturbed sleep, poor memory, anxiety, a tendency to be easily startled, mental restlessness, uneasiness, 'feeling hot and bothered', night sweating, normal-coloured tongue without coating or with rootless coating, Floating-Empty pulse, especially on the left Front position.

Liver-Yin deficiency

Slight thirst with a desire to drink in small sips, dry cough, weak voice, dry throat, hoarse voice, night sweating, tiredness, tongue without coating in the front, Floating-Empty pulse.

Kidney-Yin deficiency

Slight thirst with a desire to drink in small sips, dizziness, tinnitus, hardness of hearing, poor memory, night sweating, dry mouth and throat at night, lower backache, constipation, scanty dark urine, tiredness, normal-coloured tongue without coating, Floating-Empty pulse.

Lung-Yin deficiency

Slight thirst with a desire to drink in small sips, dry cough, weak voice, dry throat, hoarse voice, night sweating, tiredness, tongue without coating in the front, Floating-Empty pulse.

Stomach-Yin deficiency

Slight thirst with a desire to drink in small sips, dry mouth, dull epigastric pain, poor appetite, tongue of a normal colour without coating in the centre.

Clinical note

- It is often difficult to establish whether a patient suffers from excessive 'thirst' owing to the widespread habit of forcing oneself to drink large amounts of water.

DRY MOUTH

Interrogation, Chapter 32

Yin deficiency

Dry mouth with a desire to drink in small sips, dry throat in the evening, night sweating, scanty dark urine, dry stools, normal-coloured tongue without

coating, Floating-Empty pulse. Other symptoms and signs depend on the organ involved, which could be the Stomach, Lungs, Liver, Kidneys, Heart, or Spleen.

Damp-Heat in the Stomach and Spleen

Dry mouth with no desire to drink, thirst without a desire to drink, a feeling of fullness and pain of the epigastrium and lower abdomen, poor appetite, a feeling of heaviness, nausea, loose stools with offensive odour, a feeling of heat, dull-yellow complexion, sticky taste, Red tongue with sticky yellow coating, Slippery-Rapid pulse.

Phlegm-Heat in the Stomach

Dry mouth with no desire to drink, thirst, foul breath, burning epigastric pain, mental restlessness, bleeding gums, dry stools, mouth ulcers, sour regurgitation, nausea, vomiting soon after eating, excessive hunger, a feeling of heat, a feeling of oppression of the chest and epigastrium, insomnia, tongue Red in the centre with a sticky yellow coating and a Stomach crack with a rough, sticky yellow coating inside it, Slippery-Rapid pulse.

ABSENCE OF THIRST

Interrogation, Chapter 32

Deficiency of Yang of the Spleen and Stomach

Absence of thirst, poor appetite, slight abdominal distension after eating, uncomfortable feeling in the epigastrium, tiredness, lassitude, pale complexion, weakness of the limbs, loose stools, feeling cold, cold limbs, oedema. Pale and wet tongue, Deep-Weak pulse.

Cold in the Stomach

Absence of thirst, severe pain in the epigastrium, a feeling of cold, cold limbs, preference for warmth, vom-iting of clear fluids (which may alleviate the pain), nausea, feeling worse after swallowing cold fluids (which are quickly vomited), thick white tongue coating, Deep-Tight-Slow pulse.

Dampness in the Stomach and Spleen

Lack of desire to drink, sticky taste, a feeling of fullness and pain of the epigastrium and lower abdomen, poor appetite, a feeling of heaviness, nausea, loose stools, a feeling of heat, dull-yellow complexion, tongue with sticky coating, Slippery pulse.

Clinical note

- Remember always to ask about 'absence of thirst': no patient will report that spontaneously. This is also often difficult to establish owing to the widespread habit of drinking vast amounts of water.

INCREASED SALIVATION

Stomach and Spleen deficient and cold

Increased salivation, preference for warm drinks and foods, discomfort or dull pain in the epigastrium, better after eating and with pressure or massage, no appetite, vomiting of clear fluid, no thirst, cold and weak limbs, tiredness, pale complexion, Pale and wet tongue, Deep-Weak-Slow pulse.

Kidney-Yang deficiency, Water overflowing

Increased salivation, oedema especially of the legs and ankles, a feeling of cold generally or in the legs and back, fullness and distension of abdomen, soreness of the lower back, scanty clear urination, palpitations, breathlessness, cold hands, Pale and Swollen tongue with a wet white coating, Deep-Weak-Slow pulse.

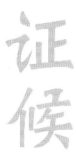

Chapter **71**

ABDOMEN

Chapter contents

INTRODUCTION   735

PAIN   736
  Area below the xyphoid process   736
  Epigastric pain   737
  Hypochondrial pain   738
  Umbilical pain   738
  Central-lower abdominal pain   739
  Lateral-lower abdominal pain   740

DISTENSION AND FULLNESS   740
  Abdominal distension   740
  Abdominal fullness   741

ABNORMAL FEELINGS IN THE ABDOMEN   741
  Feeling of cold in the abdomen   741
  Feeling of pulsation under the umbilicus   742
  Feeling of energy rising in the abdomen   742

BORBORYGMI   742

FLATULENCE   743

SKIN SIGNS   743
  Distended abdominal veins   743
  Lines   743
  Maculae   743

ABDOMINAL MASSES   744
  Small hypochondrial lumps   744
  Lumps in the epigastrium   744

OEDEMA OF THE ABDOMEN   745

ABDOMINAL SIZE   745
  Thin abdomen   745
  Large abdomen   745

SAGGING LOWER ABDOMEN   745

UMBILICUS   745
  Protruding umbilicus   745
  Sunken umbilicus   745

INTRODUCTION

Although the headings below refer primarily to pain in various areas of the abdomen, other sensations may be experienced in each of those areas; these are primarily distension, oppression, fullness or stuffiness.

The clinical significance of these sensations is briefly explained below. For a fuller explanation, see Part 2, Chapter 38.

Distension

A feeling of abdominal distension (usually called 'bloating' in English) may indicate the following patterns:

> • Qi stagnation – severe distension
> • Spleen-Qi deficiency – mild distension
> • Damp-Phlegm.

Besides the subjective feeling of bloating, distension is also characterized by an objective, distended, drum-like feeling on palpation.

Oppression

A feeling of oppression (called *men* in Chinese) usually indicates Phlegm, but it may also indicate severe Qi stagnation. The feeling of oppression is purely subjective.

Fullness

A feeling of fullness in the abdomen is usually caused by Dampness or retention of food. Subjectively the patient feels full as if having had a large meal and there is a very slight feeling of nausea; objectively the abdomen feels hard on palpation.

Stuffiness

'Stuffiness' is a translation of the Chinese term *pi* (although this term has a broader meaning than simply 'feeling of stuffiness'). A feeling of stuffiness in the abdomen is characterized by a subjective mild feeling of fullness, together with an objective soft feeling of the abdomen on palpation. This symptom is usually due either to Dampness or Heat occurring against a background of Deficiency.

PAIN

The regions of abdominal pain in Chinese medicine are as follows:

- area under the heart (this is the small area immediately below the xyphoid process extending approximately 2 inches and bordered by the ribs)
- epigastric (this is the area between the xyphoid process and the umbilicus but excluding the hypochondrial area)
- hypochondrial (these are the two areas below the rib cage)
- umbilical (this is the area around the umbilicus)
- central-lower abdominal (this is the central area of the abdomen between the umbilicus and the symphysis pubis)
- lateral-lower abdominal (these are the lateral areas of the lower abdomen).

Figure 16.7 on p. 145 illustrates these areas.

Area below the xyphoid process

Interrogation, Chapter 38

Rebellious Qi of the Penetrating Vessel

Pain below the xyphoid process with a feeling of tightness, a feeling of heat in the face, a feeling of a lump in the throat, palpitations, anxiety, a feeling of tightness of the chest, nausea, slight breathlessness, epigastric fullness or stuffiness, umbilical and abdominal fullness, irregular/painful periods, a feeling of energy rising in the abdomen to the chest, Firm pulse.

Stomach-Heat

Pain below the xyphoid process, burning epigastric pain, thirst, sour regurgitation, nausea, excessive hunger, foul breath, a feeling of heat, Red tongue with a yellow coating, Overflowing-Rapid pulse.

Stomach-Qi stagnation

Pain below the xyphoid process with a feeling of distension, epigastric pain and distension, belching, nausea, vomiting, hiccup, irritability, pulse Wiry on the right Middle position.

Heart-Qi stagnation

Pain below the xyphoid process with a feeling of distension, palpitations, a feeling of oppression of the chest, depression, a slight feeling of a lump in the throat, slight shortness of breath, sighing, poor appetite, chest and epigastric distension, a dislike of lying down, weak and cold limbs, slightly purple lips, pale complexion, tongue slightly Pale-Purple on the sides in the chest area, pulse Empty but very slightly Overflowing on the left Front position.

Retention of Food in the Stomach

Pain below the xyphoid process with feelings of fullness, fullness, pain and distension of the epigastrium which are relieved by vomiting, nausea, vomiting of sour fluids, foul breath, sour regurgitation, belching, insomnia, loose stools or constipation, poor appetite, thick tongue coating, Full-Slippery pulse.

Stomach- and Spleen-Qi deficiency with Heart-Heat

Pain below the xyphoid process with a feeling of stuffiness, poor appetite, slight abdominal distension after eating, tiredness, lassitude, pale complexion, weakness of the limbs, loose stools, an uncomfortable feeling in the epigastrium, loss of sense of taste, palpitations, thirst, mouth and tongue ulcers, mental restlessness, feeling agitated, insomnia, dream-disturbed sleep, a feeling of heat, red face, bitter taste, Red tongue with redder tip and yellow coating, Overflowing and Rapid pulse.

Phlegm in the Stomach

Pain below the xyphoid process with a feeling of oppression, a feeling of oppression in the epigastrium or the chest, nausea, sputum in the throat, nausea, Swollen tongue with sticky coating, Slippery pulse.

Qi stagnation and Phlegm

Pain below the xyphoid process with a feeling of oppression and distension, a feeling of oppression of the chest, a feeling of a lump in the throat, sighing, sputum in the throat, irritability, Swollen tongue, Wiry or Slippery pulse.

> ### Clinical note
>
> - In my experience, repressed feelings are often 'stored' in the area below the xyphoid process; this often manifests with a hardness in this area on palpation.

Epigastric pain

Interrogation, Chapter 38

Stomach- and Spleen-Qi deficiency

Dull epigastric pain that is alleviated by eating and pressure coming in bouts, poor appetite, slight abdominal distension after eating, tiredness, lassitude, pale complexion, weakness of the limbs, loose stools, lack of sense of taste, Pale tongue, Empty pulse.

Stomach-Yin deficiency

Dull epigastric pain, poor appetite, poor digestion, retching, gnawing hunger, loss of sense of taste, dry mouth, dry lips, dry stools, thin body, sallow complexion with possibly a red tip of the nose, night sweating, tongue with transversal cracks on the sides, Weak or Floating-Empty pulse.

Liver-Qi invading the Stomach

Epigastric pain and distension extending to the hypochondrium, irritability, a feeling of oppression of the epigastrium, sour regurgitation, hiccup, belching, nausea, vomiting, sighing, weak limbs, normal-coloured tongue (or slightly Red on the sides in severe cases of Liver-Qi stagnation), pulse Wiry on the left and Weak on the right.

Cold in the Stomach

Severe, sudden-onset, spastic epigastric pain that is alleviated by drinking warm liquids and aggravated by drinking cold liquids, a feeling of cold, cold limbs, preference for warmth, vomiting of clear fluids (which may alleviate the pain), nausea, feeling worse after swallowing cold fluids (which are quickly vomited), preference for warm liquids, thick white tongue coating, Deep-Tight-Slow pulse.

Stomach-Heat

Burning epigastric pain, thirst, sour regurgitation, nausea, excessive hunger, foul breath, a feeling of heat, Red tongue with a yellow coating, Overflowing-Rapid pulse.

Stomach-Fire

Burning epigastric pain, intense thirst with a desire to drink cold liquids, mental restlessness, dry mouth, mouth ulcers, bleeding gums, dry stools, sour regurgitation, foul breath, nausea, vomiting soon after eating, a feeling of heat, sour regurgitation, tongue Red with a thick, dry dark-yellow coating, Deep-Full-Rapid pulse.

Cold-Dampness in the Stomach

Epigastric pain that is aggravated by drinking cold liquids and ameliorated by drinking warm liquids, poor appetite, a feeling of fullness or cold in the epigastrium, a feeling of heaviness of the head and body, a sweetish taste or absence of taste, no thirst, loose stools, tiredness, lassitude, nausea, oedema, dull-white complexion, excessive white vaginal discharge, Pale tongue with sticky white coating, Slippery-Slow pulse.

Damp-Heat in the Stomach

Epigastric pain, a feeling of fullness of the epigastrium, a feeling of heaviness, facial pain, stuffed nose or thick sticky nasal discharge, thirst without a desire to drink, nausea, a feeling of heat, dull-yellow complexion, a sticky taste, Red tongue with sticky yellow coating, Slippery-Rapid pulse.

Blood stasis in the Stomach

Severe, stabbing epigastric pain that may be worse at night, a dislike of pressure, nausea, vomiting, possibly of blood, or food looking like coffee grounds, Purple tongue, Wiry pulse.

Phlegm-Heat in the Stomach

Burning epigastric pain, thirst without a desire to drink, mental restlessness, bleeding gums, dry stools, dry mouth, mouth ulcers, sour regurgitation, nausea, vomiting soon after eating, excessive hunger, foul breath, a feeling of heat, a feeling of oppression of the chest and epigastrium, insomnia, tongue Red in the centre with a sticky yellow coating and a Stomach crack with a rough, sticky yellow coating inside it, Slippery-Rapid pulse.

Retention of Food

Epigastric pain, distension and fullness which are relieved by vomiting, nausea, vomiting of sour fluids, foul breath, sour regurgitation, belching, insomnia, loose stools or constipation, poor appetite, thick tongue coating, Full-Slippery pulse.

Liver-Fire invading the Stomach

Burning epigastric pain, distension and fullness, irritability, sour regurgitation, hiccup, belching, nausea, vomiting, sighing, weak limbs, tongue Red on the sides, pulse Wiry-Rapid and Weak on the right.

Phlegm-Fluids in the Stomach

Dull epigastric pain, abdominal fullness and distension, nausea, vomiting of watery fluids, dry mouth without a desire to drink, shortness of breath, dizziness, a feeling of oppression of the chest, swelling of the limbs, expectoration of thin watery sputum, inability to lie down, Swollen tongue with sticky coating, Deep-Wiry or Deep-Slippery pulse.

> **Clinical note**
>
> - Liver-Qi invading the Stomach is probably the commonest cause of epigastric pain.

Hypochondrial pain

Interrogation, Chapter 38

These are the two lateral areas of the upper abdomen below the rib cage.

Liver-Qi stagnation

Hypochondrial pain and distension without a fixed location and coming and going according to the emotional state, irritability, moodiness, a feeling of a lump in the throat, premenstrual tension, Wiry pulse.

Liver-Blood stasis

Stabbing hypochondrial pain with fixed location which is worse at night, painful periods, dark and clotted menstrual blood, masses in the abdomen, purple nails and lips, purple or dark complexion, Purple tongue, Wiry or Firm pulse.

Damp-Heat in Liver and Gall-Bladder

Hypochondrial pain distension and fullness, bitter taste, poor appetite, nausea, a feeling of heaviness of the body, yellow vaginal discharge, vaginal itching, mid-cycle bleeding/pain, burning on urination, dark urine, yellow complexion and eyes, vomiting, Red tongue with redder sides and unilateral or bilateral sticky yellow coating, Wiry-Slippery-Rapid pulse.

Liver-Yin deficiency

Dull hypochondrial pain that is alleviated by rest, dizziness, numbness/tingling of the limbs, insomnia, blurred vision, floaters in the eyes, dry eyes, diminished night vision, scanty menstruation or amenorrhoea, dull-pale complexion without lustre but with red cheekbones, muscular weakness, cramps, withered and brittle nails, very dry skin and hair, night sweating, depression, a feeling of aimlessness, normal-coloured tongue without coating, Fine or Floating-Empty pulse.

Lesser-Yang syndrome

Hypochondrial pain and distension, alternation of chills and a feeling of heat, bitter taste, dry throat, blurred vision, irritability, nausea, unilateral sticky tongue coating, Wiry pulse.

Phlegm-Fluids in the hypochondrium

Hypochondrial pain that is worse on coughing and breathing, a feeling of distension and pulling of the hypochondrium, shortness of breath, Swollen tongue with sticky coating, Deep-Slippery-Wiry pulse.

> **Clinical note**
>
> - Never ask a patient about pain in the 'hypochondrium' but instead point to the area you mean.

Umbilical pain

Interrogation, Chapter 38

Pain in the area around the umbilicus is common in children.

Stagnation of Qi in the Stomach and Intestines

Umbilical pain and distension, epigastric pain and distention, belching, nausea, vomiting, hiccup, irritability, pulse Wiry on the right Middle position.

Cold in the Intestines

Spastic umbilical pain that is aggravated by cold liquids and alleviated by hot liquids, diarrhoea with pain,

feeling of cold, a cold sensation in abdomen, thick white tongue coating, Deep-Wiry pulse.

Damp-Heat in the Intestines

Umbilical pain that is not relieved by a bowel movement, diarrhoea, mucus and blood in stools, offensive odour of stools, burning in the anus, scanty dark urine, fever, sweating which does not decrease the fever, a feeling of heat, thirst without a desire to drink, a feeling of heaviness of the body and limbs, Red tongue with sticky yellow coating, Slippery-Rapid pulse.

Spleen- and Kidney-Yang deficiency

Dull umbilical pain that comes and goes, lower backache, cold and weak knees, a feeling of cold, bright-white complexion, impotence, decreased libido, tiredness, lassitude, abundant clear urination, urination at night, loose stools, poor appetite, a desire to lie down, early-morning diarrhoea, Pale and wet tongue, Deep-Weak pulse.

Food poisoning

Severe umbilical pain, belching, nausea, vomiting, loose stools, thick tongue coating, Slippery pulse.

Heat in Bright Yang

Burning umbilical pain, intense thirst with a desire to drink cold liquids, mental restlessness, dry mouth, mouth ulcers, bleeding gums, dry stools, sour regurgitation, foul breath, nausea, vomiting soon after eating, a feeling of heat, sour regurgitation, tongue Red with a thick, dry dark-yellow coating, Deep-Full-Rapid pulse.

This corresponds to either the organ pattern of the Bright-Yang Heat within the identification of patterns according to the Six Stages or to the pattern of Dry-Heat in the Intestines within the identification of patterns according to the Four Levels.

> ## Clinical note
>
> - Umbilical pain is more common in children than in adults.

Central-lower abdominal pain

Interrogation, Chapter 38

In Chinese this area is called *xiao fu* which means 'small abdomen'. It is influenced by the channels of the Kidneys, Bladder, Small Intestine and Directing Vessel.

The symptoms and signs discussed here are only the non-gynaecological ones. Pain in the central-lower abdominal area may of course also be due to various pathologies affecting the Uterus and the Directing Vessel. These are discussed in Chapters 84–89.

Damp-Heat in the Bladder

Central-lower abdominal pain and fullness, frequency and difficulty in urination, burning on urination, dark urine, thirst with no desire to drink, sticky yellow tongue coating on the root, Slippery-Rapid pulse.

Stagnation of Qi in the Bladder

Central-lower abdominal pain and distension, a pronounced feeling of distension in the area immediately over the symphysis pubis, frequent but scanty urination, Wiry pulse.

Intestines deficient and cold

Dull central-lower abdominal pain that comes and goes and is alleviated by warm liquids and the application of heat and aggravated by cold liquids, abdomen cold when touched, cold limbs, loose stools, pale urine, Pale tongue, Deep-Weak pulse.

Stasis of Blood in the Bladder

Stabbing central-lower abdominal pain, blood in the urine, pain on urination, Purple tongue, Deep-Wiry pulse.

Liver-Qi stagnation

Pain and distension of the central-lower abdominal area, urinary difficulty, a pronounced feeling of distension before urination, Wiry pulse.

Liver-Blood stasis

Severe pain of the central-lower abdominal area, urinary difficulty, blood in the urine, Purple tongue, Wiry pulse.

Liver-Fire

Pain of the central-lower abdominal area, urinary difficulty, burning on urination, headaches, dizziness, tinnitus, irritability, propensity to outbursts of anger, red face, thirst, bitter taste, constipation, dark urine, Red tongue with redder sides and dry yellow coating, Wiry-Rapid pulse.

Retention of food and Cold

Pain of the central-lower abdominal area, a pronounced feeling of distension which is worse after eating and with cold, a feeling of fullness, abdomen cold to the touch, Deep-Slippery pulse, tongue with thick sticky coating.

Spleen-Qi deficiency

Pain of the central-lower abdominal area, poor appetite, tiredness, slight abdominal distension, pale complexion, loose stools, Pale tongue, Empty pulse.

Kidney-Yin deficiency

Pain of the central-lower abdominal area, dizziness, tinnitus, night sweating, dry mouth with a desire to sip water, backache, poor memory, dark-scanty urine, tongue without coating, Floating-Empty pulse.

Kidney-Yang deficiency

Pain of the central-lower abdominal area, backache, dizziness, tinnitus, feeling cold, weak knees, bright-white complexion, tiredness, abundant clear urination, Pale and wet tongue, Deep-Weak pulse.

Lateral-lower abdominal pain

Interrogation, Chapter 38

In Chinese the lateral-lower abdominal areas are called *shao fu* which means 'lesser abdomen'. They are under the influence of the channels of the Liver, Large Intestine and Penetrating Vessel. As a rule of thumb, when a problem occurs in the right lateral-lower abdominal area, it is likely to be caused by the gynaecological system; when it occurs in the left lateral-lower abdominal area, it is more likely to be the result of a Large Intestine pathology. However, this is only a broad rule and subject to exceptions.

Liver-Qi stagnation

Lateral-lower abdominal pain and distension, pain coming and going according to emotional mood, irritability, moodiness, constipation with small stools, Wiry pulse.

Damp-Heat in the Large Intestine

Lateral-lower abdominal pain, loose stools with mucus and blood, a feeling of heaviness, thirst with no desire to drink, burning in the anus, tongue with sticky yellow coating, Slippery-Rapid pulse.

Cold-Dampness in the Large Intestine

Lateral-lower abdominal pain, loose stools with mucus, a feeling of heaviness, sticky white tongue coating, Slippery-Slow pulse.

Liver-Blood stasis

Stabbing lateral-lower abdominal pain, a feeling of abdominal mass, hypochondrial pain, painful periods, dark complexion, Purple tongue, Wiry pulse.

Large Intestine deficient and cold

Dull lateral-lower abdominal pain that comes and goes and is better with rest, loose stools, a feeling of cold, cold limbs, pale complexion, tiredness, abdomen cold to the touch, Pale tongue, Deep-Weak pulse.

Girdle Vessel pain 👤

Lateral-lower abdominal pain radiating to the back, or backache radiating to the lateral-lower abdominal area, Wiry pulse.

Stagnation of Qi and stasis of Blood in the Penetrating Vessel 👤

Lateral-lower abdominal pain, a feeling of fullness in the abdomen and umbilical region, a feeling of tightness of the chest, palpitations, anxiety, painful periods, a feeling of lump in the throat, a feeling of heat in the face, Purple tongue, Firm pulse.

Stagnation of Cold in the Liver channel

Lateral-lower abdominal pain radiating to the testis or vagina, contraction of the scrotum or vagina, pain alleviated by the application of heat, pale complexion, cold hands and feet, white tongue coating, Deep-Wiry-Slow pulse.

DISTENSION AND FULLNESS

Abdominal distension

Observation, Chapter 16; Interrogation, Chapter 38

'Distension' (in Chinese called *zhang*) is a word frequently used by Chinese patients; Western patients will seldom use this word and in Anglo-Saxon countries they might say 'bloating' or 'bursting' to express this symptom. Distension is a subjective feeling of the patient but also an objective sign, that is, the abdomen feels distended and hard like a drum on palpation.

Distension is the classic symptom of Qi stagnation; indeed, if there is a feeling of distension there is Qi stagnation. However, a feeling of distension may also be associated with Damp-Phlegm and, in a few cases, with a deficiency of Qi.

Liver-Qi stagnation

Abdominal distension that comes and goes according to emotional moods, hypochondrial or epigastric distension, irritability, moodiness, Wiry pulse.

Spleen-Qi deficiency

Slight abdominal distension after eating, poor appetite, tiredness, pale complexion, loose stools, Pale tongue, Empty pulse.

Damp-Phlegm obstructing the Spleen

Abdominal distension, a pronounced feeling of distension and oppression of the chest and epigastrium, sputum in the throat, a feeling of heaviness, Swollen tongue with sticky coating, Slippery pulse.

Liver-Yin deficiency

Slight abdominal and hypochondrial distension, dizziness, blurred vision, floaters, dry eyes, dry hair, dry nails, insomnia, tongue without coating, Floating-Empty pulse.

Clinical note

- Abdominal distension is one of the most common symptoms of all. Remember that no patient will use the word 'distension' but usually 'bloating'.

Abdominal fullness

Interrogation, Chapter 38

'Fullness' (called *man* in Chinese) indicates a feeling of fullness in the abdomen or epigastrium; this is different from the feeling of distension, from both a subjective and an objective point of view. 'Distension' indicates a subjective feeling of bloating, while the abdomen feels distended and hard like a drum on palpation; 'fullness' indicates a subjective feeling of fullness and obstruction similar to what one feels after eating too much. With 'fullness', the abdomen feels hard on palpation but *not* distended like a drum.

A feeling of fullness generally indicates Dampness or retention of food.

Cold-Dampness in the Intestines

Abdominal fullness, hardness and coldness of the abdomen on palpation, cold limbs, nausea, vomiting, loose stools, sticky white tongue coating, Soft-Slow or Slippery-Slow pulse.

Damp-Heat in the Intestines

Abdominal fullness, hardness of the abdomen on palpation, nausea, vomiting, irritability, thirst with no desire to drink, foul-smelling stools, mucus in stools, dark urine, sticky yellow tongue coating, Slippery-Rapid pulse.

Retention of food

Epigastric fullness, epigastrium feels hard on palpation, nausea, sour regurgitation, belching, thick sticky tongue coating, Slippery pulse.

Stomach and Spleen deficient and cold

Slight abdominal fullness that comes and goes, abdomen not too hard on palpation, tiredness, poor appetite, loose stools, Pale tongue, Weak pulse.

Heat in Bright Yang (Organ pattern)

Umbilical fullness and pain, fever, sweating, intense thirst, constipation, dry stools, Red tongue with dry yellow or brown coating, Deep-Full-Rapid pulse. This corresponds to either the Organ pattern of the Bright-Yang Heat within the identification of patterns according to the Six Stages or to the pattern of Dry-Heat in the Intestines within the identification of patterns according to the Four Levels.

Clinical note

- It is important to explain to patients what we mean by 'fullness' and how it differs from 'distension'.

ABNORMAL FEELINGS IN THE ABDOMEN

Feeling of cold in the abdomen

Interrogation, Chapter 38

This indicates both a subjective feeling of cold and an objective feeling of cold of the abdomen on palpation.

Yang deficiency of the Stomach and Spleen

A feeling of cold of the epigastrium and abdomen, dull epigastric pain, poor appetite, loose stools, tiredness, cold limbs, Pale tongue, Deep-Weak pulse.

Kidney-Yang deficiency

A feeling of cold generally or in the lower abdomen, backache, dizziness, tinnitus, weak knees, bright-white complexion, tiredness, abundant clear urination, Pale and wet tongue, Deep-Weak pulse.

Directing and Penetrating Vessels deficient and cold

A feeling of cold in the lower abdomen (centrally in the case of the Directing Vessel and laterally in the case of the Penetrating Vessel), irregular periods, painful periods, infertility, excessive white vaginal discharge, dark rings under the eyes, Pale tongue, Weak pulse.

Stagnation of Cold in the Liver channel

A feeling of cold in the central-lower abdomen extending to the scrotum, contraction of the scrotum or vagina, cold hands and feet, white tongue coating, Deep-Wiry pulse.

Feeling of pulsation under the umbilicus

Rebellious Qi in the Penetrating Vessel

A feeling of pulsation under the umbilicus, abdominal distension, epigastric fullness and discomfort, a feeling of tightness of the chest, palpitations, anxiety, a feeling of a lump in the throat, a feeling of heat in the face, Firm pulse.

Kidneys not receiving Qi

A feeling of pulsation under the umbilicus, breathlessness, wheezing, sighing, sweating, Pale tongue, Weak pulse.

Phlegm-Fluids in the abdomen

A feeling of pulsation under the umbilicus, abdominal fullness and distension, vomiting of watery fluids, a feeling of oppression of the chest, loose stools, Swollen tongue with sticky coating, Deep-Wiry pulse.

Feeling of energy rising in the abdomen

Western patients will seldom report this symptom as such, but it does occur frequently and must be elicited on interrogation. In Chinese medicine this symptom occurs in the so-called 'Running Piglet' pattern: the patient feels a sensation of energy rising all the way from the lower abdomen to the throat as if there were a running piglet in the abdomen. The most common pathology causing this symptom is rebellious Qi in the Penetrating Vessel.

Rebellious Qi in the Penetrating Vessel

A feeling of energy rising in the abdomen, abdominal distension or fullness, epigastric fullness and discomfort, 'butterflies in the stomach', a feeling of tightness of the chest, palpitations, anxiety, a feeling of a lump in the throat, a feeling of heat in the face, Firm pulse.

Stagnant Liver-Qi turned into Heat rebelling upwards

A feeling of energy rushing up from the abdomen to the throat and face from the lower abdomen, a feeling of heat in the face, anxiety, a tendency to be easily startled, a feeling as if one were going to die, palpitations, abdominal pain, a bitter taste, vomiting, mental restlessness, a feeling of hot and cold, tongue with red sides and yellow coating, Wiry-Rapid pulse.

Yin-Cold in the abdomen

A feeling of energy rising in the abdomen, abdominal fullness, distension and pain, vomiting of watery fluids, a feeling of oppression of the chest, loose stools, a feeling of cold, cold limbs, lower backache, Pale and Swollen tongue with sticky coating, Deep-Tight pulse.

BORBORYGMI

'Borborygmi' indicates a gurgling sound in the intestines.

Liver-Qi invading the Spleen

Borborygmi that come and go according to emotional moods and are not relieved after diarrhoea, abdominal distension, alternation of constipation and diarrhoea, irritability, sighing, pulse Wiry on the left and Weak on the right.

Damp-Heat in the Intestines

Borborygmi, loose stools with foul smell and mucus, burning sensation in the anus, thirst with no desire to drink, sticky taste, sticky yellow tongue coating, Slippery-Rapid pulse.

Damp-Phlegm in the Intestines

Borborygmi, loose stools, a feeling of abdominal fullness, a feeling of oppression of the chest, nausea, vomiting, mucus in the stools, Swollen tongue with sticky coating, Slippery pulse.

Spleen- and Kidney-Yang deficiency

Slight borborygmi, loose stools, backache, dizziness, cold limbs, tiredness, abundant pale urination, Pale and wet tongue, Deep-Weak pulse.

Stomach and Spleen deficient and cold

Slight borborygmi, a feeling of cold in abdomen and epigastrium, loose stools, cold limbs, tiredness, Pale and wet tongue, Deep-Weak pulse.

FLATULENCE

Spleen-Qi deficiency

Flatulence, slight abdominal distension, loose stools, poor appetite, tiredness, pale complexion, Pale tongue, Empty pulse.

Liver-Qi invading the Spleen

Flatulence, hypochondrial and abdominal distension, alternation of constipation and diarrhoea, irritability, tiredness, poor appetite, Pale tongue, pulse Wiry on the left and Weak on the right.

Liver-Qi stagnation

Flatulence, hypochondrial or epigastric distension, irritability, moodiness, Wiry pulse.

SKIN SIGNS

Distended abdominal veins

Observation, Chapter 16

Stasis of Blood in the Liver and Spleen

Blue veins on abdomen, abdominal pain, hypochondrial pain, blood in stools, dark complexion, spider naevi on the throat and chest, Purple tongue, Wiry pulse.

Qi stagnation with Dampness

Blue veins on abdomen, abdominal distension and fullness, a feeling of heaviness, sticky tongue coating, Wiry-Slippery pulse.

Spleen- and Kidney-Yang deficiency

Pale-blue veins on abdomen, abdominal distension, oedema, cold limbs, frequent pale urination, tiredness, weak knees, loose stools, darkish complexion, Pale and wet tongue, Deep-Weak pulse.

Liver- and Kidney-Yin deficiency

Blue veins on abdomen, dizziness, tinnitus, dry eyes, backache, night sweating, tongue without coating, Floating-Empty pulse.

Blood-Heat

Red veins on the abdomen, abdomen hot to the touch, a feeling of heat, skin diseases with red eruptions, dry mouth, bleeding, Red tongue, Rapid pulse.

Stagnation of Cold

Dark blue veins on the abdomen, abdominal pain and distension worse for cold liquids and better for warmth, tongue with white coating, Deep-Slow pulse.

Lines

Observation, Chapter 16

Blood stasis deriving from Cold

Blue lines on the abdomen, abdominal pain, blood in the stools worse with cold liquids and better for warmth, Pale-Purple tongue, Wiry-Slow pulse.

Blood stasis with Blood-Heat

Purple lines on the abdomen, abdominal pain aggravated by exposure to heat, blood in the stools, Reddish-purple tongue, Wiry-Rapid pulse.

Maculae

Observation, Chapter 16

Blood-Heat

Red maculae on the abdomen aggravated by exposure to heat, blood in the stools, skin eruptions, Red tongue, Rapid pulse.

Blood stasis

Purple maculae on the abdomen, abdominal pain, abdomen hard on palpation, Purple tongue, Wiry or Choppy pulse.

ABDOMINAL MASSES

Observation, Chapter 16

Abdominal masses are called *Ji Ju*. *Ji* indicates actual abdominal masses which are fixed and immovable; if there is an associated pain, its location is fixed. These masses are due to stasis of Blood and I call them 'Blood masses'. *Ju* indicates abdominal masses which come and go, do not have a fixed location and are movable. If there is an associated pain, it too comes and goes and changes location. Such masses are due to stagnation of Qi and I call them 'Qi masses'.

Actual abdominal lumps therefore pertain to the category of abdominal masses and specifically *Ji* masses (i.e. Blood masses).

Another name for abdominal masses was *Zheng Jia*, *Zheng* being equivalent to *Ji* (i.e. fixed masses) and *Jia* being equivalent to *Ju* (i.e. non-substantial masses from stagnation of Qi). The two terms *Zheng Jia* normally referred to abdominal masses occurring only in women, but although these masses are more frequent in women they do occur in men as well.

Liver-Qi stagnation

Movable abdominal masses which come and go, abdominal distension and pain which come and go with the masses, irritability, depression, hypochondrial or epigastric distension, irritability, moodiness, Wiry pulse.

Liver-Blood stasis

Hard and immovable abdominal masses, abdominal distension and pain, irritability, painful periods, dark complexion, Purple tongue, Wiry pulse.

Phlegm and retention of food

Masses in the epigastrium or umbilical area, a feeling of fullness, oppression and pain of the epigastrium, Swollen tongue with thick coating, Slippery pulse.

Stomach- and Spleen-Qi deficiency

Soft masses in the epigastrium or umbilical area, slight abdominal distension, poor appetite, tiredness, pale complexion, loose stools, Pale tongue, Empty pulse.

Kidney-Yang deficiency with Liver-Blood stasis

Abdominal masses, backache, dizziness, tinnitus, a feeling of cold, weak knees, bright-white complexion, tiredness, abundant clear urination, Pale and wet tongue, Deep-Weak pulse.

Damp-Phlegm

Abdominal masses which are relatively soft on palpation, a feeling of heaviness, a feeling of oppression of the chest, Swollen tongue with thick sticky coating, Slippery pulse.

Damp-Heat

Abdominal masses, pain, tenderness on palpation, thirst, a feeling of heat, a feeling of heaviness, tongue with sticky yellow coating, Slippery-Rapid pulse.

Small hypochondrial lumps

Observation, Chapter 16

Liver-Blood stasis

Small, hypochondrial lumps, hypochondrial pain, abdominal pain, painful periods, dark complexion, Purple tongue, Wiry pulse.

Lumps in the epigastrium

Observation, Chapter 16

Damp-Phlegm in the Middle Burner

Lumps in the epigastrium which are soft, epigastric distension, a feeling of heaviness, poor appetite, Swollen tongue, Slippery pulse.

Blood stasis

Lumps in the epigastrium which are hard and immovable, epigastric pain, vomiting of blood, dark complexion, Purple tongue, Wiry or Choppy pulse.

Phlegm and Blood stasis in the Middle Burner

Lumps in the epigastrium which are hard and immovable, epigastric distension and pain, vomiting of blood,

dark complexion, Purple and Swollen tongue, Wiry-Slippery pulse.

OEDEMA OF THE ABDOMEN

Observation, Chapter 16

Spleen-Yang deficiency

Oedema of the abdomen, poor appetite, slight abdominal distension after eating, tiredness, lassitude, pale complexion, weakness of the limbs, loose stools, feeling cold, cold limbs, Pale and wet tongue, Deep-Weak pulse.

Kidney-Yang deficiency

Oedema of the abdomen and ankles, lower backache, cold knees, a feeling of cold generally or in the lower back, weak legs, bright-white complexion, weak knees, tiredness, lassitude, abundant clear or scanty clear urination, urination at night, apathy, loose stools, impotence, decreased libido, Pale and wet tongue, Deep-Weak pulse.

ABDOMINAL SIZE

Thin abdomen

Observation, Chapter 16

Qi and Blood deficiency

Thin abdomen, loose stools, tiredness, weak limbs, Pale tongue, Weak or Choppy pulse.

Yin deficiency

Thin abdomen, poor appetite, dizziness, tinnitus, night sweating, dry mouth with a desire to sip water, backache, poor memory, scanty dark urine, tongue without coating, Floating-Empty pulse.

Large abdomen

Observation, Chapter 16

Phlegm obstructing the Spleen

Large abdomen, abdominal distension, oppression of the chest, dizziness, poor appetite, Swollen and Pale tongue, Slippery pulse.

SAGGING LOWER ABDOMEN

Observation, Chapter 16

Damp-Phlegm in the Lower Burner

Sagging lower abdomen, swollen and soft abdomen, abdominal distension, a feeling of heaviness, Swollen tongue, Slippery pulse.

Severe Spleen- and Kidney-Yang deficiency

Sagging lower abdomen, tiredness, lethargy, feeling cold, frequent clear urination, lower backache, Pale and Wet tongue, Deep-Weak pulse.

UMBILICUS

Protruding umbilicus

Observation, Chapter 16

Empty-Cold with Qi stagnation

Protruding umbilicus worse with cold liquids, better for warmth, worse with emotional upsets, Pale tongue, Deep-Weak-Slow and slightly Wiry pulse.

Blood stasis with oedema

Protruding umbilicus, pain around the umbilicus, swollen abdomen, blood in the stools, Purple tongue, Wiry or Choppy pulse.

Spleen- and Kidney-Yang deficiency

Protruding umbilicus worse with cold, loose stools, tiredness, Pale and Wet tongue, Deep-Weak pulse.

Sunken umbilicus

Observation, Chapter 16

Blood stasis with Spleen-Qi sinking

Sunken umbilicus, pain around the umbilicus, a feeling of bearing down, tiredness, blood in the stools, Pale-Purple tongue, Wiry or Choppy pulse.

Damp-Heat in the abdomen

Sunken umbilicus, umbilical area tender on palpation, abdominal distension, swollen abdomen, tongue with sticky yellow coating, Slippery-Rapid pulse.

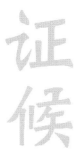

Chapter **72**

DEFECATION

Chapter contents

DIARRHOEA OR LOOSE STOOLS   *747*

DIARRHOEA WITH VOMITING   *748*

CONSTIPATION   *748*

ALTERNATION OF CONSTIPATION AND LOOSE STOOLS   *749*

INCONTINENCE OF FAECES   *750*

BLOOD AND MUCUS IN THE STOOLS   *750*

MUCUS IN THE STOOLS   *751*

BLOOD IN THE STOOLS   *751*

DIFFICULTY IN DEFECATION   *751*

STRAINING IN DEFECATION   *752*

DIARRHOEA OR LOOSE STOOLS

Interrogation, Chapter 31

Spleen-Qi deficiency

Loose stools, slight abdominal distension, poor appetite, tiredness, pale complexion, Pale tongue, Empty pulse.

Kidney-Yang deficiency

Early-morning diarrhoea, lower backache, cold knees, a feeling of cold, bright-white complexion, weak knees, tiredness, lassitude, abundant clear urination, urination at night, impotence, decreased libido, Pale and wet tongue, Deep-Weak pulse.

Liver-Qi invading the Spleen

Loose stools or alternation of loose stools and constipation, stools sometimes dry and bitty and sometimes loose, flatulence, irritability, abdominal distension and pain, tiredness, poor appetite, normal-coloured tongue (or slightly Red on the sides in severe cases of Liver-Qi stagnation), pulse Wiry on the left and Weak on the right.

Damp-Heat in the Intestines

Loose stools with foul smell and mucus and possibly blood, offensive odour of stools, burning in the anus, abdominal pain that is not relieved by a bowel movement, scanty dark urine, fever, sweating which does not decrease the fever, a feeling of heat, thirst without a desire to drink, a feeling of heaviness of the body and limbs, Red tongue with sticky yellow coating, Slippery-Rapid pulse.

Cold-Dampness in the Intestines

Loose stools with mucus and without smell, abdominal pain, abdominal fullness, undigested food in the stools,

a feeling of cold, cold limbs, a feeling of heaviness, sticky white tongue coating, Slippery-Slow pulse.

Spleen-Qi deficient and sinking

Chronic loose stools or normal but very frequent stools, urgency, a dragging-down feeling, tiredness, depression, poor appetite, weak limbs, Pale tongue with teethmarks, Weak pulse.

Retention of food

Loose stools, fullness, pain and distension of the epigastrium which are relieved by vomiting, nausea, vomiting of sour fluids, foul breath, sour regurgitation, belching, insomnia, poor appetite, thick tongue coating, Full-Slippery pulse.

DIARRHOEA WITH VOMITING

Food poisoning

Violent diarrhoea and vomiting with sudden onset, nausea at the smell of food, epigastric fullness, sour regurgitation, thick tongue coating, Slippery pulse.

Cold-Dampness in the Stomach and Intestines

Diarrhoea without smell, and vomiting, mucus in the stools, abdominal pain that is alleviated by application of heat, epigastric and abdominal fullness, a feeling of heaviness of the head and body, a feeling of cold, cold limbs, sticky white tongue coating, Slippery-Slow pulse.

Stomach and Intestines deficient and cold

Diarrhoea and vomiting of watery fluids, dull abdominal pain, discomfort or dull pain in the epigastrium, better after eating and with pressure or massage, no appetite, preference for warm drinks and foods, vomiting of clear fluid, absence of thirst, cold and weak limbs, tiredness, pale complexion, Pale and wet tongue, Deep-Weak-Slow pulse.

Retention of food

Diarrhoea with vomiting, fullness, pain and distension of the epigastrium which are relieved by vomiting, nausea, vomiting of sour fluids, foul breath, sour regurgitation, belching, insomnia, loose stools or constipation, poor appetite, thick tongue coating, Full-Slippery pulse.

Invasion of Summer-Heat

Sudden diarrhoea and vomiting, epigastric pain, sour regurgitation, aversion to cold, fever, thirst, irritability, a feeling of oppression of the chest, headache, cold hands and feet, dark urine, Floating-Rapid pulse.

CONSTIPATION

Interrogation, Chapter 31

The term 'constipation' is used to describe the slow movement of unduly firm contents through the large bowel leading to infrequent passing of small hard stools. Thus, constipation may indicate several different symptoms, among which are:

- bowel movements which do not occur daily
- dry stools
- difficult defecation
- abnormal shape of stools.

Views on what constitutes a normal frequency of bowel movement vary widely. From the point of view of Chinese medicine the bowel movement should occur at least once a day. This view runs counter to the Western medical view, according to which the frequency of bowel movement is not that important so long so they occur regularly.

Heat in the Intestines

Constipation with dry stools, burning sensation in the mouth, dry tongue, burning and swelling in anus, scanty dark urine, thick, dry yellow (or brown or black) tongue coating, Full-Rapid pulse.

Liver-Fire

Constipation with dry stools, headaches, dizziness, tinnitus, irritability, propensity to outbursts of anger, red face, thirst, bitter taste, dark urine, Red tongue with redder sides and dry yellow coating, Wiry-Rapid pulse.

Heat in Bright Yang (organ syndrome)

Constipation with dry stools, abdominal pain and fullness, fever, burning epigastric pain, intense thirst with a desire to drink cold liquids, mental restlessness, dry mouth, mouth ulcers, bleeding gums, sour regurgitation, foul breath, nausea, vomiting soon after eating, a feeling of heat, tongue Red with a thick, dry dark-yellow coating, Deep-Full-Rapid pulse.

This corresponds either to the organ pattern of Heat in Bright Yang within the identification of patterns according to the Six Stages or to the pattern of Dry-Heat in the Intestines within the identification of patterns according to the Four Levels.

Liver-Qi stagnation

Constipation with small stools, or alternation of constipation with diarrhoea, difficulty in defecation, hypochondrial or epigastric distension, irritability, moodiness, a feeling of a lump in the throat, premenstrual tension, Wiry pulse.

Kidney-Yang deficiency

Chronic constipation, exhaustion after bowel movement, stools not dry, lower backache, cold knees, a feeling of cold, bright-white complexion, weak knees, tiredness, lassitude, abundant clear urination, urination at night, impotence, decreased libido, Pale and wet tongue, Deep-Weak pulse.

Blood deficiency

Dry stools, difficulty in defecation, dizziness, blurred vision, floaters, numbness/tingling of the limbs, scanty menstruation, dull-pale complexion, Pale tongue, Choppy or Fine pulse.

Yin deficiency of the Stomach and Intestines

Constipation, dry stools, no appetite or slight hunger but no desire to eat, dull or slightly burning epigastric pain, abdominal pain, dry mouth and throat especially in the afternoon, thirst but no desire to drink, or a desire to drink in small sips, a slight feeling of fullness after eating, normal-coloured tongue without coating, or without coating, in the centre, Floating-Empty pulse.

Kidney- and Liver-Yin deficiency

Dry stools, dizziness, tinnitus, hardness of hearing, lower backache, dull occipital or vertical headache, insomnia, numbness/tingling of the limbs, dry eyes, blurred vision, dry throat, dry hair and skin, brittle nails, night sweating, scanty menstruation or amenorrhoea, normal-coloured tongue without coating, Floating-Empty pulse.

Spleen- and Lung-Qi deficiency

Constipation with difficulty in opening the bowels with a feeling of exhaustion afterwards, thin and long stools that are not dry, poor appetite, slight abdominal distension after eating, tiredness, lassitude, pale complexion, weakness of the limbs, slight shortness of breath, slight cough, weak voice, spontaneous daytime sweating, a dislike of speaking, bright-white complexion, tendency to catch colds, tiredness, dislike of cold, Pale tongue, Empty pulse.

Cold in the Intestines

Constipation, stools not dry, absence of bowel movement for several days, spastic abdominal pain, a cold sensation in abdomen, thick white tongue coating, Deep-Wiry pulse.

Dampness in the Intestines

Constipation, a feeling of fullness and heaviness of the abdomen, abdominal pain, sticky taste, thick sticky tongue coating on the root, pulse Slippery on both Rear positions.

Retention of food in the Intestines

Constipation, abdominal pain alleviated by evacuation, a feeling of fullness of the abdomen, thick sticky tongue coating on the root, pulse that is Slippery on both rear positions.

Clinical note

- When a patient complains about 'constipation', always establish clearly what they are referring to (i.e. frequency of stool, consistency of it or difficulty in passing a stool).

ALTERNATION OF CONSTIPATION AND LOOSE STOOLS

Alternation of constipation and loose stools means that the patient goes through periods of constipation (by which is meant that the stools are infrequent or rather difficult and bitty) followed by a period of loose stools; these periods may last days or weeks.

Interrogation, Chapter 31

Stagnant Liver-Qi invading the Spleen

Alternation of periods of constipation and loose stools, small and bitty stools, straining on defecation during the periods of constipation, abdominal distension, abdominal pain that is not relieved by the bowel movement, hypochondrial or epigastric distension,

irritability, moodiness, a feeling of a lump in the throat, premenstrual tension, tongue that may have Red sides (if Liver-Qi stagnation predominates) or Pale sides (if Spleen-Qi deficiency predominates), pulse that is Wiry on the left and Weak on the right.

Stagnant Liver-Qi invading the Spleen, Dampness

Alternation of periods of constipation and loose stools, small and bitty stools, mucus in the stools, straining on defecation during the periods of constipation, abdominal distension and fullness, abdominal pain that may be relieved by the bowel movement (if Dampness predominates), hypochondrial or epigastric distension, irritability, moodiness, a feeling of a lump in the throat, premenstrual tension, a feeling of heaviness of the abdomen, tongue that may have Red sides (if Liver-Qi stagnation predominates) or Pale sides (if Spleen-Qi deficiency predominates) with a sticky coating, pulse that is Wiry on the left and Soggy on the right.

Severe Spleen-Qi deficiency

Alternation of constipation and loose stools, no abdominal pain or fullness, poor appetite, slight abdominal distension after eating, tiredness, lassitude, pale complexion, weakness of the limbs, loose stools, Pale tongue, Empty pulse.

> ### Clinical note
>
> - I find nearly always that the so-called 'irritable bowel syndrome' characterized by alternation of constipation and loose stools is due to three pathogenic conditions in varying proportions:
>   —Liver-Qi stagnation
>   —Spleen-Qi deficiency
>   —Dampness.

INCONTINENCE OF FAECES

Spleen- and Kidney-Yang deficiency

Incontinence of faeces, early-morning diarrhoea, lower backache, cold and weak knees, a feeling of cold, bright-white complexion, impotence, decreased libido, tiredness, lassitude, abundant clear urination, urination at night, loose stools, poor appetite, slight abdominal distension, a desire to lie down, Pale and wet tongue, Deep-Weak pulse.

Spleen- and Lung-Qi deficiency

Incontinence of faeces, poor appetite, slight abdominal distension after eating, tiredness, pale complexion, weakness of the limbs, loose stools, slight shortness of breath, slight cough, weak voice, spontaneous daytime sweating, a dislike of speaking, tendency to catch colds, dislike of cold, Pale tongue, Empty pulse.

This pattern usually occurs only in the elderly.

BLOOD AND MUCUS IN THE STOOLS

Interrogation, Chapter 31

Damp-Heat in the Intestines

Diarrhoea with blood and mucus, a burning sensation of the anus, a feeling of heaviness, abdominal pain, a feeling of heat, Red tongue with sticky yellow coating, Slippery-Rapid pulse.

Deficiency of Yin of the Stomach and Intestines with Empty-Heat

Blood and mucus in the stools, dull abdominal pain, dull or burning epigastric pain, a feeling of heat in the afternoon, dry mouth and throat especially in the afternoon, thirst with a desire to drink in small sips, feeling of hunger but no desire to eat, night sweating, five-palm heat, bleeding gums, Red tongue (or Red centre only) without coating in the centre, Floating-Empty and Rapid pulse.

Cold-Dampness in the Intestines

Diarrhoea with a lot of mucus and a little blood, abdominal pain and fullness, nausea, vomiting, a feeling of heaviness, cold limbs, Pale tongue with sticky white coating, Slippery-Slow pulse.

Large Intestine deficient and cold

Diarrhoea with little mucus and blood, dull abdominal pain that is relieved by the application of heat, a feeling of cold, cold limbs, tiredness, Pale tongue, Deep-Weak pulse.

Toxic Heat in the Intestines

Diarrhoea with mucus and blood, foul-smelling stools, a burning sensation of the anus, fever, a feeling of heat, abdominal pain, Red tongue with red points and thick, sticky yellow coating, Overflowing-Slippery-Rapid pulse.

Clinical note

- Blood and mucus in the stools may indicate ulcerative colitis and the patient should always be referred for a colonoscopy.

MUCUS IN THE STOOLS

Interrogation, Chapter 31

Dampness in the Intestines

Mucus in the stools, loose stools, abdominal fullness/pain, a feeling of heaviness of the abdomen, a sticky taste, sticky tongue coating, Slippery pulse.

Damp-Heat in the Intestines

Mucus in the stools, loose stools with foul smell, a burning sensation of the anus, abdominal fullness and pain, a feeling of heaviness of the abdomen, a sticky taste, thirst without desire to drink, sticky yellow tongue coating, Slippery-Rapid pulse.

BLOOD IN THE STOOLS

Interrogation, Chapter 31

Chinese medicine differentiates this symptom according to the colour of the blood to identify the pattern without consideration of the site of bleeding. In this instance, however, it is important to ask the patient to obtain a Western diagnosis as well. In fact, blood in the stools can be caused by bleeding haemorrhoids or anal fissures, or by bleeding within the large intestine; obviously these two symptoms are very different in pathology and severity.

Damp-Heat in the Intestines

Fresh blood in the stools, loose stools, smelly stools, abdominal pain, a burning sensation in the anus, a feeling of heaviness, abdominal fullness, Red tongue with sticky yellow coating and red spots on the root, Slippery-Rapid pulse.

Stomach- and Spleen-Qi deficiency

Profuse fresh blood in the stools, no smell, loose stools, slight abdominal pain, poor appetite, slight abdominal distension after eating, tiredness, lassitude, pale complexion, weakness of the limbs, an uncomfortable feeling in the epigastrium, lack of taste sensation, Pale tongue, Empty pulse.

Heat in the Intestines

Dark blood in the stools, abdominal pain, constipation, a feeling of heat, thirst, Red tongue with dry yellow coating, Deep-Full-Rapid pulse.

Toxic Heat in the Intestines

Diarrhoea with mucus and blood, foul-smelling stools, a burning sensation of the anus, fever, feeling of heat, abdominal pain, Red tongue with red points and thick, sticky yellow coating, Overflowing-Slippery-Rapid pulse.

Blood stasis in the Intestines

Dark blood in the stools, abdominal pain, dark complexion, anxiety, Purple tongue, Wiry pulse.

Liver- and Kidney-Yin deficiency with Empty-Heat

Fresh blood in the stools, constipation, dizziness, tinnitus, dull occipital or vertical headache, insomnia, numbness/tingling of limbs, malar flush, dry eyes, blurred vision, lower backache, dry throat, dry hair and skin, brittle nails, dry vagina, night sweating, scanty menstruation, five-palm heat, a feeling of heat in the evening, Red tongue without coating, Floating-Empty and Rapid pulse.

DIFFICULTY IN DEFECATION

Interrogation, Chapter 31

'Difficulty in defecation' is a translation of the complex Chinese symptom called *li ji hou zhong*. This symptom is composed of two parts: *li ji* means that the patient has abdominal pain and the urge to defecate but is unable to; *hou zhong* means that the patient does defecate eventually but the abdominal discomfort is not relieved by it and there is a feeling of heaviness after defecation.

Stagnation of Qi in the Intestines

Difficulty in defecation, abdominal distension, abdominal pain before defecation not relieved after defecation, small, bitty stools, Wiry pulse.

Damp-Heat in the Intestines

Difficulty in defecation, abdominal pain relieved by defecation, burning sensation in the anus, mucus in the stools, foul-smelling stools, a feeling of heaviness, sticky yellow tongue coating, Slippery-Rapid pulse.

Spleen-Qi deficiency

Difficulty in defecation or loose stools, tiredness after defecation, slight abdominal distension, poor appetite, tiredness, pale complexion, Pale tongue, Empty pulse.

Intestines Dryness and Liver-Blood deficiency

Difficulty in defecation, dry stools, dull abdominal pain, dry skin, dizziness, blurred vision, floaters, numbness/tingling of limbs, scanty menstruation, dull-pale complexion, Pale tongue, Choppy or Fine pulse.

STRAINING IN DEFECATION

Interrogation, Chapter 31

'Straining in defecation' means that the patient does have a bowel movement every day but the movement takes a long time and involves straining. 'Straining in defecation' differs from 'constipation' in three respects:

> 1. With 'straining in defecation', unlike 'constipation', there is a bowel movement every day
> 2. With 'straining in defecation', unlike 'constipation' the stools are not dry
> 3. With 'straining in defecation', unlike 'constipation', there are no other obvious abdominal symptoms such as pain, fullness or distension.

Liver-Qi invading the Spleen

Straining in defecation, small stools, alternation of constipation and diarrhoea, stools sometimes dry and bitty and sometimes loose, abdominal distension, flatulence, tiredness, poor appetite, normal-coloured tongue (or slightly Red on the sides in severe cases of Liver-Qi stagnation), pulse Wiry on the left and Weak on the right.

Spleen- and Lung-Qi deficiency

Straining in defecation with a feeling of exhaustion afterwards, poor appetite, slight abdominal distension after eating, tiredness, pale complexion, weakness of the limbs, slight shortness of breath, slight cough, weak voice, spontaneous daytime sweating, dislike of speaking, tendency to catch colds, dislike of cold, Pale tongue, Empty pulse.

This pattern usually occurs in the elderly.

Spleen- and Kidney-Yang deficiency

Straining in defecation, occasionally loose stools, exhaustion after defecation, slight abdominal distension, lower backache, cold and weak knees, a feeling of cold, bright-white complexion, impotence, decreased libido, tiredness, lassitude, abundant clear urination, urination at night, poor appetite, a desire to lie down, early-morning diarrhoea, Pale and wet tongue, Deep-Weak pulse.

This pattern usually occurs in the elderly.

Kidney- and Liver-Yin deficiency

Straining in defecation, dry stools, dizziness, tinnitus, weak knees, hardness of hearing, lower backache, dull occipital or vertical headache, insomnia, numbness/tingling of the limbs, dry eyes, blurred vision, dry throat in the evening, dry hair and skin, brittle nails, night sweating, scanty menstruation or amenorrhoea, normal-coloured tongue without coating, Floating-Empty pulse.

Damp-Heat in the Intestines

Straining in defecation, mucus in the stools, foul-smelling stools, burning sensation in the anus, abdominal pain and fullness, a feeling of heaviness, sticky yellow tongue coating, Slippery-Rapid pulse.

Heat in the Intestines

Straining in defecation, small stools, a feeling of heat, thirst, red face, Red tongue with dry yellow coating, Deep-Full-Rapid pulse.

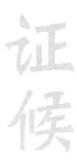

Chapter **73**

URINATION

Chapter contents

DARK URINE   753

PALE AND ABUNDANT URINE   754

TURBID URINE   754

PAINFUL URINATION   754

SCANTY AND DIFFICULT URINATION   755

DIFFICULT URINATION   755

FREQUENT URINATION   756

DRIBBLING OF URINE   756

INCONTINENCE OF URINE   757

NOCTURNAL ENURESIS   757

URINATION AT NIGHT   758

BLOOD IN THE URINE   758

SPERM IN THE URINE   759

DARK URINE

Interrogation, Chapter 31

Damp-Heat in the Bladder

Dark urine, frequent and urgent urination, burning on urination, difficult urination, dark-yellow/turbid urine, thirst with no desire to drink, hypogastric fullness and pain, feeling of heat, thick, sticky yellow coating on the tongue root with red spots, Slippery-Rapid pulse.

Kidney-Yin deficiency with Empty-Heat

Dark and scanty urine, slight burning on urination, dizziness, tinnitus, hardness of hearing, night sweating, dry mouth at night, five-palm heat, a feeling of heat in the evening, malar flush, thirst with a desire to drink in small sips, lower backache, insomnia, Red tongue without coating, Floating-Empty and Rapid pulse.

Heat in the Heart and Small Intestine

Dark urine which may contain blood, burning on urination, a feeling of heat, anxiety, red face, insomnia, palpitations, tongue ulcers, excessive dreaming, Red tongue with redder tip and yellow coating, Rapid-Overflowing pulse.

Damp-Heat in the Liver

Dark and scanty urine, urinary difficulty, burning on urination, fullness of the hypochondrium, abdomen or hypogastrium, bitter taste, nausea, a feeling of heaviness of the body, yellow vaginal discharge, vaginal itching, mid-cycle bleeding/pain, genital papular or vesicular shin rashes and itching, Red tongue with redder sides and sticky yellow coating, Slippery-Wiry-Rapid pulse.

Heat in the Intestines

Dark and scanty urine, thirst, abdominal pain, constipation, abdominal fullness, Red tongue with dry yellow coating, Overflowing-Rapid pulse.

Cold-Dampness in the Intestines

Dark and turbid urine coloured like tea, *not* scanty, difficulty in urination, mucus in the stools, abdominal fullness and pain, pale complexion, a feeling of heaviness, cold limbs, sticky white tongue coating on the root, Slippery-Slow pulse.

In this pattern, it is the Dampness, rather than the Cold, that makes the urine darkish and turbid.

> ### Clinical note
>
> - In women it is often difficult to establish the colour of the urine as they often do not look after micturition to take notice of the colour.

PALE AND ABUNDANT URINE

Interrogation, Chapter 31

Kidney-Yang deficiency

Pale and abundant urine, urination at night, lower backache, cold knees, feeling cold, bright-white complexion, weak knees, tiredness, lassitude, impotence, decreased libido, Pale and wet tongue, Deep-Weak pulse.

Cold in the Bladder

Pale and abundant urine, a feeling of cold, cold limbs, lower backache, central-lower abdominal pain that is alleviated by the application of heat, Pale tongue, Deep-Weak pulse.

TURBID URINE

Interrogation, Chapter 31

Dampness in the Bladder

Turbid urine like rice soup, difficult urination, pain on urination, a feeling of heaviness, sticky tongue coating on the root, Slippery pulse.

Other symptoms and signs depend on whether the Dampness is associated with Cold or Heat.

Kidney-Yin deficiency

Turbid and dilute urine like a sauce, scanty urine, dizziness, tinnitus, hardness of hearing, poor memory, night sweating, dry mouth and throat at night, lower backache, constipation, tiredness, normal-coloured tongue without coating, Floating-Empty pulse.

Kidney-Yang deficiency

Turbid and abundant urine, dribbling after urination, urination at night, lower backache, cold knees, a feeling of cold, bright-white complexion, weak knees, tiredness, lassitude, impotence, decreased libido, Pale and wet tongue, Deep-Weak pulse.

Spleen-Qi deficiency

Turbid urine, dribbling after urination, poor appetite, slight abdominal distension after eating, tiredness, pale complexion, weakness of the limbs, loose stools, Pale tongue, Empty pulse.

PAINFUL URINATION

Interrogation, Chapter 31

'Painful urination' comes under the Chinese medicine heading of *Lin* disease, which, by definition, is characterized by painful urination. There are six types of *Lin* diseases: Heat, Stone, Qi, Blood, Sticky and Fatigue *Lin*, all of which present with painful and difficult urination.

Damp-Heat in the Bladder

Pain during urination, difficult urination, burning on urination, dark urine, turbid urine, frequent and urgent urination, thirst with no desire to drink, hypogastric fullness and pain, a feeling of heat, thick, sticky yellow coating on the root with red spots, Slippery-Rapid pulse.

Heat-Fire 👤

Pain during urination, burning on urination, dark urine, occasionally blood in the urine, palpitations, thirst, mouth and tongue ulcers, mental restlessness, feeling agitated, insomnia, dream-disturbed sleep, a feeling of heat, red face, bitter taste, Red tongue with redder tip and yellow coating, Overflowing-Rapid pulse.

Liver-Fire 👤

Burning pain during urination, dark urine, hypogastric distension, headache, red face, dizziness, tinni-

tus, irritability, propensity to outbursts of anger, thirst, bitter taste, constipation, Red tongue with redder sides and dry yellow coating, Wiry-Rapid pulse.

Liver-Qi stagnation

Pain before urination, hypogastric distension, hypochondrial or epigastric distension, irritability, moodiness, a feeling of a lump in the throat, premenstrual tension, Wiry pulse.

Stasis of Blood in the Bladder

Painful before urination, blood in the urine, stabbing hypogastric pain, lower abdominal pain, Purple tongue, Wiry pulse.

Kidney-Yin deficiency with Empty-Heat

Slight pain during urination, scanty and dark urine, dizziness, tinnitus, hardness of hearing, night sweating, dry mouth at night, five-palm heat, a feeling of heat in the evening, malar flush, thirst with a desire to drink in small sips, lower backache, scanty dark urine, insomnia, Red tongue without coating, Floating-Empty and Rapid pulse.

SCANTY AND DIFFICULT URINATION

Interrogation, Chapter 31

Damp-Heat in the Bladder

Scanty, difficult and painful urination, dark urine, turbid urine, frequent and urgent urination, thirst with no desire to drink, hypogastric fullness and pain, a feeling of heat, thick, sticky yellow coating on the root with red spots, Slippery-Rapid pulse.

Liver-Qi stagnation

Scanty and difficult urination, absence of pain during urination, pain and distension of the hypogastrium before urination, hypochondrial or epigastric distension, irritability, moodiness, a feeling of lump in the throat, premenstrual tension, Wiry pulse.

Kidney-Yin deficiency

Scanty and difficult urination, dark urine, dizziness, tinnitus, hardness of hearing, poor memory, night sweating, dry mouth and throat at night, lower backache, constipation, tiredness, normal-coloured tongue without coating, Floating-Empty pulse.

Kidney-Yang deficiency

Scanty and difficult urination, pale urine, absence of pain on urination, urination at night, lower backache, cold knees, a feeling of cold, bright-white complexion, weak knees, tiredness, lassitude, impotence, decreased libido, Pale and wet tongue, Deep-Weak pulse.

Normally, Kidney-Yang deficiency causes the urination to be abundant; however, in rare cases, Kidney-Yang may be so deficient that it fails to move fluids at all and therefore the urine becomes scanty.

Spleen-Yang deficiency with Dampness

Scanty and difficult urination, absence of pain on urination, pale, slightly turbid urine, poor appetite, slight abdominal distension after eating, abdominal fullness, a sticky taste, tiredness, excessive vaginal discharge, lassitude, pale complexion, weakness of the limbs, loose stools, a feeling of cold, cold limbs, Pale and wet tongue, Deep-Weak pulse.

Deficient Lung-Qi not descending

Scanty and difficult urination, absence of pain on urination, oedema of face, slight shortness of breath, slight cough, weak voice, spontaneous daytime sweating, dislike of speaking, bright-white complexion, tendency to catch colds, tiredness, a dislike of cold, Pale tongue, Empty pulse.

DIFFICULT URINATION

Interrogation, Chapter 31

Damp-Heat in the Bladder

Difficult and painful urination, dark and turbid urine, frequent and urgent urination, thirst with no desire to drink, hypogastric fullness and pain, a feeling of heat, thick, sticky yellow coating on the root with red spots, Slippery-Rapid pulse.

Lung-Qi deficiency

Difficult urination but absence of pain, slight shortness of breath, slight cough, weak voice, spontaneous daytime sweating, dislike of speaking, bright-white complexion, tendency to catch colds, tiredness, a dislike of cold, Pale tongue, Empty pulse.

This condition generally occurs only in the elderly.

Stomach- and Spleen-Qi deficiency

Difficult urination but absence of pain, poor appetite, slight abdominal distension after eating, tiredness, lassitude, pale complexion, weakness of the limbs, loose stools, an uncomfortable feeling in the epigastrium, loss of sense of taste, Pale tongue, Empty pulse.

Kidney-Yang deficiency

Difficult urination pale urine, absence of pain on urination, lower backache, cold knees, a feeling of cold, bright-white complexion, weak knees, tiredness, lassitude, abundant clear urination, urination at night, impotence, decreased libido, Pale and wet tongue, Deep-Weak pulse.

Liver-Qi stagnation

Difficult urination but absence of pain, pain and distension of the hypogastrium before urination, hypochondrial or epigastric distension, irritability, moodiness, a feeling of a lump in the throat, premenstrual tension, Wiry pulse.

Stasis of Blood in the Lower Burner

Difficult urination, pain before micturition, urination stops and starts, hypogastric pain, Purple tongue, Wiry pulse.

FREQUENT URINATION

Interrogation, Chapter 31

'Frequent urination' indicates excessive frequency of micturition. This varies between men and women as women have a larger bladder and need to urinate less frequently than men; thus 'frequent urination' could be defined as urinating more than three times a day for women and more than about five to six times for men. Urinating at night is never normal and is also a type of frequent urination, which will be discussed separately below.

Kidney-Yang deficiency

Frequent, abundant and pale urination, urination at night, lower backache, cold knees, a feeling of cold, bright-white complexion, weak knees, tiredness, lassitude, impotence, decreased libido, Pale and wet tongue, Deep-Weak pulse.

Lung- and Spleen-Qi deficiency

Frequent urination, a feeling of bearing down, slight incontinence of urine, poor appetite, slight abdominal distension after eating, tiredness, pale complexion, weakness of the limbs, loose stools, slight shortness of breath, slight cough, weak voice, spontaneous daytime sweating, dislike of speaking, tendency to catch colds, Pale tongue, Empty pulse.

Damp-Heat in the Bladder

Frequent, scanty and dark urination, burning on urination, difficulty in urination, thirst with no desire to drink, hypogastric fullness and pain, a feeling of heat, thick, sticky yellow coating on the root with red spots, Slippery-Rapid pulse.

Kidney-Yin deficiency

Frequent, scanty and dark urine, dizziness, tinnitus, hardness of hearing, poor memory, night sweating, dry mouth and throat at night, lower backache, constipation, tiredness, normal-coloured tongue without coating, Floating-Empty pulse.

> ### Clinical note
>
> - We should not ask patients whether urination is frequent but should ask specifically how many times they urinate in a day. This information is often of no clinical value if the patient is forcing himself or herself to drink large amounts of water.

DRIBBLING OF URINE

Interrogation, Chapter 31

Kidney-Qi not firm

Dribbling of urine which is worse after sex, clear frequent urination, weak-stream urination, abundant urination, incontinence of urine, urination at night, soreness and weakness of the lower back, weak knees, premature ejaculation, in women prolapse of uterus, chronic white vaginal discharge, tiredness, a dragging-down feeling in the lower abdomen, a feeling of cold, cold limbs, Pale tongue, Deep-Weak pulse.

Stomach- and Spleen-Qi deficiency

Dribbling of urine, poor appetite, slight abdominal distension after eating, tiredness, lassitude, pale complexion, weakness of the limbs, loose stools, an uncomfortable feeling in the epigastrium, loss of sense of taste, Pale tongue, Empty pulse.

Damp-Heat in the Bladder

Dribbling of urine, difficult urination, burning on urination, dark urine, turbid urine, frequent and urgent urination, thirst with no desire to drink, hypogastric fullness and pain, feeling of heat, thick sticky yellow coating on the tongue root with red spots, Slippery-Rapid pulse.

INCONTINENCE OF URINE

Interrogation, Chapter 31

'Incontinence of urine' should be differentiated from 'enuresis' (see below): the former indicates involuntary urination with the person conscious of it happening, whereas enuresis, usually occurring at night, indicates involuntary urination of which the person is not conscious.

Kidney-Qi not firm

Incontinence of urine which is worse after sex, clear frequent urination, weak-stream urination, abundant urination, incontinence of urine, urination at night, soreness and weakness of the lower back, weak knees, premature ejaculation, in women prolapse of uterus, chronic white vaginal discharge, tiredness, a dragging-down feeling in the lower abdomen, a feeling of cold, cold limbs, Pale tongue, Deep-Weak pulse.

Lung- and Spleen-Qi deficiency

Incontinence of urine, poor appetite, slight abdominal distension after eating, tiredness, pale complexion, weakness of the limbs, loose stools, slight shortness of breath, slight cough, weak voice, spontaneous daytime sweating, dislike of speaking, tendency to catch colds, Pale tongue, Empty pulse.

This usually occurs in old people.

Heat in the Bladder

Incontinence of urine, scanty dark urination, burning on urination, thirst, dry yellow tongue coating, pulse Wiry on the left Rear position and Rapid.

Liver- and Kidney-Yin deficiency

Incontinence of urine, scanty urination, dark urine, dizziness, tinnitus, weak knees, hardness of hearing, lower backache, dull occipital or vertical headache, insomnia, numbness/tingling of the limbs, dry eyes, blurred vision, dry throat in the evening, dry hair and skin, brittle nails, night sweating, dry stools, scanty menstruation or amenorrhoea, normal-coloured tongue without coating, Floating-Empty pulse.

NOCTURNAL ENURESIS

Interrogation, Chapter 31

'Nocturnal enuresis' should be differentiated from 'incontinence of urine': the former occurs at night and the person is obviously unaware of it; the latter occurs at any time and the person is aware it is happening. Nocturnal enuresis should also be differentiated from urination at night (or nocturia): the former occurs when the person is asleep and is obviously not conscious of it; the latter occurs when the patient wakes and gets up at night to urinate. Nocturnal enuresis is much more frequent in children.

Kidney-Yang deficiency

Nocturnal enuresis, abundant clear urination, urination at night, lower backache, cold knees, a feeling of cold, bright-white complexion, weak knees, tiredness, lassitude, impotence, decreased libido, Pale and wet tongue, Deep-Weak pulse.

In children, this is usually a constitutional Kidney-Yang deficiency and due to their age, there will not be many symptoms of Kidney deficiency. Indeed, if a child suffers from nocturnal enuresis and the tongue is Pale and the Kidney pulse is Weak, these signs are enough to diagnose a constitutional Kidney-Yang deficiency. This child will usually be a quiet, shy child without much energy.

Liver-Fire

Nocturnal enuresis, dark urine, headache, red face, dizziness, tinnitus, irritability, propensity to outbursts of anger, thirst, bitter taste, constipation, dark urine, Red tongue with redder sides and dry yellow coating, Wiry-Rapid pulse.

This is fairly common in children and this child will be tense and highly strung, in contrast to the previous condition of constitutional Kidney-Yang deficiency. As in the former pattern, a child may have very few symptoms of Liver-Fire such as red sides of the tongue, irritability and thirst.

Spleen-Qi deficient and sinking

Nocturnal enuresis, tiredness, poor appetite, loose stools, slight abdominal distension, a bearing-down

feeling, prolapse of the uterus, Pale tongue, Weak pulse.

Lung-Qi deficiency

Nocturnal enuresis, slight shortness of breath, slight cough, weak voice, spontaneous daytime sweating, a dislike of speaking, bright-white complexion, tendency to catch colds, tiredness, a dislike of cold, Pale tongue, Empty pulse.

Kidney-Yin deficiency

Nocturnal enuresis, dizziness, tinnitus, hardness of hearing, poor memory, night sweating, dry mouth and throat at night, lower backache, constipation, scanty dark urine, tiredness, normal-coloured tongue without coating, Floating-Empty pulse.

URINATION AT NIGHT

Interrogation, Chapter 31

'Urination at night' should be differentiated from 'nocturnal enuresis': the difference has been explained above under 'Nocturnal enuresis'.

In Chinese medicine, any degree of urination at night is considered abnormal, that is, a person should not get up to urinate at night at all. Thus, even if the patient gets up only once, this would still be considered as 'urination at night'. Obviously the more times the patient gets up to urinate, the more serious is the condition. In Western medicine, frequent urination at night may indicate prostate hypertrophy.

Kidney-Yang deficiency

Urination at night, abundant pale urination, lower backache, cold knees, a feeling of cold, bright-white complexion, weak knees, tiredness, lassitude, impotence, decreased libido, Pale and wet tongue, Deep-Weak pulse.

Spleen- and Kidney-Yang deficiency

Urination at night, abundant clear urination, lower backache, cold and weak knees, a feeling of cold, bright-white complexion, impotence, decreased libido, tiredness, lassitude, loose stools, poor appetite, slight abdominal distension, a desire to lie down, early-morning diarrhoea, Pale and wet tongue, Deep-Weak pulse.

BLOOD IN THE URINE

Interrogation, Chapter 31

'Blood in the urine' should be differentiated from 'Blood Painful-Urination Syndrome' (*Lin* disease): the former simply indicates the presence of blood in the urine without pain, whereas the latter indicates painful urination with blood in the urine.

Damp-Heat in the Bladder

Blood in the urine, difficult urination, turbid urine, frequent and urgent urination, burning on urination, dark-yellow/turbid urine, thirst with no desire to drink, hypogastric fullness and pain, a feeling of heat, thick, sticky yellow coating on the tongue root with red spots, Slippery-Rapid pulse.

Damp-Heat in the Liver

Blood in the urine, dark urine, urinary difficulty, burning on urination, fullness of the hypochondrium, abdomen or hypogastrium, bitter taste, nausea, feeling of heaviness of the body, yellow vaginal discharge, vaginal itching, mid-cycle bleeding/pain, Red tongue with redder sides and sticky yellow coating, Slippery-Wiry-Rapid pulse.

Heart-Fire

Blood in the urine, palpitations, thirst, mouth and tongue ulcers, mental restlessness, feeling agitated, insomnia, dream-disturbed sleep, a feeling of heat, red face, bitter taste, Red tongue with redder tip and yellow coating, Overflowing-Rapid pulse.

Kidney-Yin deficiency with Empty-Heat

Blood in the urine, dizziness, tinnitus, hardness of hearing, poor memory, night sweating, dry mouth and throat at night, lower backache, constipation, scanty dark urine, tiredness, normal-coloured tongue without coating, Floating-Empty pulse.

Spleen- and Kidney-Yang deficiency

Pale blood in the urine, abundant clear urination, urination at night, lower backache, cold and weak knees, a feeling of cold, bright-white complexion, impotence, decreased libido, tiredness, lassitude, loose stools, poor appetite, slight abdominal distension, a desire to lie down, early-morning diarrhoea, Pale and wet tongue, Deep-Weak pulse.

SPERM IN THE URINE

Damp-Heat in the Bladder

Sperm in the urine, burning on urination, difficult urination, frequent and urgent urination, dark-yellow/ turbid urine, thirst with no desire to drink, hypogastric fullness and pain, a feeling of heat, thick, sticky yellow coating on the tongue root with red spots, Slippery-Rapid pulse.

Kidney-Yin deficiency with Empty-Heat

Sperm in the urine, dark-scanty urine, dizziness, tinnitus, night sweating, dry mouth with a desire to drink in small sips, lower backache, poor memory, five-palm heat, malar flush, a feeling of heat in the evening, Red tongue without coating, Floating-Empty and Rapid pulse.

Kidney-Qi not firm

Sperm in the urine, dribbling of urine which is worse after sex, frequent clear urination, weak-stream urination, abundant urination, incontinence of urine, urination at night, soreness and weakness of the lower back, weak knees, premature ejaculation,

Chapter **74**

ANUS

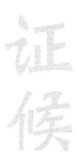

Chapter contents

ITCHING OF THE ANUS   *761*

HAEMORRHOIDS   *761*

ANAL PROLAPSE   *762*

ANAL FISSURE   *762*

ANAL FISTULA   *762*

ANAL ULCERS   *763*

ITCHING OF THE ANUS

Damp-Heat in the Bladder channel

Intense itching of the anus, haemorrhoids, frequent and urgent urination, burning on urination, difficult urination, dark-yellow turbid urine, thirst with no desire to drink, hypogastric fullness and pain, a feeling of heat, thick, sticky yellow tongue coating on the root with red spots, Slippery-Rapid pulse.

Cold-Dampness in the Bladder channel

Itching of the anus, haemorrhoids, frequent and urgent urination, difficult urination, a feeling of heaviness in the hypogastrium and urethra, pale and turbid urine, sticky white tongue coating on root, Slippery-Slow pulse.

Damp-Heat in the Governing Vessel

Itchy anus, haemorrhoids, stiffness and pain of the spine, lower backache, headache, painful urination, sticky yellow tongue coating on the root, Pulse Floating and Long on all three positions of the left side.

Blood deficiency generating Empty-Wind

Slight itching of the anus, dryness of the anus, anal fissures, no pain or burning, dry skin, facial tic, dizziness, blurred vision, numbness/tingling of the limbs, Pale and Thin tongue, Choppy or Fine and slightly Wiry pulse.

HAEMORRHOIDS

Damp-Heat in the Bladder channel

Bleeding haemorrhoids, pain, redness and swelling of the anus, fresh red blood, frequent and urgent urina-

tion, burning on urination, difficult urination, dark-yellow/ turbid urine, thirst with no desire to drink, hypogastric fullness and pain, a feeling of heat, thick, sticky yellow coating on the tongue root with red spots, Slippery-Rapid pulse.

Stagnation of Qi and stasis of Blood in the Bladder channel

Bleeding haemorrhoids, dark blood, pain and swelling, difficulty in defecation, hypogastric distension and pain, Purple tongue, Wiry pulse.

Spleen-Qi deficient and sinking

Haemorrhoids, may be bleeding with fresh red blood but absence of pain, poor appetite, slight abdominal distension after eating, tiredness, lassitude, pale complexion, weakness of the limbs, loose stools, depression, a bearing-down feeling, prolapse of the uterus, Pale tongue, Empty pulse.

Liver-Fire

Bleeding haemorrhoids, fresh or dark red blood, burning, pain and swelling, headache, red face, dizziness, tinnitus, irritability, propensity to outbursts of anger, thirst, bitter taste, constipation, dark urine, Red tongue with redder sides and dry yellow coating, Wiry-Rapid pulse.

ANAL PROLAPSE

Spleen-Qi deficient and sinking

Anal prolapse which may come and go, no redness, no pain, no swelling, loose stools, poor appetite, slight abdominal distension after eating, tiredness, lassitude, pale complexion, weakness of the limbs, depression, a bearing-down feeling, prolapse of the uterus, Pale tongue, Empty pulse.

Kidney-Yang deficiency

Anal prolapse, lower backache, cold knees, a feeling of cold, bright-white complexion, weak knees, tiredness, lassitude, abundant clear urination, urination at night, impotence, decreased libido, Pale and wet tongue, Deep-Weak pulse.

Damp-Heat in the Bladder channel

Anal prolapse, swelling, redness and pain of the anus, frequent and urgent urination, burning on urination, difficult urination, dark-yellow/turbid urine, thirst with no desire to drink, hypogastric fullness and pain, a feeling of heat, thick, sticky yellow coating on the root with red spots, Slippery-Rapid pulse.

ANAL FISSURE

Damp-Heat in the Bladder

Anal fissure, redness, swelling and itching of the anus, fresh red blood in the stools, frequent and urgent urination, burning on urination, difficult urination, dark-yellow/turbid urine, thirst with no desire to drink, hypogastric fullness and pain, a feeling of heat, thick, sticky yellow coating on the tongue root with red spots, Slippery-Rapid pulse.

Blood deficiency and Intestines Dryness

Anal fissure, dryness of the anus, dry stools, pain in the anus, difficulty in defecation, dizziness, blurred vision, floaters, numbness/tingling of the limbs, scanty menstruation, dull-pale complexion, Pale and dry tongue, Choppy or Fine pulse.

Fire in the Intestines

Anal fissure, constipation, dry stools, redness and burning of the anus, burning abdominal pain, intense thirst with a desire to drink cold liquids, mental restlessness, dry mouth, a feeling of heat, tongue Red with a thick, dry dark-yellow coating, Deep-Full-Rapid pulse.

ANAL FISTULA

Full-Heat

Anal fistula, swelling and burning of the anus, oozing of a yellow fluid, constipation, mental restlessness, a feeling of heat, thirst, Red tongue with yellow coating, Overflowing-Rapid pulse.

Empty-Heat

Anal fistula, burning of the anus, oozing of a thin fluid, a feeling of heat in the evening, night sweating, five-palm heat, Red tongue without coating, Floating-Empty and Rapid pulse.

Empty-Cold

Anal fistula, absence of burning, pain or swelling, a feeling of cold, oozing of a thin fluid, cold limbs, Pale tongue, Deep-Weak-Slow pulse.

ANAL ULCERS

Deficiency of Lungs, Spleen and Kidneys

Anal ulcers that are not painful or raised, pale red in colour, no burning, oozing a thin fluid, loose stools, slight shortness of breath, weak voice, spontaneous daytime sweating, dislike of speaking, bright-white complexion, tiredness, poor appetite, slight abdominal distension after eating, weakness of the limbs, lower backache, cold knees, a feeling of cold, weak knees, abundant clear urination, urination at night, impotence, decreased libido, Pale and wet tongue, Deep-Weak pulse.

Toxic Heat

Anal ulcers, swelling, pain, redness of the anus, thirst, a feeling of heat, Red tongue with red points and sticky yellow coating on the root, Overflowing-Slippery-Rapid pulse.

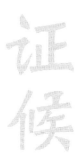

Chapter **75**

MEN'S SEXUAL AND GENITAL SYMPTOMS

Chapter contents

IMPOTENCE 765

LACK OF LIBIDO 766

EJACULATION 766
Premature ejaculation 766
Nocturnal emissions 767
Inability to ejaculate 767
Blood in the sperm 768
Cold watery sperm 768
Tiredness and dizziness after ejaculation 768

PRIAPISM 768

COLD GENITALS 769

SCROTUM 769
Contraction of the scrotum 769
Loose scrotum 769
Scrotum drooping to one side 769
Swollen scrotum 770
Swollen and oozing scrotum 770
Pale scrotum 770
Red scrotum 770
Purple scrotum 770
Dark scrotum 771
Itchy scrotum 771

PENIS 771
Pain and itching of the penis 771
Soft and withered penis 771
Redness and swelling of the glans penis 772
Peyronie's disease 772
Ulcers 772

SWELLING AND PAIN OF THE TESTICLES 773

PUBIC HAIR 773
Loss of pubic hair 773
Excessive pubic hair 773

IMPOTENCE

Interrogation, Chapter 45

'Impotence' should be differentiated from 'lack of libido': the former indicates an inability to sustain or obtain an erection while the sexual desire is normal; the latter indicates lack of sexual desire while the erection is normal.

Kidney-Yang deficiency

Impotence, lower backache, cold knees, a feeling of cold, bright-white complexion, weak knees, tiredness, lassitude, abundant clear urination, urination at night, Pale and wet tongue, Deep-Weak pulse.

Spleen- and Heart-Yang deficiency

Impotence, premature ejaculation, poor appetite, slight abdominal distension after eating, tiredness, lassitude, pale complexion, weakness of the limbs, loose stools, a feeling of cold, cold limbs, oedema, palpitations, shortness of breath on exertion, spontaneous sweating, a slight feeling of discomfort or stuffiness in the heart region, Pale and wet tongue, Deep-Weak pulse.

This type of impotence is very common, probably more so than the type from Kidney deficiency.

Damp-Heat in the Lower Burner

Impotence, burning on urination, sperm in the urine, difficult urination, sticky yellow tongue coating, Slippery-Rapid pulse.

Liver- and Kidney-Yin deficiency

Impotence, dizziness, tinnitus, weak knees, hardness of hearing, lower backache, dull occipital or vertical headache, insomnia, numbness/tingling of the limbs, dry eyes, blurred vision, dry throat in the evening, dry

hair and skin, brittle nails, night sweating, dry stools, normal-coloured tongue without coating, Floating-Empty pulse.

Kidney-Essence deficiency

Impotence, softening of bones in adults, deafness, weakness of knees and legs, poor memory, loose teeth, falling hair or premature greying of the hair, weakness of sexual activity, lower backache, infertility, sterility, dizziness, tinnitus, normal-coloured tongue and Floating-Empty or Leather pulse if Kidney-Essence deficiency occurs against a background of Kidney-Yin deficiency, or Pale tongue and Deep-Weak pulse if against a background of Kidney-Yang deficiency.

> ### Clinical note
>
> - In my experience, impotence is due more often to a Heart disharmony than to a deficiency of Kidney-Yang.
> - In treatment with acupuncture, I treat the Heart (HE-7 Shenmen, Du-24 Shenting and Ren-15 Jiuwei with Ren-4 Guanyuan).
> - In treatment with herbal medicine do not forget to add one or two herbs to invigorate Blood, especially Dan Shen *Radix Salviae milthiorrhizae*.

LACK OF LIBIDO

Interrogation, Chapter 45

In Chinese medicine, libido depends on the state of the Fire of the Gate of Life (*Ming Men*), which represents the Fire within the Kidneys and is also called the Minister Fire. A deficiency of this Fire may cause lack of libido in both men and women (and also infertility), whereas an excess of this Fire may cause excessive sexual desire.

Kidney-Yang deficiency

Lack of libido, lower backache, cold knees, a feeling of cold, bright-white complexion, weak knees, tiredness, lassitude, abundant clear urination, urination at night, Pale and wet tongue, Deep-Weak pulse.

Heart-Yang deficiency

Lack of libido, premature ejaculation, palpitations, shortness of breath on exertion, spontaneous sweating, a slight feeling of discomfort or stuffiness in the heart region, Pale and wet tongue, Deep-Weak pulse.

Heart-Blood deficiency

Lack of libido, palpitations, dizziness, insomnia, dream-disturbed sleep, poor memory, anxiety, tendency to be easily startled, dull-pale complexion, pale lips, Pale and Thin tongue, Choppy or Fine pulse.

Heart- and Spleen-Blood deficiency

Lack of libido, palpitations, dizziness, insomnia, dream-disturbed sleep, poor memory, anxiety, tendency to be easily startled, dull-pale complexion, pale lips, poor appetite, loose stools, tiredness, Pale and Thin tongue, Choppy or Fine pulse.

Liver-Qi stagnation

Lack of libido, hypochondrial or epigastric distension, irritability, moodiness, a feeling of a lump in the throat, Wiry pulse.

> ### Clinical note
>
> - In my experience, lack of libido in men is often caused by a Heart deficiency, whereas in women a Kidney deficiency is more common.

EJACULATION

Premature ejaculation

Interrogation, Chapter 45

Kidney-Qi not firm

Premature ejaculation, dribbling of urine which is worse after sex, frequent clear urination, weak-stream urination, incontinence of urine, soreness and weakness of the lower back, weak knees, tiredness, a dragging-down feeling in the lower abdomen, a feeling of cold, cold limbs, Pale tongue, Deep-Weak pulse.

Damp-Heat in the Liver channel

Premature ejaculation, burning on urination, urinary difficulty, dark urine, genital papular or vesicular skin rashes and itching, fullness of the hypochondrium, abdomen or hypogastrium, bitter taste, nausea, a feeling of heaviness of the body, Red tongue with redder sides and sticky yellow coating, Slippery-Wiry-Rapid pulse.

Spleen- and Heart-Yang deficiency

Premature ejaculation, poor appetite, slight abdominal distension after eating, tiredness, lassitude, pale com-

plexion, weakness of the limbs, loose stools, a feeling of cold, cold limbs, oedema, palpitations, shortness of breath on exertion, spontaneous sweating, a slight feeling of discomfort or stuffiness in the heart region, Pale and wet tongue, Deep-Weak pulse.

> ### Clinical note
>
> • Heart-Qi descending plays a role in ejaculation. Therefore premature ejaculation may be due to Heart-Qi deficiency. For this reason, I treat the Heart and Kidneys.

Nocturnal emissions

Interrogation, Chapter 45

'Nocturnal emissions' indicates ejaculation during sleep. This symptom always has 'pride of place' among Kidney-deficiency symptoms in Chinese books. In the West, this symptom is relatively rare and it is not even considered a 'symptom' unless it occurs very frequently (e.g. once a week or more). There are cultural reasons why this symptom always has a prominent place among Kidney-deficiency symptoms in Chinese books because in ancient times ejaculation during sleep, especially if with sexual dreams, was considered to be due to the man having intercourse with female ghosts at night; such ghosts were considered very dangerous because they robbed men of their vital Essence.

Heart-Fire

Nocturnal emissions with dreams, premature ejaculation, palpitations, thirst, mouth and tongue ulcers, mental restlessness, a feeling of agitation, insomnia, dream-disturbed sleep, a feeling of heat, red face, bitter taste, Red tongue with redder tip and yellow coating, Overflowing-Rapid pulse.

Spleen-Qi and Heart-Blood deficiency

Nocturnal emissions without dreams, poor appetite, slight abdominal distension after eating, tiredness, weakness of the limbs, loose stools, palpitations, dizziness, insomnia, dream-disturbed sleep, poor memory, anxiety, tendency to be easily startled, dull-pale complexion, pale lips, Pale and Thin tongue, Choppy or Fine pulse.

Heart- and Kidney-Yin deficiency with Empty-Heat

Nocturnal emissions with dreams, premature ejaculation, excessive sexual desire, palpitations, mental rest-lessness, insomnia, dream-disturbed sleep, anxiety, poor memory, dizziness, tinnitus, hardness of hearing, lower backache, nocturnal emissions with dreams, a feeling of heat in the evening, night sweating, five-palm heat, scanty dark urine, dry stools, Red tongue with redder tip and a Heart crack, Floating-Empty and Rapid pulse.

Minister Fire blazing upwards

Nocturnal emissions with dreams, premature ejaculation, excessive sexual desire, thirst, a feeling of agitation, a feeling of heat, red face, Red tongue with yellow coating, Overflowing-Rapid pulse.

Kidney-Qi not firm

Nocturnal emissions without dreams, premature ejaculation, dribbling of urine which is worse after sex, frequent clear urination, weak-stream urination, incontinence of urine, soreness and weakness of the lower back, weak knees, tiredness, a dragging-down feeling in the lower abdomen, a feeling of cold, cold limbs, Pale tongue, Deep-Weak pulse.

Damp-Heat in the Lower Burner

Nocturnal emissions with dreams, burning on urination, dark and turbid urine, itchy scrotum, sticky yellow tongue coating, Slippery-Rapid pulse.

Kidney-Essence deficiency

Nocturnal emissions without dreams, lack of libido, impotence, softening of bones in adults, deafness, weakness of knees and legs, poor memory, loose teeth, falling hair or premature greying of the hair, weakness of sexual activity, lower backache, infertility, sterility, dizziness, tinnitus, normal-coloured tongue and Floating-Empty or Leather pulse if Kidney-Essence deficiency occurs against a background of Kidney-Yin deficiency, or Pale tongue and Deep-Weak pulse if against a background of Kidney-Yang deficiency.

Inability to ejaculate
Kidney-Yin deficiency with Empty-Heat

Inability to ejaculate, dizziness, tinnitus, hardness of hearing, night sweating, dry mouth at night, five-palm heat, a feeling of heat in the evening, malar flush, thirst with a desire to drink in small sips, lower backache, scanty dark urine, insomnia, Red tongue without coating, Floating-Empty and Rapid pulse.

Blood stasis in the Lower Burner

Inability to ejaculate, abdominal pain, mental restlessness, pain in the testis, Purple tongue, Wiry pulse.

Blood in the sperm
Kidney-Yin deficiency with Empty-Heat

Blood in the sperm, dizziness, tinnitus, hardness of hearing, night sweating, dry mouth at night, five-palm heat, a feeling of heat in the evening, malar flush, thirst with a desire to drink in small sips, lower backache, scanty dark urine, insomnia, Red tongue without coating, Floating-Empty and Rapid pulse.

Damp-Heat in the Lower Burner

Blood in the sperm, turbid sperm, burning on urination, hypogastric fullness and pain, pain and swelling of the scrotum, dark urine, sticky yellow tongue coating, Slippery-Rapid pulse.

Toxic Heat in the Lower Burner

Blood in the sperm, a feeling of heaviness and pain of the perineum, urethral discharge, abdominal pain, Red tongue with sticky, thick yellow coating and red points, Slippery-Overflowing-Rapid pulse.

Blood stasis in the Lower Burner

Blood in the sperm, pain in the perineum, difficulty in urination, abdominal pain, purple complexion, Purple tongue, Firm pulse.

Cold-watery sperm
Kidney-Qi not firm

Cold-watery sperm, premature ejaculation, impotence, dribbling of urine which is worse after sex, frequent clear urination, weak-stream urination, incontinence of urine, soreness and weakness of the lower back, weak knees, tiredness, a dragging-down feeling in the lower abdomen, a feeling of cold, cold limbs, Pale tongue, Deep-Weak pulse.

Cold in the Lower Burner

Cold-watery sperm, impotence, lack of libido, abdominal pain, a feeling of cold in the scrotum, cold limbs, a feeling of cold, lower backache, pale face, abundant pale urination, white tongue coating, Deep-Weak-Slow pulse.

Tiredness and dizziness after ejaculation

Interrogation, Chapter 45

Kidney-Yang deficiency

Tiredness and dizziness after ejaculation, impotence, decreased libido, tinnitus, lower backache, cold knees, a feeling of cold, bright-white complexion, weak knees, tiredness, lassitude, abundant clear urination, urination at night, Pale and wet tongue, Deep-Weak pulse.

Kidney-Yin deficiency

Tiredness and dizziness after ejaculation, impotence, decreased libido, nocturnal emissions, tinnitus, hardness of hearing, poor memory, night sweating, dry mouth and throat at night, lower backache, constipation, scanty dark urine, tiredness, normal-coloured tongue without coating, Floating-Empty pulse.

Spleen-Blood and Heart-Blood deficiency

Tiredness and dizziness after ejaculation, palpitations, dizziness, insomnia, dream-disturbed sleep, poor memory, anxiety, tendency to be easily startled, dull-pale complexion, pale lips, poor appetite, slight abdominal distension after eating, weakness of the limbs, loose stools, Pale tongue, Choppy pulse.

PRIAPISM

Observation, Chapter 17

'Priapism' indicates persistent abnormal erection of the penis accompanied by pain and tenderness.

Damp-Heat in the Liver channel

Persistent erection, pain in the testis, fullness of the hypochondrium, abdomen or hypogastrium, bitter taste, nausea, a feeling of heaviness of the body, genital papular or vesicular skin rashes and itching, urinary difficulty, burning on urination, dark urine, Red tongue with redder sides and sticky yellow coating, Slippery-Wiry-Rapid pulse.

Kidney-Yin deficiency with Empty-Heat

Persistent erection, dizziness, tinnitus, hardness of hearing, night sweating, dry mouth at night, five-palm heat, a feeling of heat in the evening, malar flush,

thirst with a desire to drink in small sips, lower backache, scanty dark urine, insomnia, Red tongue without coating, Floating-Empty and Rapid pulse.

COLD GENITALS

Deficiency of Minister Fire

Cold genitals, backache, lack of libido, impotence, a feeling of cold, dizziness, depression, pale-abundant urination, Pale tongue, Deep-Weak pulse.

Stagnation of Cold in the Liver channel

Cold genitals, contracted scrotum, fullness and distension of the hypogastrium, with pain which refers downwards to the scrotum and testis and upwards to the hypochondrium, alleviation of the pain by warmth, straining of the testis or contraction of the scrotum, vertical headache, a feeling of cold, cold hands and feet, vomiting of clear watery fluids or dry vomiting, Pale and wet tongue with white coating, Deep-Wiry-slow pulse.

Cold-Dampness in the Lower Burner

Cold genitals, abdominal fullness, turbid urine, abdominal pain, a feeling of heaviness, a feeling of cold, cold limbs, sticky white tongue coating, Slippery-Slow pulse.

SCROTUM

Contraction of the scrotum

Observation, Chapter 17

Stagnation of Cold in the Liver channel

Contraction of the scrotum, fullness and distension of the hypogastrium with pain, which refers downwards to the scrotum and testis and upwards to the hypochondrium, alleviation of the pain by warmth, straining of the testis or contraction of the scrotum, vertical headache, a feeling of cold, cold hands and feet, vomiting of clear watery fluids, or dry vomiting, Pale and wet tongue with white coating, Deep-Wiry-slow pulse.

Deficiency of Qi and Blood

Contraction of the scrotum, poor appetite, loose stools, weak voice, tiredness, blurred vision, dizziness, numbness/tingling of the limbs, palpitations, dull-pale complexion, Pale tongue, Weak or Choppy pulse.

Chinese books explain that this condition is due to overexertion after an acute disease.

Collapse of Yang

Contraction of the scrotum, chilliness, cold limbs, weak breathing, profuse sweating with sweat-like pearls, absence of thirst, profuse pale urination or incontinence of urine, loose stools, incontinence of faeces, mental confusion or unconsciousness, Pale-Wet-Short tongue, Deep-Minute pulse.

Collapse of Yin

Contraction of the scrotum, abundant perspiration, skin hot to the touch, hot limbs, dry mouth, retention of urine, constipation, Red, Short tongue without coating, Floating-Empty-Rapid pulse.

Loose scrotum

Observation, Chapter 17

Kidney-Yang deficiency

Loose scrotum, lower backache, cold knees, a feeling of cold, bright-white complexion, weak knees, tiredness, lassitude, abundant clear urination, urination at night, impotence, decreased libido, Pale and wet tongue, Deep-Weak pulse.

Spleen-Qi sinking

Loose scrotum, a feeling of bearing down, poor appetite, slight abdominal distension after eating, tiredness, lassitude, pale complexion, weakness of the limbs, loose stools, Pale tongue, Empty pulse.

Scrotum drooping to one side

Observation, Chapter 17

Empty-Cold in the Lower Burner

Scrotum drooping on side, a feeling of cold in the abdomen, abundant clear urination, lack of libido, Pale tongue, Deep-Weak-Slow pulse.

Damp-Phlegm in the Lower Burner

Scrotum drooping on side, a feeling of heaviness in the abdomen, obesity, urethral discharge, Swollen tongue, Slippery pulse.

Swollen scrotum

Observation, Chapter 17

Spleen- and Kidney-Yang deficiency

Swollen scrotum, lower backache, cold and weak knees, a feeling of cold, bright-white complexion, impotence, decreased libido, tiredness, lassitude, abundant clear urination, urination at night, loose stools, poor appetite, slight abdominal distension, a desire to lie down, early-morning diarrhoea, Pale and wet tongue, Deep-Weak pulse.

Heart-Yang deficiency

Swollen scrotum, palpitations, shortness of breath on exertion, tiredness, listlessness, depression, spontaneous sweating, a slight feeling of discomfort or stuffiness in the heart region, a feeling of cold, cold hands, bright-pale face, Pale tongue, Deep-Weak pulse.

Liver-Blood deficiency with Empty internal Wind

Swollen scrotum, dizziness, blurred vision, floaters, numbness or tingling of limbs, scanty menstruation, dull-pale complexion, tremors, tic, Pale tongue, Choppy or Fine pulse.

Swollen and oozing scrotum

Observation, Chapter 17

Damp-Heat in the Liver channel

Red and swollen scrotum oozing a sticky fluid, pain in the testicles, genital, papular or vesicular skin rashes and itching, urinary difficulty, burning on urination, dark urine, fullness of the hypochondrium, abdomen or hypogastrium, bitter taste, poor appetite, nausea, a feeling of heaviness of the body, Red tongue with redder sides and a sticky yellow coating, Slippery-Wiry-Rapid pulse.

Toxic Heat in the Liver channel

Red, swollen and painful scrotum oozing a sticky fluid, ulcers on the penis, pain in the testicles and perineum, genital papular skin rash and itching, burning on urination, dark urine, Red tongue with thick, sticky yellow coating and red spots on the root and sides, Slippery-Overflowing-Rapid pulse.

Pale scrotum

Observation, Chapter 17

Spleen- and Kidney-Yang deficiency

Pale scrotum, lower backache, cold and weak knees, a feeling of cold, bright-white complexion, impotence, decreased libido, tiredness, lassitude, abundant clear urination, urination at night, loose stools, poor appetite, slight abdominal distension, a desire to lie down, early-morning diarrhoea, Pale and wet tongue, Deep-Weak pulse.

Red scrotum

Observation, Chapter 17

Damp-Heat in the Liver channel

Red scrotum, pain in the testis, fullness of the hypochondrium, abdomen or hypogastrium, bitter taste, nausea, a feeling of heaviness of the body, genital papular or vesicular skin rashes and itching, urinary difficulty, burning on urination, dark urine, Red tongue with redder sides and sticky yellow coating, Slippery-Wiry-Rapid pulse.

Toxic Heat in the Liver channel

Red scrotum, pain, swelling, redness and itching of the testis, dark urine, burning on urination, hypogastric fullness and distension, painful penis, thick, sticky yellow tongue coating, Overflowing-Slippery-Rapid pulse.

Purple scrotum

Observation, Chapter 17

Liver-Blood stasis

Purple scrotum, hypochondrial/abdominal pain, masses in the abdomen, purple nails and lips, purple or dark complexion, Purple tongue, Wiry or Firm pulse.

Damp-Heat with Blood stasis in the Liver channel

Purple scrotum, persistent erection, pain in the testis, tenderness and pain of penis, genital papular or vesicular skin rashes and itching, urinary difficulty, burning on urination, dark urine, fullness of the hypochon-

drium, abdomen or hypogastrium, bitter taste, nausea, a feeling of heaviness of the body, hypochondrial/abdominal pain, masses in the abdomen, purple nails and lips, purple or dark complexion, Red tongue with purplish sides and sticky yellow coating, Wiry-Slippery-Rapid pulse.

Dark scrotum

Observation, Chapter 17

Stagnation of Cold in the Liver channel

Dark scrotum, straining of the testis or contraction of the scrotum, fullness and distension of the hypogastrium with pain, which refers downwards to the scrotum and testis and upwards to the hypochondrium, alleviation of the pain by warmth, vertical headache, a feeling of cold, cold hands and feet, vomiting of clear watery fluids or dry vomiting, Pale and wet tongue with white coating, Deep-Wiry-Slow pulse.

Kidney-Yang deficiency

Dark scrotum, lower backache, cold knees, a feeling of cold, bright-white complexion, weak knees, tiredness, lassitude, abundant clear urination, urination at night, impotence, decreased libido, Pale and wet tongue, Deep-Weak pulse.

Itchy scrotum

Damp-Heat in the Lower Burner

Itchy and burning of the scrotum, sweaty scrotum, burning on urination, dark urine, sticky yellow tongue coating, Slippery-Rapid pulse.

Kidney-Yin deficiency with Empty-Heat

Itchy scrotum, dry skin, bleeding on scratching, dizziness, tinnitus, hardness of hearing, night sweating, dry mouth at night, five-palm heat, a feeling of heat in the evening, malar flush, thirst with a desire to drink in small sips, lower backache, scanty dark urine, insomnia, Red tongue without coating, Floating-Empty and Rapid pulse.

Cold-Dampness in the Lower Burner

Itchy and sweaty scrotum, a feeling of heaviness of the scrotum, turbid urine, sticky white tongue coating, Slippery-Slow pulse.

PENIS

Pain and itching of the penis

Damp-Heat in the Lower Burner

Pain and itching of the penis, dark urine, burning on urination, turbid urine, irritability, sticky yellow tongue coating, Slippery-Rapid pulse.

Blood stasis in the Lower Burner

Pain in the penis, hypogastric pain, blood in the urine, abdominal pain, Purple tongue, Wiry pulse.

Kidney-Yin deficiency with Empty-Heat

Pain and itching of the penis, dizziness, tinnitus, hardness of hearing, night sweating, dry mouth at night, five-palm heat, a feeling of heat in the evening, malar flush, thirst with a desire to drink in small sips, lower backache, scanty-dark urine, insomnia, Red tongue without coating, Floating-Empty and Rapid pulse.

Heart-Fire

Pain and itching of the penis, dark urine, burning on urination, premature ejaculation, palpitations, thirst, mouth and tongue ulcers, mental restlessness, feeling agitated, insomnia, dream-disturbed sleep, a feeling of heat, red face, bitter taste, Red tongue with redder tip and yellow coating, Overflowing-Rapid pulse.

Soft and withered penis

Observation, Chapter 17

Liver-Qi deficiency

Soft and withered penis, timidity, tendency to being easily startled, difficulty in making decisions, sighing, depression, inability to make plans, nervousness, lack of courage and initiative, restless dreams, dizziness, blurred vision, floaters, mild hypochondrial discomfort, Pale tongue, pulse Empty on the left.

Kidney-Yin deficiency

Soft and withered penis, dizziness, tinnitus, night sweating, dry mouth with a desire to sip water, lower backache, poor memory, scanty dark urine, tongue without coating, Floating-Empty pulse.

Kidney-Yang deficiency

Soft and withered penis, lower backache, cold knees, a feeling of cold, bright-white complexion, weak knees,

tiredness, lassitude, abundant clear urination, urination at night, impotence, decreased libido, Pale and wet tongue, Deep-Weak pulse.

Phlegm and Blood stasis in the Lower Burner

Soft and withered penis, inability to ejaculate, abdominal pain, a feeling of heaviness in the abdomen, mental restlessness, pain in the testis, Swollen and Purple tongue, Wiry-Slippery pulse.

Redness and swelling of the glans penis

Observation, Chapter 17

Toxic Heat in the Liver channel

Redness and swelling of the glans penis, painful urination, thick urethral discharge, hypogastric pain, Red tongue with red points on the side and thick, sticky yellow coating, Overflowing-Slippery-Rapid pulse.

Damp-Heat in the Liver channel

Redness and swelling of the glans penis, persistent erection, pain in the testis, tenderness and pain of penis, genital papular or vesicular skin rashes and itching, urinary difficulty, burning on urination, dark urine, fullness of the hypochondrium, abdomen or hypogastrium, bitter taste, nausea, a feeling of heaviness of the body, Red tongue with redder sides and sticky yellow coating, Slippery-Wiry-Rapid pulse.

Peyronie's disease

Observation, Chapter 17

Peyronie's disease is an unnatural curvature of the penis, which is noticeable during an erection. It may prevent a complete erection, owing to plaque or scar tissue inside the penis. The curvature may also cause a painful erection which may be so severe as to make intercourse impossible.

Blood stasis in the Liver channel

Peyronie's disease, painful curvature of the penis, painful erection, hypogastric pain, painful urination, hypochondrial/abdominal pain, purple nails and lips, purple or dark complexion, Purple tongue, Wiry or Firm pulse.

Dampness in the Lower Burner with Blood stasis in the Liver channel

Peyronie's disease, painful curvature of the penis, painful erection, swelling and hardening under the skin of the penis, a feeling of heaviness and fullness of the lower abdomen, urethral discharge, hypogastric pain, painful urination, hypochondrial/abdominal pain, purple nails and lips, purple or dark complexion, Purple tongue with sticky coating, Wiry-Slippery or Firm-Slippery pulse.

Blood stasis in the Liver channel with Kidney-Yang deficiency

Peyronie's disease, curvature of the penis, soft erection, hypogastric pain, painful urination, hypochondrial/abdominal pain, purple nails and lips, purple or dark complexion, lower backache, cold knees, a feeling of cold, bright-white complexion, weak knees, tiredness, lassitude, abundant clear urination, urination at night, impotence, decreased libido, Pale and wet tongue with purplish sides, Deep-Weak pulse.

Cold in the Liver channel with Blood stasis

Peyronie's disease, painful curvature of the penis, painful erection, straining of the testis or contraction of the scrotum, fullness and distension of the hypogastrium, with pain which refers downwards to the scrotum and testis and upwards to the hypochondrium, alleviation of the pain by warmth, vertical headache, a feeling of cold, cold hands and feet, vomiting of clear watery fluids or dry vomiting, hypochondrial/abdominal pain, purple nails and lips, purple or dark complexion, Bluish-Purple tongue, white coating, Deep-Wiry-Slow pulse.

Ulcers

Observation, Chapter 17

Damp-Heat in the Liver channel

Red ulcers on the penis, oozing of fluid, swelling and pain of the penis, genital papular or vesicular skin rashes and itching, urinary difficulty, burning on urination, dark urine, fullness of the hypochondrium, abdomen or hypogastrium, bitter taste, nausea, a feeling of heaviness of the body, Red tongue with redder sides and sticky yellow coating, Slippery-Wiry-Rapid pulse.

Liver-Fire

Painful, red ulcers on the penis oozing a sticky yellow fluid, swelling and redness of the penis, headache, red face, dizziness, tinnitus, irritability, propensity to outbursts of anger, thirst, bitter taste, constipation, dark urine, Red tongue with redder sides and dry yellow coating, Wiry-Rapid pulse.

Kidney deficiency with Dampness

Ulcers on the penis, itching and oozing a sticky fluid, lower backache, dizziness, tinnitus, a feeling of fullness and heaviness of the lower abdomen, sticky yellow tongue coating, Deep-Weak and slightly Slippery pulse.

Liver- and Kidney-Yin deficiency with Empty-Heat

Ulcers on the penis, edges of the ulcers not raised, not painful, dizziness, tinnitus, dull occipital or vertical headache, insomnia, numbness/tingling of the limbs, malar flush, dry eyes, blurred vision, lower backache, dry throat, dry hair and skin, brittle nails, dry vagina, night sweating, dry stools, scanty dark urine, scanty menstruation, five-palm heat, a feeling of heat in the evening, Red tongue without coating, Floating-Empty and Rapid pulse.

Toxic Heat

Ulcers on the penis, with itching, heat and pain, thirst, a feeling of heat, skin rashes, Red tongue with thick, sticky yellow coating, Overflowing-Slippery-Rapid pulse.

SWELLING AND PAIN OF THE TESTICLES

Cold in the Lower Burner

Swelling and pain of the testicles, abdominal pain, pale urine, a feeling of cold, white tongue coating, Deep-Tight pulse.

Cold-Dampness in the Lower Burner

Swelling of the testicles with slight pain, abdominal fullness and pain, a feeling of heaviness, turbid urine, sticky white tongue coating, Slippery-Slow pulse.

Damp-Heat in the Lower Burner

Swelling and pain of the testicles, abdominal fullness and pain, a feeling of heaviness, dark and turbid urine, burning on urination, sticky yellow tongue coating, Slippery-Rapid pulse.

Stagnation of Qi in the Lower Burner

Swelling and pain of the testicles that come and go, abdominal distension, irritability, Wiry pulse.

Toxic Heat in the Lower Burner

Swelling, pain and hardness of the testicles, hypogastric pain, burning on urination, swelling of scrotum, fever, thirst, Red tongue with thick, sticky yellow coating and red spots on the root, Slippery-Overflowing-Rapid pulse.

PUBIC HAIR

Loss of pubic hair

Observation, Chapter 17

Kidney-Essence deficiency

Loss of pubic hair, softening of bones in adults, deafness, weakness of knees and legs, poor memory, loose teeth, falling hair or premature greying of the hair, weakness of sexual activity, lower backache, sterility, dizziness, tinnitus, normal-coloured tongue and Floating-Empty or Leather pulse if Kidney-Essence deficiency occurs against a background of Kidney-Yin deficiency, or Pale tongue and Deep-Weak pulse if against a background of Kidney-Yang deficiency.

Spleen- and Kidney-Yang deficiency

Loss of pubic hair, lower backache, cold and weak knees, a feeling of cold, bright-white complexion, impotence, decreased libido, tiredness, lassitude, abundant clear urination, urination at night, loose stools, poor appetite, slight abdominal distension, a desire to lie down, early-morning diarrhoea, Pale and wet tongue, Deep-Weak pulse.

Excessive pubic hair

Observation, Chapter 17

Phlegm and Blood stasis

Excessive pubic hair, pain in the genital area, a feeling of oppression of the chest, Swollen and Purple tongue, Slippery-Wiry pulse.

Kidney-Yin deficiency with Empty-Heat

Excessive pubic hair, dizziness, tinnitus, night sweating, dry mouth with a desire to sip water, backache, poor memory, scanty dark urine, five-palm heat, malar flush, a feeling of heat in the evening, Red tongue without coating, Floating-Empty and Rapid pulse.

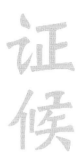

Chapter **76**

SWEATING

Chapter contents

SPONTANEOUS SWEATING   775

NIGHT SWEATING   776

SWEATING FROM COLLAPSE   776

YELLOW SWEAT   777

LOCALIZED SWEATING   777
   Unilateral sweating   777
   Sweating on the head   778
   Sweating on the chest   778
   Sweating of hands and feet   778
   Sweating of the palms   779
   Sweating in the axillae   779

ABSENCE OF SWEATING   780

SPONTANEOUS SWEATING

Interrogation, Chapter 41

Lung-Qi deficiency

Spontaneous sweating which is worse on exercise, slight shortness of breath, slight cough, weak voice, dislike of speaking, bright-white complexion, tendency to catch colds, tiredness, a dislike of cold, Pale tongue, Empty pulse.

Lung-Yang deficiency

Spontaneous sweating which is worse on exercise, slight shortness of breath, slight cough, weak voice, dislike of speaking, bright-white complexion, tendency to catch colds, tiredness, dislike of cold, a feeling of cold, cold hands, Pale and wet tongue, Weak pulse.

Full-Heat

Profuse spontaneous sweating, a feeling of heat, thirst, mental restlessness, Red tongue with yellow coating, Overflowing-Rapid pulse.

   This may be Full-Heat in the Heart, Liver, Lungs, or Stomach.

Phlegm-Heat

Profuse daytime sweating, a feeling of oppression of the chest, sputum in the throat, mental restlessness, thirst with no desire to drink, Red and Swollen tongue with sticky yellow coating, Slippery-Rapid pulse.

   This can be Phlegm-Heat affecting the Lungs, Stomach or Heart.

Invasion of Wind-Cold with prevalence of Wind

Slight sweating, aversion to cold, fever, cough, itchy throat, slight breathlessness, stuffed or runny nose

with clear watery discharge, sneezing, occipital head-ache, body aches, thin white tongue coating, Floating-Slow pulse.

This is due to a disharmony between Nutritive and Defensive Qi.

Wind-Dampness on the Exterior

Spontaneous sweating, aversion to cold, fever, swollen glands, nausea, occipital stiffness, body aches, muscle ache, a feeling of heaviness of the body, swollen joints, a feeling of heaviness of the limbs, headache, sticky white tongue coating, Floating-Slippery pulse.

Invasion of Summer-Heat

Slight sweating, fever, aversion to cold, headache, a feeling of heaviness, an uncomfortable sensation in the epigastrium, irritability, thirst, tongue Red in the front or sides with a sticky white coating, Soggy and Rapid pulse.

NIGHT SWEATING

Interrogation, Chapter 41

Night sweating is called in Chinese *dao han*, which literally means 'thief sweating'; this name probably refers to the fact that night-time sweating is very depleting of the body's energies and it 'robs' the body of its Qi. Both daytime and night-time sweating deplete the body's energy: the former depletes Qi and Yang, and the latter Yin. Thus both daytime and night-time sweating start a pathological vicious circle because they can derive from a deficiency but they also aggravate that deficiency.

Yin deficiency

Night sweating, dry mouth with a desire to drink in small sips, dry throat in the evening, scanty dark urine, dry stools, normal-coloured tongue without coating, Floating-Empty pulse.

This may be Yin deficiency of several different organs: the Lungs, Heart, Stomach, Liver, Kidneys or Spleen.

Yin deficiency with Empty-Heat

Profuse night sweating, five-palm heat, feeling of heat in the evening, dry mouth at night with a desire to drink in small sips, malar flush, Red tongue without coating, Floating-Empty and Rapid pulse.

Damp-Heat in Stomach and Spleen

Night sweating, a feeling of fullness and pain of the epigastrium and lower abdomen, poor appetite, a feeling of heaviness, thirst without a desire to drink, nausea, loose stools with an offensive odour, a feeling of heat, dull-yellow complexion, sticky taste, Red tongue with sticky yellow coating, Slippery-Rapid pulse.

Deficiency of Qi and Blood of the Heart

Night sweating, palpitations, shortness of breath on exertion, pale face, tiredness, slight depression, spontaneous sweating, dizziness, insomnia, dream-disturbed sleep, poor memory, anxiety, tendency to be easily startled, dull-pale complexion, pale lips, Pale and Thin tongue, Choppy or Fine pulse.

This is less common than the night sweating from Yin deficiency and it usually occurs in women.

Lesser-Yang pattern

Night sweating, bitter taste, hypochondrial discomfort, dry throat, alternation of hot and cold feeling, irritability, unilateral coating on the tongue, Wiry pulse.

This can be either the Lesser-Yang pattern within the Six Stages identification of patterns (in which there is a prevalence of cold feeling) or the Gall-Bladder Heat pattern within the Four Levels identification of patterns (in which there is a prevalence of hot feeling). This type of night sweating usually follows a febrile disease.

> ### Clinical note
> - **Remember**: night sweating is *not* always caused by Yin deficiency!

SWEATING FROM COLLAPSE

Interrogation, Chapter 41

Collapse of Qi and Yin

Profuse sweating like oil drops, a feeling of heat, body hot to the touch, thirst, collapse, Red tongue without coating, Deep-Minute-Rapid pulse.

Collapse of Yang

Profuse sweating like pearls, watery sweat, body cold to the touch, a feeling of cold, cold limbs, unconscious-

ness, pale face, weak breathing, Pale tongue, Hidden pulse.

YELLOW SWEAT

Observation, Chapter 20; Interrogation, Chapter 41

Yellow sweat was first mentioned in the 'Synopsis of Prescriptions from the Golden Cabinet' (*Jin Gui Yao Lue*, c. AD200). In Chapter 14, where yellow sweat is mentioned three times, it says: '*With Yellow Sweat disease there is swelling, fever, thirst and yellow sweat like Phellodendron sap [i.e. bright-yellow]'.*[1]

Damp-Heat

Yellow sweat like *Phellodendron* sap all over the body, fever, swelling, a feeling of heaviness, sticky/bitter taste, sticky yellow tongue coating, Slippery pulse.

Other symptoms and signs depend on the organ involved, which may be the Stomach, Spleen, Liver or Gall-Bladder.

Nutritive and Defensive Qi obstructed

Fever, sweat like *Phellodendron* sap, swelling, a feeling of heaviness of the body, a feeling as if there were insects crawling under the skin, thirst, difficult urination, white tongue coating, Deep pulse.

This pattern is characterized by a deficiency of the Defensive Qi and a stagnation of the Nutritive Qi (this is the exact opposite of the Greater-Yang Wind pattern); fluids are retained, Qi is obstructed and the Bladder's function is impaired. This cause of yellow sweat is less frequent than the previous one.

Stagnant Liver-Qi turned into Heat

Yellow sweat which stains the clothing particularly in the axilla, hypochondrium or genital region, hypochondrial or epigastric distension, a slight feeling of oppression of the chest, irritability, premenstrual tension, irregular periods, premenstrual breast distension, a feeling of a lump in the throat, a feeling of heat, red face, thirst, propensity to outbursts of anger, heavy periods, tongue Red on the sides, Wiry and slightly Rapid pulse.

Spleen- and Lung-Qi deficiency

Yellow sweat in the upper back, hypochondrium or head worse after exertion, slight shortness of breath, weak voice, spontaneous daytime sweating, dislike of speaking, bright-white complexion, tendency to catch colds, tiredness, poor appetite, slight abdominal distension after eating, weakness of the limbs, loose stools, Pale tongue, Empty pulse.

This pattern is more common in the elderly.

Yin deficiency with Empty-Heat and Dampness

Yellow sweat that stains the clothing in the axilla or genital region, greasy skin, dry throat at night, a feeling of heat in the evening, night sweating, five-palm heat, malar flush, insomnia, anxiety, dry mouth with a desire to drink in small sips, excessive vaginal discharge, a feeling of heaviness, Red tongue without coating, Floating-Empty and slightly Slippery pulse.

LOCALIZED SWEATING

Unilateral sweating

Unilateral sweating can occur on the left or the right side of the body. From an acupuncture perspective, this symptom is often due to an imbalance within the Yin or Yang Heel vessels. Unilateral sweating was mentioned in the 'Yellow Emperor's Classic of Internal Medicine – Simple Questions' (*Huang Di Nei Jing Su Wen*), which says in Chapter 3: '*Unilateral sweating is due to a withering of the channels on that side of the body'.*[2] A 'withering' or weakness of the channels on one side of the body may occur as a result of an accident to that side or after a high fever which injures the Yin fluids and leads to malnourishment of the channel of that side.

Wind-Phlegm

Unilateral sweating, severe dizziness, blurred vision, tremors, unilateral numbness or tingling of a limb, tinnitus, nausea, sputum in the throat, a feeling of oppression of the chest, Stiff or Deviated and Swollen tongue, Wiry-Slippery pulse.

Phlegm with Blood stasis

Unilateral sweating, unilateral numbness of a limb, dizziness, nausea, phlegm in the throat, a feeling of oppression of the chest, pain in the limbs, Purple and Swollen tongue, Slippery-Wiry pulse.

Deficiency of Qi and Blood

Unilateral sweating, poor appetite, loose stools, weak voice, tiredness, blurred vision, dizziness, numbness/

tingling of limbs, palpitations, dull-pale complexion, Pale tongue, Weak or Choppy pulse.

Cold-Dampness

Unilateral sweating, contraction of tendons, contraction of hands, a feeling of heaviness of the limbs, epigastric fullness, a feeling of heaviness of the head and body, a feeling of cold, cold limbs, sticky white tongue coating, Slippery-Slow pulse.

Nutritive- and Defensive-Qi not harmonized

Unilateral sweating, fever, occipital headache, aversion to cold, stiff neck, Floating-Slow pulse.

Wind-Dampness in the Girdle Vessel

Sweating of the upper or lower half of the body, numbness of the legs, a feeling of heaviness of the abdomen and legs, cold feet, pulse that is Wiry on both Middle positions.

Sweating on the head

Observation, Chapter 20; Interrogation, Chapter 41

Stomach Damp-Heat steaming upwards

Sweating on the head, facial pain, stuffed nose or thick, sticky nasal discharge, a feeling of fullness and pain of the epigastrium, a feeling of heaviness, thirst without a desire to drink, nausea, a feeling of heat, dull-yellow complexion, sticky taste, Red tongue with sticky yellow coating, Slippery-Rapid pulse.

In this case, Dampness does not accumulate in the limbs but 'steams' upwards to the head; this is more likely to happen when Heat is pronounced.

Liver-Fire

Sweating on the head, headache, red face, dizziness, tinnitus, irritability, propensity to outbursts of anger, thirst, bitter taste, constipation, dark urine, Red tongue with redder sides and dry yellow coating, Wiry-Rapid pulse.

Deficient Yang floating upwards

Sweating on the head, pale complexion, cold limbs, shortness of breath, a feeling of cold, tiredness, Weak-Deep pulse.

Retention of food with Stomach-Heat in children

Sweating on the head at night, restless sleep, waking up with crying during the night, vomiting, fullness, pain and distension of the epigastrium which are relieved by vomiting, nausea, vomiting of sour fluids, foul breath, sour regurgitation, belching, loose stools or constipation, poor appetite, thirst, a feeling of heat, thick, sticky yellow tongue coating, Slippery-Rapid pulse.

Sweating on the chest

Observation, Chapter 20; Interrogation, Chapter 41

Sweating on the chest is also called 'heart region sweating'.

Heart- and Spleen-Qi deficiency

Sweating on the chest, palpitations, shortness of breath on exertion, pale face, tiredness, slight depression, spontaneous sweating, poor appetite, slight abdominal distension after eating, weakness of the limbs, loose stools, Pale tongue, Empty pulse.

Heart- and Kidney-Yin deficiency

Sweating on the chest especially in the evening or night, palpitations, insomnia, dream-disturbed sleep, anxiety, poor memory, dizziness, tinnitus, hardness of hearing, lower backache, night sweating, scanty dark urine, normal-coloured tongue without coating, Floating-Empty pulse.

This is a common cause of sweating in the chest area.

Sweating of hands and feet

Observation, Chapters 14 and 20; Interrogation, Chapter 41

Damp-Heat in Stomach and Spleen

Sweating of hands and feet, hot hands, swollen fingers and toes, a feeling of fullness and pain of the epigastrium and lower abdomen, poor appetite, a feeling of heaviness, thirst without a desire to drink, nausea, loose stools with an offensive odour, a feeling of heat, dull-yellow complexion, sticky taste, Red tongue with sticky yellow coating, Slippery-Rapid pulse.

Stomach- and Spleen-Qi deficiency

Sweating of hands and feet, cold hands, poor appetite, slight abdominal distension after eating, tiredness, las-

situde, pale complexion, weakness of the limbs, loose stools, uncomfortable feeling in the epigastrium, loss of sense of taste, Pale tongue, Empty pulse.

Stomach- and Spleen-Yin deficiency

Sweating of hands and feet, dry mouth that is worse after sleep, dry lips, no appetite or slight hunger but no desire to eat, constipation (dry stools), dull or slightly burning epigastric pain, dry mouth and throat especially in the afternoon, thirst but with no desire to drink, or a desire to drink in small sips, slight feeling of fullness after eating, normal-coloured tongue without coating, or without coating in the centre, Floating-Empty pulse.

Sweating of the palms

Observation, Chapters 14 and 20; Interrogation, Chapter 41

Lung-Qi deficiency

Sweating of the hands, slight shortness of breath, slight cough, weak voice, spontaneous daytime sweating, dislike of speaking, bright-white complexion, tendency to catch colds, tiredness, dislike of cold, Pale tongue, Empty pulse.

Lung-Yin deficiency

Sweating of the hands in the afternoon, cough which is dry or with scanty, sticky sputum, weak/hoarse voice, dry mouth and throat, tickly throat, tiredness, dislike of speaking, thin body or thin chest, night sweating, normal-coloured tongue without coating (or with rootless coating) in the front part, Floating-Empty pulse.

Heart-Qi deficiency

Sweating of the hands, palpitations, shortness of breath on exertion, pale face, tiredness, slight depression, spontaneous sweating, Pale tongue, Empty pulse.

Heart-Yang deficiency

Profuse sweating of the hands, cold hands, palpitations, shortness of breath on exertion, tiredness, spontaneous sweating, a slight feeling of discomfort or stuffiness in the heart region, a feeling of cold, cold hands, bright-pale face, slightly dark lips, Pale tongue, Deep-Weak pulse.

Heart-Yin deficiency

Sweating of the hands in the evening, palpitations, insomnia, dream-disturbed sleep, poor memory, anxiety, tendency to be easily startled, mental restlessness, uneasiness, 'feeling hot and bothered', dry mouth and throat, night sweating, normal-coloured tongue without coating or with rootless coating, Floating-Empty pulse, especially on the left Front position.

Sweating in the axillae

The Liver and Heart channels influence the axilla.

Liver-Yin deficiency with Empty-Heat

Sweating in axillae, dizziness, numbness/tingling of limbs, insomnia, blurred vision, floaters, dry eyes, scanty menstruation or heavy bleeding (if Empty-Heat is severe), malar flush, cramps, withered and brittle nails, dry hair and skin, a feeling of heat in the evening, night sweating, five-palm heat, thirst with a desire to drink in small sips, Red tongue without coating, Floating-Empty and slightly Rapid pulse.

Damp-Heat in Liver and Gall-Bladder

Smelly sweating in axillae, fullness/pain of the hypochondrium, abdomen or epigastrium, bitter taste, poor appetite, nausea, a feeling of heaviness of the body, yellow vaginal discharge, vaginal itching, mid-cycle bleeding/pain, burning on urination, dark urine, yellow complexion and eyes, vomiting, Red tongue with redder sides and unilateral or bilateral sticky yellow coating, Wiry-Slippery-Rapid pulse.

Heart-Yin deficiency with Empty-Heat

Sweating in axillae, palpitations, insomnia, dream-disturbed sleep, poor memory, anxiety, tendency to be easily startled, mental restlessness, dry mouth and throat, thirst with a desire to sip fluids, a feeling of heat in the evening, malar flush, night sweating, five-palm heat, Red tongue, redder on the tip with no coating, Floating-Empty and Rapid pulse.

Heart-Fire

Sweating in axillae, palpitations, thirst, mouth and tongue ulcers, mental restlessness, a feeling of agitation, insomnia, dream-disturbed sleep, a feeling of heat, red face, bitter taste, Red tongue with redder tip and yellow coating, Overflowing-Rapid pulse.

ABSENCE OF SWEATING

Interrogation, Chapter 41

In exterior invasions of Wind, it is always important to ask about sweating, as absence of sweating indicates invasion of Wind-Cold with the prevalence of Cold and this corresponds to the Greater-Yang stage within the Six Stages identification of patterns. The Greater-Yang stage is always caused by the invasion of Wind-Cold, of which there are two types: one with the prevalence of Cold (in which there is no sweating), the other with the prevalence of Wind (in which there is sweating). Thus, it is very important in the initial stages of invasion of external Wind to ask about the presence or absence of sweating, especially if herbal medicine is used because there are two quite distinct prescriptions depending on whether there is a prevalence of Cold or Wind. These are Gui Zhi Tang *Ramulus Cinnamomi Decoction* for prevalence of Wind and Ma Huang Tang *Ephedra Decoction* for prevalence of Cold.

In other exterior conditions, absence of sweating usually indicates Cold or Cold-Dampness in the superficial layers of the body (the space between skin and muscles).

Invasion of Wind-Cold

Absence of sweating, aversion to cold, fever, cough, itchy throat, slight breathlessness, stuffed or runny nose with clear watery discharge, sneezing, occipital headache, body aches, thin white tongue coating, Floating-Tight pulse.

Cold on the Exterior, Heat in the Interior

Absence of sweating in any part of the body, aversion to cold, fever, restless legs, mental restlessness, thirst, sore throat, cough with yellow sputum.

Cold-Dampness on the Exterior

Absence of sweating, headache, a feeling of heaviness of the head and limbs, muscle ache, painful joints, dislike of cold.

NOTES

1. He Ren 1981 A New Explanation of the Synopsis of Prescriptions from the Golden Cabinet *Jin Gui Yao Lue Xin Jie* 金匮要略新解), Zhejiang Science Publishing House, Zhejiang, p. 120.
2. 1979 The Yellow Emperor's Classic of Internal Medicine – Simple Questions (*Huang Di Nei Jing Su Wen* 黄帝内经素问), People's Health Publishing House, Beijing, p. 17. First published c. 100BC.

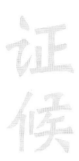

Chapter **77**

SKIN SIGNS

Chapter contents

GREASY SKIN   *781*

DRY SKIN   *782*

ERUPTIONS   *782*
  Eczema   *782*
  Psoriasis   *783*
  Acne   *783*
  Urticaria   *784*
  Rosacea   *785*
  Rash in the axillae   *785*
  Red, itchy and swollen fingers   *785*

INFECTIONS   *785*
  Herpes simplex   *785*
  Herpes zoster   *786*
  Tinea   *786*
  Candida   *787*

GROWTHS AND MASSES   *787*
  Warts   *787*
  Naevi (moles)   *787*
  Malignant melanoma   *788*
  Furuncle (boil) on the head   *788*
  Carbuncles on the neck   *788*
  Carbuncles on the upper back   *788*
  Nodules under the skin   *788*

NECK ULCERS   *789*

Due to the nature of skin diseases, in most cases only the skin signs will be given for each pattern without the other accompanying symptoms and signs pertaining to the Internal Organs.

GREASY SKIN

Dampness

Greasy skin, tendency to spots, a feeling of heaviness of the head and body, epigastric fullness, a sticky taste, a feeling of oppression of the chest, excessive vaginal discharge, sticky tongue coating, Slippery or Soggy pulse.

Other symptoms and signs depend on the organ involved and on whether Dampness is associated with Cold or Heat.

Damp-Phlegm

Greasy skin, puffy face, dark rings under the eyes in chronic cases, blackheads, greasy hair, tendency to sinus problems, chronic cough with expectoration of profuse, sticky white sputum which is easy to expectorate, a feeling of oppression of the chest, dizziness, blurred vision, somnolence, nausea, sputum in the throat, muzziness of the head, Swollen tongue with sticky coating, Slippery pulse.

Other symptoms and signs depend on the organ involved.

Phlegm-Heat

Greasy skin, tendency to red papules, dark rings under the eyes in chronic cases, blackheads, greasy hair, tendency to sinus problems, red face, puffy face, a feeling of heaviness and muzziness of the head, a feeling of heat, thirst with no desire to drink, a feeling of oppression of the chest, sputum in the throat, expectoration of yellow sputum, dizziness, nausea, Red and Swollen

tongue with sticky yellow coating, Slippery-Rapid pulse.

DRY SKIN

Observation, Chapter 21

Liver-Blood deficiency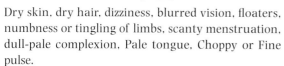

Dry skin, dry hair, dizziness, blurred vision, floaters, numbness or tingling of limbs, scanty menstruation, dull-pale complexion, Pale tongue, Choppy or Fine pulse.

Lung-Yin deficiency

Dry skin, thin hair, dry cough, weak voice, dry throat with a desire to sip water, hoarse voice, night sweating, tiredness, tongue without coating in the front, Floating-Empty pulse.

Kidney-Yin deficiency

Dry skin, dry hair, dry eyes, dizziness, tinnitus, hardness of hearing, poor memory, night sweating, dry mouth and throat at night, lower backache, constipation, scanty dark urine, tiredness, normal-coloured tongue without coating, Floating-Empty pulse.

Liver-Yin deficiency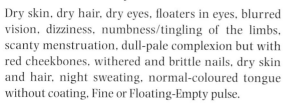

Dry skin, dry hair, dry eyes, floaters in eyes, blurred vision, dizziness, numbness/tingling of the limbs, scanty menstruation, dull-pale complexion but with red cheekbones, withered and brittle nails, dry skin and hair, night sweating, normal-coloured tongue without coating, Fine or Floating-Empty pulse.

Lung Dryness

Dry skin with acute onset, dry cough, dry throat, hoarse voice, dry tongue.

Wind-Dryness invading the Lungs

Dry skin with acute onset, aversion to cold, fever, dry cough, dry throat, itchy throat, hoarse voice, sore throat, Floating pulse.

Severe, chronic Blood stasis

Dry skin, dark face, dark rings under the eyes, abdominal pain, abdominal masses, painful periods, purple lips, Purple tongue, Wiry or Choppy pulse.

Other symptoms and signs depend on the organ involved. Blood stasis causes a dry skin only in severe and chronic cases.

Full-Heat

Dry skin, red face, a feeling of heat, thirst, mental restlessness, insomnia, Red tongue with dry yellow coating, Overflowing-Rapid pulse.

Other symptoms and signs depend on the organ involved.

Empty-Heat

Dry skin, scaly skin, malar flush, a feeling of heat in the evening, thirst with a desire to drink in small sips, mental restlessness, five-palm heat, night sweating, scanty dark urine, dry stools, Red tongue without coating, Floating-Empty and Rapid pulse.

Other symptoms and signs depend on the organ involved.

Wind in the skin

Dry skin, itchy skin, numbness/tingling of the limbs, skin eruptions that move around, come and go quickly and affect the top part of the body.

This is neither an external Wind, such as that seen in common colds and flu, nor internal Wind but simply 'Wind' in the skin, a condition frequently seen in skin diseases.

Liver-Blood deficiency with Empty-Wind

Chronic dry skin, itchy skin, scaly skin with white scales, slight tremor of the head/hand, facial tic, dizziness, blurred vision, unilateral numbness/tingling of a limb, Pale and Thin tongue, Choppy or Fine and slightly Wiry pulse.

ERUPTIONS

Eczema

Observation, Chapter 21

Damp-Heat with predominance of Heat

Red papular rash, vesicles, exudate, erosion, itching, a feeling of heat in the limbs, swollen, red and painful joints, epigastric fullness, sticky and bitter taste, thirst with no desire to drink, a feeling of heaviness of the head and body, a feeling of heat, Red tongue with sticky yellow coating, Slippery-Rapid pulse.

Damp-Heat with predominance of Dampness ⌘

Red papular rash, vesicles, exudate, weeping skin eruptions, thickening of the skin, itching, epigastric fullness, sticky taste, thirst with no desire to drink, a feeling of heaviness of the head and body, sticky yellow tongue coating, Slippery-Rapid pulse.

Blood deficient and dry

Chronic eczema, pale-red skin eruptions, dry skin, erosion, itching, thickening of the skin, ridges on the skin, dry hair, brittle nails, dizziness, blurred vision, floaters, numbness/tingling of limbs, scanty menstruation, dull-pale complexion, Pale tongue, Choppy or Fine pulse.

Spleen-Qi deficiency with Dampness

Chronic eczema, pale-red papular rash, vesicles, exudate, weeping skin eruptions, slight itching, poor appetite, slight abdominal distension after eating, tiredness, lassitude, pale or sallow complexion, weakness of the limbs, loose stools, abdominal fullness, a feeling of heaviness, sticky taste, poor digestion, undigested food in the stools, nausea, dull frontal headache, excessive vaginal discharge, Pale tongue with sticky coating, Soggy pulse.

Clinical note

- In my opinion, atopic eczema in children is caused by a congenital deficiency of the Defensive-Qi systems of the Lungs and Kidneys.

Psoriasis

Observation, Chapter 21

Blood-Heat

Red skin eruptions, hot limbs, itching with a feeling of heat, thirst, Red tongue, Overflowing-Rapid pulse.

Blood-Heat with Wind and Dryness

Red skin eruptions, red scales, dry skin, hot limbs, intense itching with feeling of heat, thirst,

Blood deficient and dry with Wind in the skin

Pale-red skin eruptions, dry and scaly skin with white scales, thickening of the skin, itching, dizziness, blurred vision, floaters, numbness/tingling of limbs, scanty

menstruation, dull-pale complexion, Pale tongue, Choppy or Fine pulse.

Blood stasis

Purple skin eruptions (often nummular or verrucous), chronic condition, dry skin, thickening of the skin, itching, purplish limbs, dark complexion, Purple tongue, Wiry or Choppy pulse.

Blood stasis with Wind and Dryness

Purple skin eruptions (often nummular or verrucous), chronic condition, dry scales, dry skin, thickening of the skin, intense itching, purplish limbs, dark complexion, Purple tongue, Wiry or Choppy pulse.

Wind and Heat in the skin

Acute red skin eruptions, itching, itchy area changing from day to day, hot limbs, a feeling of heat, thirst, Overflowing-Rapid pulse.

Blood-Heat with Wind and Dampness in the skin

Red, papular or vesicular skin eruptions often in skin creases, puffy skin, exudate, scaly skin, itching, Red and Swollen tongue, Overflowing-Rapid-Slippery pulse.

Liver- and Kidney-Yin deficiency with Empty-Heat ⚕

Pale-red macules covered by a thin layer of greyish-white scales, dry hair and skin, numbness/tingling of limbs, brittle nails, dizziness, tinnitus, dull occipital or vertical headache, insomnia, malar flush, dry eyes, blurred vision, lower backache, dry throat, dry vagina, night sweating, dry stools, scanty dark urine, scanty menstruation, five-palm heat, a feeling of heat in the evening, Red tongue without coating, Floating-Empty and Rapid pulse.

Acne

Observation, Chapter 21

Damp-Heat in the skin

Acne with red, papular eruptions, greasy skin, puffy face, sticky yellow tongue coating, Slippery-Rapid pulse.

Toxic Heat in the skin

Acne with large, red, pustular eruptions that are painful, a feeling of heat, red face, red eyes, Red tongue

with red points and thick, sticky yellow coating, Slippery-Overflowing-Rapid pulse.

Toxic Heat with Blood stasis in the skin

Acne with large, dark red or purple, pustular eruptions that are painful, a feeling of heat, dark face, red eyes, Reddish-Purple tongue with red points and thick, sticky yellow coating, Slippery-Overflowing-Wiry-Rapid pulse.

Spleen-Qi deficiency with Dampness

Chronic acne with pale-red, papular or vesicular eruptions which take a long time to come to a head, greasy skin, dull-pale complexion, Pale tongue with sticky coating, Soggy pulse.

Heat in the Stomach and Lungs

Acne with small, red, papular eruptions, on the face, chest and upper back, dry skin, blackheads, red face, a feeling of heat, Red tongue with dry yellow coating, Overflowing-Rapid pulse.

Damp-Phlegm in the skin

Acne with large, pale, vesicular eruptions, greasy skin, puffy face, greasy hair, Swollen tongue with sticky coating, Slippery pulse.

Damp-Phlegm with Blood stasis in the skin

Acne with large, dark, purple, papular eruptions, dark complexion, puffy face, dry skin if Blood stasis predominates, greasy skin if Damp-Phlegm predominates, Purple and Swollen tongue, Slippery-Wiry pulse.

Disharmony of Penetrating and Directing Vessels 👤

Acne that starts with puberty, greasy skin, papular eruptions which are aggravated before the period in females.

The essential characteristics of this condition are its onset at puberty and its aggravation before the period in females. This condition can manifest with any of the above patterns.

Clinical note

- When I treat acne, especially in women, I always harmonize the Penetrating and Directing Vessels, irrespective of the pattern.

Urticaria

Observation, Chapter 21

Wind-Heat in the skin

Urticaria with acute onset, red wheals with distinct margins, intense, generalized itching, itchy area changing from day to day, Red tongue, Floating-Rapid pulse.

Wind-Cold in the skin

Urticaria with acute onset, pale or pale-red wheals, itching, Floating pulse.

Heart-Fire

Urticaria with large, red wheals which could be cord shaped rather than round, swelling and discoloration of the skin on scratching, itching worse at night, mental restlessness, insomnia, Red tongue with redder tip and dry yellow coating, Overflowing-Rapid pulse.

Liver-Blood deficiency with internal Wind

Chronic urticaria that comes and goes with pale-red wheals, aggravated by overexertion, slight itching, dry skin, dry hair, Pale and dry tongue, Fine or Choppy pulse.

Toxic Heat in the skin

Urticaria with bright-red or dark-red wheals which may join together to form large patches, acute onset, severe itching, a feeling of heat, mental restlessness, Red tongue with red points and thick, sticky yellow coating, Overflowing-Slippery-Rapid pulse.

Wind-Heat in the skin with Stomach- and Spleen-Qi deficiency

Chronic urticaria with pale or pale-red wheals with indistinct margins, aggravated by overexertion, slight itching, aggravated by eating certain foods, loose stools, tiredness, poor appetite, Pale tongue, Empty pulse.

Disharmony of the Penetrating and Directing Vessels 👤

Urticaria which is worse before the periods and better after, and worse in the lower part of the body and legs, slight itching.

Blood stasis in the skin

Urticaria with large, dark-red or purple wheals, itching, worse at night, Purple tongue, Wiry or Choppy pulse.

Stomach-Heat

Urticaria with red wheals with distinct margins, elicited by eating certain foods, itching, burning epigastric pain, thirst, sour regurgitation, nausea, excessive hunger, foul breath, a feeling of heat, Red tongue with a yellow coating, Overflowing-Rapid pulse.

Blood-Heat

Urticaria with wheals which are very large and bright red, itching, an intense feeling of heat, skin very hot to the touch, mental restlessness, insomnia, thirst, Red tongue, Overflowing-Rapid pulse.

Rosacea

Observation, Chapter 21

Heat in Lungs and Stomach

Erythema of the face, especially like two large butterfly wings to the sides of the nostrils, a feeling of heat, thirst, Red tongue with yellow coating, Overflowing-Rapid pulse.

Blood-Heat

Erythema of the face with papular skin eruptions, a feeling of heat, mental restlessness, Red tongue, Overflowing-Rapid pulse.

Blood stasis

Chronic erythema of the face with dark colour, dark papular skin eruptions, dark complexion, Purple tongue, Wiry or Choppy pulse.

Toxic Heat

Pustular red, rash of the cheeks with swelling of the nose, a feeling of heat, insomnia, thirst, mental restlessness, Red tongue with red points and thick, sticky yellow coating, Overflowing-Slippery-Rapid pulse.

Rash in the axillae

Liver-Qi stagnation with Blood-Heat

Rash in the armpit, swelling and pain, a feeling of heat, headache, Red tongue with redder sides and yellow coating, Wiry-Rapid pulse.

Toxic Heat

Red rash in the armpit, oozing pus, painful, swollen, skin hard, fever, thirst, Red tongue with red points and sticky yellow coating, Overflowing-Slippery-Rapid pulse.

Damp-Heat in the Gall-Bladder

Rash in the armpit with pustular or papular eruptions, hypochondrial pain, fullness and distension, nausea, vomiting, inability to digest fats, yellow complexion and eyes, dizziness, tinnitus, irritability, a feeling of heaviness, unilateral or bilateral thick, sticky yellow coating, Slippery-Rapid pulse.

Heart-Fire

Red papular rash in the armpit, palpitations, thirst, agitation, insomnia, dream-disturbed sleep, feeling of heat, red face, bitter taste, Red tongue with redder tip and yellow coating, Overflowing-Rapid pulse.

Red, itchy and swollen fingers

Observation, Chapter 14

Toxic Heat in the Stomach

Red, itchy and swollen fingers, swelling of the fingers, numbness, a feeling of heat, thirst, Red tongue with red points and thick, sticky yellow coating, Overflowing-Slippery-Rapid pulse.

Damp-Heat in the Stomach

Red, itchy and swollen fingers, swelling of the fingers, epigastric fullness, sticky taste, thirst with no desire to drink, sticky yellow tongue coating, Slippery-Rapid pulse.

Invasion of external Toxic Heat

Red, swollen and painful fingers to the side of the nails with acute onset, white fingers, shivers, fever, Floating-Rapid pulse.

INFECTIONS

Herpes simplex

Observation, Chapter 21

Damp-Heat in the skin

Red papular or vesicular skin eruptions around the mouth or nostrils, erythema, itching, pain, sticky yellow tongue coating, Slippery-Rapid pulse.

Damp-Heat in the skin with Spleen-Qi deficiency

Chronic, red, papular or vesicular skin eruptions around the mouth or nostrils which come and go, aggravated by overexertion, erythema, slight itching, Pale tongue with sticky yellow coating, Soggy-Rapid pulse.

Damp-Heat with Toxic Heat in the skin

Dark-red, papular or pustular skin eruptions around the mouth or nostrils, itching, pain, a feeling of heat, thirst, mental restlessness, Red tongue with red points and thick, sticky yellow coating, Overflowing-Slippery-Rapid pulse.

Invasion of Toxic Heat

Acute, red, papular eruptions around the mouth or eyes in newborn babies and infants, crying at night.

Damp-Heat with invasion of Wind-Heat

Acute, red, papular eruptions in the top part of the body, especially face, with intense itching, aversion to cold, fever, headache, eye pain, tongue Red on the sides/front, Floating-Slippery-Rapid pulse.

Damp-Heat in the Liver channel

Papular or pustular herpes eruptions in the genital area, itching, a feeling of heaviness, malaise, fever, sticky taste, tongue Red on the sides with sticky yellow coating, Slippery-Wiry-Rapid pulse.

Yin deficiency with Empty-Heat and Damp-Heat

Chronic, recurrent, lingering, pale-red, papular eruptions, exudate, puffy skin, night sweating, a feeling of heat in the evening, dry mouth, desire to drink in small sips, five-palm heat, Red tongue without coating, Floating-Empty and Rapid pulse.

Herpes zoster

Observation, Chapter 21

Wind-Heat in the skin

Papular skin eruptions in the upper part of the body preceded by intense itching, later turning into vesicles oozing a clear fluid, tongue Red on the sides/front with red points, Floating-Rapid pulse.

Damp-Heat in the skin

Vesicular skin eruptions oozing a sticky fluid, itching, tongue Red on the sides/front with red points and sticky yellow coating, Slippery-Rapid pulse.

Damp-Heat in the Gall-Bladder and Liver

Papular skin eruptions later turning into vesicles oozing a sticky yellow fluid, itching, fullness/pain of the hypochondrium, abdomen or epigastrium, bitter taste, a feeling of heaviness of the body, yellow vaginal discharge, vaginal itching, burning on urination, dark urine, Red tongue with redder sides and unilateral or bilateral sticky yellow coating, Wiry-Slippery-Rapid pulse.

Stagnation of Qi and stasis of Blood

Late stage of herpes zoster infection, dark, papular rash, intense pain.

Toxic Heat

Painful, pustular eruptions, a feeling of heat, thirst, mental restlessness, insomnia, Red tongue with red points and thick, sticky yellow coating, Overflowing-Slippery-Rapid pulse.

Blood stasis

Large, painful, dark-red or purple, pustular eruptions which last a long time, mental restlessness, Purple tongue, Wiry pulse.

Tinea

Observation, Chapter 21

Damp-Heat

Tinea with redness and swelling of the skin, pustular swelling of the scalp (tinea capitis), itchy vesicular rash of the feet (tinea pedis), Red tongue with sticky yellow coating, Slippery-Rapid pulse.

Toxic Heat

Tinea with redness, pain and pronounced swelling of the skin, pustular swelling of the scalp (tinea capitis), painful pustular rash of the feet (tinea pedis), Red tongue with thick, sticky yellow coating and red points, Slippery-Overflowing-Rapid pulse.

Wind-Heat

Tinea with sudden onset, with redness, itching and papular rash of the scalp, tongue Red on the sides/front, Floating-Rapid pulse.

Dampness with chronic Spleen-Qi deficiency

Chronic tinea, characterized by a pale-red rash with a white ring around the lesions with scaling, excessive vaginal discharge, poor appetite, slight abdominal distension after eating, tiredness, lassitude, pale or sallow complexion, weakness of the limbs, loose stools, abdominal fullness, a feeling of heaviness, a sticky taste, poor digestion, undigested food in the stools, nausea, Pale tongue with sticky coating, Soggy pulse.

Candida

Observation, Chapter 21

Damp-Heat

Candida with weepy rash in the flexures of the body (under breasts in women, axilla, groin or between fingers and toes), redness and itching of the skin, itchiness, soreness and redness of the vulva, vagina or penis, white plaques and swelling of the inside of the mouth, epigastric fullness, sticky taste, thirst with no desire to drink, a feeling of heaviness of the head and body, a feeling of heat, sticky yellow tongue coating, Slippery-Rapid pulse.

Dampness

Candida with weepy rash in the flexures of the body (under breasts in women, axilla, groin or between fingers and toes), itching of the skin, itchiness and soreness of the vulva, vagina or penis, white plaques and swelling of the inside of the mouth, epigastric fullness, sticky taste, a feeling of heaviness of the head and body, a feeling of heat, sticky white tongue coating, Slippery pulse.

Dampness with chronic Spleen-Qi deficiency

Chronic candida with weepy rash in the flexures of the body (under breasts in women, axilla, groin or between fingers and toes), itching of the skin, itchiness and soreness of the vulva, vagina or penis, excessive vaginal discharge, white plaques and swelling of the inside of the mouth, epigastric fullness, a sticky taste, a feeling of heaviness of the head and body, poor appetite, slight abdominal distension after eating, tiredness, pale complexion, weakness of the limbs, loose stools, Pale tongue with a sticky white coating, Soggy pulse.

GROWTHS AND MASSES

Warts

Observation, Chapter 21

Blood deficiency and Dryness

Common warts usually on the hands, dry and pale brown in colour, dry skin, dry hair, blurred vision, Pale and dry tongue, Choppy or Fine pulse.

Blood-Heat

Reddish or brown warts, a feeling of heat, mental restlessness, insomnia, thirst, Red tongue, Overflowing-Rapid pulse.

Blood stasis

Dark-brown warts, dark complexion, mental restlessness, dry skin, Purple tongue, Wiry pulse.

Damp-Heat in the Liver channel

Genital warts on the penis or vulva and vagina, genital itching and pain, Red tongue with redder sides and sticky yellow coating, Wiry-Slippery-Rapid pulse.

Damp-Heat with Toxic Heat

Painful genital warts with pustular eruption, a feeling of heat, thirst, mental restlessness, Red tongue with red points and thick, sticky yellow coating, Overflowing-Slippery-Rapid pulse.

Naevi (moles)

Observation, Chapter 21

Blood-Heat

Red or light brown moles, Red tongue, Overflowing-Rapid pulse.

Damp-Heat

Brown moles in the lower part of the body, Red tongue with sticky yellow coating, Slippery-Rapid pulse.

Blood stasis

Dark-brown naevi, dark complexion, mental restlessness, dry skin, Purple tongue, Wiry pulse.

Malignant melanoma

Observation, Chapter 21

Blood-Heat

Red or bright-brown moles, Red tongue, Overflowing-Rapid pulse.

Blood stasis

Dark-red or dark-brown moles with nodules, dark complexion, Purple tongue, Wiry pulse.

Blood-Heat with Damp-Heat

Brown moles with plaques, Red tongue with sticky yellow coating, Overflowing-Slippery-Rapid pulse.

Furuncle (boil) on the head
Damp-Heat in the Stomach and Spleen

Painful furuncle on the head oozing pus, greasy skin, facial pain, stuffed-up nose or thick sticky nasal discharge, a feeling of fullness and pain of the epigastrium and lower abdomen, a feeling of heaviness especially of the head, thirst without desire to drink, dull-yellow complexion, Red tongue with sticky yellow coating, Slippery-Rapid pulse.

Summer-Heat with Toxic Heat

White, movable furuncle on the head shaped like an egg or a plum, of acute onset in summertime and oozing pus, Red tongue with sticky white coating, Rapid pulse.

Carbuncles on the neck
Damp-Heat in Stomach and Spleen

Painful carbuncle on the neck, shaped like a honeycomb, oozing yellow pus, fever, with higher fever when the carbuncle breaks and oozes pus, headache, a feeling of heaviness, sticky taste, nausea, epigastric fullness, thirst, constipation, dark urine, Red tongue with sticky yellow coating and Slippery-Rapid pulse.

Empty-Heat with Toxic Heat in the Stomach

Carbuncle on the neck that is dark in colour, not oozing pus until late stages, skin slow in healing after breaking, a feeling of heat in the evening, dry throat, dry stools, night sweating, five-palm heat, insomnia, Red tongue without coating, Floating-Empty and Rapid pulse.

Deficiency of Qi and Blood

Carbuncle on the neck that is light in colour, not oozing pus until late stages, skin slow to heal after breaking, oozing thin dilute pus, poor appetite, loose stools, weak voice, palpitations, tiredness, blurred vision, dull-pale complexion, dizziness, Pale tongue, Weak or Choppy pulse.

Carbuncles on the upper back
Toxic Heat in Stomach and Lungs

Carbuncles on the upper back, red, swollen, painful, fever, thirst, Red tongue with red points and thick, sticky yellow coating, Rapid-Slippery-Overflowing pulse.

Summer-Heat

Carbuncles on the upper back, sudden onset in summer time, red, swollen, painful, dizziness, fever, insomnia, Red tongue with thin yellow coating, Floating-Rapid pulse.

Nodules under the skin

Soft nodules under the skin are, by definition, due to Phlegm. Generally they are not red, not painful, not hot and not hard; they are usually shaped like a plum and are movable. They do not break and produce pus.

Spleen-Qi deficiency with Phlegm

Soft, movable nodules under the skin, tiredness, poor appetite, loose stools, Pale and Swollen tongue with sticky coating, Weak and slightly Slippery pulse.

Phlegm-Heat

Soft nodules under the skin that are slightly red, expectoration of yellow sputum, a feeling of oppression of the chest, a feeling of heat, Red and Swollen tongue with sticky yellow coating, Slippery-Rapid pulse.

Wind-Phlegm

Nodules under the skin, headache, giddiness, possibly hypertension, blurred vision, numbness of the limbs, a feeling of oppression of the chest, nausea, headache, Swollen and Stiff tongue, Slippery-Wiry pulse.

This condition is more common in the elderly.

NECK ULCERS

Heat in Liver and Stomach

Neck ulcers that are hard and shaped like an egg, red in colour, painful, burning, headache, bitter taste, thirst, Red tongue with dry yellow coating, Overflowing-Rapid pulse.

Toxic Heat in Lungs and Stomach

Ulcers on the neck, red, swollen, painful, thirst, headache, cough, Red tongue with dry yellow coating, Overflowing-Slippery-Rapid pulse.

Liver-Qi and Liver-Blood stagnation

Ulcers on the neck on both sides, hard like a stone, shaped like a plum or an egg, dark in colour, or no change in skin colour, painful, no feeling of heat, not oozing pus until late stages, Purple tongue, Wiry pulse.

Liver-Qi stagnation and Liver-Blood stasis with Phlegm

Ulcers on the neck behind the ear, shaped like a plum, not hard, immovable, no skin colour changes, no feeling of heat, no pain, Purple and Swollen tongue, Wiry-Slippery pulse.

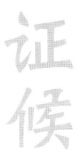

Chapter **78**

EMOTIONAL SYMPTOMS

Chapter contents

PROPENSITY TO ANGER   *791*

PROPENSITY TO WORRY   *791*

SADNESS   *792*

FEAR/ANXIETY   *792*

TENDENCY TO BE EASILY STARTLED   *793*

EXCESS JOY   *794*

MENTAL RESTLESSNESS   *794*

SEVERE TIMIDITY   *795*

INAPPROPRIATE LAUGHTER   *795*

PROPENSITY TO ANGER

Interrogation, Chapter 44

Liver-Qi stagnation

Repressed anger with occasional outbursts, hypochondrial or epigastric distension, irritability, moodiness, a feeling of a lump in the throat, premenstrual tension, Wiry pulse.

Liver-Yang rising

Propensity to outbursts of anger, irritability, headache, dizziness, tinnitus, irritability, propensity to outbursts of anger, Wiry pulse.

Liver-Fire

Propensity to severe outbursts of anger, irritability, aggressiveness, insomnia, headache, red face, dizziness, tinnitus, irritability, propensity to outbursts of anger, thirst, bitter taste, constipation, dark urine, Red tongue with redder sides and dry yellow coating, Wiry-Rapid pulse.

Clinical note

- Venting one's anger helps only if there is Liver-Qi stagnation; with Liver-Yang rising and Liver-Fire, venting one's anger will only fan it more.

PROPENSITY TO WORRY

Interrogation, Chapter 44

Heart- and Spleen-Qi deficiency

Worry, slightly obsessive thinking, slight depression, overthinking, palpitations, shortness of breath on exertion, pale face, tiredness, spontaneous sweating,

poor appetite, slight abdominal distension after eating, weakness of the limbs, loose stools, Pale tongue, Empty pulse.

Lung-Qi deficiency

Worry, depression, dislike of speaking, slight shortness of breath, slight cough, weak voice, spontaneous daytime sweating, bright-white complexion, tendency to catch colds, tiredness, dislike of cold, Pale tongue, Empty pulse.

Lung-Qi stagnation

Worry, mild irritability, depression, a feeling of a lump in the throat, difficulty in swallowing, a feeling of oppression or distension of the chest, slight breathlessness, sighing, tongue slightly Red on the sides in the chest areas, pulse very slightly Tight on the right Front position.

Heart-Blood deficiency

Worry, depression, insomnia, poor memory, anxiety, dream-disturbed sleep, poor memory, tendency to be easily startled, palpitations, dizziness, dull-pale complexion, pale lips, Pale and Thin tongue, Choppy or Fine pulse.

Liver-Blood deficiency

Worry which increases after the period in women, dizziness, blurred vision, floaters, numbness/tingling of limbs, scanty menstruation, dull-pale complexion, Pale tongue, Choppy or Fine pulse.

Heart-Yin deficiency

Worry, insomnia, dream-disturbed sleep, poor memory, anxiety, tendency to be easily startled, mental restlessness, uneasiness, 'feeling hot and bothered', palpitations, dry mouth and throat, night sweating, normal-coloured tongue without coating or with rootless coating, Floating-Empty pulse especially on the left Front position.

Heart-Yin deficiency with Empty-Heat

Worry, especially in the evening, insomnia, dream-disturbed sleep, poor memory, anxiety, tendency to be easily startled, mental restlessness, uneasiness, 'feeling hot and bothered', palpitations, dry mouth and throat, thirst with a desire to sip fluids, a feeling of heat in the evening, malar flush, night sweating, five-palm heat, Red tongue, redder on the tip with no coating, Floating-Empty and Rapid pulse.

> ### Clinical note
> - Worry is one of the most pervasive emotional causes of disease in Western patients. It affects the Lungs and Heart and it causes pathology of the chest and breasts.

SADNESS

Interrogation, Chapter 44

This includes a sad emotional state with frequent crying.

Lung- and Heart-Qi deficiency

Sadness, crying, depression, dislike of speaking, palpitations, shortness of breath on exertion, pale face, tiredness, weak voice, spontaneous daytime sweating, bright-white complexion, tendency to catch colds, dislike of cold, Pale tongue, Empty pulse.

Liver-Blood deficiency

Sadness, crying, mental confusion, aimlessness, poor memory, dizziness, blurred vision, floaters, numbness/tingling of limbs, scanty menstruation, dull-pale complexion, Pale tongue, Choppy or Fine pulse.

This pattern is more common in women and is due to sadness affecting the Liver.

Heart-Blood deficiency

Sadness, crying, depression, insomnia, dream-disturbed sleep, anxiety, tendency to be easily startled, poor memory, palpitations, dizziness, dull-pale complexion, pale lips, Pale and Thin tongue, Choppy or Fine pulse.

Lung-Qi stagnation

Sadness, mild irritability, depression, a feeling of a lump in the throat, difficulty in swallowing, a feeling of oppression or distension of the chest, slight breathlessness, sighing, tongue slightly Red on the sides in the chest areas, pulse very slightly Tight on the right Front position.

FEAR/ANXIETY

Interrogation, Chapter 44

Deficiency of Qi and Blood

Mild anxiety, timidity, poor appetite, loose stools, weak voice, tiredness, blurred vision, dizziness, numbness/

tingling of limbs, palpitations, dull-pale complexion, Pale tongue, Weak or Choppy pulse.

Kidney-Yin deficiency

Fearfulness, anxiety, depression, lack of will-power and motivation, insomnia, poor memory, dizziness, tinnitus, hardness of hearing, night sweating, dry mouth and throat at night, lower backache, constipation, scanty dark urine, tiredness, normal-coloured tongue without coating, Floating-Empty pulse.

Kidney-Yang deficiency

Mild anxiety, depression, timidity, lower backache, cold knees, a feeling of cold, bright-white complexion, weak knees, tiredness, lassitude, abundant clear urination, urination at night, impotence, decreased libido, Pale and wet tongue, Deep-Weak pulse.

Liver-Blood deficiency

Mild anxiety, fear of the future, depression, a feeling of aimlessness, dizziness, blurred vision, floaters, numbness/tingling of limbs, scanty menstruation, dull-pale complexion, Pale tongue, Choppy or Fine pulse.

Gall-Bladder deficiency

Fearfulness, timidity, irresoluteness and indecisiveness when something crops up, tendency to be easily startled, dislike of speaking, lack of courage, fluster, sighing, restless dreams, insomnia, nervousness, excessive dreaming, dizziness, blurred vision, floaters, Pale tongue.

Liver-Qi deficiency

Fear and timidity, lack of resolve, depression, unhappiness, nervousness, tendency to be easily startled, lack of courage and initiative, indecision, sighing, restless dreams, irritability, weak tendons, dizziness, blurred vision, floaters, hypochondrial distension, irregular periods, Pale or normal tongue, Weak pulse.

TENDENCY TO BE EASILY STARTLED

Most of the causes of this symptom are due to Heart patterns and the patient is likely to have a Heart crack on the tongue.

Heart-Blood deficiency

Tendency to be easily startled, insomnia, poor memory, anxiety, dream-disturbed sleep, palpitations, dizziness,

dull-pale complexion, pale lips, Pale and Thin tongue, Choppy or Fine pulse.

Heart-Yin deficiency

Tendency to be easily startled that is worse in the evening, mental restlessness, uneasiness, 'feeling hot and bothered', poor memory, anxiety, insomnia, dream-disturbed sleep, palpitations, dry mouth and throat, night sweating, normal-coloured tongue without coating or with rootless coating, Floating-Empty pulse especially on the left Front position.

Deficiency of Heart and Gall-Bladder

Tendency to be easily startled, timidity, dislike of speaking, lack of courage and initiative, indecisiveness, fluster, sighing, restless dreams, insomnia, nervousness, excessive dreaming, dizziness, blurred vision, floaters, Pale tongue.

This is an unusual pattern, which actually describes the character of a person rather than a pattern; and it is based on the idea of the Gall-Bladder being the seat of courage and decisiveness.

Heart-Fire

Tendency to be easily startled, agitation, mental restlessness, insomnia, dream-disturbed sleep, palpitations, thirst, mouth and tongue ulcers, a feeling of heat, red face, dark urine or blood in the urine, bitter taste (after a bad night's sleep), Red tongue with redder tip and yellow coating, Overflowing and Rapid pulse.

Phlegm-Fire harassing the Heart

Tendency to be easily startled whilst in bed, agitation, insomnia, dream-disturbed sleep, mental confusion, mental restlessness, depression, manic behaviour, rash behaviour, tendency to hit or scold people, palpitations, thirst, red face, a feeling of oppression of the chest, dark urine, expectoration of phlegm, rattling sound in the throat, bitter taste, Red tongue with redder swollen tip and Heart crack with a sticky yellow coating inside it, Slippery-Rapid or Slippery-Overflowing-Rapid pulse.

Liver-Qi stagnation and Blood deficiency

Tendency to be easily startled, irritability, propensity to anger, hypochondrial or epigastric distension, irritability, moodiness, a feeling of a lump in the throat, premenstrual tension, dizziness, blurred

vision, floaters, numbness/tingling of limbs, scanty menstruation, dull-pale complexion, Pale tongue, Choppy or Fine pulse that is also slightly Wiry on the left.

EXCESS JOY

Interrogation, Chapter 44

A normal state of joy is obviously not a cause of disease. Several emotional states are included under the term of 'excess joy'. First, it includes the sudden state of extreme elation deriving from joyful news; this makes Qi rise and it expands the Heart. Secondly, excess joy can be interpreted as a life characterized by excessive excitement and stimulation; this also causes Qi to rise and may lead to Heart-Fire. Thirdly, excess joy is seen in certain mental conditions such as hypomania or manic behaviour.

Heart-Fire

Excess joy, permanently elated mood, excessive laughter, mental restlessness, a feeling of agitation, dream-disturbed sleep, insomnia, palpitations, thirst, mouth and tongue ulcers, a feeling of heat, red face, bitter taste, Red tongue with redder tip and yellow coating, Overflowing-Rapid pulse.

Heart Empty-Heat

Excess joy, a permanently elated feeling as if being driven, anxiety, tendency to be easily startled, mental restlessness, uneasiness, 'feeling hot and bothered', insomnia, dream-disturbed sleep, palpitations, poor memory, dry mouth and throat, thirst with a desire to sip fluids, a feeling of heat in the evening, malar flush, night sweating, five-palm heat, Red tongue redder on the tip with no coating, Floating-Empty and Rapid pulse.

Phlegm-Fire harassing the Heart

Excess joy, mental confusion, excessive and inappropriate laughter, mental restlessness, insomnia, dream-disturbed sleep, a feeling of agitation, palpitations, thirst, red face, a feeling of oppression of the chest, dark urine, expectoration of phlegm, rattling sound in the throat, bitter taste, shouting, Red tongue with redder swollen tip and Heart crack with a sticky yellow coating inside it, Slippery-Rapid or Slippery-Overflowing-Rapid pulse.

MENTAL RESTLESSNESS

Interrogation, Chapter 44

'Mental restlessness' is a translation of the term *fan zao*, which literally means 'vexation and restlessness'. It also includes restless legs. The term *fan zao* encompasses two different symptoms: *fan* (vexation) is due to Full-Heat and pertains to the Lungs, whereas *zao* (restlessness) is due to Empty-Heat and pertains to the Kidneys. *Fan* is Yang, whereas *Zao* is Yin.

Yin deficiency with Empty-Heat

Vague mental restlessness, insomnia, restless legs, excessive dreaming, anxiety, dry throat at night, a feeling of heat in the evening, night sweating, five-palm heat, malar flush, dry mouth with a desire to drink in small sips, Red tongue without coating, Floating-Empty and Rapid pulse.

This is a general pattern of Yin deficiency with Empty-Heat, which may affect the Kidneys, Heart or Lungs.

Phlegm-Heat in the Stomach and Heart

Mental restlessness, mental confusion, insomnia, dream-disturbed sleep, agitation, rash behaviour, tendency to hit or scold people, shouting, depression, manic behaviour, palpitations, thirst, red face, a feeling of oppression of the chest and epigastrium, dark urine, expectoration of phlegm, rattling sound in the throat, bitter taste, burning epigastric pain, bleeding gums, dry mouth, mouth ulcers, sour regurgitation, nausea, vomiting soon after eating, excessive hunger, foul breath, a feeling of heat, tongue Red in the centre with a sticky-yellow coating and a Stomach/Heart crack with a rough, sticky yellow coating inside it, Slippery-Rapid pulse.

Heart-Fire

Pronounced mental restlessness, agitation, insomnia, dream-disturbed sleep, palpitations, thirst, mouth and tongue ulcers, a feeling of heat, red face, bitter taste, Red tongue with redder tip and yellow coating, Overflowing-Rapid pulse.

Lung-Heat

Mental restlessness, worry, cough, slight breathlessness, a feeling of heat, chest ache, flaring of nostrils, thirst, red face, Red tongue with yellow coating, Overflowing-Rapid pulse.

SEVERE TIMIDITY

Gall-Bladder deficiency

Severe timidity, indecisiveness, tendency to be easily startled, lack of resolve, dislike of speaking, lack of courage, fluster, fear, irresoluteness and indecisiveness when something crops up, sighing, restless and excessive dreaming, insomnia, nervousness, dizziness, blurred vision, floaters, Pale tongue.

Liver-Qi deficiency

Severe timidity, lack of resolve, unhappiness, weak tendons, fear, depression, nervousness, tendency to being easily startled, lack of courage and initiative, indecision, sighing, restless dreams, irritability, weak tendons, dizziness, blurred vision, floaters, hypochondrial distension, irregular periods, Pale or normal tongue, Weak pulse.

Kidney-Yang deficiency

Severe timidity, lack of will-power or confidence, lower backache, cold knees, a feeling of cold, bright-white complexion, weak knees, tiredness, lassitude, abundant clear urination, urination at night, impotence, decreased libido, Pale and wet tongue, Deep-Weak pulse.

Heart- and Spleen-Qi deficiency

Severe timidity, worry, inappropriate eagerness to please others, slight depression, palpitations, shortness of breath on exertion, pale face, tiredness, spontaneous sweating, poor appetite, slight abdominal distension after eating, weakness of the limbs, loose stools, Pale tongue, Empty pulse.

Heart- and Spleen-Blood deficiency

Severe timidity, anxiety, lack of confidence, worry, slightly obsessive thinking, slight depression, overthinking, palpitations, shortness of breath on exertion, pale face, tiredness, spontaneous sweating, poor appetite, slight abdominal distension after eating, weakness of the limbs, loose stools, Pale tongue, Empty pulse.

INAPPROPRIATE LAUGHTER

This includes a mental state that may range from mild hypomania to full-blown manic behaviour.

Heart-Fire

Inappropriate laughter, manic behaviour, mental restlessness, a feeling of agitation, insomnia, dream-disturbed sleep, palpitations, thirst, mouth and tongue ulcers, a feeling of heat, red face, bitter taste, Red tongue with redder tip and yellow coating, Overflowing-Rapid pulse.

Phlegm-Fire harassing the Heart

Inappropriate laughter, mental confusion, a feeling of agitation, mental restlessness, insomnia, dream-disturbed sleep, rash behaviour, tendency to hit or scold people, shouting, depression, manic behaviour, palpitations, thirst, red face, a feeling of oppression of the chest, dark urine, expectoration of phlegm, rattling sound in the throat, bitter taste, Red tongue with redder swollen tip and Heart crack with a sticky, dry yellow coating inside it, Slippery-Rapid or Slippery-Overflowing-Rapid pulse.

Kidney- and Heart-Yin deficiency with Heart Empty-Heat

Inappropriate laughter, insomnia, excessive dreaming, mental restlessness, anxiety, poor memory, palpitations, dizziness, tinnitus, hardness of hearing, lower backache, nocturnal emissions with dreams, a feeling of heat in the evening, night sweating, five-palm heat, scanty dark urine, dry stools, Red tongue with redder tip and a Heart crack, Floating-Empty and Rapid pulse, or a pulse that is Deep and Weak on both Rear positions and Overflowing on both Front positions.

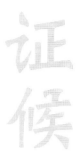

MENTAL AND EMOTIONAL SYMPTOMS

Chapter contents

DEPRESSION   *797*

DEPRESSION AND MANIC BEHAVIOUR   *798*
Depressive phase   *798*
Manic phase   *799*

ANXIETY   *799*

IRRITABILITY   *800*

SCHIZOPHRENIA   *802*

DEPRESSION

Interrogation, Chapter 44

Liver-Qi stagnation

Depression, moodiness, irritability, anxiety, frustration, nervous tension, hypochondrial or epigastric distension, a feeling of a lump in the throat, premenstrual tension, Wiry pulse.

Stagnant Liver-Qi turned into Heat rebelling upwards

Depression, anxiety, insomnia, moodiness, irritability, propensity to outbursts of anger, hypochondrial or epigastric distension, a slight feeling of oppression of the chest, premenstrual tension, irregular periods, premenstrual breast distension, a feeling of a lump in the throat, a feeling of heat, red face, thirst, heavy periods, tongue Red on the sides, Wiry and slightly Rapid pulse.

Liver-Qi stagnation with Qi-Phlegm

Depression, moodiness, irritability, a feeling of a lump in the throat, hypochondrial or epigastric distension, premenstrual tension, sputum in the throat, Swollen tongue, Wiry-Slippery pulse.

Kidney-Yang deficiency

Depression, lack of motivation, lack of will-power, lack of initiative, exhaustion, desire to curl up, lower backache, cold knees, a feeling of cold, bright-white complexion, weak knees, tiredness, lassitude, abundant clear urination, urination at night, impotence, decreased libido, Pale and wet tongue, Deep-Weak pulse.

Heart-Blood deficiency

Depression, tearfulness, sadness, insomnia, dream-disturbed sleep, poor memory, anxiety, tendency to be

easily startled, palpitations, dizziness, dull-pale complexion, pale lips, Pale and Thin tongue, Choppy or Fine pulse.

Liver-Blood deficiency

Depression, sadness, lack of direction, dizziness, blurred vision, floaters, numbness/tingling of limbs, scanty menstruation, dull-pale complexion, Pale tongue, Choppy or Fine pulse.

Spleen- and Heart-Blood deficiency

Depression, brooding, slightly obsessive thinking, anxiety, insomnia, dream-disturbed sleep, poor memory, tendency to be easily startled, palpitations, dizziness, dull-pale complexion, pale lips, tiredness, weak muscles, loose stools, poor appetite, scanty periods, Pale and Thin tongue, Choppy or Fine pulse.

Heart-Yang deficiency

Depression, lack of motivation, tendency to be easily startled, palpitations, shortness of breath on exertion, tiredness, spontaneous sweating, a slight feeling of discomfort or stuffiness in the heart region, a feeling of cold, cold hands, bright-pale face, slightly dark lips, Pale tongue, Deep-Weak pulse.

Heart- and Kidney-Yin deficiency with Empty-Heat

Depression, anxiety in the evening, mental restlessness, insomnia, dream-disturbed sleep, anxiety, poor memory, palpitations, dizziness, tinnitus, hardness of hearing, lower backache, nocturnal emissions with dreams, a feeling of heat in the evening, night sweating, five-palm heat, scanty dark urine, dry stools, Red tongue with redder tip and a Heart crack, Floating-Empty and Rapid pulse.

Phlegm-Fire harassing the Heart

Depression, mental restlessness, anxiety, agitation, phobias, insomnia, excessive dreaming, mental confusion, rash behaviour, shouting, manic behaviour, a feeling of heat in the heart region, palpitations, thirst, red face, a feeling of oppression of the chest, expectoration of phlegm, sputum in the throat, bitter taste, Red tongue with redder swollen tip and Heart crack with a sticky, dry yellow coating inside it, Slippery-Rapid or Slippery-Overflowing-Rapid pulse.

Heart-Blood stasis

Depression, mental restlessness, insomnia, a feeling of agitation in the evening, excessive dreaming, palpitations, stabbing or pricking chest pain which may radiate to the inner aspect of the left arm or to the shoulder, a feeling of oppression or constriction of the chest, cyanosis of lips and nails, cold hands, tongue entirely Purple or Purple only on the sides in the chest areas, Choppy or Wiry pulse.

Heat in the Gall-Bladder

Depression, mental restlessness, short temper, irritability, nausea, dry throat, bitter taste, a feeling of fullness of the hypochondrium, blurred vision, unilateral yellow tongue coating, Wiry pulse.

Worry injuring the Mind

Depression, feeling like in a trance, absentmindedness, lack of initiative, sadness, worry, crying, yawning, Pale tongue, Weak pulse.

Diaphragm-Heat

Depression, mental restlessness, a feeling of anxiety in the chest, a feeling of heat in the heart region, a feeling of stuffiness of the chest, thirst, nausea, yellow tongue coating, Rapid pulse.

This is a short-term depression caused by residual Heat following an invasion of Wind-Heat.

> ### Clinical note
>
> - In chronic depression I often use BL-23 Shenshu and BL-52 Zhishi to stimulate will-power irrespective of the pattern.

DEPRESSION AND MANIC BEHAVIOUR

Interrogation, Chapter 44

Depressive phase
Stagnation of Qi and Phlegm

Depression, apathy, dull thinking, incoherent speech, muttering to oneself, irritability, moodiness, not remembering to eat, hypochondrial or epigastric distension, a feeling of a lump in the throat, premenstrual tension, Swollen tongue with sticky coating, Wiry-Slippery pulse.

Heart- and Spleen-Blood deficiency

Depression, excessive dreaming, mental confusion, tendency to be easily startled, sadness, crying, shouting, shutting of windows, muttering to oneself, brooding, slightly obsessive thinking, anxiety, insomnia, dream-disturbed sleep, poor memory, tendency to be easily startled, palpitations, dizziness, dull-pale complexion, pale lips, tiredness, weak muscles, loose stools, poor appetite, scanty periods, Pale and Thin tongue, Choppy or Fine pulse.

Manic phase
Phlegm-Fire harassing the Mind

Manic behaviour, insomnia, dream-disturbed sleep, propensity to outbursts of anger, shouting, scolding or hitting people, overspending of money, exceptional physical strength, having several projects on the go simultaneously, staying up all night, forgetting to eat, singing, mental restlessness, a feeling of agitation, mental confusion, incoherent speech, rash behaviour, uncontrolled laughter, shouting, palpitations, thirst, red face, a feeling of oppression of the chest, expectoration of phlegm, sputum in the throat, bitter taste, Red tongue with redder-swollen tip and Heart crack with a sticky, dry yellow coating inside it, Slippery-Rapid or Slippery-Overflowing-Rapid pulse.

Stomach Phlegm-Fire affecting the Heart

Manic behaviour, desire to climb to high places, shouting, laughing, singing, taking off of one's clothes, insomnia, mental restlessness, burning epigastric pain, thirst without a desire to drink, bleeding gums, dry stools, dry mouth, mouth ulcers, sour regurgitation, nausea, vomiting soon after eating, excessive hunger, foul breath, a feeling of heat, a feeling of oppression of the chest and epigastrium, tongue Red in the centre with a sticky yellow coating and a Stomach crack with a rough, sticky yellow coating inside it, Slippery-Rapid pulse.

Stomach and Pericardium Fire

Manic behaviour, mental restlessness, inability to lie down, hallucinations, incoherent speech, excessive dreaming, red face, hot hands, palpitations, burning epigastric pain, intense thirst with a desire to drink cold liquids, dry mouth, mouth ulcers, bleeding gums, dry stools, sour regurgitation, foul breath, nausea, vomiting soon after eating, a feeling of heat, tongue Red with a thick, dry dark-yellow coating, Deep-Full-Rapid pulse.

Fire injuring Yin

Chronic manic behaviour, excessive talking, tendency to be easily startled, mental restlessness, loss of weight, malar flush, a feeling of heat in the evening, Red tongue without coating, Fine-Rapid pulse.

> ## Clinical note
> - **Remember**: 'manic' behaviour does not occur only in its extreme form but also to a mild degree in many patients.

ANXIETY

Interrogation, Chapter 44

Heart-Blood deficiency

Mild anxiety, insomnia, dream-disturbed sleep, poor memory, anxiety, tendency to be easily startled, palpitations, dizziness, dull-pale complexion, pale lips, Pale and Thin tongue, Choppy or Fine pulse.

Heart-Yin deficiency

Vague anxiety that is worse in the evening, insomnia, poor memory, anxiety, mental restlessness, dream-disturbed sleep, tendency to be easily startled, uneasiness, 'feeling hot and bothered', palpitations, dry mouth and throat, night sweating, normal-coloured tongue without coating or with rootless coating, Floating-Empty pulse, especially on the left Front position.

Heart-Yin deficiency with Empty-Heat

Anxiety that is worse in the evening, mental restlessness, insomnia, dream-disturbed sleep, poor memory, uneasiness, 'feeling hot and bothered', palpitations, dry mouth and throat, a feeling of heat in the evening, malar flush, night sweating, five-palm heat, Red tongue with redder tip and without coating, Floating-Empty and Rapid pulse.

Heart-Fire

Severe anxiety, mental restlessness, a feeling of agitation, insomnia, dream-disturbed sleep, palpitations, thirst, mouth and tongue ulcers, a feeling of heat, red

face, dark urine or blood in the urine, bitter taste, Red tongue with redder tip and yellow coating, Overflowing and Rapid pulse.

Heart-Blood stasis

Severe anxiety, agitation, palpitations, stabbing or pricking chest pain which may radiate to the inner aspect of the left arm or to the shoulder, a feeling of oppression or constriction of the chest, cyanosis of lips and nails, cold hands, tongue entirely Purple or Purple only on the sides in the chest areas, Choppy or Wiry pulse.

Phlegm-Fire harassing the Heart

Severe anxiety, agitation, mental restlessness, manic behaviour, phobias, insomnia, dream-disturbed sleep, mental confusion, depression, palpitations, thirst, red face, a feeling of oppression of the chest, dark urine, expectoration of phlegm, rattling sound in the throat, bitter taste, Red tongue with redder swollen tip, and Heart crack with a sticky yellow coating inside it, Slippery-Rapid or Slippery-Overflowing-Rapid pulse.

Heart- and Kidney-Yin deficiency with Empty-Heat

Anxiety, mental restlessness, a feeling of agitation that is worse in the evening, insomnia, dream-disturbed sleep, poor memory, palpitations, dizziness, tinnitus, hardness of hearing, lower backache, nocturnal emissions with dreams, a feeling of heat in the evening, night sweating, five-palm heat, scanty dark urine, dry stools, Red tongue with redder tip and a Heart crack, Floating-Empty and Rapid pulse.

Liver-Blood deficiency

Mild anxiety, mild depression, lack of direction, insomnia, excessive dreaming, dizziness, blurred vision, floaters, numbness/tingling of limbs, scanty menstruation, dull-pale complexion, Pale tongue, Choppy or Fine pulse.

Liver-Yin deficiency

Vague anxiety, depression, lack of direction, insomnia, excessive dreaming, dizziness, blurred vision, floaters, dry eyes, dry hair, dry nails, insomnia, numbness/tingling of the limbs, scanty menstruation, tongue without coating, Floating-Empty pulse.

Liver-Qi stagnation

Anxiety, depression, irritability, moodiness, hypochondrial or epigastric distension, a feeling of a lump in the throat, premenstrual tension, Wiry pulse.

Liver-Fire

Severe anxiety, irritability, propensity to outbursts of anger, headache, red face, dizziness, tinnitus, thirst, bitter taste, constipation, dark urine, Red tongue with redder sides and dry yellow coating, Wiry-Rapid pulse.

Liver-Yang rising

Anxiety, headache, dizziness, tinnitus, irritability, propensity to outbursts of anger, Wiry pulse.

Kidney-Yin deficiency

Vague anxiety that is worse in the evening, dizziness, tinnitus, hardness of hearing, poor memory, night sweating, dry mouth and throat at night, lower backache, constipation, scanty dark urine, tiredness, normal-coloured tongue without coating, Floating-Empty pulse.

Deficiency of Qi of the Heart and Gall-Bladder

Mild anxiety, insomnia, timidity, absentmindedness, indecisiveness, tendency to be easily startled, palpitations, slight breathlessness, tiredness, Pale tongue, Weak pulse.

Diaphragm-Heat

Anxiety, a feeling of heat and stuffiness in the region under the heart, thirst, dry mouth, irritability, insomnia, Red tongue, Rapid pulse.

This pattern is caused by residual Heat following an invasion of Wind-Heat.

IRRITABILITY

Interrogation, Chapter 44

Irritability is a common emotional complaint. It includes feeling irritable frequently, flying off the handle easily, feeling frustrated and similar emotional states. Of the traditional seven emotions, irritability is akin to 'anger' but it encompasses a broader range of emotional states than 'anger' and is generally not so intense. A propensity to anger is generally due to Liver patterns, whereas irritability may be caused by many different patterns affecting most organs.

Liver-Qi stagnation

Irritability, moodiness, premenstrual irritability, hypochondrial or epigastric distension, irritability, moodiness, a feeling of a lump in the throat, premenstrual tension, Wiry pulse, 'I feel extremely irritable before my periods and take it out on my family.'

Lung-Qi stagnation

Mild irritability, bouts of crying, sighing, sadness, depression, a feeling of a lump in the throat, difficulty in swallowing, a feeling of oppression or distension of the chest, slight breathlessness, tongue slightly Red on the sides in the chest areas, pulse very slightly Tight on the right Front position, 'I feel this lump in the throat, I am on edge and feel like bursting into tears.'

Liver-Blood stasis

Severe irritability, agitation at night, hypochondrial/abdominal pain, painful periods, dark and clotted menstrual blood, masses in the abdomen, purple nails and lips, purple or dark complexion, Purple tongue, Wiry or Firm pulse, 'I seethe with resentment.'

Heart-Blood stasis

Irritability, obsessive thinking, palpitations, stabbing or pricking chest pain which may radiate to the inner aspect of the left arm or to the shoulder, a feeling of oppression or constriction of the chest, cyanosis of lips and nails, cold hands, tongue entirely Purple or Purple only on the sides in the chest areas, Choppy or Wiry pulse, 'My mind is constantly judging and I feel resentful.'

Liver-Yang rising

Severe irritability, propensity to outbursts of anger, headache, dizziness, tinnitus, Wiry pulse, 'I fly off the handle easily.'

Liver-Fire

Severe irritability, propensity to outbursts of anger, headache, red face, dizziness, tinnitus, thirst, bitter taste, constipation, dark urine, Red tongue with redder sides and dry yellow coating, Wiry-Rapid pulse, 'I explode into a rage.'

Heart-Fire

Severe irritability, rage, agitation, insomnia, dream-disturbed sleep, palpitations, thirst, mouth and tongue ulcers, mental restlessness, a feeling of heat, red face, bitter taste, Red tongue with redder tip and yellow coating, Overflowing-Rapid pulse, 'I feel irritable, impatient and angry.'

Lung-Heat

Irritability, bouts of crying, restlessness, cough, slight breathlessness, a feeling of heat, chest ache, flaring of nostrils, thirst, red face, Red tongue with yellow coating, Overflowing-Rapid pulse, 'I feel frustrated, weepy and irritable.'

Stomach-Heat

Irritability, insomnia, dream-disturbed sleep, restlessness, burning epigastric pain, thirst, sour regurgitation, nausea, excessive hunger, foul breath, a feeling of heat, Red tongue with a yellow coating, Overflowing-Rapid pulse, 'I feel often angry and obsessive.'

Liver-Blood deficiency

Mild irritability, mild impatience, vague anxiety, dizziness, blurred vision, floaters, numbness/tingling of limbs, scanty menstruation, dull-pale complexion, Pale tongue, Choppy or Fine pulse, 'I feel lost, overwhelmed and on edge.'

Kidney-Yin deficiency

Mild irritability, vague anxiety and fear which is worse in the evening, lack of will-power, tendency to be easily annoyed, dizziness, tinnitus, hardness of hearing, poor memory, night sweating, dry mouth and throat at night, lower backache, constipation, scanty dark urine, tiredness, normal-coloured tongue without coating, Floating-Empty pulse, 'I feel helpless, unmotivated and on edge in the evening.'

Heart-Blood deficiency

Mild irritability, sadness, vague anxiety, insomnia, dream-disturbed sleep, poor memory, tendency to be easily startled, palpitations, dizziness, dull-pale complexion, pale lips, Pale and Thin tongue, Choppy or Fine pulse, 'I feel sad and on edge.'

Kidney-Yin deficiency with Empty-Heat

Vague irritability, mental restlessness that is worse in the evening, a feeling of being on edge, 'feeling hot and bothered', depression, anxiety, insomnia, dizziness, tinnitus, vertigo, poor memory, hardness of hearing, night sweating, dry mouth at night, five-palm heat, a

feeling of heat in the evening, thirst with a desire to sip fluids, lower backache, constipation, scanty dark urine, tiredness, Red tongue without coating, Floating-Empty and Rapid pulse, 'I feel hot and bothered.'

Heart-Yin deficiency with Empty-Heat

Irritability, mental restlessness that is worse in the evening, a feeling of being on edge, sadness, anxiety, insomnia, dream-disturbed sleep, anxiety, tendency to be easily startled, uneasiness, 'feeling hot and bothered', palpitations, poor memory, dry mouth and throat, thirst with a desire to sip fluids, a feeling of heat in the evening, malar flush, night sweating, five-palm heat, Red tongue, redder on the tip with no coating, Floating-Empty and Rapid pulse, 'I feel sad and hot and bothered.'

Damp-Heat

Irritability, mental restlessness, slightly obsessive thinking, a feeling of heaviness and fullness of the epigastrium, sticky taste, feeling of heat, sticky yellow tongue coating, Slippery-Rapid pulse, 'I feel heavy, yucky and irritable.'

Other manifestations depend on the organ involved.

SCHIZOPHRENIA

Heart- and Spleen-Blood deficiency

Absentmindedness, insomnia, excessive dreaming, inability to concentrate, forgetfulness, anxiety, sadness, hearing of voices, depression, mental confusion, tendency to be easily startled, sadness, crying, shouting, muttering to oneself, brooding, obsessive thinking, palpitations, dizziness, dull-pale complexion, pale lips, tiredness, weak muscles, loose stools, poor appetite, scanty periods, Pale and Thin tongue, Choppy or Fine pulse.

Stagnation of Qi and Phlegm

Melancholy, apathy, mental dullness, incoherent speech, mumbling to onself, hearing of voices, moodiness, irritability, inappropriate laughing and crying, hypochondrial or epigastric distension, a feeling of a lump in the throat, premenstrual tension, sputum in the throat, a feeling of oppression of the chest, Wiry-Slippery pulse.

Phlegm-Fire harassing the Heart

Acute onset, hallucinations, hearing voices, violent behaviour, abusiveness, insomnia, dream-disturbed sleep, destructive behaviour, a feeling of agitation, mental confusion, incoherent speech, rash behaviour, tendency to hit or scold people, uncontrolled laughter or crying, shouting, muttering to oneself, palpitations, thirst, red face, a feeling of oppression of the chest, dark urine, expectoration of phlegm, rattling sound in the throat, bitter taste, Red tongue with redder swollen tip and Heart crack with a sticky yellow coating inside it, Slippery-Rapid or Slippery-Overflowing-Rapid pulse.

Phlegm-Fire and Yin deficiency with Empty-Heat

Hallucinations, hearing voices, abusiveness, insomnia, dream-disturbed sleep, destructive behaviour, agitation, mental confusion, incoherent speech, rash behaviour, tendency to hit or scold people, uncontrolled laughter or crying, shouting, muttering to oneself, palpitations, thirst, red face, a feeling of oppression of the chest, dark urine, expectoration of phlegm, rattling sound in the throat, a feeling of heat in the evening, malar flush, thirst with a desire to drink in small sips, dry throat at night, night sweating, five-palm heat, Red and Swollen tongue with redder tip and without coating and Heart crack with rough, dry yellow coating inside it, Slippery-Floating-Empty-Rapid pulse.

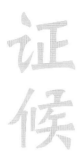

Chapter **80**

MENTAL DIFFICULTIES

Chapter contents

POOR MEMORY *803*

DIFFICULTY IN CONCENTRATION *804*

LEARNING DIFFICULTY IN CHILDREN *804*

HYPERACTIVITY *804*

POOR MEMORY

Qi and Blood deficiency of the Heart and Spleen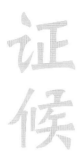

Poor memory of distant events, excessive dreaming, insomnia, anxiety, poor memory, tendency to be easily startled, palpitations, dizziness, dull-pale complexion, pale lips, tiredness, weak muscles, loose stools, poor appetite, scanty periods, Pale and Thin tongue, Choppy or Fine pulse.

Kidney deficiency

Poor memory of recent events, absentmindedness, slow thinking, premature greying of the hair or balding, dizziness, tinnitus, lower backache.

Other symptoms or signs depend on whether there is Kidney-Yin or Kidney-Yang deficiency.

Heart- and Kidney-Yin deficiency with Empty-Heat

Poor memory, excessive dreaming, insomnia, anxiety, mental restlessness, dream-disturbed sleep, poor memory, palpitations, dizziness, tinnitus, hardness of hearing, lower backache, nocturnal emissions with dreams, a feeling of heat in the evening, night sweating, five-palm heat, scanty dark urine, dry stools, Red tongue with redder tip and a Heart crack, Floating-Empty and Rapid pulse.

Turbid Phlegm in the Heart

Poor memory, somnolence, absentmindedness, insomnia, poor memory and concentration, a feeling of muzziness of the head, sputum in the throat, a feeling of oppression of the chest, nausea, Swollen tongue with sticky coating, Slippery pulse.

Heart-Blood stasis

Poor memory, insomnia, agitation, palpitations, stabbing or pricking chest pain which may radiate to the inner aspect of the left arm or to the shoulder, a feeling of oppression or constriction of the chest, cyanosis of lips and nails, cold hands, tongue entirely Purple or Purple only on the sides in the chest areas, Choppy or Wiry pulse.

> ## Clinical note
> - Du-24 Shenting is an important point to stimulate memory.

DIFFICULTY IN CONCENTRATION

Spleen-Qi and Spleen-Blood deficiency

Poor concentration, difficulty in applying oneself to study, poor appetite, slight abdominal distension after eating, tiredness, pale complexion, weakness of the limbs, loose stools, scanty menstruation, Pale tongue, Choppy pulse.

Heart-Blood deficiency

Poor concentration, poor memory, insomnia, dream-disturbed sleep, anxiety, tendency to be easily startled, palpitations, dizziness, dull-pale complexion, pale lips, Pale and Thin tongue, Choppy or Fine pulse.

Kidney deficiency

Poor concentration, poor memory, a feeling of emptiness of the head, dizziness, tinnitus, lower backache.

Other symptoms and signs depend on whether there is Kidney-Yang or Kidney-Yin deficiency.

Phlegm

Poor concentration that is worse in the morning, a feeling of heaviness and muzziness of the head, dizziness, blurred vision, sticky taste, dull frontal headache, a feeling of oppression of the chest, sputum in the throat, Swollen tongue with a sticky coating, Slippery pulse.

Dampness

Poor concentration that is worse in the morning, a feeling of heaviness of the head, sticky taste, dull frontal headache, sticky tongue coating, Slippery pulse.

> ## Clinical note
> - I use Du-20 Baihui to stimulate concentration.

LEARNING DIFFICULTY IN CHILDREN

Spleen- and Heart-Blood deficiency

Learning difficulty, difficulty in concentration, poor memory, mental dullness, insomnia, dream-disturbed sleep, tendency to be easily startled, flaccid muscles, lassitude, apathy, palpitations, dizziness, dull-pale complexion, pale lips, tiredness, weak muscles, loose stools, poor appetite, Pale and Thin tongue, Choppy or Fine pulse.

Emptiness of the Sea of Marrow

Learning difficulty, childhood weakness, mental dullness, slow growth, slow development (in walking, speech, teeth, hair), dizziness, poor memory, deafness, a feeling of emptiness of the head, blurred vision.

HYPERACTIVITY

The discussion of hyperactivity below is centred on children, but it is applicable to adults as well.

Liver- and Kidney-Yin deficiency with Liver-Yang rising

Hyperactivity, insomnia, thin body, slow development, restlessness, propensity to outbursts of anger, clumsiness, dizziness, dull occipital or vertical headache, numbness/tingling of the limbs, dry eyes, blurred vision, dry throat in the evening, dry hair and skin, brittle nails, night sweating, dry stools, headache, normal-coloured tongue without coating, Floating-Empty and slightly Wiry pulse.

Qi deficiency of Spleen and Heart with floating Yang

Hyperactivity, fat body, slow development, poor memory, poor concentration, mental dullness, poor sleep, difficulty in speech, stuttering, lassitude, poor appetite, slight abdominal distension after eating, tiredness, pale complexion, weakness of the limbs, loose stools, palpitations, shortness of breath on exertion, Pale tongue, Empty pulse.

Liver-Fire

Hyperactivity, thin body, insomnia, headache, red face, dizziness, tinnitus, irritability, propensity to outbursts of anger, thirst, bitter taste, constipation, dark urine, Red tongue with redder sides and dry yellow coating, Wiry-Rapid pulse.

Phlegm-Fire

Hyperactivity, expectoration of sputum, catarrh, chronic 'glue ear', poor concentration, a feeling of heaviness, restlessness, difficulty in speaking, sputum in the throat, chronic catarrh, a feeling of heat, thirst without a desire to drink, Swollen tongue with sticky coating, Slippery-Rapid pulse.

Blood stasis leading to obstruction of the upper orifices

Hyperactivity, mental restlessness, agitation, poor sleep, dark complexion, history of difficult birth, propensity to outbursts of anger, Purple tongue, Wiry pulse.

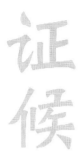

Chapter **81**

SLEEP PROBLEMS

Chapter contents

INSOMNIA   *807*

EXCESSIVE DREAMING   *808*

SOMNOLENCE   *810*

SLEEP TALKING   *810*

SLEEP WALKING   *810*

SNORING   *811*

INSOMNIA

Interrogation, Chapter 40

Insomnia includes difficulty in falling or staying asleep.

Heart-Blood deficiency

Insomnia with difficulty in falling asleep, dream-disturbed sleep, poor memory, anxiety, tendency to be easily startled, palpitations, dizziness, dull-pale complexion, pale lips, Pale and Thin tongue, Choppy or Fine pulse.

Deficiency of Qi and Blood of the Spleen and Heart

Insomnia, anxiety, dream-disturbed sleep, poor memory, anxiety, tendency to be easily startled, palpitations, dizziness, dull-pale complexion, pale lips, tiredness, weak muscles, loose stools, shortness of breath on exertion, slight abdominal distension, poor appetite, scanty periods, Pale and Thin tongue, Choppy or Fine pulse.

Heart-Yin deficiency

Insomnia, dream-disturbed sleep, anxiety, tendency to be easily startled, mental restlessness, uneasiness, 'feeling hot and bothered', poor memory, palpitations, dry mouth and throat, night sweating, normal-coloured tongue without coating or with rootless coating, Floating-Empty pulse especially on the left Front position.

Liver-Blood deficiency

Insomnia, difficulty in falling asleep, dizziness, blurred vision, floaters, numbness/tingling of limbs, scanty menstruation, dull-pale complexion, Pale tongue, Choppy or Fine pulse.

Liver-Yin deficiency

Insomnia, difficulty in falling asleep, dreaming, dizziness, numbness/tingling of the limbs, blurred vision, floaters in the eyes, dry eyes, scanty menstruation, dull-pale complexion but with red cheekbones, withered and brittle nails, dry skin and hair, night sweating, normal-coloured tongue without coating, Fine or Floating-Empty pulse.

Heart- and Kidney-Yin deficiency

Insomnia with difficulty in falling asleep, dream-disturbed sleep, anxiety, poor memory, palpitations, dizziness, tinnitus, hardness of hearing, lower backache, night sweating, scanty dark urine, normal-coloured tongue without coating, dizziness, tinnitus, backache, tongue without coating, Floating-Empty pulse.

Heart- and Kidney-Yin deficiency with Heart Empty-Heat

Insomnia, frequent waking during the night, dream-disturbed sleep, mental restlessness, anxiety, poor memory, palpitations, dizziness, tinnitus, hardness of hearing, lower backache, nocturnal emissions with dreams, a feeling of heat in the evening, night sweating, five-palm heat, scanty dark urine, dry stools, Red tongue with redder tip and a Heart crack, Floating-Empty and Rapid pulse or a pulse that is Deep and Weak on both Rear positions and Overflowing on both Front positions.

Liver-Fire

Insomnia, excessive dreaming, restless sleep, headache, red face, dizziness, tinnitus, irritability, propensity to outbursts of anger, thirst, bitter taste, constipation, dark urine, Red tongue with redder sides and dry yellow coating, Wiry-Rapid pulse.

Phlegm-Fire harassing the Heart

Restless sleep, insomnia, dream-disturbed sleep, mental restlessness, a feeling of agitation, mental confusion, palpitations, thirst, red face, a feeling of oppression of the chest, dark urine, expectoration of phlegm, rattling sound in the throat, bitter taste, Red tongue with redder swollen tip and Heart crack with a sticky yellow coating inside it, Slippery-Rapid or Slippery-Overflowing-Rapid pulse.

Heart-Fire

Restless sleep, dream-disturbed sleep, mental restlessness, a feeling of agitation, palpitations, thirst, mouth and tongue ulcers, red face, dark urine or blood in the urine, bitter taste, Red tongue with redder tip and yellow coating, Overflowing and Rapid pulse.

Gall-Bladder deficiency

Tendency to be easily awakened at night and easily startled with difficulty in going back to sleep or waking up early in the morning, restless sleep, depression, timidity, tendency to be easily startled, lack of courage and initiative, indecision, sighing, dizziness, blurred vision, floaters, nervousness, Weak pulse.

Residual Heat in the diaphragm

Restless sleep, preference for sleeping propped up, inability to fall asleep, mental restlessness, a feeling of oppression of the diaphragm, dry throat, epigastric discomfort, red points in the front or around the centre of the tongue, slightly Rapid pulse.

> **Clinical note**
>
> - If a patient suffers from insomnia and headaches, these will never improve until the insomnia is treated.

EXCESSIVE DREAMING

Interrogation, Chapter 40

Liver-Fire

Excessive dreaming, nightmares, restless sleep, headache, red face, dizziness, tinnitus, irritability, propensity to outbursts of anger, thirst, bitter taste, constipation, dark urine, Red tongue with redder sides and dry yellow coating, Wiry-Rapid pulse.

Heart-Fire

Excessive dreaming, restless sleep, mental restlessness, a feeling of agitation, insomnia, palpitations, thirst, mouth and tongue ulcers, a feeling of heat, red face, bitter taste, Red tongue with redder tip and yellow coating, Overflowing-Rapid pulse.

Phlegm-Fire harassing the Heart

Excessive dreaming, restless sleep, insomnia, waking up from nightmares, mental restlessness, agitation, mental confusion, palpitations, thirst, red face, a

feeling of oppression of the chest, dark urine, expectoration of phlegm, bitter taste, insomnia, Red tongue with redder swollen tip and a Heart crack with a sticky yellow coating inside it, Slippery-Rapid or Slippery-Overflowing-Rapid pulse.

Phlegm-Fire in the Stomach

Excessive dreaming, restless sleep, insomnia, mental restlessness, burning epigastric pain, thirst without a desire to drink, bleeding gums, dry stools, dry mouth, mouth ulcers, sour regurgitation, nausea, vomiting soon after eating, excessive hunger, foul breath, a feeling of heat, a feeling of oppression of the chest and epigastrium, mucus in the stools, expectoration of phlegm, Red tongue with a sticky yellow coating and a Stomach crack with a rough, sticky yellow coating inside it, Slippery-Rapid and slightly Overflowing pulse.

Heart-Yin deficiency with Empty-Heat

Dream-disturbed sleep with dreams that are not too agitated, poor memory, anxiety, tendency to be easily startled, mental restlessness, uneasiness, 'feeling hot and bothered', palpitations, dry mouth and throat, thirst with a desire to sip fluids, a feeling of heat in the evening, malar flush, night sweating, five-palm heat, Red tongue redder on the tip with no coating, Floating-Empty and Rapid pulse.

Liver-Yin deficiency with Empty-Heat

Dream-disturbed sleep, insomnia, depression, a feeling of aimlessness, dizziness, numbness of the limbs, blurred vision, 'floaters' in the eyes, dry eyes, diminished night vision, scanty menstruation or amenorrhoea, dull-pale complexion without 'spirit' but with red cheekbones, muscular weakness, cramps, withered and brittle nails, very dry hair and skin, a feeling of heat in the evening, night sweating, five-palm heat, thirst with a desire to sip fluids, Red tongue without coating, Floating-Empty and slightly Rapid pulse.

Heart- and Kidney-Yin deficiency with Empty-Heat

Dream-disturbed sleep, palpitations, mental restlessness, insomnia, anxiety, poor memory, dizziness, tinnitus, deafness, backache, nocturnal emissions with dreams, a feeling of heat in the evening, night sweating, five-palm heat, scanty dark urine, dry stools, Red tongue with redder tip without coating and midline Heart crack, Floating-Empty and Rapid pulse, or Deep-

Weak pulse on both Rear positions and relatively Overflowing on both Front positions.

Heart and Gall-Bladder deficiency

Excessive dreaming, waking up easily from dreaming, absentmindedness, emotional instability, anxiety and palpitations.

Box 81.1 is a list of dreams and the patterns that cause them, according to the 'Simple Questions' and 'Spiritual Axis'.

Box 81.1 Dreams and their significance

- flying: Emptiness in the Lower Burner[1]
- falling: Fullness in the Lower Burner[2]
- floods and fear: Excess of Yin[3]
- fire: Excess of Yang[4]
- killing and destruction: Yin and Yang both in Excess[5]
- giving away things: Excess condition[6]
- receiving things: Deficiency condition[7]
- being angry: Liver in Excess[8]
- crying, weeping: Lungs in Excess[9]
- crowds: roundworms in the intestines[10]
- attack and destruction: tapeworms in the intestines[11]
- fires: Heart deficiency[12]
- volcanic eruptions (if the dream takes place in summer): Heart deficiency[13]
- laughing: Heart in Excess[14]
- mountains, fire and smoke: Heart deficiency[15]
- very fragrant mushrooms: Liver deficiency[16]
- lying under a tree being unable to get up (if the dream takes place in spring): Liver deficiency[17]
- forests on mountains: Liver deficiency[18]
- white objects or bloody killings: Lung deficiency[19]
- battles and war (dream taking place in the autumn): Lung deficiency[20]
- worry, fear, crying, flying: Lungs in Excess[21]
- flying and seeing strange objects made of gold or iron: Lung deficiency[22]
- being hungry: Spleen deficiency[23]
- building a house (dream taking place in late summer): Spleen deficiency[24]
- singing and feeling very heavy: Spleen in Excess[25]
- abysses in mountains and marshes: Spleen deficiency[26]
- swimming after a shipwreck: Kidney deficiency[27]
- plunging into water and being scared (dream taking place in winter): Kidney deficiency[28]
- spine being detached from the body: Kidneys in Excess (i.e. Dampness in Kidneys)[29]
- being immersed in water: Kidney deficiency[30]
- having a large meal: Stomach deficiency[31]
- large cities: Small Intestine deficiency[32]
- open fields: Large Intestine deficiency[33]
- fights, trials, suicide: Gall-Bladder deficiency[34]
- voyages: Bladder deficiency[35]
- crossing the sea and being scared: Excess of Yin[36]

SOMNOLENCE

Interrogation, Chapter 44

Spleen-Yang deficiency with Dampness

Somnolence especially after a meal, tiredness, a feeling of heaviness and muzziness of the head, a feeling of heaviness of the limbs, poor appetite, epigastric fullness, sticky taste, absence of thirst, loose stools, a feeling of cold, cold limbs, Pale and wet tongue with sticky coating, Soggy pulse.

This is the most common cause of somnolence.

Spleen-Qi deficiency with Phlegm

Somnolence, poor memory, slight depression, mental confusion, a feeling of heaviness and muzziness of the head, a feeling of oppression of the chest, dizziness, poor appetite, slight abdominal distension after eating, tiredness, lassitude, pale complexion, weakness of the limbs, loose stools, tendency to obesity, Pale-Swollen tongue with sticky coating, Slippery-Weak pulse.

Spleen- and Heart-Qi deficiency

Somnolence, poor memory, slight depression, poor appetite, slight abdominal distension after eating, tiredness, lassitude, pale complexion, weakness of the limbs, loose stools, palpitations, shortness of breath on exertion, Pale tongue, Empty pulse.

Kidney-Yang deficiency

Somnolence, poor memory, lower backache, cold knees, a feeling of cold, bright-white complexion, weak knees, tiredness, lassitude, abundant clear urination, urination at night, impotence, decreased libido, Pale and wet tongue, Deep-Weak pulse.

> **Clinical note**
> • I use Du-20 Baihui for somnolence.

SLEEP TALKING

Heart-Fire

Talking or shouting in one's sleep, restless sleep, dream-disturbed sleep with dreams of laughing and fires, insomnia, palpitations, thirst, mouth and tongue ulcers, mental restlessness, a feeling of agitation, a feeling of heat, red face, bitter taste, Red tongue with redder tip and yellow coating, Overflowing-Rapid pulse.

Heart-Yin deficiency with Empty-Heat

Talking in one's sleep, waking up during the night, dream-disturbed sleep with dreams of laughing and fires, palpitations, insomnia, poor memory, anxiety, mental restlessness, dry mouth and throat, a feeling of heat in the evening, malar flush, night sweating, five-palm heat, Red tongue with redder tip and without coating, Floating-Empty and Rapid pulse.

Liver-Yin deficiency

Talking in one's sleep, excessive dreaming, a feeling of floating just before falling asleep, insomnia, dizziness, blurred vision, floaters, night sweating, dry eyes, dry hair, dry nails, tongue without coating, Floating-Empty pulse.

Liver-Yin deficiency with Empty-Heat

Talking in one's sleep, excessive dreaming, a feeling of floating just before falling asleep, insomnia, dizziness, blurred vision, floaters, night sweating, dry eyes, dry hair, dry nails, five-palm heat, Red tongue without coating, Floating-Empty and Rapid pulse.

Gall-Bladder Heat

Talking in one's sleep, dizziness, tinnitus, bitter taste, dry throat, irritability, red face and ears, hypochondrial fullness, tongue with unilateral or bilateral yellow coating, Wiry pulse.

Stomach-Heat

Talking in one's sleep, restless sleep, burning epigastric pain, thirst, sour regurgitation, nausea, excessive hunger, foul breath, a feeling of heat, Red tongue with a yellow coating, Overflowing-Rapid pulse.

Heart-Blood deficiency

Talking in one's sleep, palpitations, dizziness, insomnia, poor memory, anxiety, dull-pale complexion, Pale tongue, Choppy or Fine pulse.

SLEEP WALKING

Liver-Yin deficiency

Sleep walking, excessive dreaming, a feeling of floating just before falling asleep, insomnia, dizziness, blurred

vision, floaters, dry eyes, night sweating, dry hair, dry nails, tongue without coating, Floating-Empty pulse.

Liver-Yin deficiency with Empty-Heat

Sleep walking, excessive dreaming, a feeling of floating just before falling asleep, insomnia, dizziness, blurred vision, floaters, night sweating, dry eyes, dry hair, dry nails, five-palm heat, Red tongue without coating, Floating-Empty and Rapid pulse.

Liver-Blood stasis

Sleep walking, excessive dreaming, mental restlessness, abdominal pain, painful periods, Purple tongue, Firm pulse.

SNORING

Hearing, Chapter 53; Symptoms and Signs, Chapter 83

Phlegm-Heat in the Lungs

Loud snoring, dry throat, thirst with no desire to drink, barking cough with profuse, sticky yellow or green sputum, shortness of breath, wheezing, a feeling of oppression of the chest, a feeling of heat, thirst, Red and Swollen tongue with a sticky yellow coating, Slippery-Rapid pulse.

Damp-Phlegm in the Lungs

Soft snoring, a feeling of oppression of the chest, cough with expectoration of sticky sputum, a feeling of heaviness, thirst with no desire to drink, Swollen tongue with sticky coating, Slippery pulse.

Dry-Phlegm in the Lungs

High-pitched snoring, dry cough with occasional, difficult expectoration of scanty sputum, thirst with no desire to drink, dry mouth and throat, Swollen tongue with sticky, dry coating, Slippery pulse.

Phlegm in the Lungs with Lung- and Spleen-Qi deficiency

Soft snoring, a feeling of oppression of the chest, a feeling of heaviness, weak voice, tendency to catch colds, poor appetite, loose stools, tiredness, Pale tongue with teeth marks, Soggy pulse.

NOTES

1. 1979 The Yellow Emperor's Classic of Internal Medicine – Simple Questions (*Huang Di Nei Jing Su Wen* 黄帝内经素问), People's Health Publishing House, Beijing, p. 102. First published c. 100BC.
2. Ibid., p. 102.
3. Ibid., p. 102.
4. Ibid., p. 102.
5. Ibid., p. 102.
6. Ibid., p. 102.
7. Ibid., p. 102.
8. Ibid., p. 102.
9. Ibid., p. 102.
10. Ibid., p. 102.
11. Ibid., p. 103.
12. Ibid., p. 569.
13. Ibid., p. 569.
14. 1981 Spiritual Axis (*Ling Shu Jing* 灵枢经), People's Health Publishing House, Beijing, p. 84. First published c. 100BC.
15. Ibid., p. 84.
16. Simple Questions, p. 569.
17. Ibid., p. 569.
18. Spiritual Axis, p. 85.
19. Simple Questions, p. 569.
20. Ibid., p. 569.
21. Spiritual Axis, p. 85.
22. Ibid., p. 85.
23. Simple Questions, p. 569.
24. Ibid., p. 569.
25. Spiritual Axis, p. 85.
26. Ibid., p. 85.
27. Simple Questions, p. 569.
28. Ibid., p. 569.
29. Spiritual Axis, p. 85.
30. Ibid., p. 85.
31. Ibid., p. 85.
32. Ibid., p. 85.
33. Ibid., p. 85.
34. Ibid., p. 85.
35. Ibid., p. 85.
36. Ibid., p. 85.

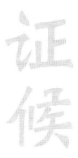

Chapter **82**

FEELING OF COLD, FEELING OF HEAT, FEVER

Chapter contents

FEELING OF COLD, SHIVERING   *813*
   Exterior   *813*
   Interior   *814*

FEVER   *814*
   Acute fever   *814*
   Chronic fever   *815*
   Tidal fever   *816*
   Fever in cancer   *816*
   Fever after chemotherapy   *817*

FIVE-PALM HEAT   *817*

CONTRADICTORY FEELINGS OF COLD AND HEAT   *817*

FEELING OF COLD, SHIVERING

Interrogation, Chapter 43

Exterior

Invasion of exterior Wind

Aversion to cold, hot dorsum of the hands, fever, occipital stiffness, occipital headache, Floating pulse.

Lesser-Yang pattern

Alternation of cold and hot feeling, mental restlessness, bitter taste, dry throat, blurred vision, hypochondrial discomfort, unilateral tongue coating, Wiry pulse.

Lesser-Yang pattern with predominance of Heat

Alternation of cold and hot feeling with a predominance of the latter, sweating, a feeling of oppression of the chest, vomiting, headache, mental restlessness, dry mouth, dark urine, Red tongue with a unilateral sticky yellow coating, Wiry pulse.

This is also a Lesser-Yang pattern but with the predominance of Heat and with some Dampness. Within the Four Levels identification of patterns, it is called Heat in the Gall-Bladder.

Exterior Cold and interior Heat

Aversion to cold, fever, cold limbs, body aches, headache, thirst, mental restlessness, dark urine, dry stools, Red tongue.

This situation occurs after an invasion of external Wind when interior Heat is generated but the exterior Cold is still there; thus exterior Cold and interior Heat coexist. This pattern is not common.

Long-lasting invasion of Wind-Heat

Aversion to cold, fever, sweating, hot dorsum of the hands. The pulse becomes quiet after sweating, the patient desires to lie down and the limbs are cold.

Interior
Internal Cold

Cold feeling, no fever, dorsum of the hands not hot, cold feet, cold limbs.

Deficiency of Yang of the Heart/Lungs

Cold hands, a feeling of cold, shortness of breath, palpitations, Weak pulse.

Yang deficiency of the Stomach and Spleen

Cold limbs and abdomen, poor appetite, tiredness, slight abdominal distension, bright-white complexion, loose stools, a feeling of cold, Pale and wet tongue, Deep-Weak pulse.

Kidney-Yang deficiency

Cold legs, knees, feet and back, lower backache, dizziness, tinnitus, a feeling of cold, weak knees, bright-white complexion, tiredness, abundant clear urination, Pale and wet tongue, Deep-Weak pulse.

Qi stagnation

Cold hands and feet (especially fingers and toes), irritability, depression, hypochondrial discomfort, sighing, Wiry pulse.

Heart-Blood deficiency

Cold hands, a feeling of cold, palpitations, dizziness, insomnia, poor memory, anxiety, dull-pale complexion, Pale tongue, Choppy or Fine pulse.

Liver-Blood deficiency

Cold feet and hands, a feeling of cold, dizziness, blurred vision, floaters, numbness/tingling of limbs, dull-pale complexion, Pale tongue, Choppy or Fine pulse.

Phlegm in the Interior

A feeling of cold, cold limbs, a feeling of heaviness of the limbs, a feeling of oppression of the chest, sputum in the throat, Slippery pulse.

Often Phlegm may cause a cold feeling and cold limbs because it may obstruct the circulation of the Defensive Qi; this may happen even in the case of Phlegm-Heat and may account for contradictory hot and cold signs.

Heat stagnating in the Interior (True Heat–False Cold)

A feeling of cold, cold limbs, thirst, mental restlessness, dry throat, dry stools, red tongue, deep pulse.

This is due to interior Heat blocking Yang Qi in the Interior so that it cannot extend towards the Exterior; however, this situation is quite rare.

> **Clinical note**
>
> - Apart from obvious differences in patterns, the cold feeling from exterior invasions manifests with typical 'waves' of feelings of cold and shivering.

FEVER

Interrogation, Chapter 43

Acute fever

In acute fevers the identification of patterns according to the Four Levels provides the best framework of interpretation. Within the Four Levels, the Defensive-Qi level is the only exterior one and therefore there is fever and shivering with a slight feeling of cold simultaneously. At the other three levels (Qi, Nutritive Qi and Blood), Heat is in the Interior and the fever is interior. The identification of patterns according to the Four Levels describes the symptomatology of invasions of Wind-Heat. However, fever, to a lesser degree, may be present also in invasions of Wind-Cold, for which the identification of patterns according to the Six Stages is used.

Invasion of external Wind-Heat in the Lungs Defensive-Qi portion

Fever with a slight aversion to cold, cough, sore throat, stuffed or runny nose with yellow discharge, headache, body aches, slight sweating, slight thirst, swollen tonsils, tongue slightly Red on the sides in the chest area or on the front part, Floating-Rapid pulse.

Invasion of external Wind-Cold

A slight fever with a pronounced cold feeling and possibly shivering, cough, itchy throat, slight breathlessness, stuffed or runny nose with clear watery discharge,

sneezing, occipital headache, body aches, thin white tongue coating, Floating-Tight pulse.

Invasion of Summer-Heat

Fever, a slight feeling of cold, absence of sweating, headache, a feeling of heaviness, an uncomfortable feeling of the epigastrium, irritability, thirst, Red tongue, with white coating, Weak-Floating and Rapid pulse.

Heat in the Lungs (Qi level)

Fever, cough, slight breathlessness, a feeling of heat, chest ache, flaring of the nostrils, thirst, red face, Red tongue with yellow coating, Overflowing-Rapid pulse.

Heat in Bright Yang – channel pattern

Fever, sweating, intense thirst, burning epigastric pain, thirst, sour regurgitation, nausea, excessive hunger, foul breath, a feeling of heat, Red tongue with a yellow coating, Overflowing-Rapid pulse.

This corresponds to Heat in the Stomach channel and is described by the Stomach-Heat level within the Four Levels or the Bright-Yang channel pattern within the Six Stages.

Heat in Bright Yang – organ pattern

Fever, burning epigastric pain, intense thirst with a desire to drink cold liquids, mental restlessness, bleeding gums, dry stools, abdominal pain, tongue Red with a thick, dry dark-yellow coating, Deep-Full-Rapid pulse.

This is Dry-Heat in the Intestines level within the Four Levels and is the same as the Bright-Yang organ pattern within the Six Stages.

Damp-Heat in the Stomach and Intestines

Low-grade fever, sweating which does not relieve the fever and does not lead to the clearing of Heat, a feeling of fullness of the epigastrium/abdomen, epigastric/abdominal pain, poor appetite, sticky taste, a feeling of heaviness of the body, thirst without a desire to drink, nausea, vomiting, loose stools with offensive odour, burning sensation of the anus, a feeling of heat, scanty dark urine, headache with a feeling of heaviness of the head, dull-yellow complexion like tangerine peel, yellow sclera of the eyes, oily sweat, bitter taste, Red tongue with sticky yellow coating, Slippery-Rapid pulse.

Heat at Nutritive-Qi level

Fever at night, thirst, dry mouth with no desire to drink, mental restlessness.

This is Heat at the Nutritive-Qi level within the Four Levels.

Heat at Blood level

Fever at night, thirst, mental restlessness, macular rash, bleeding.

This is Heat in the Blood level within the Four Levels.

Chronic fever
Empty-Heat from Yin deficiency

Low-grade fever or feeling of heat in the afternoon or evening, five-palm heat, malar flush, thirst with a desire to drink in small sips, dry mouth and throat at night, mental restlessness, night sweating, insomnia, dream-disturbed sleep, dry stools, scanty dark urination, a thin red line on the inside of the lower eyelid, Red tongue without coating and with cracks, Fine-Rapid pulse.

These are the general symptoms of Empty-Heat deriving from Yin deficiency; they may arise from the Lungs, Heart, Stomach, Spleen, Liver or Kidneys.

Qi deficiency

Low-grade fever or feeling of heat that is aggravated by overwork, dizziness, tiredness, depression, muscular weakness, spontaneous sweating, shortness of breath, loose stools, poor appetite, weak voice, Pale tongue, Weak or Empty pulse.

Blood deficiency

Low-grade fever or feeling of heat in the afternoon, dizziness, blurred vision, floaters, numbness/tingling of limbs, scanty menstruation, dull-pale complexion, Pale tongue, Choppy or Fine pulse.

Stagnant Liver-Qi turned into Heat rebelling upwards

Chronic low-grade fever or feeling of heat that comes and goes according to the emotional state (it comes when the person is upset), volatile mood, irritability, a feeling of distension of the chest and hypochondrium, moodiness, a feeling of a lump in the throat, premenstrual tension, a bitter taste, tongue Red on the sides and thin yellow coating, Rapid-Wiry pulse.

Blood stasis

Low-grade fever or feeling of heat in the afternoon or evening, abdominal pain, dry skin and nails, dark

complexion, purple lips, Purple tongue, Choppy or Firm pulse.

Tidal fever

Tidal fever is a fever that rises and decreases at regular intervals. It is usually seen only in interior patterns.

Yin deficiency

Fever that is higher in the afternoon or only in the afternoon, hot palms and soles, night sweating, dry mouth with a desire to drink in small sips, dry throat in the evening, scanty dark urine, dry stools, normal-coloured tongue without coating, Floating-Empty pulse.

Stomach- and Spleen-Qi deficiency

Fever in the mornings, decreasing in the afternoon, poor appetite, slight abdominal distension after eating, an uncomfortable sensation of the epigastrium, tiredness, lassitude, pale complexion, weakness of the limbs, loose stools, Pale tongue, Empty pulse.

This pattern is relatively rare and is due to a severe deficiency of Stomach and Spleen Qi occurring after a febrile disease. It was described by Li Dong Yuan in his 'Discussion of Stomach and Spleen' (see Bibliography) and for which he used the famous prescription Bu Zhong Yi Qi Tang *Tonifying the Centre and Benefiting Qi Decoction*. This condition is what he called Yin Fire, which is not Full-Heat nor Empty-Heat from Yin deficiency but a kind of Empty-Heat from Qi deficiency.

Blood stasis

Fever in the afternoon or night, dry throat, abdominal pain, dry skin and nails, dark rings under the eyes, Purple tongue, Choppy or Wiry pulse.

This is unusual and it is more likely to occur in the elderly; it is often seen in the late stages of cancer due to Blood stasis.

Bright-Yang organ pattern

Fever that is higher in the afternoon, sweating of the hands and feet, abdominal pain and fullness, constipation, Red tongue and black tongue coating, Deep-Full pulse.

This is the Bright-Yang organ pattern within the Six Stages identification of patterns.

Summer-Heat

Fever in the morning, cold feeling at dusk or vice versa, thirst, irritability.

This corresponds to invasion of Summer-Heat injuring Qi. This occurs only in children and is relatively rare.

Fever in cancer

Fever in cancer may present with symptoms that are different from the norm and may also be caused by patterns that do not normally cause fever such as Liver-Qi stagnation and Yang deficiency.

Blood stasis

Fever, cancer characterized by pain and a mass, dark complexion, Purple tongue, Wiry pulse.

This may be cancer of the stomach, lung, intestines, uterus or breast.

Phlegm

Fever in the afternoon, cancer characterized by relatively soft masses, a feeling of oppression of the chest, Swollen tongue with sticky coating, Slippery pulse.

This may be cancer of the breast, lymphoma, Hodgkin's disease or thyroid cancer.

Damp-Heat

Afternoon fever, which may be high with delirium, headache, night sweating, mental restlessness, a feeling of oppression of the chest, oedema, nausea, Red tongue with sticky yellow coating, Slippery-Rapid pulse.

This may be cancer of the bladder, intestines, prostate or skin.

Toxic Heat

High fever, shivers, whole body hot to touch, cancer mass growing rapidly, purulent discharges, dark complexion, Red tongue with red points and thick, sticky, dry brown coating, Overflowing-Rapid pulse.

This may be cancer of oesophagus, lungs, stomach, intestines, breast or uterus.

Yin deficiency with Empty-Heat

Low-grade afternoon fever, late stage of cancer, five-palm heat, night sweating, malar flush, Red tongue without coating, Fine-Rapid pulse.

Stagnant Liver-Qi turned into Heat rebelling upwards

Low-grade afternoon fever, breast cancer, irritability, hypochondrial distension, sighing, Wiry pulse, tongue with Red sides.

Heat in Nutritive-Qi level

High fever, delirium, stage of rapid deterioration, mental confusion, maculae, dark-Red tongue without coating, Fine-Rapid pulse.

Yang deficiency

Midday low-grade fever, late stage of cancer, tiredness, chilliness, Pale tongue, Weak pulse.

Fever after chemotherapy
Stagnation of Qi and stasis of Blood

Low-grade fever, with no sweating, starts 3–5 days after the end of chemotherapy, Purple tongue, Wiry-Slow pulse.

Deficiency of Qi and Blood

Low-grade fever in the afternoon, poor appetite, loose stools, weak voice, palpitations, tiredness, blurred vision, dull-pale complexion, dizziness, Pale tongue, Weak or Choppy pulse.

Blood-Heat

Low-grade fever, thirst, mouth ulcers, blood in urine, red complexion, Red tongue, Rapid pulse.

FIVE-PALM HEAT

This is a feeling of heat in the palms, soles and chest, which is also sometimes called five-centre heat or five-heart heat. It may or may not be accompanied by an actual fever. It is usually accompanied by mental restlessness, night sweating and insomnia. This is frequently seen in practice; however, it may sometimes manifest only in the soles and palms, or in the palms and chest.

Yin deficiency with Empty-Heat

Five-palm heat in the afternoon, a desire to grasp cold objects, a desire to stretch hands and feet out of the blankets, dry throat at night, a feeling of heat in the evening, night sweating, malar flush, insomnia, anxiety, dry mouth with a desire to drink in small sips, Red tongue without coating, Floating-Empty and Rapid pulse.

This can be Yin deficiency of the Lungs, Heart, Liver, Kidneys, Stomach or Spleen.

Blood deficiency

Five-palm heat in the afternoon which is worse when tense or tired, dizziness, blurred vision, floaters, numbness/tingling of limbs, scanty menstruation, dull-pale complexion, Pale tongue, Choppy or Fine pulse.

Blood deficiency, like Yin deficiency, may also cause Empty-Heat and it usually occurs only in women, especially after the age of 40.

Liver-Fire

Five-palm heat, headaches, dizziness, tinnitus, irritability, propensity to outbursts of anger, red face, thirst, bitter taste, constipation, dark urine, Red tongue with redder sides and dry yellow coating, Wiry-Rapid pulse.

Although five-palm heat is nearly always associated with Yin deficiency, it may also be caused by Liver-Fire, but this is not common.

Latent Heat in Lesser Yin

Five-palm heat, low-grade fever, cold in the morning and hot at dusk, mental restlessness, insomnia, Red tongue without coating.

> ### Clinical note
> - Although five-palm heat involves three areas (the chest, the palms and the soles), the clinical significance would be the same if only two areas are involved, e.g. chest and palms, or chest and soles, or palms and soles.

CONTRADICTORY FEELINGS OF COLD AND HEAT

Simultaneous deficiency of Kidney-Yin and Kidney-Yang with prevalence of Kidney-Yin

Dizziness, tinnitus, night sweating, malar flush, a feeling of heat in the evening, but possibly also cold feet.

Simultaneous deficiency of Kidney-Yin and Kidney-Yang with prevalence of Kidney-Yang

Dizziness, backache, tinnitus, frequent urination, a pronounced feeling of cold, cold feet, but possibly also a feeling of heat in the afternoon.

Blood deficiency

Cold hands or feet, a feeling of cold, blurred vision, dizziness, tingling, dull ache in hands and feet, a feeling of heat in the face.

Disharmony of the Penetrating Vessel

Cold feet, a feeling of heat in the face, palpitations, anxiety, a feeling of tightness of the chest, a feeling of energy rising from the abdomen, irregular periods, painful period, Firm pulse.

Coexistence of a Heat and a Cold pattern in different organs

Example:

Kidney-Yang deficiency with Heart-Heat   Lower backache, a feeling of cold in the back or generally, cold feet, frequent pale urination, dizziness, anxiety, red face, a feeling of heat in the face, insomnia, palpitations, Pale tongue but with a Red tip, Deep-Weak pulse.

This is just an example of a coexistence of a Cold and Heat pattern. This situation may arise in connection with many other organs, for example Kidney-Yang deficiency with Liver-Yang rising, Spleen-Yang deficiency with Heart-Heat, Kidney-Yang deficiency with Damp-Heat in the Bladder, Spleen-Yang deficiency with Liver-Fire, Spleen- and Kidney-Yang deficiency with Phlegm-Heat, etc.

Lesser-Yang pattern (Six Stages)

Alternation of aversion to cold and fever, bitter taste, dry throat, blurred vision, hypochondrial fullness and distension, absence of desire to eat or drink, irritability, nausea, vomiting, unilateral thin white tongue coating, Wiry-Fine pulse.

Gall-Bladder Heat (Four Levels)

Alternating hot and cold feeling with a prevalence of heat, bitter taste, thirst, dry throat, hypochondrial pain, nausea, a feeling of fullness in the epigastrium, Red tongue with unilateral sticky yellow coating, Wiry-Rapid pulse.

Clinical note

- In women over the age of 45, a simultaneous deficiency of Kidney-Yin and Kidney-Yang is more the rule than the exception.

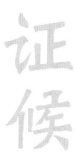

Chapter **83**

VOICE, SPEECH AND SOUNDS

Chapter contents

LOUD VOICE   819

WEAK VOICE   820

MUFFLED VOICE   820

HOARSE VOICE   820

NASAL VOICE   820

SNORING   821

SLURRED SPEECH   821

INCOHERENT, INCESSANT SPEECH   821

MUTTERING TO ONESELF   821

DELIRIOUS SPEECH   822

DIFFICULTY IN FINDING WORDS   822

STUTTERING   822

GROANING   822

CRYING OUT   822

LOUD VOICE

Hearing, Chapter 53

Heart-Fire

Loud voice, speaking a lot, speech punctuated by frequent bursts of laughter, palpitations, thirst, agitation, insomnia, dream-disturbed sleep, a feeling of heat, red face, bitter taste, Red tongue with redder tip and yellow coating, Overflowing-Rapid pulse.

Liver-Fire

Loud voice with a trembling, angry sound, headaches, dizziness, tinnitus, irritability, propensity to outbursts of anger, red face, thirst, bitter taste, constipation, dark urine, Red tongue with redder sides and dry yellow coating, Wiry-Rapid pulse.

Liver-Qi stagnation

Loud voice which comes and goes according to the emotional state, hypochondrial or epigastric distension, irritability, moodiness, Wiry pulse.

Lung-Heat

Loud voice, cough, slight breathlessness, a feeling of heat, chest ache, flaring of the nostrils, thirst, red face, Red tongue with yellow coating, Overflowing-Rapid pulse.

Lung-Qi stagnation

Trembling, loud voice sounding as if the person is on the brink of tears, sighing, sadness, worry, depression, slight breathlessness, a feeling of tightness of the chest.

WEAK VOICE

Hearing, Chapter 53

Lung-Qi deficiency

Weak voice, dislike of speaking, slight shortness of breath, spontaneous daytime sweating, bright-white complexion, tendency to catch colds, tiredness, dislike of cold, Pale tongue, Empty pulse.

Spleen-Qi deficiency

Weak voice, dislike of speaking, poor appetite, tiredness, slight abdominal distension, pale complexion, loose stools, Pale tongue, Empty pulse.

Kidney-Yang deficiency

Weak, slightly groaning voice, backache, dizziness, tinnitus, a feeling of cold, weak knees, bright-white complexion, tiredness, abundant clear urination, Pale and wet tongue, Deep-Weak pulse.

Severe depletion of Qi

Very feeble voice with speech frequently interrupted, great difficulty in starting to speak again after stopping, exhaustion, Pale tongue with teethmarks, Weak-Hidden pulse.

MUFFLED VOICE

Invasion of Wind

Muffled voice with acute onset, nasal sound, aversion to cold, fever, headache, body aches, Floating pulse.

Other symptoms and signs depend on whether it is Wind-Heat or Wind-Cold.

Deficiency of Qi and Blood

Muffled voice with slow onset, weak voice, poor appetite, loose stools, palpitations, tiredness, blurred vision, dull-pale complexion, dizziness, Pale tongue, Weak or Choppy pulse.

HOARSE VOICE

Hearing, Chapter 53

Invasion of Wind-Heat

Hoarse voice with acute onset, sore throat, aversion to cold, fever, headache, body aches, slight sweating, tongue with Red sides/front, Floating-Rapid pulse.

Liver/Lung-Qi stagnation

Hoarse voice that comes and goes according to the emotional state, irritability, depression, moodiness, a feeling of a lump in the throat, sighing.

Lung- and Kidney-Yin deficiency

Hoarse voice with slow onset, dry throat, thirst with a desire to drink in small sips, dry cough which is worse in the evening, thin body, breathlessness on exertion, lower backache, night sweating, dizziness, tinnitus, hardness of hearing, scanty urination, normal-coloured tongue without coating, Floating-Empty pulse.

Phlegm and Blood stasis

Hoarse voice in a chronic condition, swelling of the pharynx, sputum in the throat, a feeling of oppression of the chest, abdominal pain, mental restlessness, dark complexion, Reddish-Purple and Swollen tongue with sticky coating, Wiry-Slippery pulse.

Collapse of Yin or Yang

Hoarse voice with sudden onset in the course of a serious, chronic disease. Other symptoms and signs depend on whether there is collapse of Yin or collapse of Yang.

Kidney channel pathology in pregnancy

Hoarse voice towards the end of term; this is due to pathology in the Kidney Connecting channel from the Uterus to the throat and it does not require treatment.

NASAL VOICE

Hearing, Chapter 53

Invasion of Wind-Cold

Nasal voice with sudden onset, itchy throat, aversion to cold, fever, occipital headache, stiff neck, sneezing, body aches, tongue with thin white coating, Floating-Tight pulse.

Invasion of Wind-Dampness

Nasal voice with sudden onset, aversion to cold, fever, a feeling of heaviness of the body, nausea, epigastric pain, vomiting, body aches, tongue with sticky white coating, Floating-Slippery pulse.

Phlegm in the nasal passages

Nasal voice, blocked nose, snoring, a feeling of oppression of the chest, a feeling of heaviness, sputum in the throat, Swollen tongue with sticky coating, Slippery pulse.

Dampness in the nasal passages

Nasal voice, blocked nose, facial pain, sinusitis, sticky taste, a feeling of heaviness, sticky tongue coating, Slippery pulse.

Spleen- and Lung-Qi deficiency with Phlegm/Dampness in the nasal passages

Nasal voice, blocked nose, runny nose in the morning, chronic sinusitis, tiredness, poor appetite, loose stools, weak voice, tendency to catch colds, Pale and Swollen tongue with teethmarks and a sticky coating, Soggy pulse.

> **Clinical note**
>
> • A nasal voice is relatively common in children with residual Dampness in the sinuses.

SNORING

Hearing, Chapter 53; Symptoms and Signs, Chapter 81

Phlegm-Heat in the Lungs

Loud snoring, dry throat, thirst with no desire to drink, barking cough with profuse, sticky yellow sputum, shortness of breath, wheezing, a feeling of oppression of the chest, a feeling of heat, thirst, Red and Swollen tongue with a sticky yellow coating, Slippery-Rapid pulse.

Damp-Phlegm in the Lungs

Soft snoring, a feeling of oppression of the chest, cough with expectoration of sticky sputum, a feeling of heaviness, sputum in the throat, thirst with no desire to drink, Swollen tongue with sticky coating, Slippery pulse.

Dry-Phlegm in the Lungs

High-pitched snoring, dry cough with occasional, difficult expectoration of scanty sputum, thirst with no desire to drink, dry mouth and throat, Swollen tongue with sticky dry coating, Slippery pulse.

Phlegm in the Lungs with Lung- and Spleen-Qi deficiency

Soft snoring, a feeling of oppression of the chest, feeling of heaviness, weak voice, tendency to catch colds, poor appetite, loose stools, tiredness, Pale tongue with teethmarks, Soggy pulse.

SLURRED SPEECH

Phlegm

Slurred speech, difficulty in finding words, inverting words, a feeling of heaviness of the head, dizziness, blurred vision, a feeling of oppression of the chest, Swollen tongue with sticky coating, Slippery pulse.

Wind-Phlegm

Slurred speech following a stroke, hemiplegia, severe dizziness, blurred vision, tremors, unilateral numbness of a limbs, tinnitus, nausea, sputum in the throat, a feeling of oppression of the chest, Stiff or Deviated and Swollen tongue, Wiry-Slippery pulse.

Heart-Blood deficiency

Slurred speech, palpitations, dizziness, insomnia, dream-disturbed sleep, poor memory, anxiety, tendency to be easily startled, dull-pale complexion, pale lips, Pale and Thin tongue, Choppy or Fine pulse.

INCOHERENT, INCESSANT SPEECH

Phlegm-Fire harassing the Heart

Incoherent, incessant speech, agitation, mental confusion, palpitations, manic behaviour, mental restlessness, thirst, red face, a feeling of oppression of the chest, dark urine, expectoration of phlegm, rattling sound in the throat, bitter taste, insomnia, dream-disturbed sleep, Red tongue with redder swollen tip and Heart crack with a sticky yellow coating inside it, Slippery-Rapid or Slippery-Overflowing-Rapid pulse.

MUTTERING TO ONESELF

Phlegm obstructing the Mind's orifices

Muttering to oneself, mental confusion, sputum in the throat, a feeling of oppression of the chest, Swollen tongue with sticky coating, Slippery pulse.

DELIRIOUS SPEECH

Heat in the Pericardium

Delirious speech, fever at night, mental confusion, incoherent speech or aphasia, delirium, body hot, cold hands and feet, macules, Red tongue without coating, Fine-Rapid pulse.

DIFFICULTY IN FINDING WORDS

Phlegm

Difficulty in finding words, inverting words, a feeling of heaviness and muzziness of the head, dizziness, blurred vision, a feeling of oppression of the chest, Swollen tongue with sticky coating, Slippery pulse.

Heart-Blood deficiency

Difficulty in finding words, poor concentration, palpitations, dizziness, insomnia, dream-disturbed sleep, poor memory, anxiety, tendency to be easily startled, dull-pale complexion, pale lips, Pale and Thin tongue, Choppy or Fine pulse.

Kidney deficiency

Difficulty in finding words, dizziness, tinnitus, poor memory, lower backache.

Other symptoms and signs depend on whether there is Kidney-Yang or Kidney-Yin deficiency.

STUTTERING

Hearing, Chapter 53

Heart-Blood deficiency

Stuttering, nervous tension, palpitations, dizziness, insomnia, dream-disturbed sleep, poor memory, anxiety, tendency to be easily startled, dull-pale complexion, pale lips, Pale and Thin tongue, Choppy or Fine pulse.

Heart-Fire

Stuttering, palpitations, thirst, mouth and tongue ulcers, mental restlessness, a feeling of agitation, insomnia, dream-disturbed sleep, a feeling of heat, red face, bitter taste, Red tongue with redder tip and yellow coating, Overflowing-Rapid pulse.

GROANING

Hearing, Chapter 53

Dampness

Groaning, acute pain, a feeling of heaviness, tongue with thick sticky coating, Slippery pulse.

Other symptoms and signs depend on the location of the Dampness causing the pain.

Qi stagnation

Groaning, acute pain and distension, Wiry pulse.

Other symptoms and signs depend on the location of the Qi stagnation causing the pain.

CRYING OUT

Hearing, Chapter 53

Blood stasis

Crying out, severe, acute pain which is stabbing in character, Wiry pulse.

Other symptoms and signs depend on the location of the Blood stasis causing the pain.

Damp-Heat

Crying out, severe, acute pain, a feeling of fullness and heaviness, thick, sticky yellow tongue coating, Slippery-Wiry pulse.

Toxic Heat

Crying out, severe, acute pain, a feeling of heat, swelling and redness, thick sticky dark-yellow tongue coating with red spots, Overflowing-Slippery-Rapid pulse.

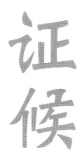

SECTION 2

GYNAECOLOGICAL SYMPTOMS AND SIGNS

Section contents

84 Menstrual symptoms *825*
85 Problems at period time *831*
86 Problems during pregnancy *837*
87 Problems after childbirth *843*
88 Breast signs *849*
89 Miscellaneous gynaecological symptoms *855*

INTRODUCTION

This section of Part 5 lists gynaecological symptoms and signs. These are extremely important not only in gynaecological conditions, but also to help us reach a diagnosis in women for non-gynaecological conditions. Questions about menstrual problems or problems arising at period time are very important in every female patient, even after the menopause; this is because, even after the menopause, we need to find out about the menstrual history to build a picture of the constitution of the patient.

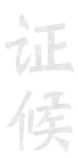

Chapter **84**

MENSTRUAL SYMPTOMS

Chapter contents

MENSTRUAL BLOOD *825*
  Pale menstrual blood *825*
  Purple menstrual blood *825*
  Menstrual clots *826*
  Sticky menstrual blood *826*
  Watery menstrual blood *826*

PERIODS *827*
  Early periods (short cycle) *827*
  Late periods (long cycle) *827*
  Irregular periods *827*
  Heavy periods *827*
  Scanty periods *828*
  Painful periods *828*
  Absence of periods *829*
  Mid-cycle bleeding *829*
  Periods that stop and start *830*
  Periods that return after the menopause *830*

MENSTRUAL BLOOD

Pale menstrual blood

Interrogation, Chapter 46

Blood deficiency

Pale and dilute menstrual blood, scanty periods, dull-pale complexion, dizziness, Pale tongue, Choppy pulse.

Qi deficiency

Pale menstrual blood, heavy bleeding, shortness of breath, tiredness, pale complexion, Pale tongue, Empty pulse.

Spleen- and Kidney-Yang deficiency

Pale and dilute menstrual blood, tiredness, loose stools, poor appetite, backache, dizziness, a feeling of cold, Pale tongue, Weak pulse.

Damp-Phlegm in the Uterus

Pale and sticky menstrual blood, excessive vaginal discharge, a feeling of heaviness, infertility, Swollen tongue with sticky coating, Slippery pulse.

Purple menstrual blood

Interrogation, Chapter 46

Qi stagnation and Blood stasis in the Uterus

Purple menstrual blood with dark clots, abdominal distension and pain, Purple tongue, Wiry pulse.

Blood stasis with Heat in the Uterus

Reddish-purple menstrual blood, purple clots, abdominal pain, mental restlessness, thirst, Reddish-Purple tongue, Wiry-Rapid pulse.

Blood stasis with Cold in the Uterus

Bluish-purple menstrual blood, small, stringy dark clots, abdominal pain, a feeling of cold, painful periods alleviated by the application of heat, Bluish-Purple tongue, Wiry-Tight-Slow pulse.

Blood deficiency with Cold in the Uterus

Pale-purplish menstrual blood, scanty periods, painful periods alleviated by the application of heat, a feeling of cold, dizziness, blurred vision, Pale tongue with white coating, Choppy pulse.

Menstrual clots

Interrogation, Chapter 46

Blood stasis in the Uterus

Dark menstrual blood with large dark clots, painful periods relieved by the passage of clots, periods starting with a brownish discharge, periods stopping and starting, painful periods, irregular periods, infertility, Purple tongue, Wiry pulse.

Blood-Heat

Dark but fresh-looking clots, heavy periods, a feeling of heat, red face, Red tongue, Overflowing-Rapid pulse.

Cold in the Uterus

Small, stringy clots with bright-red blood, painful periods alleviated by the application of heat, a feeling of cold during the periods, dilute menstrual blood, Pale tongue, Deep-Tight pulse.

Qi deficiency

Small, pale-red, fresh-looking clots, heavy periods with bright-red and dilute blood, pale face, tiredness, dizziness, Pale tongue, Weak pulse.

Sticky menstrual blood

Interrogation, Chapter 46

Damp-Heat in the Uterus

Sticky menstrual blood with offensive odour, excessive vaginal discharge, hypogastric fullness, vaginal itching, sticky yellow tongue coating, Slippery-Rapid pulse.

Damp-Phlegm in the Uterus

Sticky menstrual blood of pale colour, a feeling of oppression of the chest, dizziness, nausea, excessive vaginal discharge, infertility, Swollen tongue with sticky coating, Slippery pulse.

Liver- and Heart-Fire

Sticky menstrual blood, early periods, heavy periods, mental restlessness, insomnia, thirst, red face, palpitations, headaches, bitter taste, burning on urination, Red tongue with redder sides and tip and dry yellow coating, Wiry-Rapid pulse.

Blood stasis in the Uterus with Heat

Sticky menstrual blood, dark clots, a feeling of heat, abdominal pain, painful periods, Reddish-Purple tongue, Wiry-Rapid pulse.

Watery menstrual blood

Interrogation, Chapter 46

Qi deficiency

Watery pale menstrual blood, heavy periods, tiredness, pale face, shortness of breath, Pale tongue, Empty pulse.

Blood deficiency

Watery menstrual blood, scanty periods, late periods, blurred vision, dull-pale face, Pale-Thin tongue, Choppy pulse.

Cold-Dampness in the Uterus

Watery menstrual blood, a feeling of heaviness and cold in the hypogastrium, painful periods alleviated by the application of heat, late periods, abdominal pain, excessive vaginal discharge, sticky white tongue coating, Slippery-Slow or Tight-Slow pulse.

Spleen- and Kidney-Yang deficiency

Watery pale menstrual blood, heavy periods, tiredness, a feeling of cold, backache, loose stools, dizziness, Pale and Swollen tongue, Deep-Weak pulse.

Liver- and Kidney-Yin deficiency

Watery menstrual blood that is scarlet red, late periods, scanty periods, backache, dizziness, tinnitus, night sweating, tongue without coating, Floating-Empty pulse.

PERIODS

Early periods (short cycle)

Interrogation, Chapter 46

Qi deficiency

Early periods, heavy bleeding, pale blood, tiredness, poor appetite, loose stools, pale complexion, Pale tongue, Empty pulse.

Blood-Heat

Early period, heavy bleeding, bright-red or dark-red blood, a feeling of heat, thirst, mental restlessness, red face, Red tongue with yellow coating, Overflowing-Rapid pulse.

Liver- and Kidney-Yin deficiency

Early periods, scanty periods, dizziness, tinnitus, backache, night sweating, tongue without coating, Floating-Empty pulse.

Blood stasis in the Uterus

Early periods, painful periods with dark blood and clots, Purple tongue, Wiry pulse.

Late periods (long cycle)

Interrogation, Chapter 46

Blood deficiency

Late period, scanty periods, blurred vision, dizziness, Pale tongue, Choppy or Fine pulse.

Cold in the Uterus

Late periods, scanty bleeding, painful periods alleviated by the application of heat, small, stringy dark clots, a feeling of cold, Pale tongue, Deep-Tight-Slow pulse.

Damp-Phlegm in the Uterus

Late periods, sticky menstrual blood, a feeling of heaviness, excessive vaginal discharge, Swollen tongue with sticky coating, Slippery pulse.

Kidney deficiency

Late periods, backache, dizziness, tinnitus, tongue without coating.

Other symptoms and signs depend on whether there is a deficiency of Kidney-Yin or Kidney-Yang.

Irregular periods

Interrogation, Chapter 46

'Irregular periods' indicates periods that come sometimes early and sometimes late. It is important to bear in mind that many women refer to 'irregular periods' when the periods are either consistently late or consistently early, in which case they fall under the headings of 'late periods' or 'early periods' respectively.

Liver-Qi stagnation

Irregular periods, premenstrual tension, hypochondrial or epigastric distension, irritability, moodiness, Wiry pulse.

Kidney deficiency

Irregular periods, backache, dizziness, tinnitus, infertility.

Other manifestations, including the pulse and tongue, depend on whether there is Kidney-Yang or Kidney-Yin deficiency.

Heart- and Spleen-Blood deficiency

Irregular periods, scanty bleeding, pale blood, palpitations, tiredness, Pale-Thin tongue, Choppy pulse.

Heavy periods

Interrogation, Chapter 46

'Heavy periods' indicates heavy menstrual blood that occurs at the proper time; that is, the period comes regularly, it lasts approximately 4 or 5 days and the bleeding is heavy during that time. There is another condition characterized by heavy bleeding called 'Flooding and trickling' (*Beng Lou*): this indicates heavy menstrual blood outside the proper time; that is, the period may come early with a sudden flood (*Beng*), or it may continue with a trickle after the proper period time (*Lou*), or both. The various pathological conditions indicated below apply to both 'Heavy periods' and 'Flooding and trickling'.

Qi deficiency

Heavy menstrual bleeding that may come early with a flood, pale blood, tiredness, pale face, poor appetite, palpitations, Pale tongue, Empty pulse.

Blood-Heat

Heavy menstrual bleeding, bright-red or dark-red blood, a feeling of heat, mental restlessness, red face,

thirst, Red tongue with yellow coating, Overflowing-Rapid pulse.

Liver-Fire

Heavy menstrual bleeding, headaches, dizziness, tinnitus, irritability, propensity to outbursts of anger, red face, thirst, bitter taste, constipation, dark urine, Red tongue with redder sides and dry yellow coating, Wiry-Rapid pulse.

Spleen- and Kidney-Yang deficiency

Heavy menstrual bleeding, pale blood, irregular periods, backache, a feeling of cold, loose stools, tiredness, infertility, Pale and Swollen tongue, Deep-Weak pulse.

Liver- and Kidney-Yin deficiency

Heavy menstrual bleeding, trickling after the proper time, irregular periods, infertility, dizziness, tinnitus, night sweating, tongue without coating, Floating-Empty pulse.

Liver- and Kidney-Yin deficiency with Blood Empty-Heat

Heavy menstrual bleeding, irregular periods, trickling after the proper time, infertility, dizziness, tinnitus, night sweating, a feeling of heat in the evening, five-palm heat, Red tongue without coating, Floating-Empty and Rapid pulse.

Blood stasis in the Uterus

Heavy menstrual bleeding, painful periods with dark blood and dark clots, periods that stop and start, abdominal pain, Purple tongue, Wiry pulse.

Clinical note

- In my opinion, most practitioners tend to have a bias towards Qi deficiency as a cause of heavy menstrual bleeding. However, in my experience, roughly half the cases are due to Blood-Heat.

Scanty periods

Interrogation, Chapter 46

Blood deficiency

Scanty periods with pale-dilute blood, late periods, dizziness, blurred vision, Pale-Thin tongue, Choppy pulse.

Kidney-Yang deficiency

Scanty periods with pale blood, late periods, infertility, irregular periods, backache, dizziness, tinnitus, a feeling of cold, weak knees, bright-white complexion, tiredness, abundant clear urination, Pale and wet tongue, Deep-Weak pulse.

Kidney-Yin deficiency

Scanty periods, irregular periods, late periods, infertility, dizziness, tinnitus, night sweating, dry mouth with a desire to drink in small sips, backache, poor memory, scanty dark urine, tongue without coating, Floating-Empty pulse.

Blood stasis in the Uterus

Scanty periods with dark blood and clots, painful periods, Purple tongue, Wiry pulse.

Phlegm obstructing the Uterus

Scanty periods with a brownish discharge, excessive vaginal discharge, a feeling of heaviness, obesity, Swollen tongue, Slippery pulse.

Cold in the Uterus

Scanty periods, late periods, painful periods alleviated by the application of heat, a feeling of cold, abdominal pain, white tongue coating, Tight-Slow pulse.

Painful periods

Interrogation, Chapter 46

Liver-Qi stagnation

Abdominal distension and pain before or during the periods, premenstrual tension, distension of the breasts, no clots, hypochondrial or epigastric distension, irritability, moodiness, Wiry pulse.

Liver-Blood stasis

Severe period pain which is alleviated by the passage of clots, hypochondrial pain, abdominal pain, dark complexion, Purple tongue, Wiry pulse.

Stagnation of Cold in the Uterus

Severe spastic cramp-like menstrual pain that is alleviated by the application of heat, small, stringy clots of bright red blood, a feeling of cold during the period, Pale tongue, Deep-Tight pulse.

Damp-Heat in the Uterus

Painful periods with a feeling of heaviness extending to the sacrum, mid-cycle pain, small red clots, excessive vaginal discharge, dark urine, Red tongue with sticky yellow coating, Slippery-Rapid pulse.

Stagnant Liver-Qi turning to Liver-Fire

Painful periods, heavy periods, irritability, thirst, bitter taste, dry stools, Red tongue with redder sides and yellow coating, Rapid-Wiry pulse.

Deficiency of Qi and Blood

Dull menstrual pain towards the end of or after the period, pain relieved by pressure, scanty periods, poor appetite, loose stools, weak voice, palpitations, tiredness, blurred vision, dull-pale complexion, dizziness, Pale tongue, Weak or Choppy pulse.

Spleen-Yang and Liver-Blood deficiency

Dull period pain during or after the period, scanty bleeding without clots, dull headache, blurred vision, tiredness, loose stools, Pale and Swollen tongue, Choppy or Fine pulse.

Liver- and Kidney-Yin deficiency

Dull period pain during or after the period, scanty period, backache, dizziness, tinnitus, night sweating, tongue without coating, Floating-Empty pulse.

Absence of periods

Interrogation, Chapter 46

Blood deficiency

Menstruation stops after several months of decreasing periods, blurred vision, dizziness, Pale tongue, Choppy or Fine pulse.

Liver and Kidney deficiency

Menstruation not started by the age of 18, or stopped after becoming scanty, backache, dizziness, tiredness.

Other manifestations, including pulse and tongue, depend on whether there is Kidney-Yin or Kidney-Yang deficiency.

Spleen- and Kidney-Yang deficiency

Absence of periods, tiredness, loose stools, backache, dizziness, a feeling of cold, Pale and swollen tongue, Deep-Weak pulse.

Liver- and Kidney-Yin deficiency

Absence of periods, dizziness, tinnitus, backache, blurred vision, dry eyes, tongue without coating, Floating-Empty pulse.

This is usually secondary amenorrhoea in older women.

Lung-Yin and Blood deficiency

Absence of periods, dry cough, shortness of breath, malar flush, depression, sighing, dizziness, sadness, tongue without coating in the front, Floating-Empty pulse.

Heart- and Kidney-Yin deficiency

Absence of periods, palpitations, insomnia, backache, dizziness, tinnitus, depression, anxiety, night sweating, Red tongue with redder tip and without coating, Floating-Empty pulse.

Heart- and Spleen-Blood deficiency

Absence of periods, palpitations, depression, insomnia, pale-dull complexion, tiredness, loose stools, poor appetite, Pale tongue, Weak or Choppy pulse.

Stagnation of Qi and stasis of Blood

Periods that stop suddenly, irritability, abdominal distension and pain, depression, Wiry pulse.

Damp-Phlegm in the Uterus

Periods that stop after gradually decreasing in amount, obesity, excessive vaginal discharge, a feeling of heaviness, abdominal fullness, Swollen tongue with sticky coating, Slippery pulse.

Mid-cycle bleeding

Interrogation, Chapter 46

Liver- and Kidney-Yin deficiency with Empty-Heat

Mid-cycle bleeding that is scanty, scarlet-red blood, dizziness, tinnitus, night sweating, backache, five-palm heat, malar flush, Red tongue without coating, Floating-Empty pulse.

Damp-Heat

Mid-cycle bleeding that may be heavy or scanty, sticky blood, fatigue, ache in the joints, a feeling of heaviness, poor appetite, vaginal discharge, sticky yellow tongue coating, Slippery-Rapid pulse.

Blood stasis

Mid-cycle bleeding with pain, scanty blood, dark blood with dark clots, abdominal pain, Purple tongue, Wiry pulse.

Spleen- and Kidney-Yang deficiency

Mid-cycle bleeding that may be profuse, dilute bright-red blood, dizziness, tinnitus, backache, loose stools, tiredness, depression, a feeling of cold, frequent urination, Pale and Swollen tongue, Deep-Weak pulse.

Periods that stop and start

Interrogation, Chapter 46

Blood stasis in the Uterus

Periods that stop and start, painful periods with dark blood and clots, Purple tongue, Wiry pulse.

Cold in the Uterus

Periods that stop and start, painful periods with small, stringy dark clots, scanty periods, abdominal pain alleviated by the application of heat, white tongue coating, Deep-Tight pulse.

Liver-Qi stagnation

Periods that stop and start, hypochondrial or epigastric distension, irritability, moodiness, Wiry pulse.

Periods that return after the menopause

This symptom occurs only in menopausal women, when the periods stop for at least a year and then suddenly return; in ancient times this was called 'inverted opening flower'.

Liver- and Kidney-Yin deficiency with Empty Heat

Periods that return suddenly after 1 year of climacterium, scanty in volume, fresh red blood, malar flush, dizziness, tinnitus, night sweating, insomnia, dry mouth with a desire to drink in small sips, five-palm heat, Red tongue without coating, Floating-Empty pulse.

Stagnant Liver-Qi turned into Liver-Fire

Periods that return suddenly after 1 year of climacterium, heavy period, dark-red blood with red clots, propensity to outbursts of anger, thirst, bitter taste, insomnia, Red tongue with redder sides and yellow coating, Wiry-Rapid pulse.

Spleen-Qi deficiency

Periods that return suddenly after 1 year of climacterium, heavy period, dilute bright-red blood, poor appetite, tiredness, slight abdominal distension, pale complexion, loose stools, Pale tongue, Empty pulse.

Toxic Heat in the Uterus

Periods that return suddenly after 1 year of climacterium, bloody vaginal discharge with offensive odour, five-colour vaginal discharge, foul breath, constipation, Red tongue with sticky yellow coating and red spots, Rapid-Overflowing pulse.

This condition may correspond to carcinoma of the uterus in Western medicine; therefore a bloody vaginal discharge with offensive odour in a woman after the menopause always requires a gynaecological examination.

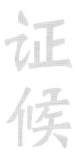

Chapter **85**

PROBLEMS AT PERIOD TIME

Chapter contents

PREMENSTRUAL TENSION   *831*

HEADACHE   *832*

BREAST DISTENSION   *832*

FEVER   *833*

BODY ACHES   *833*

OEDEMA   *833*

DIARRHOEA   *833*

CONSTIPATION   *834*

NOSEBLEED   *834*

MOUTH ULCERS   *834*

SKIN ERUPTIONS   *834*

DIZZINESS   *835*

VOMITING   *835*

INSOMNIA   *835*

EYE PAIN   *835*

PREMENSTRUAL TENSION

Interrogation, Chapter 46

Liver-Qi stagnation

Irritability, depression, moodiness, propensity to outbursts of anger, impatience, irregular periods, breast distension, hypochondrial or epigastric distension, a feeling of a lump in the throat, Wiry pulse.

Liver- and Heart-Fire

Propensity to outbursts of anger, irritability, mental restlessness, shouting, anxiety, insomnia, breast distension, heavy periods, a feeling of heat, headache, red face, dizziness, tinnitus, thirst, bitter taste, constipation, dark urine, palpitations, mouth and tongue ulcers, Red tongue with redder sides and tip and yellow coating, Overflowing-Wiry-Rapid pulse.

Heart-Fire

Mental restlessness, anxiety, insomnia, dream-disturbed sleep, breast distension, heavy periods, palpitations, thirst, mouth and tongue ulcers, a feeling of heat, red face, bitter taste, Red tongue with redder tip and yellow coating, Overflowing-Rapid pulse.

Phlegm-Fire harassing upwards

Mental restlessness, anxiety, insomnia, hyperactivity, dream-disturbed sleep, mental confusion, breast distension, swelling and pain, a feeling of heaviness and muzziness of the head, a feeling of heat, red face, greasy skin, a feeling of oppression of the chest, sputum in the throat, expectoration of yellow sputum, dizziness, nausea, Red and Swollen tongue with sticky yellow coating, Slippery-Rapid pulse.

Liver-Blood deficiency with secondary Liver-Qi stagnation

Weepiness, crying, depression, mild irritability, mild breast distension, dizziness, blurred vision, floaters, numbness/tingling of limbs, scanty menstruation, dull-pale complexion, Pale tongue, Choppy or Fine pulse.

Liver- and Kidney-Yin deficiency

Weepiness, crying, depression, lack of motivation, insomnia, scanty menstruation or amenorrhoea, dizziness, tinnitus, lower backache, dull occipital or vertical headache, numbness/tingling of the limbs, dry eyes, blurred vision, dry throat in the evening, dry hair and skin, brittle nails, night sweating, dry stools, normal-coloured tongue without coating, Floating-Empty pulse.

Spleen- and Kidney-Yang deficiency

Weepiness, crying, depression, lack of motivation, tiredness, lassitude, scanty or heavy periods, lower backache, a sensation of cold in the back, a feeling of cold, bright-white complexion, decreased libido, tiredness, lassitude, abundant clear or scanty clear urination, urination at night, apathy, oedema of the lower legs, loose stools, poor appetite, slight abdominal distension, a desire to lie down, Pale and wet tongue, Deep-Weak pulse.

Spleen-Qi deficiency with Dampness and secondary Liver-Qi stagnation

Weepiness, depression, tiredness, lassitude, feeling of heaviness, swelling of the breasts, mild irritability, poor appetite, slight abdominal distension after eating, pale complexion, weak limbs, loose stools, abdominal fullness, sticky taste, nausea, excessive vaginal discharge, Pale tongue with sticky coating, Soggy pulse.

Clinical note

- **Remember**: premenstrual tension is not always due to a Liver disharmony. For example, Heart-Fire can also cause it.

HEADACHE

Interrogation, Chapter 46

Liver-Blood deficiency

Dull vertical headache during or after the period, scanty period, dizziness, blurred vision, Pale tongue, Choppy or Fine pulse.

Liver-Yang rising

Throbbing headache on the temples before or during the period, dizziness, tinnitus, irritability, propensity to outbursts of anger, red face, Wiry pulse.

Liver-Fire

Throbbing headache on the temples or eyes during the period, bloodshot eyes, red face, thirst, bitter taste, headaches, dizziness, tinnitus, irritability, propensity to outbursts of anger, constipation, dark urine, Red tongue with redder sides and dry yellow coating, Wiry-Rapid pulse.

Blood stasis

Stabbing headache on the temples during the period, painful periods with dark blood and clots, Purple tongue, Wiry pulse.

BREAST DISTENSION

Interrogation, Chapter 46

Liver-Qi stagnation

Premenstrual breast distension, hypochondrial or epigastric distension, irritability, moodiness, Wiry pulse.

Liver-Blood stasis

Premenstrual breast distension and pain, painful period with dark blood and clots, hypochondrial pain, abdominal pain, dark complexion, Purple tongue, Wiry pulse.

Phlegm with stagnation of Qi

Premenstrual breast distension, breast nodularity, swollen and painful breasts, a feeling of oppression of the chest, sighing, obesity, Swollen tongue, Slippery-Wiry pulse.

Liver- and Kidney-Yin deficiency with Liver-Qi stagnation

Slight premenstrual breast distension, scanty periods, dizziness, tinnitus, irregular periods, tongue without coating, Fine and slightly Wiry pulse.

Stagnant Liver-Qi turning to Liver-Fire

Premenstrual breast distension and pain, abdominal distension, bitter taste, thirst, insomnia, irritability, Red tongue with redder sides and yellow coating, Wiry-Rapid pulse.

Spleen- and Kidney-Yang deficiency with Liver-Qi stagnation

Slight premenstrual breast distension, late periods, irregular periods, infertility, backache, dizziness, tiredness, loose stools, Pale and Swollen tongue, Weak pulse.

Liver-Blood and Kidney-Yang deficiency

Slight breast distension before or during the period, irregular periods, dizziness, tinnitus, blurred vision, backache, pale face, Pale tongue, Deep-Weak pulse.

Lung-Qi stagnation

Premenstrual breast distension, a feeling of oppression or distension of the chest, slight breathlessness, sighing, a feeling of a lump in the throat, difficulty in swallowing, sadness, irritability, depression, tongue slightly Red on the sides in the chest areas, pulse very slightly Tight on the right Front position.

Phlegm with Lung-Qi stagnation

Phlegm in the throat, a feeling of a lump in the throat, a feeling of oppression or distension of the chest, slight breathlessness, difficulty in swallowing, sighing, sadness, irritability, depression, sputum in the throat, tongue slightly Swollen on the sides in the chest areas, Slippery pulse that is also very slightly Tight on the right Front position.

Clinical note

- **Remember**: premenstrual breast distension is not always due to a Liver disharmony. Stagnation of Lung-Qi (with or without Phlegm) also affects the breasts.

FEVER

Blood-Heat

Fever before or during the period, heavy period, mental restlessness, thirst, hot nose, red lips, Red tongue, Rapid-Overflowing pulse.

Kidney- and Liver-Yin deficiency with Empty-Heat

Low-grade fever during the period, five-palm heat, night sweating, mental restlessness, dizziness, tinnitus, Red tongue without coating, Floating-Empty and Rapid pulse.

Qi and Blood deficiency with disharmony of Nutritive and Defensive Qi

Low-grade fever during or after the period, pale complexion, dizziness, tiredness, Pale-Thin tongue, Fine-Rapid pulse.

Blood stasis in the Uterus

Fever during the period that is worse in the evening, painful periods, dark blood with clots, Purple tongue, Wiry-Rapid pulse.

BODY ACHES

Blood deficiency

Aches during or after the period, mostly in the limbs, numbness/tingling of the limbs, tiredness, dizziness, Pale-Thin tongue, Choppy pulse.

Blood stasis

Severe aches during or before the period, painful periods with dark blood and clots, Purple tongue, Wiry pulse.

OEDEMA

Interrogation, Chapter 46

Spleen- and Kidney-Yang deficiency

Oedema during or after the period especially of the ankles, backache, tiredness, loose stools, heavy periods, Pale and wet tongue, Deep-Weak pulse.

Qi stagnation

Non-pitting oedema during or before the periods, abdominal and breast distension, premenstrual tension, irritability, Wiry pulse.

DIARRHOEA

Interrogation, Chapter 46

Spleen-Qi deficiency

Diarrhoea during or after the period, slight abdominal distension, poor appetite, tiredness, pale complexion, loose stools, Pale tongue, Empty pulse.

Stagnant Liver-Qi invading the Spleen

Diarrhoea before the period, alternating constipation and diarrhoea, premenstrual tension, breast distension, irritability, Wiry pulse.

Kidney-Yang deficiency

Diarrhoea after the period, irregular periods, backache, dizziness, tinnitus, a feeling of cold, weak knees, bright-white complexion, tiredness, abundant clear urination, Pale and wet tongue, Deep-Weak pulse.

CONSTIPATION

Interrogation, Chapter 46

Stagnant Liver-Qi invading the Intestines

Constipation with bitty stools, abdominal distension, premenstrual irritability, irregular periods, hypochondrial or epigastric distension, irritability, moodiness, a feeling of a lump in the throat, Wiry pulse.

Liver-Blood deficiency

Constipation with dry stools, premenstrual weepiness and depression, dizziness, blurred vision, floaters, numbness/tingling of limbs, scanty menstruation, dull-pale complexion, Pale tongue, Choppy or Fine pulse.

Kidney-Yang deficiency

Constipation with infrequent bowel movements, lower backache, cold knees, a sensation of cold in the lower back, a feeling of cold, weak legs, bright-white complexion, weak knees, tiredness, lassitude, abundant clear or scanty clear urination, urination at night, oedema of the lower legs, depression, decreased libido, Pale and wet tongue, Deep-Weak pulse.

NOSEBLEED

Stagnant Liver-Qi turning into Fire

Nosebleed before or during the period, heavy bleeding, abdominal distension, bitter taste, thirst, irritability, headache, Red tongue with redder sides and yellow coating, Wiry-Rapid pulse.

Lung- and Kidney-Yin deficiency with Empty-Heat

Nosebleed during or after the period, dry cough, scanty period, night sweating, dizziness, tinnitus, five-palm heat, Red tongue without coating, Floating-Empty and Rapid pulse.

Stomach-Fire

Nosebleed during the period, bleeding gums, burning epigastric pain, intense thirst with a desire to drink cold liquids, mental restlessness, dry stools, sour regurgitation, foul breath, a feeling of heat, tongue Red with a thick, dry dark-yellow coating, Deep-Full-Rapid pulse.

Spleen-Qi deficiency

Nosebleed during the period, poor appetite, tiredness, slight abdominal distension, pale complexion, loose stools, Pale tongue, Empty pulse.

MOUTH ULCERS

Kidney-Yin deficiency with Empty-Heat

Mouth or tongue ulcers during the period, dizziness, tinnitus, night sweating, dry mouth with a desire to drink in small sips, backache, poor memory, scanty-dark urine, five-palm heat, malar flush, a feeling of heat in the evening, Red tongue without coating, Floating-Empty and Rapid pulse.

Stomach-Fire

Mouth ulcers during the period, bleeding gums, burning epigastric pain, intense thirst with a desire to drink cold liquids, mental restlessness, dry stools, sour regurgitation, foul breath, a feeling of heat, tongue Red with a thick, dry dark-yellow coating, Deep-Full-Rapid pulse.

Stomach Damp-Heat with Spleen-Qi deficiency

Mouth ulcers, cold sores around the lips, abdominal distension, loose stools, thirst with no desire to drink, a sticky taste, poor appetite, Pale tongue but with a sticky yellow coating in the centre, Weak and Slippery pulse.

SKIN ERUPTIONS

Blood deficiency

Itchy papular skin eruptions during or after the period, insomnia, dizziness, scanty periods, Pale-Thin tongue, Choppy pulse.

Wind-Heat invading Blood

Itchy skin eruptions during or before the period, irritability, dry mouth, Red tongue with red points, Rapid pulse.

DIZZINESS

Blood deficiency

Dizziness during or after the period, blurred vision, scanty periods, Pale-Thin tongue, Choppy pulse.

Kidney- and Liver-Yin deficiency with Liver-Yang rising

Severe dizziness during or before the period, tinnitus, scanty periods, insomnia, dizziness, tinnitus, night sweating, tongue without coating, Floating-Empty pulse.

Phlegm with Spleen-Qi deficiency

Severe dizziness during or before the period, a feeling of heaviness and muzziness of the head, excessive vaginal discharge, swelling of the breasts before the period, Pale and Swollen tongue, Slippery and slightly Weak pulse.

VOMITING

Interrogation, Chapter 46

Stagnant Liver-Qi invading the Stomach

Vomiting before or during the period, belching, epigastric distension and pain, irritability, Wiry pulse.

Stomach- and Spleen-Qi deficiency

Vomiting of thin fluids or nausea during or after the periods, dull epigastric pain, poor appetite, tiredness, slight abdominal distension, pale complexion, loose stools, Pale tongue, Empty pulse.

Phlegm with Spleen-Qi deficiency

Vomiting during the periods, nausea, a feeling of oppression of the chest, tiredness, loose stools, poor appetite, Pale and Swollen tongue, Slippery and slightly Weak pulse.

INSOMNIA

Liver-Yang rising

Insomnia before the periods, anxiety, dizziness, headache, dry throat, irregular periods.

Other symptoms and signs, including pulse and tongue, depend on the condition underlying the Liver-Yang rising, which may be Liver-Blood deficiency, Liver-Yin deficiency or Kidney-Yin deficiency.

Liver- and Heart-Fire

Insomnia during the period, dream-disturbed sleep, agitation, anxiety, bitter taste, thirst, palpitations, bloodshot eyes, propensity to outbursts of anger, dizziness, headache, epistaxis, heavy periods, red face, Red tongue with redder sides and yellow coating, Wiry and Rapid pulse.

Heart- and Spleen-Blood deficiency

Insomnia during or after the period, slight anxiety, depression, tiredness, blurred vision, dizziness, poor appetite, Pale-Thin tongue, Choppy pulse.

EYE PAIN

Liver-Blood deficiency

Dull eye pain at period time, dull headache, dizziness, blurred vision, floaters, numbness/tingling of limbs, dull-pale complexion, Pale tongue, Choppy or Fine pulse.

Liver-Blood deficiency giving rise to internal Wind

Eye pain at period time, facial tic, giddiness, vertigo, headache, sallow complexion, blurred vision, floaters, Pale-Thin tongue, Wiry pulse.

Liver-Fire

Eye pain at period time, bloodshot eyes, premenstrual tension, heavy periods, red face, thirst, bitter taste, headaches, dizziness, tinnitus, irritability, propensity to outbursts of anger, constipation, dark urine, Red tongue with redder sides and dry yellow coating, Wiry-Rapid pulse.

Liver-Blood stasis

Stabbing eye pain at period time, painful periods with dark clotted blood, hypochondrial pain, abdominal pain, dark complexion, Purple tongue, Wiry pulse.

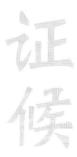

Chapter **86**

PROBLEMS DURING PREGNANCY

Chapter contents

MORNING SICKNESS *837*

VAGINAL BLEEDING *838*

ABDOMINAL PAIN *838*

OEDEMA *838*

URINATION PROBLEMS *839*
    Painful urination *839*
    Retention of urine *839*
    Blood in the urine *839*

CONSTIPATION *839*

ANXIETY *840*

DIZZINESS *840*

COUGH *840*

LOSS OF VOICE *840*

FEELING OF SUFFOCATION *841*

CONVULSIONS (ECLAMPSIA) *841*

PROBLEMS WITH THE FETUS *841*
    Threatened miscarriage *841*
    Fetus not growing *842*
    Breech presentation *842*
    Habitual miscarriage *842*

MORNING SICKNESS

Interrogation, Chapter 46

Stomach-Qi deficiency with Empty-Cold

Slight morning sickness, absence of vomiting or vomiting of dilute fluids, tiredness, a feeling of cold, poor appetite, Pale tongue, Weak pulse.

Stomach-Yin deficiency

Morning sickness, dry mouth with a desire to drink in small sips, poor appetite, tongue without coating in the centre.

Stagnant Liver-Qi invading the Stomach

Morning sickness, retching, belching, vomiting of food with sour taste, epigastric distension, irritability, Wiry pulse.

Stomach-Heat

Severe morning sickness that may persist beyond the first 3 months, vomiting of food soon after eating, burning epigastric pain, thirst, sour regurgitation, excessive hunger, foul breath, a feeling of heat, Red tongue with a yellow coating, Overflowing-Rapid pulse.

Accumulation of Phlegm

Morning sickness, profuse vomiting, occasional vomiting of clear fluids with mucus, a feeling of oppression of the chest and epigastrium, dizziness, Swollen tongue with sticky coating, Slippery pulse.

Heart-Qi deficiency

Slight morning sickness, palpitations, anxiety, depression, Pale tongue, Empty pulse on the left Front position.

Heart-Fire

Morning sickness which may persist beyond the first 3 months, palpitations, thirst, agitation, insomnia, dream-disturbed sleep, a feeling of heat, red face, bitter taste, Red tongue with redder tip and yellow coating, Overflowing-Rapid pulse.

Clinical note

- Simple, straightforward cases of morning sickness react well to P-6 Neiguan, Ren-13 Shangwan and ST-36 Zusanli. If they do not react to this treatment, it often indicates that there is a pre-existing, underlying Stomach pathology.

VAGINAL BLEEDING

Spleen-Qi deficiency

Vaginal bleeding early in the pregnancy, scanty fresh-red blood, poor appetite, tiredness, slight abdominal distension, pale complexion, loose stools, Pale tongue, Empty pulse.

Liver-Blood deficiency

Vaginal bleeding early in the pregnancy, scanty pale blood, dull-pale complexion, blurred vision, palpitation, insomnia, Pale tongue, Choppy or Fine pulse.

Kidney-Yang deficiency

Vaginal bleeding during the first 3 months, scanty fresh-red blood, backache, dizziness, tinnitus, a feeling of cold, weak knees, bright-white complexion, tiredness, abundant clear urination, Pale and wet tongue, Deep-Weak pulse.

Blood-Heat

Vaginal bleeding which may occur beyond the first 3 months, bright-red or dark-red blood, red face, anxiety, insomnia, dark urine, Red tongue with yellow coating, Rapid-Overflowing pulse.

Kidney-Yin deficiency with Empty-Heat

Vaginal bleeding during pregnancy, scanty blood, dizziness, tinnitus, night sweating, dry mouth with a desire to drink in small sips, backache, poor memory, scanty dark urine, five-palm heat, malar flush, a feeling of heat in the evening, Red tongue without coating, Floating-Empty and Rapid pulse.

Trauma

Vaginal bleeding after a fall or trauma, backache.

ABDOMINAL PAIN

Liver-Blood deficiency

Mild abdominal pain that comes and goes, dull-pale complexion, dizziness, blurred vision, Pale tongue, Choppy or Fine pulse.

Liver-Qi stagnation

Abdominal pain and distension, hypochondrial pain and distension, irritability, Wiry pulse.

Empty-Cold in the Uterus

Dull abdominal pain that improves with the application of heat and drinking warm liquids, a feeling of cold, white complexion, cold limbs, Pale tongue, Deep-Weak pulse.

OEDEMA

Interrogation, Chapter 46

In some cases, oedema during pregnancy may be the first symptom heralding a pre-eclampsia state.

Spleen-Yang deficiency

Oedema early in the pregnancy, swelling of face or whole body, yellowish and shiny skin, poor appetite, tiredness, slight abdominal distension, bright-white complexion, loose stools, feeling cold, cold limbs, Pale and wet tongue, Deep-Weak pulse.

Kidney-Yang deficiency

Oedema early in the pregnancy, worse in the ankles, cold legs, backache, dizziness, tinnitus, feeling cold, weak knees, bright-white complexion, tiredness, abundant-clear urination, Pale and wet tongue, Deep-Weak pulse.

Qi stagnation

Oedema beginning towards the fourth month of pregnancy, starting in the feet, not pitting, abdominal distension, irritability, Wiry pulse.

URINATION PROBLEMS

Painful urination
Heart-Fire

Burning on urination, scanty-dark urine, palpitations, thirst, agitation, insomnia, dream-disturbed sleep, feeling of heat, red face, bitter taste, Red tongue with redder tip and yellow coating, Overflowing-Rapid pulse.

Damp-Heat in the Bladder

Burning on urination, difficult urination, slight retention, turbid urine, thirst with no desire to drink, a feeling of heaviness, a sticky taste, sticky yellow tongue coating, Slippery-Rapid pulse.

Kidney-Yin deficiency with Empty-Heat

Slight burning on urination, scanty dark urine, dizziness, tinnitus, night sweating, dry mouth with a desire to drink in small sips, backache, poor memory, scanty dark urine, five-palm heat, malar flush, a feeling of heat in the evening, Red tongue without coating, Floating-Empty and Rapid pulse.

Spleen-Qi deficiency

Slight pain after urination, pale urine, slight incontinence of urine, pale face, tiredness, poor appetite, loose stools, Pale tongue, Weak pulse.

Retention of urine
Spleen-Qi deficient and sinking

Scanty but frequent urination, a feeling of bearing down, loose stools, pale complexion, tiredness, Pale tongue, Weak pulse.

Kidney-Qi deficient and sinking

Scanty but frequent urination, pale urine, interrupted flow of micturition, an uncomfortable sensation in the hypogastrium which is worse when sitting, a feeling of cold, backache, dizziness, Pale tongue, Deep-Weak pulse.

Damp-Heat in the Bladder

Difficult urination, dark/turbid urine, a feeling of heaviness in the lower abdomen, sticky taste, sticky yellow tongue coating, Slippery-Rapid pulse.

Liver-Qi stagnation

Urinary difficulty in the seventh or eighth month, hypochondrial or epigastric distension, irritability, moodiness, Wiry pulse.

Blood in the urine
Heart-Fire

Blood in the urine during pregnancy, dark urine, palpitations, thirst, a feeling of agitation, insomnia, dream-disturbed sleep, a feeling of heat, red face, bitter taste, Red tongue with redder tip and yellow coating, Overflowing-Rapid pulse.

Kidney-Yin deficiency with Empty-Heat

Blood in the urine during pregnancy, dizziness, tinnitus, night sweating, dry mouth with a desire to drink in small sips, backache, poor memory, scanty dark urine, five-palm heat, malar flush, a feeling of heat in the evening, Red tongue without coating, Floating-Empty and Rapid pulse.

Liver-Yin deficiency with Empty-Heat

Blood in the urine in pregnancy, blurred vision, dry eyes, dizziness, night sweating, Red tongue without coating, Floating-Empty pulse that is slightly Wiry on the left.

CONSTIPATION

Liver-Blood deficiency

Constipation, difficult defecation, dry stools, pale complexion, dizziness, blurred vision, tiredness, Pale tongue, Choppy or Fine pulse.

Kidney-Yang deficiency

Constipation, difficulty in defecation, stools not dry, exhaustion after defecation, backache, dizziness, tinnitus, a feeling of cold, weak knees, bright-white complexion, tiredness, abundant clear urination, Pale and wet tongue, Deep-Weak pulse.

Kidney-Yin deficiency

Constipation, dry stools, dizziness, tinnitus, night sweating, dry mouth with a desire to drink in small sips, backache, poor memory, scanty dark urine, tongue without coating, Floating-Empty pulse.

Liver-Qi stagnation

Constipation, bitty stools, desire to open the bowels but difficulty in doing so, belching, hypochondrial or epigastric distension, irritability, moodiness, Wiry pulse.

ANXIETY

Liver-Fire

Severe anxiety, irritability, propensity to outbursts of anger, headaches, dizziness, tinnitus, red face, thirst, bitter taste, constipation, dark urine, Red tongue with redder sides and dry yellow coating, Wiry-Rapid pulse.

Liver- and Kidney-Yin deficiency with Empty-Heat

Anxiety, worse in the evening, dry mouth with a desire to drink in small sips, malar flush, night sweating, five-palm heat, backache, dizziness, tinnitus, Red tongue without coating, Floating-Empty and Rapid pulse.

Phlegm-Fire harassing the Mind

Anxiety, mental restlessness, agitation, mental confusion, phobias, irritability, a feeling of oppression of the chest, dizziness, nausea, Red and Swollen tongue with sticky yellow coating, Slippery-Rapid pulse.

Heart-Fire

Severe anxiety, palpitations, thirst, agitation, insomnia, dream-disturbed sleep, a feeling of heat, red face, bitter taste, Red tongue with redder tip and yellow coating, Overflowing-Rapid pulse.

Liver-Qi stagnation

Anxiety, hypochondrial or epigastric distension, irritability, moodiness, Wiry pulse.

DIZZINESS

Liver- and Kidney-Yin deficiency with Liver-Yang rising

Severe dizziness towards the latter stages of pregnancy, tinnitus, insomnia, a feeling of heat in the evening, night sweating, Red tongue without coating, Floating-Empty pulse.

Spleen deficiency with Liver-Yang rising and Phlegm

Dizziness with early onset during the pregnancy, swelling of the fingers and ankles, tiredness, a feeling of oppression of the chest, blurred vision, tingling of the limbs, insomnia, Pale tongue, Choppy pulse if Liver-Blood deficiency predominates, or Slippery and slightly Weak if Phlegm predominates.

Deficiency of Qi and Blood

Slight dizziness in pregnancy, poor appetite, loose stools, weak voice, palpitations, tiredness, blurred vision, dull-pale complexion, dizziness, Pale tongue, Weak or Choppy pulse.

COUGH

Lung-Yin deficiency

Dry cough that starts during the second trimester and is worse in the evenings, dry cough, weak voice, dry throat with a desire to drink in small sips, hoarse voice, night sweating, tiredness, tongue without coating in the front, Floating-Empty pulse.

Phlegm-Heat in the Lungs

Cough with expectoration of profuse yellow sputum, a feeling of oppression of the chest, a feeling of heat, mental restlessness, Red and Swollen tongue with sticky yellow coating, Slippery-Rapid pulse.

Damp-Phlegm in the Lungs

Cough with expectoration of profuse white sputum, a feeling of oppression of the chest, cold limbs, a feeling of heaviness, a sticky taste, Swollen tongue with sticky white coating, Slippery pulse.

LOSS OF VOICE

Kidney-Yin deficiency

Loss of voice or hoarseness of voice towards the end of pregnancy, dry throat, dizziness, tinnitus, night sweating, dry mouth with a desire to drink in small sips, backache, poor memory, scanty dark urine, tongue without coating, Floating-Empty pulse.

Phlegm-Heat

Loss of voice or hoarseness of voice, dry cough with occasional expectoration of scanty phlegm, a feeling of

oppression of the chest, sticky taste, mental restlessness, Swollen tongue with sticky yellow coating, Slippery-Rapid pulse.

Lung-Yin deficiency

Loss of voice or hoarseness of the voice, preceded by a weakening of the voice, dry cough, weak voice, dry throat with a desire to drink in small sips, hoarse voice, night sweating, tiredness, tongue without coating in the front, Floating-Empty pulse.

FEELING OF SUFFOCATION

Qi stagnation with disharmony of the Liver and Spleen

A feeling of suffocation and anxiety, a feeling of tightness of the chest, irritability, insomnia, inability to lie down, a feeling of energy rising from the lower abdomen towards the chest and throat, a feeling of breathlessness, Pale tongue with slightly red sides, pulse that is Wiry on the left and Weak on the right.

Qi stagnation with deficiency of Blood and Kidneys

Feeling of suffocation and anxiety, a feeling of tightness of the chest, mental restlessness, insomnia, inability to lie down, tiredness, blurred vision, dizziness, backache, frequent urination, Pale tongue, pulse that is Weak in general, especially on both the Rear positions, and slightly Wiry on the left.

CONVULSIONS (ECLAMPSIA)

Interrogation, Chapter 46

Liver-Wind agitating within

Tremor of limbs, hypertension late in the pregnancy, headache, malar flush, a feeling of heat in the afternoon, convulsions, unconsciousness.

The pulse and tongue depend on the condition underlying the Liver-Wind.

Phlegm-Fire harassing upwards

Slight tremor of limbs, hypertension, oedema, mental confusion, unconsciousness, a feeling of oppression of the chest, Swollen tongue with a sticky coating, Wiry-Slippery-Rapid pulse.

Empty-Wind

Slight tremor and twitching of limbs especially if occurring after delivery, dizziness, palpitations, sweating, pale face, Pale and Short tongue, Fine-Scattered pulse.

Blood deficiency

Mild convulsions of the legs that are worse in the evening, insomnia, palpitations, blurred vision, dizziness, Pale and Thin tongue, Choppy pulse.

PROBLEMS WITH THE FETUS

Threatened miscarriage

Interrogation, Chapter 46

Kidney deficiency

Threatened miscarriage early in the pregnancy, backache, scanty vaginal bleeding, dizziness, exhaustion.

Other symptoms, including pulse and tongue, depend on whether there is a Kidney-Yang or Kidney-Yin deficiency.

Deficiency of Qi and Blood

Threatened miscarriage towards the end of pregnancy or beyond the first 3 months, backache, scanty vaginal bleeding, poor appetite, loose stools, weak voice, palpitations, tiredness, blurred vision, dull-pale complexion, dizziness, Pale tongue, Weak or Choppy pulse.

Blood-Heat

Threatened miscarriage early in the pregnancy, backache, scanty vaginal bleeding, a feeling of heat, thirst, anxiety, insomnia, Red tongue with yellow coating, Rapid pulse.

Liver-Qi stagnation

Threatened miscarriage in the first 3 months, backache, scanty vaginal bleeding, hypochondrial or epigastric distension, irritability, moodiness, Wiry pulse.

Falls, trauma

Threatened miscarriage following a fall or a trauma, backache, abdominal pain, scanty vaginal bleeding, tongue and pulse normal.

Clinical note

- **Remember**: threatened miscarriage can be due to causes within the mother or causes within the fetus. If within the fetus, Chinese medicine is unlikely to help; if within the mother, it can help.

Fetus not growing
Deficiency of Qi and Blood

Slow fetal growth, poor appetite, loose stools, weak voice, palpitations, tiredness, blurred vision, dull-pale complexion, dizziness, Pale tongue, Weak or Choppy pulse.

Spleen- and Kidney-Yang deficiency

Slow fetal growth in the fifth and sixth months, tiredness, loose stools, poor appetite, backache, dizziness, Pale and Swollen tongue, Deep-Weak pulse.

Breech presentation
Liver-Qi stagnation

Breech presentation, hypochondrial or epigastric distension, irritability, moodiness, Wiry pulse.

Spleen-Qi deficiency with Dampness

Breech presentation, obesity, a feeling of heaviness of the body, tiredness, poor appetite, loose stools, Pale and Swollen tongue, Soft pulse.

Deficiency of Qi and Blood

Breech presentation, poor appetite, loose stools, weak voice, palpitations, tiredness, blurred vision, dull-pale complexion, dizziness, Pale tongue, Weak or Choppy pulse.

Habitual miscarriage
Interrogation, Chapter 46

Kidney-Yang deficiency

A history of miscarriage early in the pregnancy, backache, dizziness, tinnitus, a feeling of cold, weak knees, bright-white complexion, tiredness, abundant clear urination, Pale and wet tongue, Deep-Weak pulse.

Kidney-Yin deficiency

A history of repeated miscarriage (usually in the first 3 months) and infertility, dizziness, tinnitus, night sweating, dry mouth with a desire to drink in small sips, backache, poor memory, scanty dark urine, tongue without coating, Floating-Empty pulse.

Blood-Heat

A history of repeated miscarriages, often beyond the first 3 months, thirst, a feeling of heat, mental restlessness, a history of heavy periods, Red tongue with yellow coating, Overflowing and Rapid pulse.

Spleen-Qi deficiency

A history of repeated miscarriages after the first 3 months, poor appetite, tiredness, slight abdominal distension, pale complexion, loose stools, Pale tongue, Empty pulse.

Blood deficiency

A history of repeated miscarriages, dizziness, blurred vision, a history of scanty periods, insomnia, depression, dry hair and skin, Pale and Thin tongue, Choppy pulse.

Blood stasis

A history of repeated miscarriages, abdominal pain, a history of painful periods, Purple tongue, Wiry pulse.

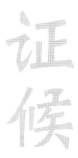

Chapter **87**

PROBLEMS AFTER CHILDBIRTH

Chapter contents

RETENTION OF PLACENTA   843

LOCHIA   843
  Persistent lochial discharge   843
  Retention of lochia   844

PAIN   844
  Abdominal pain   844
  Joint pain   844
  Hypochondrial pain   844

VAGINAL BLEEDING   845
  Vaginal bleeding after childbirth   845
  Amenorrhoea after miscarriage   845

URINARY DIFFICULTY   845

CONSTIPATION   845

SWEATING   846

DIZZINESS   846

OEDEMA   846

FEVER   846

BREAST MILK   847
  Breast milk not flowing   847
  Spontaneous flow of milk after childbirth   847

POSTNATAL DEPRESSION/PSYCHOSIS   847

COLLAPSE   847

CONVULSIONS   848

Clinical note

- Remember to pay attention to invigorating Blood after childbirth. The closer to the childbirth, the more one needs to invigorate Blood. As a rule of thumb, within 3 weeks from childbirth place the emphasis on invigorating Blood (and nourishing Blood secondarily); after 3 weeks place the emphasis on nourishing Blood (and invigorating Blood secondarily).

RETENTION OF PLACENTA

Kidney-Qi deficiency

Retention of placenta, abdominal distension, abdominal pain that is better with pressure, abundant lochia, pale complexion, tiredness, breathlessness, backache, Pale tongue, Weak pulse.

Liver-Blood stasis

Retention of placenta, abdominal pain, retention of lochia, Purple tongue, Wiry pulse.

Cold in the Uterus

Retention of placenta, abdominal pain that is alleviated by application of heat, a feeling of cold, scanty lochia, pale complexion, Pale tongue, Tight pulse.

LOCHIA

Persistent lochial discharge

Observation, Chapter 20

Kidney-Qi deficiency

Persistent lochial discharge that is red, profuse, dilute and without odour, dizziness, exhaustion, breathlessness, backache, sweating, Pale tongue, Weak pulse.

Liver-Blood stasis

Persistent lochial discharge that is dark, scanty and with clots, abdominal pain that is alleviated by passing clots, Purple tongue, Wiry pulse.

Blood-Heat

Persistent lochial discharge that is dark in colour, red face, thirst, a feeling of heat, anxiety, abdominal pain, dry stools, Red tongue with yellow coating, Overflowing-Rapid pulse.

Kidney-Yin deficiency with Empty-Heat

Persistent lochial discharge that is dilute and scarlet red, dizziness, tinnitus, night sweating, dry mouth with a desire to drink in small sips, backache, poor memory, scanty dark urine, five-palm heat, malar flush, a feeling of heat in the evening, Red tongue without coating, Floating-Empty and Rapid pulse.

Retention of lochia

Observation, Chapter 20

Qi stagnation and Blood stasis

Absence of lochial discharge, or scanty discharge with clots, or discharge that stops and starts, abdominal pain, Purple tongue, Wiry pulse.

Stagnation of Cold and stasis of Blood

Absent or scanty dark lochial discharge with small stringy clots, abdominal pain relieved by the application of heat, cold limbs, Bluish-Purple tongue, Tight pulse.

Deficiency of Qi and Blood

Retention of lochia, no abdominal pain, poor appetite, loose stools, weak voice, palpitations, tiredness, blurred vision, dull-pale complexion, dizziness, Pale tongue, Weak or Choppy pulse.

PAIN

Abdominal pain
Liver-Blood deficiency

Dull abdominal pain after childbirth that is relieved by pressure and after eating, scanty but continuous uterine bleeding with pale blood, dizziness, tiredness, blurred vision, constipation, Pale tongue, Choppy or Fine pulse.

Liver-Blood stasis

Severe abdominal pain after childbirth that is worse with pressure and after eating, discharge of dark lochia, dark complexion, Purple tongue, Wiry pulse.

Retention of food

Abdominal and epigastric pain after childbirth, a feeling of fullness of the abdomen and epigastrium, foul breath, belching, thick tongue coating, Slippery pulse.

Cold in the Uterus

Severe abdominal pain that is alleviated by the application and by drinking warm liquids, cold limbs, dark lochia, Bluish-Purple tongue, Tight pulse.

Joint pain
Liver-Blood deficiency

Dull ache in the joints after childbirth, tingling of the limbs, dizziness, blurred vision, insomnia, depression, tiredness, Pale tongue, Choppy or Fine pulse.

Invasion of Wind

Pain in the joints after childbirth with sudden onset, contraction of the joints, fever, shivers, Floating pulse.

Liver-Blood stasis

Severe joint pain after childbirth, stiffness of the joints, contraction of the limbs, abdominal pain, scanty lochial discharge, dark complexion, Purple tongue, Wiry pulse.

Liver-Blood and Kidney-Yang deficiency

Dull joint pain after childbirth especially in the knees and lower back, tiredness, dizziness, backache, frequent urination, a feeling of cold, Pale tongue, Deep-Weak and Choppy pulse.

Hypochondrial pain
Liver-Blood deficiency

Bilateral dull hypochondrial pain aggravated by exertion and alleviated by rest, palpitations, blurred vision, dizziness, tiredness, Pale tongue, Choppy or Fine pulse.

Liver-Qi stagnation

Right-sided hypochondrial pain and distension, irritability, moodiness, Wiry pulse.

Liver-Blood stasis

Left-sided, stabbing hypochondrial pain, retention of lochia, hypochondrial pain, abdominal pain, dark complexion, Purple tongue, Wiry pulse.

VAGINAL BLEEDING

Vaginal bleeding after childbirth
Kidney-Qi deficiency

Profuse bleeding after childbirth, dilute pale blood, sweating, tiredness, exhaustion, pale complexion, palpitations, backache, Pale tongue, Empty pulse.

Liver-Blood stasis

Bleeding after childbirth, dark blood with clots, abdominal pain, Purple tongue, Wiry pulse.

Amenorrhoea after miscarriage
Deficiency of Qi and Blood

Amenorrhoea after miscarriage, abdomen soft to touch, absence of abdominal distension or pain, absence of vaginal discharge, poor appetite, loose stools, weak voice, palpitations, tiredness, blurred vision, dull-pale complexion, dizziness, Pale tongue, Weak or Choppy pulse.

Liver-Blood stasis

Amenorrhoea after miscarriage, abdominal pain, dark complexion, Purple tongue, Wiry pulse.

Liver-Qi stagnation

Amenorrhoea after miscarriage, abdominal distension, hypochondrial or epigastric distension, breast distension, depression, irritability, moodiness, Wiry pulse.

URINARY DIFFICULTY

This may include pain on urination, difficult urination, frequent urination or slight retention of urine.

Spleen-Qi deficiency

Frequency/incontinence of urine, or retention of urine after childbirth, a feeling of fullness and distension in the hypogastrium, poor appetite, tiredness, slight abdominal distension, pale complexion, loose stools, Pale tongue, Empty pulse.

Kidney-Qi deficiency

Frequency/incontinence of urine, or retention of urine after childbirth, backache, dizziness, a feeling of cold, pale complexion, Pale and wet tongue, Deep-Weak pulse.

Liver-Qi stagnation

Difficult urination after childbirth, a feeling of distension in the lower abdomen, hypochondrial or epigastric distension, irritability, moodiness, Wiry pulse.

Kidney-Yin deficiency with Bladder-Heat

Frequency of urination after childbirth, blood in the urine, burning on urination, anxiety, a feeling of heat, dry lips, dry mouth with a desire to drink in small sips, night sweating, Red tongue without coating, Floating-Empty and Rapid pulse.

Lung- and Spleen-Qi deficiency

Urinary retention after childbirth, absence of abdominal distension or pain, dizziness, breathlessness, sweating, dislike of speaking, depression, tiredness, poor appetite, pale complexion, Pale tongue, Weak pulse.

Injury to the Bladder

Incontinence of urine after childbirth, blood in the urine, Wiry pulse on the left Rear position.

CONSTIPATION

Liver-Blood deficiency

Constipation after childbirth, difficult defecation with dry stools, dull-pale complexion, dizziness, blurred vision, tiredness, depression, Pale tongue, Choppy or Fine pulse.

Kidney-Yang deficiency

Constipation after childbirth, difficulty in defecation, exhaustion and sweating after defecation, backache, dizziness, tinnitus, a feeling of cold, weak knees, bright-white complexion, tiredness, abundant clear urination, Pale and wet tongue, Deep-Weak pulse.

Kidney-Yin deficiency

Constipation after childbirth with dry stools, dizziness, tinnitus, night sweating, dry mouth with a desire to drink in small sips, backache, poor memory, scanty dark urine, tongue without coating, Floating-Empty pulse.

Cold in the Uterus

Constipation after childbirth, difficult defecation, abdominal pain relieved by the application of heat, scanty lochia, Bluish-Purple tongue, Tight pulse.

SWEATING

Interrogation, Chapter 46

Kidney-Qi deficiency

Daytime sweating after childbirth, pale complexion, breathlessness, weak voice, tiredness, backache, Pale tongue, Empty pulse.

Kidney-Yin deficiency

Night-time sweating after childbirth, insomnia, dry throat, dry mouth with a desire to drink in small sips, dizziness, tinnitus, tongue without coating, Floating-Empty pulse.

DIZZINESS

Liver-Blood deficiency

Dizziness after childbirth, scanty lochia, blurred vision, tingling, dull-pale complexion, palpitations, insomnia, depression, Pale tongue, Choppy or Fine pulse.

Blood stasis

Dizziness after childbirth, dark lochia, abdominal pain, mental restlessness, palpitations, Purple tongue, Wiry pulse.

Kidney deficiency

Dizziness after childbirth, backache, tinnitus, tiredness.

Other symptoms and signs, including tongue and pulse, depend on whether there is a Kidney-Yin or a Kidney-Yang deficiency.

OEDEMA

Deficiency of Qi and Blood

Oedema after childbirth, more on the face or abdomen, poor appetite, loose stools, weak voice, palpitations, tiredness, blurred vision, dull-pale complexion, dizziness, Pale tongue, Weak or Choppy pulse.

Qi stagnation and Blood stasis

Oedema after childbirth, abdominal pain, joint pain, Purple tongue, Wiry pulse.

Spleen-Qi deficiency

Oedema of the limbs after childbirth, poor appetite, tiredness, slight abdominal distension, pale complexion, loose stools, Pale tongue, Empty pulse.

Kidney-Yang deficiency

Oedema of the ankles after childbirth, backache, dizziness, tinnitus, a feeling of cold, weak knees, bright-white complexion, tiredness, abundant clear urination, Pale and wet tongue, Deep-Weak pulse.

Damp-Heat

Oedema of the limbs after childbirth, swelling and heat of the joints, feeling of heaviness, a feeling of oppression of the chest, sticky taste, dark urine, difficult urination, sticky yellow tongue coating, Slippery-Rapid pulse.

FEVER

Interrogation, Chapter 46

Invasion of external toxins

High fever after childbirth, lower abdominal pain that is worse with pressure, scanty lochial discharge that is dark and offensive, mental restlessness, thirst, delirium, convulsions, scanty dark urine, constipation, Red tongue with a thick, sticky yellow coating and red points, Overflowing-Slippery-Rapid pulse.

Invasion of Wind-Cold

Fever after childbirth, aversion to cold, fever, occipital headache, stiff neck, sneezing, body aches, tongue with thin white coating, Floating-Tight pulse.

Invasion of Wind-Heat

Fever after childbirth, aversion to cold, fever, sore throat, headache, body aches, slight sweating, tongue with Red sides front, Floating-Rapid pulse.

Spleen-Qi deficiency

Low-grade fever after childbirth, sweating, exhaustion, pallor, poor appetite, loose stools, Pale tongue, Empty pulse.

Liver-Blood deficiency

Continuous low-grade fever after childbirth, sweating, blurred vision, palpitations, dizziness, tiredness, insomnia, tingling of the limbs, Pale tongue, Choppy or Fine pulse.

Liver-Blood stasis

Fever after childbirth, a feeling of heat, scanty lochial discharge, abdominal pain, Purple tongue, Wiry pulse.

Steaming breast

Low-grade fever 2 or 3 days after childbirth, breast milk which does not flow freely or no milk at all, irritability, distension, hardness and pain of the breasts, which feel lumpy, sticky yellow tongue coating, Wiry-Slippery pulse.

Retention of food

Low-grade fever 3 or 4 days after childbirth, fever that is higher in the afternoon, bad digestion, a feeling of fullness and distension of the epigastrium, sour regurgitation, belching, foul breath, thick sticky tongue coating, Slippery pulse.

BREAST MILK

Breast milk not flowing

Interrogation, Chapter 46

Deficiency of Qi and Blood

Insufficient or absent breast milk, watery milk, absence of feeling of distension of the breasts, poor appetite, loose stools, weak voice, palpitations, tiredness, blurred vision, dull-pale complexion, dizziness, Pale tongue, Weak or Choppy pulse.

Liver-Qi stagnation

Absent or scanty breast milk, a feeling of distension, hardness and pain of the breasts, hypochondrial distension, sighing, irritability, tongue Red on the sides, Wiry pulse.

Spontaneous flow of milk after childbirth

Interrogation, Chapter 46

Stomach- and Spleen-Qi deficiency

Spontaneous flow of milk a few days after childbirth, scanty but constant flow of watery milk, soft breasts, absence of feeling of distension of the breasts, dull epigastric pain, poor appetite, tiredness, slight abdominal distension, pale complexion, loose stools, Pale tongue, Empty pulse.

Liver-Fire

Spontaneous trickling of milk after childbirth, dense milk, a feeling of distension of the breasts, hypochondrial distension, headaches, dizziness, tinnitus, irritability, propensity to outbursts of anger, red face, thirst, bitter taste, constipation, dark urine, Red tongue with redder sides and dry yellow coating, Wiry-Rapid pulse.

POSTNATAL DEPRESSION/PSYCHOSIS

Interrogation, Chapter 46

Liver- and Heart-Blood deficiency

Postnatal depression, palpitations, dizziness, insomnia, poor memory, anxiety, dull-pale complexion, blurred vision, floaters, numbness/tingling of limbs, scanty menstruation, Pale tongue, Choppy or Fine pulse.

Liver- and Heart-Yin deficiency

Postnatal depression, poor memory, anxiety, mental restlessness, scanty breast milk, loss of libido, palpitations, dizziness, insomnia, night sweating, dry throat, numbness/tingling of the limbs, blurred vision, floaters, dry eyes, scanty menstruation or amenorrhoea, dull-pale complexion, withered and brittle nails, dry skin and nails, tongue without coating, Floating-Empty pulse.

Heart-Blood stasis

Postnatal psychosis, manic behaviour, aggressive behaviour, delusions, hallucinations, suicidal, palpitations, chest pain, purple lips, dark complexion, Purple tongue, Choppy pulse.

COLLAPSE

Collapse of Qi with deficiency of Blood

Profuse bleeding after childbirth, sudden vertigo, pale complexion, palpitations, fainting, cold limbs, profuse sweating, Pale and Short tongue, Fine or Scattered pulse.

Blood stasis

Retention of lochia or scanty lochia, abdominal pain, a feeling of fullness under the heart, chest pain, cough,

fainting, mouth closed, dark complexion, Purple-Stiff tongue, Wiry pulse.

CONVULSIONS

Blood and Yin deficiency with Empty-Wind

Profuse loss of blood during childbirth, tremor of limbs, rigidity of the spine, pale complexion or malar flush, tongue without coating, pulse Choppy or Floating-Empty.

Exterior invasion of toxin

Shivers and fever soon after childbirth, headache, stiff neck, rigidity of the spine, lock jaw, convulsions, in severe cases opisthotonos, Red-Stiff tongue with yellow coating and red points, Wiry pulse.

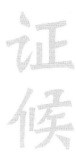

Chapter **88**

BREAST SIGNS

Chapter contents

BREAST DISTENSION AND SWELLING *849*
  Breast distension *849*
  Swollen breasts *850*
  Redness and swelling of the breasts *850*

BREAST PAIN *850*

BREAST LUMPS *850*

NIPPLES *851*
  Milky nipple discharge *851*
  Sticky yellow nipple discharge *851*
  Bloody discharge from the nipple *851*
  Cracked nipples *852*
  Inverted nipples *852*

PEAU D'ORANGE SKIN *852*

SMALL BREASTS *852*

BREAST DISTENSION AND SWELLING

Breast distension

Observation, Chapter 12; Interrogation, Chapter 46

Liver-Qi stagnation

Breast distension which may be unilateral or bilateral, more obvious on the lateral side, decreasing after the period, breasts relatively hard, premenstrual tension, hypochondrial distension, moodiness, irritability, Wiry pulse.

Phlegm and Qi stagnation

Swelling and distension of the breasts that is relatively soft, obesity, a feeling of oppression of the chest, expectoration of sputum, Swollen tongue with sticky coating, Slippery-Wiry pulse.

Deficiency of Qi and Blood

Slight distension of the breasts, no pain, poor appetite, loose stools, weak voice, palpitations, tiredness, blurred vision, dull-pale complexion, dizziness, Pale tongue, Weak or Choppy pulse.

Spleen- and Kidney-Yang deficiency

Slight breast distension which occasionally may even occur *after* the period, tiredness, lethargy, a feeling of cold, lower backache, cold limbs, weak limbs, Pale and wet tongue, Deep-Weak pulse.

Lung-Qi stagnation

A feeling of a lump in the throat, difficulty in swallowing, a feeling of oppression or distension of the chest, slight breathlessness, sighing, sadness, irritability, depression, tongue slightly Red on the sides in the chest areas, pulse very slightly Tight on the right Front position.

Phlegm with Lung-Qi stagnation

Phlegm in the throat, a feeling of a lump in the throat, a feeling of oppression or distension of the chest, slight breathlessness, difficulty in swallowing, sighing, sadness, irritability, depression, sputum in the throat, tongue slightly Swollen on the sides in the chest areas, Slippery pulse that is also very slightly Tight on the right Front position.

Swollen breasts

Observation, Chapter 12

Liver-Qi stagnation with Phlegm

Severe breast distension and swelling, breast pain, premenstrual tension, irritability, hypochondrial distension, a feeling of oppression of the chest, sputum in the throat, Swollen tongue with sticky coating, Wiry-Slippery pulse.

Liver-Qi stagnation with Phlegm-Heat

Severe breast distension and swelling, breast pain, premenstrual tension, irritability, hypochondrial distension, a feeling of oppression of the chest, sputum in the throat, a feeling of heat, thirst with no desire to drink, red face, Swollen tongue with sticky yellow coating, Wiry-Slippery-Rapid pulse.

Spleen- and Kidney-Yang deficiency with Phlegm

Slight breast distension and swelling, a feeling of oppression of the chest, sputum in the throat, obesity, tiredness, a feeling of cold, lower backache, cold limbs, lethargy, loose stools, Pale and wet tongue, Deep-Weak and slightly Slippery pulse.

Redness and swelling of the breasts

Stagnant Liver-Qi turning into Heat with Blood stasis

Breasts red, hard, painful and swollen, irregular periods, heavy periods, irritability, tongue with Reddish-Purple sides, Wiry-Rapid pulse.

Toxic Heat

Red, swollen, painful breasts, thirst, a feeling of heat, mental restlessness, Red tongue with red points and sticky yellow coating, Overflowing-Slippery-Rapid pulse.

Stagnant Liver-Qi turning into Heat

Red, swollen and distended breasts, hypochondrial distension, irritability, premenstrual tension, heavy periods, tongue with Red sides, Wiry-Rapid pulse.

BREAST PAIN

Severe Liver-Qi stagnation

Breast pain and distension that is worse premenstrually, irregular periods, premenstrual tension, hypochondrial distension, moodiness, irritability, Wiry pulse.

Liver-Qi stagnation with Phlegm

Breast pain and distension, swollen breasts, a feeling of a lump in the throat, phlegm in the throat, premenstrual tension, hypochondrial distension, a feeling of oppression of the chest, irritability, irregular periods, Swollen tongue, Wiry-Slippery pulse.

Liver-Blood stasis

Stabbing breast pain, chest pain, period pain, dark menstrual blood with dark clots, irregular periods, hypochondrial pain, abdominal pain, dark complexion, Purple tongue, Wiry pulse.

Toxic Heat

Redness, pain and swelling of the breast, a feeling of heat, fever, thirst, Red tongue with red points and dry, sticky yellow coating, Overflowing-Slippery-Rapid pulse.

BREAST LUMPS

Observation, Chapter 12; Interrogation, Chapter 46; Palpation, Chapter 51

Liver-Qi stagnation

Lumpy breasts, small nodules that are not hard and decrease in size after the period, severe premenstrual breast distension, premenstrual tension, pain in the breasts, depression, irritability, moodiness, Wiry pulse.

Liver-Qi stagnation with Blood stasis

Hard breast lumps which are immovable and may be painful, chest pain, irregular periods, painful periods, premenstrual tension, Purple tongue, Wiry pulse.

Phlegm and Qi stagnation

Soft, painless, breast lumps, movable and slipping under the finger on palpation, premenstrual breast distension and swelling, premenstrual tension, a feeling of a lump in the throat, a feeling of oppression and distension of the chest, irritability, depression, Swollen tongue with sticky coating, Wiry-Slippery pulse.

Spleen- and Kidney-Yang deficiency with Phlegm

Lumpy breasts, soft nodules, a feeling of heaviness, a feeling of oppression of the chest, tiredness, a feeling of cold, poor appetite, loose stools, dizziness, tinnitus, backache, profuse pale urination, urination at night, irregular periods, Pale, Swollen and wet tongue with sticky coating, Deep-Weak and slightly Slippery pulse.

Disharmony of Directing and Penetrating Vessels

Lumpy breasts, small hard nodules, swollen breasts, premenstrual breast distension, late cycle, infertility, irregular periods, anxiety, abdominal pain, backache, cold feet, Pale tongue, Fine-Wiry pulse.

Stagnant Liver-Qi turned into Fire

Single large and hard breast lump, painful breasts, thirst, bitter taste, headaches, irritability, red face, dark urine, dry stools, Red tongue with redder sides, Wiry-Rapid pulse.

Phlegm with Lung-Qi stagnation

Soft and movable breast lumps, phlegm in the throat, a feeling of a lump in the throat, a feeling of oppression and distension of the chest, slight breathlessness, sighing, sadness, worry, irritability, depression, tongue slightly swollen on the sides in the chest areas, pulse that is Slippery and very slightly Tight on the right Front position.

Toxic Heat

Large breast lump with discharge of yellow fluid, pain in the breast, thirst, bitter taste, dark urine, Red tongue with redder sides and thick, sticky, dry yellow coating, Overflowing-Slippery-Rapid pulse.

Liver- and Kidney-Yin deficiency

Chronic breast lumps, loss of weight, dark complexion, tiredness, irregular periods, dizziness, tinnitus, night sweating, dry eyes, tongue without coating, Floating-Empty pulse.

NIPPLES

Milky nipple discharge
Severe deficiency of Qi and Blood

Slight milky nipple discharge that is aggravated by exertion and ameliorated by rest, poor appetite, loose stools, weak voice, palpitations, tiredness, blurred vision, dull-pale complexion, dizziness, Pale tongue, Weak or Choppy pulse.

Spleen- and Kidney-Yang deficiency

Slight milky nipple discharge that is aggravated by exertion and ameliorated by rest, heavy or scanty periods, premenstrual oedema, tiredness, lower backache, a feeling of cold, cold limbs, loose stools, Pale and wet tongue, Deep-Weak pulse.

Liver-Qi stagnation

Premenstrual milky nipple discharge, breast distension, premenstrual tension, hypochondrial or epigastric distension, irritability, moodiness, Wiry pulse.

Sticky yellow nipple discharge
Damp-Heat in the Liver channel

Sticky yellow nipple discharge, breast distension and pain, irregular periods, painful periods, mid-cycle pain, yellow vaginal discharge, urinary discomfort, tongue with sticky yellow coating, Wiry-Slippery pulse.

Toxic Heat

Sticky yellow nipple discharge, redness, swelling and pain of the breasts, feeling of heat, thirst, mental restlessness, Red tongue with red points on the sides and sticky yellow coating, Overflowing-Slippery-Rapid pulse.

Bloody discharge from the nipple
Toxic Heat

Bloody discharge from the nipple, redness, swelling and pain of the breasts, a feeling of heat, thirst, mental restlessness, Red tongue with red points on the sides and sticky yellow coating, Overflowing-Slippery-Rapid pulse.

Stagnant Liver-Qi turning into Heat

Intermittent bloody discharge from the nipple, premenstrual breast distension, premenstrual tension, irritability, irregular periods, a feeling of heat, red face, tongue with Red sides, Wiry-Rapid pulse.

Deficiency of the Liver and Kidneys and of the Penetrating Vessel

Intermittent bloody discharge from the nipple that is aggravated by exertion and ameliorated by rest, heavy or scanty periods, tiredness, dizziness, tinnitus, backache, Deep-Weak pulse.

Other symptoms and signs depend on whether there is a Yin or a Yang deficiency.

Cracked nipples

Observation, Chapter 12

Stagnant Liver-Qi turning into Fire

Cracked nipples, flaking skin over the nipples, stabbing pain in the nipple, irritability, thirst, bitter taste, Red tongue with redder sides and yellow coating, Wiry-Rapid pulse.

Yin deficiency with Blood-Heat

Cracked nipple with dry skin, slight pain, bleeding from the nipple, crusts on the nipple, a feeling of heat in the evening, night sweating, mental restlessness, thirst with a desire to drink in small sips, dry mouth, Red tongue without coating, Floating-Empty and Rapid pulse.

Inverted nipples

Liver-Qi stagnation and Liver-Blood stasis with Phlegm

Inverted nipples, distended and painful breasts, premenstrual tension, irregular periods, a feeling of oppression of the chest, hypochondrial distension and pain, painful periods, tongue Swollen and with Purple sides, Wiry-Slippery pulse.

Toxic Heat with Blood stasis

Inverted nipples, redness, pain and swelling of the breasts, hypochondrial pain, feeling of heat, mental restlessness, thirst, irregular periods, painful periods, Red tongue with Reddish-Purple sides, red points and a sticky yellow coating, Overflowing-Wiry-Rapid pulse.

PEAU D'ORANGE SKIN

'Peau d'orange' means orange skin and it refers to an area of the breast with many small dimples resembling an orange skin.

Liver-Qi stagnation and Liver-Blood stasis with Phlegm

Peau d'orange, distended and painful breasts, premenstrual tension, irregular periods, a feeling of oppression of the chest, hypochondrial distension and pain, painful periods, tongue Swollen and with Purple sides, Wiry-Slippery pulse.

Toxic Heat with Blood stasis

Peau d'orange, redness, pain and swelling of the breasts, hypochondrial pain, a feeling of heat, mental restlessness, thirst, irregular periods, painful periods, Red tongue with Reddish-Purple sides and red points and a sticky yellow coating, Overflowing-Wiry-Rapid pulse.

SMALL BREASTS

Observation, Chapter 12

Qi and Blood deficiency

Gradual decrease in breast size, poor appetite, loose stools, weak voice, tiredness, blurred vision, dizziness, numbness/tingling of the limbs, palpitations, dull-pale complexion, Pale tongue, Weak or Choppy pulse.

Liver- and Kidney-Yin deficiency

Gradual decrease in breast size, dry vagina, scanty menstruation or amenorrhoea, delayed cycle, infertility, dizziness, tinnitus, hardness of hearing, lower backache, dull occipital or vertical headache, insomnia, numbness/tingling of the limbs, dry eyes, blurred vision, dry throat, dry hair and skin, brittle nails, night sweating, dry stools, normal-coloured tongue without coating, Floating-Empty pulse.

Stomach-Qi deficiency

Sagging breasts, an uncomfortable feeling in the epigastrium, no appetite, lack of sense of taste, loose stools, tiredness especially in the morning, weak limbs, Pale tongue, Empty pulse.

Blood deficient and dry

Gradual decrease in breast size, dizziness, blurred vision, floaters, numbness/tingling of limbs, scanty menstruation, dull-pale complexion, dry eyes, dry skin and hair, dry nails, Pale tongue, Choppy or Fine pulse.

Chapter **89**

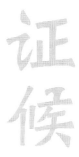

MISCELLANEOUS GYNAECOLOGICAL SYMPTOMS

Chapter contents

INFERTILITY   855

MENOPAUSAL SYNDROME   856

ABDOMINAL MASSES   856

VAGINAL DISCHARGE   857
  White   857
  Yellow   857
  Red-white   857
  Five-colour   857

INFLAMMATION AND SWELLING   858
  Vaginal itching   858
  Genital eczema   858
  Vulvar sores   858
  Swelling of the vulva   858

PROLAPSE   859
  Prolapse of uterus   859
  Prolapse of vagina   859

LEUKOPLAKIA   859

DYSPAREUNIA   859

BLEEDING ON INTERCOURSE   859

LACK OF LIBIDO   860

PUBIC HAIR   860
  Loss of pubic hair   860
  Excessive pubic hair   860

INFERTILITY

Interrogation, Chapter 46

Kidney deficiency

Primary or secondary infertility, late periods, scanty periods, backache, dizziness, tinnitus.

Other symptoms, including tongue and pulse, depend on whether there is Kidney-Yang or Kidney-Yin deficiency. This is the most common cause of infertility, accounting for over half the cases.[1]

Blood deficiency

Secondary infertility, scanty periods or amenorrhoea, late periods, tiredness, dizziness, blurred vision, pale complexion, Pale-Thin tongue, Choppy pulse.

Cold in the Uterus

Primary infertility, late periods, painful periods, bright-red blood with small, dark clots, a feeling of cold during the period, cold limbs, backache, Pale tongue, Tight pulse.

Dampness in the Lower Burner

Secondary infertility, excessive vaginal discharge, late periods, mid-cycle pain and bleeding, a feeling of heaviness, obesity, sticky tongue coating, Slippery pulse.

Blood-Heat

Secondary infertility, early periods, heavy periods, a feeling of heat, thirst, anxiety, Red tongue, Rapid-Overflowing pulse.

Qi stagnation

Secondary infertility, irregular periods, premenstrual tension, breast distension, irritability, Wiry pulse.

Blood stasis

Secondary infertility, painful periods, dark blood with large, dark clots, Purple tongue, Wiry pulse.

Kidney-Yin deficiency with Blood Empty-Heat

Secondary infertility, heavy periods, dizziness, tinnitus, night sweating, dry mouth with a desire to drink in small sips, backache, poor memory, scanty dark urine, five-palm heat, malar flush, a feeling of heat in the evening, Red tongue without coating, Floating-Empty and Rapid pulse.

> ### Clinical note
> - More than half of the cases of infertility are due to a Kidney deficiency.
> - This means that nearly half of cases are due to a Full condition and especially Damp-Phlegm in the Uterus.

MENOPAUSAL SYNDROME

Interrogation, Chapter 46

Kidney-Yin deficiency

Hot flushes, dryness of the vagina, dizziness, tinnitus, night sweating, dry mouth with a desire to drink in small sips, backache, poor memory, scanty dark urine, tongue without coating, Floating-Empty pulse.

Kidney-Yang deficiency

Hot flushes, backache, dizziness, tinnitus, a feeling of cold, weak knees, bright-white complexion, tiredness, abundant clear urination, Pale and wet tongue, Deep-Weak pulse.

Kidney-Yin and Kidney-Yang deficiency

Hot flushes, night sweating, dryness of the vagina, backache, dizziness, tinnitus, cold feet, frequent urination. The tongue is Pale if Kidney-Yang deficiency predominates and Red if Kidney-Yin deficiency predominates.

Kidney- and Liver-Yin deficiency with Liver-Yang rising

Hot flushes, dryness of the vagina, dry eyes, blurred vision, headache, irritability, insomnia, Red tongue without coating, pulse Floating-Empty and slightly Wiry on the left.

Heart- and Kidney-Yin deficiency

Hot flushes, dryness of the vagina, night sweating, palpitations, insomnia, dizziness, tinnitus, anxiety, mental restlessness, depression, a feeling of heat in the evening, dry mouth and throat, poor memory, tongue without coating, pulse Floating-Empty.

Accumulation of Phlegm and stagnation of Qi

Hot flushes, obesity, a feeling of oppression of the chest, expectoration of scanty phlegm, a feeling of distension of the breasts, irritability, sighing, nausea, depression, tongue slightly Red on the sides, Wiry-Slippery pulse.

This pattern frequently appears in early menopause.

Blood stasis

Hot flushes, night sweating, anxiety, mental restlessness, a feeling of agitation, menopause preceded by a period of time when menses are very irregular, stopping for a long time and then starting again, insomnia, possibly hypertension, Purple tongue, Wiry pulse.

> ### Clinical note
> - **Remember**: menopausal symptoms are not always due to Kidney-Yin deficiency. A simultaneous deficiency of both Kidney-Yin and Kidney-Yang (in varying proportions) is the most common situation.

ABDOMINAL MASSES

Observation, Chapter 16; Symptoms and Signs, Chapter 71

Liver-Qi stagnation

Movable abdominal masses which come and go, abdominal distension and pain, hypochondrial or epigastric distension, depression, irritability, moodiness, Wiry pulse.

Stagnation of Qi and stasis of Blood

Hard and immovable abdominal masses, abdominal distension and pain, late periods, Purple tongue, Wiry pulse.

Blood stasis knotted in the Interior

Hard, immovable and painful abdominal masses, dark complexion, dry skin, a feeling of cold, amenorrhoea,

painful periods, late periods, Purple tongue, Choppy pulse.

Damp-Phlegm

Relatively soft abdominal masses, sputum in the throat, excessive vaginal discharge, ovarian cysts, sputum in the throat, a feeling of oppression of the chest, Swollen tongue with sticky coating, Slippery pulse.

VAGINAL DISCHARGE

Interrogation, Chapter 46; Hearing and Smelling, Chapter 54

White
Spleen-Qi deficiency

Profuse white vaginal discharge that is aggravated by exertion, sticky without offensive odour, poor appetite, tiredness, slight abdominal distension, pale complexion, loose stools, Pale tongue, Empty pulse.

Kidney-Yang deficiency

Profuse and dilute, white vaginal discharge, without offensive odour, backache, dizziness, tinnitus, a feeling of cold, weak knees, bright-white complexion, tiredness, abundant clear urination, Pale and wet tongue, Deep-Weak pulse.

Cold-Dampness

Profuse and sticky white vaginal discharge, a feeling of heaviness, abdominal fullness, sticky taste, thick, sticky white tongue coating, Slippery-Slow pulse.

Damp-Heat

White vaginal discharge that may look like curdled milk, offensive odour, a feeling of heaviness, thirst with no desire to drink, vaginal itching and redness, sticky yellow tongue coating, Slippery-Rapid pulse.

Yellow
Damp-Heat

Yellow, profuse vaginal discharge, sticky with strong odour, vaginal redness and itching, a feeling of heaviness, abdominal fullness, thirst with no desire to drink, sticky yellow tongue coating, Slippery-Rapid pulse.

Spleen-Qi deficiency

Chronic, pale-yellow vaginal discharge, abundant and dilute, without strong odour, irregular periods, heavy periods, poor appetite, tiredness, slight abdominal distension, pale complexion, loose stools, Pale tongue, Empty pulse.

Red-white
Damp-Heat

Red-white vaginal discharge, abundant and sticky, vaginal redness, itching and swelling, abdominal pain, painful urination, abdominal fullness, a feeling of heaviness, thirst with no desire to drink, sticky yellow tongue coating, Slippery-Rapid pulse.

Liver-Qi stagnation with Damp-Heat in the Liver channel

Red-white vaginal discharge, predominantly red, abundant and sticky with strong odour, vaginal itching, abdominal distension and pain, irritability, dizziness, hypochondrial pain, unilateral sticky yellow coating, Wiry-Slippery pulse.

Liver- and Kidney-Yin deficiency with Empty-Heat

Red-white vaginal discharge, scanty and dilute, vaginal burning and itching, difficult urination, dizziness, tinnitus, night sweating, five-palm heat, Red tongue without coating, Floating-Empty and Rapid pulse.

Five-colour

The 'five-colour vaginal discharge' may be watery like rice soup, like bloody water or like pus, usually with an offensive odour. The five colours are white, yellow, red, green and dark brown (like soya sauce).

Damp-Heat

Five-colour vaginal discharge, abundant and sticky, with an offensive odour, a feeling of heaviness, abdominal fullness, thirst with no desire to drink, a sticky taste, sticky yellow tongue coating, Slippery-Rapid pulse.

Liver- and Kidney-Yin deficiency with Empty-Heat

Five-colour vaginal discharge, scanty without odour, vaginal itching and redness, dizziness, tinnitus, night sweating, five-palm heat, Red tongue without coating, Floating-Empty and Rapid pulse.

Cold in the Lower Burner

Five-colour vaginal discharge that is watery and with an offensive odour, a feeling of cold, abdominal pain, painful periods, Pale tongue, Tight pulse.

Liver-Qi stagnation with Damp-Heat in the Liver channel

Five-colour vaginal discharge without odour, abdominal distension, hypochondrial pain, bitter taste, thirst with no desire to drink, irritability, tongue with unilateral sticky yellow coating, Wiry-Slippery pulse.

Toxic Heat

Profuse yellow, blood-stained vaginal discharge, offensive odour, a feeling of heat, thirst, dark urine, Red tongue with a sticky yellow coating, Overflowing-Slippery-Rapid pulse.

INFLAMMATION AND SWELLING

Vaginal itching
Damp-Heat in the Liver channel

Intense vaginal itching, yellow vaginal discharge, pain on intercourse, irritability, insomnia, dark urine, Red tongue with redder sides and sticky yellow coating, Wiry-Slippery pulse.

Spleen-Qi deficiency with Dampness

Slight vaginal itching, white vaginal discharge, tiredness, poor appetite, loose stools, a feeling of heaviness, Pale tongue with sticky white coating, Weak and slightly Slippery pulse.

Liver- and Kidney-Yin deficiency

Vaginal itching with a burning sensation, dryness of the vagina, night sweating, dizziness, tinnitus, a feeling of heat in the evening, tongue without coating, Floating-Empty pulse.

Genital eczema

Observation, Chapter 21; Symptoms and Signs, Chapter 77

Damp-Heat in the Liver channel

Genital eczema with papules that ooze a fluid, red and moist genital area, vaginal itching, difficult urination, tongue with Red sides and sticky yellow coating, Slippery-Wiry pulse.

Blood deficient and dry

Genital eczema with thickening of the skin, dryness of the vagina, dry red rash, vaginal itching, Pale and dry tongue, Choppy or Fine pulse.

Vulvar sores
Toxic Heat with Liver-Fire and Damp-Heat

Vulvar sores, redness, swelling, heat and pain of the external genitalia, oozing of yellow fluid, Red tongue with redder sides with thick, sticky yellow coating and red spots, Slippery-Wiry-Rapid pulse.

Toxic Heat with Blood stasis in the Liver channel

Vulvar sores, redness, swelling, heat and pain of the external genitalia, dyspareunia, oozing of yellow fluid, Reddish-Purple tongue with thick sticky yellow coating and red spots, Slippery-Wiry-Rapid pulse.

Retention of Cold

Vulvar erosion and pain, pale lesions in genital area, chronic condition with repeated attacks, lassitude, Pale tongue, Weak pulse.

Swelling of the vulva
Toxic Heat with Blood stasis in the Liver channel

Swelling of the vulva, pain in the perineum, genital papular eruptions, sticky yellow vaginal discharge, hypogastric pain, a feeling of heat, mental restlessness, Reddish-Purple tongue with thick, sticky yellow coating and red spots on the root and sides, Slippery-Rapid-Firm pulse.

Damp-Phlegm in the Lower Burner

Swelling of the vulva, a feeling of heaviness of the abdomen, abdominal fullness, ovarian cysts, painful periods, excessive vaginal discharge, Swollen tongue with sticky coating, Slippery pulse.

Damp-Heat and Toxic Heat in the Liver channel

Swelling of the vulva, pain in the perineum, genital papular eruptions, sticky yellow vaginal discharge, vaginal itching, vulvar eczema or sores, genital papular skin rashes and itching, mid-cycle bleeding/pain, fullness of the hypochondrium, abdomen or hypogastrium, bitter taste, poor appetite, nausea, a

feeling of heaviness of the body, urinary difficulty, burning on urination, dark urine, Red tongue with redder sides and red points and a thick, sticky yellow coating, Slippery-Wiry-Rapid pulse.

PROLAPSE

Prolapse of uterus

Spleen-Qi sinking

Prolapse of the uterus, a feeling of bearing down in the lower abdomen, tiredness, poor appetite, loose stools, Pale tongue, Weak pulse.

Kidney-Qi deficient and sinking

Prolapse of the uterus, frequent urination, bearing-down sensation, backache, frequent urination, slight incontinence of urine, Pale tongue, Deep-Weak pulse.

Prolapse of vagina

Spleen-Qi sinking

Prolapse of vagina, feeling of bearing down in the abdomen, poor appetite, tiredness, slight abdominal distension, pale complexion, loose stools, Pale tongue, Empty pulse.

Kidney-Qi not firm

Prolapse of vagina, soreness and weakness of the lower back, weak knees, frequent clear urination, weak-stream urination, abundant urination, dribbling after urination, incontinence of urine, urination at night, prolapse of uterus, chronic white vaginal discharge, tiredness, a dragging-down feeling in the lower abdomen, recurrent miscarriage, a feeling of cold, cold limbs, Pale tongue, Deep-Weak pulse.

LEUKOPLAKIA

Damp-Heat in the Liver channel

Leukoplakia, vaginal itching and swelling, yellow vaginal discharge, difficult urination, bitter taste, a feeling of heaviness, irritability, tongue with Red sides and sticky yellow coating, Wiry-Slippery pulse.

Spleen-Qi deficiency with Dampness

Leukoplakia, thickening of the skin, ulcers, white vaginal discharge, sticky white tongue coating, Weak and Slippery pulse.

Liver-Blood deficiency

Leukoplakia, dryness and itching of the vagina that is worse at night, dull complexion, blurred vision, dizziness, scanty periods, Pale tongue, Choppy or Fine pulse.

Liver- and Kidney-Yin deficiency

Leukoplakia, dryness of the vagina, backache, tinnitus, dizziness, tongue without coating, Floating-Empty pulse.

Kidney-Yang deficiency

Leukoplakia, vaginal itching, scanty periods, backache, dizziness, tinnitus, a feeling of cold, weak knees, bright-white complexion, tiredness, abundant clear urination, Pale and wet tongue, Deep-Weak pulse.

DYSPAREUNIA

Liver-Blood stasis

Dyspareunia, hypochondrial pain, abdominal pain, painful periods, dark complexion, Purple tongue, Wiry pulse.

Dampness in the Lower Burner

Dyspareunia, a feeling of heaviness of the abdomen, excessive vaginal discharge, painful periods, sticky tongue coating, Slippery pulse.

Liver-Fire

Dyspareunia, heavy periods, headaches, dizziness, tinnitus, irritability, propensity to outbursts of anger, red face, thirst, bitter taste, constipation, dark urine, Red tongue with redder sides and dry yellow coating, Wiry-Rapid pulse.

Liver- and Kidney-Yin deficiency

Dyspareunia, heavy periods, irregular periods, dizziness, blurred vision, floaters, dry eyes, dry hair, dry nails, insomnia, tinnitus, night sweating, dry mouth with a desire to sip water, backache, poor memory, scanty dark urine, tongue without coating, Floating-Empty pulse.

BLEEDING ON INTERCOURSE

Kidney- and Liver-Yin deficiency

Bleeding on intercourse with fresh blood, backache, dizziness, tinnitus, a feeling of heat in the evening,

night sweating, tongue without coating, Floating-Empty pulse.

Damp-Heat in the Directing and Penetrating Vessels

Bleeding on intercourse with sticky dark blood, yellow or white-red vaginal discharge, backache, abdominal pain and fullness, sticky yellow tongue coating, Slippery pulse.

Spleen-Qi deficiency

Bleeding on intercourse with pale dilute blood, poor appetite, tiredness, slight abdominal distension, pale complexion, loose stools, Pale tongue, Empty pulse.

LACK OF LIBIDO

Interrogation, Chapter 45

Heart-Qi deficiency

Lack of libido, palpitations, shortness of breath on exertion, pale complexion, tiredness, Pale tongue, Empty pulse.

Heart- and Kidney-Yin deficiency with Heart Empty-Heat

Lack of libido, palpitations, mental restlessness, anxiety, dizziness, tinnitus, night sweating, dry mouth with a desire to sip water, backache, poor memory, scanty dark urine, tongue without coating, Floating-Empty pulse.

Kidney-Yang deficiency

Lack of libido, backache, dizziness, tinnitus, a feeling of cold, weak knees, bright-white complexion, tiredness, abundant clear urination, Pale and wet tongue, Deep-Weak pulse.

Liver-Blood deficiency

Lack of libido, dizziness, blurred vision, floaters, numbness/tingling of the limbs, dull-pale complexion, Pale tongue, Choppy or Fine pulse.

Liver-Qi stagnation

Lack of libido, hypochondrial or epigastric distension, irritability, moodiness, Wiry pulse.

Dampness in the Lower Burner

Lack of libido, excessive vaginal discharge, a feeling of heaviness in the abdomen, painful periods, tongue with sticky coating, Slippery pulse.

PUBIC HAIR

Loss of pubic hair
Kidney-Essence deficiency

Loss of pubic hair, backache, dizziness, tinnitus, weak knees, poor memory, loose teeth, premature greying of hair, infertility, sterility, Leather pulse.

Spleen- and Kidney-Yang deficiency

Loss of pubic hair, poor appetite, tiredness, slight abdominal distension, bright-white complexion, loose stools, a feeling of cold, cold limbs, backache, dizziness, tinnitus, weak knees, abundant clear urination, Pale and wet tongue, Deep-Weak pulse.

Excessive pubic hair
Phlegm and Blood stasis

Excessive pubic hair, pain in the genital area, irregular and painful periods, a feeling of oppression of the chest, Swollen and Purple tongue, Slippery-Wiry pulse.

Kidney-Yin deficiency with Empty-Heat

Excessive pubic hair, dizziness, tinnitus, night sweating, dry mouth with a desire to sip water, backache, poor memory, scanty dark urine, five-palm heat, malar flush, a feeling of heat in the evening, Red tongue without coating, Floating-Empty and Rapid pulse.

NOTES

1. Gynaecology Department of the Long Hua Hospital Affiliated to the Shanghai College of Traditional Chinese Medicine 1987 Report on the differentiation and treatment of 257 cases of infertility. Journal of Chinese Medicine (*Zhong Yi Za Zhi* 中 医 杂 志), vol. 28, no. 10, p. 38.

证
候

SECTION 3

PAEDIATRIC SYMPTOMS AND SIGNS

Section contents

90 Children's problems *863*

INTRODUCTION

Section 3 of Part 5 deals with the symptoms and signs that are typical of children. The symptoms and signs of children are often quite distinct from those of adults, for example crying at night, Accumulation Disorder, nocturnal enuresis, late closure of the fontanelles and various childhood diseases. In order to ask the right questions, we should therefore be familiar with the general principles of Chinese paediatrics.

Particularly important symptoms and signs are those revolving around digestion and the respiratory system as these are the two areas of most common illness in children. Indeed, there is a link between these two as many respiratory problems of children (especially those linked to residual pathogenic factor) are often due to Phlegm, which itself is generally formed when there is a disharmony in the digestive system.

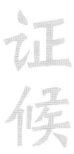

Chapter **90**

CHILDREN'S PROBLEMS

Chapter contents

FEVER   *863*
  Low-grade fever   *864*

VOMITING   *864*

DIARRHOEA   *865*

RESPIRATORY PROBLEMS   *865*
  Cough   *865*
  Wheezing   *865*

EAR PROBLEMS   *865*
  Earache   *865*
  Glue ear   *866*

HOT PALMS AND SOLES   *866*

CONSTITUTIONAL WEAKNESS   *866*

CONSTIPATION IN INFANCY   *867*

URINATION PROBLEMS   *867*
  Retention of urine in infancy   *867*
  Nocturnal enuresis   *867*

CRYING   *868*
  Crying at night in babies   *868*

DISTURBED SLEEP   *868*

ACCUMULATION DISORDER   *868*

WORMS   *869*
  Pinworms   *869*
  Roundworms   *869*

FIVE FLACCIDITIES   *869*

FIVE RETARDATIONS   *869*

INFLAMMATION   *869*
  Acute skin rash   *869*
  Erysipelas   *870*

JAUNDICE   *870*

INFECTIONS   *870*
  Chickenpox   *870*
  Mumps   *870*

FLAPPING OF NOSTRILS   *870*

CONVULSIONS   *870*
  Acute   *870*
  Chronic   *871*

FETUS TOXIN   *871*

FONTANELLES   *871*
  Sunken fontanelles   *871*
  Raised fontanelles   *871*
  Late closure of fontanelles   *872*

WHITE SPOTS ON THE PALATE AND TONGUE   *872*

LONG PENIS   *872*

For problems such as learning difficulty and hyper-activity, see Chapter 80.

FEVER

External invasion of Wind-Cold

Low fever, aversion to cold, occipital headache, stiff neck, sneezing, body aches, tongue with thin white coating, Floating-Tight pulse.

External invasion of Wind-Heat

Fever, aversion to cold, fever, sore throat, headache, body aches, slight sweating, tongue with Red sides/front, Floating-Rapid pulse.

Heat in Bright Yang

High fever, a feeling of heat, throwing off of the bed clothes, thirst, irritability, crying, sweating, Red tongue with yellow coating, Rapid-Overflowing pulse.

This corresponds to the Bright-Yang channel pattern within the identification of patterns according to the Six Stages, which is equivalent to the Stomach-Heat pattern within the identification of patterns according to the Four Levels.

Dry-Heat in the Intestines

High fever that is worse in the afternoon, a feeling of heat, throwing off of the bed clothes, constipation, abdominal fullness and pain, thirst, sweating, Red tongue with thick, dry yellow coating, Deep-Full-Rapid pulse.

This corresponds to the Bright-Yang organ pattern within the identification of patterns according to the Six Stages, which is equivalent to the Intestines Dry-Heat pattern within the identification of patterns according to the Four Levels.

Heat at the Ying level

High fever that is worse at night, delirium, fainting, dry mouth, macules, Red tongue without coating, Fine-Rapid pulse.

This corresponds to the patterns of Heat in the Pericardium or Heat in the Ying within the identification of patterns according to the Four Levels.

Heat at the Blood level

High fever that is worse at night, delirium, fainting, dry mouth, pronounced and numerous dark macules, epistaxis, blood in the stools, blood in the urine, mental confusion, Reddish-Purple tongue without coating, Fine-Rapid pulse.

This corresponds to the Blood-Heat pattern at the Blood level within the identification of patterns according to the Four Levels.

Low-grade fever
Retention of food

Recurrent low-grade fever, epigastric fullness, loose stools, sour regurgitation, foul breath, abdominal pain, thick sticky tongue coating, Slippery pulse.

Residual Heat in the Lungs

Low-grade fever, dry cough, a feeling of heat, irritability, tongue Red in the front, Fine-Rapid pulse.

Damp-Heat

Low-grade fever that is worse in the afternoon, sweating, a feeling of heaviness, thirst with no desire to drink, nausea, loose stools, sticky yellow tongue coating, Slippery-Rapid pulse.

Qi deficiency

Low-grade fever, sweating, listlessness, shortness of breath, pale complexion, poor appetite, Pale tongue, Empty pulse.

Yin deficiency

Low-grade fever in the afternoon, night sweating, dry throat, mental restlessness, malar flush, Red tongue without coating, Floating-Empty and Rapid pulse.

VOMITING

Accumulation of breast milk from overfeeding in infants

Vomiting of curdled milk with offensive odour, crying, better after vomiting, epigastric fullness and distension, stools with offensive odour.

Damp-Heat in the Stomach and Spleen

Vomiting, nausea, sticky taste, skin rashes, a feeling of fullness and pain of the epigastrium and lower abdomen, poor appetite, a feeling of heaviness, thirst without a desire to drink, loose stools with offensive odour, a feeling of heat, dull-yellow complexion, Red tongue with sticky yellow coating, Slippery-Rapid pulse.

Stomach-Qi deficiency

Vomiting of fluids, cold limbs, pale complexion, listlessness, Pale tongue, Weak pulse.

Stomach-Yin deficiency

Vomiting of thin fluids, retching, dry lips, dry mouth with a desire to drink in small sips, irritability, crying, tongue without coating in the centre, Floating-Empty pulse.

Spleen- and Kidney-Yang deficiency

Vomiting of thin fluids, dull-pale complexion, cold limbs, listlessness, loose stools, Pale-Swollen tongue, Deep-Weak pulse.

Invasion of Cold in the Stomach

Sudden vomiting, epigastric pain, desire to drink warm liquids, thick white tongue coating, Tight pulse.

DIARRHOEA

Spleen-Qi deficiency

Chronic diarrhoea, poor appetite, tiredness, slight abdominal distension, pale complexion, Pale tongue, Empty pulse.

Retention of food

Loose stools, epigastric fullness and pain, foul breath, sour regurgitation, nausea, thick sticky tongue coating, Slippery pulse.

Invasion of Cold in the Spleen

Sudden diarrhoea, abdominal pain, a feeling of heat and cold, thick white tongue coating, Tight pulse.

Invasion of Damp-Heat

Sudden diarrhoea with offensive odour, abdominal pain and fullness, irritability, a feeling of heat, dark urine, sticky yellow tongue coating, Slippery-Rapid pulse.

RESPIRATORY PROBLEMS

Cough

Interrogation, Chapter 47

Invasion of Wind-Cold

Cough with expectoration of white sputum, aversion to cold, fever, occipital headache, stiff neck, sneezing, body aches, tongue with thin white coating, Floating-Tight pulse.

Invasion of Wind-Heat

Cough with expectoration of yellow sputum, aversion to cold, fever, sore throat, headache, body aches, slight sweating, tongue with Red sides/front, Floating-Rapid pulse.

Phlegm-Heat in the Lungs

Barking cough with expectoration of profuse sticky yellow or green sputum, shortness of breath, wheezing, a feeling of oppression of the chest, a feeling of heat, thirst, Red and Swollen tongue with a sticky yellow coating, Slippery-Rapid pulse.

Lung- and Spleen-Qi deficiency

Slight cough with low sound, expectoration of thin sputum, shortness of breath, pale complexion, poor appetite, loose stools, Pale tongue, Weak pulse.

Wheezing

Interrogation, Chapter 47

Cold-Phlegm in the Lungs

Acute wheezing, cough with expectoration of white sputum, pale face, shortness of breath, a feeling of tightness of the chest, sticky white coating, Slippery-Slow pulse.

Phlegm-Heat in the Lungs

Acute wheezing, cough with expectoration of yellow sputum, a feeling of oppression of the chest, slightly red face, shortness of breath, sticky yellow coating, Slippery-Rapid pulse.

Residual Phlegm in the Lungs with Lung-Qi deficiency

Chronic wheezing, cough with occasional expectoration of scanty sputum, insomnia, a feeling of oppression of the chest, tiredness, pale face, shortness of breath, Pale tongue with swelling in the Lung area, Empty pulse.

Residual Phlegm in the Lungs with Spleen-Qi deficiency

Chronic wheezing, cough with occasional expectoration of scanty sputum, insomnia, a feeling of oppression of the chest, tiredness, pale face, shortness of breath, poor appetite, loose stools, a desire to lie down, Pale tongue with swelling in the Lung area, Empty pulse.

Deficiency of the Defensive-Qi system of the Lungs and Kidneys

Chronic wheezing, allergic asthma, history of eczema, hay fever, Pale tongue, Empty pulse.

EAR PROBLEMS

Earache

Interrogation, Chapter 47

Invasion of Wind-Heat in the Lesser-Yang channels

Acute earache, aversion to cold, fever, sore throat, headache, body aches, slight sweating, tongue with Red sides/front, Floating-Rapid pulse.

Invasion of Damp-Heat in the Lesser-Yang channels

Acute earache, discharge from the ear, swollen glands, fever, aversion to cold, headache, irritability, body aches, nausea, indigestion, tongue with unilateral sticky yellow coating, Slippery-Rapid pulse.

Residual Damp-Heat in the Lesser-Yang channels with Spleen-Qi deficiency

Chronic earache which comes and goes, a feeling of pressure in the ear, blocked ears, periodically slightly swollen glands, irritability, insomnia, poor appetite, listlessness, pale face, Pale tongue with unilateral sticky yellow coating, Soggy pulse.

Damp-Heat in the Gall-Bladder and Liver channels

Chronic earache, loss of hearing, feeling of pressure in the ear, blocked ears, slight bleeding of the ear drum on examination, swollen glands, insomnia, irritability, hyperactivity, red face, nervous child, Red tongue with redder sides and sticky yellow coating, Wiry-Rapid pulse.

Glue ear

'Glue ear' is a condition characterized by accumulation of fluid behind the ear drum, which causes a blockage of the Eustachian tube with the result that air cannot enter the middle ear. When this occurs, the cells lining the middle ear begin to produce fluid, which can be runny or thick, eventually filling the middle ear; this may cause a severe decrease in hearing. Glue ear is most common in children between 2 and 4 years old. Glue ear may be associated with ear infections but it may also occur without.

Damp-Phlegm

Glue ear, decreased hearing, dull headaches, sinus problems, poor concentration, listlessness, chronic catarrh, Swollen tongue with a sticky coating, Slippery pulse.

Dampness

Glue ear, decreased hearing, dull frontal headaches, sinus problems, listlessness, tongue with sticky coating, Slippery pulse.

Other symptoms and signs depend on whether Dampness is associated with Cold or Heat.

Clinical note

- Both earache and glue ear in children are nearly always due to residual Dampness in the ears.
- This usually occurs when a child suffers repeated invasions of Wind which are treated with antibiotics.

HOT PALMS AND SOLES

Accumulation Disorder with Spleen deficiency

Hot palms and soles, thin body, sallow complexion, withered hair, a desire to lie down, an increased desire to suckle, abdominal distension and fullness, red face, irritability, a feeling of heat in the afternoon, night sweating, restlessness at night, loose stools, turbid urine, sticky tongue coating, Weak-Soft pulse.

'Accumulation Disorder' is a paediatric condition characterized by accumulation of food in the stomach; it is equivalent to 'retention of food' in adults.

Blood and Yin deficiency

Hot palms and soles, listlessness, thin body, dry cough, dry mouth, a feeling of heat in the afternoon, malar flush, night sweating, mental restlessness, dry stools, tongue without coating, Floating-Empty pulse.

CONSTITUTIONAL WEAKNESS

Constitutional weakness in children may manifest with slow mental development, early-onset asthma, early-onset myopia, thin body, poor muscle development, early-onset whooping cough, fearfulness, or crying at night.

Heart deficiency

Quiet child, bluish tinge on the forehead, fearful, crying at night, pale-bluish cheeks, palpitations, cold limbs.

This condition may be due to the mother eating Wind-producing foods, which dry out the fetus's Blood and weaken its Heart. Wind-producing foods include shrimps, prawns, crab, lobster and all shellfish, spinach and mushrooms. A constitutional Heart deficiency may also be due to the mother suffering a severe shock during pregnancy.

Liver deficiency

Tense child, early-onset myopia and headaches, sinewy body, greenish complexion, crying, a history of convulsions in infancy, twitching during sleep, crying at night, desire to suckle frequently, contraction of the tendons, ridged nails.

This condition may be due to the mother suffering an emotional upset and anger during pregnancy.

Spleen deficiency

Quiet child, poor muscle development, flaccid muscles, sallow complexion, pale lips, cold limbs, poor digestion, poor appetite, crying with a low sound, loose stools, vomiting, diarrhoea.

This condition may be due to the mother eating too many Phlegm-producing foods or to overworking during pregnancy.

Lung deficiency

Quiet child, fearful, pale complexion, shortness of breath, crying with weak sound, moaning, weeping, cold hands, lustreless flaccid skin, thin chest, early-onset asthma/eczema, Lung cracks on the tongue.

This condition may be due to the mother suffering from sadness or grief during pregnancy.

Kidney deficiency

Quiet child, lassitude, thin body, slow mental and physical development, early-onset myopia, weak limbs, early-onset asthma/eczema, frequent urination, feeling cold, nocturnal enuresis after the age of 3 years. This condition is usually due to a Kidney-Essence deficiency of both parents.

CONSTIPATION IN INFANCY

Fetus Heat

Constipation in infancy, no desire to suckle, crying, crying at night, irritability, red face, dry lips, abdominal pain, dark urine.

Constitutional weakness

Constipation in infancy, listlessness, poor appetite, tendency to be easily startled, crying at night with weak sound, pale complexion.

URINATION PROBLEMS

Retention of urine in infancy

Heat in the Bladder

Retention of urine, dark urine, irritability, crying, dry lips.

Deficiency of Original Qi

Retention of urine, quiet child, pale face, listlessness, crying with a low sound, pale complexion, pale lips, slow development.

Nocturnal enuresis

Urination in bed at night in children constitutes 'nocturnal enuresis' only in children over the age of 3 years.

Kidney-Yang deficiency

Nocturnal enuresis, quiet child, a feeling of cold, bright-white complexion, tiredness, abundant clear urination, Pale and wet tongue, Deep-Weak pulse.

In children, this is usually a constitutional Kidney-Yang deficiency and, due to their age, there will not be many Kidney-deficiency symptoms. Indeed, if a child suffers from nocturnal enuresis and the tongue is Pale and the Kidney pulse is Weak, these signs are enough to diagnose a constitutional Kidney-Yang deficiency. This child will usually be a quiet, shy child without much energy.

Liver-Fire

Nocturnal enuresis, tense and highly-strung child, headaches, dizziness, tinnitus, irritability, propensity to outbursts of anger, red face, thirst, bitter taste, constipation, dark urine, Red tongue with redder sides and dry yellow coating, Wiry-Rapid pulse.

Spleen- and Lung-Qi deficiency

Nocturnal enuresis, tiredness, poor appetite, loose stools, poor digestion, chronic weak cough, weak voice, sweating, Pale tongue, Weak pulse.

> ### Clinical note
>
> - **Remember**: nocturnal enuresis is not always due to a constitutional Kidney deficiency. In a tense, nervous child with a Red tongue, think of Liver-Fire as a possible cause. If so, use HE-7 Shenmen and LIV-2 Xingjian.

CRYING

Spleen deficient and cold

Crying with a weak sound, arching of the back, crying without tears, a desire to lie down, pale bluish complexion, abdominal pain, poor appetite, pale lips, Pale tongue, Deep- Weak-Slow pulse.

Heart-Heat

Crying with a loud sound, irritability, insomnia, crying at night, crying as soon as the light is switched on, dark urine, red face, red lips, Red tongue with yellow coating.

Heart deficiency

Crying with a low sound, crying at night, tendency to be easily startled, pale-bluish complexion, quietness, thin body, pale lips, Pale tongue.

Shock

Crying, crying at night, grimacing, tendency to be easily startled, bluish tinge on the forehead, crying when left alone, white foam emerging from the corners of the mouth, bluish lips, clinging to the mother.

Retention of food

Crying with a loud sound, crying after eating, crying at night, abdominal fullness and hardness, vomiting, absence of desire to suckle, loose stools with foul smell.

Crying at night in babies

Spleen deficient and cold

Crying at night with low sound, a preference for lying on the stomach, falling asleep easily but waking up, arching the back whilst crying, cold limbs, poor appetite, loose stools, bright-white complexion.

Heart-Heat

Crying at night with loud sound, a preference for sleeping on the back, difficulty in falling asleep, crying and then stopping when lights are turned on, irritability, dark urine, red face, red lips.

Shock

Crying at night, tendency to be easily frightened, fear of going to sleep, waking up frightened during the night, bluish tinge on forehead, pale-bluish face and lips, clinging to the mother.

DISTURBED SLEEP

Liver-Fire

Disturbed sleep, waking up during the night, excessive dreaming, nightmares, night sweating, headaches, irritability, propensity to outbursts of anger, red face, thirst, bitter taste, constipation, dark urine, Red tongue with redder sides and dry yellow coating, Wiry-Rapid pulse.

Heart-Fire

Disturbed sleep, waking up during the night, excessive dreaming, nightmares, palpitations, thirst, agitation, a feeling of heat, red face, bitter taste, Red tongue with redder tip and yellow coating, Overflowing-Rapid pulse.

Residual pathogenic factor (Heat)

Disturbed sleep after a febrile episode, a feeling of tightness of the chest, irritability, hypochondrial pain, tongue Red in the front, Wiry-Rapid pulse.

Retention of food

Disturbed sleep, excessive dreaming, night sweating, epigastric fullness, undigested food in the stools, sour regurgitation, vomiting, thick sticky tongue coating, Slippery pulse.

Stomach-Heat

Disturbed sleep, excessive dreaming, night sweating, burning epigastric pain, thirst, sour regurgitation, nausea, excessive hunger, foul breath, a feeling of heat, Red tongue with a yellow coating, Overflowing-Rapid pulse.

Shock

Disturbed sleep, tendency to be easily frightened, fear of going to sleep, waking up frightened during the night, bluish tinge on forehead, pale-bluish face and lips, clinging to the mother.

ACCUMULATION DISORDER

'Accumulation Disorder' is a typical children's problem characterized by retention of food and slow digestion. It is very common early in life because the Spleen and Stomach energy are always weak in small children and they get stronger as they grow up. Accumulation Disorder is equivalent to 'retention of food' in adults and is characterized by poor digestion, abdominal full-

ness and pain, poor appetite, vomiting and diarrhoea. Accumulation Disorder in babies is usually due to not breast-feeding, breast-feeding for too short a time or weaning too early.

Stagnation of food

Babies: vomiting of curdled milk, no appetite, milky film on palate, foul-smelling stools, restlessness, whining, red cheeks.

Children: vomiting of undigested food, abdominal pain relieved by bowel movement, irritability, crying, low-grade fever, sweating at night, sallow complexion, a burning sensation in the palms, thick sticky tongue coating, Slippery pulse.

Spleen-Qi deficiency with retention of food

Sallow complexion, poor digestion, poor appetite, listlessness, slight abdominal pain and fullness, loose stools, vomiting, restless sleep, sleepiness during the daytime, Pale tongue with sticky coating, Weak-Slippery pulse.

WORMS

Pinworms

Abdominal pain that comes and goes, gurgling in the intestines, vomiting, profuse urination, itching of the anus at night, sweaty perineum, vaginal itching in girls, sallow complexion, thin body, poor appetite, a desire to eat strange objects such as soil, raw rice, tea leaves or paper, white spots on the face, small grey spots in the eyes, small spots under the lips, red points on the tongue.

Roundworms

Abdominal pain, vomiting, listlessness, thin body, sallow complexion, white spots on the face, small grey spots in the eyes, darkness under the eyes, itchy nose, small spots below the lips, red points on the tongue, a desire to eat strange objects, constipation or loose stools, abdominal distension.

FIVE FLACCIDITIES

'Five Flaccidities' is called *wu ruan* in Chinese, which literally means 'five softnesses': these are flaccidity of the head and neck (cannot keep the head up), flaccidity of the mouth (dribbling and difficulty in chewing), flaccid-

ity of the arms (cannot hold objects), flaccidity of the legs (cannot stand up), and flaccidity of the muscles.

Constitutional Kidney deficiency

Five Flaccidities, cannot hold the head up or straight, head leaning to one side, difficulty in walking, mental retardation, inability to stand up, frequent urination, inability to grasp objects, pale lips, Pale tongue, Deep-Weak pulse.

Constitutional Spleen deficiency

Five Flaccidities, especially flaccid muscles, poor digestion, poor appetite, listlessness, sleepiness, inability to grasp objects, difficulty in speaking, open mouth, slow development, difficulty in walking, mental retardation, sallow complexion, Pale tongue, Weak pulse.

FIVE RETARDATIONS

The 'Five Retardations' indicate late development in children, in standing, walking, teeth development, growth of hair and speech. The slow development is due to a combination of prenatal and postnatal deficiency. The Five Retardations are called *wu chi* in Chinese. The organs involved in the pathology of the Five Retardations are the Kidneys (lateness in being able to stand, slow teeth and hair development), Liver (lateness in being able to stand and walk), Heart (slowness in speech development) and Stomach (lateness in being able to walk).

Cold fetus

Five Retardations, a feeling of cold, cold body, cold limbs, lying stiff, pale-bluish complexion, shortness of breath, crying with low sound, difficulty in suckling, pale lips, Pale and wet tongue, Deep-Slow pulse.

Liver and Spleen deficiency

Five Retardations, poor appetite, abdominal distension, blue veins in the abdomen, flaccid muscles, pale-greenish complexion, Pale tongue, Weak pulse.

INFLAMMATIONS

Acute skin rash
Wind-Heat at Defensive-Qi level

Acute skin rash that starts on the head and then spreads rapidly to the trunk and finally to the limbs, red

papules, low fever, itching, swelling behind the ears, swollen tonsils, cough, sneezing, yellow nasal discharge, sore throat, red eyes, tongue Red in the front/sides with red points, Floating-Rapid pulse.

Heat at the Qi level

Acute rash, high fever, red papules with dense distribution, intense thirst, sweating, mental restlessness, dry stools, dark urine, Red tongue with yellow coating, Overflowing pulse.

Erysipelas
Toxic Heat on the Exterior

Erysipelas, fever, sticky discharge in the corner of the eyes, convulsions, crying, bright-red macular rash, hardened skin that is hot and painful to touch, restlessness, Red tongue with red points and with yellow coating.

Toxic Heat in the Interior

Erysipelas, high fever at night, mental restlessness, crying, dry mouth, a feeling of fullness of the chest, delirium, fainting, coarse breathing, blurred vision, dull dark-red or purple macular rash, skin hot and painful to touch, Red tongue with red points and without coating.

JAUNDICE

Damp-Heat

Jaundice, bright-yellow skin, bright-yellow eyes like tangerine peel, sweating, dark urine, fever, thirst, abdominal fullness and distension, pale stools, listlessness, poor appetite, sticky yellow tongue coating.

Cold-Dampness

Jaundice, dull-yellow skin, dull-yellow eyes, listlessness, a desire to lie down, poor appetite, abdominal fullness and distension, pale stools, loose stools, pale urine, sticky white tongue coating.

INFECTIONS

Chickenpox
Wind-Heat at the Defensive-Qi level

Chickenpox, vesicles like dew filled with clear fluid, headache, fever, runny nose with white discharge, cough, sneezing, tongue Red on the sides/front with white coating, Floating-Rapid pulse.

Toxic Heat

Chickenpox, dull-coloured vesicles which are red around the edge, filled with a turbid fluid and with a dense distribution, fever, mental restlessness, thirst, red face, red lips, tongue ulcers, dark urine, Red tongue with thick, dry yellow coating and red points, Deep-Rapid pulse.

Mumps
Invasion of Wind-Heat

Mumps, fever, shivers, headache, cough, sore throat, pain, redness and swelling behind the ears, tongue Red on the sides/front with red points, Floating-Rapid pulse.

Toxic Heat at the Qi level

Mumps, high fever, a feeling of heat, irritability, headache, thirst, red lips, vomiting, swelling, redness, pain and hardness behind the ears, sore throat, swollen tonsils, constipation, dark urine, Red tongue with thick yellow coating and red points, Deep-Full-Slippery pulse.

FLAPPING OF NOSTRILS

Wind-Heat in the Lung Defensive-Qi portion

Flapping of nostrils, sore throat, cough, fever, shivers, slight thirst, slight sweating, tongue Red on the sides or front with white coating, Floating-Rapid pulse.

Phlegm-Heat in the Lungs

Flapping of nostrils, barking cough with profuse, sticky yellow or green sputum, shortness of breath, wheezing, a feeling of oppression of the chest, a feeling of heat, thirst, Red and Swollen tongue with a sticky yellow coating, Slippery-Rapid pulse.

Lung and Kidney deficiency

Flapping of nostrils, shortness of breath, shallow breathing, dull-pale complexion, listlessness, sweating, cold limbs, Pale tongue, Deep-Weak pulse.

CONVULSIONS

Acute

An old paediatric book mentions eight characteristics of 'acute convulsions': twitching of the limbs, open

hands, pulling of the head towards the shoulder, tremor of the limbs, arching of the body, stretching of the hands, the eyes turning up, and blurred vision.

Invasion of Wind with penetration of Heat at the Qi level

Acute convulsions, tremor of the limbs, high fever, sweating, headache, cough, red face, irritability, mental confusion, delirium, dark urine, constipation, abdominal fullness and pain, Red tongue with yellow coating and red spots, Deep-Full pulse.

Phlegm-Heat

Acute convulsions, fever, hot body, red face, irritability, thirst, cough with expectoration of yellow sputum, shortness of breath, wheezing, clenching of teeth, dark urine, dry stools, Red tongue with sticky yellow coating, Slippery-Rapid pulse.

Retention of food

Acute convulsions, sallow complexion, vomiting, abdominal fullness and pain, constipation, foul breath, rattling sound in the throat, thick, sticky yellow tongue coating, Slippery-Rapid pulse.

Shock

Acute convulsions, no fever, bluish complexion, cold hands, tendency to be easily startled, insomnia or sleepiness with difficulty in being aroused and crying after waking up, crying at night, Moving pulse.

Chronic
Liver- and Kidney-Yin deficiency with Empty-Heat

Chronic convulsions, slight tremor of limbs which comes and goes, thin body, malar flush, mental restlessness, insomnia, five-palm heat, night sweating, Red tongue without coating, Floating-Empty and Rapid pulse.

Stomach- and Spleen-Yang deficiency

Chronic convulsions, eyes turning up, sleepiness, wet glazed eyes, mental confusion, listlessness, sallow complexion, cold limbs, loose stools, Pale tongue, Deep-Weak pulse.

Spleen- and Kidney-Yang deficiency

Chronic convulsions, slight tremor of the limbs which comes and goes, listlessness, sleepiness, sallow com-

plexion, sunken fontanelle, sweating, cold limbs, loose stools, weak breathing, Pale tongue, Deep-Weak pulse.

FETUS TOXIN

According to Chinese medicine, most fetuses absorb toxin in the uterus and develop Toxic Heat: this is all the more likely to happen when the mother eats too many hot and spicy foods, suffers an invasion of Toxic Heat or has a shock during pregnancy.

Fetus Toxin Heat

Fever, hot body, red face and eyes, mouth closed, noisy breathing, swollen eyes, shortness of breath, crying, tendency to be easily startled, dark urine, dry stools.

Fetus Toxin Cold

Pale face, mental confusion, sleepiness, shortness of breath, cold body, cold limbs, abdominal pain, crying, mouth open.

Fetus Toxin convulsions

Convulsions, body hot, face bluish, clenched teeth, shortness of breath, wheezing, stiffness of body, eyes turning up, grimacing.

Fetus Toxin jaundice

Jaundice, golden-yellow skin and eyes, hot body, dark urine, crying.

FONTANELLES

Sunken fontanelles
Spleen- and Kidney-Yang deficiency

Sunken fontanelle, late closure of fontanelle, quiet child, cold limbs, listlessness, poor appetite.

Exhaustion of Qi and Fluids

Sunken fontanelle, dry skin, listlessness, crying at night.

Raised fontanelles
Toxic Heat

Raised and swollen fontanelle like a heap, soft to touch, red skin over the fontanelle, headache, thirst, crying, sweating, red face and lips, shortness of breath, dark

urine, Red tongue with red points and dry, thick yellow coating, Rapid-Overflowing pulse.

Cold in the Interior

Raised fontanelle, which is hard to touch, white skin over the fontanelle, dull-pale complexion, cold limbs, possibly twitching of the limbs, Pale tongue, Deep-Tight pulse.

Late closure of fontanelles

Observation, Chapter 5

The posterior fontanelle usually closes about 2 months after birth; the sphenoid fontanelle closes at about 3 months, the mastoid one closes near the end of the first year, and the anterior fontanelle may not close completely until the middle or end of the second year.

Kidney-Essence deficiency

Late closure of fontanelle, listlessness, weak and quiet child, slow mental and physical development.

Spleen deficiency

Late closure of fontanelle, listlessness, poor digestion, poor appetite, quiet child, loose stools.

WHITE SPOTS ON THE PALATE AND TONGUE

Heat in Spleen and Heart

White spots on the palate and tongue like snow, red face, red lips, thirst, irritability, insomnia, crying, palpitations, dark urine, Red tongue with yellow coating, Overflowing-Rapid pulse.

Spleen- and Kidney-Yin deficiency

White spots on palate and tongue like snow, listlessness, poor development, malar flush, dry mouth, tongue without coating, Floating-Empty pulse.

LONG PENIS

Observation, Chapter 17

Congenital Kidney-Yin deficiency

Long penis, slow development, lateness in walking and standing, slow growth of the teeth, normal coloured tongue without coating, Floating-Empty pulse.

Spleen-Qi sinking

Long penis, a feeling of bearing down in the abdomen, tiredness, lassitude, poor appetite, loose stools, failure to thrive, Pale tongue, Empty pulse.

Phlegm and Blood stasis in the Lower Burner

Long penis, sputum in the throat, slow mental and speech development, a feeling of oppression of the throat, abdominal pain, Purple and Swollen tongue, Wiry-Slippery pulse.

Damp-Heat in the Liver channel

Long penis, fullness of the hypochondrium, abdomen or hypogastrium, bitter taste, poor appetite, nausea, a feeling of heaviness of the body, pain, redness and swelling of the scrotum, genital, papular or vesicular skin rashes and itching, urinary difficulty, burning on urination, dark urine, Red tongue with redder sides and a sticky yellow coating, Slippery-Wiry-Rapid pulse.

PART 6

IDENTIFICATION OF PATTERNS

辩
证

Part contents

SECTION 1
IDENTIFICATION OF PATTERNS ACCORDING TO THE INTERNAL ORGANS
91 Heart   *879*
92 Spleen   *885*
93 Liver   *891*
94 Lungs   *899*
95 Kidneys   *905*
96 Small Intestine   *911*
97 Stomach   *913*
98 Gall-Bladder   *917*
99 Large Intestine   *921*
100 Bladder   *925*

SECTION 2
IDENTIFICATION OF PATTERNS ACCORDING TO QI, BLOOD AND BODY FLUIDS
101 Identification of patterns according to Qi, Blood, Yang and Yin   *929*
102 Identification of patterns according to Body Fluids   *935*

SECTION 3
IDENTIFICATION OF PATTERNS ACCORDING TO PATHOGENIC FACTORS, FOUR LEVELS, SIX STAGES AND THREE BURNERS
103 Identification of patterns according to pathogenic factors   *943*
104 Identification of patterns according to the Four Levels   *953*
105 Identification of patterns according to the Six Stages   *965*
106 Identification of patterns according to the Three Burners   *969*
107 Residual pathogenic factor   *973*

SECTION 4
IDENTIFICATION OF PATTERNS ACCORDING TO THE EIGHT PRINCIPLES, 12 CHANNELS, EIGHT EXTRAORDINARY VESSELS AND FIVE ELEMENTS
108 Identification of patterns according to the Eight Principles   *983*
109 Identification of patterns according to the 12 channels   *993*
110 Identification of patterns according to the Eight Extraordinary Vessels   *997*
111 Identification of patterns according to the Five Elements   *1007*

INTRODUCTION

'Identification of patterns' indicates the process of identifying the basic disharmony that underlies all clinical manifestations. This is the essence of Chinese medical diagnosis and pathology. By considering the picture that is formed by all the symptoms and signs, we discern and identify the underlying pattern of disharmony.

Identification of patterns thus involves forming an overall picture of disharmony taking all symptoms and signs into consideration. In this respect, Chinese medicine does not look for causes but patterns. When we say that a patient presents with the pattern of disharmony of Kidney-Yin deficiency, this is not the cause of the disease (which has to be looked for in the person's life), but the disharmony underlying the disease. Of course, in other respects, after identifying the pattern Chinese medicine does go a step further in trying to identify a cause for the disharmony.

In the context of identification of patterns, 'symptoms' and 'signs' should be interpreted in a broad way. Included among them are manifestations that are not 'symptoms' or 'signs' in Western medicine (e.g. timidity, a weak voice, incapacity of making decisions, lack of thirst, etc.).

In identifying patterns we follow the typical Chinese medical philosophy of looking for relationships rather

than linear causes. Each symptom or sign has a meaning only in relation to all other manifestations; therefore, a particular symptom can mean different things in different situations. For example, the sign of 'dry hair' accompanied by night sweating, a feeling of heat in the evening, a dry throat at night and a Red tongue without coating indicates Yin deficiency, whereas 'dry hair' accompanied by blurred vision, scanty periods and a Pale tongue indicates Blood deficiency.

Identifying the pattern of disharmony blends diagnosis, pathology and treatment principle all in one. When we say that a certain pattern is characterized by Spleen-Yang deficiency with retention of Dampness, we are defining the nature of the condition (Yang deficiency), the site (Spleen) and, by implication, the treatment principle, that is, tonify and warm the Spleen and resolve Dampness.

In the particular case of external invasions, by identifying the pattern we indentify the cause of the disharmony (e.g. external Wind), the nature of the condition (invasion of Wind), the site (the Exterior of the body) and the treatment principle, that is, release the Exterior and expel Wind. Thus, identifying the pattern (or patterns) allows us to identify the nature and character of the condition, the site of the disease, the treatment principle and the prognosis (Fig. P6.1).

When identifying patterns, we should not only identify the pattern but also understand how it arose and how different aspects of it interact with each other. For example, if we identify a pattern of Liver-Qi stagnation and also a pattern of Spleen-Qi deficiency, we should go a step further and find out which pattern started first, how the two patterns interact, which is primary and whether one can be considered the cause of the other.

Patterns may be identified according to different aspects. These are applicable in different situations and were formulated at different times in the development of Chinese medicine. The various modes of identifying patterns are:

- identification of patterns according to Internal Organs
- identification of patterns according to Qi, Blood and Body Fluids
- identification of patterns according to pathogenic factors
- identification of patterns according to the Four Levels
- identification of patterns according to the Six Stages
- identification of patterns according to the Three Burners
- identification of patterns according to the Eight Principles
- identification of patterns according to the channels
- identification of patterns according to the Five Elements.

Each of these methods is applicable in different cases.

Identification of patterns according to Internal Organs

The identification of patterns according to the Internal Organs is the most important means of diagnosing internal, chronic diseases when the organs are involved. This identification of patterns is the mainstay of everyday clinical practice.

Identification of patterns according to Qi, Blood and Body Fluids

The identification of patterns according to Qi, Blood and Body Fluids describes the patterns emerging from a pathology in the transformation, production and movement of Qi and Blood and in the transformation, transportation and excretion of Body Fluids.

The pathology of Qi includes Qi deficiency, Qi stagnation, Qi sinking and rebellious Qi. The pathology of Blood includes Blood deficiency, Blood stasis, Blood-Heat, Cold in the Blood and bleeding. The pathology of Body Fluids includes deficiency of Body Fluids, Oedema and Phlegm (Dampness is discussed under the identification of patterns according to pathogenic factors).

The identification of patterns according to Qi, Blood and Body Fluids overlaps with that according to the Eight Principles and that according to the Internal Organs. For example, the pattern of Qi

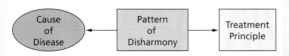

Fig. P6.1 Relationship between the cause of a disease, the pattern of disharmony and the treatment principle

deficiency is the same as the eponymous one in the identification of patterns according to the Eight Principles.

The identification of patterns according to Qi, Blood and Body Fluids is useful to give a general idea about the state of Qi, Blood and Body Fluids; it is complementary to the patterns of the Internal Organs, which provide further detail. For example, the pattern of Blood deficiency within the Qi, Blood and Body Fluids patterns gives only the general symptoms and signs of Blood deficiency and the Internal Organs patterns of Liver-Blood and Heart-Blood deficiency identify the organ involved.

Identification of patterns according to pathogenic factors

The identification of patterns according to pathogenic factors describes the patterns formed when the body is invaded by external pathogenic factors such as Dampness, Wind, Cold, Dryness and Summer-Heat. However, since the symptoms and signs of the corresponding internal pathogenic factors are similar, these are usually discussed within this type of identification of pattern, which also includes the discussion of Fire as an internal pathogenic factor.

Identification of patterns according to the Four Levels

The identification of patterns according to the Four Levels was formulated primarily by Ye Tian Shi and described in his book 'Discussion of Warm Diseases' (*Wen Bing Lun*, 1746). It describes the patterns arising when the patient is invaded by external Wind-Heat. The patterns consist of Four Levels: the Defensive-Qi, Qi, Nutritive-Qi and Blood levels. They describe four levels of Heat, the first being external Wind-Heat and the other three internal Heat.

Identification of patterns according to the Six Stages

This pattern identification is also very old as it is derived from Zhang Zhong Jing's 'Discussion of Cold-induced Diseases' (c. AD220) (see Bibliography, Shang Han Lang Research Group). It describes the patterns arising when the patient is invaded by external Wind and especially Wind-Cold. It consists of six patterns, which are the Greater Yang, Lesser Yang, Bright Yang, Greater Yin, Lesser Yin and Terminal Yin.

Identification of patterns according to the Three Burners

The identification of patterns according to the Three Burners is quite similar to that according to the Four Levels. It was formulated by Wu Ju Tong in the Qing dynasty. Many of the patterns are essentially the same as those of the Four Levels, except that they are seen from the perspective of the Three Burners, that is, the patterns of the Upper Burner, Middle Burner and Lower Burner. The Middle Burner patterns correspond to the Qi level, whereas those of the Lower Burner correspond to the Nutritive-Qi and Blood levels. By contrast, the patterns of the Upper Burner encompass the Defensive-Qi, Qi and Nutritive-Qi levels.

Identification of patterns according to the Eight Principles

Elements of this method of identification of patterns are found throughout Chinese medical texts starting from the 'Yellow Emperor's Classic of Internal Medicine' and the 'Discussion of Cold-induced Disorders'. In its present form, this method of identifying patterns was formulated by Cheng Zhong Ling in the early Qing dynasty.

Identification of patterns according to the Eight Principles is based on the categories of Interior/Exterior, Heat/Cold, Full/Empty and Yin/Yang. It is the summarization of all other modes of identifying patterns and is applicable in all cases for both interior and exterior diseases.

Identification of patterns according to the channels

This is actually the oldest of the methods of pattern identification as it is described in Chapter 10 of the 'Spiritual Axis'. It describes the symptoms and signs arising from the channel, when the organs are not affected.

Identification of patterns according to the Five Elements

The identification of patterns according to the Five Elements describes the patterns of disharmony purely from the point of view of the Five Elements. This is useful as a general indication for two reasons: first, it can help us to plot the progression of a pathological condition from one Element to the other (bearing in mind that a progression along the Controlling cycle is more serious); secondly, the Five-Element patterns are sometimes useful to form a picture of the mental–spiritual condition of the patient.

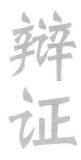

SECTION 1

IDENTIFICATION OF PATTERNS ACCORDING TO THE INTERNAL ORGANS

Section contents

91 Heart *879*
92 Spleen *885*
93 Liver *891*
94 Lungs *899*
95 Kidneys *905*
96 Small Intestine *911*
97 Stomach *913*
98 Gall-Bladder *917*
99 Large Intestine *921*
100 Bladder *925*

INTRODUCTION

The identification of patterns according to the Internal Organs is based on the clinical manifestations arising when the Qi and Blood of the Internal Organs are out of balance. This method of identification is used mostly for interior and chronic conditions but it also includes a few exterior and acute conditions.

The Internal Organs patterns are an application of the Eight-Principle method of identification to the particular disharmonies of specific Internal Organs. For example, according to the Eight-Principle pattern identification, the symptoms and signs of Qi deficiency are shortness of breath, a weak voice, a pale face, tiredness and poor appetite. Although useful to diagnose a condition of Qi deficiency, this is not detailed enough and does not identify the organ involved. It is therefore too general to give an indication of the treatment needed. According to the Internal-Organ pattern identification, the above symptoms can be further classified as Lung-Qi deficiency (shortness of breath and a weak voice) and

Spleen-Qi deficiency (tiredness and poor appetite). This is more useful in clinical practice because it gives an indication as to which organ needs to be treated.

Let us now look at some of the characteristics and points of attention of the identification of patterns according to the Internal Organs.

1. In the following pages, the Internal Organs are described in as much detail as possible. It is important to remember, however, that not all symptoms and signs listed need to be present to diagnose those patterns. The patterns listed actually describe advanced cases of Internal Organs patterns. As such a case develops gradually over several years, in the beginning stages there will be relatively few symptoms and signs. Sometimes, just a few symptoms are enough to diagnose a certain pattern. For example, scanty periods and blurred vision in a woman may be enough to diagnose Liver-Blood deficiency; similarly if she suffers from blurred vision and her tongue is Pale on the sides.

2. It should not be forgotten that the pulse is a sign that is part of the constellation of symptoms and signs forming a pattern. Indeed, the pulse is a very important sign and one can sometimes diagnose a pattern simply on the basis of the pulse. For example, if the Kidney pulse on both left and right positions is *consistently* Weak, I interpret that as a sign of a Kidney deficiency even in the absence of any other symptom and sign.

3. Within the Yin-deficiency patterns, I list two separate patterns, that is, a pattern of Yin deficiency without Empty-Heat and a pattern of Yin deficiency with Empty-Heat. Although Empty-Heat does eventually arise from Yin deficiency, in the beginning stages there is usually Yin deficiency without Empty-Heat. Besides the symptoms of Heat, the tongue is an important sign indicating whether there is Empty-Heat or not: if it is Red (without coating), this indicates that there is Empty-Heat; if it is without coating (but is not Red), this indicates Yin deficiency without Empty-Heat. In other words, it is important to remember that the Yin deficiency on the tongue is indicated by the lack of coating (*not* its redness) and Empty-Heat is indicated by its redness (of course associated with the lack of coating).

4. The organ patterns are not 'pigeon holes' into which we fit symptoms and signs. In practice, it is essential to have an understanding of the aetiology, pathology and interaction of patterns. The aim of the identification of patterns according to Internal Organs, therefore, is to understand how symptoms and signs arose and how they interact with each other.

5. There is absolutely no direct correspondence between Internal Organ patterns and Western diseases. Each Western disease may manifest itself with many different patterns and each pattern may give rise to various Western diseases.

Furthermore, there is no direct correspondence between an organ pattern in Chinese medicine and an organ disease in Western medicine. For example, a person may suffer from Kidney-Yin deficiency without any sign of kidney disease in Western medicine; vice versa, a person may suffer from a kidney inflammation from a Western point of view but a pattern of Bladder Damp-Heat from the perspective of Chinese medicine.

6. Most patients suffer from a combination of Internal Organs patterns. The most frequent ones are:
   (a) two or more patterns from the same organs, either Yin or Yang (e.g. Liver-Qi stagnation with Liver-Yang rising, and Stomach-Yin deficiency with rebellious Stomach-Qi)
   (b) two or more patterns from different organs, either Yin or Yang (e.g. Liver-Fire and Heart-Fire, and Stomach-Heat with Gall-Bladder Damp-Heat)
   (c) one or more patterns of a Yin organ with one or more of a Yang organ (e.g. Spleen-Qi deficiency with Bladder Damp-Heat)
   (d) an interior with an exterior pattern (e.g. Damp-Phlegm in the Lungs with invasion of exterior Wind in the Lungs Defensive-Qi portion)
   (e) an organ pattern with a channel pattern of the related channel (e.g. Dampness in the Large Intestine with Painful Obstruction Syndrome of the Large Intestine channel)
   (f) an organ pattern with a channel pattern of an unrelated channel (e.g. Lung-Qi deficiency with stagnation of Qi in the Bladder channel).

Chapter **91**

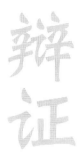

HEART

Chapter contents

HEART-QI DEFICIENCY *879*

HEART-YANG DEFICIENCY PATTERNS *879*
  Heart-Yang deficiency *879*
  Heart-Yang deficiency with Phlegm *880*

HEART-YANG COLLAPSE *880*

HEART-BLOOD DEFICIENCY *880*

HEART-QI AND HEART-BLOOD DEFICIENCY *880*

HEART-YIN DEFICIENCY PATTERNS *880*
  Heart-Yin deficiency *880*
  Heart-Yin deficiency with Empty Heat *881*

HEART-QI AND HEART-YIN DEFICIENCY *881*

DEfiCIENCY OF BOTH HEART-YANG AND HEART-YIN *881*

HEART-QI STAGNATION *881*

HEART-FIRE BLAZING *881*

PHLEGM PATTERNS *882*
  Phlegm-Fire harassing the Heart *882*
  Phlegm misting the Mind *882*

HEART-BLOOD STASIS **882**

HEART-VESSEL OBSTRUCTION *882*

WATER OVERFLOWING TO THE HEART *883*

TURBID DAMPNESS SURROUNDING THE HEART *883*

COMBINED PATTERNS *883*

HEART-QI DEFICIENCY

Clinical manifestations

Palpitations, shortness of breath on exertion, pale face, tiredness, slight depression, spontaneous sweating.
Tongue Pale.
Pulse Empty.

Acupuncture

HE-5 Tongli, P-6 Neiguan, BL-15 Xinshu, Ren-17 Shanzhong, Ren-6 Qihai.

Prescription

Bao Yuan Tang *Preserving the Source Decoction.*

HEART-YANG DEFICIENCY PATTERNS

Heart-yang deficiency
Clinical manifestations

Palpitations, shortness of breath on exertion, tiredness, slight depression, spontaneous sweating, a slight feeling of discomfort or stuffiness in the heart region, a feeling of cold, cold hands, bright-pale face, slightly dark lips.
Tongue Pale.
Pulse Deep-Weak, in severe cases Knotted.

Acupuncture

HE-5 Tongli, P-6 Neiguan, BL-15 Xinshu, Ren-17 Shanzhong, Ren-6 Qihai, Du-14 Dazhui.

Prescription

Rou Fu Bao Yuan Tang *Cinnamomum-Aconitum Preserving the Source Decoction.*

Heart-Yang deficiency with Phlegm
Clinical manifestations

Palpitations, a feeling of oppression of the chest, sputum in the throat, dizziness, tiredness, cold hands, numbness of the limbs, oedema of the hands, muzziness (fuzziness) of the head, poor memory, a feeling of heaviness, depression.
Tongue Pale, wet and Swollen.
Pulse Weak but slightly Slippery.

Acupuncture

Ren-6 Qihai, Ren-4 Guanyuan, Ren-8 Shenque, Du-4 Mingmen, ST-36 Zusanli, P-6 Neiguan, BL-23 Shenshu, Du-14 Dazhui, BL-15 Xinshu, ST-40 Fenglong, Ren-12 Zhongwan, P-5 Jianshi, Ren-17 Shanzhong.

Prescription

Ling Gui Zhu Gan Tang *Poria-Ramulus Cinnamomi-Atractylodes-Glycyrrhiza Decoction* plus Yi Yi Ren *Semen Coicis lachryma jobi.*

HEART-YANG COLLAPSE

Clinical manifestations

Palpitations, shortness of breath, weak and shallow breathing, profuse sweating, cold limbs, cyanosis of the lips, greyish-white complexion, in severe cases coma.
Tongue Very Pale or Bluish-Purple, Short.
Pulse Hidden-Minute.

Acupuncture

Ren-6 Qihai, Ren-4 Guanyuan, Ren-8 Shenque, Du-4 Mingmen, ST-36 Zusanli, P-6 Neiguan, BL-23 Shenshu, Du-20 Baihui, Du-14 Dazhui, BL-15 Xinshu. Moxa is applicable.

Prescription

Shen Fu Tang *Ginseng-Aconitum Decoction.*

HEART-BLOOD DEFICIENCY

Clinical manifestations

Palpitations, dizziness, insomnia, dream-disturbed sleep, poor memory, anxiety, tendency to be easily startled, dull-pale complexion, pale lips.

Tongue Pale and Thin.
Pulse Choppy or Fine.

Acupuncture

HE-7 Shenmen, P-6 Neiguan, Ren-14 Juque, Ren-15 Jiuwei, Ren-4 Guanyuan, BL-17 Geshu (with moxa), BL-20 Pishu.

Prescription

Shen Qi Si Wu Tang *Ginseng-Astragalus Four Substances Decoction.*

HEART-QI AND HEART-BLOOD DEFICIENCY

Clinical manifestations

Palpitations, shortness of breath, spontaneous sweating, depression, anxiety, tiredness, dull-pale complexion, insomnia.
Tongue Pale and Thin.
Pulse Weak or Choppy.

Acupuncture

HE-5 Tongli, HE-7 Shenmen, P-6 Neiguan, Ren-14 Juque, Ren-15 Jiuwei, Ren-4 Guanyuan, BL-17 Geshu (with moxa), BL-20 Pishu, BL-15 Xinshu.

Prescription

Ba Zhen Tang *Eight Precious Decoction*
Gui Pi Tang *Tonifying the Spleen Decoction.*

HEART-YIN DEFICIENCY PATTERNS

Heart-Yin deficiency
Clinical manifestations

Palpitations, insomnia, dream-disturbed sleep, poor memory, anxiety, tendency to be easily startled, mental restlessness, uneasiness, dry mouth and throat in the afternoon or evening.
Tongue Normal-coloured without coating or with rootless coating.
Pulse Floating-Empty, especially in the left- Front position.

Acupuncture

HE-7 Shenmen, P-6 Neiguan, Ren-14 Juque, Ren-15 Jiuwei, Ren-4 Guanyuan, HE-6 Yinxi, SP-6 Sanyinjiao, KI-7 Fuliu, KI-6 Zhaohai.

Prescription

Tian Wang Bu Xin Dan *Heavenly Emperor Tonifying the Heart Pill.*

Heart-Yin deficiency with Empty-Heat
Clinical manifestations

Palpitations, insomnia, dream-disturbed sleep, poor memory, anxiety, tendency to be easily startled, mental restlessness, uneasiness, 'feeling hot and bothered', dry mouth and throat in the evening, thirst with a desire to drink in small sips, a feeling of heat in the evening, malar flush, night sweating, five-palm heat.

Tongue   Red, redder on the tip, without coating.
Pulse   Floating-Empty, especially on the left-Front position and Rapid.

Acupuncture

HE-7 Shenmen, P-6 Neiguan, Ren-14 Juque, Ren-15 Jiuwei, Ren-4 Guanyuan, HE-6 Yinxi, SP-6 Sanyinjiao, KI-7 Fuliu, KI-6 Zhaohai, P-7 Daling, LI-11 Quchi, HE-9 Shaochong.

Prescription

Tian Wang Bu Xin Dan *Heavenly Emperor Tonifying the Heart Pill* plus Mu Dan Pi *Cortex Moutan radicis.*

HEART-QI AND HEART-YIN DEFICIENCY

Clinical manifestations

Palpitations, anxiety, tendency to be easily startled, slight breathlessness, tiredness, insomnia, mental restlessness, sweating on exertion, dry throat, night sweating.

Tongue   Normal-coloured without coating.
Pulse   Floating-Empty.

Acupuncture

HE-5 Tongli, HE-7 Shenmen, P-6 Neiguan, Ren-14 Juque, Ren-15 Jiuwei, Ren-4 Guanyuan, HE-6 Yinxi, SP-6 Sanyinjiao, BL-15 Xinshu.

Prescription

Zhi Gan Cao Tang *Glycyrrhiza Decoction*
Sheng Mai San *Generating the Pulse Powder.*

DEFICIENCY OF BOTH HEART-YANG AND HEART-YIN

Clinical manifestations

Palpitations, tendency to be easily startled, shortness of breath, a slight feeling of oppression of the chest, a feeling of cold, cold limbs, mental restlessness, night sweating, poor memory, malar flush.

Tongue   Pale or Red without coating depending on whether Yang or Yin deficiency predominates.
Pulse   Weak or Floating-Empty.

Acupuncture

HE-5 Tongli, HE-7 Shenmen, Ren-17 Shanzhong, BL-15 Xinshu, Ren-15 Jiuwei, SP-6 Sanyinjiao, ST-36 Zusanli.

Prescription

Zhi Gan Cao Tang *Glycyrrhiza Decoction.*

HEART-QI STAGNATION

Clinical manifestations

Palpitations, a feeling of distension or oppression of the chest, depression, a slight feeling of a lump in the throat, slight shortness of breath, sighing, poor appetite, chest and upper epigastric distension, dislike of lying down, weak and cold limbs, slightly purple lips, pale complexion.

Tongue   Slightly Pale-Purple on the sides in the chest area.
Pulse   Empty but very slightly Overflowing on the left Front position.

Acupuncture

HE-5 Tongli, HE-7 Shenmen, P-6 Neiguan, Ren-15 Jiuwei, Ren-17 Shanzhong, LU-7 Lieque, ST-40 Fenglong, LI-4 Hegu.

Prescription

Mu Xiang Liu Qi Yin *Aucklandia Flowing Qi Decoction*
Ban Xia Hou Po Tang *Pinellia-Magnolia Decoction.*

HEART-FIRE BLAZING

Clinical manifestations

Palpitations, thirst, mouth and tongue ulcers, mental restlessness, a feeling of agitation, insomnia,

dream-disturbed sleep, a feeling of heat, red face, dark urine or blood in the urine, bitter taste (after a bad night's sleep).

Tongue   Red with redder tip and yellow coating. In more severe cases the tip could also be swollen.

Pulse   Overflowing-Rapid especially on the left Front position. It could also be Hasty (rapid and stopping at irregular intervals).

Acupuncture

HE-9 Shaochong, HE-8 Shaofu, HE-7 Shenmen, Ren-15 Jiuwei, SP-6 Sanyinjiao, KI-6 Zhaohai, LI-11 Quchi, Du-24 Shenting, Du-19 Houding.

Prescription

Xie Xin Tang *Draining the Heart Decoction.*

PHLEGM PATTERNS

Phlegm-Fire harassing the Heart
Clinical manifestations

Palpitations, mental restlessness, thirst, red face, a feeling of oppression of the chest, dark urine, expectoration of phlegm, rattling sound in the throat, bitter taste, insomnia, dream-disturbed sleep, a feeling of agitation, mental confusion, incoherent speech, rash behaviour, tendency to hit or scold people, uncontrolled laughter or crying, shouting, muttering to oneself, depression, manic behaviour.

Tongue   Red with redder and swollen tip and a sticky yellow coating. In severe cases there will be a deep Heart crack with a sticky, dry yellow coating inside it.

Pulse   Slippery-Rapid or Slippery-Overflowing-Rapid.

Acupuncture

P-5 Jianshi, HE-7 Shenmen, HE-8 Shaofu, HE-9 Shaochong, P-7 Daling, Ren-15 Jiuwei, BL-15 Xinshu, Ren-12 Zhongwan, ST-40 Fenglong, SP-6 Sanyinjiao, BL-20 Pishu, Du-20 Baihui, GB-13 Benshen, GB-17 Zhengying, Du-24 Shenting.

Prescription

Wen Dan Tang *Warming the Gall-Bladder Decoction.*

Phlegm misting the Mind
Clinical manifestations

Mental confusion, lethargic stupor, unconsciousness, incoherent speech, vomiting of phlegm, rattling sound in the throat, aphasia, mental depression, emotional lability, very dull eyes.

Tongue   Swollen with sticky coating.

Pulse   Slippery.

Acupuncture

HE-9 Shaochong, P-5 Jianshi, BL-15 Xinshu, ST-40 Fenglong, Du-26 Renzhong, Ren-12 Zhongwan, BL-20 Pishu, Du-20 Baihui, Du-14 Dazhui.

Prescription

Di Tan Tang *Scouring Phlegm Decoction*
Gun Tan Wan *Vapourizing Phlegm Pill.*

HEART-BLOOD STASIS

Clinical manifestations

Palpitations, stabbing or pricking chest pain which may radiate to the inner aspect of the left arm or to the shoulder, a feeling of oppression or constriction of the chest, cyanosis of lips and nails, cold hands.

Tongue   Purple in its entirety or only on the sides in the chest areas.

Pulse   Choppy, Wiry or Knotted. The pulse will be Knotted if Heart-Blood stasis occurs against a background of severe Heart-Yang deficiency.

Acupuncture

P-6 Neiguan, P-4 Ximen, HE-7 Shenmen, Ren-17 Shanzhong, BL-14 Jueyinshu, BL-17 Geshu, SP-10 Xuehai, KI-25 Shencang.

Prescription

Xue Fu Zhu Yu Tang *Blood-Mansion Eliminating Stasis Decoction.*

HEART VESSEL OBSTRUCTION

Clinical manifestations

Palpitations, shortness of breath with an inability to lie down, depression, mental restlessness, a feeling of stuffiness under the hypochondrium, a flustered feeling, a feeling of oppression of the chest, stabbing or pricking pain in the heart region which comes and goes, and which may radiate to the upper back or shoulder, pain aggravated by exposure to cold and alleviated by heat, expectoration of phlegm, epigastric or hypochondrial distension, a feeling of heaviness, dislike of speaking, cold hands, sighing, purple lips, face and nails.

Tongue Purple on the sides in the chest areas, Swollen with a sticky coating.
Pulse Wiry, Choppy or Knotted. It could also be Slippery if Phlegm is predominant.

This is a complex pattern due to Qi stagnation, Blood stasis, Cold and Phlegm occurring simultaneously.

Acupuncture

P-6 Neiguan, LU-7 Lieque, P-5 Jianshi, Ren-17 Shanzhong, LI-4 Hegu, ST-40 Fenglong, Ren-12 Zhongwan, Ren-15 Jiuwei, Ren-14 Juque, BL-17 Geshu, BL-14 Jueyinshu, Du-14 Dazhui (with moxa).

Prescription

Zhi Shi Gua Lou Gui Zhi Tang *Citrus-Trichosantes-Ramulus Cinnamomi Decoction* plus Dan Shen *Radix Salviae miltiorrhizae*.

WATER OVERFLOWING TO THE HEART

Clinical manifestations

Palpitations, dizziness, nausea, vomiting of watery, frothy white fluid, a feeling of cold, cold limbs, severe shortness of breath, a feeling of fullness and stuffiness of the chest and epigastrium, thirst with no desire to drink, urinary retention.
Tongue Pale, Swollen and wet.
Pulse Deep-Wiry or Deep-Fine-Slippery.

This pattern is seen only in the elderly.

Acupuncture

HE-5 Tongli, HE-6 Yinxi, BL-15 Xinshu, Ren-12 Zhongwan, Ren-9 Shuifen, KI-7 Fuliu, Ren-17 Shanzhong. Moxa is applicable.

Prescription

Ling Gui Zhu Gan Tang *Poria-Ramulus Cinnamomi-Atractylodes-Glycyrrhiza Decoction*.
Zhen Wu Tang *True Warrior Decoction*.

TURBID DAMPNESS SURROUNDING THE HEART

Clinical manifestations

Palpitations, cold hands, scanty urination, oedema of the ankles, sleepiness, mental confusion, sallow complexion, dizziness, frontal headache, blurred vision, nausea, vomiting, a feeling of oppression of the chest, poor appetite, abdominal fullness, loose stools, excessive salivation.
Tongue Pale, Swollen with sticky white coating.
Pulse Soggy or Deep-Slippery.

Acupuncture

HE-5 Tongli, BL-15 Xinshu, Ren-17 Shanzhong, Ren-12 Zhongwan, Ren-9 Shuifen, ST-28 Shuidao, SP-9 Yinlingquan, SP-6 Sanyinjiao.

Prescription

Wen Pi Tang *Warming the Spleen Decoction* plus Su He Xiang Wan *Styrax Pill*.

COMBINED PATTERNS

The Heart combined patterns are:

- Heart- and Liver-Blood deficiency (see under Liver combined patterns)
- Heart- and Spleen-Blood deficiency (see under Spleen combined patterns)
- Heart- and Kidney-Yin deficiency with Heart Empty-Heat (see 'Heart and Kidneys not harmonized' under Kidney combined patterns)
- Heart- and Lung-Qi deficiency (see under Lung combined patterns).

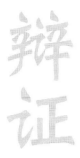

Chapter **92**

SPLEEN

Chapter contents

SPLEEN-QI DEFICIENCY PATTERNS   *885*
  Spleen-Qi deficiency   *885*
  Spleen-Qi deficiency with Dampness   *885*
  Spleen-Qi deficiency with Phlegm   *886*

SPLEEN-YANG DEFICIENCY   *886*

SPLEEN-BLOOD DEFICIENCY   *886*

SPLEEN-QI SINKING   *886*

SPLEEN NOT CONTROLLING BLOOD   *886*

SPLEEN-YIN DEFICIENCY PATTERNS   *887*
  Spleen-Yin deficiency   *887*
  Spleen-Yin deficiency with Empty-Heat   *887*

COLD-DAMPNESS IN THE SPLEEN   *887*

DAMP-HEAT IN THE SPLEEN   *887*

SPLEEN-HEAT   *888*

PHLEGM OBSTRUCTING THE MIDDLE BURNER   *888*

YIN FIRE FROM DEFICIENCY OF THE STOMACH AND SPLEEN
AND ORIGINAL QI   *888*

COMBINED PATTERNS   *888*
  Spleen- and Stomach-Qi deficiency   *888*
  Spleen- and Heart-Blood deficiency   *888*
  Spleen- and Lung-Qi deficiency   *889*
  Spleen- and Liver-Blood deficiency   *889*
  Obstruction of the Spleen by Dampness with
   stagnation of Liver-Qi   *889*

SPLEEN-QI DEFICIENCY PATTERNS

Spleen-Qi deficiency
Clinical manifestations

Poor appetite, slight abdominal distension after eating, tiredness, lassitude, pale complexion, weakness of the limbs, loose stools, slight depression, tendency to obesity.
Tongue   Pale.
Pulse   Empty.

Acupuncture

Ren-12 Zhongwan, ST-36 Zusanli, SP-3 Taibai, SP-6 Sanyinjiao, BL-20 Pishu, BL-21 Weishu.

Prescription

Si Jun Zi Tang *Four Gentlemen Decoction.*

Spleen-Qi deficiency with dampness
Clinical manifestations

Poor appetite, slight abdominal distension after eating, tiredness, lassitude, pale or sallow complexion, weakness of the limbs, loose stools, slight depression, tendency to obesity, abdominal fullness, a feeling of heaviness, a sticky taste, poor digestion, undigested food in the stools, nausea, dull frontal headache, excessive vaginal discharge.
Tongue   Pale with sticky coating.
Pulse   Soggy.

Acupuncture

Ren-12 Zhongwan, ST-36 Zusanli, SP-3 Taibai, SP-6 Sanyinjiao, BL-20 Pishu, BL-21 Weishu, SP-9 Yinlingquan, BL-22 Sanjiaoshu, ST-28 Shuidao.

Prescription

Si Jun Zi Tang *Four Gentlemen Decoction* plus Yi Yi Ren *Semen Coicis lachryma jobi*
Shi Pi Yin *Bolster the Spleen Decoction.*

Spleen-Qi deficiency with Phlegm
Clinical manifestations

Nausea, vomiting of watery fluids, a feeling of oppression of the chest and epigastrium, tiredness, poor appetite, a feeling of heaviness, weak limbs, loose stools, dull-pale complexion, cold limbs.
Tongue Pale, Swollen with sticky coating.
Pulse Soggy or Weak and slightly Slippery.

Acupuncture

Ren-12 Zhongwan, Ren-9 Shuifen, ST-36 Zusanli, SP-9 Yinglingquan, ST-40 Fenglong, BL-20 Pishu, BL-22 Sanjiaoshu.

Prescription

Liu Jun Zi Tang *Four Gentlemen Decoction* plus Er Chen Tang *Two Old Decoction.*

SPLEEN-YANG DEFICIENCY

Clinical manifestations

Poor appetite, slight abdominal distension after eating, tiredness, lassitude, pale complexion, weakness of the limbs, loose stools, slight depression, tendency to obesity, a feeling of cold, cold limbs, oedema.
Tongue Pale and wet.
Pulse Deep-Weak.

Acupuncture

Ren-12 Zhongwan, ST-36 Zusanli, SP-3 Taibai, SP-6 Sanyinjiao, BL-20 Pishu, BL-21 Weishu, SP-9 Yinlingquan, Ren-9 Shuifen, BL-22 Sanjiaoshu, ST-28 Shuidao, Ren-11 Jianli, ST-22 Guanmen. Moxa is applicable.

Prescription

Li Zhong Tang *Regulating the Centre Decoction.*

SPLEEN-BLOOD DEFICIENCY

Clinical manifestations

Poor appetite, slight abdominal distension after eating, tiredness, lassitude, dull-pale complexion, weakness of

the limbs, loose stools, depression, thin body, scanty periods or amenorrhoea, insomnia, joint ache.
Tongue Pale and Thin.
Pulse Choppy or Fine.

Acupuncture

Ren-12 Zhongwan, ST-36 Zusanli, SP-3 Taibai, SP-6 Sanyinjiao, BL-20 Pishu, BL-21 Weishu, Ren-4 Guanyuan, BL-17 Geshu (with direct moxa).

Prescription

Gui Pi Tang *Tonifying the Spleen Decoction.*

SPLEEN-QI SINKING

Clinical manifestations

Poor appetite, slight abdominal distension after eating, tiredness, lassitude, pale complexion, weakness of the limbs, loose stools, depression, tendency to obesity, a bearing-down sensation in the abdomen, prolapse of the stomach, uterus, anus or bladder, frequency and urgency of urination.
Tongue Pale.
Pulse Weak.

Acupuncture

Ren-12 Zhongwan, ST-36 Zusanli, SP-3 Taibai, SP-6 Sanyinjiao, BL-20 Pishu, BL-21 Weishu, Du-20 Baihui, Ren-6 Qihai, ST-21 Liangmen, Du-1 Chengqiang. Moxa is applicable.

Prescription

Bu Zhong Yi Qi Tang *Tonifying the Centre and Benefiting Qi Decoction.*

SPLEEN NOT CONTROLLING BLOOD

Clinical manifestations

Poor appetite, slight abdominal distension after eating, tiredness, lassitude, pale complexion, weakness of the limbs, loose stools, depression, tendency to obesity, blood spots under the skin, blood in the urine or stools, excessive uterine bleeding, sallow complexion.
Tongue Pale.
Pulse Weak or Fine.

Acupuncture

Ren-12 Zhongwan, ST-36 Zusanli, SP-3 Taibai, SP-6 Sanyinjiao, BL-20 Pishu, BL-21 Weishu, Du-20

Baihui, Ren-6 Qihai, BL-17 Geshu, SP-10 Xuehai, SP-1 Yinbai.

Prescription

Gui Pi Tang *Tonifying the Spleen Decoction*.

SPLEEN-YIN DEFICIENCY PATTERNS

Spleen-Yin deficiency
Clinical manifestations

Poor appetite, poor digestion, retching, gnawing hunger, loss of sense of taste, slight epigastric pain, dry mouth, dry lips, dry stools, thin body, night sweating, sallow complexion with possibly red tip of the nose.
Tongue   Without coating, transversal cracks on the sides.
Pulse   Weak or Floating-Empty.

Acupuncture

ST-36 Zusanli, Ren-12 Zhongwan, SP-6 Sanyinjiao.

Prescription

Ma Zi Ren Wan *Cannabis Pill*
Wu Ren Wan *Five-Seed Pill*
Shen Ling Bai Zhu San *Ginseng-Poria-Atractylodes Powder*.

Spleen-Yin deficiency with Empty-Heat
Clinical manifestations

Poor appetite, poor digestion, retching, gnawing hunger, loss of sense of taste, slight epigastric pain, dry mouth, dry lips, dry stools, thin body, sallow complexion with possibly red tip of the nose, malar flush, a feeling of heat in the evening, night sweating.
Tongue   Red without coating, transversal cracks on the sides.
Pulse   Floating-Empty and Rapid.

Acupuncture

ST-36 Zusanli, Ren-12 Zhongwan, SP-6 Sanyinjiao.

Prescription

Ma Zi Ren Wan *Cannabis Pill*
Wu Ren Wan *Five-Seed Pill*
Shen Ling Bai Zhu San *Ginseng-Poria-Atractylodes Powder*
plus (for any of the above prescriptions): Zhi Mu *Radix Anemarrhenae asphodeloidis*.

COLD-DAMPNESS IN THE SPLEEN

Clinical manifestations

Poor appetite, a feeling of fullness of the epigastrium/abdomen, a feeling of cold in the epigastrium which improves with the application of heat, a feeling of heaviness of the head and body, a sweetish taste or absence of taste, absence of thirst, loose stools, lassitude, tiredness, nausea, oedema, dull-white complexion, excessive white vaginal discharge.
Tongue   Pale with a sticky white coating.
Pulse   Slippery-Slow.

Acupuncture

SP-9 Yinlingquan, SP-6 Sanyinjiao, Ren-12 Zhongwan, SP-3 Taibai, ST-8 Touwei, BL-22 Sanjiaoshu, BL-20 Pishu, Ren-9 Shuifen, Ren-11 Jianli, ST-22 Guanmen, ST-28 Shuidao.

Prescription

Ping Wei San *Balancing the Stomach Powder*.

DAMP-HEAT IN THE SPLEEN

Clinical manifestations

A feeling of fullness of the epigastrium/lower abdomen, epigastric/abdominal pain, poor appetite, a feeling of heaviness, thirst without a desire to drink, nausea, vomiting, loose stools with an offensive odour, burning sensation in the anus, a feeling of heat, scanty dark urine, low-grade fever, dull headache with a feeling of heaviness of the head, dull-yellow complexion like tangerine peel, yellow sclera of the eyes, oily sweat, bitter taste, itchy skin or skin eruptions (papules or vesicles), sweating which does not relieve the fever and does not lead to the clearing of Heat.
Tongue   Red with sticky yellow coating.
Pulse   Slippery-Rapid.

Acupuncture

SP-9 Yinlingquan, SP-6 Sanyinjiao, Du-9 Zhiyang, LI-11 Quchi, BL-20 Pishu, GB-34 Yanglingquan, Ren-9 Shuifen, Ren-11 Jianli, ST-22 Guanmen, ST-28 Shuidao, BL-22 Sanjiaoshu.

Prescription

Lian Po Yin *Coptis-Magnolia Decoction*.

SPLEEN-HEAT

Clinical manifestations

Burning epigastric/abdominal pain, excessive hunger, red tip of the nose, dry lips, mouth ulcers, thirst, dry stools, a feeling of heat, scanty dark urine, yellow complexion.
Tongue Red with dry yellow coating.
Pulse Overflowing-Rapid.

Acupuncture

SP-9 Yinlingquan, SP-6 Sanyinjiao, SP-2 Dadu, LI-11 Quchi, ST-44 Neiting, Ren-11 Jianli, BL-20 Pishu.

Prescription

Xie Huang San *Draining the Yellow Powder*.

PHLEGM OBSTRUCTING THE MIDDLE BURNER

Clinical manifestations

A feeling of oppression of the chest and epigastrium, poor appetite, sour regurgitation, nausea, vomiting, gnawing hunger, dizziness, a feeling of heaviness, loose stools.
Tongue Swollen with a thick sticky coating in the centre.
Pulse Slippery on the right Middle position.

Acupuncture

Ren-10 Xiawan, ST-21 Liangmen, Ren-9 Shuifen, ST-22 Guanmen, ST-40 Fenglong, SP-9 Yinglingquan.

Prescription

Er Chen Tang *Two Old Decoction*.

YIN FIRE FROM DEFICIENCY OF THE STOMACH AND SPLEEN AND ORIGINAL QI

Clinical manifestations

Tiredness, a feeling of heat in the face but a feeling of cold in general, alternating feelings of heat and cold, dry mouth, dry lips, thirst, a feeling as if coming down with a cold, mouth ulcers, insomnia, poor appetite, loose stools, weak limbs.

Tongue Pale
Pulse Empty or slightly Overflowing but Empty.

Acupuncture

Ren-4 Guanyuan (moxa is applicable), Ren-12 Zhongwan, ST-36 Zusanli, SP-6 Sanyinjiao, TB-5 Waiguan, BL-20 Pishu, BL-21 Weishu, P-6 Neiguan.

Prescription

Bu Zhong Yi Qi Tang *Tonifying the Centre and Benefiting Qi Decoction*.

COMBINED PATTERNS

The Spleen Combined Patterns are:

> - Spleen- and Stomach-Qi deficiency
> - Spleen- and Heart-Blood deficiency
> - Spleen- and Lung-Qi deficiency
> - Spleen- and Liver-Blood deficiency
> - obstruction of the Spleen by Dampness with stagnation of Liver-Qi (Spleen insulting the Liver).

Spleen- and Stomach-Qi deficiency
Clinical manifestations

Poor appetite, slight abdominal distension after eating, tiredness, lassitude, pale complexion, weakness of the limbs, loose stools, an uncomfortable feeling in the epigastrium, lack of sense of taste.
Tongue Pale.
Pulse Empty, especially on the right Middle position.

Acupuncture

Ren-12 Zhongwan, ST-36 Zusanli, SP-3 Taibai, SP-6 Sanyinjiao, BL-20 Pishu, BL-21 Weishu, Ren-6 Qihai. Moxa is applicable.

Prescription

Si Jun Zi Tang *Four Gentlemen Decoction*
Shen Ling Bai Zhu San *Ginseng-Poria-Atractylodes Powder*.

Spleen- and heart-blood deficiency
Clinical manifestations

Palpitations, dizziness, insomnia, dream-disturbed sleep, poor memory, anxiety, tendency to be easily star-

tled, dull-pale complexion, pale lips, tiredness, weak muscles, loose stools, poor appetite, scanty periods.
Tongue   Pale and Thin.
Pulse   Choppy or Fine.

Acupuncture

HE-7 Shenmen, P-6 Neiguan, Ren-14 Juque, Ren-15 Jiuwei, Ren-4 Guanyuan, BL-17 Geshu (with moxa), BL-20 Pishu, Ren-12 Zhongwan, ST-36 Zusanli, SP-6 Sanyinjiao.

Prescription

Gui Pi Tang *Tonifying the Spleen Decoction.*

Spleen- and Lung-Qi deficiency
Clinical manifestations

Poor appetite, slight abdominal distension after eating, tiredness, lassitude, pale complexion, weakness of the limbs, loose stools, slight depression, tendency to obesity, slight shortness of breath, slight cough, weak voice, spontaneous daytime sweating, dislike of speaking, tendency to catch colds, dislike of cold.
Tongue   Pale.
Pulse   Empty, especially on the right side.

Acupuncture

LU-9 Taiyuan, LU-7 Lieque, Ren-6 Qihai, BL-13 Feishu, Du-12 Shenzhu, ST-36 Zusanli, Ren-12 Zhongwan, SP-3 Taibai, SP-6 Sanyinjiao, BL-20 Pishu, BL-21 Weishu.

Prescription

Si Jun Zi Tang *Four Gentlemen Decoction* plus Huang Qi *Radix Astragali membranacei.*

Spleen- and Liver-Blood deficiency
Clinical manifestations

Poor appetite, slight abdominal distension after eating, tiredness, lassitude, dull-pale complexion, weakness of the limbs, loose stools, thin body, scanty periods or amenorrhoea, insomnia, dizziness, numbness of the limbs, blurred vision, 'floaters' in eyes, diminished night vision, pale lips, muscular weakness, cramps, withered and brittle nails, dry hair and skin, slight depression, a feeling of aimlessness.
Tongue   Pale body especially on the sides, which in extreme cases can assume an orange colour, and Dry.
Pulse   Choppy or Fine.

Acupuncture

LIV-8 Ququan, SP-6 Sanyinjiao, Ren-4 Guanyuan, BL-18 Ganshu, BL-23 Shenshu, Ren-12 Zhongwan, ST-36 Zusanli, SP-3 Taibai, BL-20 Pishu, BL-21 Weishu, BL-17 Geshu (with direct moxa).

Prescription

Gui Pi Tang *Tonifying the Spleen Decoction.*

Obstruction of the Spleen by Dampness with stagnation of Liver-Qi
Clinical manifestations

A feeling of oppression and fullness of the epigastrium, nausea, lack of appetite, loose stools, a feeling of heaviness, dry mouth without a desire to drink, sallow complexion, hypochondrial pain, bitter taste, a sticky taste, epigastric and hypochondrial distension, irritability.
Tongue   Thick, sticky yellow coating.
Pulse   Slippery-Wiry.

Acupuncture

Ren-12 Zhongwan, SP-6 Sanyinjiao, SP-3 Taibai, BL-20 Pishu, LIV-13 Zhangmen, LIV-14 Qimen, GB-24 Riyue, GB-34 Yanglingquan, LIV-3 Taichong, ST-19 Burong, SP-9 Yinlingquan.

Prescription

Ping Wei San *Balancing the Stomach Powder* plus Mu Xiang *Radix Aucklandiae lappae* and Xiang Fu *Rhizoma Cyperi rotundi*
Huo Xiang Zheng Qi San *Agastache Upright Qi Powder* plus Mu Xiang *Radix Aucklandiae lappae* and Xiang Fu *Rhizoma Cyperi rotundi*
Yi Jia Jian Zheng Qi San *First Variation of Upright Qi Powder.*

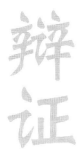

Chapter **93**

LIVER

Chapter contents

LIVER-QI STAGNATION PATTERNS   *891*
    Stagnation of Liver-Qi   *891*
    Stagnant Liver-Qi turning into Heat   *891*
    Liver-Qi stagnation with Phlegm   *892*

REBELLIOUS LIVER-QI   *892*

LIVER-YANG RISING   *892*

LIVER-BLOOD STASIS   *892*

LIVER-FIRE BLAZING UPWARDS   *893*

DAMP-HEAT   *893*
    Damp-Heat in the Liver   *893*
    Damp-Heat in the Liver and Gall-Bladder   *893*

LIVER-WIND   *893*
    Extreme Heat generating Wind   *893*
    Liver-Yang rising generating Wind   *894*
    Liver-Fire generating Wind   *894*
    Liver-Blood deficiency giving rise to Wind   *894*
    Liver-Wind harbouring Phlegm   *895*

LIVER-BLOOD DEFICIENCY PATTERNS   *895*
    Liver-Blood deficiency   *895*
    Liver-Blood deficiency with Phlegm   *895*

STAGNATION OF COLD IN THE LIVER CHANNEL   *895*

LIVER-YIN DEFICIENCY PATTERNS   *895*
    Liver-Yin deficiency   *895*
    Liver-Yin deficiency with Empty-Heat   *896*

LIVER-QI DEFICIENCY   *896*

LIVER PHLEGM-FIRE   *896*

LIVER-YANG DEFICIENCY   *896*

COMBINED PATTERNS   *897*
    Rebellious Liver-Qi invading the Spleen   *897*
    Rebellious Liver-Qi invading the Stomach   *897*
    Liver-Fire insulting the Lungs   *897*
    Liver- and Heart-Blood deficiency   *898*

LIVER-QI STAGNATION PATTERNS

Stagnation of Liver-Qi
Clinical manifestations

Hypochondrial or epigastric distension, a slight feeling of oppression of the chest, irritability, melancholy, depression, moodiness, premenstrual tension, irregular periods, premenstrual breast distension, a feeling of a lump in the throat.
Tongue   In light cases the tongue-body colour may not change; in severe cases the sides will be red.
Pulse   Wiry, especially on the left side.

Acupuncture

P-6 Neiguan, GB-34 Yanglingquan, LIV-13 Zhangmen, LIV-14 Qimen, LIV-3 Taichong, TB-6 Zhigou.

Prescription

Yue Ju Wan *Gardenia-Ligusticum Pill*
Xiao Yao San *Free and Easy Wanderer Powder*.

Stagnant Liver-Qi turning into Heat
Clinical manifestations

Hypochondrial or epigastric distension, a slight feeling of oppression of the chest, irritability, melancholy, depression, moodiness, premenstrual tension, irregular periods, premenstrual breast distension, a

feeling of a lump in the throat, a feeling of heat, red face, thirst, propensity to outbursts of anger, heavy periods.

Tongue   Red on the sides.

Pulse   Wiry, especially on the left side and slightly Rapid.

Acupuncture

P-6 Neiguan, GB-34 Yanglingquan, LIV-13 Zhangmen, LIV-14 Qimen, LIV-3 Taichong, TB-6 Zhigou, LIV-2 Xingjian.

Prescription

Dan Zhi Xiao Yao San *Moutan-Gardenia Free and Easy Wanderer Powder*.

Liver-Qi stagnation with Phlegm

Clinical manifestations

Mental depression, irritability, moodiness, a feeling of oppression of the chest, a feeling of a lump in the throat, difficulty in swallowing, sighing, cough with expectoration of phlegm, hypochondrial distension, premenstrual breast distension, swelling and pain.

Tongue   Swollen with a sticky coating.

Pulse   Wiry-Slippery.

Acupuncture

LIV-3 Taichong, ST-40 Fenglong, LI-4 Hegu, Du-24 Shenting, GB-13 Benshen, P-7 Daling, P-6 Neiguan.

Prescription

Yue Ju Wan *Gardenia-Ligusticum Pill*
Ban Xia Hou Po Tang *Pinellia-Magnolia Decoction*
Ju He Wan *Citrus Seed Pill*
Si Hai Shu Yu Wan *Fours Seas Soothe Stagnation Pill* (specific for goitre from Qi stagnation and Phlegm).

REBELLIOUS LIVER-QI

Clinical manifestations

Hypochondrial or epigastric distension, hiccup, sighing, nausea, vomiting, belching, 'churning feeling in the stomach', irritability, breast distension in women.

Tongue   In light cases the tongue-body colour may not change; in severe cases the sides will be Red.

Pulse   Wiry. It may be particularly Wiry on the Liver and Stomach positions.

Acupuncture

LIV-14 Qimen, P-6 Neiguan, GB-34 Yanglingquan, LIV-3 Taichong, TB-6 Zhigou, LI-4 Hegu, ST-21 Liangmen, ST-19 Burong.

Prescription

Chai Hu Shu Gan Tang *Bupleurum Soothing the Liver Decoction*
Yi Gan San *Restrain the Liver Powder*.

LIVER-YANG RISING

Clinical manifestations

Headache which may be on the temples, eyes or lateral side of the head, dizziness, tinnitus, deafness, blurred vision, dry mouth and throat, insomnia, irritability, a feeling of being worked-up, propensity to outbursts of anger, stiff neck.

Tongue   The tongue presentation may vary widely depending on the underlying condition causing Liver-Yang rising. If this derives from Liver-Blood deficiency the tongue-body colour will be Pale; if it derives from Liver-Yin deficiency the tongue-body colour will be slightly Red on the sides and without coating. In some cases, Liver-Yang rising may develop from rebellious Liver-Qi; in this case the tongue-body colour may be normal or slightly red on the sides.

Pulse   Wiry. However, if there is a background of Liver-Blood or Liver-Yin deficiency, the pulse may be Wiry only on one side, or it may also be Wiry but Fine.

Acupuncture

LIV-3 Taichong, TB-5 Waiguan, P-6 Neiguan, LI-4 Hegu, GB-43 Xiaxi, GB-38 Yangfu, BL-2 Zanzhu, Taiyang extra point, GB-20 Fengchi, GB-9 Tianchong, GB-8 Shuaigu, GB-6 Xuanli. In cases of Liver-Blood or Liver-Yin deficiency: SP-6 Sanyinjiao, KI-3 Taixi, LIV-8 Ququan, ST-36 Zusanli.

Prescription

Tian Ma Gou Teng Yin *Gastrodia-Uncaria Decoction*
Ling Jiao Gou Teng Tang *Cornu Antelopis-Uncaria Decoction*.

LIVER-BLOOD STASIS

Clinical manifestations

Hypochondrial pain, abdominal pain, vomiting of blood, epistaxis, painful periods, irregular periods, dark

and clotted menstrual blood, infertility, masses in the abdomen, purple nails, purple lips, purple or dark complexion, dry skin (in severe cases), purple petechiae.
Tongue Purple especially, or only, on the sides. In severe cases, there will be purple spots on the sides.
Pulse Wiry or Firm.

Acupuncture

GB-34 Yanglingquan, LIV-3 Taichong, BL-18 Ganshu, BL-17 Geshu, SP-10 Xuehai, Ren-6 Qihai, SP-4 Gongsun and P-6 Neiguan (opening points of the Penetrating Vessel), ST-29 Guilai, KI-14 Siman, LIV-5 Ligou, LIV-6 Zhongdu.

Prescription

Ge Xia Zhu Yu Tang *Eliminating Stasis below the Diaphragm Decoction*
Shi Xiao San *Breaking into a Smile Powder*
Yan Hu Suo Tang *Corydalis Decoction*.

LIVER-FIRE BLAZING UPWARDS

Clinical manifestations

Irritability, propensity to outbursts of anger, tinnitus/deafness (with sudden onset), temporal headache, dizziness, red face and eyes, thirst, bitter taste, dream-disturbed sleep, constipation with dry stools, dark-yellow urine, epistaxis, haematemesis, haemoptysis.
Tongue Red with redder sides and dry yellow coating.
Pulse Wiry-Rapid.

Acupuncture

LIV-2 Xingjian, LIV-3 Taichong, GB-20 Fengchi, Taiyang extra point, GB-13 Benshen, LI-11 Quchi, GB-1 Tongziliao, GB-9 Tianchong, GB-8 Shuaigu, GB-6 Xuanli, Du-24 Shenting, SP-6 Sanyinjiao, LIV-1 Dadun.

Prescription

Long Dan Xie Gan Tang *Gentiana Draining the Liver Decoction*
Dang Gui Long Hui Tang *Angelica-Gentiana-Aloe Decoction*.

DAMP-HEAT

Damp-Heat in the Liver
Clinical manifestations

Fullness of the hypochondrium, abdomen or hypogastrium, bitter taste, poor appetite, nausea, a feeling of heaviness of the body, yellow vaginal discharge, vaginal itching, vulvar eczema or sores, mid-cycle bleeding/pain, pain, redness and swelling of the scrotum, genital, papular or vesicular skin rashes and itching, urinary difficulty, burning on urination, dark urine.
Tongue Red body with redder sides, sticky-yellow coating.
Pulse Slippery-Wiry-Rapid.

Prescription

Long Dan Xie Gan Tang *Gentiana Draining the Liver Decoction*.

Damp-Heat in the Liver and Gall-Bladder
Clinical manifestations

Fullness of the hypochondrium, abdomen or hypogastrium, bitter taste, poor appetite, nausea, a feeling of heaviness of the body, yellow vaginal discharge, vaginal itching, vulvar eczema or sores, mid-cycle bleeding/pain, pain, redness and swelling of the scrotum, genital, papular or vesicular skin rashes and itching, urinary difficulty, burning on urination, dark urine, hypochondrial pain, fever, yellow complexion and eyes, vomiting.
Tongue Red body with redder sides, unilateral or bilateral sticky yellow coating.
Pulse Slippery-Wiry-Rapid.

Acupuncture

LIV-14 Qimen, GB-24 Riyue, GB-34 Yanglingquan, BL-18 Ganshu, BL-19 Danshu, Du-9 Zhiyang, Ren-12 Zhongwan, SP-9 Yinlingquan, SP-6 Sanyinjiao, SP-3 Taibai, LI-11 Quchi, LIV-2 Xingjian, LIV-3 Taichong.

Prescription

Long Dan Xie Gan Tang *Gentiana Draining the Liver Decoction*.

LIVER-WIND

Extreme Heat generating Wind
Clinical manifestations

High temperature, convulsions, rigidity of the neck, tremor of the limbs, opisthotonos, in severe cases coma.
Tongue Deep-Red, Stiff, dry yellow coating.
Pulse Wiry-Rapid.

Acupuncture

LIV-3 Taichong, LIV-2 Xingjian, Shixuan extra points, SI-3 Houxi, Du-20 Baihui, Du-16 Fengfu, GB-20 Fengchi, Du-8 Jinsuo, Du-14 Dazhui.

Prescription

Ling Jiao Gou Teng Tang *Cornu Antelopis-Uncaria Decoction.*

Liver-Yang rising generating Wind

Liver-Yang rising deriving from Liver-Yin deficiency

Clinical manifestations

Tremor, facial tic, severe dizziness, tinnitus, headache, hypertension, dry throat, dry eyes, blurred vision, numbness/tingling of the limbs, poor memory.
Tongue   Normal-coloured without coating.
Pulse   Wiry-Fine.

Acupuncture

LIV-3 Taichong, GB-20 Fengchi, LI-4 Hegu, TB-5 Waiguan, Du-19 Houding, SP-6 Sanyinjiao, LIV-8 Ququan, KI-3 Taixi.

Prescription

Da Ding Feng Zhu *Big Stopping Wind Pearl* (for febrile-disease Heat injuring Yin)
San Jia Fu Mai Tang *Three Carapaces Restoring the Pulse Decoction.*

Liver-Yang rising deriving from Liver- and Kidney-Yin deficiency

Clinical manifestations

Tremor, facial tic, severe dizziness, tinnitus, headache, hypertension, dry throat, dry eyes, blurred vision, numbness/tingling of the limbs, poor memory, backache, scanty urination, night sweating.
Tongue   Normal coloured without coating.
Pulse   Wiry-Fine.

Acupuncture

LIV-3 Taichong, GB-20 Fengchi, LI-4 Hegu, TB-5 Waiguan, Du-19 Houding, SP-6 Sanyinjiao, LIV-8 Ququan, KI-3 Taixi, KI-6 Zhaohai, Ren-4 Guanyuan.

Prescription

Zhen Gan Xi Feng Tang *Pacifying the Liver and Subduing Wind Decoction*
Jian Ling Tang *Constructing Roof Tiles Decoction.*

Liver-Yang rising deriving from Liver-Blood deficiency

Clinical manifestations

Tremor, dizziness, tinnitus, headache, hypertension, dry throat, blurred vision, numbness/tingling of the limbs, poor memory, insomnia.
Tongue   Pale and Thin.
Pulse   Wiry-Fine.

Acupuncture

LIV-3 Taichong, GB-20 Fengchi, LI-4 Hegu, TB-5 Waiguan, Du-19 Houding, SP-6 Sanyinjiao, LIV-8 Ququan, KI-3 Taixi, BL-17 Geshu, Ren-4 Guanyuan.

Prescription

E Jiao Ji Zi Huang Tang *Gelatinum Corii Asini-Egg Yolk Decoction.*

Liver-Fire generating Wind

Clinical manifestations

Tremor, irritability, propensity to outbursts of anger, tinnitus/deafness (with sudden onset), temporal headache, dizziness, red face and eyes, thirst, bitter taste, dream-disturbed sleep, constipation with dry stools, dark-yellow urine, epistaxis, haematemesis, haemoptysis.
Tongue   Red with redder sides and dry yellow coating.
Pulse   Wiry-Rapid.

Acupuncture

LIV-2 Xingjian, LIV-3 Taichong, GB-20 Fengchi, Taiyang extra point, GB-13 Benshen, LI-11 Quchi, GB-1 Tongziliao, GB-9 Tianchong, GB-8 Shuaigu, GB-6 Xuanli, Du-24 Shenting, SP-6 Sanyinjiao, LIV-1 Dadun, Du-8 Jinsuo.

Prescription

Ling Jiao Gou Teng Tang *Cornu Antelopis-Uncaria Decoction* plus Long Dan Cao *Radix Gentianae scabrae.*

Liver-Blood deficiency giving rise to Wind

Clinical manifestations

Fine tremor, facial tic, dizziness, blurred vision, numbness/tingling of the limbs, poor memory, insomnia, scanty periods.
Tongue   Pale and Thin.
Pulse   Wiry-Fine.

Acupuncture

LIV-3 Taichong, GB-20 Fengchi, LI-4 Hegu, TB-5 Waiguan, Du-19 Houding, SP-6 Sanyinjiao, LIV-8 Ququan, KI-3 Taixi, BL-17 Geshu, Ren-4 Guanyuan.

Prescription

E Jiao Ji Zi Huang Tang *Gelatinum Corii Asini-Egg Yolk Decoction.*

Liver-Wind harbouring Phlegm
Clinical manifestations

Headache, dizziness, blurred vision, a feeling of heaviness and muzziness (fuzziness) of the head, occipital stiffness, tinnitus, nausea, cough with profuse sputum, insomnia, dream-disturbed sleep.
Tongue Stiff, Swollen with sticky coating.
Pulse Wiry-Slippery.

Acupuncture

LIV-3 Taichong, ST-40 Fenglong, LI-4 Hegu, GB-20 Fengchi, ST-8 Touwei, Ren-12 Zhongwan, SP-6 Sanyinjiao.

Prescription

Ban Xia Bai Zhu Tian Ma Tang *Pinellia-Atractylodes-Gastrodia Decoction.*

LIVER-BLOOD DEFICIENCY PATTERNS

Liver-Blood deficiency
Clinical manifestations

Dizziness, numbness/tingling of the limbs, insomnia, blurred vision, 'floaters' in the eyes, diminished night vision, scanty menstruation or amenorrhoea, dull-pale complexion without lustre, pale lips, muscular weakness, cramps, withered and brittle nails, dry hair and skin, depression, a feeling of aimlessness.
Tongue Pale body especially on the sides which, in extreme cases, can assume an orange colour, and Dry.
Pulse Choppy or Fine.

Acupuncture

LIV-8 Ququan, SP-6 Sanyinjiao, ST-36 Zusanli, Ren-4 Guanyuan, BL-18 Ganshu, BL-20 Pishu, BL-23 Shenshu, BL-17 Geshu, Yuyao extra point.

Prescription

Bu Gan Tang *Tonifying the Liver Decoction.*

Liver-Blood deficiency with Phlegm
Clinical manifestations

Mental depression, dizziness, blurred vision, tingling of the limbs, brittle nails, sputum in the throat, a feeling of oppression of the chest, a feeling of muzziness (fuzziness) of the head, irregular periods, late periods.
Tongue Pale with a sticky coating.
Pulse Choppy on the left, Slippery on the right.

Acupuncture

LIV-8 Ququan, SP-6 Sanyinjiao, ST-36 Zusanli, Ren-4 Guanyuan, ST-40 Fenglong, SP-9 Yinlingquan.

Prescription

Ba Zhen Tang *Eight Precious Decoction* plus Er Chen Tang *Two Old Decoction.*

STAGNATION OF COLD IN THE LIVER CHANNEL

Clinical manifestations

Fullness and distension of the hypogastrium with pain, which refers downwards to the scrotum and testis and upwards to the hypochondrium, alleviation of the pain by warmth, straining of the testis or contraction of the scrotum, vertical headache, a feeling of cold, cold hands and feet, vomiting of clear watery fluid or dry vomiting. In women there can be shrinking of the vagina.
Tongue Pale and wet with a white coating.
Pulse Deep-Wiry-Slow.

Acupuncture

Ren-3 Zhongji, LIV-5 Ligou, LIV-1 Dadun, LIV-3 Taichong. Moxa is applicable.

Prescription

Nuan Gan Jian *Warming the Liver Decoction.*

LIVER-YIN DEFICIENCY PATTERNS

Liver-Yin deficiency
Clinical manifestations

Dizziness, numbness/tingling of the limbs, insomnia, blurred vision, 'floaters' in the eyes, dry eyes, diminished night vision, scanty menstruation or amenorrhoea, dull-pale complexion without lustre but with

red cheekbones, muscular weakness, cramps, withered and brittle nails, very dry hair and skin, depression, a feeling of aimlessness.
Tongue Normal coloured without coating or with rootless coating.
Pulse Floating-Empty.

Acupuncture

LIV-8 Ququan, SP-6 Sanyinjiao, ST-36 Zusanli, Ren-4 Guanyuan, KI-3 Taixi, KI-6 Zhaohai, Yuyao extra point.

Prescription

Yi Guan Jian *One Linking Decoction*.

Liver-Yin deficiency with Empty-Heat

Clinical manifestations

Dizziness, numbness/tingling of the limbs, insomnia, blurred vision, 'floaters' in the eyes, dry eyes, diminished night vision, scanty menstruation, or heavy menstrual bleeding (if Empty-Heat is severe), red cheekbones, muscular weakness, cramps, withered and brittle nails, very dry hair and skin, depression, a feeling of aimlessness, anxiety, a feeling of heat in the evening, night sweating, five-palm heat, thirst with a desire to drink in small sips.
Tongue Red without coating.
Pulse Floating-Empty and slightly Rapid.

Acupuncture

LIV-8 Ququan, SP-6 Sanyinjiao, ST-36 Zusanli, Ren-4 Guanyuan, KI-3 Taixi, KI-6 Zhaohai, Yuyao extra point, LIV-2 Xingjian, LI-11 Quchi.

Prescription

Yi Guan Jian *One Linking Decoction* plus Zhi Mu *Radix Anemarrhenae asphodeloidis* and Mu Dan Pi *Cortex Moutan radicis*
Qing Hao Bie Jia Tang *Artemisia Annua-Carapax Amydae Decoction*
Qing Gu San *Clearing the Bones Powder*.

LIVER-QI DEFICIENCY

Clinical manifestations

Dizziness, blurred vision, floaters, nervousness, timidity, tendency to be easily startled, lack of courage and initiative, indecision, sighing, restless dreams, depres-

sion, irritability, hypochondrial distension, irregular periods.
Tongue Pale or normal.
Pulse Weak.

Acupuncture

LIV-8 Ququan, GB-40 Qiuxu, ST-36 Zusanli, SP-6 Sanyinjiao, Ren-4 Guanyuan, BL-18 Ganshu.

Prescription

Empirical prescription by Dr Chen Jia Xu.[1]

LIVER PHLEGM-FIRE

Clinical manifestations

Irritability, propensity to outbursts of anger, tinnitus/deafness (with sudden onset), temporal headache, dizziness, red face and eyes, thirst, bitter taste, dream-disturbed sleep, constipation with dry stools, dark-yellow urine, epistaxis, haematemesis, haemoptysis, a feeling of oppression of the chest, rattling sound in the throat, a feeling of muzziness (fuzziness) of the head, expectoration of sputum, hypertension.
Tongue Red with redder sides, Swollen and with sticky yellow coating.
Pulse Wiry-Slippery-Rapid.

Acupuncture

LIV-2 Xingjian, LIV-3 Taichong, GB-20 Fengchi, Taiyang extra point, GB-13 Benshen, LI-11 Quchi, GB-1 Tongziliao, GB-9 Tianchong, GB-8 Shuaigu, GB-6 Xuanli, Du-24 Shenting, SP-6 Sanyinjiao, LIV-1 Dadun, Ren-12 Zhongwan, ST-40 Fenglong, SP-9 Yinlingquan, LI-4 Hegu.

Prescription

Wen Dan Tang *Warming the Gall-Bladder Decoction*
Ling Jiao Gou Teng Tang *Cornu Antelopis-Uncaria Decoction*.

LIVER-YANG DEFICIENCY

Clinical manifestations

Tendency to worry, fearfulness, moroseness, depression, floaters, blurred vision, a feeling of cold, hypochondrial pain and distension, cold legs, numbness of the head and body, tingling of the limbs, greenish complexion, pale and withered nails, contraction of

the tendons, inability to grasp, lack of libido, impotence, cold penis, damp scrotum, nocturnal emissions without dreams, contraction of the vagina, a feeling of cold and pain in the abdomen in women, late periods, trickling of periods, a feeling of cold in the waist, infertility.

Tongue Pale.

Pulse Deep-Fine or Wiry-Slow but Weak on the left Middle position.

Acupuncture

LIV-8 Ququan, LIV-3 Taichong, BL-18 Ganshu, HE-7 Shenmen, TB-3 Zhongzhu, Du-20 Baihui. Moxa is applicable.

Prescription

Long Chi Qing Hun Tang *Dens Draconis Clearing the Ethereal Soul Decoction*

Wen Yang Bu Gan Jian *Warming Yang and Tonifying the Liver Decoction* plus Ren Shen *Radix Ginseng*, Huang Qi *Radix Astragali membranacei*, Chai Hu *Radix Bupleuri*, Sheng Ma *Rhizoma Cimicifugae*.

COMBINED PATTERNS

The Liver combined patterns are:

- rebellious Liver-Qi invading the Spleen
- rebellious Liver-Qi invading the Stomach
- Liver-Fire insulting the Lungs
- Liver- and Kidney-Yin deficiency (see Chapter 95, 'Kidneys' under combined patterns)
- Liver- and Kidney-Yin deficiency with Empty-Heat (see Chapter 95, 'Kidneys' under combined patterns)
- Liver- and Heart-Blood deficiency.

Rebellious Liver-Qi invading the Spleen
Clinical manifestations

Irritability, abdominal distension and pain, alternation of constipation and diarrhoea, stools sometimes dry and bitty (small pieces) and sometimes loose, flatulence, tiredness.

Tongue Normal coloured or slightly Red on the sides.

Pulse Wiry on the left and Weak on the right.

Acupuncture

LIV-13 Zhangmen, LIV-14 Qimen, LIV-3 Taichong, GB-34 Yanglingquan, Ren-6 Qihai, ST-25 Tianshu, SP-15 Daheng, Ren-12 Zhongwan, TB-6 Zhigou, ST-36 Zusanli, SP-6 Sanyinjiao, P-6 Neiguan.

Prescription

Xiao Yao San *Free and Easy Wanderer Powder*.

Rebellious Liver-Qi invading the Stomach
Clinical manifestations

Irritability, epigastric and hypochondrial distension and pain, a feeling of oppression in the epigastrium, sour regurgitation, hiccup, belching, nausea, vomiting, sighing, weak limbs.

Tongue Normal coloured or slightly Red on the sides.

Pulse Wiry on the left and Weak on the right or Wiry on both Middle positions.

Acupuncture

LIV-14 Qimen, GB-34 Yanglingquan, Ren-13 Shangwan, Ren-10 Xiawan, ST-21 Liangmen, ST-19 Burong, ST-36 Zusanli, ST-34 Liangqiu, BL-21 Weishu.

Prescription

Si Mo Tang *Four Milled-Herb Decoction*
Xuan Fu Dai Zhe Tang *Inula-Haematite Decoction*
Ju Pi Zhu Ru Tang *Citrus-Bambusa Decoction*
Ding Xiang Shi Di Tang *Caryophyllum-Diospyros Decoction*
Ban Xia Hou Po Tang *Pinellia-Magnolia Decoction* plus Zuo Jin Wan *Left Metal Pill*.

Liver-Fire insulting the Lungs
Clinical manifestations

Breathlessness, asthma, a feeling of fullness and distension of the chest and hypochondrium, cough with a yellow or blood-tinged sputum, headache, dizziness, red face, thirst, bitter taste, bloodshot eyes, scanty dark urine, constipation.

Tongue Red with redder sides and dry yellow coating.

Pulse Wiry.

Acupuncture

LIV-2 Xingjian, LIV-3 Taichong, LIV-14 Qimen, Ren-17 Shanzhong, Ren-22 Tiantu, P-6 Neiguan, LU-7 Lieque, LI-11 Quchi.

Prescription

Long Dan Xie Gan Tang *Gentiana Draining the Liver Decoction* plus Su Zi *Fructus Perillae frutescentis*, Sang Bai Pi *Cortex Mori albae radicis* and Zhu Ru *Caulis Bambusae in Taeniis*.

Liver- and Heart-Blood deficiency
Clinical manifestations

Palpitations, dizziness, insomnia, dream-disturbed sleep, poor memory, anxiety, tendency to be easily startled, dull-pale complexion, pale lips, blurred vision, 'floaters' in the eyes, diminished night vision, numbness/tingling of the limbs, scanty periods or amenorrhoea, cramps, muscular weakness, dry hair and skin, depression, a feeling of aimlessness, withered and brittle nails.
Tongue   Pale and Thin.
Pulse   Choppy or Fine, especially on the left.

Acupuncture

HE-7 Shenmen, P-6 Neiguan, Ren-14 Juque, Ren-4 Guanyuan, Ren-15 Jiuwei, BL-17 Geshu, BL-18 Ganshu, BL-20 Pishu, LIV-8 Ququan, SP-6 Sanyinjiao, ST-36 Zusanli.

Prescription

Gui Pi Tang *Tonifying the Spleen Decoction*
Sheng Yu Tang *Sage Healing Decoction*
Bu Gan Tang *Tonifying the Liver Decoction*
Dang Gui Ji Xue Teng Tang *Angelica-Ji Xue Teng Decoction*.

NOTES

1. Chen Jia Xu, Discussion on the syndrome of Liver-Qi deficiency, in Journal of Chinese Medicine (*Zhong Yi Za Zhi* 中 医 杂 志), Beijing, 5, 1994, pp. 264–267.

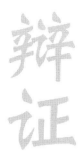

Chapter **94**

LUNGS

Chapter contents

LUNG-QI DEFICIENCY PATTERNS   899
  Lung-Qi deficiency   899
  Lung-Qi deficiency with Phlegm   899

LUNG-YANG DEFICIENCY   900

LUNG-YIN DEFICIENCY PATTERNS   900
  Lung-Yin deficiency   900
  Lung-Yin deficiency with Empty-Heat   900
  Lung-Yin deficiency with Phlegm   900

LUNG-QI AND LUNG-YIN DEFICIENCY   900

LUNG-DRYNESS   901

INVASION OF LUNGS BY WIND   901
  Invasion of Lungs by Wind-Cold   901
  Invasion of Lungs by Wind-Heat   901
  Invasion of Lungs by Wind-Dryness   901
  Invasion of Lungs by Wind-Water   901

LUNG-HEAT   902

PHLEGM PATTERNS   902
  Damp-Phlegm in the Lungs   902
  Cold-Phlegm in the Lungs   902
  Phlegm-Heat in the Lungs   902
  Phlegm-Dryness in the Lungs   902
  Phlegm-Fluids in the Lungs   903

LUNG-QI STAGNATION   903

LUNG-QI COLLAPSE   903

COMBINED PATTERNS   903
  Lung- and Heart-Qi deficiency   903

LUNG-QI DEFICIENCY PATTERNS

Lung-Qi deficiency
Clinical manifestations
Slight shortness of breath, slight cough, weak voice, spontaneous daytime sweating, dislike of speaking, bright-white complexion, tendency to catch colds, tiredness, dislike of cold.
Tongue   Pale.
Pulse   Empty, especially on the right Front position.

Acupuncture
LU-9 Taiyuan, LU-7 Lieque, Ren-6 Qihai, BL-13 Feishu, Du-12 Shenzhu, ST-36 Zusanli, Ren-12 Zhongwan.

Prescription
Ren Shen Bu Fei Tang *Ginseng Tonifying the Lungs Decoction.*

Lung-Qi deficiency with Phlegm
Clinical manifestations
Chronic cough which is worse on exertion, scanty phlegm that is difficult to expectorate or dilute watery phlegm, spontaneous sweating, a feeling of cold, shortness of breath, a feeling of oppression of the chest, weak voice.
Tongue   Pale and slightly Swollen in the front.
Pulse   Empty on the right Front position and slightly Slippery.

Acupuncture
LU-9 Taiyuan, ST-36 Zusanli, Ren-12 Zhongwan, ST-40 Fenglong, Ren-17 Shanzhong, BL-13 Feishu.

Prescription

Bu Fei Tang *Tonifying the Lungs Decoction* plus Er Chen Tang *Two Old Decoction*.

LUNG-YANG DEFICIENCY

Clinical manifestations

Slight shortness of breath, slight cough with profuse watery sputum, weak voice, spontaneous daytime sweating, dislike of speaking, bright-white complexion, tendency to catch colds, tiredness, dislike of cold, a feeling of cold, cold hands, a feeling of cold of the upper back, absence of thirst.

Tongue   Pale and slightly wet.
Pulse   Weak, especially on the right Front position.

Acupuncture

LU-9 Taiyuan, LU-7 Lieque, Ren-6 Qihai, BL-13 Feishu, Du-12 Shenzhu, ST-36 Zusanli, Ren-12 Zhongwan. Moxa must be used.

Prescription

Sheng Mai San *Generating the Pulse Powder* combined with Gan Cao Gan Jiang Tang *Glycyrrhiza-Zingiber Decoction* plus Huang Qi *Radix Astragali membranacei*.

LUNG-YIN DEFICIENCY PATTERNS

Lung-Yin deficiency
Clinical manifestations

Cough which is dry or with scanty sticky sputum, weak/hoarse voice, dry mouth and throat, tickly throat, tiredness, dislike of speaking, thin body or thin chest, night sweating.

Tongue   Normal coloured, dry without coating (or with rootless coating) in the front part.
Pulse   Floating-Empty.

Acupuncture

LU-9 Taiyuan, Ren-17 Shanzhong, BL-43 Gaohuangshu, BL-13 Feishu, Du-12 Shenzhu, Ren-4 Guanyuan, KI-6 Zhaohai, Ren-12 Zhongwan, SP-6 Sanyinjiao.

Prescription

Bai He Gu Jin Tang *Lilium Consolidating Metal Decoction*.

Lung-Yin deficiency with Empty-Heat
Clinical manifestations

Dry cough or with scanty sticky sputum which could be blood tinged, dry mouth and throat at night, weak/hoarse voice, tickly throat, night sweating, tiredness, malar flush, dislike of speaking, a feeling of heat or a low-grade fever in the evening, five-palm heat, thirst with a desire to drink in small sips, insomnia, anxiety, thin body, thin chest.

Tongue   Red without coating.
Pulse   Floating-Empty and Rapid.

Acupuncture

LU-9 Taiyuan, Ren-17 Shanzhong, BL-43 Gaohuangshu, BL-13 Feishu, Du-12 Shenzhu, Ren-4 Guanyuan, KI-6 Zhaohai, Ren-12 Zhongwan, SP-6 Sanyinjiao, LU-10 Yuji, LI-11 Quchi.

Prescription

Yang Yin Qing Fei Tang *Nourishing Yin and Clearing the Lungs Decoction*.

Lung-Yin deficiency with Phlegm
Clinical manifestations

Bouts of dry cough followed by expectoration of scanty sputum, a feeling of oppression of the chest, night sweating, a feeling of heat in the afternoon, dry throat.

Tongue   Peeled in the front, Swollen, sticky coating in the centre.
Pulse   Weak on the right Front position and slightly Slippery.

Acupuncture

LU-9 Taiyuan, ST-36 Zusanli, SP-6 Sanyinjiao, Ren-12 Zhongwan, ST-40 Fenglong, BL-43 Gaohuangshu.

Prescription

Bai He Gu Jin Tang *Lilium Consolidating Metal Decoction* plus Er Chen Tang *Two Old Decoction*.

LUNG-QI AND LUNG-YIN DEFICIENCY

Clinical manifestations

Slight cough, shortness of breath, weak/hoarse voice, spontaneous daytime sweating, night sweating, dry mouth and throat at night, tiredness, pale complexion, tendency to catch colds.

Tongue Pale if Qi deficiency predominates, normal coloured and without coating if Yin deficiency predominates. The tongue could also be Pale in general but without coating in the front.
Pulse Empty if Qi deficiency predominates, Floating-Empty on the right Front position if Yin deficiency predominates.

Acupuncture

LU-9 Taiyuan, Ren-12 Zhongwan, Ren-6 Qihai, BL-13 Feishu, BL-43 Gaohuangshu, ST-36 Zusanli, SP-6 Sanyinjiao.

Prescription

Sheng Mai San *Generating the Pulse Powder*
Mai Men Dong Tang *Ophipogon Decoction*
Zhu Ye Shi Gao Tang *Lophatherus-Gypsum Decoction* if there is injury of Lung-Yin following a febrile disease and with a pre-existing Lung-Qi deficiency.

LUNG-DRYNESS

Clinical manifestations

Dry cough, dry skin, dry throat, dry mouth, thirst, hoarse voice.
Tongue Dry.
Pulse Empty especially on the right Front position.

Acupuncture

LU-9 Taiyuan, Ren-4 Guanyuan, KI-6 Zhaohai, SP-6 Sanyinjiao, Ren-12 Zhongwan, ST-36 Zusanli.

Prescription

Bai He Gu Jin Tang *Lilium Consolidating Metal Decoction*
Mai Men Dong Tang *Ophiopogon Decoction*
Zeng Ye Tang *Increasing Fluids Decoction*.

INVASION OF LUNGS BY WIND

Invasion of Lungs by Wind-Cold
Clinical manifestations

Aversion to cold, fever, cough, itchy throat, slight breathlessness, stuffed or runny nose with clear watery discharge, sneezing, occipital headache, body aches.
Tongue Thin white coating.
Pulse Floating-Tight.

Acupuncture

LU-7 Lieque, BL-12 Fengmen (with cupping), Du-16 Fengfu.

Prescription

Ma Huang Tang *Ephedra Decoction*.

Invasion of Lungs by Wind-Heat
Clinical manifestations

Aversion to cold, fever, cough, sore throat, stuffed or runny nose with yellow discharge, headache, body aches, slight sweating, slight thirst, swollen tonsils.
Tongue Slightly Red on the sides in the chest areas or on the front part.
Pulse Floating-Rapid.

Acupuncture

LI-4 Hegu, LI-11 Quchi, LU-11 Shaoshang, Du-14 Dazhui, BL-12 Fengmen (with cupping), Du-16 Fengfu, GB-20 Fengchi, TB-5 Waiguan.

Prescription

Sang Ju Yin *Morus-Chrysanthemum Decoction*
Yin Qiao San *Lonicera-Forsythia Powder*.

Invasion of Lungs by Wind-Dryness
Clinical manifestations

Dry cough, aversion to cold, fever, dry throat, tickly throat, dry nose, discomfort in the chest.
Tongue Thin dry white coating.
Pulse Floating.

Acupuncture

LU-7 Lieque, LI-4 Hegu, TB-5 Waiguan, Ren-12 Zhongwan, SP-6 Sanyinjiao, BL-12 Fengmen (with cupping), BL-13 Feishu.

Prescription

Sang Xing Tang *Morus-Prunus Decoction*
Qing Zao Jiu Fei Tang *Clearing Dryness and Rescuing the Lungs Decoction*.

Invasion of Lungs by Wind-Water
Clinical manifestations

Sudden swelling of eyes and face gradually spreading to the whole body, bright shiny complexion, scanty and

palc urination, aversion to wind, fever, cough, slight breathlessness.
Tongue   Sticky white coating.
Pulse   Floating-Slippery.

Acupuncture

LU-7 Lieque, LI-6 Pianli, LI-7 Wenli, LI-4 Hegu, BL-12 Fengmen, Ren-9 Shuifen, BL-13 Feishu.

Prescription

Xiao Qing Long Tang *Small Green Dragon Decoction.*

LUNG-HEAT

Clinical manifestations

Cough, slight breathlessness, a feeling of heat, chest ache, flaring of the nostrils, thirst, red face.
Tongue   Red with yellow coating
Pulse   Overflowing-Rapid.

Acupuncture

LU-5 Chize, LU-10 Yuji, LU-7 Lieque, LI-11 Quchi, LU-1 Zhongfu, BL-13 Feishu.

Prescription

Qing Bai San *Clearing White Powder.*

PHLEGM PATTERNS

Damp-Phlegm in the Lungs
Clinical manifestations

Chronic cough coming in bouts with profuse sticky white sputum which is easy to expectorate, pasty-white complexion, a feeling of oppression in the chest, shortness of breath, dislike of lying down, wheezing, nausea.
Tongue   Swollen with a sticky white coating.
Pulse   Slippery

Acupuncture

LU-5 Chize, LU-7 Lieque, LU-1 Zhongfu, Ren-17 Shanzhong, ST-40 Fenglong, P-6 Neiguan, Ren-22 Tiantu, Ren-12 Zhongwan, Ren-9 Shuifen, BL-20 Pishu, BL-13 Feishu.

Prescription

Er Chen Tang *Two Old Decoction.*

Cold-Phlegm in the Lungs
Clinical manifestations

Cough with expectoration of watery white sputum, aggravated by exposure to cold, a feeling of cold, cold hands, phlegm in the throat, dizziness, a feeling of oppression of the chest, a feeling of cold of the chest.
Tongue   Swollen and wet tongue with a sticky white coating.
Pulse   Slippery-Slow.

Acupuncture

LU-5 Chize, LU-7 Lieque, Ren-17 Shangzhong, Ren-12 Zhongwan, BL-13 Feishu, BL-20 Pishu. Moxa must be used.

Prescription

She Gan Ma Huang Tang *Belamcanda-Ephedra Decoction*
Ling Gui Zhu Gan Tang *Poria-Ramulus Cinnamomi-Atractylodes-Glycyrrhiza Decoction*
Ling Gan Wu Wei Jiang Xin Tang *Poria-Glycyrrhiza-Schisandra-Zingiberis-Asarum Decoction*
San Zi Yang Qin Tang *Three-Seed Nourishing the Ancestors Decoction.*

Phlegm-Heat in the Lungs
Clinical manifestations

Barking cough with profuse sticky yellow or green sputum, shortness of breath, wheezing, a feeling of oppression of the chest, a feeling of heat, thirst, insomnia, agitation.
Tongue   Red, Swollen with a sticky yellow coating.
Pulse   Slippery-Rapid.

Acupuncture

LU-5 Chize, LU-7 Lieque, LU-10 Yuji, LI-11 Quchi, LU-1 Zhongfu, BL-13 Feishu, Ren-12 Zhongwan, ST-40 Fenglong.

Prescription

Wen Dan Tang *Warming the Gall-Bladder Decoction*
Qing Qi Hua Tan Tang *Clearing Qi and Resolving Phlegm Decoction.*

Phlegm-Dryness in the Lungs
Clinical manifestations

Dry cough but with occasional, difficult expectoration of scanty sputum, shortness of breath, a feeling of

oppression of the chest, dry throat, wheezing, pasty dry complexion.
Tongue Swollen with a dry sticky coating.
Pulse Fine-Slippery.

Acupuncture

LU-9 Taiyuan, LU-7 Lieque and KI-6 Zhaohai in combination, Ren-12 Zhongwan, ST-36 Zusanli, SP-6 Sanyinjiao, ST-40 Fenglong, BL-13 Feishu, Ren-17 Shanzhong.

Prescription

Bei Mu Gua Lou San *Fritillaria-Trichosanthes Powder*.

Phlegm-Fluids in the Lungs
Clinical manifestations

Cough with expectoration of watery white mucus, breathlessness, splashing sound in the chest, vomiting of watery, frothy white sputum, a feeling of cold, cough which may be elicited by a scare.
Tongue Pale with thick, sticky white coating.
Pulse Fine-Slippery or Weak-Floating.

Acupuncture

LU-5 Chize, LU-9 Taiyuan, Ren-17 Shanzhong, BL-13 Feishu, ST-40 Fenglong, BL-43 Gaohuangshu, Ren-12 Zhongwan, ST-36 Zusanli, Ren-9 Shuifen, SP-9 Yinlingquan.

Prescription

Ling Gan Wu Wei Jiang Xin Tang *Poria-Glycyrrhiza-Schisandra-Zingiberis-Asarum Decoction*
San Zi Yang Qin Tang *Three-Seed Nourishing the Ancestors Decoction*.

LUNG-QI STAGNATION

Clinical manifestations

A feeling of a lump in the throat, difficulty in swallowing, a feeling of oppression or distension of the chest, slight breathlessness, sighing, sadness, slight anxiety, depression.
Tongue Slightly Red on the sides in the chest areas.
Pulse Very slightly Tight on the right Front position.

Acupuncture

LU-7 Lieque, ST-40 Fenglong, Ren-15 Jiuwei, P-6 Neiguan.

Prescription

Ban Xia Hou Po Tang *Pinella-Magnolia Decoction*.

LUNG-QI COLLAPSE

Clinical manifestations

Weak and interrupted breathing, profuse sweating, sweat drops like pearls, extreme cold feeling, very cold hands, bright-pale complexion.
Tongue Pale or Bluish-Purple.
Pulse Floating-Scattered or Weak-Minute.

Acupuncture

Ren-12 Zhongwan, LU-9 Taiyuan, Ren-6 Qihai, Ren-4 Guanyuan, BL-13 Feishu. Moxa must be used; indirect moxibustion with moxa cones on slices of aconite on Ren-6 is particularly applicable.

Prescription

Sheng Mai San *Generating the Pulse Powder* in higher doses than normal.

COMBINED PATTERNS

The combined patterns of the Lungs are:

- Lung-Qi and Kidney-Yang deficiency (see 'Kidney-Yang deficiency, Water overflowing' or 'Kidneys failing to receive Qi' patterns in Chapter 95, 'Kidneys').
- Lung- and Kidney-Yin deficiency (see Chapter 95, 'Kidneys' under combined patterns).
- Liver-Fire insulting the Lungs (see Chapter 93, 'Liver' under combined patterns).
- Lung- and Spleen-Qi deficiency (see Chapter 92, 'Spleen' under combined patterns).
- Lung- and Heart-Qi deficiency.

Lung- and Heart-Qi Deficiency
Clinical manifestations

Slight breathlessness, slight cough, weak voice, dislike of speaking, bright-white complexion, tendency to catch colds, tiredness, dislike of cold, palpitations, shortness of breath on exertion, listlessness, depression, spontaneous sweating, sighing.

Tongue   Pale.
Pulse   Empty, especially on both Front positions.

Acupuncture

LU-9 Taiyuan, LU-7 Lieque, Ren-6 Qihai, BL-13 Feishu, Du-12 Shenzhu, ST-36 Zusanli, Ren-12 Zhongwan, HE-5 Tongli, P-6 Neiguan, BL-15 Xinshu, Ren-17 Shanzhong.

Prescription

Si Jun Zi Tang *Four Gentlemen Decoction* plus Huang Qi *Radix Astragali membranacei*
Bao Yuan Tang *Preserving the Source Decoction*
Bu Fei Tang *Tonifying the Lungs Decoction*
Sheng Mai San *Generating the Pulse Powder*.

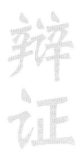

Chapter **95**

KIDNEYS

Chapter contents

KIDNEY-QI DEFICIENCY   *905*

KIDNEY-YANG DEFICIENCY PATTERNS   *905*
Kidney-Yang deficiency   *905*
Kidney-Yang deficiency, Water overflowing   *906*

KIDNEY-YIN DEFICIENCY PATTERNS   *906*
Kidney-Yin deficiency   *906*
Kidney-Yin deficiency with Empty-Heat   *906*
Kidney-Yin deficiency, Empty-Heat blazing   *906*
Kidney-Yin deficiency with Phlegm   *907*

KIDNEY-YANG AND KIDNEY-YIN DEFICIENCY PATTERNS   *907*
Kidney-Yang and Kidney-Yin deficiency –
    predominance of Kidney-Yin deficiency   *907*
Kidney-Yang and Kidney-Yin deficiency –
    predominance of Kidney-Yang deficiency   *907*

KIDNEY-QI NOT FIRM   *907*

KIDNEYS FAILING TO RECEIVE QI   *908*

KIDNEY-ESSENCE DEFICIENCY   *908*

COMBINED PATTERNS   *908*
Kidney- and Liver-Yin deficiency   *908*
Kidney- and Liver-Yin deficiency with
    Empty-Heat   *909*
Kidney and Heart not harmonized (Kidney- and
    Heart-Yin deficiency with Heart Empty-Heat)   *909*
Kidney- and Lung-Yin deficiency   *909*
Kidney- and Lung-Yin deficiency with
    Empty-Heat   *909*
Kidney- and Spleen-Yang deficiency   *910*

KIDNEY-QI DEFICIENCY

Clinical manifestations

Diminished hearing, dizziness, tinnitus, backache, frequent urination, urination at night, premature ejaculation, heavy periods.
Tongue   Slightly Pale.
Pulse   Weak on the right Rear position.

Acupuncture

BL-23 Shenshu, Du-4 Mingmen, Ren-4 Guanyuan, Ren-6 Qihai, KI-3 Taixi, KI-7 Fuliu. Moxa is applicable.

Prescription

Qing E Wan *Young Maiden Pill*.

KIDNEY-YANG DEFICIENCY PATTERNS

Kidney-Yang deficiency
Clinical manifestations

Lower backache, cold and weak knees, a sensation of cold in the lower back, a feeling of cold, weak legs, bright-white complexion, tiredness, lassitude, abundant clear urination, urination at night, apathy, oedema of the legs, infertility in women, loose stools, depression, impotence, premature ejaculation, low sperm count, cold and thin sperm, decreased libido.
Tongue   Pale and wet.
Pulse   Deep-Weak.

Acupuncture

BL-23 Shenshu, Du-4 Mingmen, Ren-4 Guanyuan, Ren-6 Qihai, KI-3 Taixi, KI-7 Fuliu, BL-52 Zhishi, Jinggong extra point (0.5 cun lateral to BL-52 Zhishi). Moxa must be used.

Prescription

You Gui Wan *Restoring the Right [Kidney] Pill*
Jin Gui Shen Qi Wan *Golden Chest Kidney-Qi Pill*.

Kidney-Yang deficiency, Water overflowing
Clinical manifestations

Oedema especially of the legs and ankles, a cold feeling in the legs and back, fullness and distension of the abdomen, soreness of the lower back, a feeling of cold, scanty clear urination.

> 1. Water overflowing to the Heart: the above symptoms plus palpitations, breathlessness, cold hands.
> 2. Water overflowing to the Lungs: the above symptoms plus thin, watery, frothy sputum, cough, asthma and breathlessness on exertion.

Tongue   Pale, Swollen and wet with a white coating.
Pulse   Deep-Weak-Slow.

Acupuncture

Du-4 Mingmen, BL-23 Shenshu, BL-22 Sanjiaoshu, BL-20 Pishu, Ren-9 Shuifen, ST-28 Shuidao, SP-9 Yinlingquan, SP-6 Sanyinjiao, KI-7 Fuliu.

> 1. For Water overflowing to the Heart: Du-14 Dazhui (moxa), BL-15 Xinshu.
> 2. For Water overflowing to the Lungs: LU-7 Lieque, BL-13 Feishu, Du-12 Shenzhu.

Prescription

Jin Gui Shen Qi Wan *Golden Chest Kidney-Qi Pill* plus Wu Ling San *Five 'Ling' Powder*.

KIDNEY-YIN DEFICIENCY PATTERNS

Kidney-Yin deficiency
Clinical manifestations

Dizziness, tinnitus, vertigo, poor memory, hardness of hearing, night sweating, dry mouth and throat at night, lower backache, ache in bones, nocturnal emissions, constipation, scanty dark urine, infertility, premature ejaculation, tiredness, lassitude, depression, slight anxiety.

Tongue   Normal-coloured without coating.
Pulse   Floating-Empty.

Acupuncture

Ren-4 Guanyuan, KI-3 Taixi, KI-6 Zhaohai, KI-10 Yingu, KI-9 Zhubin, SP-6 Sanyinjiao, Ren-7 Yinjiao, LU-7 Lieque and KI-6 Zhaohai in combination (opening points of the Directing Vessel).

Prescription

Zuo Gui Wan *Restoring the Left [Kidney] Pill*
Liu Wei Di Huang Wan *Six-Ingredient Rehmannia Pill*.

Kidney-Yin deficiency with Empty-Heat
Clinical manifestations

Dizziness, tinnitus, vertigo, poor memory, hardness of hearing, night sweating, dry mouth at night, five-palm heat, a feeling of heat in the evening, malar flush, menopausal hot flushes, thirst with a desire to drink in small sips, lower backache, ache in the bones, nocturnal emissions with dreams, constipation, scanty dark urine, infertility, premature ejaculation, tiredness, depression, anxiety, insomnia, excessive menstrual bleeding.
Tongue   Red without coating; in severe cases also cracked.
Pulse   Floating-Empty and slightly Rapid.

Acupuncture

Ren-4 Guanyuan, KI-3 Taixi, KI-6 Zhaohai, KI-10 Yingu, KI-9 Zhubin, SP-6 Sanyinjiao, Ren-7 Yinjiao, LU-7 Lieque and KI-6 Zhaohai in combination (opening points of the Directing Vessel), KI-2 Rangu, HE-6 Yinxi.

Prescription

Zhi Bo Di Huang Wan *Anemarrhena-Phellodendron-Rehmannia Pill*
Da Bu Yin Wan *Great Tonifying Yin Pill*
Er Zhi Wan *Two Solstices Pill*.

Kidney-Yin deficiency, Empty-Heat blazing
Clinical manifestations

Malar flush, mental restlessness, night sweating, low-grade fever, afternoon fever, a feeling of heat in the afternoon/evening, insomnia, scanty dark urine, blood

in the urine, dry throat especially at night, thirst with a desire to drink in small sips, dizziness, tinnitus, hardness of hearing, lower backache, nocturnal emissions with dreams, excessive sexual desire, dry stools.
Tongue Red-Peeled, cracked with a red tip.
Pulse Floating-Empty and Rapid.

Acupuncture

KI-3 Taixi, KI-6 Zhaohai, KI-2 Rangu, KI-9 Zhubin, Ren-4 Guanyuan, KI-10 Yingu, SP-6 Sanyinjiao, HE-5 Tongli, LU-7 Lieque, LU-10 Yuji, HE-6 Yinxi, Du-24 Shenting, LI-11 Quchi.

Prescription

Liu Wei Di Huang Wan *Six-Ingredient Rehmannia Pill* plus Di Gu Pi *Cortex Lycii radicis* and Zhi Mu *Radix Anemarrhenae asphodeloidis*.

Kidney-Yin deficiency with Phlegm
Clinical manifestations

Sputum in the throat, bouts of dry cough followed by expectoration of scanty sputum, breathlessness, a feeling of oppression in the chest, dizziness, tinnitus, hardness of hearing, night sweating.
Tongue Red with rootless sticky yellow coating.
Pulse Floating-Empty and slightly Slippery.

Acupuncture

KI-3 Taixi, Ren-4 Guanyuan, SP-6 Sanyinjiao, SP-9 Yinlingquan, ST-40 Fenglong, KI-6 Zhaohai.

Prescription

Zuo Gui Wan *Restoring the Left [Kidney] Pill* plus Bei Mu Gua Lou Tang *Fritillaria-Trichosanthes Decoction*.

KIDNEY-YANG AND KIDNEY-YIN DEFICIENCY PATTERNS

Kidney-Yang and Kidney-Yin deficiency – predominance of Kidney-Yin deficiency
Clinical manifestations

Dizziness, tinnitus, vertigo, poor memory, hardness of hearing, night sweating, dry mouth and throat at night, lower backache, ache in the bones, nocturnal emissions, infertility, premature ejaculation, tiredness, lassitude, depression, slight anxiety, cold feet, abundant pale urine.

Tongue Normal-coloured without coating or with rootless coating.
Pulse Floating-Empty or Weak on both Kidney positions.

Acupuncture

Ren-4 Guanyuan, KI-3 Taixi, KI-6 Zhaohai, KI-10 Yingu, KI-9 Zhubin, SP-6 Sanyinjiao, Ren-7 Yinjiao, LU-7 Lieque and KI-6 Zhaohai in combination (opening points of the Directing Vessel). Moderate use of moxa is applicable (e.g. moxa on the needle on KI-3 Taixi).

Prescription

Zuo Gui Wan *Restoring the Left [Kidney] Pill* plus Ba Ji Tian *Radix Morindae officinalis*.

Kidney-Yang and Kidney-Yin deficiency – predominance of Kidney-Yang deficiency
Clinical manifestations

Lower backache, cold knees, a sensation of cold in the back, a feeling of cold in general but also occasionally one of heat in the face, menopausal hot flushes, night sweating, weak legs, bright-white complexion, weak knees, impotence, premature ejaculation, low sperm count, cold and thin sperm, decreased libido, tiredness, lassitude, abundant clear or scanty clear urination, urination at night, apathy, oedema of the legs, infertility in women, loose stools, depression.
Tongue Pale.
Pulse Deep-Weak.

Acupuncture

BL-23 Shenshu, Du-4 Mingmen, Ren-4 Guanyuan, Ren-6 Qihai, KI-3 Taixi, KI-7 Fuliu, BL-52 Zhishi, Jinggong extra point (0.5 cun lateral to BL-52 Zhishi). Moxa is applicable, but less than in Kidney-Yang deficiency.

Prescription

You Gui Wan *Restoring the Right [Kidney] Pill* plus Sheng Di Huang *Radix Rehmanniae glutinosae* and Tian Men Dong *Tuber Asparagi cochinchinensis*.

KIDNEY-QI NOT FIRM

Clinical manifestations

Soreness and weakness of the lower back, weak knees, clear frequent urination, weak-stream urination,

abundant urination, dribbling after urination, incontinence of urine, enuresis, urination at night, nocturnal emissions without dreams, premature ejaculation, spermatorrhoea, prolapse of the uterus in women chronic white vaginal discharge, tiredness, a dragging-down feeling in the lower abdomen, recurrent miscarriage, a feeling of cold, cold limbs.

Tongue Pale.
Pulse Deep-Weak especially in the Rear positions.

Acupuncture

BL-23 Shenshu, Du-4 Mingmen, KI-3 Taixi, BL-52 Zhishi, Ren-4 Guanyuan, Jinggong extra point, Ren-6 Qihai, Du-20 Baihui, KI-13 Qixue, BL-32 Ciliao. Moxa is applicable.

Prescription

You Gui Yin *Restoring the Right [Kidney] Decoction* plus Huang Qi *Radix Astragali membranacei* and Qian Shi *Semen Euryales ferocis*
Jin Suo Gu Jing Wan *Metal Lock Consolidating the Essence Pill*
Fu Tu Dan *Poria-Cuscuta Pill*.

KIDNEYS FAILING TO RECEIVE QI

Clinical manifestations

Shortness of breath on exertion, rapid and weak breathing, difficulty in inhaling, chronic cough asthma, spontaneous sweating, cold limbs, cold limbs after sweating, swelling of the face, thin body, mental listlessness, clear urination during asthma attack, lower backache, dizziness, tinnitus.

Tongue Pale.
Pulse Deep-Weak-Tight.

Acupuncture

KI-7 Fuliu, KI-3 Taixi, LU-7 Lieque and KI-6 Zhaohai in combination (opening points of the Directing Vessel), ST-36 Zusanli, BL-23 Shenshu, Du-4 Mingmen, Ren-6 Qihai, Ren-17 Shanzhong, KI-25 Shencang, Du-12 Shenzhu, BL-13 Feishu, Ren-4 Guanyuan, KI-13 Qixue. Moxa is applicable.

Prescription

You Gui Yin *Restoring the Right [Kidney] Decoction* plus Dong Chong Xia Cao *Sclerotium Cordicipitis chinensis* and Wu Wei Zi *Fructus Schisandrae chinensis*.

Shen Ge San *Ginseng-Gecko Powder*
Su Zi Jiang Qi Tang *Perilla-Seed Subduing Qi Decoction*.

KIDNEY-ESSENCE DEFICIENCY

Clinical manifestations

In children: poor bone development, late closure of the fontanelles, deafness, mental dullness or retardation.
In adults: softening of the bones, weakness of the knees and legs, poor memory, loose teeth, falling hair or premature greying of hair, weakness from sexual activity, lower backache, infertility, sterility, primary amenorrhoea, dizziness, tinnitus, deafness, blurred vision, absentmindedness, decreased mental sharpness.

Tongue Without coating if this pattern occurs against a background of Kidney-Yin deficiency; Pale if against a background of Kidney-Yang deficiency.
Pulse Floating-Empty or Leather.

Acupuncture

KI-3 Taixi, KI-6 Zhaohai, Ren-4 Guanyuan, KI-13 Qixue, BL-23 Shenshu, Du-4 Mingmen, GB-39 Xuanzhong, Du-20 Baihui, Du-14 Dazhui, BL-15 Xinshu, BL-11 Dashu, Du-17 Naohu, Du-16 Fengfu.

Prescription

Zuo Gui Yin *Restoring the Left [Kidney] Decoction*
Zuo Gui Wan *Restoring the Left [Kidney] Pill*.

COMBINED PATTERNS

The Kidneys Combined Patterns are:

- Kidney- and Liver-Yin deficiency
- Kidney- and Liver-Yin deficiency with Empty-Heat
- Kidney and Heart not Harmonized
- Kidney- and Lung-Yin deficiency
- Kidney- and Lung-Yin deficiency with Empty-Heat
- Kidney- and Spleen-Yang deficiency.

Kidney- and Liver-Yin deficiency
Clinical manifestations

Dizziness, tinnitus, hardness of hearing, lower backache, dull occipital or vertical headache, insomnia,

numbness/tingling of the limbs, dry eyes, blurred vision, dry throat, dry hair and skin, brittle nails, dry vagina, night sweating, dry stools, nocturnal emissions, scanty menstruation or amenorrhoea, delayed cycle, infertility.
Tongue normal coloured without coating or with rootless coating.
Pulse Floating-Empty.

Acupuncture

KI-3 Taixi, KI-6 Zhaohai, LIV-8 Ququan, Ren-4 Guanyuan, BL-23 Shenshu, KI-13 Qixue, SP-6 Sanyinjiao.

Prescription

Zuo Gui Wan *Restoring the Left [Kidney] Pill*
Qi Ju Di Huang Wan *Lycium-Chrysanthemum-Rehmannia Pill*.

Kidney- and Liver-Yin deficiency with Empty-Heat
Clinical manifestations

Dizziness, tinnitus, hardness of hearing, dull occipital or vertical headache, insomnia, numbness/tingling of the limbs, dry eyes, blurred vision, lower backache, dry throat at night, thirst with a desire to drink in small sips, dry hair and skin, brittle nails, dry vagina, night sweating, dry stools, nocturnal emissions, scanty menstruation or amenorrhoea, delayed cycle, infertility, five-palm heat, a feeling of heat in the evening, malar flush, menopausal hot flushes.
Tongue Red without coating.
Pulse Floating-Empty and slightly Rapid.

Acupuncture

KI-3 Taixi, KI-6 Zhaohai, LIV-8 Ququan, Ren-4 Guanyuan, BL-23 Shenshu, KI-13 Qixue, SP-6 Sanyinjiao, KI-2 Rangu, LI-11 Quchi, HE-6 Yinxi, LIV-2 Xingjian.

Prescription

Liu Wei Di Huang Wan *Six-Ingredient Rehmannia Pill* plus Di Gu Pi *Cortex Lycii radicis* and Zhi Mu *Radix Anemarrhenae asphodeloidis*.

Kidney and Heart not harmonized (Kidney- and Heart-Yin deficiency with Heart Empty-Heat)
Clinical manifestations

Palpitations, mental restlessness, insomnia, dream-disturbed sleep, anxiety, poor memory, dizziness, tinni-

tus, hardness of hearing, lower backache, nocturnal emissions with dreams, a feeling of heat in the evening, dry throat at night, thirst with a desire to drink in small sips, night sweating, five-palm heat, scanty dark urine, dry stools.
Tongue Red with redder tip without coating, midline Heart crack.
Pulse Floating-Empty and Rapid or Deep-Weak on both Rear positions and relatively Overflowing on both Front positions.

Acupuncture

HE-7 Shenmen, HE-6 Yinxi, HE-5 Tongli, Yintang extra point, BL-15 Xinshu, Ren-15 Jiuwei, Du-24 Shenting, KI-3 Taixi, KI-6 Zhaohai, KI-10 Yingu, KI-9 Zhubin, Ren-4 Guanyuan, SP-6 Sanyinjiao.

Prescription

Tian Wang Bu Xin Dan *Heavenly Emperor Tonifying the Heart Pill*.

Kidney- and Lung-Yin deficiency
Clinical manifestations

Dry cough which is worse in the evening, dry throat and mouth, thin body, breathlessness on exertion, lower backache, night sweating, dizziness, tinnitus, hardness of hearing, scanty urination.
Tongue Normal coloured without coating or with rootless coating.
Pulse Floating-Empty.

Acupuncture

KI-3 Taixi, KI-6 Zhaohai, LU-7 Lieque and KI-6 Zhaohai in combination (opening points of the Directing Vessel), Ren-4 Guanyuan, KI-13 Qixue, LU-9 Taiyuan, LU-1 Zhongfu, SP-6 Sanyinjiao, BL-43 Gaohuangshu.

Prescription

Ba Xian Chang Shou Wan *Eight Immortals Longevity Pill*.

Kidney- and Lung-Yin deficiency with Empty-Heat
Clinical manifestations

Dry cough which is worse in the evening, dry throat and mouth at night, thirst with a desire to drink in small sips, thin body, breathlessness on exertion, lower

backache, night sweating, dizziness, tinnitus, hardness of hearing, scanty urination, a feeling of heat in the evening, five-palm heat, malar flush.

Tongue   Red without coating.
Pulse   Floating-Empty and slightly Rapid.

Acupuncture

KI-3 Taixi, KI-6 Zhaohai, LU-7 Lieque and KI-6 Zhaohai in combination (opening points of the Directing Vessel), Ren-4 Guanyuan, KI-13 Qixue, LU-9 Taiyuan, LU-1 Zhongfu, SP-6 Sanyinjiao, BL-43 Gaohuangshu, KI-2 Rangu, LU-10 Yuji, LI-11 Quchi.

Prescription

Ba Xian Chang Shou Wan *Eight Immortals Longevity Pill* plus Di Gu Pi *Cortex Lycii radicis*.

Kidney- and Spleen-Yang deficiency
Clinical manifestations

Lower backache, cold and weak knees, a sensation of cold in the back, a feeling of cold, weak legs, bright-white complexion, impotence, premature ejaculation, low sperm count, cold and thin sperm, decreased libido, tiredness, lassitude, abundant clear or scanty clear urination, urination at night, apathy, oedema of the legs, infertility in women, loose stools, depression, poor appetite, slight abdominal distension, a desire to lie down, early-morning diarrhoea, chronic diarrhoea.

Tongue   Pale and wet.
Pulse   Deep-Weak.

Acupuncture

BL-23 Shenshu, Du-4 Mingmen, Ren-4 Guanyuan, Ren-6 Qihai, KI-3 Taixi, KI-7 Fuliu, BL-52 Zhishi, Jinggong extra point (0.5 cun lateral to BL-52 Zhishi), Ren-12 Zhongwan, Ren-9 Shuifen, ST-36 Zusanli, SP-3 Taibai, BL-20 Pishu, BL-21 Weishu, ST-37 Shangjuxu, ST-25 Tianshu, BL-25 Dachangshu. Moxa is applicable.

Prescription

Li Zhong Wan *Regulating the Centre Pill* plus Jin Gui Shen Qi Wan *Golden Chest Kidney-Qi Pill*.

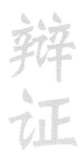

Chapter **96**

SMALL INTESTINE

Chapter contents

FULL-HEAT IN THE SMALL INTESTINE   *911*

SMALL INTESTINE QI PAIN   *911*

SMALL INTESTINE QI TIED   *912*

SMALL INTESTINE DEFICIENT AND COLD   *912*

INFESTATION OF WORMS IN THE SMALL INTESTINE   *912*

FULL-HEAT IN THE SMALL INTESTINE

Clinical manifestations

Mental restlessness, insomnia, tongue/mouth ulcers, pain in the throat, deafness, an uncomfortable feeling and sensation of heat in the chest, abdominal pain, thirst with a desire to drink cold liquids, scanty dark urine, burning pain on urination, blood in urine.
Tongue Red with redder and swollen tip, yellow coating.
Pulse Overflowing-Rapid, especially in the Front position. If there are urinary symptoms the pulse would be Wiry on the left Rear position.

Acupuncture

SI-2 Qiangu, SI-5 Yanggu, HE-5 Tongli, HE-8 Shaofu, ST-39 Xiajuxu.

Prescription

Dao Chi San *Eliminating Redness Powder*
Dao Chi Qing Xin Tang *Eliminating Redness and Clearing the Heart Decoction.*

SMALL INTESTINE QI PAIN

Clinical manifestations

Lower abdominal twisting pain which may extend to back, abdominal distension, dislike of pressure on abdomen, borborygmi, flatulence, abdominal pain relieved by emission of wind, pain in the testis.
Tongue White coating.
Pulse Deep-Wiry, especially on the Rear positions.

Acupuncture

Ren-6 Qihai, GB-34 Yanglingquan, LIV-13 Zhangmen, ST-27 Daju, ST-29 Guilai, SP-6 Sanyinjiao, LIV-3 Taichong, ST-39 Xiajuxu.

Prescription

Chai Hu Shu Gan Tang *Bupleurum Soothing the Liver Decoction.*

SMALL INTESTINE QI TIED

Clinical manifestations

Violent abdominal pain, dislike of pressure, abdominal distension, constipation, vomiting, borborygmi, flatulence.
Tongue Thick white coating.
Pulse Deep-Wiry.

Acupuncture

ST-39 Xiajuxu, extra point Lanweixue, Ren-6 Qihai, GB-34 Yanglingquan, ST-25 Tianshu, SP-6 Sanyinjiao, LIV-3 Taichong.

Prescription

Zhi Shi Dao Zhi Wan *Citrus Eliminating Stagnation Pill*
Tian Tai Wu Yao San *Top-Quality Lindera Powder.*

SMALL INTESTINE DEFICIENT AND COLD

Clinical manifestations

Dull abdominal pain alleviated by pressure, a desire for hot drinks, borborygmi, diarrhoea, pale and abundant urination, cold limbs.

Tongue Pale body, white coating.
Pulse Deep-Weak-Slow.

Acupuncture

Ren-6 Qihai, ST-25 Tianshu, ST-39 Xiajuxu, ST-36 Zusanli, BL-20 Pishu, BL-27 Xiaochangshu. Moxa is applicable.

Prescription

Xiao Jian Zhong Tang *Small Strengthening the Centre Decoction*
Shen Ling Bai Zhu San *Ginseng-Poria-Atractylodis Powder.*

INFESTATION OF WORMS IN THE SMALL INTESTINE

Clinical manifestations

Abdominal pain and distension, bad taste in mouth, sallow complexion.
Roundworms (ascarid) Abdominal pain, vomiting of roundworms, cold limbs.
Hookworms Desire to eat strange objects such as soil, wax, uncooked rice or tea leaves.
Pinworms Itchy anus, worse in the evening.
Tapeworms Constant hunger.

Acupuncture

Acupuncture is not applicable in this pattern.

Prescription

Li Zhong An Hui Tang *Regulating the Centre and Calming Roundworms Decoction*
Lian Mei An Hui Tang *Picrorhiza-Mume Calming Roundworms Decoction*
Hua Chong Wan *Dissolving Parasites Pill*
Qu Tiao Tang *Expelling Tapeworms Decoction.*

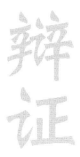

Chapter **97**

STOMACH

Chapter contents

STOMACH-QI DEFICIENCY   *913*

STOMACH DEFICIENT AND COLD (STOMACH-YANG DEFICIENCY)   *913*

STOMACH-YIN DEFICIENCY PATTERNS   *914*
Stomach-Yin deficiency   *914*
Stomach-Yin deficiency with Empty-Heat   *914*

DEFICIENCY OF STOMACH-YIN AND STOMACH-YANG   *914*

STOMACH-QI STAGNATION   *914*

BLOOD STASIS IN THE STOMACH   *915*

STOMACH-HEAT   *915*

STOMACH-FIRE   *915*

STOMACH PHLEGM-FIRE   *915*

STOMACH DAMP-HEAT   *916*

COLD INVADING THE STOMACH   *916*

STOMACH-QI REBELLING UPWARDS   *916*

RETENTION OF FOOD IN THE STOMACH   *916*

STOMACH-QI DEFICIENCY

Clinical manifestations

An uncomfortable feeling in the epigastrium, lack of appetite, lack of sense of taste, loose stools, tiredness especially in the morning, weak limbs.
Tongue   Pale.
Pulse   Empty, especially on the right Middle position.

Acupuncture

ST-36 Zusanli, Ren-12 Zhongwan, BL-21 Weishu, Ren-6 Qihai. Moxa is applicable.

Prescription

Si Jun Zi Tang *Four Gentlemen Decoction*.

STOMACH DEFICIENT AND COLD (STOMACH-YANG DEFICIENCY)

Clinical manifestations

Discomfort or a dull pain in the epigastrium, better after eating and with pressure or massage, lack of appetite, preference for warm drinks and foods, vomiting of clear fluid, absence of thirst, cold and weak limbs, tiredness, pale complexion.
Tongue   Pale and wet.
Pulse   Deep-Weak-Slow, especially on the right Middle position.

Acupuncture

ST-36 Zusanli, Ren-12 Zhongwan, BL-20 Pishu, BL-21 Weishu, Ren-6 Qihai. Moxa is applicable.

Prescription

Huang Qi Jian Zhong Tang *Astragalus Strengthening the Centre Decoction*
Xiao Jian Zhong Tang *Small Strengthening the Centre Decoction.*

STOMACH-YIN DEFICIENCY PATTERNS

Stomach-Yin deficiency
Clinical manifestations

No appetite or slight hunger but no desire to eat, constipation (dry stools), dull or slightly burning epigastric pain, dry mouth and throat especially in the afternoon, slight feeling of fullness after eating.
Tongue   Peeled in the centre, or with rootless coating, normal body colour.
Pulse   Floating-Empty on the right Middle position.

Acupuncture

Ren-12 Zhongwan, ST-36 Zusanli, SP-6 Sanyinjiao, SP-3 Taibai.

Prescription

Sha Shen Mai Dong Tang *Glehnia-Opheopogan Decoction*
Shen Ling Bai Zhu San *Ginseng-Poria-Atractylodis Powder*
Yi Wei Tang *Benefiting the Stomach Decoction.*

Stomach-Yin deficiency with Empty-Heat
Clinical manifestations

Dull or burning epigastric pain, a feeling of heat in the afternoon, constipation (dry stools), dry mouth and throat especially in the afternoon, thirst with a desire to drink in small sips, feeling of hunger but no desire to eat, a slight feeling of fullness after eating, night sweating, five-palm heat, bleeding gums, a feeling of heat in the evening.
Tongue   Red and Peeled in the centre.
Pulse   Floating-Empty on the right Middle position and slightly Rapid.

Acupuncture

Ren-12 Zhongwan, ST-36 Zusanli, SP-6 Sanyinjiao, SP-3 Taibai, ST-44 Neiting, ST-21 Liangmen, LI-11 Quchi.

Prescription

Sha Shen Mai Dong Tang plus Zhi Mu *Radix Anemarrhenae asphodeloidis* and Shi Hu *Herba Dendrobii.*

DEFICIENCY OF STOMACH-YIN AND STOMACH-YANG

Clinical manifestations

Dull or burning epigastric pain, dry throat and mouth, poor appetite, sour regurgitation, tiredness, sweating, night sweating, five-palm heat, cold fingers.
Tongue   Red in the centre without coating.
Pulse   Floating-Empty.
   This is essentially a Stomach-Yin deficiency which has developed from a Stomach-Yang deficiency.

Acupuncture

Ren-12 Zhongwan, ST-36 Zusanli, SP-6 Sanyinjiao, SP-3 Taibai, ST-21 Liangmen, ST-44 Neiting. Generally no moxa but moxa on the needle on ST-36 may be used.

Prescription

Si Jun Zi Tang *Four Gentlemen Decoction* or Huang Qi Jian Zhong Tang *Astragalus Strengthening the Centre Decoction* combined with Yi Wei Tang *Benefiting the Stomach Decoction* or Sha Shen Mai Dong Tang *Glehnia-Ophiopogan Decoction.*

STOMACH-QI STAGNATION

Clinical manifestations

Epigastric pain and distension, belching, nausea, vomiting, hiccup, irritability.
Tongue   No particular signs on the tongue except that in severe cases it may be Red on the sides in the central section.
Pulse   Wiry on the right Middle position.

Acupuncture

ST-34 Liangqiu, ST-21 Liangmen, ST-19 Burong, KI-21 Youmen, TB-6 Zhigou, SP-4 Gongsun with P-6 Neiguan (opening points of the Penetrating Vessel), GB-34 Yanglingquan with Ren-12 Zhongwan, ST-40 Fenglong.

Prescription

Chen Xiang Jiang San *Aquilaria Subduing Qi Powder*
Ban Xia Hou Po Tang *Pinellia-Magnolia Decoction*
Zuo Jin Wan *Left Metal Pill*.

BLOOD STASIS IN THE STOMACH

Clinical manifestations

Severe, stabbing epigastric pain that may be worse at night, dislike of pressure, nausea, vomiting, possibly of blood, or of food looking like coffee grounds.
Tongue Purple.
Pulse Wiry.

Acupuncture

ST-34 Liangqiu, ST-21 Liangmen, ST-19 Burong, KI-21 Youmen, TB-6 Zhigou, SP-4 Gongsun with P-6 Neiguan (opening points of the Penetrating Vessel), GB-34 Yanglingquan with Ren-12 Zhongwan, ST-40 Fenglong, BL-17 Geshu, SP-10 Xuehai, LI-4 Hegu, Ren-11 Jianli.

Prescription

Shi Xiao San *Breaking into a Smile Powder*
Dan Shen Yin *Salvia Decoction*
Ge Xia Zhu Yu Tang *Eliminating Stasis below the Diaphragm Decoction*
Tong You Tang *Penetrating the Depth Decoction*.

STOMACH-HEAT

Clinical manifestations

Burning epigastric pain, thirst, sour regurgitation, nausea, vomiting soon after eating, excessive hunger, foul breath, a feeling of heat.
Tongue Red in the centre with a yellow coating.
Pulse Rapid and slightly Overflowing on the right Middle position.

Acupuncture

ST-44 Neiting, ST-34 Liangqiu, ST-21 Liangmen, Ren-12 Zhongwan, Ren-13 Shangwan, LI-11 Quchi, LI-4 Hegu, Ren-11 Jianli.

Prescription

Bai Hu Tang *White Tiger Decoction*
Yu Nu Jian *Jade Woman Decoction*
Qing Wei San *Clearing the Stomach Powder*.

STOMACH-FIRE

Clinical manifestations

Burning epigastric pain, intense thirst with a desire to drink cold liquids, mental restlessness, bleeding gums, dry stools, dry mouth, mouth ulcers, sour regurgitation, nausea, vomiting soon after eating, excessive hunger, foul breath, a feeling of heat.
Tongue Red in the centre with a dry yellow or dark-yellow (or even black) coating.
Pulse Rapid and slightly Overflowing on the right Middle position.

Acupuncture

ST-44 Neiting, ST-34 Liangqiu, ST-21 Liangmen, Ren-12 Zhongwan, Ren-13 Shangwan, LI-11 Quchi, LI-4 Hegu, Ren-11 Jianli, SP-15 Daheng.

Prescription

Tiao Wei Cheng Qi Tang *Regulating the Stomach Conducting Qi Decoction*
Qing Wei San *Clearing the Stomach Powder*
Liang Ge San *Cooling the Diaphragm Powder*.

STOMACH PHLEGM-FIRE

Clinical manifestations

Burning epigastric pain, thirst without a desire to drink, mental restlessness, bleeding gums, dry stools, dry mouth, mouth ulcers, sour regurgitation, nausea, vomiting soon after eating, excessive hunger, foul breath, a feeling of heat, a feeling of oppression of the chest and epigastrium, mucus in the stools, insomnia, excessive dreaming, expectoration of phlegm.
Tongue Red in the centre with a sticky yellow or dark-yellow (or even black) coating, Stomach crack with a rough, sticky yellow coating inside it.
Pulse Slippery-Rapid and slightly Overflowing on the right Middle position.

Acupuncture

ST-44 Neiting, ST-34 Liangqiu, ST-21 Liangmen, Ren-12 Zhongwan, Ren-13 Shangwan, LI-11 Quchi, LI-4 Hegu, Ren-11 Jianli, SP-15 Daheng, ST-40 Fenglong, SP-9 Yinlingquan, Ren-9 Shuifen, SP-6 Sanyinjiao.

Prescription

Wen Dan Tang *Warming the Gall-Bladder Decoction*.

STOMACH DAMP-HEAT

Clinical manifestations

A feeling of fullness and pain of the epigastrium, a feeling of heaviness, facial pain, stuffed nose or thick, sticky nasal discharge, thirst without a desire to drink, nausea, a feeling of heat, dull-yellow complexion, a sticky taste.
Tongue Red tongue with sticky yellow coating.
Pulse Slippery-Rapid.

Acupuncture

ST-44 Neiting, ST-34 Liangqiu, ST-21 Liangmen, Ren-12 Zhongwan, Ren-13 Shangwan, LI-11 Quchi, LI-4 Hegu, Ren-11 Jianli, ST-25 Tianshu, ST-40 Fenglong, SP-9 Yinlingquan, Ren-9 Shuifen.

Prescription

Lian Po Yin *Coptis-Magnolia Decoction*.

COLD INVADING THE STOMACH

Clinical manifestations

Sudden severe pain in the epigastrium, a feeling of cold, cold limbs, preference for warmth, vomiting of clear fluids (which may alleviate the pain), nausea, feeling worse after swallowing cold fluids (which are quickly vomited), preference for warm liquids.
Tongue Thick white coating.
Pulse Deep-Tight-Slow.

Acupuncture

ST-21 Liangmen, SP-4 Gongsun, Ren-13 Shangwan, ST-34 Liangqiu. Moxa must be used.

Prescription

Liang Fu Wan *Alpinia-Cyperus Pill*.

STOMACH-QI REBELLING UPWARDS

Clinical manifestations

Nausea, difficulty in swallowing, belching, vomiting, hiccup.
Tongue No changes.
Pulse Tight or Wiry on the right Middle position.

Acupuncture

Ren-13 Shangwan, Ren-10 Xiawan, P-6 Neiguan, SP-4 Gongsun, ST-21 Liangmen, ST-19 Burong.

Prescription

Ding Xiang Shi Di Tang *Caryophyllum-Diospyros Decoction*
Huo Xiang Zheng Qi San *Agastaches Upright-Qi Powder*
Ban Xia Hou Po Tang *Pinellia-Magnolia Decoction*.

RETENTION OF FOOD IN THE STOMACH

Clinical manifestations

Fullness, pain and distension of the epigastrium which are relieved by vomiting, nausea, vomiting of sour fluids, foul breath, sour regurgitation, belching, insomnia, loose stools or constipation, poor appetite.
Tongue Thick coating (which could be white or yellow).
Pulse Full-Slippery.

Acupuncture

Ren-13 Shangwan, Ren-10 Xiawan, ST-21 Liangmen, ST-44 Neiting, ST-45 Lidui, SP-4 Gongsun, P-6 Neiguan, ST-40 Fenglong, ST-19 Burong, KI-21 Youmen, Ren-12 Zhongwan.

Prescription

Bao He Wan *Preserving and Harmonizing Pill*
Zhi Shi Dao Zhi Wan *Citrus Eliminating Stagnation Pill*.

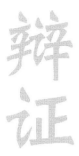

Chapter **98**

GALL-BLADDER

Chapter contents

DAMP-HEAT PATTERNS *917*
  Damp-Heat in the Gall-Bladder and Liver *917*
  Damp-Heat in the Gall-Bladder *917*

DAMP-COLD IN THE GALL-BLADDER *918*

GALL-BLADDER HEAT *918*

GALL-BLADDER DEFICIENT *918*

STAGNATION OF THE GALL-BLADDER WITH PHLEGM-HEAT *918*

DAMP-HEAT PATTERNS

Damp-Heat in the Gall-Bladder and Liver

Clinical manifestations

Hypochondrial pain, fullness and distension, nausea, vomiting, inability to digest fats, yellow complexion, scanty and dark yellow urine, fever, thirst without a desire to drink, bitter taste, dizziness, yellow sclera, tinnitus, irritability, a feeling of heaviness of the body, numbness of the limbs, swelling of the feet, burning on urination, difficulty in urinating, excessive vaginal discharge, loose stools or constipation, alternation of hot and cold feeling, a feeling of heat, genital papular skin rashes and itching, swelling and heat of the scrotum.
Tongue Thick, sticky yellow coating, either bilateral or only on one side.
Pulse Slippery-Wiry-Rapid.

Acupuncture

GB-24 Riyue, LIV-14 Qimen, Ren-12 Zhongwan, GB-34 Yanglingquan, extra point Dannangxue, Du-9 Zhiyang, BL-19 Danshu, BL-20 Pishu, LI-11 Quchi, TB-6 Zhigou, ST-19 Burong, LIV-3 Taichong, LIV-5 Ligou.

Prescription

Long Dan Xie Gan Tang *Gentiana Draining the Liver Decoction.*

Damp-Heat in the Gall-Bladder

Clinical manifestations

Hypochondrial pain, fullness and distension, nausea, vomiting, inability to digest fats, yellow complexion, scanty and dark yellow urine, fever, thirst without a

desire to drink, bitter taste, dizziness, tinnitus, irritability, a feeling of heaviness of the body, numbness of the limbs, swelling of the feet, loose stools or constipation, an alternation of hot and cold feeling, yellow sclera, a feeling of heat.

Tongue Thick, sticky yellow coating, either bilateral in two strips or unilateral.

Pulse Slippery-Wiry-Rapid.

Acupuncture

GB-24 Riyue, LIV-14 Qimen, Ren-12 Zhongwan, GB-34 Yanglingquan, extra point Dannangxue, Du-9 Zhiyang, BL-19 Danshu, BL-20 Pishu, LI-11 Quchi, TB-6 Zhigou, ST-19 Burong.

Prescription

Yin Chen Hao Tang *Artemisia Capillaris Decoction*.

DAMP-COLD IN THE GALL-BLADDER

Clinical manifestations

Jaundice, dull-yellow eyes and skin, hypochondrial pain, fullness and distension, nausea, vomiting, inability to digest fats, dull-yellow sclera, turbid urine, absence of thirst, sticky taste, dull headache, a feeling of heaviness of the body, a feeling of cold.

Tongue Thick, sticky white coating, either bilateral in two strips or unilateral.

Pulse Slippery-Wiry-Slow.

Acupuncture

GB-24 Riyue, LIV-14 Qimen, Ren-12 Zhongwan, GB-34 Yanglingquan, extra point Dannangxue, Du-9 Zhiyang, BL-19 Danshu, BL-20 Pishu, TB-6 Zhigou, ST-19 Burong.

Prescription

San Ren Tang *Three Seeds Decoction* plus Yin Chen Hao *Herba Artemisiae capillaris*.

GALL-BLADDER HEAT

Clinical manifestations

Dizziness, tinnitus, bitter taste, dry throat, irritability, red face and ears, hypochondrial fullness.

Tongue Unilateral or bilateral yellow coating.

Pulse Wiry-Rapid.

Acupuncture

GB-24 Riyue, GB-34 Yanglingquan, extra point Dannangxue, Du-9 Zhiyang, BL-19 Danshu, LI-11 Quchi, TB-6 Zhigou, ST-19 Burong, GB-43 Xiaxi.

Prescription

Jin Ling Zi San *Melia Powder* combined with Zuo Jin Wan *Left Metal Pill*.

GALL-BLADDER DEFICIENT

Clinical manifestations

Dizziness, blurred vision, 'floaters', nervousness, timidity, tendency to be easily startled, lack of courage and initiative, indecision, sighing, waking up early in the morning, restless dreams.

Tongue Pale or normal.

Pulse Weak.

Acupuncture

GB-40 Qiuxu. Moxa is applicable.

Prescription

Wen Dan Tang *Warming the Gall-Bladder Decoction*. This formula, originally by Sun Si-Miao, was used for irritability and insomnia deriving from Cold in the Gall-Bladder after a severe illness. The original formula omitted Fu Ling and contained Sheng Jiang in a larger dosage (12 g).

An Shen Ding Zhi Wan *Calming the Spirit and Settling the Will-Power Pill*.

STAGNATION OF THE GALL-BLADDER WITH PHLEGM-HEAT

Clinical manifestations

Hypochondrial distension and pain, dizziness, blurred vision, irritability, insomnia, palpitations, a feeling of oppression of the chest and hypochondrium, sighing, slight breathlessness, excessive dreaming, bitter taste, nausea.

Tongue Sticky yellow coating.

Pulse Wiry-Slippery.

Acupuncture

GB-24 Riyue, GB-34 Yanglingquan, SP-9 Yinglingquan, ST-19 Burong, Ren-12 Zhongwan, ST-40

Fenglong, LU-7 Lieque, TB-6 Zhigou, P-6 Neiguan, LI-11 Quchi.

Prescription

Wen Dan Tang plus Yin Chen Hao *Herba Artemisiae capillaris*, Mu Xiang *Radix Aucklandiae lappae* and Xiang Fu *Rhizoma Cyperi rotundi*.

COMBINED PATTERNS

For combined Liver and Gall-Bladder patterns, see Chapter 93, 'Liver'.

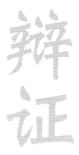

Chapter **99**

LARGE INTESTINE

Chapter contents

DAMP-HEAT IN THE LARGE INTESTINE   *921*

HEAT PATTERNS   *921*
   Heat in the Large Intestine   *921*
   Heat obstructing the Large Intestine   *922*

COLD PATTERNS   *922*
   Cold invading the Large Intestine   *922*
   Large Intestine Cold   *922*

LARGE INTESTINE DRYNESS   *922*

DAMPNESS IN THE LARGE INTESTINE   *922*

LARGE INTESTINE DEFICIENT AND COLD   *923*

LARGE INTESTINE DEFICIENT AND DAMP   *923*

COLLAPSE OF LARGE INTESTINE   *923*

DAMP-HEAT IN THE LARGE INTESTINE

Clinical manifestations

Abdominal pain that is not relieved by a bowel movement, diarrhoea, mucus and blood in the stools, offensive odour of the stools, burning in the anus, scanty dark urine, fever, sweating which does not decrease the fever, a feeling of heat, thirst without a desire to drink, a feeling of heaviness of the body and limbs.

Tongue   Red with sticky yellow coating.
Pulse   Slippery-Rapid.

Acupuncture

SP-9 Yinlingquan, SP-6 Sanyinjiao, BL-22 Sanjiaoshu, ST-25 Tianshu, ST-27 Daju, Ren-6 Qihai, BL-25 Dachangshu, LI-11 Quchi, Ren-12 Zhongwan, ST-37 Shangjuxu, BL-20 Pishu.

Prescription

Ge Gen Qin Lian Tang *Pueraria-Scutellaria-Coptis Decoction*
Bai Tou Weng Tang *Pulsatilla Decoction*
Shao Yao Tang *Paeonia Decoction*.

HEAT PATTERNS

Heat in the Large Intestine
Clinical manifestations

Constipation with dry stools, a burning sensation in the mouth, dry tongue, burning and swelling in the anus, scanty dark urine.

Tongue   Thick yellow (or brown or black) dry coating.
Pulse   Full-Rapid.

Acupuncture

ST-25 Tianshu, BL-25 Dachangshu, LI-11 Quchi, ST-37 Shangjuxu, ST-44 Neiting, LI-2 Erjian, SP-6 Sanyinjiao, KI-6 Zhaohai.

Prescription

Ma Zi Ren Wan *Cannabis Pill.*

Heat Obstructing the Large Intestine
Clinical manifestations

Constipation, burning in the anus, abdominal distension and pain which is worse with pressure, high fever or tidal fever (fever that rises in the afternoon), sweating especially on limbs, vomiting, thirst, delirium.
Tongue   Thick, dry yellow (or brown-black) coating, Red body.
Pulse   Deep-Full.

Acupuncture

LI-11 Quchi, LI-4 Hegu, SP-15 Daheng, TB-6 Zhigou, SP-6 Sanyinjiao, LI-2 Erjian, ST-44 Neiting, ST-25 Tianshu, BL-25 Dachangshu.

Prescription

Tiao Wei Cheng Qi Tang *Regulating the Stomach Conducting Qi Decoction.*

COLD PATTERNS

Cold invading the Large Intestine
Clinical manifestations

Sudden abdominal pain, diarrhoea with pain, a feeling of cold, a cold sensation in the abdomen.
Tongue   Thick white coating.
Pulse   Deep-Wiry.

Acupuncture

ST-37 Shangjuxu, ST-25 Tianshu, ST-36 Zusanli, SP-6 Sanyinjiao, LIV-3 Taichong, ST-27 Daju. Moxa is applicable.

Prescription

Liang Fu Wan *Alpinia Cyperus Pill* plus Zheng Qi Tian Xiang San *Upright Qi Heavenly Fragrance Powder.*

Large Intestine Cold
Clinical manifestations

Loose stools like duck droppings, dull abdominal pain, borborygmi, pale urine, cold limbs.
Tongue   Pale.
Pulse   Deep-Weak.

Acupuncture

ST-25 Tianshu, Ren-6 Qihai, ST-36 Zusanli, ST-37 Shangjuxu, BL-25 Dachangshu, BL-20 Pishu. Moxa is applicable.

Prescription

Liang Fu Wan *Alpinia Cyperus Pill.*

LARGE INTESTINE DRYNESS

Clinical manifestations

Dry stools which are difficult to discharge, dry mouth and throat, thin body, foul breath, dizziness.
Tongue   Dry, either Pale or Red without coating.
Pulse   Fine.

Acupuncture

ST-36 Zusanli, SP-6 Sanyinjiao, KI-6 Zhaohai, Ren-4 Guanyuan, ST-25 Tianshu.

Prescription

Zeng Ye Tang *Increasing Fluids Decoction*
Qing Zao Run Chang Tang *Clearing Dryness and Moistening the Intestines Decoction*
Wu Ren Wan *Five-Seeds Pill*
Tian Di Jian *Heaven and Earth Decoction*
Si Wu Ma Ren Wan *Four-Substance Cannabis Pill*
Ma Zi Ren Wan *Cannabis Pill.*

DAMPNESS IN THE LARGE INTESTINE

Clinical manifestations

Abdominal distension and fullness, difficulty in urination, scanty urination, loose stools, borborygmi, sticky taste, nausea, vomiting, mucus in the stools.
Tongue   Sticky white coating.
Pulse   Soggy on the right Rear position.

Acupuncture

ST-25 Tianshu, BL-25 Dachangshu, ST-37 Shangjuxu, ST-27 Daju, SP-6 Sanyinjiao, SP-9 Yinlingquan, Ren-12 Zhongwan, BL-22 Sanjiaoshu.

Prescription

Wei Ling Tang *Stomach 'Ling' Decoction.*

LARGE INTESTINE DEFICIENT AND COLD

Clinical manifestations

Chronic dull abdominal pain that is alleviated by pressure, application of heat and ingestion of warm liquids, borborygmi, loose stools, in some cases constipation, cold limbs especially the legs, pale stools.
Tongue Pale and wet.
Pulse Deep-Weak especially on both Rear positions.

Acupuncture

ST-25 Tianshu, BL-25 Dachangshu, ST-37 Shangjuxu, ST-27 Daju, SP-6 Sanyinjiao, Ren-6 Qihai, ST-36 Zusanli. Moxa should be used.

Prescription

Fu Zi Li Zhong Wan *Aconitum Regulating the Centre Pill* Zhen Ren Yang Zang Tang *True Man Nourishing the Organs Decoction.*

LARGE INTESTINE DEFICIENT AND DAMP

Clinical manifestations

Dull abdominal pain that is alleviated by pressure or application of heat, and aggravated by exposure to cold or ingestion of cold foods, loose stools, possibly mucus in the stools, a feeling of heaviness, incontinence of the stools, abdominal fullness, tiredness.
Tongue Pale with a sticky coating.
Pulse Weak and slightly Slippery.

Acupuncture

ST-25 Tianshu, BL-25 Dachangshu, ST-37 Shangjuxu, ST-27 Daju, SP-6 Sanyinjiao, SP-9 Yinlingquan, Ren-12 Zhongwan, BL-22 Sanjiaoshu, Ren-6 Qihai, ST-36 Zusanli.

Prescription

Shen Ling Bai Zhu San *Ginseng-Poria-Atractylodes Powder* plus Xiang Fu *Rhizoma Cyperi rotundi.*

COLLAPSE OF LARGE INTESTINE

Clinical manifestations

Chronic diarrhoea, prolapse ani, haemorrhoids, tiredness after bowel movements, cold limbs, lack of appetite, mental exhaustion, a desire to drink warm liquids, a desire to have the abdomen massaged.
Tongue Pale.
Pulse Deep-Fine-Weak.

Acupuncture

Ren-6 Qihai, ST-25 Tianshu, ST-36 Zusanli, SP-3 Taibai, BL-20 Pishu, BL-21 Weishu, Du-20 Baihui.

Prescription

Bu Zhong Yi Qi Tang *Tonifying the Centre Benefiting Qi Decoction.*

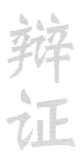

Chapter **100**

BLADDER

Chapter contents

DAMP-HEAT IN THE BLADDER *925*

DAMP-COLD IN THE BLADDER *925*

BLADDER DEFICIENT AND COLD *926*

For combined Kidney and Bladder patterns, please refer to Chapter 95, 'Kidney'.

DAMP-HEAT IN THE BLADDER

Clinical manifestations

Frequent and urgent urination, burning on urination, difficult urination (stopping in the middle of flow), dark-yellow/turbid urine, blood in the urine, fever, thirst with no desire to drink, hypogastric fullness and pain, a feeling of heat.
Tongue   Thick, sticky yellow coating on the root with red spots.
Pulse   Slippery-Rapid and slightly Wiry on the left Rear position.

Acupuncture

SP-9 Yinlingquan, SP-6 Sanyinjiao, BL-22 Sanjiaoshu, BL-28 Pangguangshu, Ren-3 Zhongji, BL-63 Jinmen, BL-66 Tonggu, ST-28 Shuidao.

Prescription

Ba Zheng Tang *Eight Upright Powder*.

DAMP-COLD IN THE BLADDER

Clinical manifestations

Frequent and urgent urination, difficult urination (stopping in mid-stream), a feeling of heaviness in hypogastrium and urethra, pale and turbid urine.
Tongue   White sticky coating on root.
Pulse   Slippery-Slow and slightly Wiry on left Rear position.

Acupuncture

SP-9 Yinlingquan, SP-6 Sanyinjiao, BL-22 Sanjiaoshu, Ren-3 Zhongji, ST-28 Shuidao, Ren-9 Shuifen, BL-28 Pangguangshu. Moxa is applicable.

Prescription

Ba Zheng San *Eight Upright Powder*
Shi Wei San *Pyrrosia Powder.*

BLADDER DEFICIENT AND COLD

Clinical manifestations

Frequent, abundant pale urination, incontinence, enuresis, lower backache, dizziness, nocturia, white urethral discharge.

Tongue Pale, wet.
Pulse Deep-Weak.

Acupuncture

BL-23 Shenshu, Du-4 Mingmen, BL-28 Pangguang-shu, Ren-4 Guanyuan, Ren-3 Zhongji, Du-20 Baihui.

Prescription

Suo Quan Wan *Contracting the Spring Pill*
Sang Piao Xiao San *Ootheca Mantidis Pill*
Tu Si Zi Wan *Cuscuta Pill.*

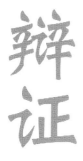

SECTION 2

IDENTIFICATION OF PATTERNS ACCORDING TO QI, BLOOD AND BODY FLUIDS

Section contents

101 Identification of patterns according to Qi, Blood, Yang and Yin *929*
102 Identification of patterns according to Body Fluids *935*

INTRODUCTION

The identification of patterns according to Qi, Blood and Body Fluids describes the patterns emerging from a pathology in the transformation, production and movement of Qi and Blood and in the transformation, transportation and excretion of Body Fluids.

The pathology of Qi includes Qi deficiency, Qi stagnation, Qi sinking and rebellious Qi. The pathology of Blood includes Blood deficiency, Blood stasis, Blood-Heat, Cold in the Blood and bleeding. The pathology of Body Fluids includes deficiency of Body Fluids, oedema and Phlegm (Dampness is discussed under the identification of patterns according to pathogenic factors).

The identification of patterns according to Qi, Blood and Body Fluids overlaps with that according to the Eight Principles and that according to the Internal Organs. For example, the pattern of Qi deficiency is the same as the eponymous one in the identification of patterns according to the Eight Principles.

The identification of patterns according to Qi, Blood and Body Fluids is useful to give a general idea about the state of Qi, Blood and Body Fluids; it is complementary to the patterns of the Internal Organs, which provide further detail. For example, the pattern of Blood deficiency within the Qi, Blood and Body Fluids patterns gives only the general symptoms and signs of Blood deficiency and the Internal Organs patterns of Liver-Blood and Heart-Blood deficiency identify the organ involved.

An understanding of the pathology of Qi, Blood, Yin and Yang is essential in practice because it reflects the way in which Qi, Blood and Body Fluids are out of harmony; this always involves a disruption of the ascending/descending and entering/exiting of Qi.

Although many of the Qi, Blood and Body Fluids patterns are found in the Internal Organ patterns, some are not and these deepen our understanding of clinical reality. For example, the pattern of 'Clear Yang not ascending' has no direct correspondent in the Internal Organ patterns.

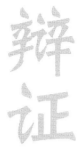

Chapter **101**

IDENTIFICATION OF PATTERNS ACCORDING TO QI, BLOOD, YANG AND YIN

Chapter contents

QI *929*
   Qi deficiency *929*
   Qi sinking *929*
   Collapse of Qi *929*
   Qi stagnation *929*
   Rebellious Qi *930*
   Qi obstructed *930*

BLOOD *930*
   Blood deficiency *930*
   Blood stasis *930*
   Blood-Heat *931*
   Blood-Dryness *931*
   Blood-Cold *931*
   Loss of Blood *931*
   Collapse of Blood *931*

YANG *932*
   Yang deficiency *932*
   Collapse of Yang *932*
   Clear Yang not ascending *932*

YIN *932*
   Yin deficiency *932*
   Yin deficiency with Empty-Heat *932*
   Collapse of Yin *932*
   Turbid Yin not descending *932*

COMBINED QI, BLOOD, YIN AND YANG *932*
   Yin and Yang both deficient *932*
   Qi and Blood both deficient *932*
   Qi and Yin both deficient *933*

QI

Qi deficiency
Clinical manifestations

Slight shortness of breath, weak voice, spontaneous sweating, poor appetite, loose stools, tiredness, pale complexion, dislike of speaking.
Pulse Empty.

Qi sinking
Clinical manifestations

Breathlessness, weak voice, spontaneous sweating, poor appetite, loose stools, tiredness, pale complexion, dislike of speaking, a feeling of bearing down, prolapse of organs (stomach, uterus, anus, bladder), listlessness, chronic diarrhoea, chronic excessive vaginal discharge, mental depression.
Pulse Empty.

Collapse of Qi
Clinical manifestations

Sudden profuse sweating, mental confusion or unconsciousness, open eyes and hands, bright-white complexion, shortness of breath, incontinence of urine and faeces.
Pulse Minute.

Qi stagnation
Clinical manifestations

A feeling of distension of chest, epigastrium or abdomen, distending pain that moves from place to place, abdominal masses that appear and disappear, abdominal distension and pain which is not relieved by a

bowel movement, premenstrual tension, breast distension, irregular periods, painful periods, mental depression, irritability, headache, constipation with bitty stools, a gloomy feeling, mood swings, frequent sighing.
Tongue   In most cases, the tongue-body colour does not change but it will be slightly Red on the sides in severe cases of Qi stagnation.
Pulse   Wiry.

Rebellious Qi

The clinical manifestations of rebellious Qi depend on the organ involved.

Clinical manifestations
Stomach-Qi rebelling upwards

Belching, hiccup, nausea, vomiting, sour regurgitation.

Liver-Qi rebelling towards Stomach

Belching, sour regurgitation, nausea, vomiting.

Liver-Qi rebelling towards Spleen

Diarrhoea, alternation of diarrhoea and constipation.

Liver-Qi rebelling upwards

Headache, dizziness, irritability, epistaxis.

Lung-Qi rebelling upwards

Cough, breathlessness, asthma.

Heart-Qi rebelling upwards

Nausea, insomnia, mental restlessness.

Kidney-Qi rebelling upwards

Breathlessness, a feeling of energy rising from the lower abdomen to the chest and throat, a feeling of tightness of the chest, a feeling of heat in the face, cold feet. This is equivalent to the Qi of the Penetrating Vessel rebelling upwards.

Qi obstructed

Qi obstructed occurs when internal pathogenic factors completely disrupt the proper flow of Qi and the balance of Yin and Yang, obstructing the orifices; this is a Full pattern seen only in acute cases, often with Phlegm, Fire, Wind and Blood stasis. The acute stage of Wind-stroke is an example of this condition.

Clinical manifestations

Sudden unconsciousness or intense, constant restlessness, red face, tinnitus, rattling sound in the throat, clenched teeth, clenched fists, constipation, retention of urine.
Tongue   Stiff and Deviated.
Pulse   Wiry.

BLOOD

Blood deficiency
Clinical manifestations

Dull complexion, dizziness, numbness tingling of the limbs, poor memory, blurred vision, insomnia, pale lips, dry eyes, white nails, floaters, palpitations, scanty periods, amenorrhoea, infertility.
Tongue   Pale and Thin.
Pulse   Choppy or Fine.

Blood stasis
Clinical manifestations

Dark complexion, purple lips, pain which is boring, fixed and stabbing in character and may be aggravated at night, abdominal masses that do not move, purple nails, purple petechiae, purple venules, bleeding with dark blood and dark clots.
Tongue   Purple.
Pulse   Wiry, Firm or Choppy.

Liver

Purple nails, dark face, painful periods with dark menstrual blood containing dark clots, abdominal pain, premenstrual pain, irregular periods, infertility.
Tongue   Purple especially on the sides.
Pulse   Wiry or Firm.

Heart

Purple lips, stabbing or pricking pain in the chest, palpitations, mental restlessness, in severe cases psychosis.
Tongue   Purple on the sides towards the front, purple and distended veins under the tongue.
Pulse   Choppy or Knotted.

Lungs

A feeling of oppression of the chest, chest pain, coughing of dark blood.

Tongue Purple in the front part or the sides in the centre section, purple and distended veins under the tongue.

Stomach

Epigastric pain, vomiting of dark blood, dark blood in the stools.
Tongue Purple in the centre.

Intestines

Severe abdominal pain, dark blood in the stools.

Uterus

Painful periods with severe stabbing pain that is usually unilateral, premenstrual pain, irregular periods, heavy periods, menstrual blood dark with clots, amenorrhoea, abdominal masses, infertility.
Tongue Purple.

Limbs

Swelling and pain of the limbs, purple extremities, purple nails, stiffness of the limbs.

Blood-Heat
Clinical manifestations

A feeling of heat, skin diseases with red eruptions, dry mouth, bleeding.
Tongue Red.
Pulse Rapid.

Heart

Red face, thirst, mental restlessness, insomnia, in severe cases manic behaviour, a feeling of heat, palpitations, blood in the urine, heavy periods.
Tongue Red.
Pulse Rapid-Full.

Liver

A feeling of heat, thirst, red skin eruptions, irritability, propensity to outbursts of anger, epistaxis, red eyes, bitter taste, heavy periods.
Tongue Red.
Pulse Rapid-Wiry.

Stomach

A feeling of heat, thirst, bleeding gums, vomiting of blood, epigastric pain.
Tongue Red.
Pulse Rapid-Overflowing.

Blood-Dryness

Blood-Dryness occurs in conjunction with Blood deficiency and it is an extreme case of it.

Clinical manifestations

Dull complexion, dizziness, numbness/tingling of the limbs, poor memory, blurred vision, insomnia, pale lips, dry eyes, white nails, 'floaters', palpitations, scanty periods with dry menstrual blood, amenorrhoea, irregular periods, dryness of the vagina, infertility, dry mouth and throat, dry skin and hair, dry, withered nails, thin body, dry stools, scanty urination, itching of the skin, very dry and scaly skin.
Tongue Pale, Thin and Dry.
Pulse Choppy or Fine.

Blood-Cold
Clinical manifestations

A feeling of cold, cold hands and feet, numbness of the limbs, dry skin, a feeling of cold and pain of the chest, epigastrium or abdomen, abdominal pain that is relieved by the application of heat, bluish or dull-white complexion, painful periods, pain alleviated by the application of heat, a feeling of cold during the periods, scanty periods, delayed cycle, menstrual blood bright red with small dark clots.
Tongue Pale or Bluish-Purple.
Pulse Choppy.

Loss of Blood
Clinical manifestations

Nosebleed, vomiting of blood, coughing of blood, blood in the stools, heavy periods, with flooding and trickling, blood in the urine.

Collapse of Blood

Collapse of Blood occurs with an acute, profuse, sudden haemorrhage.

Clinical manifestations

Sudden, profuse haemorrhage, bright-white face, sudden loss of lustre and moisture of the face, dizziness, blurred vision, 'floaters', palpitations, shortness of breath, cold hands and feet, pale lips, in severe cases unconsciousness.

Tongue Pale.
Pulse Minute or Hollow.

YANG

Yang deficiency
Clinical manifestations

Shortness of breath, weak voice, spontaneous sweating, poor appetite, loose stools, tiredness, bright-pale complexion, dislike of speaking, a feeling of cold, cold limbs, absence of thirst, desire for hot drinks, frequent pale urination.
Tongue Pale.
Pulse Deep-Weak.

Collapse of Yang
Clinical manifestations

Chilliness, cold limbs, weak breathing, profuse sweating with sweat like pearls, absence of thirst, profuse pale urination or incontinence of urine, loose stools, incontinence of faeces, mental confusion or unconsciousness.
Tongue Pale-Wet-Short.
Pulse Deep-Minute.

Clear Yang not ascending
Clinical manifestations

Dizziness, blurred vision, tinnitus, a feeling of cold, cold limbs, tiredness, weak muscles, poor appetite, loose stools.
Tongue Pale.
Pulse Weak.

In this case, the dizziness and blurred vision are not due to Blood deficiency but instead to the deficient clear Qi not ascending and therefore not brightening the orifices. For the same reason, in this case tinnitus is not due to a Kidney deficiency but rather to a failure of clear Qi to ascend and brighten the ear orifices.

YIN

Yin deficiency
Clinical manifestations

Dry mouth, dry throat at night, night sweating, dizziness, tinnitus, tiredness, thin body, insomnia.

Tongue Without coating.
Pulse Fine or Floating-Empty.

Yin deficiency with Empty-Heat
Clinical manifestations

Dry mouth, dry throat at night, night sweating, dizziness, tinnitus, tiredness, thin body, insomnia, five-palm heat, a feeling of heat in the evening, scanty dark urine, dry stools.
Tongue Red without coating.
Pulse Fine-Rapid or Floating-Empty.

Collapse of Yin
Clinical manifestations

Abundant perspiration, skin hot to the touch, hot limbs, dry mouth, retention of urine, constipation.
Tongue Red, Short without coating.
Pulse Floating-Empty-Rapid.

Turbid Yin not descending
Clinical manifestations

A feeling of distension and oppression of the epigastrium, poor appetite, loose stools or constipation, scanty urine, urine retention, a feeling of heaviness of the body, lethargy, oedema of the ankles.
Tongue Sticky coating.
Pulse Soggy.

COMBINED QI, BLOOD, YIN AND YANG

Yin and Yang both deficient
Clinical manifestations

Thin body, depression, shortness of breath, dislike of speaking, tiredness, cold limbs, a feeling of cold, sweating and a feeling of heat on slight exertion, palpitations, blurred vision, dizziness, tinnitus.
Tongue Either Pale or Red.
Pulse Fine or Weak.

Qi and Blood both deficient
Clinical manifestations

Tiredness, loose stools, poor appetite, weak muscles, weak voice, dislike of speaking, spontaneous sweat-

ing, palpitations, blurred vision, dizziness, shortness of breath, dull-pale complexion, numbness/tingling of the limbs, scanty periods, late periods, heavy periods.
Tongue Pale.
Pulse Weak or Choppy.

Qi and Yin both deficient
Clinical manifestations

Tiredness, loose stools, poor appetite, weak muscles, weak voice, dislike of speaking, spontaneous sweating, shortness of breath, dry throat, dry mouth, dry cough, dry eyes, a feeling of heat in the afternoon.
Tongue Without coating.
Pulse Fine.

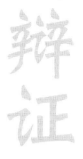

Chapter **102**

IDENTIFICATION OF PATTERNS ACCORDING TO BODY FLUIDS

Chapter contents

DEFICIENCY OF BODY FLUIDS *935*

OEDEMA *935*

PHLEGM *936*
  Wind-Phlegm *936*
  Phlegm-Heat *936*
  Cold-Phlegm *936*
  Damp-Phlegm *936*
  Dry-Phlegm *936*
  Qi-Phlegm *936*
  Food-Phlegm *936*
  Phlegm with Blood stasis *937*
  Phlegm-Fluids *937*
  Phlegm under the skin *937*
  Phlegm in the channels *937*
  Phlegm misting the Heart *937*
  Phlegm in the joints *937*
  Phlegm in the Gall-Bladder *937*
  Phlegm in the Kidneys *937*
  Shock-Phlegm *937*
  Wine-Phlegm *938*

DEFICIENCY OF BODY FLUIDS

Clinical manifestations

Dry skin, mouth, nose, lips, throat, eyes, cracked lips, dry cough, hoarse voice, absence of sweating, scanty urination, dry stools, scanty periods.
Tongue Dry.

Lungs

Dry throat, dry cough, dry skin.

Stomach

Dry mouth, thirst with a desire to sip liquids, dry tongue.

Kidneys

Dry throat, dry skin, scanty urination.

Large Intestine

Dry stools.

Liver

Dry eyes, dry skin, scanty periods.

OEDEMA

Clinical manifestations

Pitting oedema of the face, hands, abdomen, ankles or legs, a feeling of oppression of the chest, a feeling of heaviness of the body, scanty urination.
Tongue Swollen.

PHLEGM

The patterns caused by Phlegm are:

- Wind-Phlegm
- Phlegm-Heat
- Cold-Phlegm
- Damp-Phlegm
- Dry-Phlegm
- Qi-Phlegm
- Food-Phlegm
- Phlegm with Blood stasis
- Phlegm-Fluids
- Phlegm under the skin
- Phlegm in the channels
- Phlegm misting the Heart
- Phlegm in the joints
- Phlegm in the Gall-Bladder
- Phlegm in the Kidneys
- Shock-Phlegm
- Wine-Phlegm.

Wind-Phlegm
Clinical manifestations

Severe dizziness, nausea, vomiting, numbness of the limbs, coughing of phlegm, a feeling of oppression of the chest, blurred vision, a rattling sound in the throat, slurred speech.
Tongue Swollen with sticky coating.
Pulse Wiry-Slippery.

In cases of Wind-stroke, manifestations also include: aphasia, deviation of eyes and mouth, hemiplegia and a Swollen-Deviated tongue.

Phlegm-Heat
Clinical manifestations

Cough with expectoration of profuse yellow sputum, which may be blood tinged, a feeling of oppression of the chest, dark eye sockets, red cheekbones, red face, thirst, oily skin, breathlessness, chest pain, insomnia, dark urine, a feeling of heat, mental restlessness.
Tongue Red-Swollen with sticky yellow coating.
Pulse Rapid-Slippery.

Cold-Phlegm
Clinical manifestations

Cough with expectoration of watery white sputum, a feeling of cold, cold hands and feet, nausea, vomiting, a feeling of oppression of the chest and epigastrium, dull-white complexion, pale urine.
Tongue Pale-Swollen with wet-white coating.
Pulse Slippery-Slow.

Damp-Phlegm
Clinical manifestations

Cough with easy expectoration of profuse, sticky white sputum, a feeling of oppression of the chest and epigastrium, breathlessness, rattling sound in the throat, dark eye sockets, sallow-greyish complexion, a feeling of heaviness, tendency to obesity, swollen hands and feet, poor appetite, nausea, dizziness, blurred vision, oily skin.
Tongue Swollen with sticky coating.
Pulse Slippery.

Dry-Phlegm
Clinical manifestations

Sputum in the chest that is difficult to expectorate, bouts of dry cough followed by expectoration of sticky sputum, breathlessness, dull-white complexion, dark eye sockets, dry throat, dry nose and lips, dry mouth but no desire to drink.
Tongue Swollen with sticky dry coating.
Pulse Slippery.

Qi-Phlegm
Clinical manifestations

A feeling of a lump in the throat, difficulty in swallowing, a feeling of oppression of the chest and diaphragm, mental depression, irritability, nausea, sighing.
Pulse Wiry.

Food-Phlegm
Clinical manifestations

Cough with abundant sputum, nausea, vomiting, sour regurgitation, belching, a feeling of fullness in the epigastrium, a feeling of oppression of the chest and

epigastrium, epigastric pain after eating that is better after bowel movement.
Tongue   Swollen with thick sticky coating.
Pulse   Slippery.

Phlegm with Blood stasis
Clinical manifestations

A feeling of oppression of the chest, numbness/tingling of the limbs, pain in the joints, stiffness and rigidity of joints, abdominal masses, fibroids, goitre, mental restlessness, insomnia, dark eye sockets.
Tongue   Purple-Swollen with sticky coating.
Pulse   Slippery-Wiry or Slippery-Firm.

Phlegm-Fluids
Clinical manifestations
Phlegm-Fluids in Stomach and Intestines (Tan Yin)

Abdominal fullness and distension, nausea, vomiting of watery fluids, splashing sound in the stomach, dry mouth without a desire to drink, palpitations, shortness of breath, dizziness, a feeling of oppression of the chest, loose stools, loss of weight.
Tongue   Swollen with sticky coating.
Pulse   Deep-Wiry or Deep-Slippery.

Phlegm-Fluids in the hypochondrium (Xuan Yin)

Hypochondrial pain which is worse on coughing and breathing, a feeling of distension and pulling of the hypochondrium, shortness of breath.
Tongue   Swollen with sticky coating.
Pulse   Deep-Slippery-Wiry.

Phlegm-Fluids in the limbs (Yi Yin)

A feeling of heaviness of the body, pain in the muscles, absence of sweating, lack of desire to drink, cough with profuse watery sputum, swelling of the limbs, lethargy, breathlessness.
Tongue   Swollen with sticky coating.
Pulse   Wiry-Slippery or Tight-Slippery.

Phlegm-Fluids above the diaphragm (Zhi Yin)

Cough with watery white sputum, breathlessness, swelling of the limbs, dizziness, inability to lie down, swollen face, a feeling of cold.

Tongue   Swollen with sticky white coating.
Pulse   Slippery.

Phlegm under the skin
Clinical manifestations

Lumps or nodules under the skin, nerve-ganglia swellings, swelling of lymph nodes, swelling of the thyroid, lipoma.

Phlegm in the channels
Clinical manifestations

Numbness/tingling in the limbs (seen in Wind-stroke).

Phlegm misting the Heart
Clinical manifestations

Inappropriate laughter or crying, dull thinking, hypomania, manic behaviour, manic depression, psychosis.

Phlegm in the joints
Clinical manifestations

Swelling and deformities of joints seen in Chronic Painful Obstruction Syndrome (often seen in rheumatoid arthritis).

Phlegm in the Gall-Bladder
Clinical manifestations
Gall-Bladder stones.

Phlegm in the Kidneys
Clinical manifestations
Kidney stones.

Shock-Phlegm
Clinical manifestations

Pain in the heart region, a feeling of oppression in the chest, anxiety, mental restlessness following a shock.
   This pattern is supposed to occur when a severe shock displaces the Spirit from the Heart and its place is taken by Phlegm.
Pulse   Moving.

Wine-Phlegm

Clinical manifestations

Nausea, vomiting, a feeling of fullness of the epigastrium, foul breath, a rattling sound in the throat, purple nose, purple complexion, a feeling of oppression of the chest.

This pattern is seen in older people with Phlegm deriving from excessive alcohol consumption.

Tongue   Reddish-Purple and Swollen with a sticky yellow coating.

Pulse   Slippery.

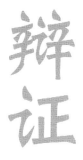

SECTION 3

IDENTIFICATION OF PATTERNS ACCORDING TO PATHOGENIC FACTORS, FOUR LEVELS, SIX STAGES AND THREE BURNERS

Section contents

103 Identification of patterns according to pathogenic factors *943*
104 Identification of patterns according to the Four Levels *953*
105 Identification of patterns according to the Six Stages *965*
106 Identification of patterns according to the Three Burners *969*
107 Residual pathogenic factor *973*

INTRODUCTION

This section includes two separate methods of pattern identification:

- the identification of patterns according to pathogenic factors
- the identification of patterns according to the Four Levels, Six Stages and Three Burners.

In addition to these, the patterns formed by residual pathogenic factors will also be discussed.

Identification of patterns according to pathogenic factors

The method of identification of patterns according to pathogenic factors describes the patterns formed when the body is invaded by external pathogenic factors such as Dampness, Wind, Cold, Dryness and Summer-Heat. However, since the symptoms and signs of the corresponding internal pathogenic factors are similar, these are usually discussed within this type of identification of pattern: this also includes the discussion of Fire, which is an internal pathogenic factor with no corresponding external factor.

Pathogenic factors invade the body in various forms, which are Wind, Cold, Dampness, Summer-Heat, Dryness and Fire. Each of these, with the exception of Fire, can be of exterior or interior origin. From the point of view of the Eight Principles, they always correspond to a Full pattern.

Although these pathogenic factors are causes of disease, and due to weather, they have a greater importance as patterns of disharmony. In fact, the diagnosis of a pathogenic factor is made not on the basis of the patient's history (i.e. whether he or she was exposed to that particular climatic factor), but on the basis of the pattern of symptoms and signs presented. Of course, when considered as causes of disease, climatic factors have a definite, direct influence on the body and they attack it in a way that corresponds to their nature. For example, a person exposed to a hot, dry climate is likely to develop a pattern of invasion of 'Wind-Dryness'. However, when considered as pathogenic factors, climatic influences are somewhat irrelevant as the diagnosis is made only on the basis of the clinical manifestations. For example, if a person has a runny nose, aversion to cold, sneezing, a headache, a stiff neck, a cough and a Floating pulse, these clinical manifestations denote a pattern of exterior Wind-Cold.

It is irrelevant whether this person was exposed to climatic cold or not and it is not usually necessary to ask.

Some internally generated pathogenic factors give rise to pathological signs and symptoms similar to those caused by exterior climatic factors. These will be discussed together with the relevant exterior pathogenic factor.

The pathogenic factors discussed are:

- Wind
- Cold
- Summer-Heat
- Dampness
- Dryness
- Fire.

Identification of patterns according to the Four Levels, Six Stages and Three Burners

These methods of identifying patterns also describe the symptomatology of pathogenic factors, but specifically those caused by acute invasions of Wind: Wind-Cold in the case of the Six Stages and Wind-Heat in the case of the Four Levels and Three Burners.

Identification of patterns according to the Six Stages

The identification of patterns according to the Six Stages is the oldest method as it is derived from Zhang Zhong Jing's 'Discussion of Cold-induced Diseases' (c. AD220) (see Shang Han Lung Research Group in Bibliography). It describes the patterns arising when the patient is invaded by external Wind and especially Wind-Cold. These six patterns are the Greater Yang, Lesser Yang, Bright Yang, Greater Yin, Lesser Yin and Terminal Yin, representing six energetic layers of penetration of external Wind. Of these, the Greater-Yang stage is the only exterior stage; that is, at that stage the pathogenic factor (Wind-Cold) is on the Exterior and in the Lungs Defensive-Qi portion.

Identification of patterns according to the Four Levels

The identification of patterns according to the Four Levels was formulated primarily by Ye Tian Shi and set out in his book 'Discussion of Warm Diseases' (*Wen*

Bing Lun, 1746). It describes the patterns arising when the patient is invaded by external Wind-Heat. These patterns consist of four levels: the Defensive-Qi, Qi, Nutritive-Qi and Blood Levels. They involve four levels of Heat, the first being external Wind-Heat and the other three internal Heat.

The identification of patterns according to the Four Levels is closely linked to the clinical entity of Warm Diseases (*Wen Bing*). Warm Diseases are caused by Wind-Heat, but not every invasion of external Wind-Heat leads to a Warm Disease. Warm Diseases have the following characteristics:

- they are all caused by external Wind-Heat
- they all present with fever
- they all have a tendency to injure Yin and Body Fluids quickly
- they are infectious (a new idea in Chinese medicine)
- they penetrate via the nose and mouth (until the development of the Warm Disease School, external Wind was thought to enter the body via the skin).

Identification of patterns according to the Three Burners

The identification of patterns according to the Three Burners is quite similar to that in relation to the Four Levels. It was formulated by Wu Ju Tong in the Qing dynasty. Many of the patterns are essentially the same as those of the Four Levels, except that they are seen from the perspective of the Three Burners, that is, patterns of the Upper Burner, Middle Burner and Lower Burner. The Middle Burner patterns correspond to the Qi level while those of the Lower Burner correspond to the Nutritive-Qi and Blood levels. By contrast, the patterns of the Upper Burner encompass the Defensive-Qi, Qi and Nutritive-Qi levels.

Table P6.S3.1 illustrates the connections between the Four Levels and the Three Burners patterns.

Figure 104.6 (p. 961) shows the relationship between the Three Burners and the Four Levels. Figure 104.7 (p. 962) shows the relationship between the Three Burners and the Six Stages. Figures 104.8 (p. 963) show the relationship between the Three Burners, the Four Levels and the Six Stages.

Table P6.S3.1 Relationship between Three Burners and Four Levels patterns

Burner	Pattern	Level
Upper Burner	Invasion of Lungs Defensive-Qi system	Defensive Qi
	Heat in Lungs	Qi
	Heat in Pericardium	Nutritive Qi
Middle Burner	Heat in Bright Yang	
	Damp-Heat in Stomach and Spleen	Qi
Lower Burner	Heat in Kidneys	
	Liver-Heat stirs Wind	Nutritive Qi, Blood
	Liver Empty-Wind	

Essential differences between the three identifications of patterns

- Six Stages: the three Yang patterns all have Full-Cold; the three Yin patterns all have Empty-Cold.
- Four Levels: mostly Full-Heat patterns.
- Three Burners: Upper Burner mostly has Heat patterns
  Middle Burner mostly has Damp-Heat patterns
  Lower Burner mostly has Yin deficiency.

Residual pathogenic factor patterns

A residual pathogenic factor occurs when the body is invaded by an external pathogen, which penetrates to the Interior. The patient appears to recover but there is a 'residual' pathogenic factor which encumbers the body's physiology of Qi and predisposes the person to a further attack of a pathogenic factor.

A residual pathogenic factor is formed mostly when the patient does not rest during an invasion of an external pathogen; this weakens Qi, the body does not react fully to the external invasion and, although the patient appears to recover, some pathogen is left in the body. This process is also often caused by the excessive use of antibiotics for relatively minor infections: antibiotics 'kill' the bacteria but they do not clear Heat, nor do they resolve Phlegm or Dampness. By killing the bacteria and eliminating the fever, antibiotics may encourage the patient to ignore the seriousness of an external invasion; as a result, the patient does not rest and returns to work too quickly, thus favouring the formation of a pathogenic factor. Antibiotics favour the formation of a residual pathogenic factor also because they injure Stomach-Qi and Stomach-Yin; by doing so, they favour the formation of Dampness or Phlegm.

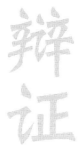

Chapter 103

IDENTIFICATION OF PATTERNS ACCORDING TO PATHOGENIC FACTORS

Chapter contents

INTRODUCTION   *943*

WIND   *943*
   Exterior Wind   *944*
   Interior Wind   *945*

COLD   *946*
   Exterior Cold   *946*
   Interior Cold   *947*

SUMMER-HEAT   *948*

DAMPNESS   *948*
   External Dampness   *949*
   Internal Dampness   *950*

DRYNESS   *950*
   External Dryness   *951*
   Internal Dryness   *951*

FIRE   *951*

INTRODUCTION

Pathogenic factors invade the body in various forms, which are Wind, Cold, Dampness, Summer-Heat, Dryness and Fire. Each of these, with the exception of Fire, can be of exterior or interior origin. From the point of view of the Eight Principles, they always correspond to a Full pattern.

Although these pathogenic factors are also causes of disease due to weather, they have greater importance as patterns of disharmony. In other words, if a person displays all the clinical manifestations of Dampness (e.g. epigastric fullness, a feeling of heaviness, sticky taste, etc.), we can safely diagnose a pattern of Dampness, irrespective of whether that person was exposed to climatic dampness or not.

Some internally generated pathogenic factors give rise to pathological signs and symptoms similar to those caused by the exterior climatic factors. These will be discussed together with the relevant exterior pathogenic factor.

The pathogenic factors are:

1. Wind
2. Cold
3. Summer-Heat
4. Dampness
5. Dryness
6. Fire.

WIND

Wind is Yang in nature and tends to injure Blood and Yin. It is often the vehicle through which other

climatic factors invade the body. For example, Cold will often enter the body as Wind-Cold and Heat as Wind-Heat.

The clinical manifestations due to Wind mimic the action of wind itself in nature, which arises quickly and changes rapidly, moves swiftly, blows intermittently and sways the top of trees.

There is a saying that captures the clinical characteristics of Wind: *'Sudden rigidity is due to Wind'*.[1] This refers to the clinical manifestations resulting from both interior and exterior Wind. In fact, interior Wind can cause paralysis (as in Wind-stroke) and exterior Wind can cause facial paralysis or simply stiffness of the neck.

The main clinical manifestations of Wind are listed in Box 103.1.

BOX 103.1 CLINICAL MANIFESTATIONS OF WIND

- Onset is rapid
- Causes rapid changes in symptoms and signs
- Causes symptoms and signs to move from place to place in the body
- Can cause tremors or convulsions, but also stiffness or paralysis
- Affects the top part of the body
- Affects the Lungs first
- Affects the skin
- Causes itching

Tremors, convulsions and paralysis apply only to interior Wind (except for facial paralysis, which can be caused by exterior Wind). Invasion of the Lungs applies only to external Wind. All the other manifestations listed apply to both exterior and interior Wind.

Exterior Wind

The symptoms and signs of invasion of exterior Wind are:

- aversion to cold or wind
- sneezing, cough
- runny nose
- possibly fever
- occipital stiffness and ache
- itchy throat
- sweating or not (depending on whether Wind or Cold is predominant)
- Floating pulse.

Besides this, exterior Wind can invade the channels of the face directly and cause deviation of mouth and eyebrows (facial paralysis).

Exterior Wind can also invade any channel, particularly the Yang channels, and can settle in the joints, causing stiffness and pain there (Painful Obstruction Syndrome). The pain would typically be 'wandering', moving from one joint to the other on different days.

Finally, Wind can also affect some Internal Organs, principally the Liver. Wind pertains to Wood and the Liver according to the Five-Element system of correspondences. The relationship can often be observed when a person prone to migraine headaches is affected by a period of windy weather (particularly an easterly wind) causing a neck ache and headache.

Box 103.2 summarizes the patterns of exterior Wind invasion.

BOX 103.2 EXTERIOR WIND

- Invasion of Wind in the Lungs Defensive-Qi portion (common cold)
- Invasion of Wind in the channels of the face (facial paralysis)
- Invasion of Wind in the channels and joints (Painful Obstruction Syndrome)
- Affliction of the Liver channel by external Wind (Liver-Yang headache elicited by external Wind)

Wind combines with other pathogenic factors and primarily Cold, Heat, Dampness and Water. Therefore, I will outline the clinical manifestation of four types of exterior Wind:

- Wind-Cold
- Wind-Heat
- Wind-Dampness
- Wind-Water.

Wind-Cold

The symptoms and signs of Wind-Cold are: aversion to cold, shivering, sneezing, cough, runny nose with watery white mucus, either no fever or only a slight fever, occipital stiffness and ache, clear urine, body aches, itchy throat, lack of thirst, tongue body colour unchanged, with thin white coating, Floating-Tight pulse.

These are the general symptoms of Wind-Cold. There are, however, two separate patterns of invasion of Wind-Cold: one with a predominance of Wind

(called Attack of Wind) and the other with a predominance of Cold (called Attack of Cold). The former is more likely to occur when the patient's Upright Qi is weak (and is treated with Gui Zhi Tang *Ramulus Cinnamomi Decoction*); the latter occurs when the patient's Upright Qi is relatively strong (and is treated with Ma Huang Tang *Ephedra Decoction*). In Attack of Wind there is slight sweating, in Attack of Cold there is no sweating.

Wind-Cold – Attack of Wind

Aversion to wind or slight aversion to cold, slight fever, slight sweating, headache, occipital stiffness, sneezing, thin white tongue coating, Floating-Slow pulse.

Wind-Cold – Attack of Cold

Aversion to cold, slight fever, severe occipital stiffness/headache, body aches, absence of sweating, sneezing, runny nose with white discharge, breathlessness, thin white tongue coating, Floating-Tight pulse.

Table 103.1 differentiates between Attack of Cold and Attack of Wind.

Wind-Heat

The symptoms and signs of Wind-Heat are: aversion to cold, sneezing, cough, runny nose with slightly yellow mucus, fever, occipital stiffness and ache, slight sweating, itchy or very sore throat, swollen tonsils, body aches, slighty dark urine, slight thirst, tongue-body colour slightly Red on the front or sides, or both (not in every case) with thin white coating, Floating-Rapid pulse.

Table 103.2 differentiates between the symptoms of Wind-Cold and those of Wind-Heat.

Wind-Dampness

The symptoms and signs of Wind-Dampness are: aversion to cold, fever, swollen glands, nausea, sweating, occipital stiffness, body aches, muscle ache, a feeling of heaviness of the body, swollen joints, Floating-Slippery pulse.

Wind-Water

The symptoms and signs of Wind-Water are: aversion to cold, fever, oedema, especially on the face, swollen face and eyes, cough with profuse white and watery mucus, sweating, absence of thirst, Floating pulse.

Interior Wind

The main clinical manifestations of interior Wind are: tremors, tics, severe dizziness, vertigo and numbness. In severe cases, they are: convulsions, unconsciousness, opisthotonos, hemiplegia and deviation of the mouth.

Interior Wind is always related to a Liver disharmony. It can arise from three different conditions:
1. Extreme Heat Extreme Heat can give rise to Liver-Wind. This happens in the late stages of febrile diseases when the Heat enters the Blood portion and generates Wind. This process is like the wind generated by a large forest fire. The clinical manifestations are a high fever, delirium, coma and opisthotonos. These signs are frequently seen in meningitis and are due to Wind in the Liver and Heat in the Pericardium.
2. Liver-Yang Liver-Yang rising can produce Liver-Wind in prolonged cases. The clinical manifestations are severe dizziness, vertigo, headache and irritability.

Table 103.1 Differentiation between Attack of Cold and Attack of Wind in Wind-Cold

	Wind-Cold – Attack of Cold	Wind-Cold – Attack of Wind
Common manifestations	Aversion to cold, occipital stiffness, Floating pulse	
Other symptoms	Pronounced aversion to cold, body aches, no sweating, pulse Floating-Tight	Aversion to wind, fever, slight sweating, pulse Floating-Slow
Treatment	Release the Exterior by causing sweating (Ma Huang Tang *Ephedra Decoction*)	Release the Exterior by adjusting the space between skin and muscles and regulating Defensive- and Nutritive-Qi (Gui Zhi Tang *Cinnamon Twig Decoction*)

Table 103.2 Differentiation between Wind-Cold and Wind-Heat manifestations

		Wind-Cold	Wind-Heat
Pathology		Wind-Cold obstructing the space between skin and muscles	Wind-Heat obstructing the space between skin and muscles and impairing the descending of Lung-Qi
Symptoms and signs	Fever	Slight	High
	Shivers	Pronounced	Slight
	Aches	Pronounced	Slight
	Thirst	No	Yes
	Urine	Clear	Slightly dark
	Headache	Occipital	Deep inside, severe
	Sweating	If sweating, in top part, head	Slight sweating
	Sore throat	Itchy throat	Very sore throat
	Tongue	No change	Slightly Red on the sides/front
	Pulse	Floating-Tight	Floating-Rapid
Treatment		Pungent-warm herbs to cause sweating	Pungent-cool herbs to release the Exterior

3. Deficiency of Liver-Blood Finally, deficiency of Liver-Blood can also give rise to Empty Liver-Wind. This is due to the deficiency of Blood creating an empty space within the blood vessels, which is taken up by interior Wind. This could be compared to the draughts generated sometimes in certain underground (subway) stations. The clinical manifestations are numbness, dizziness, blurred vision, tics and slight tremors (in Chinese called 'chicken feet Wind' as the tremors are like the jerky movements of chickens' feet when they are scouring the ground for food). Empty-Wind can also result from Liver-Yin deficiency.

Box 103.3 summarizes the patterns of interior Wind.

BOX 103.3 INTERIOR WIND

- Extreme Heat generating Wind (Blood level of Four Levels)
- Liver-Yang rising turning into Liver-Wind
- Liver-Blood (or Liver-Yin) deficiency giving rise to (Empty) Wind

---

COLD

Cold is a Yin pathogenic factor and, as such, it tends to injure Yang. Cold can be exterior or interior.

Exterior Cold

Cold, spearheaded by Wind, can invade the Exterior of the body and give rise to symptoms of Wind-Cold, already described above.

Cold can also invade the channels directly and cause Painful Obstruction Syndrome, with pain in one or more joints, chilliness and contraction of the tendons.

Apart from invading muscles, channels and joints, Cold can also invade three of the Internal Organs directly. These are the Stomach (causing epigastric pain and vomiting), the Intestines (causing abdominal pain and diarrhoea) and the Uterus (causing acute dysmenorrhoea). In all three cases the symptoms would be accompanied by chilliness and the pain would be alleviated by the application of heat.

Box 103.4 summarizes the patterns of external Cold invasion.

BOX 103.4 EXTERNAL COLD INVASION

- External Cold (with Wind) invasion in the Lung Defensive-Qi portion (common cold)
- Invasion of Cold in the channels and joints (Painful Obstruction Syndrome)
- Invasion of external Cold in organs directly (Stomach, Intestines and Uterus)
  —Stomach: vomiting and epigastric pain
  —Intestines: diarrhoea and abdominal pain
  —Uterus: acute dysmenorrhoea

Cold contracts tissues and it obstructs the circulation of Yang Qi and Blood causing pain. Hence there is a saying: *'Retention of Cold causes pain.'*[2]

Pain is therefore a frequent manifestation of Cold. Other symptoms are stiffness, contraction of tendons and chilliness. Cold can invade any part of the body and any joint, but the most common places it invades are the hands and arms, feet and knees, lower back and shoulders.

Cold is often manifested with thin, watery and clear fluid discharges, such as a clear white discharge from the nose, very pale urine, watery loose stools and clear watery vaginal discharges. Another saying clarifies this characteristic of Cold: *'A disease characterized by thin, clear, watery and cool discharges is due to Cold.'*[3]

Box 103.5 summarizes the signs of symptoms of exterior Cold.

BOX 103.5 SYMPTOMS AND SIGNS OF EXTERIOR COLD

- Severe pain (ameliorated by application of heat)
- Stiffness of muscles
- Contraction of tendons
- Feeling of cold
- Thin, watery fluid discharges

Interior Cold

Interior Cold can be Full or Empty. The clinical manifestations of Full- and Empty-Cold are very similar as they are the same in nature. The main difference is that Full-Cold is characterized by an acute onset, severe pain and a tongue and pulse of the Excess type; for example the tongue would have a thick white coating and the pulse would be Full and Tight. Empty-Cold is characterized by a gradual onset, dull pain and a tongue and pulse of the Deficiency type; for example the tongue would have a thin white coating and be Pale and the pulse would be Empty or Weak.

Interior Full-Cold

Interior Full-Cold originates from climatic cold, which either invades the channels, causing Painful Obstruction Syndrome, or invades certain organs directly. Both these cases have been mentioned above.

Generally speaking, Interior Full-Cold can last only a relatively short time. After prolonged retention, interior Cold consumes the Yang of the Spleen, giving rise

to Empty-Cold. Thus a Full-Cold pattern can turn into an Empty-Cold one.

Interior Empty-Cold

Interior Empty-Cold arises from deficiency of Yang, usually of the Spleen, Lungs or Kidneys. In this case the Cold does not come from outside the body, but is interiorly generated by deficiency of Yang.

The general symptoms are chilliness, dull pain, cold limbs, a desire to drink warm liquids, lack of thirst, a pale face, a thin white tongue coating and a Deep, Weak and Slow pulse. Other symptoms vary according to which organ is mostly affected. The Heart, Lungs, Spleen, Kidneys can all suffer from deficiency of Yang and interior Cold.

Table 103.3 lists the clinical manifestations of Full- and Empty-Cold.

Table 103.3 Differentiation between Full- and Empty-Cold

	Full-Cold	Empty-Cold
Onset	Acute	Chronic
Pain	Intense, crampy	Dull
Tongue	Thick white coating	Thin white coating, Pale body
Pulse	Full-Tight-Slow	Weak-Deep-Slow

The symptoms of Heart-Yang deficiency (in addition to the above-mentioned general symptoms) with interior Cold are stuffiness and pain in the chest, purple lips and a Knotted pulse. In Lung-Yang deficiency they are a tendency to catch colds, sweating and a cough with white mucus. In Spleen-Yang deficiency they are diarrhoea or loose stools and lack of appetite. In Kidney-Yang deficiency they are frequent, pale and profuse urination, lower backache, cold feet and knees and impotence in men or white leucorrhoea in women.

The manifestations of Yang deficiency of the various organs have been discussed in greater detail in the chapters on the identification of patterns according to the Internal Organs.

Box 103.6 summarizes the types of Empty-Cold.

BOX 103.6 EMPTY-COLD

- Heart-Yang deficiency
- Spleen-Yang deficiency
- Lung-Yang deficiency
- Kidney-Yang deficiency

SUMMER-HEAT

Summer-Heat is a Yang pathogenic factor and, as such, it tends to injure Yin. This pathogenic factor is slightly different from the others, in so far as it is definitely related to a specific season since it can occur only in summer.

The main clinical manifestations are aversion to cold, sweating, headache, scanty dark urine, dry lips, thirst, a Floating-Rapid pulse and a Red tongue on the sides and front. Note that there is aversion to cold in the beginning stages because the Summer-Heat invades the Defensive-Qi portion and Defensive Qi fails to warm the muscles.

In severe cases, Heat can invade the Pericardium and cause clouding of the mind, manifesting with delirium, slurred speech or unconsciousness.

Box 103.7 summarizes the clinical manifestations of Summer-Heat.

BOX 103.7 SUMMER-HEAT

- Aversion to cold
- Sweating
- Headache
- Scanty dark urine
- Dry lips
- Thirst
- Floating-Rapid pulse
- Tongue Red on sides and front

DAMPNESS

Dampness is a Yin pathogenic factor and it tends to injure Yang. The term refers not only to damp weather, but also to such conditions as living in a damp house. Exterior Dampness can also be caught by wearing wet clothes, wading in water, working in damp places or sitting on damp ground.

The characteristics of Dampness are that it is sticky, it is difficult to get rid of, it is heavy, it slows things down, it infuses downwards and it causes repeated attacks. When exterior Dampness invades the body, it tends to invade the lower part first, typically the legs. From the legs, it can flow upwards in the leg channels to settle in any of the pelvic cavity organs. If it settles in the female genital system it causes vaginal discharges, if it settles in the Intestines it will cause loose stools and if it settles in the Bladder it will cause difficulty, frequency and burning of urination.

The clinical manifestations of Dampness are extremely varied according to its location and nature (hot or cold), but the general ones are a feeling of heaviness of body or head, lack of appetite, a feeling of fullness of chest or epigastrium, a sticky taste, urinary difficulty, a white sticky vaginal discharge, a sticky tongue coating and a Slippery or Soggy pulse.

Box 103.8 summarizes the manifestations of Dampness.

BOX 103.8 GENERAL MANIFESTATIONS OF DAMPNESS

- Feeling of heaviness
- Poor appetite
- Feeling of fullness
- Sticky taste
- Urinary difficulty
- Vaginal discharge
- Sticky tongue coating
- Slippery or Soggy pulse

The clinical manifestations of Dampness can be classified according to its location as follows:

- Head: feeling of heaviness and muzziness of the head
- Eyes: red swollen eyelids, eyes oozing fluid, styes
- Mouth: mouth ulcers on gums, swollen-red lips
- Stomach and Spleen: feeling of fullness/oppression of epigastrium, feeling of fullness after eating, sticky taste, loose stools, poor appetite, Soggy pulse
- Lower Burner: excessive vaginal discharge, painful periods, infertility, turbid urine, difficult and painful urination, scrotal sweating or eczema, genital eczema, genital itching
- Skin: papules (Damp-Heat with more Heat), pustules, vesicles (Dampness without Heat), greasy sweat, boils, any oozing skin lesion
- Joints: swollen-painful joints (Fixed Painful Obstruction Syndrome, also Wandering Painful Obstruction Syndrome if mixed with Wind)
- Connecting channels: numbness and loss of sensation.

The various clinical manifestations can be correlated to the following main characteristics of Dampness.

Heaviness This causes a feeling of tiredness, heaviness of limbs or head, or a 'muzzy' feeling of the head. Since Dampness is heavy it causes a feeling of fullness and oppression of chest or epigastrium, and it tends to settle in the Lower Burner. However, Dampness often affects the head too causing the above-mentioned symptoms. This happens because it prevents the clear Yang from ascending to the head to brighten the sense orifices and clear the brain.

Dirtiness Dampness is dirty and is reflected in dirty discharges, such as cloudy urine, vaginal discharges or skin diseases characterized by thick and dirty fluids oozing out, such as in certain types of eczema.

Stickiness Dampness is sticky and this is reflected in a sticky tongue coating, sticky taste and Slippery pulse. The sticky nature of Dampness also accounts for its being very difficult to get rid of. It often becomes chronic, manifesting in frequent, recurrent bouts.

Dampness can also cause a large variety of diseases according to its location. There are three locations: the Internal Organs, the channels and the skin. The range of disease according to the location of Dampness is as follows.

Internal Organs In the Stomach and Spleen there may be epigastric pain and fullness, poor digestion, feeling of fullness, a sticky taste, or a poor appetite. In the Gall-Bladder hypochondrial pain and fullness are seen. In the bladder there may be difficult and painful urination, and cloudy urine. In the Uterus Dampness may cause infertility, or excessive vaginal discharge. In the Intestines there may be loose stools with mucus, abdominal pain and fullness. Dampness in the Kidneys may manifest as cloudy urine, or difficult urination. In the Liver it may cause hypochondrial fullness, distension and pain, or jaundice.

Channels In the joints Dampness can cause Painful Obstruction Syndrome. In the head there may be a feeling of heaviness of the head, or headache.

Skin Dampness is the cause of an enormous number of skin diseases manifesting with oozing skin lesions, papules, vesicles or pustules.

The classification of Dampness is quite complex and can be divided into the two broad categories of external or internal Dampness.

Within each of these are a number of subcategories. Box 103.9 summarizes the classification of Dampness.

> **BOX 103.9 CATEGORIES OF EXTERNAL AND INTERNAL DAMPNESS**
>
> **External**
> - Simple invasion of Dampness in the Internal Organs
>   —External invasion of Dampness in Bladder
>   —External invasion of Dampness in Stomach
>   —External invasion of Dampness in Intestines
>   —External invasion of Dampness in Uterus
>   —External invasion of Dampness in Gall-Bladder
> - Invasion of acute, external Dampness in channels
> - Invasion of External Damp-Heat at Defensive-Qi level
>   —External Damp-Heat
>   —External Summer-Heat with Dampness
>
> **Internal**
> *Chronic*
> - Internal Dampness in Internal Organs
>   —Dampness in Stomach and Spleen
>   —Dampness in Bladder
>   —Dampness in Intestines
>   —Dampness in Uterus
>   —Dampness in Gall-Bladder
>   —Dampness in Liver
>   —Dampness in Kidneys
> - Chronic Dampness in Channels
> - Internal Dampness in Skin
> *Acute*
> - Damp-Heat at Qi Level

External Dampness

There are three possible types of invasions of external Dampness:

> 1. A 'simple' invasion of Dampness in the Internal Organs, which may affect the Bladder, Stomach, Intestines, Uterus and Gall-Bladder
> 2. An invasion of Dampness in the channels causing Painful Obstruction Syndrome in its acute stage
> 3. An invasion of Damp-Heat of the *Wen Bing* type at the Defensive-Qi (*Wei*) level, manifesting with fever.

'Simple' invasion of external Dampness in Internal Organs
Invasion of external Dampness in Bladder

Difficulty and pain on urination, scanty but frequent urination, cloudy urine, a feeling of heaviness in the lower abdomen, tongue with a thick sticky coating on the root, pulse perhaps Slippery on the left Rear position.

If associated with Heat: burning pain on urination, dark urine, thirst but no desire to drink, yellow tongue coating and a slightly rapid pulse.

Invasion of external Dampness in the Stomach

Acute onset of vomiting/watery diarrhoea without smell, epigastric pain, a feeling of stuffiness of the epigastrium, cold limbs, no appetite, thick, sticky white tongue coating, Slippery or Soggy pulse.

Invasion of external Dampness in Intestines

Acute onset of watery diarrhoea, without smell, abdominal pain, a feeling of heaviness, tongue with a sticky, thick white coating, pulse Slippery.

Invasion of external Dampness in Uterus

Acute onset of painful periods (as a one-off when periods were not previously painful), excessive vaginal discharge, thick, sticky white tongue coating on the root, Slippery pulse.

Invasion of external Dampness in Gall-Bladder

Acute onset of hypochondrial pain, a feeling of heaviness, bitter taste, tongue with a sticky yellow coating on one side, Slippery pulse.

Invasion of acute, external Dampness in channels

This is, of course, an acute stage of Painful Obstruction Syndrome. When one joint only is affected, this is usually Cold-Dampness; when several joints are affected it is often due to Damp-Heat.

Invasion of acute, external Damp-Heat at the Defensive-Qi level

This can be external Damp-Heat or Summer-Heat mixed with Dampness.

External Damp-Heat at Defensive-Qi level

Shivers, fever, the body feels hot to touch, swollen glands, fever higher in the afternoon, headache as if wrapped, a feeling of oppression of the chest and epigastrium, a sticky taste, no thirst, tongue with a sticky white coating (it is white because it is in the beginning stage), Soggy pulse.

External Summer-Heat with Dampness

Fever, slight aversion to cold, no sweating, headache, a feeling of heaviness of the body, an uncomfortable sensation of the epigastrium, irritability, thirst, tongue body Red with a sticky coating, Weak-Floating and Rapid pulse.

Internal Dampness

Interior Dampness arises from a deficiency of the Spleen and sometimes the Kidneys. If the Spleen's function of transformation and transportation of Body Fluids fails, these will not be transformed and will accumulate to form Dampness.

There are two possible types of internal Dampness: one chronic, the other acute. Chronic internal Dampness may involve the Internal Organs, the channels or the skin. Acute internal Dampness involves Damp-Heat at the Qi Level within the 4-Level Identification of Patterns.

Chronic Dampness

Chronic Dampness derives either from acute invasion of external Dampness or from dietary causes.

Chronic Dampness in the Internal Organs

The clinical manifestations of chronic, internal Dampness in the Internal Organs have been described in the chapters on the identification of patterns according to Internal Organs (Chapters 91–100).

Chronic Dampness in the channels

Chronic retention of Dampness in the channels and joints is, of course, the main cause of Painful Obstruction Syndrome. This manifests with pain, swelling and heaviness of the joints.

Chronic Dampness in the skin

Chronic retention of Dampness in the skin is the main cause of numerous skin diseases, chiefly eczema (atopic or not). Dampness in the skin manifests with vesicles or with skin lesions oozing fluid, and with puffiness of the skin.

Acute Dampness

This is the Qi level of the identification of patterns according to the Four Levels which is described in Chapter 104.

DRYNESS

Dryness is a Yang pathogenic factor and it tends to injure Blood or Yin. It arises in very dry weather, but it

can also occur in some artificial conditions such as in very dry, centrally heated buildings.

External Dryness

The clinical manifestations of external Dryness are simply characterized by dryness and they are a dry throat, dry lips, a dry tongue, a dry mouth, dry skin, dry stools and scanty urination.

Internal Dryness

Internal Dryness arises from deficiency of Yin, particularly of the Stomach or Kidneys, or both, and the symptoms are the same as for exterior Dryness. Interior Dryness is not always the result of Yin deficiency: it may sometimes be the stage preceding it. There is a saying: *'Withering and cracking is due to Dryness.'*[4] This describes the dry skin and cracked tongue often seen in Dryness.

The Stomach is the origin of fluids and if one has an irregular diet, such as eating late at night, eating in a hurry or going back to work straight after eating, the Stomach fluids are depleted and this leads to a state of Dryness which is the precursor of Yin deficiency.

This Dryness is manifested with a dry throat and mouth and a dry tongue, possibly slightly Peeled in the centre, but not yet Red.

Box 103.10 summarizes the manifestations of Dryness.

BOX 103.10 DRYNESS

- Dry throat
- Dry lips
- Dry tongue
- Dry mouth
- Dry skin
- Dry stools
- Scanty urination

FIRE

Fire is an extreme form of Heat which can derive from any of the other exterior pathogenic factors. Strictly speaking, it is not really an exterior pathogenic factor. It either arises from the Interior or derives from other exterior pathogenic factors, but once it manifests in the body it is an interior pathogenic factor.

Heat and Fire are the same in nature but they differ in many respects. Fire is more 'solid' than Heat, it tends to move and dry out more than Heat. Heat can cause pain as well as all the other symptoms of Heat, such as a Red tongue, thirst and a Rapid pulse, but Fire moves upwards (causing mouth ulcers, for example) or damages the blood vessels (causing bleeding). Also, Fire tends to affect the mind more than Heat causing anxiety, mental agitation, insomnia or mental illness.

The differentiation between the Bright-Yang channel pattern and the Bright-Yang organ pattern of the Six Stages pattern identification illustrates the difference between Heat and Fire well; as does that between the Stomach-Heat pattern and the Intestines Dry-Heat pattern within the Four-Levels pattern identification.

The nature of Fire therefore is to rise to the head, to dry fluids, to injure Blood and Yin, to deplete Qi and to affect the Mind.

Box 103.11 summarizes the characteristics of Fire.

BOX 103.11 CHARACTERISTICS OF FIRE

- More intense than Heat (bitter taste, intense thirst)
- Dries up fluids (dark urine, constipation, dry tongue coating)
- May cause bleeding (haemoptysis, haematemesis)
- Moves upwards (red eyes, mouth ulcers)
- Affects the Mind (agitation, insomnia, restlessness)

Fire can be of the Excess (Full) or Deficient (Empty) type. The clinical manifestations of Full-Fire are a constant feeling of heat, a red face and eyes, a constantly dry mouth, a bitter taste, constipation, scanty dark urine, intense thirst, mental agitation, a Red tongue with yellow coating and a Full-Deep-Rapid pulse. When Fire enters the Blood, it may give rise to dark purple spots under the skin (macules) and vomiting of blood or other haemorrhages.

Empty-Fire arises from deficiency of Yin and is manifested with night sweating, a feeling of heat in the chest, palms and soles, red cheekbones, a dry mouth, thirst in the evening or night, a feeling of heat in the evening, a Red and peeled tongue and a Floating-Empty and Rapid pulse.

Table 103.4 differentiates Full- from Empty-Fire.

Fire (Full or Empty) can affect the Heart, Liver, Stomach, Kidneys, Lungs and Intestines; its clinical

Table 103.4 Differentiation between Full- and Empty-Fire

	Full-Fire	Empty-Fire
Feeling of heat	All the time	In the evening
Thirst	Intense, all the time	In the evening and night
Dry mouth	All the time	At night
Bitter taste	Yes	No
Mind	Intense agitation	Vague, mild restlessness in the evening
Tongue	Red with dry dark-yellow coating	Red without coating
Pulse	Full-Deep-Rapid	Floating-Empty, Rapid

manifestations related to each of these organs have been described in detail in the chapters on the identification of patterns according to the Internal Organs (Chapters 91–100).

NOTES

1. Zhai Ming Yi 1979 Clinical Chinese Medicine (*Zhong Yi Lin Chuang Ji Chu* 中医临床基础) Henan Publishing House, p. 132.
2. Ibid., p. 133.
3. Ibid., p. 133.
4. Ibid., p. 133.

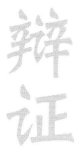

Chapter **104**

IDENTIFICATION OF PATTERNS ACCORDING TO THE FOUR LEVELS

Chapter contents

INTRODUCTION   *953*

DEFENSIVE-QI LEVEL   *954*
   Wind-Heat   *954*
   Summer-Heat   *954*
   Damp-Heat   *954*
   Dry-Heat   *955*

QI LEVEL   *955*
   Lung-Heat (Heat in chest and diaphragm)   *955*
   Stomach-Heat   *955*
   Intestines Dry-Heat (Fire)   *955*
   Gall-Bladder Heat   *955*
   Damp-Heat in Stomach and Spleen   *956*

NUTRITIVE-QI LEVEL   *956*
   Heat in Nutritive-Qi level   *956*
   Heat in the Pericardium   *956*

BLOOD LEVEL   *957*
   Heat victorious agitates Blood   *957*
   Heat victorious stirring Wind   *957*
   Empty-Wind agitating in the Interior   *957*
   Collapse of Yin   *957*
   Collapse of Yang   *957*

THE FOUR LEVELS IN A NUTSHELL   *957*

LATENT HEAT   *958*
   Lesser-Yang type   *961*
   Bright-Yang type   *961*
   Lesser-Yin type   *962*

RELATIONS BETWEEN THE FOUR LEVELS, SIX STAGES AND THREE BURNERS   *962*

INTRODUCTION

The identification of patterns according to the Four Levels was devised by Ye Tian Shi in his book 'A Study of Warm Diseases' (*Wen Bing Xue*, 1746). The identification of patterns according to the Four Levels is clinically the most useful tool to interpret the pathology and establish the treatment of infectious diseases deriving from invasion of Wind-Heat. Examples of 'Warm Diseases' are influenza, measles, German measles, chickenpox, mononucleosis, mumps, severe acute respiratory syndrome (SARS) and meningitis. However, this method of identification of patterns can be used to diagnose and treat any invasion of Wind-Heat and its consequences, whether it is a 'Warm Disease' or not. For example, if a patient suffers an acute respiratory infection from invasion of Wind-Heat and subsequently develops a chest infection, the identification of patterns according to the Four Levels provides the perfect tool to diagnose and treat this problem. In this particular example, the initial stage of the acute respiratory infection corresponds to invasion of Wind-Heat at the Defensive-Qi level; when the disease progresses and the patient suffers from a chest infection, this corresponds to internal Heat at the Qi level and specifically the pattern of Phlegm-Heat in the Lungs.

Many warm diseases often manifest with a rash; examples of exanthematous (i.e. manifesting with rash) diseases are measles, German measles and chickenpox. One must distinguish between **vesicles**, **papules** and **macules** (see Table 104.6). **Vesicles** are blister-like spots filled with a clear fluid and they always indicate Dampness. **Papules** are red, solid spots; they generally indicate Heat at the Qi Level (and especially in the Lungs and Stomach). **Macules** are spots under the

skin which, unlike vesicles and papules, cannot be felt on palpation; they always indicate Heat at the Nutritive-Qi or Blood level.

DEFENSIVE-QI LEVEL

Wind-Heat
Clinical manifestations

Fever, aversion to cold, severe deep headache, sore throat, cough, slight sweating, slight shivers, runny nose with yellow discharge, swollen tonsils, slight body aches, slightly dark urine, slight thirst.
Tongue Red in the front or sides with a thin white coating. The tongue coating is white because the pathogenic factor is on the Exterior.
Pulse Floating-Rapid.

Acupuncture

LI-4 Hegu, LI-11 Quchi, TB-5 Waiguan, Du-14 Dazhui, BL-12 Fengmen (with cupping), LU-11 Shaoshang.

Prescription

Yin Qiao San *Lonicera-Forsythia Decoction*
Sang Ju Yin *Morus-Chrysanthemum Decoction.*

Table 104.1 compares the manifestations of Wind-Heat with those of Wind-Cold (Six Stages).

Summer-Heat
Clinical manifestations

Fever, aversion to cold, absence of sweating, headache, a feeling of heaviness, an uncomfortable sensation in the epigastrium, irritability, thirst.
Tongue Red in the front or sides with a sticky white coating. The tongue coating is white because the pathogenic factor is on the Exterior.
Pulse Soggy and Rapid.

Acupuncture

LI-4 Hegu, LI-11 Quchi, TB-5 Waiguan, Du-14 Dazhui, P-9 Zhongchong.

Prescription

Qing Luo Yin *Clearing the Connecting Channels Decoction.*

Damp-Heat
Clinical manifestations

Fever that is worse in the afternoon, body hot to the touch, aversion to cold, swollen glands, headache, a feeling of heaviness, a feeling of oppression of the epigastrium, sticky taste, thirst with no desire to drink.

Table 104.1 Comparison of invasion of Wind-Cold (Six Stages) and invasion of Wind-Heat (Four Levels)

	Wind-Cold (Six Stages)	**Wind-Heat (Four Levels)**
Pathology	Wind-Cold on Exterior obstructing Defensive Qi	Wind-Heat injuring Defensive Qi and impairing descending of Lung-Qi
Penetration route	Through skin	Through nose and mouth
Fever	Slight or absent	Higher
Shivers	Severe	Slight
Aches	Severe (in prevalence of Cold)	Slight
Headache	Occipital	Deep inside, severe
Sweating	No sweating in prevalence of Cold; sweating only on top part of body in prevalence of Wind	Slight sweating
Thirst	No	Slight
Urine	Clear	Slightly dark
Tongue	Body-colour normal, thin white coating	Red sides/front, thin white coating
Pulse	Floating-Tight in prevalence of Cold; Floating-Slow in prevalence of Wind	Floating-Rapid
Treatment	Pungent-warm herbs to cause sweating	Pungent-cool herbs to release the Exterior

Tongue Sticky white coating. The tongue coating is white because the pathogenic factor is on the Exterior.
Pulse Soggy-Slow. The pulse is Slow because of the influence of Dampness.

Acupuncture

LI-4 Hegu, LI-11 Quchi, SP-9 Yinlingquan, SP-6 Sanyinjiao, Ren-12 Zhongwan.

Prescription

Huo Xiang Zheng Qi San *Agastache Upright Qi Powder*.

Dry-Heat
Clinical manifestations

Fever, slight aversion to cold, shivers, slight sweating, dry skin, nose, mouth and throat, dry cough, sore throat.
Tongue Dry with thin white coating. The tongue coating is white because the pathogenic factor is on the Exterior.
Pulse Floating-Rapid.

Acupuncture

LI-4 Hegu, LI-11 Quchi, TB-5 Waiguan, SP-6 Sanyinjiao, LU-9 Taiyuan, ST-36 Zusanli.

Prescription

Xing Su San *Prunus-Perilla Powder*
Sang Xing Tang *Morus-Prunus Decoction*.

QI LEVEL

Lung-Heat (Heat in chest and diaphragm)
Clinical manifestations

High fever, a feeling of heat, absence of aversion to cold, thirst, cough with thin yellow sputum, shortness of breath, sweating.
Tongue Red with yellow coating.
Pulse Slippery-Rapid.

Acupuncture

LU-5 Chize, LU-10 Yuji, Du-14 Dazhui, LI-11 Quchi, LU-1 Zhongfu, BL-13 Feishu.

Prescription

Ma Xing Shi Gan Tang *Ephedra-Prunus-Gypsum-Glycyrrhiza Decoction*
Xie Bai San *Draining the White Powder*
Qing Qi Hua Tan Tang *Clearing Qi and Resolving Phlegm Decoction* (if there is also Phlegm)
Wu Hu Tang *Five Tigers Decoction*.

Stomach-Heat
Clinical manifestations

High fever that is worse in the afternoon, absence of aversion to cold, a feeling of heat, intense thirst, profuse sweating.
Tongue Red with yellow coating.
Pulse Overflowing-Rapid.

Acupuncture

ST-44 Neiting, ST-34 Liangqiu, ST-21 Liangmen, ST-43 Xiangu, LI-11 Quchi, ST-25 Tianshu.

Prescription

Bai Hu Tang *White Tiger Decoction*.

Intestines Dry-Heat (Fire)
Clinical manifestations

High fever that is higher in the afternoon, constipation, dry stools, burning in the anus, abdominal fullness and pain, irritability, delirium.
Tongue Red with thick dry-yellow coating.
Pulse Deep-Full-Rapid.

Acupuncture

LI-11 Quchi, ST-25 Tianshu, SP-15 Daheng, ST-37 Shangjuxu, ST-39 Xiajuxu.

Prescription

Tiao Wei Cheng Qi Tang *Regulating the Stomach Conducting Qi Decoction*.

Table 104.2 compares Stomach-Heat with Intestines Dry-Heat (Fire) within the Qi Level. (The characteristics of Fire were covered in Chapter 103.)

Gall-Bladder Heat
Clinical manifestations

Alternating hot and cold feeling with a prevalence of heat, bitter taste, thirst, dry throat, hypochondrial pain, nausea, a feeling of fullness in the epigastrium.

Table 104.2 Comparison of Heat and Fire at the Qi level

	Stomach-Heat (Heat)	Intestines Dry-Heat (Fire)
Common manifestations	Fever, no shivers, feeling of heat, thirst, Red tongue with yellow coating, Rapid pulse	
Differences	Profuse sweating, Overflowing pulse, tongue coating not too dry	Constipation, abdominal fullness pain, mental restlessness, dry mouth, Deep-Full pulse, thick, dry tongue coating

Tongue Red with unilateral sticky yellow coating.
Pulse Wiry-Rapid.

Acupuncture

GB-34 Yanglingquan, GB-43 Xiaxi, TB-6 Zhigou, TB-5 Waiguan.

Prescription

Hao Qin Qing Dan Tang *Artemisia-Scutellaria Clearing the Gall-Bladder Decoction.*

Damp-Heat in Stomach and Spleen
Clinical manifestations

Continuous fever which decreases after sweating but soon increases again, a feeling of heaviness of the body and head, a feeling of oppression of the chest and epigastrium, nausea, loose stools.
Tongue Red with sticky yellow coating.
Pulse Soggy-Rapid.

Acupuncture

Ren-12 Zhongwan, SP-9 Yinlingquan, SP-6 Sanyinjiao, Ren-9 Shuifen, ST-36 Zusanli, LI-11 Quchi.

Prescription

Lian Po Yin *Coptis-Magnolia Decoction.*

Table 104.3 compares the Defensive-Qi level with the Qi level.

NUTRITIVE-QI LEVEL

Heat in Nutritive-Qi level
Clinical manifestations

Fever at night, dry mouth with no desire to drink, mental restlessness, insomnia, delirium, incoherent speech or aphasia, macules.
Tongue Red without coating.
Pulse Fine-Rapid.

Acupuncture

P-9 Zhongchong, P-8 Laogong, HE-9 Shaochong, KI-6 Zhaohai.

Prescription

Qing Ying Tang *Clearing the Nutritive-Qi [Heat] Decoction.*

Heat in the Pericardium
Clinical manifestations

Fever at night, mental confusion, incoherent speech or aphasia, delirium, body heat, but hands and feet cold, macules.
Tongue Red without coating.
Pulse Fine-Rapid.

Acupuncture

P-9 Zhongchong, P-8 Laogong, HE-9 Shaochong, KI-6 Zhaohai.

Prescription

Qing Ying Tang *Clearing the Nutritive-Qi [Heat] Decoction.*

Table 104.3 Comparison of Defensive-Qi and Qi levels in identification of patterns according to the Four Levels

Level	Eight Principles	Organs	Upright Qi	Location
Defensive QI	External – Heat-Full	Not affected	Strong	Exterior (Upright Qi reacts in Exterior: shivers)
QI	Internal – Heat-Full	Affected	Strong	Interior (Upright Qi reacts in Interior: no shivers)

BLOOD LEVEL

Heat victorious agitates Blood
Clinical manifestations

High fever, irritability, manic behaviour, dark macules, vomiting of blood, epistaxis, blood in stools, blood in urine.
Tongue   Dark-Red without coating.
Pulse   Wiry-Rapid.

Acupuncture

SP-10 Xuehai, LI-11 Quchi, LIV-2 Xingjian, KI-6 Zhaohai, HE-9 Shaochong.

Prescription

Xi Jiao Di Huang Tang *Cornus Rhinoceri-Rehmannia Decoction.*

Heat victorious stirring Wind
Clinical manifestations

High fever, fainting, twitching of the limbs, convulsions, rigidity of the neck, opisthotonos, eyeballs turning up, clenching of the teeth.
Tongue   Dark-Red without coating.
Pulse   Wiry-Rapid.

Acupuncture

SP-10 Xuehai, LI-11 Quchi, LIV-2 Xingjian, KI-6 Zhaohai, HE-9 Shaochong, LIV-3 Taichong, Du-16 Fengfu, GB-20 Fengchi, SI-3 Houxi and BL-62 Shenmai in combination.

Prescription

Ling Jiao Gou Teng Tang *Cornu Antelopis-Uncaria Decoction.*

Empty-Wind agitating in the Interior
Clinical manifestations

Low-grade fever, tremor of the limbs, twitching, loss of weight, malar flush, listlessness.
Tongue   Dark-Red and dry without coating.
Pulse   Fine-Rapid.

Acupuncture

LIV-3 Taichong, Du-16 Fengfu, GB-20 Fengchi, SI-3 Houxi and BL-62 Shenmai in combination, LIV-8 Ququan, KI-6 Zhaohai, KI-3 Taixi, SP-6 Sanyinjiao.

Prescription

Zhen Gan Xi Feng Tang *Pacifying the Liver and Extinguishing Wind Decoction.*

Collapse of Yin
Clinical manifestations

Low-grade fever, night sweating, mental restlessness, dry mouth with a desire to sip liquids, five-palm heat, malar flush, emaciation.
Tongue   Dark-Red and Dry without coating.
Pulse   Fine-Rapid.

Acupuncture

ST-36 Zusanli, KI-3 Taixi, SP-6 Sanyinjiao, KI-6 Zhaohai, Ren-4 Guanyuan.

Prescription

Da Bu Yin Wan *Great Tonifying the Yin Pill.*

Collapse of Yang
Clinical manifestations

A feeling of cold, cold limbs, bright-white complexion, profuse sweating on the forehead, listlessness.
Tongue   Pale-Swollen and Short.
Pulse   Hidden, Slow, Scattered.

Acupuncture

ST-36 Zusanli, Ren-6 Qihai, Ren-4 Guanyuan, Ren-8 Shenque. Moxa is applicable.

Prescription

Shen Fu Tang *Ginseng-Aconitum Decoction.*

THE FOUR LEVELS IN A NUTSHELL

Table 104.4 compares the clinical manifestations of the Four Levels, and Table 104.5 compares the tongue manifestations. Table 104.6 compares and differentiates papules, macules and vesicles. The presence of papules indicates Heat at the Qi level, whereas macules indicate that it is at the Nutritive-Qi or Blood level.

Box 104.1 summarizes the essential features of each level.

Table 104.4 Comparison of the clinical manifestations of the Four Levels

Symptoms	Defensive QI	Qi	Nutritive Qi/Blood
Fever	Slight fever, shivers	High fever, feeling of heat	Fever at night
Thirst	Slight	Intense, desire to drink cold drinks	Dry mouth, desire to sip liquids
Mental state	Unchanged	Maybe delirium, generally mind clear	Delirium, fainting, mind confused
Sweating	Slight	Profuse	Night sweating
Tongue	Red sides/front, thin white coating	Red body, thick, dry yellow coating	Red body, no coating
Pulse	Floating-Rapid	Big-Rapid, Deep-Full-Rapid or Slippery-Rapid	Fine-Rapid
Summary	Exterior pattern	Interior pattern, Upright Qi strong	Interior pattern, Upright Qi weak

Table 104.5 Comparison of tongue appearance in the Four Levels

Tongue	Defensive Qi				Qi	Nutritive Qi	Blood
	Wind-Heat	Summer-Heat	Dry-Heat	Damp-Heat			
Body	Red sides/front	Red	Dry	Red	Red	Deep-Red	Deep-Red
Coating	Thin white or yellow	Thin white	Thin white, dry	White, sticky	Thick, dry, yellow or brown (sticky in Stomach and Spleen Damp-Heat)	No coating	No coating
Remark					Coating more important	Body more important	Body more important

Table 104.6 Comparison of papules, vesicles and macules

Type	Shape	Location	Aftermath
Papule (*Zhen*)	Like small grains, sticking out from skin, red, can be felt on touch	Chest, abdomen, back, face most of all; seldom on limbs	Leave trace
Vesicle (*Bao*)	Round in shape, white, obvious, like small water vesicles, shaped like grains of rice or pearls, can be felt on touch	Chest, abdomen, axillae, neck; seldom on limbs, never on face	Leave trace
Macule (*Ban*)	Big, circular spots, level with skin, not sticking out, cannot be felt on touch	Chest, abdomen, back, face most of all; seldom on limbs	Do not leave trace

BOX 104.1 THE FOUR LEVELS IN A NUTSHELL

- Defensive-Qi level: shivers and slight fever
- Qi level: no shivers, high fever, feeling of heat
- Nutritive-Qi level: mental changes, fever at night
- Blood level: fever at night, bleeding, internal Wind

LATENT HEAT

The concept of Latent Heat is very old in Chinese medicine, having been mentioned in the 'Yellow Emperor's Classic of Internal Medicine' for the first

time. Latent Heat occurs when an external pathogenic factor such as Cold penetrates the body without causing apparent symptoms at the time; the pathogenic factor instead penetrates in the Interior and 'incubates' there turning into interior Heat. This Heat later emerges with acute symptoms of Heat; when it emerges, it is called 'Latent Heat'.

The reason that an external pathogenic factor invades the body without acute symptoms is usually to be found in a Kidney deficiency; thus, the development of Latent Heat indicates a pre-existing Kidney deficiency which induces a weakened immune response to the invasion of an external pathogenic factor.

The main clinical manifestations of the emergence of Latent Heat are listed in Box 104.2.

BOX 104.2 LATENT HEAT

- Acute onset
- Thirst
- Irritability
- Insomnia
- Sudden tiredness and lassitude
- Weary limbs
- Dark urine
- Red tongue
- Rapid pulse

Other symptoms and signs vary according to the type of Latent Heat and these are described below. Figure 104.1 illustrates the concept of Latent Heat from the 'Yellow Emperor's Classic of Internal Medicine' and Figure 104.2 compares and contrasts the movement of the pathogenic factor in an invasion of Wind-Heat with the movement of Latent Heat. Figures 104.3 and 104.4 illustrate the types of Latent Heat and patterns developing from it.

Table 104.7 compares the clinical manifestations of Wind-Heat and Latent Heat.

Latent Heat can manifest at the Qi or Blood level. There are three main patterns, two at the Qi level and one at the Blood level as follows:

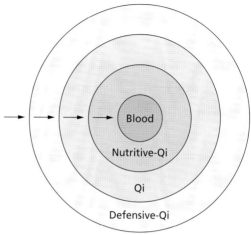

Invasion of Wind-Heat

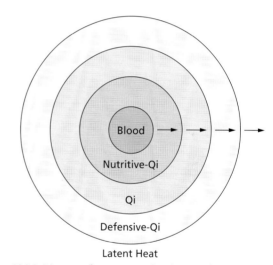

Latent Heat

Fig. 104.2 Diagram of movement of pathogenic factor in invasion of Wind-Heat compared with Latent Heat

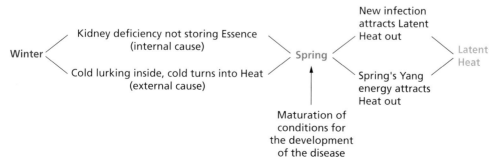

Fig. 104.1 Development of Latent Heat according to the 'Yellow Emperor's Classic of Internal Medicine'

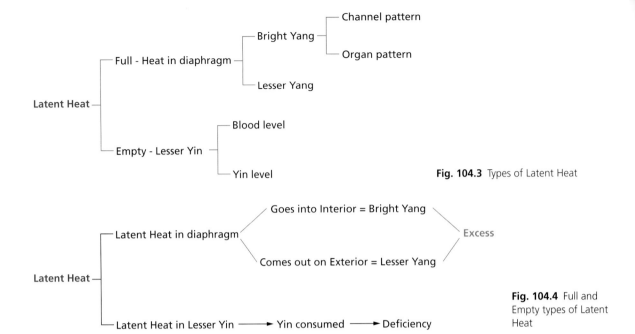

Fig. 104.3 Types of Latent Heat

Fig. 104.4 Full and Empty types of Latent Heat

Table 104.7 Comparison of invasion of Wind-Heat and Latent Heat

	Wind-Heat	Latent Heat
Symptoms	Shivers, aversion to cold, sweating, fever	No shivers, no aversion to cold (unless combined with new infection)
Cough	Cough	No cough
Pulse	Floating-Rapid	Fire-Rapid, also Wiry, Deep-full or Intermittent
Tongue	Thin white coating	Red or Deep-Red tongue from the beginning, with yellow or dry brown coating or no coating
Pathology	Easy to have abnormal transmission to Pericardium	Easy to consume Yin and dry up fluids

Fig. 104.5 Patterns developing from Latent Heat in the Lesser Yin

Table 104.8 Comparison of Qi and Blood levels in Latent Heat

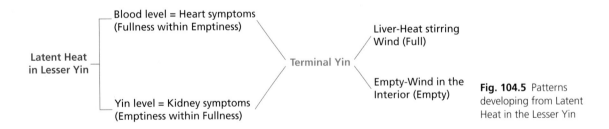

	Heat	Thirst	Skin spots	Tongue	Pulse
Qi level	Apparent	Thirst, desire to drink	Papules	Red	Big
Blood level	Not so apparent	Dry mouth, no desire to drink	Macules	Deep-Red	Fine-Rapid

Qi level: Lesser-Yang type
Bright-Yang type
Blood level: Lesser Yin type

Lesser-Yang type

Alternation of chills and fever, bitter taste, hypochondrial pain, red eyes, deafness, vomiting, a feeling of oppression of the diaphragm, Red tongue with unilateral yellow coating, Wiry pulse.

Bright-Yang type
Channel pattern

A feeling of heat, thirst, sweating, fever, Big pulse.

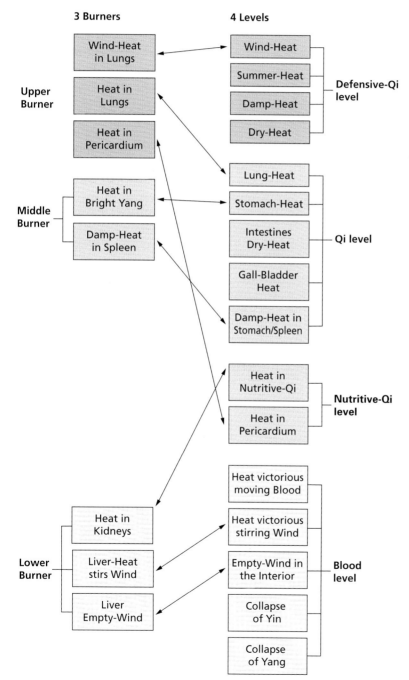

Fig. 104.6 Connections between Three Burners and Four Levels

Organ pattern

Fever, abdominal fullness and pain, constipation, Red tongue with dry brown coating, Deep-Full pulse.

Lesser-Yin type

A feeling of weariness of the limbs before the onset of other symptoms, insomnia, irritability, dry mouth and throat, scanty dark urination, headache, backache, tiredness, Red tongue, Rapid pulse.

At Blood level

Delirium, faint feeling, dry limbs, dry mouth without a desire to drink, sweating, irritability, macules, blood in urine, epistaxis, Deep-Red tongue without coating, Fine-Rapid pulse.

At Yin level

Oily beads on forehead, dry mouth and teeth, irritability, delirium, scanty urine, blood in urine, Deep-Red tongue without coating, Fine-Rapid pulse.

Figure 104.5 illustrates the pattern developing from Latent Heat of the Lesser-Yin type.

Table 104.8 compares the manifestations of Latent Heat at the Qi and Blood level.

RELATIONS BETWEEN THE FOUR LEVELS, SIX STAGES AND THREE BURNERS

Although the identification of patterns according to the Six Stages dates back to the Han dynasty and those according to the Four Levels and Three Burners to the Qing dynasty, there are many points of contact between the three methods. First of all, all three describe the symptoms of invasion of external Wind when this is on the Exterior in the beginning stages and when it is in the Interior in later stages.

The Greater-Yang stage of the Six Stages is similar to the Defensive-Qi level within the Four Levels as they both deal with invasions of external Wind: the former Wind-Cold and the latter Wind-Heat. The Bright-Yang

stage of the Six Stages is almost the same as the Qi level of the Four Levels (Heat in Bright Yang and Dry-Heat in the Stomach and Intestines patterns). The Lesser-Yang stage of the Six Stages is almost the same as the Gall-Bladder Heat at the Qi level, the former being characterized by the predominance of Cold and the latter by that of Heat.

The identification of patterns according to the Three Burners is quite similar to that according to the Four Levels (Fig. 104.6). Many of the patterns are essentially the same as those of the Four Levels, except that they are seen from the perspective of the Three Burners, (i.e. patterns of the Upper Burner, Middle Burner and Lower Burner). The Middle Burner patterns correspond to the Qi Level, and those of the Lower Burner correspond to the Nutritive-Qi and Blood levels. In contrast, the patterns of the Upper Burner encompass the Defensive-Qi, Qi and Nutritive-Qi levels.

Comparing the Three Burners and the Six Stages methods, it is apparent that the Upper Burner patterns correspond to the Greater-Yang stage. The Middle Burner patterns encompass the Bright-Yang, Lesser-Yang and Greater-Yin stages. The Lower Burner Patterns include those of the Lesser-Yin and Terminal-Yin stages (Fig. 104.7).

Further connections between the three methods of pattern identification are shown in the diagrams in Figure 104.8.

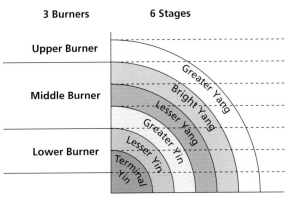

Fig. 104.7 Connections between Six Stages and Three Burners

(a)

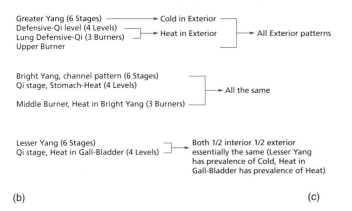

(b)   (c)

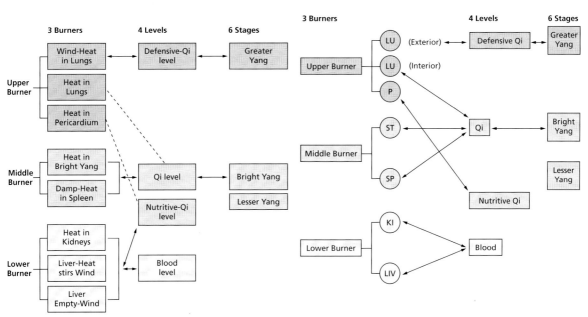

Fig. 104.8(a–d) Connections between Six Stages, Four Levels and Three Burners

(d)

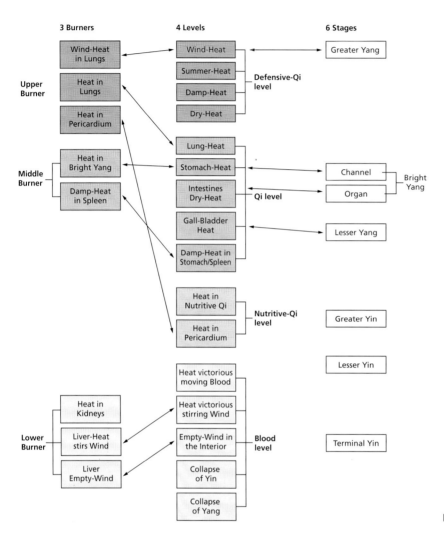

Fig. 104.8(a–d) *continued*

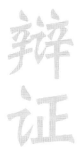

Chapter **105**

IDENTIFICATION OF PATTERNS ACCORDING TO THE SIX STAGES

Chapter contents

GREATER-YANG STAGE   *965*
 Channel patterns   *965*
 Organ patterns   *966*

BRIGHT-YANG STAGE   *967*
 Bright-Yang channel pattern   *967*
 Bright-Yang organ pattern   *967*

LESSER-YANG STAGE   *967*

GREATER-YIN STAGE   *967*

LESSER-YIN STAGE   *968*
 Cold Transformation   *968*
 Heat Transformation   *968*

TERMINAL-YIN STAGE   *968*

GREATER-YANG STAGE

Channel patterns

Invasion of Wind-Cold with prevalence of Cold (Attack of Cold)
Clinical manifestations

Aversion to cold, slight fever shivers, absence of sweating, severe headache, pronounced aching, stiff neck, sneezing, runny nose with white discharge, slight breathlessness.

Tongue   Normal tongue-body colour with thin white coating.
Pulse   Floating-Tight.

Acupuncture

BL-12 Fengmen with cupping, LU-7 Lieque, LI-4 Hegu. Moxa is applicable.

Prescription

Ma Huang Tang *Ephedra Decoction.*

Invasion of Wind-Cold with prevalence of Wind (Attack of Wind)
Clinical manifestations

Slight aversion to cold, aversion to wind, slight fever, slight sweating, mild headache, slight aching, stiff neck, sneezing.

Tongue   Normal tongue-body colour with thin white coating.
Pulse   Floating-Slow.

Acupuncture

BL-12 Fengmen with cupping, LU-7 Lieque, LI-4 Hegu, GB-20 Fengchi, ST-36 Zusanli.

Prescription

Gui Zhi Tang *Ramulus Cinnamomi Decoction.*

Table 105.1 Comparison of Attack of Cold and Attack of Wind in the Greater-Yang pattern

	Attack of Cold	Attack of Wind
Sweating	No sweating	Slight sweating
Aches	Pronounced	Slight
Headache	Severe	Mild
Aversion to cold	Pronounced	Slight
Pulse	Floating-Tight	Floating-Slow
Common symptoms	Floating pulse, headache, shivers, aversion to cold	

Table 105.1 differentiates the clinical manifestations of the Attack of Cold from those of Attack of Wind.

Invasion of Wind-Heat
Clinical manifestations

Aversion to cold, fever, slight shivers, sneezing, cough, runny nose with slightly yellow mucus, occipital stiffness and ache, slight sweating, itchy throat, sore throat, swollen tonsils, body aches, slight thirst.
Tongue Tongue-body colour slightly Red on the front/sides (not in every case), thin white coating.
Pulse Floating-Rapid.

Acupuncture

LI-4 Hegu, LI-11 Quchi, LU-7 Lieque, BL-12 Fengmen, TB-5 Waiguan.

Prescription

Yin Qiao San *Lonicera-Forsythia Powder*.

Table 105.2 differentiates the clinical manifestations of invasion of Wind-Cold (with prevalence of Wind), Wind-Cold (with prevalence of Cold) and Wind-Heat.

Organ patterns
Accumulation of Water
Clinical manifestations

Shivers, fever, aversion to cold, retention of urine, slight thirst, vomiting of fluids soon after drinking.
Pulse Floating-Rapid.

Acupuncture

Ren-9 Shuifen, Ren-3 Zhongji, LU-7 Lieque, BL-22 Sanjiaoshu, BL-39 Weiyang.

Prescription

Wu Ling San *Five 'Ling' Powder*.

Accumulation of Blood
Clinical manifestations

Hypogastric distension, fullness and urgency, urinary incontinence, blood in the urine, mental restlessness.
Tongue Reddish-Purple without coating.
Pulse Deep-Fine-Rapid.

Acupuncture

BL-62 Shenmai and SI-3 Houxi in combination, BL-39 Weiyang, SI-5 Yanggu, BL-22 Sanjiaoshu, SP-10 Xuehai, LIV-1 Dadun.

Prescription

Tao He Cheng Qi Tang *Persica Conducting Qi Decoction*.

Table 105.3 compares the manifestations of Accumulation of Water and Accumulation of Blood in the Greater-Yang organ pattern of Heat in the Bladder.

Table 105.2 Comparison of invasion of Wind-Cold with prevalence of Wind, invasion of Wind-Cold with prevalence of Cold, and invasion of Wind-Heat

	Symptoms	Tongue	Pulse
Wind-Cold with prevalence of Wind	Slight sweating	Thin white coating, body colour unchanged	Floating-Slow
Wind-Cold with prevalence of Cold	No sweating, slight breathlessness, shivers pronounced	Thin white coating, body colour unchanged	Floating-Tight
Wind-Heat invasion	Slight thirst, slight shivers	Body colour slightly Red on sides/front, thin white coating	Floating-Rapid

Table 105.3 Comparison of Accumulation of Water and Accumulation of Blood within the Greater-Yang organ pattern

	Accumulation of Water	Accumulation of Blood
Pattern	Heat in the Bladder at Qi level	Heat in the Bladder at Blood level
Symptoms	Urinary retention, no mental changes	Urinary incontinence, blood in the urine, mental restlessness

Table 105.4 Differences between channel and organ patterns in Bright-Yang pattern of the Six Stages

	Channel pattern	Organ pattern
Common manifestations	Fever, no shivers, a feeling of heat, thirst, Red tongue with yellow coating, Rapid pulse	
Differences	Profuse sweating, mental changes, Overflowing pulse, thin tongue coating	Constipation, abdominal fullness/pain, Deep-Full-Slippery pulse, thick, dry tongue coating

BRIGHT-YANG STAGE

Bright-Yang channel pattern
Clinical manifestations

High fever, profuse sweating, intense thirst, red face, a feeling of heat, irritability, delirium.
Tongue   Red with thin yellow coating.
Pulse   Overflowing-Rapid.

Acupuncture

LI-11 Quchi, Du-14 Dazhui, P-3 Quze, ST-44 Neiting, ST-43 Xiangu.

Prescription

Bai Hu Tang *White Tiger Decoction*.

Bright-Yang organ pattern
Clinical manifestations

High fever that is worse in the afternoon, profuse sweating, a feeling of heat, sweating on limbs, abdominal fullness/pain, constipation, dry stools, thirst, dark urine.
Tongue   Red with thick, dry yellow coating.
Pulse   Deep-Full-Slippery-Rapid.

Acupuncture

LI-11 Quchi, Du-14 Dazhui, P-3 Quze, ST-44 Neiting, ST-43 Xiangu, ST-25 Tianshu, SP-15 Daheng, ST-37 Shangjuxu, SP-6 Sanyinjiao.

Prescription

Tiao Wei Cheng Qi Tang *Regulating the Stomach Conducting Qi Decoction*.

Table 105.4 compares the clinical manifestations of the Bright-Yang channel pattern with those of the Bright-Yang organ pattern.

LESSER-YANG STAGE

Clinical manifestations

Alternations of shivers and fever, bitter taste, dry throat, blurred vision, hypochondrial fullness and distension, lack of desire to eat or drink, irritability, nausea, vomiting.
Tongue   Unilateral thin white coating.
Pulse   Wiry-Fine.

Acupuncture

TB-5 Waiguan, TB-6 Zhigou, GB-41 Zulinqi, Du-13 Taodao.

Prescription

Xiao Chai Hu Tang *Small Bupleurum Decoction*.

GREATER-YIN STAGE

Clinical manifestations

Abdominal fullness, a feeling of cold, vomiting, lack of appetite, diarrhoea, absence of thirst, tiredness.
Tongue   Pale with sticky white coating.
Pulse   Deep-Weak-Slow.

Acupuncture

Ren-12 Zhongwan, BL-20 Pishu, ST-36 Zusanli, SP-9 Yinlingquan. Moxa is applicable.

Prescription

Li Zhong Tang *Regulating the Centre Decoction*.

Table 105.5 Comparison of Lesser-Yin Cold transformation with Heat transformation

	Symptoms and Signs	Tongue	Pulse
Lesser-Yin Cold transformation	Chills, feeling cold, lying with body curled, listlessness, desire for sleep, cold limbs, diarrhoea, absence of thirst, frequent pale urination	Pale and wet with white coating	Deep-Weak-Slow
Lesser-Yin Heat transformation	Feeling of heat, irritability, insomnia, dry mouth and throat at night, dark urine, night sweating	Red without coating	Fine-Rapid

LESSER-YIN STAGE

Cold Transformation
Clinical manifestations

Chills, a feeling of cold, lying with the body curled, listlessness, a desire to sleep, cold limbs, diarrhoea, absence of thirst, frequent pale urination.
Tongue Pale and wet with white coating.
Pulse Deep-Weak-Slow.

Acupuncture

BL-23 Shenshu, Ren-4 Guanyuan, Ren-6 Qihai, Ren-8 Shenque, KI-7 Fuliu, KI-3 Taixi. Moxa is applicable.

Prescription

Si Ni Tang *Four Rebellious Decoction*.

Heat Transformation
Clinical manifestations

A feeling of heat, irritability, insomnia, dry mouth and throat at night, dark urine, night sweating.
Tongue Red without coating.
Pulse Fine-Rapid.

Acupuncture

Ren-4 Guanyuan, Ren-6 Qihai, KI-3 Taixi, KI-6 Zhaohai, SP-6 Sanyinjiao.

Prescription

Huang Lian E Jiao Tang *Coptis-Colla Asini Decoction*.

TERMINAL-YIN STAGE

Clinical manifestations

Persistent thirst, a feeling of energy rising to the chest, pain and a sensation of heat in the heart region, hunger but no desire to eat, cold limbs, diarrhoea, vomiting, vomiting of roundworms.
Pulse Wiry.

Acupuncture

LIV-3 Taichong, LI-4 Hegu, SP-4 Gongsun, P-6 Neiguan.

Prescription

Wu Mei Wan *Prunus Mume Decoction*.

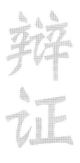

Chapter **106**

IDENTIFICATION OF PATTERNS ACCORDING TO THE THREE BURNERS

Chapter contents

UPPER BURNER   *969*
   Wind-Heat in the Lung Defensive-Qi portion   *969*
   Heat in the Lungs (Qi level)   *969*
   Heat in the Pericardium (Nutritive-Qi level)   *970*

MIDDLE BURNER   *970*
   Heat in Bright Yang   *970*
   Damp-Heat in the Spleen   *970*

LOWER BURNER   *970*
   Heat in the Kidneys   *970*
   Liver-Heat stirs Wind   *970*
   Liver Empty-Wind   *970*

UPPER BURNER

Wind-Heat in the Lung Defensive-Qi portion

Clinical manifestations

Fever, shivers, aversion to cold, headache, sore throat, slight sweating, runny nose with yellow discharge, swollen tonsils, body aches, slight thirst.

Tongue   Red in the front or sides with a thin white coating. The tongue coating is white because the pathogenic factor is on the Exterior.

Pulse   Floating-Rapid.

Acupuncture

LI-4 Hegu, LI-11 Quchi, TB-5 Waiguan, Du-14 Dazhui, BL-12 Fengmen (with cupping), LU-11 Shaoshang.

Prescription

Yin Qiao San *Honeysuckle and Forsythia Powder*
Sang Ju Yin *Mulberry Leaf and Chrysanthemum Decoction.*

Heat in the Lungs (Qi level)

Clinical manifestations

Fever, sweating, cough, breathlessness, thirst, a feeling of oppression and pain in the chest.

Tongue   Red with yellow coating.

Pulse   Rapid-Overflowing.

Acupuncture

LU-5 Chize, LU-10 Yuji, LU-1 Zhongfu, LI-11 Quchi, BL-13 Feishu.

Prescription

Ma Xing Shi Gan Tang *Ephedra-Prunus-Gypsum-Glycyrrhiza Decoction*

Wu Hu Tang *Five Tigers Decoction*
Xie Bai San *Expelling Whiteness Powder*
Qing Qi Hua Tan Tang (if there is also Phlegm) *Clearing Qi-Resolving Phlegm Decoction.*

Heat in the Pericardium (Nutritive-Qi level)

Clinical manifestations

High fever at night, a burning sensation in the epigastrium, cold limbs, delirium, aphasia.
Tongue Deep-Red and Stiff body without coating.
Pulse Fine and Rapid.

Acupuncture

P-9 Zhongchong, P-3 Quze, LI-11 Quchi.

Prescription

Qing Ying Tang *Clearing Nutritive-Qi Decoction.*

MIDDLE BURNER

Heat in Bright Yang

Clinical manifestations

High fever that is worse in the afternoon, no aversion to cold, a feeling of heat, intense thirst, profuse sweating.
Tongue Red with yellow coating.
Pulse Overflowing-Rapid.

Acupuncture

ST-44 Neiting, ST-34 Liangqiu, ST-21 Liangmen, ST-43 Xiangu, LI-11 Quchi, ST-25 Tianshu.

Prescription

Bai Hu Tang *White Tiger Decoction.*

Damp-Heat in the Spleen

Clinical manifestations

Fever, epigastric fullness, a feeling of heaviness of the body and head, nausea, vomiting.
Tongue Red with sticky yellow coating.
Pulse Soggy and Rapid.

Acupuncture

SP-9 Yinlingquan, SP-6 Sanyinjiao, Ren-12 Zhongwan, Ren-9 Shuifen, BL-22 Sanjiaoshu.

Prescription

Lian Po Yin *Coptis-Magnolia Decoction.*

LOWER BURNER

Heat in the Kidneys

Clinical manifestations

Fever in the afternoon and evening, five-palm heat, dry mouth and throat, night sweating, deafness, lassitude.
Tongue Deep-Red without coating.
Pulse Floating-Empty and Rapid.

Acupuncture

KI-3 Taixi, KI-6 Zhaohai, SP-6 Sanyinjiao, KI-2 Rangu, LI-11 Quchi.

Prescription

Xi Jiao Di Huang Tang *Cornu Rhinoceri-Rehmannia Decoction.*

Liver-Heat stirs Wind

Clinical manifestations

High fever at night, coma, convulsions, clenched teeth.
Tongue Deep-Red without coating.
Pulse Wiry-Fine-Rapid.

Acupuncture

LIV-3 Taichong, LIV-2 Xingjian, GB-20 Fengchi, Du-16 Fengfu, SI-3 Houxi and BL-62 Shenmai in combination.

Prescription

Ling Jiao Gou Teng Tang *Cornu Antelopis-Uncaria Decoction.*

Liver Empty-Wind

Clinical manifestations

Low-grade fever, cold limbs, dry and black teeth, dry and cracked lips, convulsions, tremor of the limbs.
Tongue Deep-Red without coating.
Pulse Deep-Fine-Rapid.

Acupuncture

LIV-3 Taichong, LIV-2 Xingjian, GB-20 Fengchi, Du-16 Fengfu, SI-3 Houxi and BL-62 Shenmai in combination, KI-3 Taixi, KI-6 Zhaohai, SP-6 Sanyinjiao.

Prescription

Zhen Gan Xi Feng Tang *Pacifying the Liver and Extinguishing Wind Decoction*

San Jia Fu Mai Tang *Three Carapaces Restoring the Pulse Decoction*

Da Ding Feng Zhu *Big Stopping Wind Pearl.*

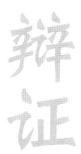

Chapter **107**

RESIDUAL PATHOGENIC FACTOR

Chapter contents

INTRODUCTION   *973*

FORMATION OF RESIDUAL PATHOGENIC FACTOR   *973*

DIAGNOSIS AND TREATMENT OF RESIDUAL PATHOGENIC
FACTOR   *975*
   How is it diagnosed?   *975*
   Types of residual pathogenic factor   *975*
   Effects of residual pathogenic factor   *975*
   Treatment of residual pathogenic factor   *975*

PHLEGM   *976*
   Damp-Phlegm in the Lungs   *976*
   Phlegm-Heat in the Lungs   *976*

DAMPNESS   *977*
   Dampness in the Stomach and Spleen   *977*
   Damp-Heat in the Stomach and Spleen   *977*
   Damp-Heat in the Gall-Bladder   *977*
   Damp-Heat in the ears   *977*
   Damp-Heat in the head   *977*

HEAT   *978*
   Heat in the Lungs   *978*
   Heat in the Lungs with Dryness   *978*
   Heat in the Stomach   *978*
   Toxic Heat in the tonsils   *979*

LESSER-YANG PATTERN   *979*
   Lesser-Yang pattern (Six Stages)   *979*
   Heat in the Gall-Bladder (Four Levels)   *979*

INTRODUCTION

A residual pathogenic factor is a pathogenic factor that is left over following an invasion or repeated invasions of Wind. I use 'Wind' here in a general sense to designate an external pathogenic factor, which may be Wind-Cold, Wind-Heat, Wind-Dryness, Heat, Dampness, Damp-Heat, Summer-Heat, or indeed any type of exterior pathogenic factor.

After an invasion of a pathogenic factor, the pathological development can have three possible outcomes:

- it may be expelled completely and the patient recovers
- it may become interior (at the Qi level of the Four levels)
- it may appear to have been expelled, and the patient appears to recover, but actually a residual pathogenic factor has been formed.

A residual pathogenic factor can also be formed after an exterior pathogenic factor has become interior (see Figure 107.1).

Thus, a residual pathogenic factor is simply a left-over pathological product when the patient *appears* to recover after an acute invasion of an exterior agent.

FORMATION OF RESIDUAL PATHOGENIC FACTOR

A residual pathogenic factor is formed in two ways: first, as described above, the original exterior pathogenic factor is not cleared and residual pathogenic factor either forms directly in the Exterior or when the

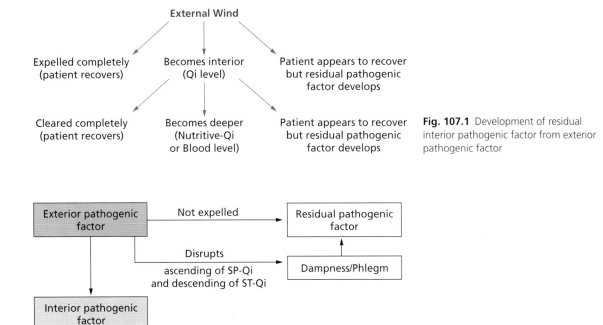

Fig. 107.1 Development of residual interior pathogenic factor from exterior pathogenic factor

Fig. 107.2 Formation of a residual pathogenic factor leading to Dampness or Phlegm

pathogenic factor penetrates the Interior (Fig. 107.1); secondly, an exterior pathogenic factor, whether at the exterior or interior level, always disrupts the ascending of Spleen-Qi and descending of Stomach-Qi thus leading to the formation of Dampness or Phlegm (Fig. 107.2).

Why is a residual pathogenic factor formed? Usually, the main reason is simply not taking care of oneself during an acute illness. Unfortunately, most people in the West have lost any idea of common sense or wisdom in looking after themselves. During an acute febrile illness, one should stop working and rest as much as possible: this is the best way to avoid a possible development of a residual pathogenic factor. Most people, however, simply go on working (or even over-working) as usual so that the body's Upright Qi (or immune system, from a Western point of view) cannot fight the pathogenic factor adequately and a residual pathogenic factor develops. Such a history is extremely common in patients suffering from ME: nearly all adults suffering from this condition report that it

started after a severe infection during which they went on working (or overworking) as before.

Another frequent reason for the development of a residual pathogenic factor is the use, or rather inappropriate use, of antibiotics. From a Chinese perspective, antibiotics kill bacteria but they do not clear Heat and, most importantly, do not resolve Dampness or Phlegm. On the contrary, they often upset the digestive system and therefore contribute to forming Dampness or Phlegm. The use of antibiotics is especially inappropriate for viral infections as these agents are not effective against viruses; in spite of this, they are still used frequently for infections that are clearly viral. It is estimated that in previously normal adults without underlying lung disease (i.e. not suffering from chronic bronchitis), up to 95% of acute episodes of lower-respiratory tract infections are caused by viral infection.[1] A meta-analysis of randomized, double-blind, placebo-controlled trials of the efficacy of antibiotics in previously healthy adults with acute bronchitis found no differences between antibiotic-

and placebo-treated groups in patient- or physician-reported symptoms, resolution of cough or fever, or return to work.[2]

Residual pathogenic factors are particularly common in children because their digestive system is still immature and easily upset, and invasions of Wind nearly always cause the formation of Dampness or Phlegm. In my experience it would not be an exaggeration to say that more than half of children's problems are due to retention of residual pathogenic factors. Box 107.1 lists conditions in children that are frequently due to retention of residual pathogenic factors.

BOX 107.1 CHILDREN'S ILLNESSES OFTEN DUE TO RETENTION OF RESIDUAL PATHOGENIC FACTOR

- Chronic earache, recurrent ear infections
- Chronic tonsillitis, swollen tonsils
- Chronic catarrh
- Chronic lymphatic congestion
- Chronic sinusitis
- Recurrent mouth ulcers
- Insomnia, restless sleep, crying at night

As children grow up, the manifestations and effects of a residual pathogenic factor may become less obvious; often, this does not mean that the residual pathogenic factor has been cleared but the Qi has got stronger. In fact, Qi and the residual pathogenic factor are like two plates of a scale: when one goes down, the other goes up and vice versa (Fig. 107.3).

DIAGNOSIS AND TREATMENT OF RESIDUAL PATHOGENIC FACTOR

How is it diagnosed?

The diagnosis of a residual pathogenic factor is made on the basis of the history and symptoms. Patients report a history of an acute febrile episode from which they appeared to recover but which left them with a chronic problem such as a cough, earache, sinusitis, catarrh, etc.

As for symptomatology, the most common forms of residual pathogenic factor are Damp-Heat and Phlegm-Heat and there will therefore be some signs of Heat and Dampness or Phlegm. Symptoms of Heat will include thirst, a feeling of heat, irritability, insomnia and dark urine. The tongue will have a sticky yellow coating and the pulse will be slightly Rapid. Figure 107.4 shows different tongue signs indicating retention of residual pathogenic factor.

Types of residual pathogenic factor

As mentioned above, Heat, Dampness and Phlegm are the most common aspects of a residual pathogenic factor; however, Dampness and Phlegm may be located in various parts of the body such as head, Stomach and Spleen, Gall-Bladder, Liver, ears, etc. All these types of residual pathogenic factor are listed and discussed below.

Effects of residual pathogenic factor

The main effect of a residual pathogenic factor is not only to give rise to a chronic condition but also to predispose the patient to further invasions of Wind, which, in turn, would reinforce the residual pathogenic factor itself, thus creating a vicious circle. For example, an invasion of Wind may lead to the formation of Phlegm in the Lungs; this obstructs the descending and diffusing of Lung-Qi and weakens the Defensive-Qi and therefore predisposes the patient to a further invasion of Wind.

Other effects of residual pathogenic factors are mostly due to Heat and Dampness/Phlegm. Lingering Heat will tend to injure Yin, which becomes a complication of a residual pathogenic factor. Dampness/Phlegm will tend to obstruct the Spleen and aggravate a Qi deficiency (Fig. 107.5).

Treatment of residual pathogenic factor

Residual pathogenic factors are treated simply as any other interior pathogenic factors, the treatment

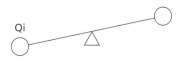

Fig. 107.3
Relationship between Upright Qi and residual pathogenic factor

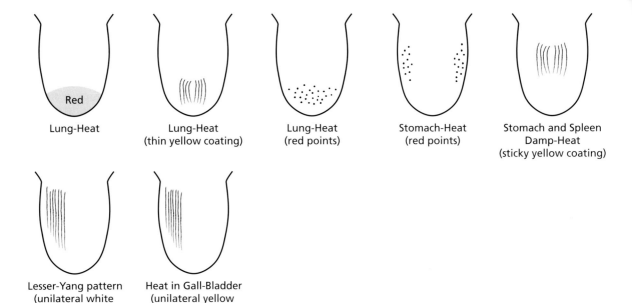

Lung-Heat	Lung-Heat (thin yellow coating)	Lung-Heat (red points)	Stomach-Heat (red points)	Stomach and Spleen Damp-Heat (sticky yellow coating)

Lesser-Yang pattern (unilateral white coating)	Heat in Gall-Bladder (unilateral yellow coating)

Fig. 107.4 Tongue signs in residual pathogenic factor

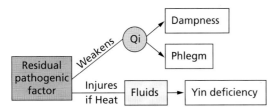

Fig. 107.5 Effects of residual pathogenic factor

principles being clearing Heat and resolving Dampness or Phlegm. What needs to be stressed, however, is the importance of diagnosing the retention of a pathogenic factor and clearing it properly before tonifying. Very often one of the main presenting symptoms will be tiredness after an invasion (or repeated invasions of Wind) and it would be easy to think that we need to tonify the Upright Qi; however, if there is a residual pathogenic factor this would definitely be a mistake. In the presence of a residual pathogenic factor, we must definitely clear it first (by clearing Heat or resolving Phlegm, or both) and, if our diagnosis is correct, the patient will feel better. Often it is not even necessary to tonify Qi afterwards as the removal of Heat and Phlegm (especially the latter) will cause Qi to move and transform better.

PHLEGM

Damp-Phlegm in the Lungs
Clinical manifestations

Persistent cough with expectoration of abundant, white sputum after an invasion of Wind, a feeling of oppression of the chest, breathlessness, wheezing, a feeling of heaviness, poor appetite, nausea.
Tongue Sticky coating.
Pulse Slippery.

Acupuncture

LU-5 Chize, LU-7 Lieque, Ren-12 Zhongwan, ST-40 Fenglong, LU-1 Zhongfu, BL-13 Feishu.

Prescription

Er Chen Tang *Two Old Decoction*.

Phlegm-Heat in the Lungs
Clinical manifestations

Persistent barking cough with expectoration of abundant yellow sputum after an invasion of Wind, a feeling of oppression of the chest, a feeling of heat, possibly low-grade fever, thirst, breathlessness, wheezing, a feeling of heaviness, irritability, nausea.

Tongue Sticky yellow coating.
Pulse Slippery-Rapid.

Acupuncture

LU-5 Chize, LU-7 Lieque, Ren-12 Zhongwan, ST-40 Fenglong, LU-1 Zhongfu, BL-13 Feishu, LI-11 Quchi, Du-14 Dazhui.

Prescription

Wen Dan Tang *Warming the Gall-Bladder Decoction*.

DAMPNESS

Dampness in the Stomach and Spleen
Clinical manifestations

Epigastric fullness and pain following an invasion of Wind, poor appetite, nausea, vomiting, loose stools, diarrhoea, a feeling of heaviness.
Tongue Sticky coating in the centre.
Pulse Slippery or Soggy.

Acupuncture

Ren-12 Zhongwan, Ren-13 Shangwan, SP-9 Yinlingquan, SP-6 Sanyinjiao, LI-4 Hegu, Ren-11 Jianli, ST-21 Liangmen, ST-34 Liangqiu, ST-25 Tianshu.

Prescription

Huo Po Xia Ling Tang *Agastache-Magnolia-Pinellia-Poria Decoction*.

Damp-Heat in the Stomach and Spleen
Clinical manifestations

Epigastric fullness and pain following an invasion of Wind, poor appetite, nausea, vomiting, loose stools with a strong odour, diarrhoea, a feeling of heaviness, thirst, a feeling of heat, bitter taste, irritability, insomnia, dark urine.
Tongue Sticky yellow coating in the centre.
Pulse Slippery and Rapid.

Acupuncture

Ren-12 Zhongwan, Ren-13 Shangwan, SP-9 Yinlingquan, SP-6 Sanyinjiao, LI-4 Hegu, Ren-11 Jianli, ST-21 Liangmen, ST-34 Liangqiu, ST-25 Tianshu, LI-11 Quchi.

Prescription

Lian Po Yin *Coptis-Magnolia Decoction*.

Damp-Heat in the Gall-Bladder
Clinical manifestations

Hypochondrial fullness and pain following an invasion of Wind, poor appetite, dry throat, bitter taste, irritability, headache.
Tongue Sticky yellow unilateral coating.
Pulse Wiry-Slippery-Rapid.

Acupuncture

LI-11 Quchi, GB-34 Yanglingquan, GB-24 Riyue, SP-9 Yinlingquan, ST-19 Burong.

Prescription

Yin Chen Hao Tang *Artemisia Yinchenhao Decoction*
Hao Qin Qing Dan Tang *Artemisia-Scutellaria Clearing the Gall-Bladder Decoction*.

Damp-Heat in the ears
Clinical manifestations

Recurrent earache following repeated invasions of Wind, especially in children, fever, irritability, insomnia, crying at night in small children, yellow discharge from the ear, deafness.
Tongue Sticky yellow coating.
Pulse Slippery-Rapid.

Acupuncture

LI-11 Quchi, TB-5 Waiguan, TB-17 Yifeng, GB-43 Xiaxi.

Prescription

Gan Lu Xiao Du Dan *Sweet Dew Dissolving Toxin Pill* plus Chai Hu *Radix Bupleuri* and Jie Geng *Radix Platycodi grandiflori*.

Damp-Heat in the head
Clinical manifestations

Recurrent sinusitis following repeated invasions of Wind, runny nose with a thick discharge, swollen adenoids, nasal voice, recurrent ear infections, irritability, insomnia, crying at night in small children, catarrh, swollen glands in the neck.
Tongue Sticky yellow coating.
Pulse Slippery.

Acupuncture

LI-11 Quchi, LI-4 Hegu, LU-7 Lieque, LI-20 Yingxiang, SP-9 Yinlingquan, Ren-12 Zhongwan.

Prescription

Cang Er Bi Dou Yan Fang *Xanthium Sinusitis Formula* (if Damp-Heat in Stomach and Spleen)

Long Dan Bi Yuan Fang *Gentiana Sinusitis Formula* or Qing Gan Tou Ding Tang *Clearing the Liver Head Calming Decoction* (if Damp-Heat in Liver and Gall-Bladder)

Xin Yi Qing Fei Yin *Flos Magnoliae Clearing the Lungs Decoction* (if Damp-Heat in the head with Lung-Heat).

Table 107.1 compares and contrasts the prescriptions for residual Damp-Heat in the head.

HEAT

Heat in the Lungs
Clinical manifestations

Cough with expectoration of scanty yellow sputum following an invasion of Wind, a feeling of heat, sweating, thirst, insomnia.

Tongue Yellow coating in the front of the tongue.
Pulse Rapid.

Acupuncture

LU-5 Chize, LU-1 Zhongfu, BL-13 Feishu, LI-11 Quchi.

Prescription

Xie Bai San *Draining the White Powder*
Zhu Ye Shi Gao Tang *Lophaterus-Gypsum Decoction.*

Heat in the Lungs with Dryness
Clinical manifestations

Dry cough with expectoration of very scanty sputum after repeated bouts of cough, following an invasion of Wind, a feeling of tightness of the chest, a dry mouth, a feeling of heat.
Tongue Dry coating.
Pulse Fine-Rapid.

Acupuncture

LU-9 Taiyuan, LU-7 Lieque, Ren-12 Zhongwan, LU-1 Zhongfu, BL-13 Feishu, ST-36 Zusanli, SP-6 Sanyinjiao.

Prescription

Qing Zao Jiu Fei Tang *Clearing Dryness Rescuing the Lungs Decoction.*

Heat in the Stomach
Clinical manifestations

Epigastric pain following an invasion of Wind, thirst, sweating, restlessness, insomnia, fever.
Tongue Yellow coating in the centre, red points around the centre.
Pulse Rapid-Overflowing.

Acupuncture

ST-44 Neiting, LI-11 Quchi, LI-4 Hegu.

Table 107.1 Comparison of formulae for residual pathogenic factor in the head (sinusitis)

Patterns	Symptoms	Tongue	Pulse	Formula
Damp-Heat in head with Damp-Heat in Stomach and Spleen	Sinusitis, epigastric fullness, sticky taste, loose stools	Sticky yellow coating in the centre	Slippery-Rapid or Weak-Floating and Rapid	Cang Er Bi Dou Yan Fang
Damp-Heat in head and Damp-Heat in Liver and Gall-Bladder, Liver-Fire	Sinusitis, headache, red eyes, constipation, irritability, thirst	Red with redder sides and a sticky yellow coating	Slippery-Wiry-Rapid	Long Dan Bi Yuan Fang
Damp-Heat in head, Liver-Yang rising, Liver-Wind	Sinusitis, headache, dizziness, vertigo, irritability	Red sides and sticky yellow coating	Wiry-Slippery-Rapid	Qing Gan Tou Ding Tang
Damp-Heat in head with Lung-Heat	Sinusitis, cough with expectoration of scanty yellow sputum, thirst	Red in the front, sticky yellow coating in the front	Rapid, Slippery	Xin Yi Qing Fei Yin

Prescription

Xie Huang San *Draining Yellowness Powder*.

Toxic heat in the tonsils
Clinical manifestations

Recurrent attacks of tonsillitis following repeated invasions of Wind, chronically swollen tonsils, difficulty in swallowing, catarrh, swollen adenoids, poor appetite, tiredness, irritability, insomnia, crying at night in small children.
Tongue Sticky yellow coating.
Pulse Slippery-Rapid.

Acupuncture

LI-11 Quchi, ST-18 Futu, ST-44 Neiting, SI-5 Yanggu, Ren-12 Zhongwan.

Prescription

Li Yan Cha plus Da Qing Ye *Folium Isatidis seu Baphicacanthi* and Shan Dou Gen *Radix Sophorae subprostratae* (caution with the latter). In children, add also Shen Qu *Massa Fermentata Medicinalis*.

LESSER-YANG PATTERN

Lesser-Yang pattern (Six Stages)
Clinical manifestations

Alternations of shivers and fever following an invasion of Wind, bitter taste, dry throat, blurred vision, hypochondrial fullness and distension, absence of desire to eat or drink, irritability, nausea, vomiting.
Tongue Unilateral thin white coating.
Pulse Wiry-Fine.

Acupuncture

TB-5 Waiguan, TB-6 Zhigou, GB-41 Zulinqi, Du-13 Taodao.

Prescription

Xiao Chai Hu Tang *Small Bupleurum Decoction*.

Heat in the Gall-Bladder (Four Levels)
Clinical manifestations

Alternating hot and cold feeling with a prevalence of heat following an invasion of Wind, swollen glands in the neck, earache, headache, bitter taste, thirst, dry throat, hypochondrial pain, nausea, a feeling of fullness in the epigastrium.
Tongue Red with unilateral sticky yellow coating.
Pulse Wiry-Rapid.

Acupuncture

GB-34 Yanglingquan, GB-43 Xiaxi, TB-6 Zhigou, TB-5 Waiguan.

Prescription

Hao Qin Qing Dan Tang *Artemisia-Scutellaria Clearing the Gall-Bladder Decoction*.

Box 107.2 summarizes the patterns of residual pathogenic factor.

BOX 107.2 TYPES OF RESIDUAL PATHOGENIC FACTOR

Phlegm
- Damp-Phlegm in Lungs
- Phlegm-Heat in Lungs

Dampness
- Dampness in Stomach and Spleen
- Damp-Heat in Stomach and Spleen
- Damp-Heat in Gall-Bladder
- Damp-Heat in ears
- Damp-Heat in Head

Heat
- Heat in Lungs
- Heat in Lungs with Dryness
- Heat in Stomach
- Toxic Heat in tonsils

Lesser-Yang patterns
- Lesser-Yang pattern (Six Stages)
- Heat in Gall-Bladder (Four Levels)

NOTES

1. San Pedro G 1998 'Bronchitis: when are antibiotics needed?', in *Infectious Medicine* 15(11), pp. 768–769.
2. Ibid.

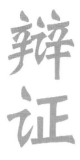

SECTION 4

IDENTIFICATION OF PATTERNS ACCORDING TO THE EIGHT PRINCIPLES, 12 CHANNELS, EIGHT EXTRAORDINARY VESSELS AND FIVE ELEMENTS

Section contents

108 Identification of patterns according to the Eight Principles *983*
109 Identification of patterns according to the 12 channels *993*
110 Identification of patterns according to the Eight Extraordinary Vessels *997*
111 Identification of patterns according to the Five Elements *1007*

INTRODUCTION

Identification of patterns according to the Eight Principles

Elements of this method of identification of patterns are found throughout Chinese medical texts starting from the 'Yellow Emperor's Classic of Internal Medicine' and the 'Discussion of Cold-induced Disorders' (see Bibliography). In its present form, this method of identifying patterns was formulated by Cheng Zhong Ling in the early Qing dynasty.

Identification of patterns according to the Eight Principles is based on the categories of Interior/ Exterior, Heat/Cold, Full/Empty and Yin/Yang. It is the summarization of all other modes of identifying patterns and is applicable in all cases for both interior and exterior diseases.

Identification of patterns according to the 12 channels

This method of pattern identification is the oldest known as it is described in Chapter 32 of the 'Simple Questions'. It describes the symptoms and signs arising from the channel, when the organs are not affected.

Identification of patterns according to the Eight Extraordinary Channels

This method of identification of patterns is based on the patterns or disharmony of the Eight Extraordinary Vessels.

Identification of patterns according to the Five Elements

The identification of patterns according to the Five Elements describes the patterns of disharmony purely from the point of view of Five Elements. This is useful as a general indication for two reasons: first, it can help us to plot the progression of a pathological condition from one Element to the other (bearing in mind that a progression along the Controlling cycle is more serious); secondly, the Five-Element patterns are sometimes useful to form a picture of the mental–emotional condition of the patient.

Chapter **108**

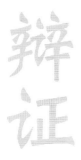

IDENTIFICATION OF PATTERNS ACCORDING TO THE EIGHT PRINCIPLES

Chapter contents

INTRODUCTION   *983*

INTERIOR–EXTERIOR   *984*
  Exterior conditions   *984*
  Interior conditions   *985*

HOT–COLD   *985*
  Hot conditions   *985*
  Cold conditions   *986*
  Combined Hot and Cold conditions   *987*

FULL–EMPTY   *988*
  Full conditions   *990*
  Empty conditions   *990*
  Combined Full–Empty conditions   *990*

YIN-YANG   *991*

INTRODUCTION

The identification of patterns according to the Eight Principles of Interior and Exterior, Full and Empty, Hot and Cold, and Yin and Yang is the foundation for all the other methods of pattern formulation. It is the basic groundwork of pattern identification in Chinese medicine, allowing the practitioner to identify the location and nature of the disharmony, as well as establish the principle of treatment.

Although the term 'Eight Principles' is relatively recent in Chinese Medicine (early Qing dynasty), their main aspects were discussed both in the 'Yellow Emperor Classic of Internal Medicine' and in the 'Discussion on Cold-induced Diseases' (see Bibliography). Both these classics contain many references to Interior/Exterior, Hot/Cold, Full/Empty and Yin/Yang characters of diseases.

Doctor Zhang Jing Yue (also called Zhang Jie Bin) (1563–1640) discussed the identification of patterns according to the above principles and called it the 'Six Changes' (*Liu Bian*), these being Interior/Exterior, Full/Empty and Hot/Cold.

During the early Qing dynasty, at the time of Emperor Kang Xi (1561–1640), doctor Cheng Zhong Ling wrote the 'Essential Comprehension of Medical Studies' (*Yi Xue Xin Wu*), in which he, for the first time, used the term 'Eight Principles' (*Ba Gang*).

The method of identification of patterns according to the Eight Principles differs from all the others in so far as it is the theoretical basis for all of them and is applicable in every case. For example, the method of identification of patterns according to the channels is applicable only in channel problems, and that according to the Internal Organs only in organ problems, but the identification of patterns according to the Eight Principles is applicable in

every case because it allows us to distinguish Exterior from Interior, Hot from Cold and Full from Empty. It therefore allows us to decide which method of identification of patterns applies to a particular case. No condition is too complex to fall outside the scope of identification according to the Eight Principles.

It is important to realize that identifying a pattern according to the Eight Principles does not mean rigidly 'categorizing' the disharmony in order to 'fit' the clinical manifestations into pigeon-holes. On the contrary, an understanding of the Eight Principles allows us to unravel complicated patterns and identify the basic contradictions within them, reducing the various disease manifestations to the bare relevant essentials. Although this process might seem rigid and somewhat forced in the beginning, after a few years of practice, it will become completely natural and spontaneous.

The Eight Principles should not be seen in terms of 'either–or'. It is not at all unusual to see conditions that are Exterior and Interior simultaneously, or Hot and Cold, or Full and Empty or Yin and Yang. It is even possible for a condition to be all of these at the same time. The purpose of applying the Eight Principles is not to categorize the disharmony, but to understand its genesis and nature. It is only by understanding this that we can decide on treatment for a particular disharmony.

Moreover, not every condition need have all four characteristics (Interior or Exterior, Hot or Cold, Full or Empty and Yin or Yang). For example, a condition need not necessarily be either Hot or Cold. Deficiency of Blood is a case in point as it does not involve any Hot or Cold symptoms.

INTERIOR–EXTERIOR

The differentiation between Exterior and Interior is made not on the basis of what caused the disharmony (aetiology), but rather on that of the location of the disease. For example, a disease may be caused by an exterior pathogenic factor, but if this is affecting the Internal Organs the condition will be classified as interior.

Exterior conditions

An exterior condition affects the skin, muscles and channels. An interior condition affects the Internal Organs and bones. Skin, muscles and channels are also called the 'Exterior' of the body, and the Internal Organs the 'Interior'. In the context of exterior diseases

from Wind, the Exterior is sometimes also called the 'Lung Defensive-Qi portion', as the Lungs control both the skin and the Defensive Qi, which circulates in the skin and muscles.

The clinical manifestations arising from invasion of the Exterior by a pathogenic factor are also called an 'exterior pattern', whereas the manifestations arising from a disharmony of the Internal Organs are called an 'interior pattern'.

When we say that an exterior condition affects the skin, muscles and channels, we mean that these areas have been invaded by an exterior pathogenic factor, giving rise to typical 'exterior' clinical manifestations. However, it would be wrong to assume that any problem manifesting on the skin is an 'exterior pattern'. In fact, most chronic skin problems are due to an interior pattern manifesting on the skin.

There are two broad types of exterior conditions: those that affect skin and muscles and are caused by an exterior pathogenic factor having an acute onset (such as in invasion of Wind-Cold or Wind-Heat); and those that affect the channels and have a slower onset (such as in Painful Obstruction Syndrome).

Acute invasion of Wind on the Exterior

When an exterior pathogenic factor invades skin and muscles it gives rise to a typical set of symptoms and signs, which are described as an 'exterior pattern'. It is difficult to generalize as to what these symptoms and signs are, as it depends on the other characteristics, that is, whether they are of the Cold or Hot type, or the Empty or Full type. However, fever and aversion to cold occurring simultaneously always indicate an invasion from an exterior pathogenic factor.

Generally speaking, we can say that the main symptoms of an exterior pattern are fever, aversion to cold, aching body, a stiff neck and a Floating pulse. The onset is acute and the correct treatment will usually induce a swift and marked improvement of the condition.

The symptoms of invasion of Wind-Cold and Wind-Heat were described in Chapter 103.

The main factors in differentiating the Hot or Cold character of an exterior pattern are listed in Box 108.1.

BOX 108.1 FACTORS DIFFERENTIATING HOT AND COLD EXTERIOR PATTERNS

- Thirst (Hot) or its absence (Cold)
- Presence (Heat) or absence (Cold) of sore throat
- Tight or Slow (Cold) or Rapid (Hot) pulse

The character of an exterior pattern will further depend on its Full or Empty character. If a person has a tendency to deficiency of Qi or Blood, the exterior pattern will have an Empty character. This is also described as an exterior pattern from Wind-Cold with prevalence of Wind (see Chapters 103 and 105).

If a person has a tendency to Fullness, the exterior pattern will have a Full character. This is also described as an exterior pattern from Wind-Cold with prevalence of Cold (see Chapter 105).

The main factors in differentiating an Empty from Full Exterior condition are listed in Box 108.2.

> **BOX 108.2 FACTORS DIFFERENTIATING EMPTY AND FULL EXTERIOR CONDITIONS**
>
> - Sweating (Empty) or its absence (Full)
> - Slowed-down pulse (Empty) or Tight pulse (Full)
> - Severe body aches (Full) or slight body aches (Empty)

It must be stressed that the terms 'Full' and 'Empty' describing the character of an exterior condition are only relative, and do not represent actual Fullness and Emptiness. In fact, an exterior pattern is characterized by Fullness by definition as it consists in an invasion by an exterior pathogenic factor. The person's Qi is still relatively intact and the pathogenic factor fights against the body's Qi. It is precisely this that defines a Full condition: that is, one characterized by the presence of a pathogenic factor and the resulting struggle with the body's Qi. Thus, an exterior condition must, by definition be Full. However, according to a person's pre-existing condition, one can further differentiate an exterior condition between Full and Empty, but only in relative terms.

Gradual invasion of external pathogenic factors in the channels (Painful Obstruction Syndrome)

The second kind of exterior pattern is that occurring when an exterior pathogenic factor invades the channels in a gradual way causing Painful Obstruction Syndrome. This is characterized by obstruction to the circulation of Qi in channels and joints by a pathogenic factor, which can be Cold, Dampness, Wind or Heat.

In obstruction from Cold, usually only one joint is affected, the pain is severe and is relieved by application of heat. In obstruction from Wind, the pain moves from joint to joint. In obstruction from Dampness,

there will be swelling of the joints. In obstruction from Heat, the pain is severe and the joints are swollen and hot.

These pathogenic factor patterns have been described in Chapter 103.

Interior conditions

A disharmony is defined as interior when the Internal Organs are affected. This may or may not have arisen from an exterior pathogenic factor, but once the disease is located in the Interior it is defined as an interior pattern, and treated as such.

It is impossible to generalize about the clinical manifestations of interior conditions as these will depend on the organ affected, and whether the condition is Hot or Cold and Full or Empty. Most of the Internal Organs patterns described in Chapters 91–100 are internal patterns.

HOT–COLD

Hot and Cold describe the nature of a pattern, and their clinical manifestations depend on whether they are combined with a Full or Empty condition.

Hot conditions
Full-Heat

The main manifestations of interior Full-Heat are fever, thirst, a feeling of heat, red face, red eyes, constipation, scanty dark urine, a Rapid-Full pulse, and a Red tongue with yellow coating. (Exterior Heat has already been discussed above.)

These are only the general symptoms of Full-Heat, however, as many others are possible depending on which organ is mostly affected. Fever need not always be present as many conditions of interior Full-Heat such as Liver-Fire or Heart-Fire do not involve fever.

Aside from the above clinical manifestations, there are other diagnostic guides which indicate Heat. Any raised, red skin eruption which feels hot indicates Heat. For example, acute urticaria normally takes this form. As for pain, any burning sensation indicates Heat, for example the burning sensation of cystitis, or a burning feeling in the stomach. Any loss of blood with large quantities of dark-red blood usually indicates Heat in the Blood (if the blood were fresh-red, the bleeding may be due to Qi deficiency). So far as the mind is

concerned, any condition of extreme restlessness or manic behaviour, indicates Heat in the Heart.

Box 108.3 summarizes the manifestations of Full-Heat.

BOX 108.3 FULL-HEAT

- Fever
- Thirst
- Feeling of heat
- Red face
- Red eyes
- Constipation
- Dark urine
- Full-Rapid pulse
- Red tongue with yellow coating
- Raised, red skin eruptions
- Burning pain
- Mental restlessness, agitation

Full-Heat arises when there is an excess of Yang energies in the body. Common causes of this are excessive consumption of hot-energy foods or long-standing emotional problems, in which the stagnation of Qi generates Heat. The former will mostly cause Stomach- or Liver-Heat, whereas the latter will mostly cause Liver- or Heart-Heat.

Full-Heat can also develop from the invasion of an exterior pathogenic factor which turns into Heat once in the body. Most pathogenic factors, including Cold, are likely to turn into Heat once in the body. A typical example of this is when exterior Cold or Heat turns into Heat and settles in the Stomach, Lung or Intestines causing high fever, sweating and thirst. The Bright Yang pattern of the Six-Stage pattern identification and the Qi level of the Four-Level pattern identification describe such situations.

From the Yin-Yang point of view, Full-Heat arises from excess of Yang.

Empty-Heat

The main manifestations of Empty-Heat are afternoon fever or a feeling of heat in the afternoon/evening, a dry mouth, a dry throat at night with a desire to drink in small sips, night sweating, a feeling of heat in the chest, palms and soles (also called 'five-palm heat'), a feeling of heat in the evening, dry stools, scanty dark urine, a Floating-Empty and Rapid pulse and a Red-Peeled tongue.

Again, these are only the general symptoms and signs; others depend on which organ is mostly affected. Aside from these manifestations, Empty-

Heat can easily be recognized from a typical feeling of mental restlessness, fidgeting and vague anxiety. The person feels that something is wrong, but is unable to describe what or how. Empty-Heat restlessness is quite different from that of Full-Heat, and one can almost visually perceive the Emptiness underlying the Heat.

Box 108.4 summarizes the manifestations of Empty-Heat.

BOX 108.4 EMPTY-HEAT

- Afternoon fever
- Feeling of heat in the afternoon/evening
- Dry mouth and throat with desire to drink in small sips
- Night sweating
- Five-palm heat
- Dry stools
- Scanty dark urine
- Mental restlessness, fidgeting, vague anxiety
- Red tongue without coating
- Floating-Empty and Rapid pulse

!

The mental restlessness from Empty-Heat differs from that from Full-Heat in so far as it is a vague feeling of anxiety, a quieter form of restlessness and a tendency to fidget.

From the Yin-Yang point of view, Empty-Heat arises from deficiency of Yin. If the Yin energy is deficient for a long period of time, the Yin is consumed and the Yang is relatively in excess. It is important to stress that Empty-Heat derives *eventually* from Yin deficiency but there will usually be a stage of Yin deficiency without Empty-Heat.

In practice, it is important to differentiate Full-Heat from Empty-Heat as the treatment method in the former case is to clear the Heat, whereas in the latter case it is to nourish Yin. The main points of differentiation between Full-Heat and Empty-Heat are listed in Table 108.1.

Cold conditions
Full-Cold

The main manifestations of Cold are chilliness, cold limbs, absence of thirst, pale face, abdominal pain aggravated by pressure and by ingestion of cold drinks and foods, a desire to drink warm liquids, loose stools, abundant clear urination, a Deep-Full-Tight pulse and

Table 108.1 Differentiation between Full-Heat and Empty-Heat

	Full-Heat	Empty-Heat
Face	Whole face red	Malar flush
Thirst	Desire to drink cold water in large amounts	Desire to drink in small sips
Eyelid	Inside of lower eyelid red	Thin red line inside lower eyelid
Taste	Bitter taste	No bitter taste
Feeling of heat	All day	In the afternoon or evening
Fever	High fever	Low-grade fever
Mind	Very restless and agitated	Vague anxiety, fidgety
Bowels	Constipation, abdominal pain	Dry stools, no abdominal pain
Bleeding	Profuse	Not so profuse
Sleep	Dream-disturbed, restless	Waking up frequently during the night
Skin	Red-hot-painful skin eruptions	Scarlet-red, not raised, painless skin eruptions
Pulse	Full-Overflowing-Rapid	Floating-Empty and Rapid
Tongue	Red with yellow coating	Red without coating
Treatment method	Clear Heat	Nourish Yin, clear Empty-Heat

a tongue with thick white coating. (These are the clinical manifestation of interior Full-Cold as exterior Cold has already been described above.)

Cold contracts and obstructs and this often causes pain. Hence pain, especially abdominal pain, is a frequent manifestation of Full-Cold. Also, anything that is white, concave (as opposed to raised), bluish-purple may indicate Cold. For example, a pale face or Pale tongue, a white tongue coating, concave very pale spots on the tongue, a Bluish-Purple tongue and bluish lips or fingers and toes.

From the Yin-Yang point of view, Full-Cold arises from excess of Yin. Interior Full-Cold can arise from direct invasion of exterior Cold into the Interior. In particular, exterior Cold can invade the Stomach causing vomiting and epigastric pain, the Intestines causing diarrhoea and abdominal pain, or the Uterus causing dysmenorrhoea. All these conditions would have an acute onset.

Cold can also invade the Liver channel causing swelling and pain of the scrotum.

Box 108.5 summarizes the general manifestations of Full-Cold.

BOX 108.5 FULL-COLD

- Feeling of cold
- Cold limbs
- Absence of thirst
- Pale (bright-white) face
- Abdominal pain aggravated by pressure and ingestion of cold drinks and foods
- Abundant clear urination
- Bluish lips, fingers, toes
- Pain of acute onset
- Pale or Bluish-Purple tongue with thick white coating
- Deep-Full-Tight pulse

Empty-Cold

The main manifestations of Empty-Cold are chilliness, cold limbs, a dull-pale face, absence of thirst, dull pain releved by pressure, listlessness, a desire to drink warm drinks, loose stools, abundant clear urination, a sallow-white face, a Deep-Weak-Slow pulse and a Pale tongue with thin white coating.

Box 108.6 summarizes the clinical manifestations of Empty-Cold.

BOX 108.6 EMPTY-COLD

- Feeling of cold
- Cold limbs
- Loose stools
- Desire to drink warm drinks
- Dull-pale face
- Absence of thirst
- Listlessness
- Abundant clear urination
- Deep-Weak-Slow pulse
- Pale tongue with thin white coating

From the Yin-Yang point of view, Empty-Cold arises from deficiency of Yang. Empty-Cold develops when Yang-Qi is weak and fails to warm the body. It is mostly related to Spleen-Yang, Kidney-Yang, Heart-Yang or Lung-Qi deficiency.

Table 108.2 differentiates the manifestations of Full-Cold from those of Empty-Cold.

Combined Hot and Cold conditions

A condition can often be characterized by the presence of both Heat and Cold. These can be Cold on the Exterior and Heat in the Interior, Heat on the Exterior and Cold in the Interior, Heat above and Cold below. Furthermore, in some cases, some of the symptoms

Table 108.2 Differentiation between Full-Cold and Empty-Cold

	Full-Cold	Empty-Cold
Face	Bright-white	Sallow-white
Pain	Strong, spastic, crampy, worse with pressure	Dull, better with pressure
Bowels	Better after bowel movement	Worse after bowel movement
Pulse	Full-Tight-Deep	Weak-Deep-Slow
Tongue	Pale or Bluish-Purple body, thick white coating	Pale body, Thin white coating

and signs may point to a false appearance of Heat whereas the true condition is Cold, or vice versa.

Cold on the Exterior–Heat in the Interior

This condition is found when a person has a pre-existing condition of interior Heat and is subsequently invaded by exterior Wind-Cold.

The symptoms and signs would include a fever with aversion to cold, absence of sweating, a headache and stiff neck, aches throughout the body (manifestations of exterior Cold), irritability and thirst (manifestations of interior Heat).

The situation also occurs in attacks of Latent Heat combined with a new invasion of Wind-Cold.

Heat on the Exterior–Cold in the Interior

This situation simply occurs when a person with a Cold condition is attacked by exterior Wind-Heat. There will therefore be some symptoms of exterior invasion of Wind-Heat (such as a fever with aversion to cold, a sore throat, thirst, a headache and a Floating-Rapid pulse) and some symptoms of interior Cold (such as loose stools, chilliness and profuse pale urine).

Heat above–Cold below

In some cases there is Heat above (as Heat tends to rise) and Cold below. The manifestations of this situation might be thirst, irritability, sour regurgitation, bitter taste, mouth ulcers (manifestations of Heat above), loose stools, borborygmi and profuse pale urine (manifestations of Cold below).

True Cold–false Heat and true Heat–false Cold

In some cases there may be contradictory signs and symptoms, some pointing to Heat and some to Cold. This usually happens only in extreme conditions and is quite rare. It is important not to confuse this phenomenon with common situations when Heat and Cold are simply combined.

For example, it is perfectly possible for someone to have a condition of Damp-Heat in the Bladder and Cold in the Spleen. This is simply a combination of Hot and Cold signs in two different organs, and does not fall under the category of false Heat and true Cold or vice versa.

It is important to stress also that the situation of false Heat or false Cold is quite different to the situation characterized by a simultaneous deficiency of both Yin and Yang and therefore Heat and Cold. For example, it is very common in women of menopausal age to suffer from a simultaneous deficiency of Kidney-Yin and Kidney-Yang (and therefore have simultaneous symptoms of Heat and Cold); in this case, the Heat and Cold are purely simultaneous and co existing and they are both 'true'.

In cases of false Heat and false Cold, tongue diagnosis shows its most useful aspect as the tongue-body colour nearly always reflects the true condition. If the tongue-body colour is Red this indicates Heat; if it is Pale it indicates Cold.

> **!**
>
> The tongue-body colour is the most important factor in differentiating true from false Heat and true from false Cold: if the tongue-body colour is Pale this indicates true Cold; if it is Red, it indicates true Heat.

It is worth mentioning here that false Heat and false Cold are definitely not the same as Empty-Heat and Empty-Cold. Empty-Heat and Empty-Cold arise from deficiency of Yin or Yang respectively, but are nevertheless true Heat or Cold conditions. In false Heat and false Cold, the appearance is false, that is, there is no Heat or no Cold respectively.

The manifestations of false Heat and false Cold are illustrated in Table 108.3.

FULL–EMPTY

The differentiation between Full and Empty is an extremely important one. The distinction is made according to the presence or absence of a pathogenic factor and to the strength of the body's energies.

A Full condition is characterized by the presence of a pathogenic factor (which may be interior or exterior) of

Table 108.3 Differentiation between True Cold–False Heat and True Heat–False Cold

Diagnostic methods	True Cold–False Heat	True Heat–False Cold
By looking	Red cheeks but red colour is like powder, while rest of face is white, irritability but also listlessness, a desire to lie with the body curled up, Pale and wet tongue	Dark face, bright eyes with lustre, dry red lips, irritability, strong body, Red tongue
By hearing	Breathing quiet, low voice	Breathing noisy, loud voice
By asking	Thirst but no desire to drink or a desire to drink warm fluids, body feels hot but patient likes to be covered, sore throat but without redness or swelling, pale urine	Thirst with a desire to drink cold fluids, scanty dark urine, constipation, a burning sensation in anus
By palpation	Rapid and Overflowing pulse, but Empty	Deep-Full pulse, limbs cold, chest hot

any kind and by the fact that the body's Qi is relatively intact. It therefore battles against the pathogenic factor and this results in the rather plethoric character of the symptoms and signs.

An Empty condition is characterized by weakness of the body's Qi and the absence of a pathogenic factor.

If the body's Qi is weak but a pathogenic factor lingers on, the condition is one of Empty character complicated with Fullness.

The distinction between Full and Empty is one which is more than any other made on the basis of observation (Table 108.4). A strong, loud voice, an excruciating pain, a very red face, profuse sweating, restlessness, throwing off the bedclothes and outbursts of temper are all signs of a Full condition. A weak voice, a dull lingering pain, a very pale face, slight sweating, listlessness, curling up in bed and quiet disposition are all signs of an Empty condition.

The pulse is another very important factor in differentiating Full from Empty conditions: in Full conditions the pulse is of the Full type, whereas in Empty conditions it is of the Empty type.

Box 108.7 summarizes the characteristics of Full, Empty and Full–Empty conditions.

Table 108.4 Comparison of Empty and Full conditions

	Empty	Full
Course	Chronic	Acute
Mind	Listlessness, apathy, poor memory	Restlessness, irritability
Voice	Weak	Strong
Breathing	Weak	Coarse
Face	Pale	Red
Tinnitus	Low pitched	High pitched
Pain	Dull, alleviated by pressure	Excruciating, aggravated by pressure
Sweating	Slight	Profuse
Stools	Loose	Constipation
Urination	Normal	Scanty
Other signs/ symptoms	Lying curled up	Throwing off of bedclothes
Pulse	Empty	Excess

BOX 108.7 CHARACTERISTICS OF FULL, EMPTY AND FULL-EMPTY CONDITIONS

Full
- A Full condition is characterized by the presence of a pathogenic factor (which may be internal or external) while the body's Qi is still intact and reacting against the pathogenic factor

Empty
- An Empty condition is characterized by a deficiency of the body's Qi and the absence of a pathogenic factor

Full–Empty
- A mixed Full–Empty condition is characterized by the presence of a pathogenic factor (generally internal) and a deficiency of the body's Qi which is reacting inadequately against the pathogenic factor; in some cases, the deficiency of the body's Qi itself leads to the formation of a pathogenic factor

Full conditions

The main clinical manifestations of a Full condition are acute disease, restlessness, irritability, a red face, a strong voice, coarse breathing, pain aggravated by pressure, high-pitched tinnitus, profuse sweating, scanty urination, constipation and a pulse of the Excess type.

As usual, it is difficult to generalize and some of the above symptoms cannot, strictly speaking, be categorized as Full symptoms. Just to give one example, constipation is included among the Full symptoms because it is often caused by stagnation or by Heat, but there are also Empty causes of constipation, such as Blood or Yin deficiency. Moreover, the above symptoms are broad generalizations, indeed too general to be of use in clinical practice.

Many examples could be given of Full conditions. First of all, any exterior condition due to invasion of exterior Cold, Wind, Damp or Heat is Full by definition, as it is characterized by the presence of those exterior pathogenic factors.

Any interior pathogenic factor also gives rise to a Full condition, provided the body's Qi is strong enough to engage in a struggle against such pathogenic factors. Examples of these are interior Cold, Heat, Dampness, Wind, Fire and Phlegm. Stagnation of Qi and stasis of Blood are also Full conditions.

Empty conditions

The main clinical manifestations of an Empty condition are chronic disease, listlessness, apathy, lying curled up, a weak voice, weak breathing, low-pitch tinnitus, pain alleviated by pressure, poor memory, slight sweating, frequent urination, loose stools and a pulse of the Empty type.

We can distinguish four types of Emptiness: Empty-Qi, Empty-Yang, Empty-Blood and Empty-Yin.

Empty-Qi

The clinical manifestations of Empty-Qi are slight shortness of breath, weak voice, spontaneous sweating, poor appetite, loose stools, tiredness, pale complexion, a dislike of speaking and an Empty pulse.

These are only the symptoms of Lung- and Spleen-Qi Deficiency, which are those customarily given in Chinese books, as it is the Spleen that produces Qi and the Lungs that govern Qi. However, there can be many other symptoms of emptiness of Qi, according to which organ is involved, in particular the Heart or Kidneys. These were described in Chapters 91 to 100.

Empty-Yang

The main clinical manifestations of Empty-Yang are: shortness of breath, weak voice, spontaneous sweating, poor appetite, loose stools, tiredness, bright-pale complexion, dislike of speaking, a feeling of cold, cold limbs, absence of thirst, desire for hot drinks, frequent pale urination, Pale tongue and a Deep-Weak pulse.

The organs which most commonly suffer from Yang deficiency are the Spleen, Kidneys, Lung, Heart and Stomach. The patterns for each of these were discussed in the section on the Internal Organs patterns (Chapters 91–100).

Empty-Blood

The main manifestations of Emptiness of Blood are a dull complexion, dizziness, numbness, tingling of the limbs, poor memory, blurred vision, insomnia, pale lips, dry eyes, white nails, floaters, palpitations, scanty periods, amenorrhoea, infertility, Pale and Thin tongue, and Choppy or Fine pulse.

The above general symptoms are due to dysfunction of various organs. In addition, Emptiness of Liver-Blood causes dizziness, blurred vision, depression, tiredness, numbness and scanty periods. Emptiness of Heart-Blood causes pale face, pale lips, Pale tongue and insomnia.

The organs which are most likely to suffer from Blood Emptiness are the Liver, Heart and Spleen. These patterns were described in Chapters 91–93.

Empty-Yin

The main manifestations of Emptiness of Yin are a dry mouth, dry throat at night, night sweating, dizziness, tinnitus, tiredness, thin body, insomnia, a tongue without coating, and a Fine or Floating-Empty pulse.

Again, the above are only the general symptoms of Emptiness of Yin, other symptoms depending on which organ is mostly involved. The organs most likely to suffer from Yin deficiency are the Kidneys, Lung, Heart, Liver and Stomach.

Combined Full–Empty conditions

Conditions characterized by a combination of Emptiness and Fullness arise when there is a pathogenic

factor but while its influence is not very strong the body's Qi is weak and not reacting properly against it. Examples of conditions of Emptiness complicated with Fullness are: Kidney-Yin deficiency with rising of Liver-Yang, Kidney-Yin deficiency with flaring up of Heart Empty-Heat, Spleen-Qi deficiency with retention of Dampness or Phlegm, deficiency of Blood with stasis of Blood, and deficiency of Qi with stasis of Blood.

YIN–YANG

The categories of Yin and Yang within the Eight Principles have two meanings: in a general sense, they are a summarization of the other six principles, whereas in a specific sense they are used mostly in the patterns Emptiness of Yin and Yang and collapse of Yin and Yang.

First, in the general sense, Yin and Yang are a generalization of the other six principles since Interior, Emptiness and Cold are Yin in nature, and Exterior, Fullness and Heat are Yang in nature.

Secondly, in the specific sense, the categories of Yin and Yang can define two kinds of Emptiness and also two kinds of collapse. Emptiness of Yin and Yang have already been described above and in Chapter 101.

Collapse of Yin or Yang simply indicates an extremely severe state of Emptiness. It also implies a complete separation of Yin and Yang from each other. Collapse of Yin or Yang is often, but not necessarily, followed by death. They have already been described in Chapter 101.

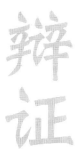

Chapter **109**

IDENTIFICATION OF PATTERNS ACCORDING TO THE 12 CHANNELS

Chapter contents

LUNGS   *993*

LARGE INTESTINE   *993*

STOMACH   *994*

SPLEEN   *994*

HEART   *994*

SMALL INTESTINE   *994*

BLADDER   *995*

KIDNEYS   *995*

PERICARDIUM   *995*

TRIPLE BURNER   *995*

GALL-BLADDER   *996*

LIVER   *996*

The clinical manifestations of the patterns according to the 12 channels are as follows.

LUNGS

Main channel

Fever, cough, nasal congestion, headache, breathlessness, chest pain, aversion to cold, a feeling of oppression of the chest, pain in the upper back, clavicle, shoulders, elbows and inner aspect of the arms, a feeling of heat in the palms.

Connecting channel
Empty

Yawning, frequent urination, shortness of breath.

Full

Hot palms.

Muscle channel

Pain, contraction and sprain of the muscles along the course of the channel, pain and contraction of the muscles of the chest and shoulder.

LARGE INTESTINE

Main channel

Sore throat, toothache, dry mouth, nosebleed, runny nose, swelling of the neck, swollen and painful gums, red, painful and swollen eyes, swelling of the throat, swelling and redness of the dorsum of the hand, shoulder pain, swelling and numbness of the thumb, pain along the course of the channel.

Connecting channel
Empty

A sensation of cold in the teeth, a feeling of tightness in diaphragm, loss of sense of smell.

Full

Toothache, deafness, tinnitus, a sensation of heat in the centre of the chest, breathlessness.

Muscle channel

Pain, stiffness or sprain of the muscles along the course of the channel, inability to raise the arm, inability to rotate the neck, shoulder ache.

STOMACH

Main channel

Pain in the eyes, nosebleed, swelling of the neck, swelling and pain of the throat, oedema, toothache, pain in the breast, thigh, knee, shin, or outer aspect of the ankle and foot, inability to raise the foot, mouth ulcers, facial paralysis, cold legs and feet, pain along the course of the channel.

Connecting channel
Empty

Flaccidity or atrophy of leg muscles, a feeling of cold in the upper teeth.

Full

Epilepsy, manic behaviour or depression, swollen and sore throat, sudden loss of voice, nosebleed.

Great Connecting channel of the Spleen

Palpitations, a feeling of fullness of the chest.

Muscle channel

Sprain of the middle toe, contraction of the muscles of the lower leg and foot, stiffness of the thigh muscles, swelling in the groin, hernia, spasm of the abdominal muscles, strained neck and cheek muscles, deviation of the eyes and mouth, inability to close the eye owing to muscle spasm, inability to open the eyes owing to flaccidity of the muscles.

SPLEEN

Main channel

Vaginal discharge, a cold feeling along the channel, pain along the channel (big toe, the inner aspect of the ankle, shin, knee, or thigh), numbness/tingling of the leg, weakness of the leg muscles, a feeling of heaviness of the legs, abdominal distension, epigastric pain, stiffness and pain of the tongue, oedema of the feet or legs.

Connecting channel
Empty

Abdominal distension.

Full

Abdominal pain, food poisoning, vomiting, diarrhoea.

Great Connecting channel of the Spleen

Pain all over the body, weakness and flaccidity of the joints of the four limbs, backache radiating to the abdomen.

Muscle channel

Strain of the big toe, pain in the inner aspect of the ankle, pain in the muscles of the medial aspect of the knee and thigh, strain of the muscles of the groin, strain of the abdominal muscles, pain in the muscles of the chest and middle back.

HEART

Main channel

Pain in the eyes, dry throat and mouth, numbness/tingling of the arm, a feeling of heat and pain of the palms, chest pain, pain on the inner side of the arm, pain of the shoulder and scapula, palpitations, stiff tongue.

Connecting channel
Empty

Aphasia.

Full

A feeling of distension and fullness of the chest and diaphragm.

Muscle channel

Pain, stiffness and sprain of the muscles along the course of the channel.

SMALL INTESTINE

Main channel

Numbness and pain in the neck, pain in the elbow, stiff neck, pain along the lateral side of the arm and

scapula, sore throat, ear ache, tinnitus, swelling of the chin.

Connecting channel
Empty

Scabies, long, finger-shaped warts.

Full

Loose joints of the shoulder, weakness of the muscles of the elbow joint.

Muscle channel

Stiffness and pain of the muscles of the little finger, arm and elbow, sprain and pain of the muscles of the scapula, pain and sprain of the neck muscles, pain from the ear to the mandible, earache radiating to the chin, swelling of the sides of the neck.

BLADDER

Main channel

Fever and aversion to cold, headache, stiff neck, pain in the lower/upper back, difficulty in bending the back, difficulty in flexing the knee, swelling and pain of the eyes, nosebleed, pain behind the leg along the channel, pain in the foot and the external aspect of the ankle, a feeling of fullness and pain of the hypogastrium.

Connecting channel
Empty

Runny nose, nosebleed.

Full

Stuffy nose, headache, backache, neck ache, shoulder ache.

Muscle channel

Pain and stiffness of the muscles of the little toe, foot, heel, knee and spine, backache and spasm of the back, stiff neck, inability to raise the shoulder, stiffness of the muscles of the axillary region, inability to twist the waist.

KIDNEYS

Main channel

Pain in the lower back, pain and a feeling of heat in the sole of the foot, pain and numbness along the channel (inner aspect of the ankle, foot, shin, knee, or thigh), swelling and pain of the throat, chest pain, breathlessness, dry throat, decreased vision, dizziness, tinnitus, dark complexion, cold feet.

Connecting channel
Empty

Lower backache.

Full

Mental restlessness, depression, retention of urine, pain in the heart region, distension and fullness of the chest.

Muscle channel

Pain, stiffness and sprain of the muscles of the toes, foot, or inner aspect of the ankle, stiffness of the muscles of the spine and neck, inability to bend forward (if the muscles of the back are affected), inability to bend backwards (if the muscles of the chest are affected, convulsions (arching of the back).

PERICARDIUM

Main channel

Stiff neck, pain along the course of the channel, contraction of elbow or hand, a feeling of heat in the palm, a feeling of fullness and pain of the chest, swelling in the axilla, red face.

Connecting channel
Empty

Stiffness of the head.

Full

Pain in the heart region, mental restlessness.

Muscle channel

Pain, stiffness and sprain of the muscles of the palms, or inner aspect of arm, elbow and axilla, pain in the heart region.

TRIPLE BURNER

Main channel

Numbness and pain along the course of the channel (fingers, wrist, elbow, or shoulder), alternation of chills and fever, deafness, tinnitus, dry throat, swelling and pain of the throat, pain in the outer canthus of the eye,

red eyes, pain around the ear, discharge from the ear, swelling and pain of the cheeks, pain in the jaw, temporal headache, dizziness.

Connecting channel
Empty

Loosening of the elbow joint.

Full

Contraction of the elbow, swollen and painful throat, dry mouth, pain of the outer aspect of the arm, inability to raise the arm.

Muscle channel

Sprain, stiffness and sprain of the muscles of the ring finger, wrist, elbow, upper arm, shoulder and neck, curling of the tongue.

GALL-BLADDER

Main channel

Alternation of chills and fever, temporal headache, deafness, pain in the hip, pain along the course of the channel (lateral aspect of thigh, knee, shin, or ankle), pain and distension of the breasts, pain in the eye, inability to raise the foot, dizziness and tinnitus, bitter taste, sighing, swelling of the sides of the neck, swelling and pain below the axilla, shoulder pain, hypochondrial pain.

Connecting channel
Empty

Weakness and flaccidity of the foot muscles, cold feet, paralysis of the legs, difficulty in standing.

Full

Fainting, hypochondrial pain.

Muscle channel

Pain, stiffness and sprain of the muscles of the fourth toe, external aspect of the ankle, or lateral aspect of leg and knee, difficulty in bending the knees, paralysis of the legs, chest and hypochondrial pain, inability to open the eyes.

LIVER

Main channel

Headache, pain and swelling of the eye, cramps in the legs, pain and numbness along the course of the channel (big toe, inner aspect of ankle, shin, knee, or thigh), pain in the genitals, hernia, abdominal pain, urinary difficulty, hypochondrial pain and distension, blurred vision, dry throat.

Connecting channel
Empty

Itching of the genital region, impotence.

Full

Swelling and pain of the testicles, colic, abnormal erection, hernia.

Muscle channel

Pain, stiffness and sprain of the muscles of the big toe, inner aspect of the ankle and leg, impotence, contraction of the scrotum or vagina, priapism (persistent erection).

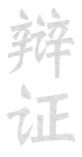

Chapter **110**

IDENTIFICATION OF PATTERNS ACCORDING TO THE EIGHT EXTRAORDINARY VESSELS

Chapter contents

INTRODUCTION   *997*

GOVERNING VESSEL (DU MAI)   *997*

DIRECTING VESSEL (REN MAI)   *998*

PENETRATING VESSEL (CHONG MAI)   *998*

COMBINED DIRECTING AND PENETRATING VESSEL
PATTERNS   *999*
  Directing and Penetrating Vessels Empty   *999*
  Directing and Penetrating Vessels unstable   *999*
  Directing and Penetrating Vessels deficient and
    cold   *999*
  Blood stasis in the Directing and Penetrating
    Vessels   *1000*
  Blood stasis and Dampness in the Directing and
    Penetrating Vessels   *1000*
  Full-Heat in the Directing and Penetrating
    Vessels   *1000*
  Empty-Heat in the Directing and Penetrating
    Vessels   *1001*
  Damp-Heat in the Directing and Penetrating
    Vessels   *1001*
  Stagnant Heat in the Directing and Penetrating
    Vessels   *1001*
  Full-Cold in the Directing and Penetrating
    Vessels   *1001*
  Uterus deficient and cold   *1002*
  Dampness and Phlegm in the Uterus   *1002*
  Stagnant Cold in the Uterus   *1002*
  Fetus Heat   *1003*
  Fetus Cold   *1003*
  Blood rebelling upwards after childbirth   *1003*

GIRDLE VESSEL (DAI MAI)   *1003*

YIN HEEL VESSEL (YIN QIAO MAI)   *1004*

YANG HEEL VESSEL (YANG QIAO MAI)   *1004*

YIN LINKING VESSEL (YIN WEI MAI)   *1005*

YANG LINKING VESSEL (YANG WEI MAI)   *1005*

INTRODUCTION

For each extraordinary vessel, the applicable pre-scriptions will be listed: the formulae indicated are general ones from Li Shi Zhen's 'Study of the Extraordinary Vessels'[1] while the ones for the combined patterns of the Directing and Penetrating Vessels are formulae specific to each pattern and are taken from 'Diagnosis, Patterns and Treatment in Chinese Medicine'.[2] As for acupuncture, given the wide variety of symptoms pertaining to each extraordinary vessel, only the opening points for each will be mentioned. The herbs and prescriptions are from a Qing dynasty book called 'The Materia Medica of Proper Combinations'.[3]

GOVERNING VESSEL (DU MAI)

Clinical manifestations

Stiffness and pain of the spine, backache, weak back, arching of the back, headache, tremors, convulsions, epilepsy, prolapse of the anus, blood in the stools, incontinence of urine, painful urination, nocturnal emissions, impotence, irregular periods, infertility, dry throat, poor memory, dizziness, tinnitus, depression, chills and fever, manic behaviour.
Pulse   Floating and Long on all three positions of the left side.

Connecting channel

Stiffness of the back, a feeling of heaviness of the head, tremor of the head.

Acupuncture

SI-3 Houxi and BL-62 Shenmai.

Herbs
Spine, Marrow, Brain

Lu Rong *Cornu Cervi parvum*
Lu Jiao *Cornu Cervi*
Lu Jiao Shuang *Cornu Cervi degelatinatum*
Marrow of beef and goat

Yang channels, Bladder, Gall-Bladder

Fu Zi *Radix Aconiti carmichaeli praeparata*
Qiang Huo *Rhizoma seu Radix Notopterygii*
Rou Gui *Cortex Cinnamomi cassiae*
Du Huo *Radix Angelicae pubescentis*
Fang Feng *Radix Ledebouriellae sesloidis*
Jing Jie *Herba seu Flos Schizonepetae tenuifoliae*
Xi Xin *Herba Asari cum radice*
Gao Ben *Rhizoma et Radix Ligustici sinensis*
Cang Er Zi *Fructus Xanthii*
Gan Jiang *Rhizoma Zingiberis officinalis*
Chuan Jiao *Pericarpium Zanthoxyli bungeani*
Gui Zhi *Ramulus Cinnamomi cassiae*
Wu Tou *Radix Aconiti carmichaeli*

Prescription

None given, but any Kidney-Yang tonic prescription containing the above herbs will strengthen the Governing Vessel.

DIRECTING VESSEL (REN MAI)

Clinical manifestations

Nocturnal emissions, incontinence of urine, retention of urine, vaginal discharge, irregular periods, infertility, pain in the genital region, epigastric and abdominal pain, abdominal masses, menopausal symptoms (night sweating, hot flushes), problems during pregnancy, amenorrhoea, oedema.
Pulse   Fine-Tight-Long on both Front positions.

Connecting channel

Pain and itching of the abdomen.

Acupuncture

LU-7 Lieque and KI-6 Zhaohai.

Herbs
Uterus and Blood tonics

Gui Ban *Plastrum Testudinis*
Gui Ban Jiao *Colla Plastri Testudinis*

Bie Jia *Carapacis Amydae sinensis*
E Jiao *Gelatinum Corii Asini*
Zi He Che *Placenta hominis*
Zi Shi Ying *Fluoritum*
Ai Ye *Folium Artemisiae Argyi*
Clams.

Nourishing Yin and clearing Empty-Heat

Zhi Mu *Radix Anemarrhenae*
Huang Bo *Cortex Phellodendri*
Xuan Shen *Radix Scrophulariae ningpoensis*
Sheng Di Huang *Radix Rehmanniae glutinosae*
Gou Qi Zi *Fructus Lycii*.

Prescription

Da Bu Yin Wan *Great Tonifying the Yin Pill*.

PENETRATING VESSEL (CHONG MAI)

Clinical manifestations

Irregular periods, infertility, painful periods, vomiting and nausea, 'internal urgency' (*Li Ji*, feeling of anxiety), breathlessness, abdominal pain and distension, a feeling of energy rising from the abdomen to the chest, a feeling of tightness and pain of the epigastrium and chest, palpitations, anxiety, a feeling of obstruction in the throat, a feeling of heat in the face, cold and numb feet with purple colour, umbilical pain, premenstrual tension, breast distension, breast nodules, menopausal symptoms (hot flushes, anxiety, palpitations), morning sickness, spontaneous bruising, nosebleed, fungal infections of the big toe.
Pulse   Deep and Firm on all three positions of either side, or Deep and Firm on both Middle positions, or Wiry on both Middle positions.

Acupuncture

SP-4 Gongsun and P-6 Neiguan.

Herbs
Uterus tonics

Gui Ban *Plastrum Testudinis*
Bie Jia *Carapacis Amydae sinensis*
E Jiao *Gelatinum Corii Asini*
Zi He Che *Placenta hominis*.

Rebellious Qi

Yan Hu Suo *Rhizoma Corydalis Yanhusuo*
Chuan Lian Zi *Fructus Meliae toosendan*

Xiang Fu *Rhizoma Cyperi rotundi*
Yu Jin *Tuber Curcumae*
Chen Xiang *Lignum Aquilariae*
Tao Ren *Semen Persicae*
Dang Gui *Radix Angelicae sinensis*
Qing Pi *Pericarpium Citri reticulatae viridae*
Wu Zhu Yu *Fructus Evodiae rutaecarpae*
Cong Bai *Herba Allii fistulosi*
Xiao Hui Xiang *Fructus Foeniculi vulgaris*
Chong Wei Zi *Semen Leonurus heterophylli*
Wu Yao *Radix Linderae Strychnifoliae*.

Prescription

None given.

COMBINED DIRECTING AND PENETRATING VESSEL PATTERNS

Directing and Penetrating Vessels Empty

Clinical manifestations
Gynaecological manifestations

Delayed cycle, scanty periods, amenorrhoea, infertility.

Other manifestations

Dull, pale complexion, dizziness, blurred vision, tiredness, depression, backache, weakness of the back and knees, decreased libido.
Tongue Pale.
Pulse Deep and Weak, especially on both Rear positions.

Acupuncture

LU-7 Lieque on the right and KI-6 Zhaohai on the left, Ren-4 Guanyuan, KI-13 Qixue, BL-23 Shenshu. Moxa is applicable.

Prescription

Da Bu Yuan Jian *Great Tonifying the Origin Decoction*
Gui Shen Wan *Tonifying the Kidneys Pill*
Shou Tai Wan *Fetus Longevity Pill*.

Directing and Penetrating Vessels unstable

Clinical manifestations
Gynaecological manifestations

Early periods, shortened cycle, heavy periods, irregular periods, persistent, chronic vaginal discharge, miscarriage, persistent lochial discharge after childbirth.

Other manifestations

Dull-pale complexion, depression, backache, weak knees, a bearing-down feeling, frequent urination, incontinence of urine, urination at night.
Tongue Pale.
Pulse Deep and Weak especially on both Rear positions.

Acupuncture

LU-7 Lieque on the right and KI-6 Zhaohai on the right, Ren-4 Guanyuan, KI-13 Qixue, BL-23 Shenshu, Du-20 Baihui, Ren-6 Qihai, extra point Zigong. Moxa is applicable.

Prescription

Gu Chong Tang *Consolidating the Penetrating Vessel Decoction*
An Chong Tang *Calming the Penetrating Vessel Decoction*
Yi Qi Gu Chong Tang *Benefiting Qi and Consolidating the Penetrating Vessel Decoction*
Bu Shen Gu Chong Wan *Tonifying the Kidneys and Consolidating the Penetrating Vessel Pill*
Lu Jiao Tu Si Zi Wan *Cornus Cervi-Cuscuta Pill*.

Directing and Penetrating Vessels deficient and cold

Clinical manifestations
Gynaecological manifestations

Early or late periods, abdominal pain, amenorrhoea, infertility, dull abdominal pain after childbirth, prolonged trickling after the period, pale and dilute menstrual blood.

Other manifestations

Dull abdominal pain alleviated by pressure and the application of heat, cold limbs, a feeling of cold, a pronounced feeling of cold during the period, decreased libido.
Tongue Pale and wet.
Pulse Deep, Weak and Slow.

Acupuncture

LU-7 Lieque on the right and KI-6 Zhaohai on the right, Ren-4 Guanyuan, KI-13 Qixue, BL-23 Shenshu, extra point Zigong. Moxa must be used.

Prescription

Wen Jing Tan *Warming the Menses Decoction*
Dang Gui Jian Zhong Tang *Angelica Warming the Centre Decoction*

Wen Shen Tiao Qi Tang *Warming the Kidneys and Regulating Qi Decoction*
Yu Yun Tang *Promoting Pregnancy Decoction*
Bu Shen Yang Xue Tang *Tonifying the Kidneys and Nourishing Blood Decoction.*

Blood stasis in the Directing and Penetrating Vessels

Clinical manifestations
Gynaecological manifestations

Irregular cycle, brown spotting before the period, painful periods with dark blood and clots, amenorrhoea (from blood stasis), infertility, retention of lochia after childbirth.

Other manifestations

Lower abdominal pain, umbilical pain, pain and distension of the breasts, anxiety, irritability, mental restlessness, tendency to worry, breast lumps, abdominal masses.
Tongue   Purple.
Pulse   Wiry or Choppy.

Acupuncture

SP-4 Gongsun on the right and P-6 Neiguan on the left, KI-14 Siman, ST-29 Guilai, SP-6 Sanyinjiao, LIV-3 Taichong, KI-5 Shuiquan.

Prescription

Xiao Yao San *Free and Easy Wanderer Powder*
Yue Ju Wan *Ligusticum-Gardenia Pill*
Wu Yao San *Lindera Powder*
Ge Xia Zhu Tang *Eliminating Stasis below the Diaphragm Decoction*
Gui Zhi Fu Ling Wan *Ramulus-Cinnamomi-Puria Pill*
Xiang Leng Wan *Aucklandia-Sparganium Pill.*

Blood stasis and Dampness in the Directing and Penetrating Vessels

Clinical manifestations
Gynaecological manifestations

Irregular cycle, heavy periods, dark menstrual blood with clots, brown spotting before the period, painful periods, chronic vaginal discharge, abdominal masses, ovarian cysts, endometriosis, infertility.

Other manifestations

Lower abdominal pain, a feeling of heaviness of the abdomen.

Tongue   Purple, Swollen with sticky coating.
Pulse   Wiry and Slippery.

Acupuncture

SP-4 Gongsun on the right and P-6 Neiguan on the left, KI-14 Siman, ST-29 Guilai, SP-6 Sanyinjiao, LIV-3 Taichong, KI-5 Shuiquan, SP-9 Yinlingquan, ST-28 Shuidao, Ren-3 Zhongji, BL-22 Sanjiaoshu.

Prescription

Tao Hong Si Wu Tang *Prunus-Carthamus Four Substances Decoction*
Shao Fu Zhu Yu Tang *Lower Abdomen Eliminating Stasis Decoction*
San Miao Hong Teng Tang *Three Wonderful Sargentodoxa Decoction*
Qing Re Tiao Xue Tang *Clearing Heat and Regulating Blood Decoction*
Cang Fu Dao Tan Wan *Atractylodes-Cyperus Conducting Phlegm Pill*
Yin Jia Wan *Lonicera-Amyda Pill.*

Full-Heat in the Directing and Penetrating Vessels

Clinical manifestations
Gynaecological manifestations

Early cycle, heavy periods, bright-red or dark-red menstrual blood, flooding and trickling, mid-cycle bleeding, nosebleed during the period, profuse lochial discharge after childbirth, fever after childbirth.

Other manifestations

Red face, a feeling of heat, thirst, irritability, insomnia.
Tongue   Red with yellow coating.
Pulse   Rapid-Overflowing, Full at the middle level.

Acupuncture

LU-7 Lieque on the right and KI-6 Zhaohai on the left, LI-11 Quchi, SP-10 Xuehai, Ren-3 Zhongji, LIV-3 Taichong, SP-6 Sanyinjiao.

Prescription

Qing Jing Tang *Clearing the Menses Powder*
Bao Yin Jian *Protecting the Yin Decoction*
Qing Re Gu Jing Tang *Clearing Heart and Consolidating the Menses Decoction*
Qing Gan Yin Jing Tang *Clearing the Liver and Guiding the Period Decoction*

Jie Du Huo Xue Tang *Expelling Poison and Invigorating Blood Decoction*
Jing Fang Si Wu Tang *Schizonepeta-Ledebouriella Four Substances Decoction*.

Empty-Heat in the Directing and Penetrating Vessels
Clinical manifestations
Gynaecological manifestations

Early cycle, long periods, trickling after the period, mid-cycle bleeding, scanty or heavy periods.

Other manifestations

A feeling of heat in the afternoon, malar flush, night sweating, five-palm heat, insomnia, mental restlessness, dry throat at night.
Tongue Red without coating.
Pulse Floating-Empty or Fine and Rapid.

Acupuncture

LU-7 Lieque on the right and KI-6 Zhaohai on the left, Ren-4 Guanyuan, KI-2 Rangu, SP-6 Sanyinjiao.

Prescription

Liang Di Tang *Two 'Di' Decoction*
Yi Yin Jian *One Yin Decoction*.

Damp-Heat in the Directing and Penetrating Vessels
Clinical manifestations
Gynaecological manifestations

Excessive yellow or red sticky vaginal discharge with offensive odour, mid-cycle bleeding/pain, heavy periods, painful periods, long periods.

Other manifestations

Abdominal pain, a feeling of heaviness in the abdomen, pain on urination, mucus in the stools, a feeling of heat, low-grade fever, cloudy urine.
Tongue Sticky yellow coating.
Pulse Slippery and Rapid.

Acupuncture

LU-7 Lieque on the right and KI-6 Zhaohai on the left, Ren-3 Zhongji, ST-28 Shuidao, Ren-9 Shuifen, SP-9 Yinlingquan, SP-6 Sanyinjiao, LI-11 Quchi, BL-22 Sanjiaoshu.

Prescription

Zhi Dai Wan *Stopping Vaginal Discharge Pill*
Long Dan Xie Gan Tang *Gentiana Draining the Liver Decoction*.

Stagnant Heat in the Directing and Penetrating Vessels
Clinical manifestations
Gynaecological manifestations

Early cycle, scanty or heavy periods, premenstrual tension, periods stopping and starting, red clots.

Other manifestations

Abdominal distension, breast distension, irritability, propensity to outbursts of anger, a feeling of heat, dry throat.
Tongue Red sides.
Pulse Wiry.
This is Heat deriving from long-term stagnation of Qi.

Acupuncture

LU-7 Lieque on the right and KI-6 Zhaohai on the left if the pulse is Wiry, or SP-4 Gongsun on the right and P-6 Neiguan on the left if the pulse is Firm, LIV-3 Taichong, Ren-6 Qihai, KI-14 Siman, LIV-2 Xingjian, LIV-14 Qimen.

Prescription

Dan Zhi Xiao Yao San *Moutan-Gardenia Free and Easy Wanderer Powder*
Hua Gan Jian *Transforming the Liver Decoction*.

Full-Cold in the Directing and Penetrating Vessels
Clinical manifestations
Gynaecological manifestations

Delayed cycle, painful periods with severe cramping pain and a pronounced feeling of cold during the period, bright-red blood with small dark clots, infertility, abdominal pain after childbirth.

Other manifestations

Abdominal pain that is aggravated by pressure and alleviated by the application of heat, a feeling of cold, cold limbs, bright-white complexion.
Tongue Pale or Bluish-Purple.
Pulse Deep, Slow, Tight.

Acupuncture

LU-7 Lieque on the right and KI-6 Zhaohai on the left, Ren-4 Guanyuan, Ren-3 Zhongji, ST-28 Shuidao, KI-14 Siman, extra point Zigong, ST-36 Zusanli, SP-6 Sanyinjiao, KI-5 Shuiquan. Moxa must be used.

Prescription

Shao Fu Zhu Yu Tang *Lower Abdomen Eliminating Stasis Decoction*
Wen Jing Tang *Warming the Menses Decoction*
Suo Gong Zhu Yu Tang *Contracting the Uterus and Eliminating Stasis Decoction*.

Uterus deficient and cold
Clinical manifestations
Gynaecological manifestations

Irregular cycle, scanty period, painful period with dull pain that is alleviated by the application of heat, excessive vaginal discharge, infertility, miscarriage, threatened miscarriage, abdominal pain during childbirth, retention of lochia after childbirth.

Other manifestations

Chronic dull, lower abdominal pain that is alleviated by pressure and the application of heat, a soft feeling of the abdomen on palpation, a feeling of cold, cold limbs, loose stools, frequent and pale urination.
Tongue Pale.
Pulse Deep and Weak.

Acupuncture

LU-7 Lieque on the right and KI-6 Zhaohai on the right, Ren-4 Guanyuan, KI-13 Qixue, BL-23 Shenshu, extra point Zigong. Moxa must be used.

Prescription

Ai Fu Nuan Gong Wan *Artemisia-Cyperus Warming the Uterus Pill*
Wen Jing Tang *Warming the Menses Decoction*
Nei Bu Wan *Inner Tonification Pill*
Sheng Hua Tang *Generating and Resolving Decoction*
Shou Jiao Ai Tang *Longevity Colla Corii Asini-Artemisia Decoction*

Dampness and Phlegm in the Uterus
Clinical manifestations
Gynaecological manifestations

Delayed cycle, amenorrhoea, scanty or heavy periods, excessive vaginal discharge, infertility, ovarian cysts, myomas, polycystic ovary syndrome, phantom pregnancy.

Other manifestations

Abdominal pain, a feeling of heaviness in the abdomen, a feeling of oppression of the chest, sputum in the throat, a feeling of heaviness of the body, weariness, loose stools, dull-pale complexion, overweight.
Tongue Swollen with a sticky coating.
Pulse Slippery.

Acupuncture

LU-7 Lieque on the right and KI-6 Zhaihai on the left, Ren-3 Zhongji, ST-28 Shuidao, extra point Zigong, Ren-9 Shuifen, SP-9 Yinlingquan, SP-6 Sanyinjiao, BL-22 Sanjiaoshu.

Prescription

Cang Fu Dao Tan Wan *Atractylodes-Cyperus Conducting Phlegm Pill*
Wei Ling Tang *Stomach 'Ling' Decoction*
Wan Dai Tang *Ending Vaginal Discharge Decoction*
Qi Gong Wan *Arousing the Uterus Pill*
Tiao Zheng San *Regulating the Upright Powder*.

Stagnant Cold in the Uterus
Clinical manifestations
Gynaecological manifestations

Delayed cycle, painful periods with severe cramps, dark menstrual blood with clots, brown spotting before the period, periods stopping and starting, abdominal pain after childbirth, retention of lochia after childbirth, white vaginal discharge, a feeling of cold in the vagina, infertility.

Other manifestations

Abdominal pain that is aggravated by pressure and alleviated by the application of heat, a feeling of cold in the abdomen, a general feeling cold, cold limbs, purple lips.
Tongue Bluish-Purple and wet.
Pulse Deep-Wiry-Slow or Deep-Choppy-Slow.

Acupuncture

LU-7 Lieque on the right and KI-6 Zhaohai on the left if the pulse is Choppy, or SP-4 Gongsun on the right and P-6 Neiguan on the left if the pulse is Wiry, KI-14 Siman, ST-29 Guilai, Ren-6 Qihai, SP-10 Xuehai, ST-36 Zusanli, SP-6 Sanyinjiao, LIV-3 Taichong. Moxa should be used.

Prescription

Wen Jing Tang *Warming the Menses Decoction*
Shao Fu Zhu Yu Tang *Lower Abdomen Eliminating Stasis Decoction*
Sheng Hua Tang *Generating and Resolving Decoction*
Ai Fu Nuan Gong Wan *Artemisia-Cyperus Warming the Uterus Pill*
Hei Shen San *Black [Bean] Spirit Powder*.

Fetus Heat
Clinical manifestations
Gynaecological manifestations

Vaginal bleeding during pregnancy, threatened miscarriage, mental restlessness during pregnancy, a history of miscarriages.

Other manifestations

Red face, a feeling of heat, thirst, abdominal pain, insomnia, mental restlessness, mouth ulcers.
Tongue Red with yellow coating.
Pulse Rapid and Overflowing.

Acupuncture

LI-11 Quchi, SP-10 Xuehai, KI-2 Rangu, LIV-2 Xingjian, P-7 Daling, P-3 Quze.

Prescription

Bao Yin Jian *Protecting Yin Decoction*
Gu Tai Jian *Consolidating the Fetus Decoction*
Qing Hai Wan *Clearing the Sea Pill*
Qing Re An Tai Yin *Clearing Heat and Calming the Fetus Decoction*.

Fetus Cold
Clinical manifestations
Gynaecological manifestations

Threatened miscarriage, fetus not growing, miscarriage, a history of miscarriages.

Other manifestations

A feeling of cold, cold limbs, sour regurgitation, nausea, vomiting, abdominal pain, loose stools.
Tongue Pale.
Pulse Deep and Slow.

Acupuncture

ST-36 Zusanli, BL-23 Shenshu, KI-9 Zhubin. Moxa must be used.

Prescription

Li Yin Jian *Regulating Yin Decoction*
Chang Tai Bai Zhu San *Long [Life] Fetus Atractylodes Powder*
Bu Shen Gu Chong Wan *Tonifying the Kidneys and Consolidating the Penetrating Vessel Pill*
Bu Shen An Tai Yin *Tonifying the Kidneys and Calming the Fetus Decoction*.

Blood rebelling upwards after childbirth
Clinical manifestations
Gynaecological manifestations

Retention of lochia or scanty lochia after childbirth.

Other manifestations

Mental restlessness, manic behaviour, nosebleed, vomiting of blood, red face, coughing of blood, abdominal pain, dark complexion, stiff joints, clenched teeth.
Tongue Purple.
Pulse Wiry.

Acupuncture

SP-4 Gongsun on the right and P-6 Neiguan on the left, KI-14 Siman, SP-10 Xuehai, ST-29 Guilai, LIV-3 Taichong, SP-6 Sanyinjiao, Ren-3 Zhongji, LIV-1 Dadun, SP-1 Yinbai, P-7 Daling.

Prescription

Duo Ming San *Seizing Life Powder*
Sheng Hua Tang *Generating and Resolving Decoction*
Wu Zhi San *Five Citrus Powder*
Di Sheng Tang *Supporting the Sage Decoction*
Fo Shou San *Buddha's Hand Powder*.

GIRDLE VESSEL (DAI MAI)

Clinical manifestations

A feeling of cold and pain of the middle and lower back, mid-back pain radiating to the abdomen, abdominal pain radiating to the middle of the back, flaccidity and weakness of the lower back, abdominal distension, chronic vaginal discharge, prolapse of the uterus, weakness and atrophy of the lower limbs, miscarriage, cold feet, amenorrhoea, irregular periods, a feeling of cold in the genital area, infertility, nocturnal emissions, umbilical pain, painful periods (from Dampness), a feeling of fullness of the abdomen, a feeling of the

back as if sitting in water, a feeling of heaviness of the body, a feeling of heaviness of the abdomen as if wearing a belt 'carrying 5000 coins', hernia.

Pulse   Wiry on both Middle positions.

Acupuncture

GB-41 Zulinqi and TB-5 Waiguan.

Herbs
Astringent herbs which infuse to the Lower Burner

Wu Wei Zi *Fructus Schisandrae chinensis*
Shan Yao *Radix Dioscoreae oppositae*
Qian Shi *Semen Euryales ferocis*
Fu Pen Zi *Fructus Rubi*
Sang Piao Xiao *Ootheca mantidis.*

Herbs which consolidate the Uterus and lift Qi

Dang Gui *Radix Angelicae sinensis*
Bai Shao *Radix Paeoniae albae*
Xu Duan *Radix Dipsaci*
Long Gu *Os Draconis*
Ai Ye *Folium Artemisiae*
Sheng Ma *Rhizoma Camicifugae*
Gan Cao *Radix Glycyrrhizae uralensis.*

Prescription

Gan Jiang Ling Zhu Tang *Glycyrrhiza-Zingiberis-Poria-Atractylodes Decoction*
Dan Gui Shao Yao San *Angelica-Paeonia Powder*
Liang Shou Tang *Two Receiving Decoction*
Variation of Bu Zhong Yi Qi Tang *Tonifying the Centre and Benefiting Qi Decoction* plus Ba Ji Tian *Radix Morindae officinalis*, Du Zhong *Cortex Eucommiae ulmoidis*, Gou Ji *Rhizoma Cibotii Barometz*, Xu Duan *Radix Dipsaci Asperi*, Wu Wei Zi *Fructus Schisandrae chinensis*
Shou Tai Wan *Fetus Longevity Pill.*

YIN HEEL VESSEL (YIN QIAO MAI)

Clinical manifestations

Sleepiness, epilepsy (seizures at night), pain in the back and hip radiating to the groin and genitals, hypogastric pain, tremors of the legs, foot turning inwards, abdominal pain, tightness of the muscles of the inner aspect of the leg and flaccidity of those of the outer aspect,

abdominal masses, myomas, difficult delivery, retention of placenta.

Pulse   Wiry on both Rear positions.

Acupuncture

KI-6 Zhaohai and LU-7 Lieque.

Herbs

Yan Hu Suo *Rhizoma Corydalis yanhusuo*
Gua Lou *Fructus Trichosanthis*
Ban Xia *Rhizoma Pinelliae ternatae*
Dan Nan Xing *Rhizoma Arisaematis praeparata*
Zhi Mu *Radix Anemarrhenae asphodeloidis*
Huang Bo *Cortex Phellodendri*
Yuan Zhi *Radix Polygalea tenufoliae*
Suan Zao Ren *Semen Ziziphi spinosae*
Shi Chang Pu *Rhizoma Acori graminea.*

Prescription

Si Wu Tang *Four Substances Decoction*
Ban Xia Tang *Pinellia Decoction*

YANG HEEL VESSEL (YANG QIAO MAI)

Clinical manifestations

Insomnia, epilepsy (seizures during the day), pain and redness of the inner corner of the eye, backache, sciatica with pain along the lateral aspect of the leg, tremor of the legs, foot turning outwards, tightness of the muscles of the outer aspect of the leg and flaccidity of those of the inner aspect, Wind-stroke, hemiplegia, aphasia, facial paralysis, severe dizziness, chills and fever, headache, stiff neck, manic behaviour, manic depression, fright, 'seeing ghosts', inability to raise the leg when lying down.

Pulse   Wiry on both Front positions.

Acupuncture

BL-62 Shenmai and SI-3 Houxi.

Herbs

Ma Huang *Herba Ephedrae*
Fang Feng *Radix Ledebouriellae sesloidis*
Cang Zhu *Rhizoma Atractylodis lanceae*
Zhi Gan Cao *Radix Glycyrrhizae uralensis praeparata*
Fang Ji *Radix Stephaniae tetrandae.*

Prescription

Sheng Yang Tang *Raising the Yang Decoction.*

YIN LINKING VESSEL (YIN WEI MAI)

Clinical manifestations

Pain in the heart region, fullness and pain of the chest and hypochondrium, pain in the kidney region, dryness of the throat, anxiety, insomnia, pensiveness, obsessive thoughts, lack of will-power, loss of self-control, depression, sadness, a feeling of a knot in the chest which feels tight and full on palpation, melancholy, crying, forgetfulness, mental cloudiness, palpitations, shock.

Pulse   Wiry on the lateral side of the Rear position extending towards the medial side of the front position (Fig. 110.1).

Acupuncture

P-6 Neiguan and SP-4 Gongsun.

Herbs

Dang Gui *Radix Angelicae sinensis*
Chuan Xiong *Radix Ligustici Chuanxiong*.

Prescription

Dang Gui Si Ni Tang *Angelica Four Rebellious Decoction*
Wu Zhu Yu Tang *Evodia Decoction*
Si Ni Tang *Four Rebellious Decoction*
Li Zhong Tang *Regulating the Centre Decoction*.

YANG LINKING VESSEL (YANG WEI MAI)

Clinical manifestations

Alternations of chills and fevers, weakness of the limbs, dizziness on eye movement, earache, stiff neck, hypochondrial pain, pain in the lateral side of the leg, tinnitus, deafness, sweating.

Pulse   Wiry on the medial side of the Rear position extending towards the lateral side of the Front position (Fig. 110.1).

Acupuncture

TB-5 Waiguan and GB-41 Zulinqi.

Herbs

Gui Zhi *Ramulus Cinnamomi cassiae*
Bai Shao *Radix Paeoniae lactiflorae*
Huang Qi *Radix Astragali membranacei*.

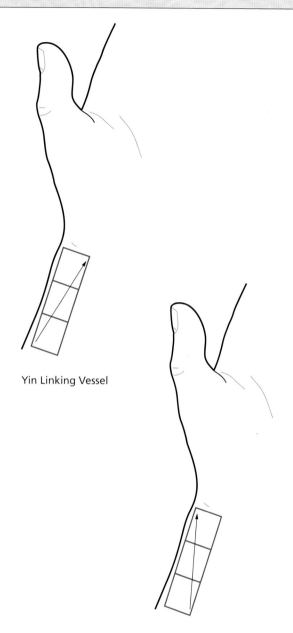

Yin Linking Vessel

Yang Linking Vessel

Fig. 110.1 Yin and Yang Linking Vessels pulses

Prescription

Dang Gui Gui Zhi Tang *Angelica-Ramulus-Cinnamomi Decoction*.

NOTES

1. Wang Luo Zhen 1985 A Compilation of the 'Study of the Eight Extraordinary Vessels' (*Qi Jing Ba Mai Kao Jiao Zhu*

奇经八脉考校注), Shanghai Science Publishing House, Shanghai. The 'Study of the Eight Extraordinary Vessels' (*Qi Jing Ba Mai Kao* 奇经八脉考) by Li Shi Zhen was published in 1578.

2. Cheng Shao En 1994 Diagnosis, Patterns and Treatment in Chinese Medicine (*Zhong Yi Zheng Hou Zhen Duan Zhi Liao Xue*), Beijing Science Publishing House, Beijing, pp. 241–278.

3. The Materia Medica of Proper Combinations (*De Pei Ben Cao*) reported in Wang Luo Zhen 1985 A Compilation of the 'Study of the Eight Extraordinary Vessels' (*Qi Jing Ba Mai Kao Jiao Zh*), Shanghai Science Publishing House, Shanghai pp. 129–131. The 'Study of the Eight Extraordinary Vessels' (*Qi Jing Ba Mai Kao*) by Li Shi Zhen was published in 1578.

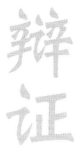

Chapter **111**

IDENTIFICATION OF PATTERNS ACCORDING TO THE FIVE ELEMENTS

Chapter contents

INTRODUCTION *1007*

GENERATING SEQUENCE PATTERNS *1007*
 Wood not generating Fire *1007*
 Fire not generating Earth *1008*
 Earth not generating Metal *1008*
 Metal not generating Water *1008*
 Water not generating Wood *1008*

OVERACTING SEQUENCE PATTERNS *1008*
 Wood overacting on Earth *1008*
 Earth overacting on Water *1008*
 Water overacting on Fire *1008*
 Fire overacting on Metal *1008*
 Metal overacting on Wood *1008*

INSULTING SEQUENCE PATTERNS *1009*
 Wood insulting Metal *1009*
 Metal insulting Fire *1009*
 Fire insulting Water *1009*
 Water insulting Earth *1009*
 Earth insulting Wood *1009*

INTRODUCTION

The identification of patterns according to the Five Elements is based on the pathological changes occurring in dysfunctions of the Generating, Overacting and Insulting sequences of the Five Elements.

These patterns are not of primary importance in practice as most of them describe clinical conditions which are better expressed by the Internal Organ patterns. In certain cases, however, some Five-Element patterns can describe conditions which fall outside the scope of the Internal Organ patterns. An example of this is the pattern of deficient Qi of Wood (manifesting with timidity and indecision), which is not included among the Internal Organ patterns.

We can distinguish the Five-Element patterns according to the Generating, Overacting and Insulting sequences.

GENERATING SEQUENCE PATTERNS

These patterns describe conditions of deficiency of each organ when this is induced by its Mother Element.

Wood not generating Fire

This pattern is sometimes also described as a pattern of deficient Gall-Bladder. It is an unusual pattern in so far as, according to the theory of the Internal Organs, Liver-Qi or the Gall-Bladder can hardly ever be deficient. This pattern describes such a situation. More than a pattern, it really describes a certain character and personality, and its salient feature

is the lack of courage and timidity. It corresponds to the Internal Organ pattern of deficient Gall-Bladder. It is also associated with Liver-Qi deficiency.

Clinical manifestations

Timidity, a lack of courage, indecision, palpitations and insomnia (in particular, waking up in the early hours of the morning).

Fire not generating Earth

This pattern basically describes a condition of Spleen-Yang deficiency due to failure of Fire in providing Heat to the Spleen to transform and transport. According to the theory of the Internal Organs, however, the Spleen derives the warmth necessary to its functions not from the Heart, but from Kidney-Yang.

Clinical manifestations

Loose stools, chilliness and weakness of the limbs.

Earth not generating Metal

This pattern describes the situation when a Spleen deficiency (causing the tiredness) leads to the formation of Phlegm, which obstructs the Lungs.

Clinical manifestations

Phlegm in the chest, cough and tiredness.

Metal not generating Water

This pattern corresponds to the Internal Organ pattern of Kidneys not receiving Qi.

Clinical manifestations

Cough, breathlessness, loss of voice and asthma.

Water not generating Wood

This pattern is the same as the Internal Organ pattern of Kidney and Liver Yin deficiency.

Clinical manifestations

Dizziness, blurred vision, headaches and vertigo.

OVERACTING SEQUENCE PATTERNS

Wood overacting on Earth

The pattern of Wood overacting on Earth is very common and it is exactly the same as the pattern of Liver invading the Spleen or Stomach.

Clinical manifestations

Hypochondrial and epigastric pain, a feeling of distension, irritability, loose stools, poor appetite and a greenish face.

When the clinical manifestations pertain to one Element and the face colour pertains to the Element which overacts on it, the face colour usually shows the origin of the disharmony. In this case, loose stools and poor appetite are symptoms of deficiency of Earth (Spleen) but the face is greenish: this indicates that the root of the problem is in Wood, that is, Wood overacting on Earth. The same principle applies to all the following cases of disharmony of the Overacting sequence.

Earth overacting on Water

This pattern occurs when a deficient Spleen fails to transform and transport fluids, which accumulate and obstruct the Kidney's function of transformation and excretion of fluids.

Clinical manifestations

Oedema, difficult urination and a yellow face.

Water overacting on Fire

There is no such pattern as the Kidneys cannot be in Excess.

Fire overacting on Metal

This pattern corresponds to Full-Heat in the Lungs.

Clinical manifestations

Cough with profuse yellow sputum, a feeling of heat and a red face.

Metal overacting on Wood
Clinical manifestations

Tiredness, irritability, a feeling of distension and a white face.

INSULTING SEQUENCE PATTERNS

Wood insulting Metal

The Liver channel influences the chest and stagnant Liver-Qi or Liver-Fire can obstruct the chest and prevent Lung-Qi from descending.

Clinical manifestations

Cough, asthma and a feeling of distension of chest and hypochondrium.

Metal insulting Fire

This pattern basically describes a condition of both Lung- and Heart-Qi deficiency.

Clinical manifestations

Palpitations, insomnia and breathlessness.

Fire insulting Water

This pattern is identical to the Internal Organ pattern of 'Kidney and Heart not harmonized', that is, Kidney-Yin deficiency giving rise to Heart Empty-Heat.

Clinical manifestations

Malar flush, dry mouth at night, insomnia, dizziness, lower backache and night sweating.

Water insulting Earth

This pattern corresponds to Spleen- and Kidney-Yang deficiency.

Clinical manifestations

Loose stools, oedema, tiredness and weakness of the limbs.

Earth insulting Wood

This pattern is caused by a failure of the Spleen in transforming fluids leading to Dampness. Dampness accumulates and obstructs the smooth flow of Liver-Qi, impeding the free flow of bile.

Clinical manifestations

Jaundice, hypochondrial pain and distension.

APPENDICES

Contents

Appendix 1 Case histories *1013*
Appendix 2 Prescriptions *1025*
Appendix 3 History of diagnosis in Chinese medicine *1051*

Appendix 1

CASE HISTORIES

There are two types of case histories in this appendix: the first group includes case histories written in a very detailed way to show the thinking process behind the interrogation of the patient and how the interrogation is integrated with observation.

The second group of case histories is used to illustrate important guidelines in diagnosis and treatment principle.

GROUP 1

Case history 1

A 41-year-old woman had been trying to conceive unsuccessfully for 1 year.

Observation: As the patient is talking, observation of her complexion and eyes is the first diagnostic clue. Her complexion is dull-pale tending to yellow, slightly without lustre and with several skin spots (pale papules). Her eyes do have lustre and her hair has a good sheen.

Deduction: The yellow colour and consistency of the complexion indicate the presence of Dampness and its dullness indicates that it occurs against a background of Spleen deficiency.

Listening: Her voice is fairly strong although it sounds slightly sad.

Deduction: The strength of her voice indicates that Lung-Qi is good and that, if there is a Qi deficiency, it does not involve the Lungs and it is therefore not too severe. However, the slightly sad tone of her voice indicates a Lung pattern due to sadness; the fact that the voice is strong indicates that, whatever the emotional problem, it is of short duration. In fact, she confirmed that she had moved to London recently from the United States and that she had been under some stress in trying to adapt to a new job and a new lifestyle.

Question: 'Have you ever been pregnant?' [Since the patient is complaining of infertility, it is important to ask whether she has ever been pregnant: if she has never been pregnant, which is called *primary infertility*, this suggests a deeper disharmony than that of a woman who cannot conceive again after having had one child.]

Answer: 'I was pregnant once 18 years ago but I had a termination and have used contraception from that time until 1 year ago.'

Question: 'Do your periods come regularly?' [At this point, it is crucial to ask about her menstrual cycle, i.e. the regularity of it, the amount of bleeding, the colour of the menstrual blood, pain and any premenstrual symptoms. These questions are important to get a preliminary idea of the main patterns involved.]

Answer: 'The periods are regular, coming every 28–30 days.'

Question: 'How many days do they last?'

Answer: '4 to 5 days.'

Question: 'Are they particularly heavy?'

Answer: 'No, they are not too heavy.'

Question: 'What colour is the blood?'

Answer: 'Dark red.'

Deduction: The regularity of the menstrual cycle, the duration of the period itself and the colour of the

menstrual blood are all normal and do not point to any pattern yet.

Question: 'Do you have any premenstrual problems?'

Answer: 'No, not really.'

Question: 'Do you suffer from lower backache?' [I now begin to ask a series of questions to establish whether there is a Kidney deficiency as this is the most common cause of infertility.]

Answer: 'Only occasionally.'

Question: 'Do you experience dizziness sometimes?'

Answer: 'No.'

Question: 'Do you experience ringing in the ears?'

Answer: 'No.'

Question: 'Do you experience night sweating?'

Answer: 'Only occasionally but it might be due to the fact that we have a very heavy duvet.'[Although she suffers from occasional backache and night sweating, which may be due to the bedding, there is not much evidence of a Kidney deficiency.]

Question: 'Do you suffer from blurred vision?' [I now begin to ask a series of questions to establish whether there is a Blood deficiency, another common Deficiency pattern in infertility.]

Answer: 'Occasionally.'

Question: 'Do you suffer from floaters?'

Answer: 'Occasionally.'

Question: 'Do you suffer from tingling in the limbs?'

Answer: 'No.'

Question: 'How is your sleep?'

Answer: 'It is disturbed but it may be due to the heavy traffic.'

Deduction: There are a few symptoms of Liver-Blood deficiency, i.e. the occasional blurred vision and floaters.

Question: 'Do you suffer from palpitations?' [Whenever a woman suffers from a pattern of Liver-Blood deficiency, I always ask questions to establish whether this has given rise to Heart-Blood deficiency as well.]

Answer: 'Yes, occasionally.'

Deduction: This confirms that there is some Heart-Blood deficiency as well.

Question: 'Do you suffer from any digestive problems, for example, pain, fullness or bloating after eating?' [Having observed that her face indicates Dampness against a background of Spleen deficiency, I ask about digestive symptoms to exclude or confirm this. However, it is always necessary to ask about any digestive symptoms to establish the state of the Stomach and Spleen, whatever the patient's main complaint.]

Answer: 'No, I have no digestive problems. My appetite is good and my digestion is good.'

Question: 'Do you have a bowel movement every day?'

Answer: 'Yes.'

Deduction: This answer contradicts what was found from observation, that is, Dampness with Spleen deficiency. However, this is not at all unusual because Dampness may settle in various parts of the body and sometimes not involve digestion itself.

Question: 'Do you have any other problems?'

Answer: 'No.'

Question: 'Are you on any medication?' [One should never forget to ask about medication because their side-effects can account for some of the presenting symptoms and signs.]

Answer: 'No.'

Observation: At this point I usually look at the tongue before taking the pulse. The tongue is Red on the sides, slightly Swollen and with a sticky yellow coating.

Deduction: The tongue appearance confirms the presence of Dampness but it adds a new dimension to the diagnosis in so far as, first of all, it does not show any deficiency and, secondly, it indicates the clear presence of Heat, which was not obvious from any of the symptoms. The tongue shows the presence of Damp-Heat in the Stomach and Spleen.

Question: 'Are you sometimes thirsty?' [I now begin to ask questions to confirm or exclude the presence of Damp-Heat in the digestive system.]

Answer: 'Yes.'

Question: 'Do you sometimes experience a strange taste in your mouth such as a sticky taste?'

Answer: 'Yes.'

Question: 'Do you experience a feeling of heaviness or bearing down in your abdomen?' [As the tongue indicates Damp-Heat, I now go back to asking more questions about the gynaecological system.]

Answer: 'Yes, sometimes during the period.'

Question: 'Do you sometimes suffer from mid-cycle pain?'

Answer: 'Yes, occasionally.'

Deduction: The sticky taste and thirst confirm the presence of Damp-Heat in the Middle Burner, while the mid-cycle pain and the bearing-down sensation indicate the presence of Damp-Heat in the Lower Burner also.

Palpation: The pulse shows no pronounced Deficiency as it is relatively normal in strength and only very slightly Slippery, confirming the presence of Dampness. The Kidney positions on the pulse are not Weak and this confirms that there is no pronounced Kidney deficiency.

Conclusion: Although the symptoms of blurred vision, occasional floaters and palpitations indicate a Liver- and Heart-Blood deficiency, this cannot be very pronounced as it is not confirmed by other symptoms or by the pulse. The prevailing pattern is that of Damp-Heat in the Middle and Lower Burners and presumably this is the cause of the infertility as Dampness may obstruct the Uterus preventing implantation of the egg. Although the Dampness was apparent from the observation of the patient's complexion, it was only observation of the tongue which changed the whole diagnosis in two ways. First, the tongue clearly indicated that Dampness was a predominant pathogenic factor and the overall condition was dominated by Excess rather than Deficiency; secondly, the tongue clearly indicated the presence of Heat, which, although not initially apparent on interrogation, was confirmed by the presence of thirst.

The main implication of this case history is that often observation of the tongue changes the diagnosis entirely and leads us to ask further questions which we may have omitted asking. The second important implication of this case history is that one should always keep an open mind during the diagnostic process and never have preconceived ideas about the causes of a condition and therefore jump to conclusions. In this case, for example, had I not looked at the tongue or misinterpreted it, it would have been easy to jump to the conclusion that the main cause of this patient's infertility lies in Liver-Blood deficiency.

Case history 2

A 40-year-old woman had been trying to conceive unsuccessfully for 18 months.

Observation: Her complexion was very slightly red on her cheeks and her eyes lacked lustre but to a very slight degree.

Listening: Her voice was strong and clear.

Question: 'Do your periods come regularly?' [At this point, it is crucial to ask about her menstrual cycle, i.e. the regularity of it, the amount of bleeding, the colour of the menstrual blood, pain and any premenstrual symptoms. These questions are important to get a preliminary idea of the main patterns involved.]

Answer: 'They come every 25 to 26 days.'

Deduction: From a Chinese perspective, this would be considered as a rather short cycle, the main causes of which can be Qi deficiency or Blood-Heat.

Question: 'How many days does your period last?'

Answer: '3 days.'

Question: 'Would you say it is rather scanty?'

Answer: 'Yes, it is quite.'

Deduction: The scanty and short period seems to indicate Blood deficiency. As the period also comes early, which may be due to Qi deficiency, this would indicate a deficiency of Qi and Blood (unless of course the short cycle is due to Blood-Heat).

Question: 'What colour is the blood?'

Answer: 'Bright red.'

Question: 'Is it painful?'

Answer: 'Yes, it was but it was greatly improved by acupuncture treatment.'

Question: 'Do you suffer from any premenstrual symptoms?'

Answer: 'I did suffer from premenstrual breast distension but that also was greatly improved by acupuncture treatment.'

Deduction: The period pain and the premenstrual breast distension seem to indicate Liver-Qi stagnation.

Question: 'Do you suffer from blurred vision or floaters?' [I now begin to ask questions to confirm or exclude the presence of Blood deficiency indicated by the short and scanty periods.]

Answer: 'No.'

Question: 'Do you suffer from dizziness?'

Answer: 'No.'

Question:: 'Do you experience tingling in your limbs sometimes?'

Answer: 'No.'

Question:: 'Do you sleep well?'

Answer: 'Yes.'

Deduction: Apart from the short and scanty periods, none of the other symptoms and signs confirm the presence of Liver-Blood deficiency.

Question: 'Do you suffer from lower backache?'

Answer: 'No.'

Question: 'Do you ever have a ringing sound in your ears?'

Answer: 'No.'

Question: 'Do your knees ever feel weak?'

Answer: 'No.'

Question: 'Do you ever suffer from night sweating?'

Answer: 'No.'

Deduction: The absence of any of these symptoms excludes the presence of a Kidney deficiency.

Question: 'Do you suffer from any digestive symptoms such as pain, fullness or bloating after eating?'

[It is always necessary to ask this question to establish the state of the Stomach and Spleen.]

Answer: 'No, none at all.'

Question: 'Do you have a bowel movement every day?'

Answer: 'I did suffer from some constipation but this was also greatly improved by acupuncture treatment.'

Deduction: The constipation could confirm either the Blood deficiency or the Liver-Qi stagnation.

Observation: At this point, I usually look at the tongue and this revealed entirely new patterns which were not obvious from interrogation. In fact, the tongue was quite Red on the sides, had a very Red tip with red points, it was Swollen and had a sticky yellow coating.

Deduction: The tongue clearly indicates the presence of Phlegm (because it is Swollen and has a sticky coating) and of Heat (because it is Red on the sides and tip). This is Phlegm-Heat affecting the Heart, which we can deduce from the very Red tip with red points. To confirm or exclude this pattern, one needs to ask questions regarding a possible affliction of the Mind by Phlegm.

Question: 'Do you suffer from anxiety or have you suffered from emotional problems in the recent or distant past?' [The slight dullness of her eyes would seem to confirm the affliction of the Heart by Phlegm, which was apparent from the tongue.]

Answer: 'I do not suffer from anxiety but I do suffer from severe mood swings.'

Deduction: The presence of severe mood swings, combined with the tongue appearance, confirms the affliction of the Heart by Phlegm-Heat.

Palpation: The pulse is Slippery on the whole and slightly Overflowing on the left Front position.

Deduction: The Slippery pulse quality confirms the presence of Phlegm, while the Overflowing quality on the Heart position confirms that the Phlegm is located in the Heart and that the Mind and Spirit are slightly disturbed.

Conclusion: The main presenting pattern is Phlegm-Heat in the Heart. Although the patient suffers from infertility, there is no Kidney deficiency, no Blood

deficiency and no evidence of Dampness or Phlegm obstructing the Lower Burner. How does Phlegm-Heat in the Heart affect fertility? The monthly menstrual cycle is like a tide determined by the ebb and flow and the mutual generation and consumption of Yin and Yang. Kidney-Yin and Kidney-Yang are the source of this Yin and Yang fluctuation in the monthly menstrual cycle. Ovulation represents a transformation of Yin to Yang, while menstruation represents a transformation of Yang to Yin; although the Kidney-Yin and Kidney-Yang are the source of the Yin and Yang in the menstrual cycle, the Heart is the agent of transformation of one into another. In particular, Heart-Qi descends and communicates with the Kidneys to control the discharge of eggs at ovulation and of menstrual blood at menstruation.

This downward movement of the Heart in ovulation and menstruation is another expression of the harmonious communication between Heart and Kidneys and Fire and Water. Heart-Fire (the physiological Emperor Fire) needs to go down to the Kidneys, while Kidney-Water needs to go up to the Heart.

When Phlegm obstructs the Heart, it prevents its Qi from descending to the Kidneys; pathological Fire affecting the Heart goes up (in contrast to the physiological Emperor Fire, which goes down to the Kidneys) and therefore the Heart cannot effect the transformation of Yin to Yang and vice versa, nor the proper discharge of eggs at ovulation; this may therefore cause infertility.

Case history 3

A 50-year-old woman had been suffering from a blocked nose, sneezing and intermittent wheezing. She took Beconase, which helped to relieve her symptoms.

Observation: She had a dull-pale complexion and her head shook when she spoke.

Listening: Her voice was very loud, almost shouting.

Deduction: A dull-pale complexion points towards a Blood deficiency. A shaking head points towards an Excess pattern of the Liver, probably Liver-Wind. The loud voice generally indicates an Excess pattern or, in health, good Lung-Qi. However, her voice had quite a high pitch with a trembling quality to it; this tends to indicate nervous tension.

Question: 'When did the problem start?'

Answer: 'My nose has been blocked for the past 3 or 4 years. Before that I had about two asthma attacks when I was about 40.'

Question: 'Did these symptoms start after childbirth?' [I asked this question as childbirth may weaken a woman's Kidney energy and they may consequently develop symptoms they have not suffered from before. In this case, it was important to determine whether childbirth had weakened the Kidney Defensive-Qi system.]

Listening: 'No, I had my last child when I was 30.'

Deduction: The patient's symptoms are not due to a weakening of the Kidney Defensive-Qi system during childbirth as they started 10 years after her last child was born.

Question: 'And did you have any allergies or asthma when you were a child?' [This question is asked to determine whether the patient has an atopic constitution and the asthma is of the allergic type or not.]

Answer: 'No, none at all.'

Deduction: The patient does not have a constitutional Kidney and Lung deficiency, which can be a cause of asthma and allergies.

Question: 'Is there a lot of white discharge when you sneeze?' [This question is important to differentiate allergic rhinitis, which is characterized by a white watery nasal discharge, from sinusitis, which is characterized by a thick yellow nasal discharge.]

Answer: 'No, there is not much discharge at all.'

Question: 'Do you sneeze all year around or just in the spring and summer?'

Answer: 'It first started in the spring but it continues all year round.'

Question: 'Are you allergic to cats and dogs?'

Answer: 'No, I am not.'

Deduction: Considering the absence of a history of childhood asthma and eczema, the absence of a

white watery nasal discharge, the absence of reaction to dogs and cats' allergens seem to indicate that this patient's rhinitis is not allergic.

Question: 'You said that apart from this you had another complaint?'

Answer: 'Yes, I have dryness and flaking around my mouth.'

Question: 'Is it all around your mouth or just on the top or the bottom?' [This is asked to determine whether the Directing Vessel is involved, which affects the area all around the mouth, or whether the Stomach and Large Intestine are involved, which affect the skin just above the mouth.]

Answer: 'It is mainly on the top and sides but a little bit on the bottom.'

Deduction: Even though the dry and flaky skin is mainly above the mouth, the fact that the areas below and to the sides of the mouth are also affected indicates a pathology of the Directing Vessel.

Question: 'Is there redness as well as dryness and flaking?' [This is asked to determine whether Heat is involved in the pathology of the symptom or whether it is caused by a deficiency of Blood and/or Yin.]

Answer: 'Yes, there is.'

Deduction: The fact that there is redness indicates that Heat (which may be Full or Empty) is present.

Question: 'How long have you had this problem?'

Answer: 'About 5 or 6 years.'

Question: 'How are your periods?' [At this point, it is crucial to ask about her menstrual cycle, i.e. the regularity of it, the amount of bleeding, the colour of the menstrual blood, pain and any premenstrual symptoms. In women these questions are crucial because the state of the gynaecological system can cause not only gynaecological problems but also other general problems. For example, in this case, the dryness, redness and flaking around the mouth may reflect a pathology of the Directing Vessel.]

Answer: 'They are regular.'

Question: 'How long do they last?'

Answer: 'About 5 or 6 days.'

Question: 'Are they particularly light or heavy?'

Answer: 'They are heavier than they used to be.'

Question: 'And are they painful?'

Answer: 'No, but they are a little uncomfortable. I get a bit of backache beforehand.'

Question: 'What colour is the blood?'

Answer: 'It is dark and there are sometimes clots.'

Question: 'Do you get any premenstrual problems?'

Answer: 'No.'

Question: 'And what about contraception? Are you on the pill or do you use the coil?' [It is important to ask about contraception as this can affect the nature of the menstrual cycle.]

Answer: 'No, I don't.'

Deduction: Her menstrual cycle is broadly normal. The periods have been heavier recently but that happens frequently in the perimenopausal years; the darkness of the blood and the clots indicates some Blood stasis but this cannot be very severe as the periods are not painful. Observation of the tongue later should confirm whether the Blood stasis is significant or not.

Question: 'Do you suffer from dizziness?' [I now begin to ask questions in order to determine whether there is any deficiency of the Kidneys involved.]

Answer: 'No.'

Question: 'Do you get any ringing in your ears?'

Answer: 'No.'

Question: 'Do you have any problems with urination?'

Answer: 'I have to go more often than I used to. I have to go at night most nights.'

Deduction: The answer to the last question implies that a Kidney deficiency may be involved as the patient's urination has become more frequent and she regularly needs to urinate at night.

Question: 'Do you feel particularly hot or cold?' [In women, Kidney-Yin and Kidney-Yang deficiency normally coexist but it is important to establish which is predominant.]

Answer: 'I feel cold at night.'

Question: 'So you never have any night sweating?'

Answer: 'No, never.'

Deduction: This points towards the fact that Kidney-Yang deficiency is predominant.

Question: 'How is your digestion?' [It is always necessary to ask this question to establish the state of the Stomach and Spleen.]

Answer: 'I don't have any problems with it.'

Question: 'You do not get any bloating after meals?'

Answer: 'No.'

Question: 'Do you have a bowel movement every day?'

Answer: 'Normally, yes.'

Question: 'And is your appetite good?'

Answer: 'Yes, I think it is quite normal.'

Deduction: There is no significant Spleen- or Stomach-Qi deficiency.

Question:: 'Do you suffer from headaches?'

Answer: 'No, but I have had sinus problems in the past. I have very blocked sinuses.'

Question: 'When did that start?'

Answer: 'When I was 30 and I was expecting my second child.'

Question: 'And do you normally sneeze more in the mornings?'

Answer: 'Yes, I have done since I was a child.'

Deduction: This contradicts slightly what the patient said earlier, that is, that she did not suffer from any allergies as a child. We must therefore discard our earlier deduction that there is no constitutional deficiency of Defensive-Qi of the Lungs and Kidneys, and conclude that actually there is. However, to complicate matters, her chronic complaint of blocked sinuses seems to point to chronic sinusitis. This is not unusual as allergic rhinitis and sinusitis can occur simultaneously.

Observation: The tongue was Pale, partially peeled and had cracks in the Stomach area.

Deduction: The Pale colour of the tongue indicates either a Qi, Yang or Blood deficiency, while the fact that it is partially peeled and with cracks in the Stomach area points towards an underlying Stomach-Yin deficiency. Most probably, the tongue indicates a simultaneous deficiency of Qi and Yin of the Stomach.

Question: 'Do you have any problems with your eyes?' [I now ask further questions to confirm or eliminate the presence of Blood deficiency.]

Answer:: 'No.'

Question: 'Do you ever feel a tingling sensation in your limbs?'

Answer: 'No, I don't.'

Question: 'Do you sleep well?'

Answer: 'Yes, I do.'

Question: 'Do you ever suffer from palpitations?'

Answer: 'No, never.'

Deduction: There is no apparent Liver- or Heart-Blood deficiency.

Palpation: The pulse is generally Wiry and the right Front position is Full.

Deduction: The overall Wiry pulse confirms what the observation of the patient indicated, that is, that there is a Full Liver pattern. The Full quality of the right Front position in this case probably reflects the congestion in the sinuses and nose, rather than a Lung pattern. It should be remembered that the pulse positions reflect areas of the body as well as the channels and organs; with reference to areas, the Front positions reflect the condition of the head.

Conclusion: The patient is suffering from a mixed condition. The Root (*Ben*) is a deficiency of the Defensive Qi of the Kidneys and Lungs (shown on the tongue which is Pale), as well as Stomach-Yin deficiency (shown by the partially peeled nature of the tongue and the cracks in the Stomach area). A geographic tongue such as this is often linked with an atopic constitution. The Manifestation (*Biao*) is Dampness in the Stomach channel and this is causing the patient's symptom of a blocked nose (shown by the Full quality of the right Front pulse).

The fact that the patient said that she has sneezed every morning since she was a child indicates that she was born with a slight deficiency of the Defensive Qi of the Lungs and Kidneys. The exacerbation of her symptoms over the last few years is probably due to the natural waning of the Kidney energy with age.

The patient also confirmed later that she had had a very stressful time over the last few years. This was reflected in the Wiry nature of her pulse and could also have been a catalyst to the worsening of her symptoms. The Wiry pulse may also reflect the beginning of a condition of Liver-Wind, which is manifested also by the slight shaking of her head. Liver-Wind could have arisen either from the Kidney deficiency or from a Blood deficiency, which is shown by the dull-pale complexion (although she has no other symptoms of it).

GROUP 2

'In confusing and complicated conditions, treat Phlegm'

Case history 4

A 35-year-old man had been suffering from a hot sensation of the palms and soles and ache of fingers and toes for about 6 months; the fingers and toes were not swollen nor hot to the touch. He had no other symptoms apart from annoying phlegm in the throat which he had to clear a few times a day. The tongue was quite normal and the pulse was very slightly Slippery. The hot sensation of palms and soles strongly suggests Yin deficiency, possibly of the Heart and Kidneys or Lung and Kidneys. However, there was no other symptom or sign of Yin deficiency at all and neither the pulse nor the tongue indicates Yin deficiency at all. The ache of the hands and feet could be a form of Painful Obstruction Syndrome (*Bi* syndrome) due to Wind, Cold or Dampness in the joints but the ache did not react to changes in weather, a symptom that is normally present in Painful Obstruction Syndrome. Furthermore, the hot sensation of palms and soles could be due to Heat Painful Obstruction Syndrome, but this was clearly not the case as the joints were not swollen or hot.

Considering that it was difficult to find a proper explanation for this patient's symptoms, I concluded that, according to the principle 'in complicated and difficult-to-explain conditions, treat Phlegm', they were due to Phlegm and the patient's need to clear his throat frequently would support this conclusion.

I therefore set out to resolve Phlegm by using the following points:

- LU-9 Taiyuan to resolve Phlegm from the Lung channel and thus affect his fingers and palms
- Ren-12 Zhongwan, ST-36 Zusanli, ST-40 Fenglong and SP-9 Yinlingquan to resolve Phlegm
- KI-3 Taixi to affect soles and toes.

Use of this combination of points four times at weekly intervals cleared the problem completely.

'Pulse determinant in diagnosis'

Case history 5

A 53-year-old woman had been suffering from hair loss for 6 years after a period of intense stress. At that time, her periods also stopped abruptly. She had no other symptoms apart from tiredness. Her tongue was Pale, slightly Purple on the right side in the breast area, and Swollen. The pulse was clearly Wiry all over.

This is a good example of the determinant importance of pulse diagnosis when there are few symptoms and signs to go by. The pulse should never be dismissed as a factor in diagnosis but even less so when there are few symptoms and signs. Falling hair may be due either to a Deficiency (usually of Liver-Blood or Kidney-Essence) or to an Excess, usually Liver-Wind. When falling hair is due to internal Wind, the hair loss occurs suddenly. The Wiry pulse definitely indicated that the hair loss was not due to a Deficiency but to Liver-Wind; this is also confirmed by the abrupt onset after a period of stress.

'Never ignore the tongue'
Case history 6

A 33-year-old woman had been suffering from otitis media for 18 months: she had a thick, yellow discharge from the ear. She had resorted to antibiotics five times but the middle-ear infection always returned. She had also suffered from asthma for 2 years and allergic rhinitis since she was 21. Her tongue was Red, Peeled in the centre and front, and had a bilateral thin white coating. Her pulse was Weak on the right and slightly Wiry on the left.

The middle-ear infection is clearly due to Damp-Heat in the Gall-Bladder channel: that it is Damp-Heat is clear from the thick, yellow discharge; that it is in the Gall-Bladder channel is clear from the bilateral coating (a sign of Gall-Bladder problems) and the Wiry pulse. However, it would be a mistake to treat her only for Damp-Heat in the Gall-Bladder channel and would be not much better than using antibiotics. In fact, the tongue shows other important patterns that cannot be ignored. The lack of coating in the centre and front indicates Stomach- and Lung-Yin deficiency while the redness of the tongue body (combined with the absence of coating) indicates Empty-Heat in these organs. Although there are no symptoms and signs of Yin deficiency with Empty-Heat of the Stomach and Lungs, the tongue appearance is enough to diagnose this condition. Thus, treatment should be aimed not only at resolving Damp-Heat from the Gall-Bladder channel, but also at nourishing Stomach- and Lung-Yin: nourishing these two organs will tonify the Upright Qi and strengthen the immune system, which should help her to fight off the ear infections.

Indeed, it could be said that the deficiency of the Stomach and Lungs is the reason that the antibiotics did not clear her condition and that it returned each time. Had the tongue shown only the retention of Damp-Heat in the Gall-Bladder with a sticky coating, it could be argued that the ear infection would not have recurred after the course of antibiotics. Thus, this case history is a good example of two principles, that is, that the tongue should never be ignored, and that the tongue may also assist in predicting the possible effect of Western medication. In this case, the deficiency of Stomach- and Lung-Yin indicated by the absence of coating clearly alerts us to a deficiency of the Upright Qi (and the immune system from a Western perspective) and therefore the possibility that the antibiotic treatment might not work.

I therefore treated this patient by simultaneously resolving Damp-Heat from the Gall-Bladder channel and nourishing Stomach- and Lung-Yin with a variation of the formula Xiao Chai Hu Tang *Small Bupleurum Decoction*:

> Chai Hu *Radix Bupleuri* 6 g
> Huang Qin *Radix Scutellariae baicalensis* 6 g
> Ban Xia *Rhizoma Pinelliae ternatae* 6 g
> Dang Shen *Radix Codonopsis pilosulae* 6 g
> Yin Chen Hao *Herba Artemisiae capillaris* 6 g
> Shan Zhi Zi *Fructus Gardeniae jasminoidis* 4 g
> Mai Men Dong *Tuber Ophiopogonis japonici* 6 g
> Tai Zi Shen *Radix Pseudostellariae* 6 g
> Shan Yao *Radix Dioscoreae oppositae* 6 g

With acupuncture, I treated the following points:

> - Ren-12 Zhongwan and SP-9 Yinlingquan to resolve Dampness in general
> - ST-36 Zusanli and SP-6 Sanyinjiao to nourish Stomach- and Lung-Yin
> - TB-5 Waiguan and GB-41 Zulinqi to resolve Damp-Heat from the Gall-Bladder channel.

'In men, the clinical manifestations sometimes mimic Yin deficiency but are not due to Yin deficiency'
Case history 7

A 31-year-old man had been suffering from tiredness, insomnia, expectoration of phlegm, nausea, backache, tinnitus and night sweating. His tongue was slightly Red and Swollen and had teethmarks and his pulse was Weak especially on the left Front position.

The tiredness, backache, tinnitus and night sweating could be easily interpreted as being due to Kidney-Yin deficiency. However, closer examination and questioning revealed that each symptom could be explained differently. The backache was due to excessive lifting, the tinnitus was due to working in a band and listening to very loud music, and the

night sweating was due to Phlegm-Heat. The symptoms of Phlegm-Heat are the expectoration of phlegm, the nausea, the insomnia, the night sweating and the Red-Swollen tongue. Thus, although the manifestations could have easily led us to diagnose Kidney-Yin deficiency, the real problem is Phlegm-Heat. The tongue was important to confirm this diagnosis.

'When the pulse contradicts the other clinical manifestations'

Case history 8

A 37-year-old woman had been suffering from a shortening of her menstrual cycle for the previous 2 years; the period was also becoming scantier in amount. Other symptoms included a gradual loss of hair, the occasional expectoration of phlegm, poor memory, poor concentration, floaters, palpitations, a feeling of cold, backache, tinnitus and night sweating. She had also been diagnosed as having the beginning of osteoporosis and a gynaecological examination revealed that she suffered from the early stages of polycystic ovary syndrome. Her tongue was Pale with a white sticky coating and her pulse was Slippery and Rapid (88 b.p.m.).

Most of her symptoms clearly show a deficiency of Blood (loss of hair, poor memory and concentration, floaters and palpitations) and of Kidney-Yang (feeling cold, backache, tinnitus, night sweating and osteoporosis). Although night sweating is a symptom of Yin deficiency, in women it often also accompanies Kidney-Yang deficiency. There are also a few manifestations of Phlegm, these being the expectoration of phlegm, the Slippery pulse, the sticky tongue coating and the polycystic ovary syndrome (usually due to Dampness and Phlegm against a background of Kidney deficiency). However, there is one symptom that does not fit all the manifestations and that is the Rapid pulse: this could conceivably be due to Phlegm-Heat but there are no signs of Heat.

A Rapid pulse in the absence of Heat symptoms is often due to shock and emotional upset. Asking the patient about this, she confirmed that this was the case.

Case history 9

A 41-year-old man complained of tiredness, sleepiness and lack of motivation. He had been feeling like that for about 1 year. He also complained of a feeling of cold 'of the skin' for about 2 years. His tongue was Red, completely Peeled, with a very deep Heart crack and Spleen cracks; his pulse was Slow (60), Empty at the deep level on the left side, especially so in the Heart position. His eyes were rather dull.

These were the presenting symptoms. On the face of it, there is a striking contradiction between the tongue, which indicates Empty-Heat from Yin deficiency, and the pulse, which indicates Cold (being Slow). The cold feeling of the skin and feet also indicates Cold and possibly Yang deficiency. When a slow pulse contradicts the other manifestations and especially the tongue, the first thing to check is whether it is due to exercise. In this case it was, as this patient had been doing a lot of vigorous exercise and many sports over many years when he was younger; thus, this could account for the slow pulse. On enquiring about other manifestations, it turned out that he felt often thirsty and drank a lot of water, his mouth was often dry, his sleep was very restless and he had a burning sensation of his feet occasionally – all symptoms which confirm the Empty-Heat. The dull *shen* of his eyes, together with the very deep Heart crack on the tongue, indicates deep emotional problems and stress, which he admitted to when asked. What to make of the cold sensation 'of the skin'? I interpreted this as being due to his mental depression and emotional stress; it is therefore neither Full- nor Empty-Cold but false Cold.

Thus, the appearance of the tongue and the symptoms of Empty-Heat (restless sleep, dry mouth and burning sensation of feet) definitely warrant a diagnosis of Empty-Heat from Yin deficiency in spite of the cold feeling of the skin and Slow pulse; furthermore, the emptiness of the pulse at deep level confirms Yin deficiency.

'Tiredness with acute onset is often due to Latent Heat'

Case history 10

A 26-year-old woman complained of sudden tiredness, a feeling of heaviness of the limbs, a feeling of muzziness of the head, loss of appetite, loose stools, a feeling of cold, headache, lack of concentration and insomnia. Her tongue was Pale and Swollen with a yellow coating and her pulse was Full and Rapid.

This is a good example of Latent Heat emerging and causing sudden tiredness and weariness. Latent Heat occurs when an external pathogenic factor invades the body without causing immediate symptoms but incubates inside and turns into interior Heat. After some weeks or months, the Latent Heat emerges from the Interior to cause symptoms similar to the above. Usually the symptoms of Latent Heat are tiredness with sudden onset, weariness, a feeling of heaviness of the legs, thirst, insomnia, irritability, Red tongue and Rapid pulse.

This patient had only some of these symptoms (there was no thirst nor irritability), while she had other symptoms not fitting the diagnosis of Latent Heat (i.e. loose stools, feeling cold, Pale tongue). The reason for this is that Latent Heat does not occur in isolation but against a pre-existing background, which in this case was Yang deficiency – hence the cold feeling and the Pale tongue. The clinching signs in this case were the yellow coating on the tongue but, most of all, the Full and Rapid pulse, which is of course normally in complete contradiction with a feeling of tiredness. In a nutshell, the essential clinching symptoms, in this case, were the sudden onset of the tiredness coupled with the Full and Rapid pulse.

The prescription used was a variation of Zhi Zi Chi Tang *Gardenia-Soja Decoction* as follows:

> Shan Zhi Zi *Fructus Gardeniae jasminoidis* 6 g
> Dan Dou Chi *Semen Sojae praeparatum* 6 g
> Ban Xia *Rhizoma Pinelliae ternatae* 6 g
> Shi Gao *Gypsum fibrosum* 6 g
> Zhu Ye *Herba Lophatheri gracilis* 4 g
> Huang Qin *Radix Scutellariae baicalensis* 6 g
> Gan Cao *Radix Glycyrrhizae uralensis* 3 g

A course of 5 days of this decoction daily cleared up the problem entirely and the patient regained her energy.

'The tongue and pulse are determinant in deciding whether to expel pathogenic factors or tonify the body's Qi in mixed Deficiency–Excess conditions'

Case history 11

A 49-year-old man complained of tiredness, insomnia, difficulty in concentrating, pain on urination, backache, recurrent sinusitis, deterioration in hearing and sight, poor memory, night sweating, and abdominal distension. His tongue was Reddish-Purple with a very sticky coating, teethmarks and a deep Heart crack; his pulse was Slippery in general and Weak on the left Rear position.

There are many symptoms of Kidney deficiency, such as tiredness, poor memory, backache, deterioration in hearing and sight, night sweating and Weak pulse on the left Kidney position. There are also a few symptoms of Spleen deficiency, such as tiredness, abdominal distension and teethmarks on the edges of the tongue. However, the pulse and tongue clearly reflect a Full rather than Empty condition; in fact, the reddish-purple colour indicates Blood stasis and the very sticky coating indicates Phlegm. Presumably, the Phlegm-Heat is causing the pain on urination and insomnia. Thus, there is a marked contrast between two Deficiency conditions (deficiency of the Spleen and Kidneys) and two Excess conditions (Blood stasis and Phlegm-Heat).

In such contradictory conditions, what should the treatment principle be? Should we concentrate on eliminating pathogenic factors or on tonifying the body's Qi? I usually prefer to eliminate pathogenic factors first, *especially* when the tongue and pulse clearly point to a Full condition as they do in this case. I therefore set out to move Qi, invigorate Blood, resolve Phlegm and clear Heat with a combination of Yue Ju Wan *Gardenia-Ligusticum Pill* and Wen Dan Tang *Warming the Gall-Bladder Decoction*.

Had his pulse been Weak in general and his tongue perhaps Peeled and with teethmarks (indicating a deficiency of Kidney-Yin and of Spleen-Qi), I would have probably concentrated my attention on tonifying the body's Qi.

'Liver patterns often occur simultaneously'

The following case history is a good example of the frequent coexistence of several Liver patterns simultaneously.

Case history 12

A 29-year-old woman had a benign lump in her left breast which grew quickly over 5 years. The lump was painful when she was angry and also before her period when she suffered from premenstrual tension. Her periods were painful and irregular, coming up to 4 days early or late; the period was rather scanty and the colour of the blood was dark red with dark clots. She also suffered from headaches on the sides of the head (along the Gall-Bladder channel). She occasionally suffered from blurred vision and dizziness. Her tongue was Pale and very slightly Purple; her pulse was Wiry.

There are four Liver patterns:

- Liver-Qi stagnation (breast lump, irregular periods, premenstrual tension)
- Liver-Blood stasis (painful breast lump, irregular and painful periods with dark clots)
- Liver-Blood deficiency (Pale tongue, blurred vision, dizziness, scanty periods)
- Liver-Yang rising (headaches, Wiry pulse).

These four Liver patterns are all interlinked. Liver-Blood deficiency leads to Liver-Qi stagnation and this, in turn, leads on the one hand to Liver-Blood stasis and on the other to Liver-Yang rising.

Appendix 2
PRESCRIPTIONS

NOTE

Please note that some of the herbs contained in the following prescriptions are banned for use in some countries. This may be either because they are toxic (in some cases wrongly perceived to be so) or because they are processed from endangered plants or endangered animal species; in some countries, no animal substances may be used at all. As the laws governing the use of these herbs (or animal substances) vary from country to country, it is the responsibility of readers to acquaint themself with the laws of their country. The inclusion of such herbs in the prescriptions below does not imply an endorsement of their use. However, I have kept the prescriptions as they are in the original source texts because this allows us to make rational substitutions for the herbs (or animal substances) which cannot be used in the West. For example, the prescription Xi Jiao Di Huang Tang *Cornus Rhinoceri-Rehmannia Decoction* contains Xi Jiao *Cornu Rhinoceri*, rhinoceros horn, which is obviously illegal; as this substance has Blood-cooling properties, we can make a rational substitution with another herb that cools Blood.

AI FU NUAN GONG WAN 艾附暖宫丸

Artemisia-Cyperus Warming the Uterus Pill
Ai Ye *Folium Artemisiae argyi* 9 g
Wu Zhu Yu *Fructus Evodiae rutaecarpae* 4.5 g
Rou Gui *Cortex Cinnamomi cassiae* 4.5 g
Xiang Fu *Rhizoma Cyperi rotundi* 9 g
Dang Gui *Radix Angelicae sinensis* 9 g
Chuan Xiong *Radix Ligustici chuanxiong* 6 g
Bai Shao *Radix Paeoniae lactiflorae* 6 g
Huang Qi *Radix Astragali membranacei* 6 g
Sheng Di Huang *Radix Rehmanniae glutinosae* 9 g
Xu Duan *Radix Dipsaci asperi* 6 g

AN SHEN DING ZHI WAN 安神定志丸

Calming the Spirit and Settling the Will-Power Pill
Fu Ling *Sclerotium Poriae cocos* 9 g
Fu Shen *Sclerotium Poriae cocos paradicis* 9 g
Ren Shen *Radix Ginseng* 9 g
Yuan Zhi *Radix Polygalae tenuifoliae* 9 g
Shi Chang Pu *Rhizoma Acori graminei* 4.5 g
Long Chi *Dens Draconis* 4.5 g

BA XIAN CHANG SHOU WAN 八仙长寿丸

Eight Immortals Longevity Pill
Mai Men Dong *Tuber Ophiopogonis japonici* 6 g
Wu Wei Zi *Fructus Schisandrae chinensis* 6 g
Shu Di Huang *Radix Rehmanniae glutinosae praeparata* 24 g
Shan Zhu Yu *Fructus Corni officinalis* 12 g
Shan Yao *Radix Dioscoreae oppositae* 12 g
Ze Xie *Rhizoma Alismatis orientalis* 9 g
Mu Dan Pi *Cortex Moutan radicis* 9 g
Fu Ling *Sclerotium Poriae cocos* 9 g

BA ZHEN TANG 八珍汤

Eight Precious Decoction
Dang Gui *Radix Angelicae sinensis* 10 g
Chuan Xiong *Radix Ligustici Chuanxiong* 5 g
Bai Shao *Radix Paeoniae lactiflorae* 8 g
Shu Di Huang *Radix Rehmanniae glutinosae praeparata* 15 g
Ren Shen *Radix Ginseng* 3g
Bai Zhu *Rhizoma Atractylodis macrocephalae* 10 g
Fu Ling *Sclerotium Poriae cocos* 8 g
Zhi Gan Cao *Radix Glycyrrhizae uralensis praeparata* 5 g

BA ZHENG SAN 八正散

Eight Rectifications Powder
Mu Tong *Caulis Mutong* 3 g
Hua Shi *Talcum* 12 g
Che Qian Zi *Semen Plantaginis* 9 g
Qu Mai *Herba Dianthi* 6 g
Bian Xu *Herba Polygoni avicularis* 6 g
Shan Zhi Zi *Fructus Gardeniae jasminoidis* 3 g
Da Huang *Radix et Rhizoma Rhei* 6 g
Deng Xin Cao *Medulla Junci effusi* 3 g
Gan Cao *Radix Glycyrrhizae uralensis* 3 g

BAI HE GU JIN TANG 白合固金汤

Lilium Consolidating Metal Decoction
Bai He *Bulbus Lilii* 15 g
Mai Men Dong *Tuber Ophiopogonis japonici* 9 g
Xuan Shen *Radix Scrophulariae ningpoensis* 9 g
Sheng Di Huang *Radix Rehmanniae glutinosae* 9 g
Shu Di Huang *Radix Rehmanniae glutinosae praeparata* 9 g
Dang Gui *Radix Angelicae sinensis* 6 g
Bai Shao *Radix Paeoniae lactiflorae* 9 g
Jie Geng *Radix Platycodi grandiflori* 6 g
Chuan Bei Mu *Bulbus Fritillariae cirrhosae* 6 g
Gan Cao *Radix Glycyrrhizae uralensis* 3 g

BAI HU TANG 白虎汤

White Tiger Decoction
Shi Gao *Gypsum fibrosum* 30 g
Zhi Mu *Radix Anemarrhenae asphodeloidis* 9 g
Zhi Gan Cao *Radix Glycyrrhizae uralensis praeparata* 3 g
Geng Mi Non-glutinous rice 9 g

BAI TOU WENG TANG 白头滃汤

Pulsatilla Decoction
Bai Tou Weng *Radix Pulsatillae chinensis* 6 g
Huang Lian *Rhizoma Coptidis* 9 g
Huang Bo *Cortex Phellodendri* 9 g
Qin Pi *Cortex Fraxini* 9 g

BAN XIA HOU PO TANG 半夏厚朴汤

Pinellia-Magnolia Decoction
Ban Xia *Rhizoma Pinelliae ternatae* 12 g
Hou Po *Cortex Magnoliae officinalis* 9 g
Zi Su Ye *Folium Perillae frutescentis* 6 g
Fu Ling *Sclerotium Poriae cocos* 12 g
Sheng Jiang *Rhizoma Zingiberis officinalis recens* 9 g

BAN XIA TANG 半夏汤

Pinelliae Decoction
Ban Xia *Rhizoma Pinelliae ternatae* 12 g
Sheng Jiang *Rhizoma Zingiberis officinalis recens* 3 slices
Jie Geng *Radix Platycodi grandiflori* 3 g
Wu Zhu Yu *Fructus Evodiae rutaecarpae* 3 g
Qiang Hu *Radix Peucedani* 6 g
Bie Jia *Carapacis Amydae sinensis* 9 g
Zhi Shi *Fructus Citri aurantii immaturus* 6 g
Ren Shen *Radix Ginseng* 9 g
Bing Lang *Semen Arecae catechu* 6 seeds

BAO HE WAN 保和丸

Preserving and Harmonizing Pill
Shan Zha *Fructus Crataegi* 9 g
Shen Qu *Massa Fermentata medicinalis* 9 g
Lai Fu Zi *Semen Raphani sativi* 6 g
Chen Pi *Pericarpium Citri reticulatae* 6 g
Ban Xia *Rhizoma Pinelliae ternatae* 9 g
Fu Ling *Sclerotium Poriae cocos* 9 g
Lian Qiao *Fructus Forsythiae suspensae* 3 g

BAO YIN JIAN 保阴煎

Protecting Yin Decoction
Sheng Di Huang *Radix Rehmanniae glutinosae* 24 g
Shu Di Huang *Radix Rehmanniae glutinosae praeparata* 15 g

Bai Shao *Radix Paeoniae lactiflorae* 12 g
Shan Yao *Radix Dioscoreae oppositae* 12 g
Huang Qin *Radix Scutellariae baicalensis* 9 g
Huang Bo *Cortex Phellodendri* 9 g
Xu Duan *Radix Dipsaci asperi* 6 g
Gan Cao *Radix Glycyrrhizae uralensis* 3 g

BAO YUAN TANG 保原汤

Preserving the Source Decoction
Huang Qi *Radix Astragali membranacei* 6 g
Ren Shen *Radix Ginseng* 6 g
Zhi Gan Cao *Radix Glycyrrhizae uralensis praeparata* 3 g
Rou Gui *Cortex Cinnamomi cassiae* 1.5 g

BEI MU GUA LOU SAN 贝母瓜蒌汤

Fritillaria-Trichosanthes Powder
Zhe Bei Mu *Bulbus Fritillariae thunbergii* 4.5 g
Gua Lou *Fructus Trichosanthis* 3 g
Tian Hua Fen *Radix Trichosanthis kirilowii* 2.4 g
Fu Ling *Sclerotium Poriae cocos* 2.4 g
Chen Pi *Pericarpium Citri reticulatae* 2.4 g
Jie Geng *Radix Platycodi grandiflori* 2.4 g

BU FEI TANG 补肺汤

Tonifying the Lungs Decoction
Ren Shen *Radix Ginseng* 9 g
Huang Qi *Radix Astragali membranacei* 24 g
Shu Di Huang *Radix Rehmanniae glutinosae praeparata* 24 g
Wu Wei Zi *Fructus Schisandrae chinensis* 6 g
Zi Wan *Radix Asteris tatarici* 9 g
Sang Bai Pi *Cortex Mori albae radicis* 12 g

BU GAN TANG 补肝汤

Tonifying the Liver Decoction
Dang Gui *Radix Angelicae sinensis* 9 g
Chuan Xiong *Radix Ligustici Chuanxiong* 6 g
Bai Shao *Radix Paeoniae lactiflorae* 9 g
Shu Di Huang *Radix Rehmanniae glutinosae praeparata* 15 g
Suan Zao Ren *Semen Ziziphi spinosae* 6 g
Mu Gua *Fructus Chaenomelis lagenariae* 6 g
Zhi Gan Cao *Radix Glycyrrhizae uralensis praeparata* 3 g

BU SHEN GU CHONG WAN 补肾固冲丸

Tonifying the Kidneys and Consolidating the Penetrating Vessel Pill
Tu Si Zi *Semen Cuscutae chinensis* 6 g
Xu Duan *Radix Dipsaci asperi* 6 g
Ba Ji Tian *Radix Morindae officinalis* 6 g
Du Zhong *Cortex Eucommiae ulmoidis* 6 g
Lu Jiao Shuang *Cornu Cervi degelatinatum* 6 g
Dang Gui *Radix Angelicae sinensis* 6 g
Shu Di Huang *Radix Rehmanniae glutinosae praeparata* 9 g
Gou Qi Zi *Fructus Lycii chinensis* 9 g
E Jiao *Gelatinum Corii asini* 6 g
Dang Shen *Radix Codonopsis pilosulae* 6 g
Bai Zhu *Rhizoma Atractylodis macrocephalae* 9 g
Da Zao *Fructus Ziziphi jujubae* 3 dates
Sha Ren *Fructus seu Semen Amomi* 3 g

BU SHEN YANG XUE TANG 补肾养血汤

Tonifying the Kidneys and Nourishing Blood Decoction
Yin Yang Huo *Herba Epimedi* 6 g
Xian Mao *Rhizoma Curculiginis orchioidis* 6 g
Zi He Che *Placenta Hominis* 6 g
Nu Zhen Zi *Fructus Ligustri lucidi* 6 g
Dang Gui *Radix Angelicae sinensis* 6 g
Bai Shao *Radix Paeoniae lactiflorae* 9 g
Dang Shen *Radix Codonopsis pilosulae* 6 g
Gou Qi Zi *Fructus Lycii* 6 g
Tu Si Zi *Semen Cuscutae chinensis* 6 g
Xiang Fu *Rhizoma Cyperi rotundi* 3 g

BU ZHONG YI QI TANG 补中益气汤

Tonifying the Centre and Benefiting Qi Decoction
Huang Qi *Radix Astragali membranacei* 12 g
Ren Shen *Radix Ginseng* 9 g
Bai Zhu *Rhizoma Atractylodis macrocephalae* 9 g
Dang Gui *Radix Angelicae sinensis* 6 g
Chen Pi *Pericarpium Citri reticulatae* 6 g
Sheng Ma *Rhizoma Cimicifugae* 3 g
Chai Hu *Radix Bupleuri* 3 g

CANG ER BI DOU YAN FANG 苍耳鼻窦炎方

Xanthium Sinusitis Formula
Cang Er Zi *Fructus Xanthii sibirici* 9 g
Huang Qin *Radix Scutellariae baicalensis* 9 g

Pu Gong Ying *Herba Taraxaci mongolici cum radice* 6 g
Ge Gen *Radix Puerariae* 9 g
Jie Geng *Radix Platycodi grandiflori* 6 g
Bai Zhi *Radix Angelicae dahuricae* 3 g
Che Qian Zi *Semen Plantaginis* 6 g
Gan Cao *Radix Glycyrrhizae uralensis* 3 g

CANG FU DAO TAN WAN 苍附导痰丸

Atractylodes-Cyperus Conducting Phlegm Pill
Cang Zhu *Rhizoma Atractylodis lanceae* 9 g
Xiang Fu *Rhizoma Cyperi rotundi* 9 g
Zhi Ke *Fructus Citri aurantii* 9 g
Fu Ling *Sclerotium Poriae cocos* 6 g
Chen Pi *Pericarpium Citri reticulatae* 6 g
Dan Nan Xing *Pulvis Arisaemae cum felle bovis* 4.5 g
Gan Cao *Radix Glycyrrhizae uralensis* 3 g
Sheng Jiang *Rhizoma Zingiberis officinalis recens* 3 slices
Shen Qu *Massa Fermentata medicinalis* 6 g

CHAI HU SHU GAN TANG 柴胡疏肝汤

Bupleurum Pacifying the Liver Decoction
Chai Hu *Radix Bupleuri* 6 g
Bai Shao *Radix Paeoniae lactiflorae* 4.5 g
Zhi Ke *Fructus Citri aurantii* 4.5 g
Zhi Gan Cao *Radix Glycyrrhizae uralensis praeparata* 1.5 g
Chen Pi *Pericarpium Citri reticulatae* 6 g
Xiang Fu *Rhizoma Cyperi rotundi* 4.5 g
Chuan Xiong *Radix Ligustici Chuanxiong* 4.5 g

CHANG TAI BAI ZHU SAN 长胎白术散

Long [Life] Fetus Atractylodes Powder
Bai Zhu *Rhizoma Atractylodis macrocephalae* 6 g
Chuan Xiong *Radix Ligustici Chuanxiong* 3 g
Chuan Jiao *Pericarpium Zanthoxyli bungeani* 3 g
Sheng Di Huang *Radix Rehmanniae glutinosae* 6 g
E Jiao *Gelatinum Corii Asini* 6 g
Mu Li *Concha Ostreae* 9 g
Fu Ling *Sclerotium Poriae cocos* 6 g

CHEN XIANG JIANG QI TANG (STOMACH-QI STAGNATION) 沉香降气汤

Aquilaria Descending Qi Decoction
Chen Xiang *Lignum Aquilariae* 9 g

Xiang Fu *Rhizoma Cyperi rotundi* 6 g
Sha Ren *Fructus seu Semen Amomi* 3 g
Gan Cao *Radix Glycyrrhizae uralensis* 3 g

DA BU YIN WAN 大补阴丸

Great Tonifying Yin Pill (Dosages for batch of pills)
Zhi Mu *Radix Anemarrhenae asphodeloidis* 120 g
Huang Bo *Cortex Phellodendri* 120 g
Shu Di Huang *Radix Rehmanniae glutinosae praeparata* 180 g
Gui Ban *Plastrum Testudinis* 180 g
Pig's bone-marrow 12 g

DA BU YUAN JIAN 大补元煎

Great Tonifying the Original [Qi] Decoction
Ren Shen *Radix Ginseng* 3 g
Shan Yao *Radix Dioscoreae oppositae* 6 g
Shu Di Huang *Radix Rehmanniae glutinosae praeparata* 9 g
Du Zhong *Cortex Eucommiae ulmoidis* 6 g
Dang Gui *Radix Angelicae sinensis* 6 g
Shan Zhu Yu *Fructus Corni officinalis* 3 g
Gou Qi Zi *Fructus Lycii chinensis* 6 g
Zhi Gan Cao *Radix Glycyrrhizae uralensis praeparata* 3 g

DA DING FENG ZHU 大定风珠

Big Stopping Wind Pearl
Ji Zi Huang *Egg yolk* 2 yolks
E Jiao *Gelatinum Corii asini* 9 g
Bai Shao *Radix Paeoniae lactiflorae* 18 g
Zhi Gan Cao *Radix Glycyrrhizae uralensis praeparata* 12 g
Wu Wei Zi *Fructus Schisandrae chinensis* 6 g
Sheng Di Huang *Radix Rehmanniae glutinosae* 18 g
Mai Men Dong *Tuber Ophiopogonis japonici* 18 g
Huo Ma Ren *Semen Cannabis sativae* 6 g
Gui Ban *Plastrum Testudinis* 12 g
Bie Jia *Carapax Amydae sinensis* 12 g
Mu Li *Concha Ostreae* 12 g

DAN SHEN YIN 丹参饮

Salvia Decoction
Dan Shen *Radix Salviae miltiorrhizae* 30 g
Tan Xiang *Lignum Santali albi* 4.5 g

Sha Ren *Fructus seu Semen et Pericarpium amomi* 4.5 g

DAN ZHI XIAO YAO SAN 丹栀逍遥散

Moutan-Gardenia Free and Easy Wanderer Powder
Dang Gui *Radix Angelicae sinensis* 3 g
Bai Shao *Radix Paeoniae lactiflorae* 3 g
Fu Ling *Sclerotium Poriae cocos* 3 g
Bai Zhu *Rhizoma Atractylodis macrocephalae* 3 g
Chai Hu *Radix Bupleuri* 34 g
Bo He *Herba Menthae haplocalycis* 3 g
Mu Dan Pi *Cortex Moutan radicis* 1.5 g
Shan Zhi Zi *Fructus Gardeniae jasminoidis* 1.5 g
Zhi Gan Cao *Radix Glycyrrhizae uralensis praeparata* 1.5 g

DANG GUI SHAO YAO SAN 当归少药散

Angelica and Peony powder
Dang Gui *Radix Angelicae sinensis* 9 g
Bai Shao *Radix Paeoniae lactiflorae* 15 g
Fu Ling *Sclerotium Poriae cocos* 12 g
Bai Zhu *Rhizoma Atractylodis macrocephalae* 12 g
Ze Xie *Rhizoma Alismatis orientalis* 12 g
Chuan Xiong *Radix Ligustici Chuanxiong* 6 g

DANG GUI SI NI TANG 当归四逆汤

Angelica Four Rebellious Decoction
Dang Gui *Radix Angelicae sinensis* 9 g
Bai Shao *Radix Paeoniae lactiflorae* 9 g
Gui Zhi *Ramulus Cinnamomi cassiae* 9 g
Xi Xin *Herba cum Radice Asari* 3 g
Zhi Gan Cao *Radix Glycyrrhizae uralensis praeparata* 3 g
Da Zao *Fructus Zizyphi jujubae* 6 dates
Mu Tong *Caulis Mutong* 3 g

DANG GUI JI XUE TENG TANG 当归鸡血藤

Angelica-Ji Xue Teng Decoction
Dang Gui *Radix Angelicae sinensis* 15 g
Shu Di Huang *Radix Rehmanniae glutinosae praeparata* 15 g
Long Yan Rou *Arillus Euphoriae longanae* 6 g
Bai Shao *Radix Paeoniae lactiflorae* 9 g
Dan Shen *Radix Salviae miltiorrhizae* 9 g
Ji Xue Teng *Radix et Caulis Jixueteng* 15 g

DANG GUI LONG HUI WAN 当归龙荟丸

Angelica Dragon Aloe Pill
Dang Gui *Radix Angelicae sinensis* 6 g
Long Dan Cao *Radix Gentianae scabrae* 6 g
Lu Hui *Herba Aloes* 6 g
Shan Zhi Zi *Fructus Gardeniae jasminoidis* 4.5 g
Huang Lian *Rhizoma Coptidis* 3 g
Huang Bo *Cortex Phellodendri* 6 g
Huang Qin *Radix Scutellariae baicalensis* 6 g
Da Huang *Radix et Rhizoma Rhei* 6 g
Mu Xiang *Radix Aucklandiae lappae* 3 g

DANG GUI GUI ZHI TANG 当归桂枝汤

Angelica-Ramulus Cinnamomi Decoction
Dang Gui *Radix Angelicae sinensis* 9 g
Gui Zhi *Ramulus Cinnamomi cassiae* 1 g
Bai Shao *Radix Paeoniae lactiflorae* 3 g
Ban Xia *Rhizoma Pinelliae ternatae* 6 g
Zhi Gan Cao *Radix Glycyrrhizae uralensis praeparata* 0.6 g
Pao Jiang *Rhizoma Zingiberis officinalis recens* (fried) 2 slices
Da Zao *Fructus Zizyphi jujubae* 3 dates

DAO CHI QING XIN TANG 导赤清心汤

Conducting Redness and Clearing the Heart Decoction
Sheng Di Huang *Radix Rehmanniae glutinosae* 6 g
Mu Tong *Caulis Mutong* 3 g
Mai Men Dong *Tuber Ophiopogonis japonici* 6 g
Fu Shen *Sclerotium Poriae cocos pararadicis* 6 g
Mu Dan Pi *Cortex Moutan radicis* 6 g
Lian Zi Xin *Plumula Nelumbinis nuciferae* 6 g
Hua Shi *Talcum* 6 g
Gan Cao *Radix Glycyrrhizae uralensis* 3 g
Hu Po *Succinum* 3 g
Zhu Ye *Herba Lophatheri gracilis* 6 g

DAO CHI SAN 导赤散

Conducting Redness Powder
Sheng Di Huang *Radix Rehmanniae glutinosae* 15 g
Mu Tong *Caulis Mutong* 3 g
Zhu Ye *Herba Lophatheri gracilis* 3 g
Gan Cao *Radix Glycyrrhizae uralensis* 3 g

DI SHENG TANG 抵圣汤

Supporting the Sage Decoction
Chi Shao *Radix Paeoniae rubra* 6 g
Ban Xia *Rhizoma Pinelliae ternatae* 6 g
Ze Lan *Herba Lycopi lucidi* 6 g
Ren Shen *Radix Ginseng* 6 g
Sheng Jiang *Rhizoma Zingiberis officinalis recens* 3 slices
Chen Pi *Pericarpium Citri reticulatae* 3 g
Gan Cao *Radix Glycyrrhizae uralensis* 3 g

DI TAN TANG 涤痰汤

Scouring Phlegm Decoction
Ban Xia *Rhizoma Pinelliae ternatae* 6.6 g
Chen Pi *Pericarpium Citri reticulatae* 6 g
Fu Ling *Sclerotium Poriae cocos* 6 g
Zhi Shi *Fructus Citri aurantii immaturus* 6 g
Zhu Ru *Caulis Bambusae in Taeniis* 2.1 g
Dan Nan Xing *Pulvis Arisaemae cum felle bovis* 6.6 g
Shi Chang Pu *Rhizoma Acori graminei* 3 g
Ren Shen *Radix Ginseng* 3 g
Gan Cao *Radix Glycyrrhizae uralensis* 1.5 g

DING XIANG SHI DI TANG 丁香柿蒂汤

Caryophyllum-Diospyros Decoction
Ding Xiang *Flos Caryophylli* 6 g
Shi Di *Calyx Diospyri Kaki* 6 g
Ren Shen *Radix Ginseng* 3 g
Sheng Jiang *Rhizoma Zingiberis officinalis recens* 6 g

DUO MING SAN 夺命散

Seizing Life Powder
Mo Yao *Myrrha* 6 g
Xue Jie *Sangui Draconis* 6 g

E JIAO JI ZI HUANG TANG 阿胶鸡子黄汤

Gelatinum Corii Asini-Egg Yolk Decoction
E Jiao *Gelatinum Corii Asini* 6 g
Ji Zi Huang Egg yolk 2 yolks
Sheng Di Huang *Radix Rehmanniae glutinosae* 12 g
Bai Shao *Radix Paeoniae lactiflorae* 9 g
Zhi Gan Cao *Radix Glycyrrhizae uralensis praeparata* 1.5 g

Gou Teng *Ramulus Uncariae* 6 g
Shi Jue Ming *Concha Haliotidis* 15 g
Mu Li *Concha Ostreae* 12 g
Fu Shen *Sclerotium Poriae cocos pararadicis* 12 g
Luo Shi Teng *Caulis Trachelospermi jasminoides* 9 g

EMPIRICAL PRESCRIPTION BY DR CHEN JIA XU FOR LIVER-QI DEFICIENCY

Huang Qi *Radix Astragali membranacei* 6 g
Dang Shen *Radix Codonopsis pilosulae* 6 g
Bai Zhu *Rhizoma Atractylodis macrocephalae* 6 g
Dang Gui *Radix Angelicae sinensis* 9 g
Chai Hu *Radix Bupleuri* 3 g
Gui Zhi *Ramulus Cinnamomi cassiae* 4 g
Fu Ling *Scleortium Poriae cocos* 6 g
Bai Shao *Radix Paeoniae lactiflorae* 9 g
Wu Wei Zi *Fructus Schisandrae chinensis* 3 g
Bai Zi Ren *Semen Biotae orientalis* 6 g
Zhi Gan Cao *Radix Glycyrrhizae uralensis praeparata* 3 g

ER CHEN TANG 二陈汤

Two Old Decoction
Ban Xia *Rhizoma Pinelliae ternatae* 15 g
Chen Pi *Pericarpium Citri reticulatae* 15 g
Fu Ling *Sclerotium Poriae cocos* 9 g
Zhi Gan Cao *Radix Glycyrrhizae uralensis praeparata* 3 g

ER ZHI WAN 二至丸

Two ultimate Pill
Nu Zhen Zi *Fructus Ligustri lucidi* 9 g
Han Lian Cao *Herba Ecliptae prostratae* 9 g

FO SHOU SAN 佛手散

Buddha's Hand Powder
Dang Gui *Radix Angelicae sinensis* 6 g
Chuan Xiong *Radix Ligustici Chuanxiong* 4 g

FU TU DAN 符菟丹

Poria-Cuscuta Pill (Dosages for batch of pills)
Tu Si Zi *Semen Cuscutae chinensis* 150 g
Wu Wei Zi *Fructus Schisandrae chinensis* 210 g
Shan Yao *Radix Dioscoreae oppositae* 60 g

Lian Zi *Semen Nelumbinis nuciferae* 60 g
Fu Ling *Sclerotium Poriae cocos* 90 g

FU ZI LI ZHONG WAN 附子理中丸

Aconitum Regulating the Centre Pill
Fu Zi *Radix lateralis Aconiti carmichaeli praeparata* 3 g
Gan Jiang *Rhizoma Zingiberis officinalis* 6 g
Ren Shen *Radix Ginseng* 6 g
Bai Zhu *Rhizoma Atractylodis macrocephalae* 6 g
Zhi Gan Cao *Radix Glycyrrhizae uralensis praeparata* 3 g

GAN CAO GAN JIANG TANG 甘草干姜汤

Glycyrrhiza-Zingiber Decoction
Zhi Gan Cao *Radix Glycyrrhizae uralensis* 12 g
Gan Jiang *Rhizoma Zingiberis officinalis* 6 g

GAN LU XIAO DU DAN 甘露消毒丹

Sweet Dew Eliminating Toxin Pill
Lian Qiao *Fructus Forsythiae suspensae* 6 g
Huang Qin *Radix Scutellariae baicalensis* 6 g
Bo He *Herba Menthae haplocalycis* 3 g
She Gan *Rhizoma Belamcandae chinensis* 4.5 g
Chuan Bei Mu *Bulbus Fritillariae cirrhosae* 3 g
Hua Shi *Talcum* 9 g
Mu Tong *Caulis Mutong* 3 g
Yin Chen Hao *Herba Artemisiae capillaris* 6 g
Huo Xiang *Herba Agastachis seu Pogostemi* 4.5 g
Shi Chang Pu *Rhizoma Acori graminei* 3 g
Bai Dou Kou *Fructus Amomi kravanh* 4.5 g

GE GEN QIN LIAN TANG 葛根芩连汤

Pueraria-Scutellaria-Coptis Decoction
Ge Gen *Radix Puerariae* 9 g
Huang Qin *Radix Scutellariae baicalensis* 9 g
Huang Lian *Rhizoma Coptidis* 4.5 g
Gan Cao *Radix Glycyrrhizae uralensis* 3 g

GE XIA ZHU YU TANG 膈下逐瘀汤

Eliminating Stasis below the Diaphragm Decoction
Dang Gui *Radix Angelicae sinensis* 9 g
Chuan Xiong *Radix Ligustici chuanxiong* 3 g
Chi Shao *Radix Paeoniae rubrae* 6 g
Hong Hua *Flos Carthami tinctorii* 9 g
Tao Ren *Semen Persicae* 9 g

Wu Ling Zhi *Excrementum Trogopteri* 9 g
Yan Hu Suo *Rhizoma Corydalis yanhusuo* 3 g
Xiang Fu *Rhizoma Cyperi rotundi* 3 g
Zhi Ke *Fructus Citri aurantii* 5 g
Wu Yao *Radix Linderae strychnifoliae* 6 g
Mu Dan Pi *Cortex Moutan radicis* 6 g
Gan Cao *Radix Glycyrrhizae uralensis* 9 g

GU TAI JIAN 固胎煎

Consolidating the Fetus Decoction
Huang Qin *Radix Scutellariae baicalensis* 6 g
Chen Pi *Pericarpium Citri reticulatae* 3 g
Bai Zhu *Rhizoma Atractylodis macrocephalae* 9 g
Dang Gui *Radix Angelicae sinensis* 6 g
Bai Shao *Radix Paeoniae lactiflorae* 9 g
E Jiao *Gelatinum Corii asini* 6 g
Sha Ren *Fructus Amomi* 3 g

GUI PI TANG 归脾汤

Tonifying the Spleen Decoction
Ren Shen *Radix Ginseng* 6 g (or **Dang Shen** *Radix Codonopsis pilosulae* 12 g)
Huang Qi *Radix Astragali membranacei* 15 g
Bai Zhu *Rhizoma Atractylodis macrocephalae* 12 g
Dang Gui *Radix Angelicae sinensis* 6 g
Fu Shen *Sclerotium Poriae cocos pararadicis* 9 g
Suan Zao Ren *Semen Ziziphi spinosae* 9 g
Long Yan Rou *Arillus Euphoriae longanae* 12 g
Yuan Zhi *Radix Polygalae tenuifoliae* 9 g
Mu Xiang *Radix Aucklandiae lappae* 3 g
Zhi Gan Cao *Radix Glycyrrhizae uralensis praeparata* 4 g
Sheng Jiang *Rhizoma Zingiberis officinalis recens* 3 slices
Hong Zao *Fructus Ziziphi jujubae* 5 dates

GUI SHEN WAN 归肾丸

Restoring the Kidneys Pill
Tu Si Zi *Semen Cuscutae chinensis* 6 g
Du Zhong *Cortex Eucommiae ulmoidis* 4 g
Gou Qi Zi *Fructus Lycii chinensis* 6 g
Shan Zhu Yu *Fructus Corni officinalis* 4 g
Dang Gui *Radix Angelicae sinensis* 6 g
Shu Di Huang *Radix Rehmanniae glutinosae praeparata* 6 g
Shan Yao *Radix Dioscoreae oppositae* 6 g
Fu Ling *Sclerotium Poriae cocos* 6 g

GUI ZHI FU LING WAN 桂枝茯苓丸

Ramulus Cinnamomi-Poria Pill
Gui Zhi *Ramulus Cinnamomi cassiae* 9 g
Fu Ling *Sclerotium Poriae cocos* 9 g
Chi Shao *Radix Paeoniae rubrae* 9 g
Mu Dan Pi *Cortex Moutan radicis* 9 g
Tao Ren *Semen Persicae* 9 g

GUI ZHI TANG 桂枝汤

Ramulus Cinnamomi Decoction
Gui Zhi *Ramulus Cinnamomi cassiae* 9 g
Bai Shao *Radix Paeoniae lactiflorae* 9 g
Sheng Jiang *Rhizoma Zingiberis officinalis recens* 9 g
Da Zao *Fructus Ziziphi jujubae* 12 dates
Zhi Gan Cao *Radix Glycyrrhizae uralensis praeparata* 6 g

GUN TAN WAN 滚痰丸

Vapourizing Phlegm Pill (Dosages for batch of pills)
Duan Meng Shi *Lapis Micae seu Chloriti* (calcined) 30 g
Da Huang *Radix et Rhizoma Rhei* 240 g
Huang Qin *Radix Scutellariae baicalensis* 240 g
Chen Xiang *Lignum Aquilariae* 15 g

HAO QIN QING DAN TANG 蒿芩清胆汤

Artemisia-Scutellaria Clearing the Gall-Bladder Decoction
Qing Hao *Herba Artemisiae apiaceae* 4.5 g
Huang Qin *Radix Scutellariae baicalensis* 4.5 g
Zhu Ru *Caulis Bambusae in Taeniis* 9 g
Zhi Shi *Fructus Citri aurantii immaturus* 4.5 g
Chen Pi *Pericarpium Citri reticulatae* 4.5 g
Ban Xia *Rhizoma Pinelliae ternatae* 4.5 g
Chi Fu Ling *Sclerotium Poriae cocos rubrae* 9 g
Bi Yu San Jasper powder:
    Hua Shi *Talcum* 6 parts
    Gan Cao *Radix Glycyrrhizae uralensis* 1 part
    Qing Dai *Indigo pulverata levis* 1 part

HEI SHEN SAN 黑神散

Black [Bean] Spirit Powder
Hei Da Dou *Semen Glycines* 6 g
Shu Di Huang *Radix Rehmanniae glutinosae praeparata* 6 g

Dang Gui *Radix Angelicae sinensis* 6 g
Rou Gui *Cortex Cinnamoni cassiae* 3 g
Bao Jiang *Rhizoma Zingiberis officinalis recens* (fried) 3 slices
Gan Cao *Radix Glycyrrhizae uralensis* 3 g
Bai Shao *Radix Paeoniae lactiflorae* 6 g
Pu Huang *Pollen Typhae* 6 g

HUA CHONG WAN 化虫丸

Dissolving Worms Pill (Dosages for batch of pills)
He Shi *Fructus Carpesii seu Daucusi* 1500 g
Bing Lang *Semen Arecae catechu* 1500 g
Ku Lian Gen Pi *Cortex Meliae radicis* 1500 g
Qian Dan *Minium* 1500 g
Ming Fan *Alumen* 375 g

HUA GAN JIAN 化肝煎

Transforming the Liver Decoction
Qing Pi *Pericarpium Citri reticulatae viride* 6 g
Chen Pi *Pericarpium Citri reticulatae* 6 g
Bai Shao *Radix Paeoniae lactiflorae* 6 g
Mu Dan Pi *Cortex Moutan radicis* 4.5 g
Shan Zhi Zi *Fructus Gardeniae jasminoidis* 4.5 g
Ze Xie *Rhizoma Alismatis orientalis* 4.5 g
Chuan Bei Mu *Bulbus Fritillariae cirrhosae* 6 g

HUANG LIAN E JIAO TANG 黄连阿胶汤

Coptis-Colla Asini Decoction
Huang Lian *Rhizoma Coptidis* 12 g
Huang Qin *Radix Scutellariae baicalensis* 6 g
E Jiao *Gelatinum Corii asini* 9 g
Bai Shao *Radix Paeoniae lactiflorae* 6 g
Ji Zi Huang egg yolk 2 yolks

HUANG QI JIAN ZHONG TANG 黄芪建中汤

Astragalus Strengthening the Centre Decoction
Huang Qi *Radix Astragali membranacei* 9 g
Yi Tang *Saccharum granorum* 18 g
Gui Zhi *Ramulus Cinnamomi cassiae* 9 g
Bai Shao *Radix Paeoniae lactiflorae* 18 g
Zhi Gan Cao *Radix Glycyrrhizae uralensis praeparata* 6 g
Sheng Jiang *Rhizoma Zingiberis officinalis recens* 9 g
Da Zao *Fructus Ziziphi jujubae* 12 dates

HUO PO XIA LING TANG 藿补下苓汤

Agastache-Magnolia-Pinellia-Poria Decoction
Huo Xiang *Herba Agastachis seu Pogostemi* 6 g
Hou Po *Cortex Magnoliae officinalis* 3 g
Ban Xia *Rhizoma Pinelliae ternatae* 4.5 g
Fu Ling *Sclerotium Poriae cocos* 9 g
Xing Ren *Semen Pruni armeniacae* 9 g
Yi Yi Ren *Semen Coicis lachryma jobi* 12 g
Bai Dou Kou *Fructus Amomi kravanh* 1.8 g
Zhu Ling *Sclerotium Polypori umbellati* 4.5 g
Dan Dou Chi *Semen Sojae praeparatum* 9 g
Ze Xie *Rhizoma Alismatis orientalis* 4.5 g

HUO XIANG ZHENG QI SAN 藿香正气散

Agastache Upright Qi Powder
Huo Xiang *Herba Agastachis seu Pogostemi* 12 g
Hou Po *Cortex Magnoliae officinalis* 9 g
Chen Pi *Pericarpium Citri reticulatae* 9 g
Zi Su Ye *Folium Perillae frutescentis* 6 g
Bai Zhi *Radix Angelicae dahuricae* 6 g
Ban Xia *Rhizoma Pinelliae ternatae* 9 g
Da Fu Pi *Pericarpium Arecae catechu* 9 g
Bai Zhu *Rhizoma Atractylodis macrocephalae* 12 g
Fu Ling *Sclerotium Poriae cocos* 9 g
Jie Geng *Radix Platycodi grandiflori* 9 g
Zhi Gan Cao *Radix Glycyrrhizae uralensis praeparata* 3 g

JIAN LING TANG 建瓴汤

Constructing Roof Tiles Decoction
Shan Yao *Radix Dioscoreae oppositae* 30 g
Huai Niu Xi *Radix Achyranthis bidentatae* 30 g
Dai Zhe Shi *Haematitum* 24 g
Long Gu *Os Draconis* 18 g
Mu Li *Concha Ostreae* 18 g
Sheng Di Huang *Radix Rehmanniae glutinosae* 18 g
Bai Shao *Radix Paeoniae lactiflorae* 12 g
Bai Zi Ren *Semen Biotae orientalis* 12 g

JIE DU HUO XUE TANG 解毒活血汤

Expelling Poison Invigorating Blood Decoction
Lian Qiao *Fructus Forsythiae suspensae* 6 g
Ge Gen *Radix Puerariae* 6 g
Chai Hu *Radix Bupleuri* 4.5 g
Gan Cao *Radix Glycyrrhizae uralensis* 6 g
Sheng Di Huang *Radix Rehmanniae glutinosae* 6 g

Chi Shao *Radix Paeoniae rubrae* 4.5 g
Dang Gui *Radix Angelicae sinensis* 6 g
Hong Hua *Flos Carthami tinctorii* 3 g
Tao Ren *Semen Persicae* 4.5 g
Zhi Ke *Fructus Citri aurantii* 6 g
Bai Shao *Radix Paeoniae lactiflorae* 6 g

JIN GUI SHEN QI WAN 金归肾气丸

Golden Chest Kidney-Qi Pill
Fu Zi *Radix lateralis Aconiti carmichaeli praeparata* 3 g
Gui Zhi *Ramulus Cinnamomi cassiae* 3 g
Shu Di Huang *Radix Rehmanniae glutinosae praeparata* 24 g
Shan Zhu Yu *Fructus Corni officinalis* 12 g
Shan Yao *Radix Dioscoreae oppositae* 12 g
Ze Xie *Rhizoma Alismatis orientalis* 9 g
Mu Dan Pi *Cortex Moutan radicis* 9 g
Fu Ling *Sclerotium Poriae cocos* 9 g

JIN LING ZI SAN 金铃子散

Melia Toosendan Powder
Jin Ling Zi *Fructus Meliae toosendan* 30 g
Yan Hu Suo *Rhizoma Corydalis yanhusuo* 30 g

JIN SUO GU JING WAN 金铃固精丸

Metal Lock Consolidating the Essence Pill
Sha Yuan Ji Li *Semen Astragali complanati* 6 g
Qian Shi *Semen Euryales ferocis* 6 g
Lian Xu *Stamen Nelumbinis nuciferae* 6 g
Long Gu *Os Draconis* 3 g
Mu Li *Concha Ostreae* 3 g
Lian Zi *Semen Nelumbinis nuciferae* 12 g

JING FANG SI WU TANG 荆防四物汤

Schizonepeta-Ledebouriella Four Substances Decoction
Jing Jie *Herba seu Flos Schizonepetae tenuifoliae* 4.5 g
Fang Feng *Radix Ledebouriellae divaricatae* 6 g
Shu Di Huang *Radix Rehmanniae glutinosae praeparata* 6 g
Dang Gui *Radix Angelicae sinensis* 6 g
Chuan Xiong *Radix Ligustici chuanxiong* 4.5 g
Bai Shao *Radix Paeoniae lactiflorae* 6 g
Zi Su Ye *Folium Perillae frutescentis* 3 g

JU HE WAN 橘核丸

Citrus Seed Pill
Ju He *Semen Citri Reticulatae* 6 g
Chuan Lian Zi *Fructus Meliae toosendan* 6 g
Mu Xiang *Radix Aucklandiae lappae* 3 g
Tao Ren *Semen Persicae* 6 g
Yan Hu Suo *Rhizoma Corydalis Yanhusuo* 3 g
Rou Gui *Cortex Cinnamomi cassiae* 3 g
Mu Tong *Caulis Mutong* 3 g
Hou Po *Cortex Magnoliae officinalis* 3 g
Zhi Shi *Fructus Citri aurantii immaturus* 3 g
Hai Zao *Herba Sargassii* 6 g
Kun Bu *Thallus Algae* 6 g
Hai Dai *Zostera marina* 6 g

JU PI ZHU RU TANG 橘皮竹茹汤

Citrus-Bambusa Decoction
Chen Pi *Pericarpium Citri reticulatae* 9 g
Zhu Ru *Caulis Bambusae in Taeniis* 9 g
Ren Shen *Radix Ginseng* 3 g
Sheng Jiang *Rhizoma Zingiberis officinalis recens* 18 g
Gan Cao *Radix Glycyrrhizae uralensis* 6 g
Da Zao *Fructus Ziziphi jujubae* 5 dates

LI YAN CHA 利咽茶

Benefiting the Throat Tea
Jin Yin Hua *Flos Lonicerae japonicae* 6 g
Ju Hua *Flos Chrysanthemi morifolii* 6 g
Jie Geng *Radix Platycodi grandiflori* 4.5 g
Mai Men Dong *Tuber Ophiopogonis japonici* 6 g
Xuan Shen *Radix Scrophulariae ningpoensis* 6 g
Mu Hu Die *Semen Oroxyli indici* 4 g
Pang Da Hai *Semen Sterculiae scaphigerae* 4.5 g
Gan Cao *Radix Glycyrrhizae uralensis* 3 g

LI YIN JIAN 理阴煎

Regulating Yin Decoction
Shu Di Huang *Radix Rehmanniae glutinosae praeparata* 9 g
Dang Gui *Radix Angelicae sinensis* 9 g
Zhi Gan Cao *Radix Glycyrrhizae uralensis praeparata* 3 g
Bao Jiang *Rhizoma Zingiberis officinalis recens* (fried) 3 slices

LI ZHONG AN HUI TANG 理中安蛔汤

Regulating the Centre and Calming Roundworms Decoction
Ren Shen *Radix Ginseng* 2.1 g
Bai Zhu *Rhizoma Atractylodis macrocephalae* 3 g
Fu Ling *Sclerotium Poriae cocos* 3 g
Chuan Jiao *Pericarpium Zanthoxyli bungeani* 0.9 g
Wu Mei *Fructus Pruni mume* 0.9 g
Gan Jiang *Rhizoma Zingiberis officinalis* 1.5 g

LI ZHONG TANG 理中汤

Regulating the Centre Decoction
Gan Jiang *Rhizoma Zingiberis officinalis* 9 g
Ren Shen *Radix Ginseng* 9 g
Bai Zhu *Rhizoma Atractylodis macrocephalae* 9 g
Zhi Gan Cao *Radix Glycyrrhizae uralensis praeparata* 3 g

LIAN MEI AN HUI TANG 连梅安蛔汤

Picrorhiza-Prunus Mume Calming Roundworms Decoction
Hu Huang Lian *Rhizoma Picrorhizae* 3 g
Chuan Jiao *Pericarpium Zanthoxyli bungeani* 1.5 g
Lei Wan *Sclerotium Omphaliae lapidescens* 9 g
Wu Mei *Fructus Pruni mume* 2 prunes
Huang Bo *Cortex Phellodendri* 2.4 g
Bing Lang *Semen Arecae catechu* 2 nuts

LIAN PO YIN 连朴饮

Coptis-Magnolia Decoction
Huang Lian *Rhizoma Coptidis* 3 g
Hou Po *Cortex Magnoliae officinalis* 6 g
Shan Zhi Zi *Fructus Gardeniae jasminoidis* 9 g
Dan Dou Chi *Semen Sojae praeparatum* 9 g
Shi Chang Pu *Rhizoma Acori graminei* 3 g
Ban Xia *Rhizoma Pinelliae ternatae* 3 g
Lu Gen *Rhizoma Phragmitis communis* 15 g

LIANG DI TANG 两地汤

Two 'Di' Decoction
Sheng Di Huang *Radix Rehmanniae glutinosae* 18 g
Di Gu Pi *Cortex Lycii chinensis radicis* 9 g
Xuan Shen *Radix Scrophulariae ningpoensis* 12 g
Mai Men Dong *Tuber Ophiopogonis japonici* 9 g

Bai Shao *Radix Paeoniae lactiflorae* 12 g
E Jiao *Gelatinum Corii asini* 9 g

LIANG FU WAN 良附丸

Alpinia-Cyperus Pill
Gao Liang Jiang *Rhizoma Alpiniae officinari* 6 g
Xiang Fu *Rhizoma Cyperi rotundi* 6 g

LIANG GE SAN 凉膈散

Cooling the Diaphragm Powder
Da Huang *Radix et Rhizoma Rhei* 600 g
Mang Xiao *Mirabilitum* 600 g
Gan Cao *Radix Glycyrrhizae uralensis* 600 g
Huang Qin *Radix Scutellariae* 300 g
Shan Zhi Zi *Fructus Gardeniae jasminoidis* 300 g
Lian Qiao *Fructus Forsythiae suspensae* 1200 g
Bo He *Herba Menthae haplocalycis* 300 g

LIANG SHOU TANG 两收汤

Two Receiving Decoction
Bai Zhu *Rhizoma Atractylodis macrocephalae* 9 g
Ren Shen *Radix Ginseng* 9 g
Chuan Xiong *Radix Ligustici chuanxiong* 6 g
Shu Di Huang *Radix Rehmanniae glutinosae praeparata* 9 g
Shan Yao *Radix Dioscoreae oppositae* 6 g
Shan Zhu Yu *Fructus Corni officinalis* 4.5 g
Qian Shi *Semen Euryales ferocis* 6 g
Bian Dou *Semen Dolichoris lablab* 6 g
Ba Ji Tian *Radix Morindae officinalis* 6 g
Du Zhong *Cortex Eucommiae ulmoidis* 6 g
Bai Guo *Semen Ginkgo bilobae* 6 g

LING GAN WU WEI JIANG XIN TANG 苓甘五味姜辛

Poria-Glycyrrhiza-Schisandra-Zingiber-Asarum Decoction
Fu Ling *Sclerotium Poriae cocos* 12 g
Gan Cao *Radix Glycyrrhizae uralensis* 9 g
Gan Jiang *Rhizoma Zingiberis officinalis* 9 g
Xi Xin *Herba Asari cum radice* 9 g
Wu Wei Zi *Fructus Schisandrae chinensis* 6 g

LING GUI ZHU GAN TANG 苓桂术甘汤

Poria-Ramulus Cinnamomi-Atractylodes-Glycyrrhiza Decoction

Fu Ling *Sclerotium Poriae cocos* 12 g
Gui Zhi *Ramulus Cinnamomi cassiae* 9 g
Bai Zhu *Rhizoma Atractylodis macrocephalae* 6 g
Zhi Gan Cao *Radix Glycyrrhizae uralensis praeparata* 3 g

LING JIAO GOU TENG TANG 羚角钩藤汤

Cornu Antelopis-Uncaria Decoction
Ling Yang Jiao *Cornu Antelopis* 4.5 g
Gou Teng *Ramulus Uncariae* 9 g
Sang Ye *Folium Mori albae* 6 g
Ju Hua *Flos Chrysanthemi morifolii* 9 g
Bai Shao *Radix Paeoniae lactiflorae* 9 g
Sheng Di Huang *Radix Rehmanniae glutinosae* 15 g
Fu Shen *Sclerotium Poriae cocos pararadicis* 9 g
Chuan Bei Mu *Bulbus Fritillariae cirrhosae* 12 g
Zhu Ru *Caulis Bambusae in Taenis* 15 g
Gan Cao *Radix Glycyrrhizae uralensis* 2.5 g

LIU JUN ZI TANG 六君子汤

Six Gentlemen Decoction
Ren Shen *Radix Ginseng* 3 g
Bai Zhu *Rhizoma Atractylodis macrocephalae* 4.5 g
Fu Ling *Sclerotium Poriae cocos* 3 g
Zhi Gan Cao *Radix Glycyrrhizae uralensis praeparata* 3 g
Chen Pi *Pericarpium Citri reticulatae* 3 g
Ban Xia *Rhizoma Pinelliae ternatae* 4.5 g

LIU WEI DI HUANG WAN 六味地黄丸

Six-Ingredient Rehmannia Pill
Shu Di Huang *Radix Rehmanniae glutinosae praeparata* 24 g
Shan Zhu Yu *Fructus Corni officinalis* 12 g
Shan Yao *Radix Dioscoreae oppositae* 12 g
Ze Xie *Rhizoma Alismatis orientalis* 9 g
Mu Dan Pi *Cortex Moutan radicis* 9 g
Fu Ling *Sclerotium Poriae cocos* 9 g

LONG CHI QING HUN TANG 龙齿清魂汤

Dens Draconis Clearing the Ethereal Soul Decoction
Long Chi *Dens Draconis* 9 g
Ren Shen *Radix Ginseng* 4.5 g
Dang Gui *Radix Angelicae sinensis* 9 g
Yuan Zhi *Radix Polygalae tenuifoliae* 4.5 g
Mai Men Dong *Tuber Ophiopogonis japonici* 9 g

Gui Xin *Cortex Cinnamomi cassiae* 3 g
Fu Shen *Sclerotium Poriae cocos pararadicis* 6 g
Xi Xin *Herba cum Radice Asari* 1.5 g

LONG DAN BI YUAN FANG 龙胆鼻渊方

Gentiana 'Nose Pool' Formula
Long Dan Cao *Radix Gentianae scabrae* 6 g
Huang Qin *Radix Scutellariae baicalensis* 6 g
Xia Ku Cao *Spica Prunellae vulgaris* 6 g
Yu Xing Cao *Herba cum Radice Houttuyniae cordatae* 6 g
Ju Hua *Flos Chrysanthemi morifolii* 6 g
Bai Zhi *Radix Angelicae dahuricae* 6 g
Cang Er Zi *Fructus Xanthii sibirici* 6 g
Huo Xiang *Herba Agastachis seu Pogostemi* 4.5 g
Yi Yi Ren *Semen Coicis lachryma jobi* 12 g
Che Qian Zi *Semen Plantaginis* 6 g
Jie Geng *Radix Platycodi grandiflori* 3 g

LONG DAN XIE GAN TANG 龙胆泻肝汤

Gentiana Draining the Liver Decoction
Long Dan Cao *Radix Gentianae scabrae* 6 g
Huang Qin *Radix Scutellariae baicalensis* 9 g
Shan Zhi Zi *Fructus Gardeniae jasminoidis* 9 g
Ze Xie *Rhizoma Alismatis orientalis* 9 g
Mu Tong *Caulis Mutong* 9 g
Che Qian Zi *Semen Plantaginis* 9 g
Sheng Di Huang *Radix Rehmanniae glutinosae* 12 g
Dang Gui *Radix Angelicae sinensis* 9 g
Chai Hu *Radix Bupleuri* 9 g
Gan Cao *Radix Glycyrrhizae uralensis* 3 g

LU JIAO TU SI ZI WAN 鹿角菟丝子丸

Cornus Cervi-Cuscuta Pill
Lu Jiao Shuang *Cornu Cervi degelatinatum* 9 g
Tu Si Zi *Semen Cuscutae chinensis* 9 g
Mu Li *Concha Ostreae* 12 g
Bai Zhu *Rhizoma Atractylodis macrocephalae* 6 g
Du Zhong *Cortex Eucommiae ulmoidis* 6 g
Lian Xu *Semen Nelumbinis nuciferae* 6 g
Bai Guo *Semen Ginkgo bilobae* 6 g
Qian Shi *Semen Euryales ferocis* 6 g

MA HUANG TANG 麻黄汤

Ephedra Decoction
Ma Huang *Herba Ephedrae* 9 g

Gui Zhi *Ramulus Cinnamomi cassiae* 6 g
Xing Ren *Semen Pruni armeniacae* 9 g
Zhi Gan Cao *Radix Glycyrrhizae uralensis praeparata* 3 g

MA XING SHI GAN TANG 麻杏石甘汤

Ephedra-Prunus-Gypsum-Glycyrrhiza Decoction
Ma Huang *Herba Ephedrae* 12 g
Shi Gao *Gypsum fibrosum* 48 g
Xing Ren *Semen Pruni armeniacae* 18 g
Zhi Gan Cao *Radix Glycyrrhizae uralensis praeparata* 6 g

MA ZI REN WAN 麻子仁丸

Cannabis Pill
Huo Ma Ren *Semen Cannabis sativae* 9 g
Da Huang *Radix et Rhizoma Rhei* 6 g
Xing Ren *Semen Pruni armeniacae* 4.5 g
Zhi Shi *Fructus Citri aurantii immaturus* 6 g
Hou Po *Cortex Magnoliae officinalis* 4.5 g
Bai Shao *Radix Paeoniae lactiflorae* 4.5 g

MAI MEN DONG TANG 麦门冬汤

Ophiopogon Decoction
Mai Men Dong *Tuber Ophiopogonis japonici* 60 g
Ban Xia *Rhizoma Pinelliae ternatae* 9 g
Ren Shen *Radix Ginseng* 6 g
Zhi Gan Cao *Radix Glycyrrhizae uralensis praeparata* 4 g
Geng Mi *Semen Oryzae sativae* 6 g
Da Zao *Fructus Ziziphi jujubae* 3 dates

MU XIANG LIU QI YIN 木香流气饮

Aucklandia Flowing Qi Decoction
Mu Xiang *Radix Aucklandiae lappae* 6 g
Ban Xia *Rhizoma Pinelliae ternatae* 6 g
Chen Pi *Pericarpium Citri reticulatae* 3 g
Hou Po *Cortex Magnoliae officinalis* 4.5 g
Qing Pi *Pericarpium Citri reticulatae viride* 3 g
Gan Cao *Radix Glycyrrhizae uralensis* 3 g
Xiang Fu *Rhizoma Cyperi rotundi* 6 g
Zi Su Ye *Folium Perillae frutescentis* 3 g
Ren Shen *Radix Ginseng* 6 g
Fu Ling *Sclerotium Poriae cocos* 6 g
Mu Gua *Fructus Chaenomelis lagenariae* 3 g
Shi Chang Pu *Rhizoma Acori graminei* 3 g

Bai Zhu *Rhizoma Atractylodis macrocephalae* 4.5 g
Bai Zhi *Radix Angelicae dahuricae* 3 g
Mai Men Dong *Tuber Ophiopogonis japonici* 6 g
Cao Guo *Fructus Amomi tsaoko* 3 g
Rou Gui *Cortex Cinnamomi cassiae* 1.5 g
E Zhu *Rhizoma Curcumae zedoariae* 3 g
Da Fu Pi *Pericarpium Arecae catechu* 3 g
Ding Xiang *Flos Caryophylli* 3 g
Bing Lang *Semen Arecae catechu* 3 g
Huo Xiang *Herba Agastachis seu Pogostemi* 3 g
Mu Tong *Caulis Mutong* 1.5 g

NEI BU WAN 内补丸

Inner Tonification Pill
Lu Rong *Cornu Cervi parvum* 3 g
Tu Si Zi *Semen Cuscutae chinensis* 6 g
Rou Cong Rong *Herba Cistanchis deserticolae* 6 g
Sha Yuan Zi *Semen Astragali complanati* 6 g
Huang Qi *Radix Astragali membranacei* 6 g
Sang Piao Xiao *Ootheca Mantidis* 6 g
Rou Gui *Cortex Cinnamomi cassiae* 2 g
Fu Zi *Radix lateralis Aconiti carmichaeli praeparata* 2 g
Bai Ji Li *Fructus Tribuli terrestris* 3 g
Zi Wan *Radix Asteris tatarici* 3 g

NUAN GAN JIAN 暖肝煎

Warming the Liver Decoction
Dang Gui *Radix Angelicae sinensis* 6 g
Gou Qi Zi *Fructus Lycii chinensis* 9 g
Xiao Hui Xiang *Fructus Foeniculi vulgaris* 6 g
Rou Gui *Cortex Cinnamomi cassiae* 3 g
Wu Yao *Radix Linderae strychnifoliae* 6 g
Chen Xiang *Lignum Aquilariae* 3 g
Fu Ling *Sclerotium Poriae cocos* 6 g
Sheng Jiang *Rhizoma Zingiberis officinalis recens* 3 slices

PING WEI SAN 平胃散

Balancing the Stomach Powder
Cang Zhu *Rhizoma Atractylodis lanceae* 12 g
Hou Po *Cortex Magnoliae officinalis* 9 g
Chen Pi *Pericarpium Citri reticulatae* 9 g
Zhi Gan Cao *Radix Glycyrrhizae uralensis praeparata* 3 g

QI JU DI HUANG WAN 杞菊地黄丸

Lycium-Chrysanthemum-Rehmannia Pill
Gou Qi Zi *Fructus Lycii chinensis* 6 g
Ju Hua *Flos Chrysanthemi morifolii* 6 g
Shu Di Huang *Radix Rehmanniae glutinosae praeparata* 24 g
Shan Zhu Yu *Fructus Corni officinalis* 12 g
Shan Yao *Radix Dioscoreae oppositae* 12 g
Ze Xie *Rhizoma Alismatis orientalis* 9 g
Mu Dan Pi *Cortex Moutan radicis* 9 g
Fu Ling *Sclerotium Poriae cocos* 9 g

QING E WAN 青娥丸

Young Maiden Pill (Dosages for batch of pills)
(Jiang Zhi Chao) Du Zhong *Cortex Eucommiae ulmoidis* (fried in ginger-juice) 480 g
(Jiu Chao) Bu Gu Zhi *Fructus et Semen Psoraleae corydifoliae* (fried in wine) 240 g
Hu Tao Rou *Semen Juglandis regiae* 20 g

QING GAN TOU DING TANG 清肝头顶汤

Clearing the Liver Penetrating the Vertex Decoction
Ling Yang Jiao *Cornu Antelopis* 6 g
Shi Jue Ming *Concha Haliotidis* 9 g
Chan Tui *Periostracum Cicadae* 6 g
Sang Ye *Folium Mori albae* 4.5 g
Bo He *Herba Menthae haplocalycis* 3 g
Xia Ku Cao *Spica Prunellae vulgaris* 6 g
Mu Dan Pi *Cortex Moutan radicis* 6 g
Xuan Shen *Radix Scrophulariae ningpoensis* 6 g
Jie Geng *Radix Platycodi grandiflori* 3 g
Chen Pi *Pericarpium Citri reticulatae* 4.5 g

QING GU SAN 清骨散

Clearing the Bones Powder
Yin Chai Hu *Radix Stellariae dichotomae* 4.5 g
Zhi Mu *Radix Anemarrhenae asphodeloidis* 3 g
Hu Huang Lian *Rhizoma Picrorhizae* 3 g
Di Gu Pi *Cortex Lycii radicis* 3 g
Qing Hao *Herba Artemisiae apiaceae* 3 g
Qin Jiao *Radix Gentianae macrophyllae* 3 g
Bie Jia *Carapax Amydae sinensis* 3 g
Gan Cao *Radix Glycyrrhizae uralensis* 1.5 g

QING HAI WAN 清海丸

Clearing the Sea Pill
Shu Di Huang *Radix Rehmanniae glutinosae praeparata* 9 g
Bai Zhu *Rhizoma Atractylodis macrocephalae* 6 g
Bai Shao *Radix Paeoniae lactiflorae* 6 g
Xuan Shen *Radix Scrophulariae ningpoensis* 6 g
Sang Ye *Folium Mori albae* 3 g
Shan Zhu Yu *Fructus Corni officinalis* 6 g
Shan Yao *Radix Dioscoreae oppositae* 6 g
Mu Dan Pi *Cortex Moutan radicis* 6 g
Di Gu Pi *Cortex Lycii radicis* 6 g
Bei Sha Shen *Radix Glehniae* 6 g
Shi Hu *Herba Dendrobii* 6 g
Mai Men Dong *Tuber Ophiopogonis japonici* 6 g
Wu Wei Zi *Fructus Schisandrae chinensis* 4.5 g
Long Gu *Os Draconis* 9 g

QING HAO BIE JIA TANG 青蒿鳖甲汤

Artemisia Annua-Carapax Amydae Decoction
Bie Jia *Carapax Amydae sinensis* 15 g
Qing Hao *Herba Artemisiae apiaceae* 6 g
Sheng Di Huang *Radix Rehmanniae glutinosae* 12 g
Zhi Mu *Radix Anemarrhenae asphodeloidis* 6 g
Mu Dan Pi *Cortex Moutan radicis* 9 g

QING JING SAN 清经散

Clearing the Menses Powder
Mu Dan Pi *Cortex Moutan radicis* 6 g
Bai Shao *Radix Paeoniae lactiflorae* 6 g
Shu Di Huang *Radix Rehmanniae glutinosae praeparata* 6 g
Di Gu Pi *Cortex Lycii radicis* 15 g
Qing Hao *Herba Artemisiae apiaceae* 6 g
Fu Ling *Sclerotium Poriae cocos* 3 g
Huang Bo *Cortex Phellodendri* 1.5 g

QING LUO YIN 清络饮

Clearing the Connecting Channels Decoction
Xian Jin Yin Hua *Flos Lonicerae japonicae recens* 6 g
Xian Bian Dou Hua *Flos Dolichoris lablab recens* 6 g
Xi Gua Shuang *Mirabilitum Praeparata citrulli* 6 g
Si Gua Pi *Pericarpium Luffae acuntagulae* 6 g
Xian He Ye *Folium Nelumbinis nuciferae recens* 6 g
Xian Zhu Ye *Herba Lophateri gracilis recens* 6 g

QING QI HUA TAN TANG 清气化痰汤

Clearing Qi and Resolving Phlegm Decoction
Dan Nan Xing *Pulvis Arisaemae cum felle bovis* 6 g
Ban Xia *Rhizoma Pinelliae ternatae* 6 g
Gua Lou Ren *Semen Trichosanthis* 6 g
Huang Qin *Radix Scutellariae baicalensis* 4.5 g
Chen Pi *Pericarpium Citri reticulatae* 3 g
Xing Ren *Semen Pruni armeniacae* 4.5 g
Zhi Shi *Fructus Citri aurantii immaturus* 4.5 g
Fu Ling *Sclerotium Poriae cocos* 6 g

QING RE AN TAI YIN 清热安胎饮

Clearing Heat and Calming the Fetus Decoction
Huang Lian *Rhizoma Coptidis* 3 g
Huang Qin *Radix Scutellariae baicalensis* 6 g
Ce Bai Ye *Cacumen Biotae orientalis* 6 g
Chun Gen Bai Pi *Cortex Ailanthi altissimae* 6 g
E Jiao *Gelatinum Corii Asini* 6 g
Shan Yao *Radix Dioscoreae oppositae* 6 g

QING RE GU JING TANG 清热固经汤

Clearing Heat and Consolidating the Menses Decoction
Huang Qin *Radix Scutellariae baicalensis* 4.5 g
Shan Zhi Zi *Fructus Gardeniae jasminoidis* (charred) 6 g
Sheng Di Huang *Radix Rehmanniae glutinosae* 9 g
Di Gu Pi *Cortex Lycii radicis* 6 g
Di Yu *Radix Sanguisorbae officinalis* 6 g
E Jiao *Gelatinum Corii asini* 6 g
Ou Jie *Nodus Nelumbinis nuciferae rhizomatis* 6 g
Zong Lu Zi *Fructus Trachycarpi fortunei* 4.5 g
Gui Ban *Plastrum Testudinis* (toasted) 12 g
Mu Li *Concha Ostreae* 12 g
Gan Cao *Radix Glycyrrhizae uralensis* 3 g

QING RE TIAO XUE TANG 清热调血汤

Clearing Heat and Regulating Blood Decoction
Mu Dan Pi *Cortex Moutan radicis* 6 g
Sheng Di Huang *Radix Rehmanniae glutinosae* 9 g
Huang Lian *Rhizoma Coptidis* 4.5 g
Dang Gui *Radix Angelicae sinensis* 9 g
Bai Shao *Radix Paeoniae lactiflorae* 9 g
Chuan Xiong *Radix Ligustici chuanxiong* 6 g
Hong Hua *Flos Carthami tinctorii* 6 g
Tao Ren *Semen Persicae* 6 g

E Zhu *Rhizoma Curcumae zedoariae* 6 g
Xiang Fu *Rhizoma Cyperi rotundi* 6 g
Yan Hu Suo *Rhizoma Corydalis yanhusuo* 6 g

QING WEI SAN 清胃散

Clearing the Stomach Powder
Huang Lian *Rhizoma Coptidis* 1.8 g
Sheng Ma *Rhizoma Cimicifugae* 3 g
Mu Dan Pi *Cortex Moutan radicis* 1.5 g
Sheng Di Huang *Radix Rehmanniae glutinosae* 0.9 g
Dang Gui *Radix Angelicae sinensis* 0.9 g

QING YING TANG 清营汤

Clearing Nutritive-Qi Decoction
Shui Niu Jiao *Cornu Bufali* 18 g
Xuan Shen *Radix Scrophulariae ningpoensis* 9 g
Sheng Di Huang *Radix Rehmanniae glutinosae* 15 g
Mai Men Dong *Tuber Ophiopogonis japonici* 9 g
Jin Yin Hua *Flos Lonicerae japonicae* 9 g
Lian Qiao *Fructus Forsythiae suspensae* 6 g
Huang Lian *Rhizoma Coptidis* 4.5 g
Zhu Ye *Herba Lophatheri gracilis* 3 g
Dan Shen *Radix Salviae miltiorrhizae* 6 g

QING ZAO JIU FEI TANG 清燥救肺汤

Clearing Dryness and Rescuing the Lungs Decoction
Sang Ye *Folium Mori albae* 9 g
Shi Gao *Gypsum fibrosum* 7.5 g
Mai Men Dong *Tuber Ophiopogonis japonici* 3.6 g
E Jiao *Gelatinum Corii asini* 2.4 g
Hei Zhi Ma *Semen Sesami indici* 3 g
Xing Ren *Semen Pruni armeniacae* 2.1 g
Pi Pa Ye *Folium Eriobotryae japonicae* 3 g
Ren Shen *Radix Ginseng* 2.1 g
Gan Cao *Radix Glycyrrhizae uralensis* 3 g

QING ZAO RUN CHANG TANG 清燥润肠汤

Clearing Dryness and Moistening the Intestines Decoction
Sheng Di Huang *Radix Rehmanniae glutinosae* 9 g
Shu Di Huang *Radix Rehmannia glutinosae praeparata* 6 g
Dang Gui *Radix Angelicae sinensis* 6 g
Huo Ma Ren *Semen Cannabis sativae* 4.5 g

Gua Lou Ren *Semen Trichosanthis* 6 g
Yu Li Ren *Semen Pruni* 6 g
Shi Hu *Herba Dendrobi* 9 g
Zhi Ke *Fructus Citri aurantii* 3 g
Qing Pi *Pericarpium Citri reticulatae viride* 3 g
Jin Ju *Fructus Fortunaellae margaritae* 4.5 g

QU TIAO TANG 去蛔汤

Expelling Tapeworms Decoction
Nan Guan Zi *Semen Cucurbitae moschatae* 60 g
Bing Lang *Semen Arecae catechu* 30 g

REN SHEN BU FEI TANG 人参补肺汤

Ginseng Tonifying the Lungs Decoction
Ren Shen *Radix Ginseng* 9 g
Huang Qi *Radix Astragali membranacei* 24 g
Shu Di Huang *Radix Rehmanniae glutinosae praeparata* 24 g
Wu Wei Zi *Fructus Schisandrae chinensis* 6 g
Zi Wan *Radix Asteris tatarici* 6 g
Sang Bai Pi *Cortex Mori albae radicis* 6 g

ROU FU BAO YUAN TANG 肉附保脉汤

Cinnamomum-Aconitum Preserving the Source Decoction
Rou Gui *Cortex Cinnamomi cassiae* 1.5 g
Fu Zi *Radix lateralis Aconiti carmichaeli praeparata* 3 g
Huang Qi *Radix Astragali membranacei* 6 g
Ren Shen *Radix Ginseng* 6 g
Zhi Gan Cao *Radix Glycyrrhizae uralensis praeparata* 3 g

SAN JIA FU MAI TANG 三甲复脉汤

Three Carapaces Restoring the Pulse Decoction
Zhi Gan Cao *Radix Glycyrrhizae uralensis praeparata* 18 g
Sheng Di Huang *Radix Rehmanniae glutinosae* 18 g
Bai Shao *Radix Paeoniae lactiflorae* 18 g
Mai Men Dong *Tuber Ophiopogonis japonici* 15 g
Huo Ma Ren *Semen Cannabis sativae* 9 g
E Jiao *Gelatinum Corii asini* 9 g
Mu Li *Concha Ostreae* 15 g
Bie Jia *Carapax Amydae sinensis* 24 g
Gui Ban *Plastrum Testudinis* 30 g

SAN MIAO HONG TENG TANG 三妙红藤汤

Three Wonderful Sargentodoxa Decoction
Cang Zhu *Rhizoma Atractylodis* 6 g
Huang Bo *Cortex Phellodendri* 6 g
Yi Yi Ren *Semen Coicis lachryma-jobi* 10 g
Hong Teng *Caulis Sargentodoxae cuneatae* 6 g
Xiao Ji *Herba Cephalanoplos* 6 g
Da Ji *Herba seu Radix Cirsii japonici* 6 g
Xian He Cao *Herba Agrimoniae pilosulae* 6 g
Yi Mu Cao *Herba Leonuri heterophylli* 6 g
Xia Ku Cao *Spica Prunellae vulgaris* 6 g
Xiang Fu *Rhizoma Cyperi rotundi* 6 g
Bai Jiang Cao *Herba cum Radice Patriniae* 6 g

SAN REN TANG 三仁汤

Three Seeds Decoction
Xing Ren *Semen Pruni armeniacae* 15 g
Hou Po *Cortex Magnoliae officinalis* 6 g
Hua Shi *Talcum* 18 g
Tong Cao *Medulla Tetrapanacis papyriferi* 6 g
Bai Dou Kou *Fructus Amomi kravanh* 6 g
Zhu Ye *Herba Lophatheri gracilis* 6 g
Yi Yi Ren *Semen Coicis lachryma jobi* 18 g
Ban Xia *Rhizoma Pinelliae ternatae* 9 g

SAN ZI YANG QIN TANG 三子养亲汤

Three-Seed Nourishing the Ancestors Decoction
Bai Jie Zi *Semen Sinapis albae* 6 g
Su Zi *Fructus Perillae frutescentis* 6 g
Lai Fu Zi *Semen Raphani sativi* 6 g

SANG JU YIN 桑菊饮

Morus-Chrysanthemum Decoction
Sang Ye *Folium Mori albae* 7.5 g
Ju Hua *Flos Chrysanthemi morifolii* 3 g
Lian Qiao *Fructus Forsythiae suspensae* 4.5 g
Bo He *Herba Menthae haplocalycis* 2.4 g
Jie Geng *Radix Platycodi grandiflori* 6 g
Xing Ren *Semen Pruni armeniacae* 6 g
Lu Gen *Rhizoma Phragmitis communis* 6 g
Gan Cao *Radix Glycyrrhizae uralensis* 3 g

SANG PIAO XIAO SAN 桑螵蛸散

Ootheca Mantidis Powder
Sang Piao Xiao *Ootheca Mantidis* 9 g
Long Gu *Os Draconis* 12 g
Ren Shen *Radix Ginseng* 9 g
Fu Shen *Sclerotium Poriae cocos paradicis* 9 g
Yuan Zhi *Radix Polygalae tenuifoliae* 3 g
Shi Chang Pu *Rhizoma Acori graminei* 6 g
Zhi Gui Ban *Plastrum Testudinis* (honey-fried) 9 g
Dang Gui *Radix Angelicae sinensis* 6 g

SANG XING TANG 桑杏汤

Morus-Prunus Decoction
Sang Ye *Folium Mori albae* 3 g
Shan Zhi Zi *Fructus Gardeniae jasminoidis* 3 g
Dan Dou Chi *Semen Sojae praeparatum* 3 g
Xing Ren *Semen Pruni armeniacae* 4.5 g
Zhe Bei Mu *Bulbus Fritillariae thunbergii* 3 g
Nan Sha Shen *Radix Adenophorae* 6 g
Li Pi *Fructus Pyri* 3 g

SHA SHEN MAI DONG TANG 沙参麦冬汤

Glehnia-Ophiopogon Decoction
Sha Shen *Radix Adenophorae seu Glehniae* 9 g
Mai Men Dong *Tuber Ophiopogonis japonici* 9 g
Yu Zhu *Rhizoma Poligonati odorati* 6 g
Sang Ye *Folium Mori albae* 4.5 g
Tian Hua Fen *Radix Trichosanthis kirilowii* 4.5 g
Bian Dou *Semen Dolichoris lablab* 4.5 g
Gan Cao *Radix Glycyrrhizae uralensis* 3 g

SHAO FU ZHU YU TANG 少腹逐瘀汤

Lower Abdomen Eliminating Stasis Decoction
Xiao Hui Xiang *Fructus Foeniculi vulgaris* 6 g
Gan Jiang *Rhizoma Zingiberis officinalis* 2 g
Rou Gui *Cortex Cinnamomi cassiae* 1.5 g
Yan Hu Suo *Rhizoma Corydalis yanhusuo* 6 g
Mo Yao *Myrrha* 6 g
Pu Huang *Pollen Typhae* 6 g
Wu Ling Zhi *Excrementum Trogopteri* 4.5 g
Dang Gui *Radix Angelicae sinensis* 9 g
Chuan Xiong *Radix Ligustici chuanxiong* 4.5 g
Chi Shao Yao *Radix Paeoniae rubrae* 6 g

SHAO YAO TANG 少药汤

Paeonia Decoction
Bai Shao *Radix Paeoniae lactiflorae* 30 g
Dang Gui *Radix Angelicae sinensis* 15 g

Gan Cao *Radix Glycyrrhizae uralensis* 6 g
Mu Xiang *Radix Aucklandiae lappae* 6 g
Bing Lang *Semen Arecae catechu* 6 g
Huang Lian *Rhizoma Coptidis* 15 g
Huang Qin *Radix Scutellariae baicalensis* 15 g
Da Huang *Radix et Rhizoma Rhei* 9 g
Guan Gui *Cortex Cinnamomi loureiroi* 7.5 g

SHE GAN MA HUANG TANG 射干麻黄汤

Belamcanda-Ephedra Decoction
She Gan *Rhizoma Belamcandae chinensis* 9 g
Ma Huang *Herba Ephedrae* 12 g
Zi Wan *Radix Asteris tatarici* 9 g
Kuan Dong Hua *Flos Tussilaginis farfarae* 9 g
Ban Xia *Rhizoma Pinelliae ternatae* 9 g
Xi Xin *Herba cum Radice Asari* 9 g
Wu Wei Zi *Fructus Schisandrae chinensis* 3 g
Sheng Jiang *Rhizoma Zingiberis officinalis recens* 12 g
Da Zao *Fructus Zizyphi jujubae* 3 pieces

SHEN FU TANG 参附汤

Ginseng-Aconitum Decoction
Ren Shen *Radix Ginseng* 30 g
Fu Zi *Radix lateralis Aconiti carmichaeli praeparata* 15 g

SHEN GE SAN 参蛤散

Ginseng-Gecko Powder
Ren Shen *Radix Ginseng* 12 g
Ge Jie *Gecko* 12 g

SHEN LING BAI ZHU SAN 参苓白术散

Ginseng-Poria-Atractylodes Powder
Ren Shen *Radix Ginseng* 10 g
Bai Zhu *Rhizoma Atractylodis macrocephalae* 10 g
Fu Ling *Sclerotium Poriae cocos* 10 g
Zhi Gan Cao *Radix Glycyrrhizae uralensis praeparata* 10 g
Shan Yao *Radix Dioscoreae oppositae* 10 g
Bian Dou *Semen Dolichoris lablab* 7.5 g
Lian Zi *Semen Nelumbinis nuciferae* 5 g
Yi Yi Ren *Semen Coicis lachryma jobi* 5 g
Sha Ren *Fructus seu Semen Amomi* 5 g
Jie Geng *Radix Platycodi grandiflori* 5 g

SHEN QI SI WU TANG 参芪四物汤

Ginseng-Astragalus Four Substances Decoction
Ren Shen *Radix Ginseng* 9 g
Huang Qi *Radix Astragali membranacei* 9 g
Dang Gui *Radix Angelicae sinensis* 6 g
Bai Shao *Radix Paeoniae lactiflorae* 9 g
Shu Du Huang *Radix Rehmanniae glutinosae praeparata* 6 g
Chuan Xiong *Radix Ligustici chuanxiong* 6 g

SHENG HUA TANG 生化汤

Generating and Resolving Decoction
Dang Gui *Radix Angelicae sinensis* 24 g
Chuan Xiong *Radix Ligustici chuanxiong* 9 g
Tao Ren *Semen Persicae* 6 g
Pao Jiang *Rhizoma Zingiberis officinalis recens* (fried) 1.5 g
Zhi Gan Cao *Radix Glycyrrhizae uralensis praeparata* 1.5 g

SHENG MAI SAN 生脉散

Generating the Pulse Powder
Ren Shen *Radix Ginseng* 1.5 g
Mai Men Dong *Tuber Ophiopogonis japonici* 1.5 g
Wu Wei Zi *Fructus Schisandrae chinensis* 7 seeds

SHENG YANG TANG 升阳汤

Raising the Yang Decoction
Zhi Gan Cao *Radix Glycyrrhizae uralensis praeparata* 6 g
Ma Huang *Herba Ephedrae* 12 g
Fang Feng *Radix Ledebouriellae divaricatae* 12 g
Qiang Huo *Rhizoma et Radix Notopterygii* 18 g

SHENG YU TANG 圣愈汤

Sage Healing Decoction
Sheng Di Huang *Radix Rehmanniae glutinosae* 9 g
Shu Di Huang *Radix Rehmanniae glutinosae praeparata* 9 g
Chuan Xiong *Radix Ligustici chuanxiong* 9 g
Ren Shen *Radix Ginseng* 9 g
Dang Gui *Radix Angelicae sinensis* 1.5 g
Huang Qi *Radix Astragali membranacei* 1.5 g

SHI PI YIN 实脾饮

Bolster the Spleen Decoction
Fu Zi *Radix lateralis Aconiti carmichaeli praeparata* 6 g
Gan Jiang *Rhizoma Zingiberis officinalis* 6 g
Fu Ling *Sclerotium Poriae cocos* 6 g
Bai Zhu *Rhizoma Atractylodis macrocephalae* 6 g
Mu Gua *Fructus Chaenomelis lagenariae* 6 g
Hou Po *Cortex Magnoliae officinalis* 6 g
Mu Xiang *Radix Aucklandiae lappae* 6 g
Da Fu Pi *Pericarpium Arecae catechu* 6 g
Cao Guo *Fructus Amomi tsaoko* 6 g
Zhi Gan Cao *Radix Glycyrrhizae uralensis praeparata* 3 g
Da Zao *Fructus Ziziphi jujubae* 3 dates

SHI XIAO SAN 失笑散

Breaking into a Smile Powder
Pu Huang *Pollen Typhae* 6 g
Wu Ling Zhi *Excrementum Trogopteri* 6 g

SHOU TAI WAN 寿胎丸

Fetus Longevity Pill
Tu Si Zi *Semen Cuscutae chinensis* 6 g
Sang Ji Sheng *Ramulus Sangjisheng* 6 g
Xu Duan *Radix Dipsaci asperi* 6 g
E Jiao *Gelatinum Corii asini* 6 g

SI HAI SHU YU WAN 四海疏郁丸

Four Seas Soothe Stagnation Pill
Mu Xiang *Radix Aucklandiae lappae* 6 g
Chen Pi *Pericarpium Citri reticulatae* 3 g
Kun Bu *Thallus Algae* 6 g
Hai Dai *Zostera marina* 6 g
Hai Zao *Herba Sargassii* 6 g
Hai Piao Xiao *Os Sepiae* 6 g
Hai Ge Ke *Concha Cyclinae sinensis* 6 g

SI JUN ZI TANG 四君子汤

Four Gentlemen Decoction
Ren Shen *Radix Ginseng* 9 g
Bai Zhu *Rhizoma Atractylodis macrocephalae* 9 g
Fu Ling *Sclerotium Poriae cocos* 9 g
Zhi Gan Cao *Radix Glycyrrhizae uralensis praeparata* 3 g

SI MO TANG 四磨汤

Four Milled-Herb Decoction
Ren Shen *Radix Ginseng* 3 g
Bing Lang *Semen Arecae catechu* 9 g
Chen Xiang *Lignum Aquilariae* 3 g
Wu Yao *Radix Linderae strychnifoliae* 9 g

SI NI TANG 四逆汤

Four Rebellious Decoction
Fu Zi *Radix lateralis Aconiti carmichaeli praeparata* 6 g
Gan Jiang *Rhizoma Zingiberis officinalis* 4.5 g
Zhi Gan Cao *Radix Glycyrrhizae uralensis praeparata* 6 g

SI WU MA ZI REN WAN 四物麻子仁丸

Four Substances Cannabis Pill
Dang Gui *Radix Angelicae sinensis* 6 g
Chuan Xiong *Radix Ligustici chuanxiong* 3 g
Shu Di Huang *Radix Rehmanniae glutinosae* 6 g
Bai Shao *Radix Paeoniae lactiflorae* 6 g
Huo Ma Ren *Semen Cannabis sativae* 9 g
Da Huang *Radix et Rhizoma Rhei* 6 g
Xing Ren *Semen Pruni armeniacae* 4.5 g
Zhi Shi *Fructus Citri aurantii immaturus* 6 g
Hou Po *Cortex Magnoliae officinalis* 4.5 g
Bai Shao *Radix Paeoniae lactiflorae* 4.5 g

SI WU TANG 四物汤

Four Substances Decoction
Shu Di Huang *Radix Rehmanniae glutinosae praeparata* 9 g
Bai Shao *Radix Paeoniae lactiflorae* 9 g
Dang Gui *Radix Angelicae sinensis* 9 g
Chuan Xiong *Radix Ligustici chuanxiong* 3 g

SU HE XIANG WAN 苏合香丸

Styrax Pill (Dosages for batch of pills)
Su He Xiang *Styrax liquidis* 30 g
She Xiang *Secretio Moschus* 60 g
Bing Pian *Borneol* 30 g
An Xi Xiang *Benzoinum* 60 g
Mu Xiang *Radix Aucklandiae lappae* 60 g
Tan Xiang *Lignum Santali albi* 60 g
Chen Xiang *Lignum Aquilariae* 60 g
Ru Xiang *Gummi Olibanum* 30 g

Ding Xiang *Flos Caryophylli* 60 g
Xiang Fu *Rhizoma Cyperi rotundi* 60 g
Bi Ba *Fructus Piperis longi* 60 g
Xi Jiao *Cornu Rhinoceri* 60 g
Zhu Sha *Cinnabaris* 60 g
Bai Zhu *Rhizoma Atractylodis macrocephalae* 60 g
He Zi *Fructus Terminaliae chebulae* 60 g
Note: She Xiang, Xi Jiao and Zhu Sha are banned substances. She Xiang can be replaced by Shi Chang Pu *Rhizoma Acori graminei* and Xi Jiao by Shui Niu Jiao *Cornu Bubali*.

SU ZI JIANG QI TANG 苏子降气汤

Perilla-Seed Subduing Qi Decoction
Su Zi *Fructus Perillae frutescentis* 9 g
Ban Xia *Rhizoma Pinelliae ternatae* 9 g
Hou Po *Cortex Magnoliae officinalis* 6 g
Qian Hu *Radix Peucedani* 6 g
Rou Gui *Cortex Cinnamomi cassiae* 3 g
Dang Gui *Radix Angelicae sinensis* 6 g
Sheng Jiang *Rhizoma Zingiberis officinalis recens* 2 slices
Su Ye *Folium Perillae* 5 leaves
Zhi Gan Cao *Radix Glycyrrhizae uralensis praeparata* 6 g
Da Zao *Fructus Ziziphi jujubae* 1 date

SUO GONG ZHU YU TANG 缩宫逐瘀汤

Contracting the Uterus and Eliminating Stasis Decoction
Dang Gui *Radix Angelicae sinensis* 9 g
Chuan Xiong *Radix Ligustici chuanxiong* 6 g
Pu Huang *Pollen Typhae* 6 g
Wu Ling Zhi *Excrementum Trogopteri seu Pteromi* 6 g
Dang Shen *Radix Codonopsis pilosulae* 6 g
Zhi Ke *Fructus Citri aurantii* 4.5 g
Yi Mu Cao *Herba Leonuri heterophylli* 6 g

SUO QUAN WAN 缩泉丸

Contracting the Spring Pill
Wu Yao *Radix Linderae strychnifoliae* 9 g
Yi Zhi Ren *Fructus Alpiniae oxyphyllae* 9 g

TAO HE CHENG QI TANG 桃核承气汤

Prunus Conducting Qi Decoction
Tao Ren *Semen Persicae* 50 pieces

Da Huang *Radix et Rhizoma Rhei* 12 g
Gui Zhi *Ramulus Cinnamomi cassiae* 6 g
Mang Xiao *Mirabilitum* 6 g
Zhi Gan Cao *Radix Glycyrrhizae uralensis praeparata* 6 g

TAO HONG SI WU TANG 桃红四物汤

Persica-Carthamus Four Substances Decoction
Shu Di Huang *Radix Rehmanniae glutinosae praeparata* 12 g
Dang Gui *Radix Angelicae sinensis* 10 g
Bai Shao *Radix Paeoniae lactiflorae* 12 g
Chuan Xiong *Radix Ligustici chuanxiong* 8 g
Tao Ren *Semen Persicae* 6 g
Hong Hua *Flos Carthami tinctorii* 4 g

TIAN DI JIAN 天地煎

Heaven and Earth Decoction
Tian Men Dong *Tuber Asparagus cochinchinensis* 9 g
Shu Di Huang *Radix Rehmanniae glutinosae praeparata* 9 g

TIAN MA GOU TENG YIN 天麻钩藤饮

Gastrodia-Uncaria Decoction
Tian Ma *Rhizoma Gastrodiae elatae* 9 g
Gou Teng *Ramulus Uncariae* 9 g
Shi Jue Ming *Concha Haliotidis* 6 g
Sang Ji Sheng *Ramulus Loranthi* 9 g
Du Zhong *Radix Eucommiae ulmoidis* 9 g
Chuan Niu Xi *Radix Cyathulae* 9 g
Shan Zhi Zi *Fructus Gardeniae jasminoidis* 6 g
Huang Qin *Radix Scutellariae baicalensis* 9 g
Yi Mu Cao *Herba Leonori heterophylli* 9 g
Ye Jiao Teng *Caulis Polygoni multiflori* 9 g
Fu Shen *Sclerotium Poriae cocos pararadicis* 6 g

TIAN TAI WU YAO SAN 天台乌药散

Top-Quality Lindera Powder
Wu Yao *Radix Linderae strychnifoliae* 15 g
Mu Xiang *Radix Aucklandiae lappae* 15 g
Xiao Hui Xiang *Fructus Foeniculi vulgaris* 15 g
Qing Pi *Pericarpium Citri reticulatae viride* 15 g
Gao Liang Jiang *Rhizoma Alpiniae officinari* 15 g
Bing Lang *Semen Arecae catechu* 2 pieces
Jin Ling Zi *Fructus Meliae toosendan* 10 pieces

TIAN WANG BU XIN DAN 天王补心丹

Heavenly Emperor Tonifying the Heart Pill
Sheng Di Huang *Radix Rehmanniae glutinosae* 12 g
Xuan Shen *Radix Scrophulariae ningpoensis* 6 g
Mai Men Dong *Tuber Ophiopogonis japonici* 6 g
Tian Men Dong *Tuber Asparagi cochinchinensis* 6 g
Ren Shen *Radix Ginseng* 6 g
Fu Ling *Sclerotium Poriae cocos* 6 g
Wu Wei Zi *Fructus Schisandrae chinensis* 6 g
Dang Gui *Radix Angelicae sinensis* 6 g
Dan Shen *Radix Salviae miltiorrhizae* 6 g
Bai Zi Ren *Semen Biotae orientalis* 6 g
Suan Zao Ren *Semen Ziziphi spinosae* 6 g
Yuan Zhi *Radix Polygalae tenuifoliae* 6 g
Jie Geng *Radix Platycodi grandiflori* 3 g

TIAO WEI CHENG QI TANG 调胃承气汤

Regulating the Stomach Conducting Qi Decoction
Da Huang *Radix et Rhizoma Rhei* 12 g
Mang Xiao *Mirabilitum* 9 g
Zhi Gan Cao *Radix Glycyrrhizae uralensis praeparata* 6 g

TIAO ZHENG SAN 调正散

Regulating the Upright Powder
Bai Zhu *Rhizoma Atractylodis macrocephalae* 6 g
Cang Zhu *Rhizoma Atractylodis* 6 g
Fu Ling *Sclerotium Poriae cocos* 6 g
Chen Pi *Pericarpium Citri reticulatae* 3 g
Zhe Bei Mu *Bulbus Fritillariae Thunbergii* 6 g
Yi Yi Ren *Semen Coicis lachryma-jobi* 12 g

TONG YOU TANG 通幽汤

Penetrating the Depth Decoction
Zhi Gan Cao *Radix Glycyrrhizae uralensis praeparata* 1.5 g
Hong Hua *Flos Carthami tinctorii* 1.5 g
Sheng Di Huang *Radix Rehmanniae glutinosae* 3 g
Shu Di Huang *Radix Rehmannia glutinosae praeparata* 3 g
Sheng Ma *Rhizoma Cimicifugae* 6 g
Tao Ren *Semen Persicae* 6 g
Dang Gui *Radix Angelicae sinensis* 6 g
Bing Lang *Semen Arecae catechu* 3 g

TU SI ZI WAN 菟丝子丸

Cuscuta Pill
Tu Si Zi *Semen Cuscutae chinensis* 6 g
Lu Rong *Cornu Cervi parvum* 3 g
Rou Cong Rong *Herba Cistanches deserticolae* 6 g
Shan Yao *Radix Dioscoreae oppositae* 3 g
Fu Zi *Radix lateralis Aconiti carmichaeli praeparata* 3 g
Wu Yao *Radix Linderae strychnifoliae* 3 g
Wu Wei Zi *Fructus Schisandrae chinensis* 3 g
Sang Piao Xiao *Ootheca Mantidis* 3 g
Yi Zhi Ren *Fructus Alpiniae oxyphyllae* 3 g
Duan Mu Li *Concha Ostreae* (calcined) 6 g
Ji Nei Jin *Endothelium cornei Gigeriae galli* 1.5 g

WEI LING SAN 胃苓散

Stomach Poria Powder
Ze Xie *Rhizoma Alismatis orientalis* 4 g
Fu Ling *Sclerotium Poriae cocos* 2.3 g
Zhu Ling *Sclerotium Polypori umbellati* 2.3 g
Bai Zhu *Rhizoma Atractylodis macrocephalae* 2.3 g
Gui Zhi *Ramulus Cinnamomi cassiae* 1.5 g
Cang Zhu *Rhizoma Atractylodis lanceae* 12 g
Hou Po *Cortex Magnoliae officinalis* 9 g
Chen Pi *Pericarpium Citri reticulatae* 9 g
Zhi Gan Cao *Radix Glycyrrhizae uralensis praeparata* 3 g

WEI LING TANG 胃苓汤

Stomach 'Ling' Decoction
Fu Ling *Sclerotium Poriae cocos* 9 g
Cang Zhu *Rhizoma Atractylodis* 6 g
Chen Pi *Pericarpium Citri reticulatae* 3 g
Bai Zhu *Rhizoma Atractylodis macrocephalae* 6 g
Gui Zhi *Ramulus Cinnamomi cassiae* 6 g
Ze Xie *Rhizoma Alismatis orientalis* 6 g
Zhu Ling *Sclerotium Polypori umbellati* 6 g
Hou Po *Cortex Magnolia officinalis* 6 g
Zhi Gan Cao *Radix Glycyrrhizae uralensis praeparata* 3 g
Da Zao *Fructus Ziziphi jujubae* 3 pieces
Sheng Jiang *Rhizoma Zingiberis officinalis recens* 3 slices

WEN DAN TANG 温胆汤

Warming the Gall Bladder Decoction
Ban Xia *Rhizoma Pinelliae ternatae* 6 g

Fu Ling *Sclerotium Poriae cocos* 5 g
Chen Pi *Pericarpium Citri reticulatae* 9 g
Zhu Ru *Caulis Bambusae in Taeniis* 6 g
Zhi Shi *Fructus Citri aurantii immaturus* 6 g
Zhi Gan Cao *Radix Glycyrrhizae uralensis praeparata* 3 g
Sheng Jiang *Rhizoma Zingiberis officinalis recens* 5 slices
Da Zao *Fructus Ziziphi jujubae* 1 date

WEN PI TANG 温脾汤

Warming the Spleen Decoction
Da Huang *Radix et Rhizoma Rhei* 12 g
Ren Shen *Radix Ginseng* 6 g
Gan Cao *Radix Glycyrrhizae uralensis* 6 g
Gan Jiang *Rhizoma Zingiberis officinalis* 6 g
Fu Zi *Radix lateralis Aconiti carmichaeli praeparata* 9 g

WEN YANG BU GAN JIAN 温阳补肝煎

Warming Yang and Tonifying the Liver Decoction
Rou Gui *Cortex Cinnamomi cassaie* 3 g
Yin Yang Huo *Herba Epimedii* 6 g
Zi Shi Ying *Fluoritum* 6 g
She Chuang Zi *Fructus Cnidii monnieri* 4.5 g
Bai Shao *Radix Paeoniae lactiflorae* 9 g
Mu Gua *Fructus Chaenomelis* 6 g

WU HU TANG 五虎汤

Five Tigers Decoction
Ma Huang *Herba Ephedrae* 2.1 g
Shi Gao *Gypsum fibrosum* 4.5 g
Xing Ren *Semen Pruni armeniacae* 3 g
Gan Cao *Radix Glycyrrhizae uralensis* 1.2 g
Sheng Jiang *Rhizoma Zingiberis officinalis recens* 3 slices
Da Zao *Fructus Ziziphi jujubae* 1 date
Xi Cha Fine green tea 2.4 g

WU LING SAN 五苓散

Five-Ingredient Poria Powder
Ze Xie *Rhizoma Alismatis orientalis* 4 g
Fu Ling *Sclerotium Poriae cocos* 2.3 g
Zhu Ling *Sclerotium Polypori umbellati* 2.3 g
Bai Zhu *Rhizoma Atractylodis macrocephalae* 2.3 g
Gui Zhi *Ramulus Cinnamomi cassiae* 1.5 g

WU MEI WAN 乌每丸

Prunus Mume Pill
Wu Mei *Fructus Pruni mume* 24 g
Chuan Jiao *Pericarpium Zanthoxyli bungeani* 1.5 g
Xi Xin *Herba Asari cum radice* 1.5 g
Huang Lian *Rhizoma Coptidis* 9 g
Huang Bo *Cortex Phellodendri* 6 g
Gan Jiang *Rhizoma Zingiberis officinalis* 6 g
Fu Zi *Radix lateralis Aconiti carmichaeli praeparata* 3 g
Gui Zhi *Ramulus Cinnamomi cassiae* 3 g
Ren Shen *Radix Ginseng* 6 g
Dang Gui *Radix Angelicae sinensis* 3 g

WU REN WAN 五仁丸

Five-Seed Pill
Tao Ren *Semen Persicae* 9 g
Xing Ren *Semen Pruni armeniacae* 9 g
Bai Zi Ren *Semen Biotae orientalis* 6 g
Song Zi Ren *Semen Pini tabulaeformis* 3 g
Yu Li Ren *Semen Pruni* 3 g
Chen Pi *Pericarpium Citri reticulatae* 9 g

WU YAO SAN 乌药散

Linderia Powder
Wu Yao *Radix Linderae strychnifoliae* 6 g
Xiang Fu *Rhizoma Cyperi rotundi* 6 g
Su Zi *Fructus Perillae frutescentis* 4.5 g
Chen Pi *Pericarpium Citri reticulatae* 3 g
Chai Hu *Radix Bupleuri* 6 g
Mu Dan Pi *Cortex Moutan radicis* 6 g
Gui Zhi *Ramulus Cinnamomi cassiae* 3 g
Mu Xiang *Radix Aucklandiae lappae* 3 g
Dang Gui *Radix Angelicae sinensis* 6 g
Chuan Xiong *Radix Ligustici chuanxiong* 3 g
Bo He *Herba Menthae haplocalycis* 3 g
Gan Cao *Radix Glycyrrhizae uralensis* 3 g

WU ZHU YU TANG 吴茱萸汤

Evodia Decoction
Wu Zhu Yu *Fructus Evodiae rutaecarpae* 9 g
Sheng Jiang *Rhizoma Zingiberis officinalis recens* 6 g
Ren Shen *Radix Ginseng* 9 g
Da Zao *Fructus Ziziphi jujubae* 3 dates

WU ZI YAN ZONG WAN 五子衍宗丸

Five-Seed Developing Ancestors Pill
Tu Si Zi *Semen Cuscutae chinensis* 240 g
Wu Wei Zi *Fructus Schisandrae chinensis* 30 g
Gou Qi Zi *Fructus Lycii chinensis* 240 g
Fu Pen Zi *Fructus Rubi chingii* 120 g
Che Qian Zi *Semen Plantaginis* 60 g

XI JIAO DI HUANG TANG 犀角地黄汤

Cornus Rhinoceri-Rehmannia Decoction
Shui Niu Jiao *Cornu Bufali* 6 g
Sheng Di Huang *Radix Rehmanniae glutinosae* 24 g
Chi Shao *Radix Paeoniae rubrae* 9 g
Mu Dan Pi *Cortex Moutan radicis* 6 g

XIANG LENG WAN 香棱丸

Aucklandia-Sparganium Pill
Mu Xiang *Radix Aucklandiae lappae* 6 g
Ding Xiang *Flos Caryophylli* 3 g
San Leng *Rhizoma Sparganii stoloniferi* 6 g
Zhi Ke *Fructus Citri aurantii* 6 g
Qing Pi *Pericarpium Citri reticulatae viride* 3 g
Chuan Lian Zi *Fructus Meliae toosendan* 3 g
Xiao Hui Xiang *Fructus Foeniculi vulgaris* 6 g
E Zhu *Rhizoma Curcumae ezhu* 6 g
Sheng Jiang *Rhizoma Zingiberis officinalis recens* 3 slices

XIAO CHAI HU TANG 小柴胡汤

Small Bupleurum Decoction
Chai Hu *Radix Bupleuri* 24 g
Huang Qin *Radix Scutellariae baicalensis* 9 g
Ban Xia *Rhizoma Pinelliae ternatae* 24 g
Sheng Jiang *Rhizoma Zingiberis officinalis recens* 9 g
Ren Shen *Radix Ginseng* 9 g
Zhi Gan Cao *Radix Glycyrrhizae uralensis praeparata* 9 g
Da Zao *Fructus Ziziphi jujubae* 12 pieces

XIAO JIAN ZHONG TANG 小建中汤

Small Strengthening the Centre Decoction
Yi Tang *Saccharum granorum* 18 g
Gui Zhi *Ramulus Cinnamomi cassiae* 9 g
Bai Shao *Radix Paeoniae lactiflorae* 18 g

Zhi Gan Cao *Radix Glycyrrhizae uralensis praeparata* 6 g
Sheng Jiang *Rhizoma Zingiberis officinalis recens* 9 g
Da Zao *Fructus Ziziphi jujubae* 12 dates

XIAO QING LONG TANG 小青龙汤

Small Green Dragon Decoction
Ma Huang *Herba Ephedrae* 9 g
Gui Zhi *Ramulus Cinnamomi cassiae* 9 g
Gan Jiang *Rhizoma Zingiberis officinalis* 9 g
Xi Xin *Herba Asari cum radice* 3 g
Wu Wei Zi *Fructus Schisandrae chinensis* 6 g
Bai Shao *Radix Paeoniae lactiflorae* 9 g
Ban Xia *Rhizoma Pinelliae ternatae* 9 g
Zhi Gan Cao *Radix Glycyrrhizae uralensis praeparata* 3 g

XIAO YAO SAN 逍遥散

Free and Easy Wanderer Powder
Bo He *Herba Menthae haplocalycis* 3 g
Chai Hu *Radix Bupleuri* 9 g
Dang Gui *Radix Angelicae sinensis* 9 g
Bai Shao *Radix Paeoniae lactiflorae* 12 g
Bai Zhu *Rhizoma Atractylodis macrocephalae* 9 g
Fu Ling *Sclerotium Poriae cocos* 15 g
Gan Cao *Radix Glycyrrhizae uralensis* 6 g
Sheng Jiang *Rhizoma Zingiberis officinalis recens* 3 slices

XIE BAI SAN 泻白散

Draining the White Powder
Sang Bai Pi *Cortex Mori albae radicis* 30 g
Di Gu Pi *Cortex Lycii radicis* 30 g
Zhi Gan Cao *Radix Glycyrrhizae uralensis praeparata* 3 g
Geng Mi Non-glutinous rice 15 g

XIE HUANG SAN 泻黄散

Draining Yellowness Powder
Shi Gao *Gypsum fibrosum* 15 g
Shan Zhi Zi *Fructus Gardeniae jasminoidis* 6 g
Fang Feng *Radix Ledebouriellae divaricatae* 12 g
Huo Xiang *Herba Agastachis seu Pogostemi* 12 g
Gan Cao *Radix Glycyrrhizae uralensis* 3 g

XIE XIN TANG 泻心汤

Draining the Heart Decoction
Da Huang *Radix et Rhizoma Rhei* 6 g
Huang Lian *Rhizoma Coptidis* 3 g
Huang Qin *Radix Scutellariae baicalensis* 3 g

XIN YI QING FEI YIN 辛荑清肺饮

Magnolia Decoction to Clear the Lung
Xin Yi Hua *Flos Magnoliae liliflorae* 6 g
Huang Qin *Radix Scutellariae baicalensis* 6 g
Shan Zhi Zi *Fructus Gardeniae jasminoidis* 4.5 g
Shi Gao *Gypsum fibrosum* 15 g
Zhi Mu *Radix Anemarrhenae asphodeloidis* 6 g
Jin Yin Hua *Flos Lonicerae japonicae* 6 g
Yu Xing Cao *Herba cum Radice Houttuyniae cordatae* 6 g
Mai Men Dong *Tuber Ophiopogonis japonici* 6 g

XING SU SAN 杏苏散

Prunus-Perilla Powder
Zi Su Ye *Folium Perillae frutescentis* 6 g
Qian Hu *Radix Peucedani* 6 g
Xing Ren *Semen Pruni armeniacae* 6 g
Jie Geng *Radix Platycodi grandiflori* 6 g
Zhi Ke *Fructus Citri aurantii* 6 g
Chen Pi *Pericarpium Citri reticulatae* 6 g
Fu Ling *Sclerotium Poriae cocos* 6 g
Ban Xia *Rhizoma Pinelliae ternatae* 6 g
Sheng Jiang *Rhizoma Zingiberis officinalis recens* 6 g
Da Zao *Fructus Ziziphi jujubae* 2 dates
Gan Cao *Radix Glycyrrhizae uralensis* 3 g

XUAN FU DAI ZHE TANG 旋复代赭汤

Inula-Hematite Decoction
Xuan Fu Hua *Flos Inulae* 9 g
Dai Zhe Shi *Haematitum* 3 g
Ban Xia *Rhizoma Pinelliae ternatae* 9 g
Sheng Jiang *Rhizoma Zingiberis officinalis recens* 6 g
Ren Shen *Radix Ginseng* 6 g
Zhi Gan Cao *Radix Glycyrrhizae uralensis praeparata* 3 g
Da Zao *Fructus Ziziphi jujubae* 12 dates

XUE FU ZHU YU TANG 血府逐瘀汤

Blood Mansion Eliminating Stasis Decoction
Dang Gui *Radix Angelicae sinensis* 9 g
Sheng Di Huang *Radix Rehmanniae glutinosae* 9 g
Chi Shao *Radix Paeoniae rubrae* 6 g
Chuan Xiong *Radix Ligustici chuanxiong* 5 g
Tao Ren *Semen Persicae* 12 g
Hong Hua *Flos Carthami tinctorii* 9 g
Chai Hu *Radix Bupleuri* 3 g
Zhi Ke *Fructus Citri aurantii* 6 g
Niu Xi *Radix Achyranthis bidentatae seu Cyathulae* 9 g
Jie Geng *Radix Platycodi grandiflori* 5 g
Gan Cao *Radix Glycyrrhizae uralensis* 3 g

YAN HU SUO TANG 延胡索汤

Corydalis Decoction
Yan Hu Suo *Rhizoma Corydalis yanhusuo* 45 g
Pu Huang *Pollen Typhae* 15 g
Chi Shao *Radix Paeoniae rubrae* 15 g
Dang Gui *Radix Angelicae sinensis* 15 g
Guan Gui *Cortex Cinnamomi loureiroi* 15 g
Jiang Huang *Rhizoma Curcumae longae* 90 g
Ru Xiang *Gummi Olibanum* 90 g
Mo Yao *Myrrha* 90 g
Mu Xiang *Radix Aucklandiae lappae* 90 g
Zhi Gan Cao *Radix Glycyrrhizae uralensis praeparata* 7.5 g

YANG YIN QING FEI TANG 养阴清肺汤

Nourishing Yin and Clearing the Lungs Decoction
Sheng Di Huang *Radix Rehmanniae glutinosae* 6 g
Xuan Shen *Radix Scrophulariae ningpoensis* 4.5 g
Mai Men Dong *Tuber Ophiopogonis japonici* 3.6 g
Bai Shao *Radix Paeoniae lactiflorae* 2.4 g
Mu Dan Pi *Cortex Moutan radicis* 2.4 g
Zhe Bei Mu *Bulbus Fritillariae thunbergii* 2.4 g
Bo He *Herba Menthae haplocalycis* 1.5 g
Gan Cao *Radix Glycyrrhizae uralensis* 1.5 g

YI GAN SAN 抑肝散

Restraining the Liver Powder
Bai Zhu (fried) *Rhizoma Atractylodis macrocephalae* 3 g
Fu Ling *Sclerotium Poriae cocos* 3 g
Dang Gui *Radix Angelicae sinensis* 3 g

Chuan Xiong *Radix Ligustici chuanxiong* 2.4 g
Gou Teng *Ramulus Uncariae* 3 g
Chai Hu *Radix Bupleuri* 1.5 g
Gan Cao *Radix Glycyrrhizae uralensis* 1.5 g

YI GUAN JIAN 一贯煎

One Linking Decoction
Bei Sha Shen *Radix Glehniae littoralis* 10 g
Mai Men Dong *Tuber Ophiopogonis japonici* 10 g
Dang Gui *Radix Angelicae sinensis* 10 g
Sheng Di Huang *Radix Rehmanniae glutinosae* 30 g
Gou Qi Zi *Fructus Lycii chinensis* 12 g
Chuan Lian Zi *Fructus Meliae toosendan* 5 g

YI JIA ZHENG QI SAN 一甲正气散

First Variation Upright Qi Powder
Huo Xiang *Herba Agastachis seu Pogostemi* 6 g
Hou Po *Cortex Magnoliae officinalis* 6 g
Xing Ren *Semen Pruni armeniacae* 6 g
Fu Ling Pi *Cortex Poriae cocos* 6 g
Chen Pi *Pericarpium Citri reticulatae* 6 g
Shen Qu *Massa Fermentata medicinalis* 4.5 g
Mai Ya *Fructus Hordei vulgaris germinatus* 4.5 g
Yin Chen Hao *Herba Artemisiae capillaris* 6 g
Da Fu Pi *Pericarpium Arecae catechu* 3 g

YI WEI TANG 益胃汤

Benefiting the Stomach Decoction
Sha Shen *Radix Adenophorae seu Glehniae* 9 g
Mai Men Dong *Tuber Ophiopogonis japonici* 15 g
Sheng Di Huang *Radix Rehmanniae glutinosae* 15 g
Yu Zhu *Rhizoma Polygonati odorati* 4.5 g
Bing Tang *Rock candy* 3 g

YI YIN JIAN 一阴煎

One Yin Decoction
Sheng Di Huang *Radix Rehmanniae glutinosae* 6 g
Shu Di Huang *Radix Rehmanniae glutinosae praeparata* 9 g
Bai Shao *Radix Paeoniae lactiflorae* 6 g
Mai Men Dong *Tuber Ophiopogonis japonici* 6 g
Gan Cao *Radix Glycyrrhizae uralensis* 3 g
Huai Niu Xi *Radix Achyranthis bidentatae* 4.5 g
Dan Shen *Radix Salviae miltiorrhizae* 6 g

YIN CHEN HAO TANG 茵陈蒿汤

Artemisia Yinchenhao Decoction
Yin Chen Hao *Herba Artemisiae capillaris* 6 g
Shan Zhi Zi *Fructus Gardeniae jasminoidis* 9 g
Da Huang *Radix et Rhizoma Rhei* 6 g

YIN JIA WAN 银甲丸

Lonicera-Amyda Pill
Jin Yin Hua *Flos Lonicerae japonicae* 6 g
Bie Jia *Carapacis Amydae sinensis* 9 g
Lian Qiao *Fructus Forsythiae suspensae* 6 g
Sheng Ma *Rhizoma Cimicifugae* 6 g
Hong Teng *Caulis Sargentodoxae cuneatae* 6 g
Pu Gong Ying *Herba Taraxaci mongolici cum Radice* 6 g
Da Qing Ye *Folium Daqingye* 6 g
Yin Chen Hao *Herba Artemisiae yinchenhao* 4.5 g
Hu Po *Succinum* 6 g
Jie Geng *Radix Platycodi grandiflori* 3 g
Zi Hua Di Ding *Herba cum Radice Violae yedoensitis* 6 g
Pu Huang *Pollen Typhae* 6 g
Chun Gen Bai Pi *Cortex Ailanthi altissimae* 6 g

YIN QIAO SAN 银翘散

Lonicera-Forsythia Powder
Jin Yin Hua *Flos Lonicerae japonicae* 9 g
Lian Qiao *Fructus Forsythiae suspensae* 9 g
Jie Geng *Radix Platycodi grandiflori* 3 g
Niu Bang Zi *Fructus Arctii lappae* 9 g
Bo He *Herba Menthae haplocalycis* 3 g
Dan Dou Chi *Semen Sojae praeparatum* 3 g
Jing Jie *Herba seu Flos Schizonepetae tenuifoliae* 6 g
Zhu Ye *Herba Lophatheri gracilis* 3 g
Lu Gen *Rhizoma Phragmitis communis* 15 g
Gan Cao *Radix Glycyrrhizae uralensis* 3 g

YOU GUI WAN 右归丸

Restoring the Right [Kidney] Pill
Fu Zi *Radix lateralis Aconiti carmichaeli praeparata* 3 g
Rou Gui *Cortex Cinnamomi cassiae* 3 g
Du Zhong *Cortex Eucommiae ulmoidis* 6 g
Shan Zhu Yu *Fructus Corni officinalis* 4.5 g
Tu Si Zi *Semen Cuscutae chinensis* 6 g
Lu Jiao Jiao *Colla Corni Cervi* 6 g

Shu Di Huang *Radix Rehmanniae glutinosae praeparata* 12 g
Shan Yao *Radix Dioscoreae oppositae* 6 g
Gou Qi Zi *Fructus Lycii chinensis* 6 g
Dang Gui *Radix Angelicae sinensis* 4.5

YU NU JIAN 玉女煎

Jade Woman Decoction
Shi Gao *Gypsum fibrosum* 15 g
Shu Di Huang *Radix Rehmanniae glutinosae praeparata* 9 g
Zhi Mu *Radix Anemarrhenae asphodeloidis* 3 g
Mai Men Dong *Tuber Ophiopogonis japonici* 6 g
Huai Niu Xi *Radix Achyranthis bidentatae* 3 g

YUE JU WAN 越鞠丸

Gardenia-Ligusticum Pill
Cang Zhu *Rhizoma Atractylodis lanceae* 6 g
Chuan Xiong *Radix Ligustici chuanxiong* 6 g
Xiang Fu *Rhizoma Cyperi rotundi* 6 g
Shan Zhi Zi *Fructus Gardeniae jasminoidis* 6 g
Shen Qu *Massa Fermentata medicinalis* 6 g

ZENG YE TANG 增液汤

Increasing Fluids Decoction
Xuan Shen *Radix Scrophulariae ningpoensis* 18 g
Mai Men Dong *Tuber Ophiopogonis japonici* 12 g
Sheng Di Huang *Radix Rehmanniae glutinosae* 12 g

ZHEN GAN XI FENG TANG 镇肝熄风汤

Pacifying the Liver and Extinguishing Wind Decoction
Huai Niu Xi *Radix Achyrantis bidentatae* 15 g
Dai Zhe Shi *Haematitum* 15 g
Long Gu *Os Draconis* 12 g
Mu Li *Concha Ostreae* 12 g
Gui Ban *Plastrum Testudinis* 12 g
Xuan Shen *Radix Scrophulariae ningpoensis* 12 g
Tian Men Dong *Tuber Asparagi cochinchinensis* 12 g
Bai Shao *Radix Paeoniae lactiflorae* 12 g
Yin Chen Hao *Herba Artemisiae capillaris* 6 g
Chuan Lian Zi *Fructus Meliae toosendan* 6 g
Mai Ya *Fructus Hordei vulgaris germinatus* 6 g
Gan Cao *Radix Glycyrrhizae uralensis* 6 g

ZHEN REN YANG ZANG TANG 真人养脏汤

True Person Nourishing the Organs Decoction
Ren Shen *Radix Ginseng* 3 g
Bai Zhu *Rhizoma Atractylodis macrocephalae* 9 g
Rou Gui *Cortex Cinnamoni cassiae* 3 g
Wei Rou Dou Kou *Semen Myristicae fragrantis* 9 g
He Zi *Fructus Terminaliae chebulae* 6 g
(Zhi) Ying Su Ke *Pericarpium Papaveris somniferi* (honey-fried) 6 g
Bai Shao *Radix Paeoniae lactiflorae* 9 g
Dang Gui *Radix Angelicae sinensis* 6 g
Mu Xiang *Radix Aucklandiae lappae* 6 g
Zhi Gan Cao *Radix Glycyrrhizae uralensis praeparata* 3 g

ZHEN WU TANG 真武汤

True Warrior Decoction
Fu Zi *Radix lateralis Aconiti carmichaeli praeparata* 9 g
Bai Zhu *Rhizoma Atractylodis macrocephalae* 6 g
Fu Ling *Sclerotium Poriae cocos* 9 g
Sheng Jiang *Rhizoma Zingiberis officinalis recens* 9 g
Bai Shao *Radix Paeoniae lactiflorae* 9 g

ZHENG QI TIAN XIANG SAN 正气天香散

Upright Qi Heavenly Fragrance Powder
Wu Yao *Radix Linderae strychnifoliae* 6 g
Gan Jiang *Rhizoma Zingiberis officinalis* 3 g
Zi Su Ye *Folium Perillae* 6 g
Chen Pi *Pericarpium Citri reticulatae* 4.5 g

ZHI BO DI HUANG WAN 知柏地黄丸

Eight-Ingredient Rehmannia Pill (Anemarrhena-Phellodendron-Rehmannia Pill)
Shu Di Huang *Radix Rehmanniae glutinosae praeparata* 24 g
Shan Zhu Yu *Fructus Corni officinalis* 12 g
Shan Yao *Radix Dioscoreae oppositae* 12 g
Ze Xie *Rhizoma Alismatis orientalis* 9 g
Fu Ling *Sclerotium Poriae cocos* 9 g
Mu Dan Pi *Cortex Moutan radicis* 9 g
Zhi Mu *Radix Anemarrhenae asphodeloidis* 9 g
Huang Bo *Cortex Phellodendri* 9 g

ZHI GAN CAO TANG 炙甘草汤

Glycyrrhiza Decoction
Zhi Gan Cao *Radix Glycyrrhizae uralensis praeparata* 12 g
Ren Shen *Radix Ginseng* 6 g
Gui Zhi *Ramulus Cinnamomi cassiae* 9 g
Sheng Di Huang *Radix Rehmanniae glutinosae* 48 g
Mai Men Dong *Tuber Ophiopogonis japonici* 9 g
E Jiao *Gelatinum Corii asini* 6 g
Huo Ma Ren *Semen Cannabis sativae* 9 g
Sheng Jiang *Rhizoma Zingiberis officinalis recens* 9 g
Da Zao *Fructus Ziziphi jujubae* 30 dates

ZHI SHI DAO ZHI WAN 枳实导滞丸

Citrus Eliminating Stagnation Pill
Zhi Shi *Fructus Citri aurantii immaturus* 12 g
Da Huang *Radix et Rhizoma Rhei* 15 g
Huang Lian *Rhizoma Coptidis* 6 g
Huang Qin *Radix Scutellariae baicalensis* 6 g
Fu Ling *Sclerotium Poriae cocos* 6 g
Ze Xie *Rhizoma Alismatis orientalis* 6 g
Bai Zhu *Rhizoma Atractylodis macrocephalae* 6 g
Shen Qu *Massa Fermentata Medicinalis* 12 g

ZHI SHI GUA LOU GUI ZHI TANG 枳实瓜蒌桂枝汤

Citrus-Trichosanthes-Ramulus Cinnamomi Decoction
Gua Lou *Fructus Trichosanthis* 12 g
Xie Bai *Bulbus Allii* 9 g
Zhi Shi *Fructus Citri aurantii immaturus* 12 g
Hou Po *Cortex Magnoliae officinalis* 12 g
Gui Zhi *Ramulus Cinnamomi cassiae* 3 g

ZHU YE SHI GAO TANG 竹叶石膏汤

Lophaterus-Gypsum Decoction
Zhu Ye *Herba Lophatheri gracilis* 9 g

Shi Gao *Gypsum fibrosum* 30 g
Ren Shen *Radix Ginseng* 6 g
Mai Men Dong *Tuber Ophiopogonis japonici* 9 g
Ban Xia *Rhizoma Pinelliae ternatae* 9 g
Gan Cao *Radix Glycyrrhizae uralensis* 3 g
Geng Mi *Semen Oryzae sativae* 12 g

ZUO GUI WAN 左归丸

Restoring the Left [Kidney] Pill
Shu Di Huang *Radix Rehmanniae glutinosae praeparata* 15 g
Shan Yao *Radix Dioscoreae oppositae* 9 g
Shan Zhu Yu *Fructus Corni officinalis* 9 g
Gou Qi Zi *Fructus Lycii chinensis* 9 g
Chuan Niu Xi *Radix Cyathulae* 6 g
Tu Si Zi *Semen Cuscutae sinensis* 9 g
Lu Jiao Jiao *Colla Cornu cervi* 9 g
Gui Ban Jiao *Colla Plastri testudinis* 9 g

ZUO GUI YIN 左归饮

Restoring the Left [Kidney] Decoction
Shu Di Huang *Radix Rehmanniae glutinosae praeparata* 6 g
Shan Yao *Radix Dioscoreae oppositae* 6 g
Gou Qi Zi *Fructus Lycii chinensis* 6 g
Fu Ling *Sclerotium Poriae cocos* 6 g
Shan Zhu Yu *Fructus Corni officinalis* 3 g
Zhi Gan Cao *Radix Glycyrrhizae uralensis praeparata* 3 g

ZUO JIN WAN 左金丸

Left Metal Pill
Huang Lian *Rhizoma Coptidis* 15 g
Wu Zhu Yu *Fructus Evodiae rutaecarpae* 2 g

Appendix 3

HISTORY OF DIAGNOSIS IN CHINESE MEDICINE

This appendix (adapted from Deng Tie Tao 1988 'Practical Chinese Medicine Diagnosis' *Shi Yong Zhong Yi Zhen Duan Xue*, Shanghai Science Publishing House, Shanghai) will give a short historical overview of the development of diagnosis in Chinese medicine.[1] I will discuss the following historical aspects of diagnosis:

- pulse diagnosis
- channel diagnosis
- tongue diagnosis.

PULSE DIAGNOSIS

Pulse diagnosis is an extremely important diagnostic method in Chinese medicine. It is an incredibly sophisticated and accurate diagnostic tool that has undergone an interrupted historical development from the Zhou dynasty (11th century–771BC) onwards.

Pulse diagnosis in early times

It is still not certain when the pulse was first referred to as a diagnostic tool. Some scholars think that pulse diagnosis was practised as early as the Zhou dynasty (11th century–771BC). The ancient book called 'Rites of Zhou' says in a chapter entitled 'Medical Matters': *'Determine the prognosis of patients according to the five kinds of Qi, five kinds of sounds and five kinds of colours; also refer to the changes of the nine orifices and the pulsation of the nine internal organs.'* Some historians interpret the expression 'refer to the pulsation' as meaning the palpation of the pulse.

Bian Que

The historian Si Ma Qian writes about the ancient doctor Bian Que in his book 'Historical Records' (*Shi Ji*) as being the earliest expert of pulse diagnosis. This view is supported in other texts. For example, Han Fei of the Warring States period (476–221BC) made similar statements in his book 'Works of Han Fei' (*Han Fei Zi*). The book 'Works of Prince Huai Nan' (*Huai Nan Zi*) by Liu An says that Bian Que could diagnose diseases by taking the pulse.

Bian Que, also known as Qin Yue Ren, lived in the 5th century BC during the transition between the Spring and Autumn period and the Warring States period. He was a well-known medical practitioner of his time, who travelled widely and became an expert in internal medicine, surgery, gynecology, paediatrics and diseases of the elderly.

Ma Wang Dui texts

Three texts unearthed from the tomb of Ma Wang Dui deal with pulse diagnosis: 'Methods of Pulse Taking' (*Mai Fa*), 'Fatal Signs of Yin and Yang Pulses' (*Yin Yang Mai Si Hou*) and 'Moxibustion Book of the 11 Channels of the Foot and Hand' (*Zu Bi Shi Yi Mai Jiu Jing*). These three classics were unearthed from the no. 3 tomb of Ma Wang Dui and, although they were written anonymously, we know that they predate the 'Yellow Emperor's Classic of Internal Medicine' (*Huang Di Nei Jing*).

'Fatal Signs of Yin and Yang Pulses' and 'Moxibustion Book of the 11 Channels of the Foot and Hand' discuss the importance of the pulse in making a prognosis. For example, the 'Moxibustion Book of the 11 Channels of the Foot and Hand' says that if the pulse is disrupted due to a disease of the three Yin, death will impend in less than 10 days; if the rhythm of the pulse feels like three people pounding grain, death will impend in less than 3 days; if the pulse feels like the one felt right after eating, death will impend in less than 3 days. The pulse described as feeling 'like three

people pounding grain' could be the earliest record of arrhythmia in China. This image gives a vivid description of the pulse felt in arrhythmia, by conjuring up the rhythm and sound produced by three people working together to pound grain.

There is a description of a similar pulse in Chapter 20 of the 'Simple Questions', namely a pulse that hits the finger like the rhythm of three people pounding grain in a mortar: this indicates that the disease is quite severe.

The Yellow Emperor's Classic of Internal Medicine (*Huang Qi Nei Jing Su Wen*)

There are many chapters in the 'Simple Questions' (*Su Wen*) and 'Spiritual Axis' (*Ling Shu*) that deal with pulse diagnosis.

For example, Chapter 17 of the 'Simple Questions' says that the pulse should be taken in the early morning '*when the Yin Qi is not disturbed, the Yang Qi is not dissipated, the stomach is empty, the Qi of the channels is not full, the Qi of the Connecting channels is even and quiet and the circulation of Qi and Blood is not disrupted yet*'.[2] Chapter 18 of the 'Simple Questions' recommends evaluating the pulse according to the breathing.

In the 'Yellow Emperor's Classic of Internal Medicine' the pulse was taken on nine different arteries in nine different locations of the body. These were called the 'nine regions' as described in Chapter 20 of the 'Simple Questions': '*There are three areas in the body, each area is divided into three which makes nine regions: these are used to determine life and death [i.e. prognosis], and in them, 100 diseases manifest, Deficiency and Excess are regulated and the pathogenic factors can be expelled.*'[3]

Chapter 19 of the 'Spiritual Axis' recommends taking the pulse at ST-9 Renying (carotid artery) and around the area of LU-9 Taiyuan, which the text called 'Portal of Qi' (*Qi Kou*) or 'Portal of Inch' (*Cun Kou*) where the radial artery runs. Renying reflects Yang Qi whereas Qi Kou reflects Yin Qi. Chapter 48 of the 'Spiritual Axis' also says that the *Cun Kou* pulse reflects the state of the Yin organs whereas the Renying pulse reflects that of the Yang organs. Later, Zhang Zhong Jing on the basis of the above theories developed pulse diagnosis at three locations, that is, at Renying (ST-9) and Fuyang (BL-59) to evaluate the Qi of the Stomach and at *Cun Kou* to evaluate the state of the 12 Channels.

There are passages in the 'Yellow Emperor's Classic of Internal Medicine' which attribute the greatest importance to the pulse of the radial artery, that is, the *Cun Kou* (or *Qi Kou*) pulse. The importance attributed to this pulse is a precursor of the division of the arterial pulse at the wrist into three sections. For example, Chapter 3 of the 'Spiritual Axis' says that we should check the quality of the *Cun Kou* pulse (big or small, slow or rapid, slippery or choppy) to find the cause of the disease. Chapter 5 of the 'Simple Questions' has a similar statement.

Chapter 21 of 'Simple Questions' says '*The balance of Qi, Blood, Yin and Yang can be gauged from the pulse at Qi Kou. Through the pulse at Qi Kou we can formulate a prognosis of the disease.*'[4] Chapter 18 of the same text says: '*We can understand a disease from the fullness or emptiness of the pulse at Cun Kou*'.[5] All these are examples of pulse diagnosis at *Qi Kou*: it is interesting to note that only the Front (*Cun*) and Rear (*Chi*) positions of the pulse are mentioned, without any mention of the Middle (*Guan*) position; moreover, the Front position is more important than the Rear one.

The 'Yellow Emperor's Classic of Internal Medicine' reports at least 30 different pulse qualities, many of which are not used nowadays. These include Big, Small, Long, Short, Slippery, Choppy, Floating, Deep, Slow, Rapid, Flourishing, Firm, Tight, Soft, Slowed-down, Abrupt, Deficient, Excessive, Scattered, Knotted, Thin, Weak, Transverse, Asthmatic, Wiry, Hook-like, Feather-like, Stone-like, Hurried, Surging, Full, Throbbing, Thick, Suspended and Feeble. There are vivid descriptions of the feeling when the pulse hits the finger: for example, the Wiry Pulse is 'rigid, straight and long', the Hook-like pulse 'surging on and fading away', the Feather-like pulse 'light and feeble like a feather', the Stone-like pulse 'like a stone being thrown', etc.

Pulse diagnosis in Han, Jin, Sui and Tang dynasties

Yi Chun Yu

Yi Chun Yu was a famous practitioner living in the beginning of the Han dynasty. He followed the theories on pulse diagnosis handed down from previous dynasties, and developed his own rich experiences in his practice. He said 'When I treat patients, I must first palpate the patient's pulse, and then give the treatment accordingly'. More than 20 different pulse qualities are found in his records such as Wiry, Big, Deep,

Intermittent, Tight, Small, Weak, Abrupt, Slippery, Rapid, Full, Firm, Scattered, etc. Yi Chun Yu palpated the pulse at the *Cun Kou* position and differentiated between the pulse felt at the superficial and deep levels.

Pulse diagnosis in the 'Classic of Difficulties' (Nan Jing)

The 'Classic of Difficulties' marked an extremely important milestone in the history of pulse diagnosis because it established for the first time pulse diagnosis based on the radial artery pulse at the wrist divided into three sections (*Cun*, *Guan* and *Chi*) and three levels. These were the new 'nine regions' of the pulse; in other words, whereas in the times of the 'Yellow Emperor's Classic of Internal Medicine' the 'nine regions' were nine different arteries in different places of the body, henceforth they were all on the radial artery at the wrist.

So, the 'Classic of Difficulties' (AD100) established for the first time the practice of taking the pulse at the radial artery: as mentioned above, this pulse was variously called *Qi Kou* ('Portal of Qi'), *Cun Kou* ('Portal of Inch [Front pulse position]') and *Mai Kou* ('Portal of Pulse'). The 'Classic of Difficulties' says: '*The 12 main channels have their own arteries but the pulse can be taken only at the Cun Kou [LU-9 position] reflecting the life and death of the 5 Yin and 6 Yang organs . . . The Cun Kou is the beginning and end point of the energy of the 5 Yin and 6 Yang organs and that is why we can take the pulse at this position only.*'[6] The last part of this statement is interesting since the description of the pulse of the *Cun Kou* is described as the 'beginning and end point of the energy of the 5 Yin and 6 Yang organs'; this seems to imply an understanding of the circulation of blood as a closed circuit.

Chapter 1 of the 'Classic of Difficulties' explains why the pulse is felt at *Cun Kou*:

Twelve channels have places where a pulse can be felt and yet one selects only the Cun Kou to determine the state of the 5 Yin and 6 Yang organs, why is this? The Cun Kou constitutes the great meeting place of the vessels, it is the place where the pulse of the Hand Greater Yin [Lungs] beats . . . the Cun Kou is the beginning and end of the 5 Yin and 6 Yang organs and therefore only the Cun Kou is used [for diagnosis].[7]

The second chapter of the 'Classic of Difficulties' explains how its author arrived at feeling the pulse at the three positions called Inch or Front, Gate or Middle and Foot or Rear (*Cun*, *Guan* and *Chi*):

The Foot and Inch sections of the pulse are the meeting point of the channels. The distance from the Gate position [LU-8, level with the radial apophysis] to the Foot position in the elbow represents the Foot-Interior and it reflects the Yin energies. The distance from the Gate position to the point Fish Margin [the thenar eminence] is the Foot-Exterior and it reflects the Yang energies. Hence, the distance of 1 inch is separated from the distance of 1 foot [from the Gate position to the elbow crease], so that the distance of 1 foot is represented by 1 inch. Hence the Yin energies are reflected within that 1-inch section of the foot-long section and the Yang energies are reflected within a 9-fen [nine-tenths of an inch] section of the Inch section. The total length of the Foot and Inch section extends over 1 inch and 9 fen; hence one speaks of Foot and Inch sections.[8]

In other words, the distance from the Gate-*Guan* (or Middle) position of the pulse (on LU-8 Jingqu) to the crease of the elbow measures 1 Chinese foot and reflects the Yin energies; the distance from the Gate-*Guan* position to the crease of the wrist is 9 *fen* (nine-tenths of an inch) and reflects the Yang energies. However, a 1-inch section is separated from the 1-foot distance from the Gate-*Guan* position to the elbow crease to represent the Yin energies; in other words, this 1-inch section is representative of the 1-foot section.

Chapter 18 of the 'Classic of Difficulties' describes the three different pressures applied to the pulse:

There are three sections, Inch, Gate and Foot, and three pressures, superficial, middle and deep [which makes] 9 regions. The Upper section pertains to Heaven and reflects diseases from the chest to the head; the Middle section pertains to Person and reflects diseases from the diaphragm to the umbilucus; the Lower section pertains to Earth and reflects diseases from the umbilicus to the feet. [One must] examine [these sections] before needling.[9]

This passage establishes clearly the principle, adopted by all successive doctors, that the Inch section of the pulse corresponds to the Upper Burner and diseases from the chest upwards, the Gate section to the Middle Burner and diseases from the diaphragm to the umbilicus, and the Foot section to the Lower Burner and diseases from the umbilicus to the feet.

Zhang Zhong Jing

Zhang Zhong Jing discusses pulse diagnosis in many passages of his celebrated 'Discussion of Cold-induced Diseases' (*Shang Han Lun*). He emphasized

paying equal attention to the pulse as to clinical manifestations when identifying patterns; in particular, he put the most emphasis on the pulse at *Cun Kou*.

In all, Zhang Zhong Jing mentions more than 20 pulse qualities in his book and he classified them into two broad groups of Yang (e.g. Big, Floating, Rapid, Slippery, etc.) and Yin pulse qualities (e.g. Deep, Choppy, Weak, etc.).

Zhang Zhong Jing was good at using pulse diagnosis to analyse the aetiology and pathology of a disease and to guide treatment. For example he says: '*When the pulse is Floating and Tight at the Cun Kou, the Floating quality indicates Wind while the Tight quality Cold*'.

Moreover, Zhang Zhong Jing also paid attention to the correlation between pulse and body shape. For example, he said '*If a fat person displays a Floating pulse and a thin person a Deep one, this should draw our attention. In general, fat people are likely to have a Deep pulse while thin people a Floating pulse.*'

Zhang Zhong Jing also made an interesting correlation between pulse quality and the emotional causes of disease. He says: '*In case of shock the pulse will be Fine and the complexion pale; in case of shame, the pulse will be Floating and the complexion red.*'

The 'Pulse Classic' (Mai Jing)

The 'Pulse Classic' (*Mai Jing*) was written by Wang Shu He at the juncture between the Han and Jin dynasties, in approximately AD280. This is the first text dedicated entirely to pulse diagnosis. This book had a great influence on the study of pulse diagnosis not only in Chinese medicine but also in Arabic and Persian medicine.

The 'Pulse Classic' consolidated and further clarified the division of the pulse in three sections and the organs assigned to each section. This book assigns the Heart and Small Intestine to the left Front position, the Liver and Gall-Bladder to the left Middle position, the Kidneys and Bladder to the left Rear position, the Lungs and Large Intestine to the right Front positions, the Spleen and Stomach to the right Middle position, and the Kidneys, Bladder and Triple Burner to the right Rear position.

The 'Pulse Classic' mentioned 24 pulse qualities and described their feeling and clinical significance in a systematic way for the first time. The pulse qualities included Floating, Hollow, Surging, Slippery, Rapid, Hurried, Wiry, Tight, Deep, Hidden, Leather-like, Full, Feeble, Choppy, Fine, Soft, Weak, Deficient, Scattered, Slowed-down, Slow, Knotted, Intermittent and Throbbing. The descriptions used for such pulse qualities became the standard for later texts on pulse diagnosis. Wang Shu He also systematically compared and contrasted similar pulse qualities to make their differentiation easier.

The 'Pulse Classic' also described the clinical significance of each pulse quality systematically. For example, it says: '*The Slow pulse indicates Cold, the Choppy pulse deficiency of Blood, the Slowed-down pulse Deficiency, and the Surging pulse Heat*'.

The 'Thousand Golden Ducats Prescriptions' (Qian Jin Fang)

The book 'Thousand Golden Ducats Prescriptions' by Sun Si Miao consolidated and expanded the 'Pulse Classic' views on the three sections of the pulse, the three depths applied to finger pressure and the assignment of organs to pulse positions. Sun Si Miao emphasized the importance of pulse diagnosis and the following excerpt is interesting and apt: '*The pulse is an important tool for practitioners of traditional Chinese medicine. How can one practise traditional Chinese medicine without a good understanding of the pulse? All practitioners of traditional Chinese medicine should study the pulse carefully.*'

Sun Si Miao associated the pulse positions only with the Yin organs, with the Heart, Liver and Kidney on the left and Lungs, Spleen and Gate of Life (*Ming Men*) on the right. He correlated the pulse to body shape and also emotional state:

It is abnormal for people of large size to have a small, Fine pulse, for thin people to have a Big pulse, for happy people to have a Deficient pulse, for unhappy people to have a Full pulse, for people of hot temper to have a Slowed-down pulse, for calm people to have an Agitated pulse, for people of strong body build to have a Fine pulse, and for people of weak body constitution to have a Big pulse.

Pulse Diagnosis in Song, Yuan, Ming and Qing dynasties

During the Song dynasty, pulse diagnosis continued to develop and many of the rhymes since used as a mnemonic aid were composed in this time. For example, a collection of rhymes to memorize pulse qualities and their clinical significance is the 'Pulse in Verse' (*Mai Jue*) by Cui Jia Yan of the Southern Song dynasty.

During the Song dynasty, illustrated books on pulse diagnosis were published for the first time. For example, Xu Shu Wei wrote the 'Illustrated Book of 36 Pulses' (*San Shi Liu Zhong Mai Fa Tu*), which is regarded as the first of these.

During the Ming dynasty, Zhang Shi Xian wrote the 'Pulse Verses with Illustrations' (*Tu Zhu Mai Jue*), which contains 22 illustrations. During the Qing Dynasty, He Sheng Ping wrote the 'Essentials of Pulse with Illustrations' (*Mai Yao Tu Zhu*).

Throughout the Song, Ming and Qing dynasties, doctors were engaged in trying to make pulse diagnosis easier to master. As there are between 28 and 32 pulse qualities, many doctors tried to find some kind of system to memorize them. The simplest classification was that into Yin and Yang pulses. Another way of classifying pulse qualities is according to various criteria, such as rate, rhythm, strength, shape and depth. A third way of systematizing the pulse qualities is to divide them up into pairs of opposite qualities (e.g. Slow-Rapid, Floating-Deep, Slippery-Choppy, Full-Empty, etc.).

The 'Pulse Classic of the Pin Hu Master' (*Pin Hu Mai Xue*) written in 1564 by Li Shi Zhen was a landmark in the history of pulse diagnosis. The book consisted of two parts. The first part was written by his father Li Yan Wen and it introduced the general theory of pulse diagnosis, whereas the second part, written by Li Shi Zhen himself, describes palpation of the pulse and the clinical significance of 27 pulse qualities. The book was written in the 'Seven-Word style', a poetic, lucid and lively style which makes it easy to learn and memorize.

Works on pulse diagnosis were quite numerous in the Ming and Qing dynasties. The most well-known of this period include the following:

- 'About the Pulse' (*Mai Yu*, 1584) by Wu Kun
- the chapter 'Discussion on the Spirit of the Pulse' in the 'Complete Works of Jing Yue' (*Jing Yue Quan Shu*, 1624) by Zhang Jie Bin
- the 'Orthodox Meaning of the Pulse Theory' (*Mai Li Zheng Yi*, 1635) by Zou Zhi Kui
- the 'Attention for Diagnosticians' (*Zhen Jia Zheng Yan*, 1642) by Li Zhong Zhi
- the 'Collection of Pulse Verses' (*Mai Jue Hui Bian*, 1667) compiled by Qu Liang

- the 'Thorough Knowledge of the Pulse' (*Mai Guan*, 1711) by Wang Xian
- the 'Pulse Studies of Hui Xi' (*Hui Xi Mai Xue*) by Xu Ling Tai
- the 'Seeking the Truth for the Theory of the Pulse' (*Mai Li Qiu Zhen*, 1769) by Huang Gong Xiu
- the 'Orthodox Classic of the Theory of the Pulse' (*Mai Li Zong Jing*, 1868) by Zhang Futian
- the 'Truth about the Theory of the Pulse' (*Mai Li Cun Zhen*, 1876) by Yu Xian Ting
- the 'Brief Discussion of the Theory of the Pulse' (*Mai Yi Jian Mo*, 1892) by Zhou Xue Hai.

During the Ming and Qing dynasties, feudal customs became very strict with regard to relations between men and women. It was considered improper for a doctor (in those times a man) to palpate the body of women. Sometimes even the interrogation of the patient was conducted through the intermediary of family members.

As for pulse diagnosis, this was often carried out by interposing a thin piece of silk on the woman's wrist to act as a barrier between her wrist and the doctor's fingers. During the Ming dynasty, Li Chan said in 'Rules for the Practice of Medicine' (*Xi Yi Gui Ge*):

When a woman is treated, her symptoms, appetite and the tongue picture were asked about through her family members. Then the treatment was given accordingly. Sometimes in a severe case, the practitioner diagnoses the patient through the bed curtain, or in a mild case, through the door curtain. In both conditions, a thin piece of silk is used to cover the wrist of the patient when the pulse is palpated. The practitioner often prepares such a piece of silk himself because sometimes it was not easy for poor families to get one.

Pulse diagnosis in modern times

In 1926, Yun Tie Jiao wrote the 'Explanation of the Pulse' (*Mai Xue Fa* Wei). This book tries to integrate the traditional Chinese view with a modern view of pulse diagnosis.

Since 1949, modern scientific methods and technology have been employed for the study of the pulse. Some doctors have researched the division of the pulse into three section and the connection of the pulse with the channel system.

CHANNEL DIAGNOSIS

Channel diagnosis is based on the observation of changes occurring on the skin overlying the channels. Since the Warring States period, the term 'channel' referred to anything which is seen on the skin, anywhere on the body. The changes observed pertain to the Connecting channel portion of the Main channels as it is only the Connecting channels that communicate with the skin through the Superficial and Minute Connecting channels. For example, visible subcutaneous veins and venules are a manifestation of the Blood Connecting channels; although they are venules from the Western point of view, they are part of the channel system from the Chinese point of view.

The blood vessels (venules) visible on the surface of the skin are always a reflection of the Connecting channels. When they become visible, the blood vessels are an expression of the percolation of the Blood Connecting channels towards the surface of the skin (the Blood Connecting vessels at the deep level of the Connecting channels).

Chapter 17 of the 'Spiritual Axis' says: '*The Main channels are in the Interior, their branches and horizontal [or crosswise] forming the Connecting channels; branching out from these are the Minute Connecting. When these are Full with stagnant Blood they should be drained with a bleeding needle; when they are deficient, they should be tonified with herbs.*'[10]

Chapter 10 of the same text says: '*The Main channels are deep and hidden between the muscles and cannot be seen; only the Spleen channel can be seen as it emerges from above the internal malleolus and it has no place to hide. The Connecting channels are superficial and can be seen.*'[11] The same chapter also says: '*When the Connecting channels are greenish-bluish it indicates Cold and pain; when they are red it indicates Heat*'.[12]

Apart from the blood vessels, the colour of the skin itself reflects the condition of the Connecting channels: red indicates Heat, green indicates pain, purple indicates Blood stasis, and bluish indicates Blood stasis and Cold.

Channel diagnosis includes several methods of diagnosis as follows:

- observation of the thenar eminence
- observation of the ear
- plucking of the vein in the inner leg
- observation of sublingual veins
- observation of the index finger in babies.

Observation of the thenar eminence

The thenar eminence shows the state of the Stomach. Chapter 10 of the 'Spiritual Axis' relates the colour of the thenar eminence to the state of the Stomach and says: '*When the Stomach has Cold, the thenar eminence is bluish; when the Stomach has Heat, the thenar eminence is reddish; if it is suddenly black, it indicates chronic Painful Obstruction Syndrome; if it is sometimes red, sometimes dark and sometimes bluish it indicates alternation of Heat and Cold; if it is bluish and short, it indicates deficiency of Qi.*'[13] Chapter 74 of the same text says: '*When the thenar eminence has bluish venules, it indicates Cold in the Stomach.*'[14]

The chapter 'Prescriptions for children, women and the elderly' in the 'Thousand Golden Ducats Prescriptions' (*Qian Jin Yao Fang*) by Sun Si Miao describes the use of the venules on the thenar eminence to diagnose epilepsy or infantile convulsions. It says: '*A black colour of the channels in the thenar eminence is a sign of epilepsy or infantile convulsions; a red colour Heat*'.

Observation of the ear

This method is based on the observation of changes in the veins on the back of the ear in small children. Chapter 74 of the 'Spiritual Axis' says: '*When an infant is sick, if the hair of the baby all stands up, it indicates a very bad prognosis. If a bluish vessel appears on the ear, it indicates abdominal pain due to spasm.*'[15] This method was further developed in later times. For example, the chapter 'Explanation of chicken pox and measles' in the 'Complete Works of Jing Yue' (*Jing Yue Quan Shu*, 1624) says: '*Chickenpox is mild if red veins appear on both ears. It is severe if they look purple*'.

During the Qing dynasty, Xia Yu Zhu noticed that the colour of the veins on the back of the ear could change according to weather, and thought that it was not, therefore, enough to make a prognosis based on the colour of these veins.

Plucking of the vein in the inner leg

The details for this method of diagnosis can be found in Chapter 20 of the 'Simple Questions'. This diagnosis is carried out by placing the fingers of the left hand gently on the skin 5 *cun* above the medial malleolus while the right hand plucks the skin above the medial malleolus gently. The results are interpreted as follows:

- if a vein appears gradually extending to 5 *cun* or more, this is normal
- if a vein appears quickly and is quite thick, this indicates a pathology
- if it appears slowly but does not reach 5 *cun*, or if it does not appear at all in response to the plucking, the prognosis is bad.

Observation of sublingual veins

This diagnostic method was first recorded in the 'Discussion on the Origin of Symptoms in Illness' (*Zhu Bing Yuan Hou Lun*, AD610) by Chao Yuan Fang.

Observation of the sublingual veins is the subject of intense research in modern China. It is believed that they may be used to determine the likelihood of future heart disease and hypertension.

Observation of the index finger in babies

This is a method of diagnosing diseases based on observation of the veins on the palmar aspect of the index finger on infants. It has a long history, probably starting in the Tang dynasty when it was first mentioned by Wang Chao in 'Verses on the Immortal's Water Mirror with Illustrations' (*Xian Ren Shui Jing Tu Jue*), and was widely used in clinical practice throughout China. It is still regarded as being a significant method of diagnosis today.

Origin of observation of the index finger in babies

Some diagnostic methods have traditionally always been applied specifically to infants; these include observation of veins on the back of the ear, observation of the root of the nose and observation of the index finger veins. These methods are generally used for children under the age of 3 years.

It is not clear when this diagnostic technique started. A book from 1750 'Complete Works of Paediatrics' (*You You Ji Cheng*) by Chen Fu Zheng dates this method back to the Song dynasty:

The diagnosis by the channels on the index finger was initiated by Qian Zhong Yang in Song Dynasty. The finger was divided into three Gates: the Gate of Wind, the Gate of Qi and the Gate of Life. The verse recited that the condition was mild if the channels reached the Gate of Wind, severe if

it reached the Gate of Qi and dangerous if it reached the Gate of Life.

Xu Shu Wei (Song dynasty) says in his 'Effective Prescriptions for Universal Relief' (*Pu Ji Ben Shi Fang*):

In infants, it is difficult to palpate the pulse and some practitioners refer to the colour in Hu Kou (the index finger) and the temperature of the limbs. A purple colour indicates Wind; a red colour indicates invasion of Cold; a blue colour indicates infantile convulsions; a white colour indicates malnutrition; a yellow colour indicates a disease of the Spleen.

Observation of the index finger in the Song and Yuan dynasties

During the Song and Yuan dynasties, the most detailed record about the observation of the colour of the channels in the index finger can be found in a book on paediatrics of the Song dynasty entitled 'A Book on Paediatrics' (*You You Xin Shu*). Liu Fang compiled the book together with Wang Li and Wang Shi. He says:

The proximal portion of the index finger is known as the Gate of Wind, the middle one is the Gate of Qi and the distal part of the finger is known as the Gate of Life. Some people emphasize using the left hand in boys and the right hand in girls. I think that it should be the same on boys and girls.

Liu Fang described eight common shapes of the veins: a shape like the skeleton of the fish, a shape like a suspended needle, a shape like the Chinese character for water, a sigmoid shape, an annular shape, a shape like an earthworm, an irregular shape and a shape like a fish-eye.

Wei Yi Lin described the clinical significance of the veins on the index finger of babies in the book 'Effective Formulae Handed down for Generations' (*Shi Yi De Xiao Fang*). He says:

Observation over the channels of the index finger should be made on the left hand for boys and on the right hand for girls. If the veins are within the Gate of Wind, it usually indicates convulsion due to fright by birds or people. If it is red and indistinct, it indicates fright by fire; if it is black, it indicates fright by water or fighting; if it is bluish, it indicates fright by thunder or animals. If there is a bluish curved line shown slightly, it is a sight of acute infantile convulsions. If the line is crooked, it is a sign of poor digestion. If the veins reach the Gate of Qi and are purple, it indicates infantile malnutrition resulting from infantile convulsions. If the veins are bluish, it indicates infantile malnutrition affecting the Liver Channel. If they are

whitish in colour, it indicates affliction of the Lung Channel. If they are black in colour, it indicates the disease is severe. If a bluish black line going through the three gates appears in the Gate of Life and runs oblique towards the fingernail, there is no hope for the patient.

Observation of the index finger in babies during the Ming and Qing dynasties

During the Ming and Qing dynasties, observation of the veins on the index finger was developed further. All pediatric books of this period include a chapter on observation of the veins of the index finger. The book 'Complete Book on Experiences in Paediatrics' (*Quan You Xin Jian I*, 1468) by Kou Ping contained detailed descriptions of the channels in the face and the three gates on the index finger. It included more than 40 pictures and the record of 13 shapes of the channels in the index finger.

Yu Tuan discusses diagnosis by the index finger in babies in his book 'Orthodox Medical Problems' (*Yi Xue Zheng Chuan*). He pointed out:

It is difficult to diagnose diseases of small children by palpating the pulse at Cun Kou at the route of the Lung Channel. For small children aged between 1 to 6 years old, the veins in the three Gates of the index finger can be used to diagnose diseases and determine their prognosis. Check the left hand for boys and right hand for girls.

It contained 19 pictures and a record of 17 abnormal shapes of the veins on the index finger.

The book 'Explanation to Questions about Paediatrics' (*You Ke Shi Mi*, 1774) by Shen Jin Ao recorded 13 abnormal appearances of the veins on the index finger, while the 'Golden Mirror of Medicine' (*Yi Zong Jin* Jian, 1742) by Wu Qian recorded 20.

Observation of the index finger in babies in modern times

Since 1949, diagnosis based on the appearance of veins on the index finger in babies has been developed further. Now it is verified by anatomy that the veins in the index finger are actually the palmar vein, which runs into the cephalic vein. Its location is superficial so that it is easily observed.

Observation shows that the vein is clearly exposed on children under 3 years old. However, some think that it can be used as a reference for diagnosis for all children under school age. The rule about observing the left hand for boys and left for girls is now considered insignificant.

Research indicates that the three Gates are significant for the understanding of diseases. Veins can appear longer when there is an increase in venous pressure, the peripheral blood vessels are dilated or there is malnutrition. This fits with the traditional view that 'a mild disease will manifest with the veins within the Gate of Wind, severe diseases with the veins within the Gate of Qi, and critical conditions with the veins reaching the Gate of Life'.

TONGUE DIAGNOSIS

Warring States period (475–221BC)

Several passages in the 'Yellow Emperor's Classic of Internal Medicine' mention tongue diagnosis. For examples:

If the tongue is loose, there is drooling and the patient is irritable, choose the Leg Lesser-Yin channel.[16]

If the Qi of the Leg Terminal Yin [Liver] is exhausted the lips turn blue and the tongue curls.[17]

This passage shows that in the 'Simple Questions' and 'Spiritual Axis', tongue diagnosis was based primarily on observation of the tongue-body shape rather than tongue-body colour. Other tongue-body shapes mentioned in these two texts are rolled, stiff, withered and short.

The tongue coating is mentioned in a few passages. For example: '*When the Lungs are invaded by Heat . . . the body hair stands up, the patient has aversion to cold, the tongue coating is yellow and the body hot.*'[18]

Han Dynasty (206BC–AD220)

During this time the most important contribution to tongue diagnosis is contained in the Zhang Zhong Jing's classics 'Discussion of Cold-induced Diseases' (*Shang Han Lun*) and 'Synopsis of Prescriptions from the Golden Cabinet' (*Jin Gui Yao Lue Fang*). For example:

A yellow tongue coating and a feeling of fullness in the intestines indicate excess Heat. If purging is applied and the Heat cleared, the yellow coating disappears.[19]

In Bright-Yang disorders with constipation, abdominal fullness and vomiting, the tongue has a white coating.[20]

If the patient has a feeling of fullness of the chest, dry lips and the tongue body colour is bluish . . . it indicates Blood stasis.[21]

Sui and Tang dynasties (AD581–907)

The two most important works containing a discussion of tongue diagnosis are the 'Discussion on the Origin of Symptoms in Illness' (*Zhu Bing Yuan Hou Lun*, 610) by Chao Yuan Fang and the 'Thousand Golden Ducats Prescriptions' (*Qian Jin Yao Fang*, 652) by Sun Si Miao. For example, the 'Discussion on the Origin of Symptoms in Illness' says: '*When the tongue has no coating, attacking methods of treatment [e.g. purgation] cannot be used.*' The 'Thousand Golden Ducats Prescriptions' says: '*In Full patterns of the Heart the tongue is cracked*'.

Song, Jin and Yuan dynasties (960–1368)

It was during this time that tongue diagnosis became a specialized subject. Li Dong Yuan attached special important to dryness of the tongue in his 'Discussion on Stomach and Spleen' (*Pi Wei Lun*).

A doctor known only by his surname, Ao, wrote the first book devoted entirely to tongue diagnosis towards the beginning of the Yuan dynasty. Later in the Yuan dynasty, Du Qing Bi revised this book and published a revised edition under the title 'Ao's Record of the Golden Mirror of Cold-induced Diseases'. The tongue-body colours mentioned are Pale, Red and Blue; tongue shapes mentioned are Flabby, Swollen and Deviated, among others.

Ming and Qing dynasties (1368–1911)

During the Ming dynasty several books on tongue diagnosis were published, all modelled on 'Ao's Record of the Golden Mirror of Cold-induced Diseases' mentioned above. The most prominent of these was Shen Dou Yuan's 'Essential Methods of Observation of the Tongue in Cold-induced Diseases', which describes 135 types of tongue.

Several texts on tongue diagnosis were written during the Qing dynasty. Zhang Dan Xian wrote the 'Mirror of the Tongue in Cold-induced Diseases' containing 120 illustrations. Fu Song Yuan wrote 'A Collection of Tongues and Coatings', which departs from the tradition of seeing tongue diagnosis only in the context of Cold-induced diseases.

In 1906, Liang Te Yan wrote the 'Differentiation of Syndromes by Examination of the Tongue', which illustrates and describes 148 types of tongues.

Modern times

Many new books on tongue diagnosis have been published since the establishment of the People's Republic of China in 1949. Chinese medical journals regularly report the results of a considerable amount of research carried out on tongue diagnosis. A particular aspect of tongue diagnosis, the sublingual veins, is the subject of considerable research which investigates the use of the sublingual veins as a diagnostic sign in heart disease.

The following are examples of articles on tongue diagnosis which have appeared in the Journal of Chinese Medicine (*Zhong Yi Za Zhi*):

- 'Clinical significance of Dark-Red tongue'[22]
- 'Tongue and patterns in hepatitis B'[23]
- 'Tongue appearance in bone fractures'[24]
- 'Tongue appearance in burns septicaemia'[25]
- 'Tongue appearance in schizophrenia'[26]
- 'Tongue appearance before and after operations'[27]
- 'Tongue changes after burns'[28]
- 'Tongue changes in cancer, chemotherapy and radiotherapy'[29]
- 'Tongue changes in diabetes'[30]
- 'Tongue coating after surgery for stomach cancer'[31]
- 'Tongue coating in lung cancer'[32]
- 'Tongue diagnosis and identification of patterns'[33]
- 'Tongue diagnosis and enteroscopy'[34]
- 'Tongue diagnosis and gastroscopy'[35]
- 'Sublingual veins in blood stasis'[36]

NOTES

1. Unless otherwise stated, all texts referred to and quotations in this appendix are cited in Deng Tie Tao 1988 Practical Chinese Medicine Diagnosis *Shi Yong Zhong Yi Zhen Duan Xue*, Shanghai Publishing House, Shanghai.
2. 1979 The Yellow Emperor's Classic of Internal Medicine – Simple Questions (*Huang Di Nei Jing Su Wen* 黄帝内经素问), People's Health Publishing House, Beijing, p. 102. First published c. 100BC.
3. Ibid., p. 130.
4. Ibid., p. 139.
5. Ibid., p. 112.
6. Nanjing College of Traditional Chinese Medicine 1979 A Revised Explanation of the Classic of Difficulties (*Nan Jing Jiao Shi* 难经校释), People's Health Publishing House, Beijing. pp. 1–2. First published c. AD100.
7. Ibid., p. 2.
8. Simple Questions, pp. 4–5.

9. Classic of Difficulties, p. 46.
10. 1981 Spiritual Axis (*Ling Shu Jing* 灵枢经), People's Health Publishing House, Beijing, p. 50. First published c. 100BC.
11. Ibid., p. 37.
12. Ibid., p. 37.
13. Ibid., p. 120, para 37.
14. Ibid., p. 133.
15. Ibid., p. 133.
16. Spiritual Axis, p. 129, para 30.
17. Ibid., p. 30.
18. Ibid., p. 186.
19. He Ren 1981 A New Explanation of the Synopsis of Prescriptions from the Golden Cabinet (*Jin Gui Yao Lue Xin Jie* 金匮要略新解), Zhejiang Science Publishing House, Zhejiang, p. 65. The Synopsis of Prescriptions from the Golden Cabinet was written by Zhang Zhong Jing c. AD200.
20. Shang Han Lun Research Group of the Nanjing College of Traditional Chinese Medicine 1980 An Explanation of the Discussion of Cold-Induced Diseases (*Shang Han Lun Jiao Shi* 伤寒论校释), Shanghai Science Publishing House, Shanghai, p. 948.
21. Synopsis of Prescriptions from the Golden Cabinet, p. 138.
22. Lan Xin Sheng et al. 1992 Journal of Chinese Medicine (*Zhong Yi Za Zhi* 中医杂志), no. 5, 1992, p. 46.
23. Chen Han Cheng and Xu Wen Da 1988 Journal of Chinese Medicine (*Zhong Yi Za Zhi*), no. 4, 1988, p. 53
24. Fractures Group of Chinese Medicine Hospital of Dang Shu City (Jiangsu Province) 1986 Journal of Chinese Medicine (*Zhong Yi Za Zhi*), no. 11, p. 41.
25. Kong Zhao Xia 1980 Journal of Chinese Medicine (*Zhong Yi Za Zhi*), no. 8, p. 26.
26. Chen Wei Ren 1995 Journal of Chinese Medicine (*Zhong Yi Za Zhi*), no. 12, p. 741.
27. Qin Ji Hua 1987 Journal of the Nanjing College of Traditional Chinese Medicine, no, 2, 1987, p. 17.
28. Han Ji Xun 1988 Journal of Chinese Medicine (*Zhong Yi Za Zhi*), no. 9, 1988, p. 45.
29. Li Su Juan 1999 Journal of Chinese Medicine (*Zhong Yi Za Zhi*), no. 10, 1999, p. 636.
30. Guo Sai Shan 1989 Journal of Chinese Medicine (*Zhong Yi Za Zhi*), no. 2, 1989, p. 33.
31. Fang Dong Xiang 1999 Journal of Chinese Medicine (*Zhong Yi Za Zhi*), no. 7, 1999, p. 433.
32. Xu Zhen Ye 1993 Journal of Chinese Medicine (*Zhong Yi Za Zhi*), no. 6, 1993, p. 334.
33. Cai Yu Qin 1993 Journal of Chinese Medicine (*Zhong Yi Za Zhi*), no. 12, 1993, p. 716.
34. Dai Wei Zheng 1994 Journal of Chinese Medicine (*Zhong Yi Za Zhi*), no. 1, 1994, p. 43.
35. Dai Hao Liang 1984 Journal of Chinese Medicine (*Zhong Yi Za Zhi*), no. 10, 1984, p. 74.
36. Jin Shi Ying 1992 Journal of Chinese Medicine (*Zhong Yi Za Zhi*), no. 3, 1992, p. 42.

Glossary of Chinese terms

GENERAL

Ba Kuo 八廓	The Eight Ramparts
Cou Li 腠里	Spaces and texture (also space between the skin and muscles)
Cun 寸	Cun (acupuncture unit of measurement)
Dan Tian 丹田	Field of Elixir
Fen Rou 分肉	Fat and Muscles
Fu 膚	Superficial layer of skin
Gao 膏	Fat tissue
Ge 革	Deep layer of skin
Huang 肓	Membranes
Ji 肌	Subcutaneous muscles
Jin 筋	Sinews
Rou 肉	Muscles or flesh
Shao Fu 少腹	Lateral-lower abdominal area
Wu Lun 五轮	The Five Wheels
Xiang 象	Image
Xiao Fu 小腹	Central-lower abdominal area
Xin Xia 心下	Area below the xyphoid process
Xu Li 虛里	Great Connecting channel of the Stomach (manifesting in apical pulse)
Xuan Fu 玄府	Pores (including sebaceous glands)
Zong Jin 宗筋	Ancestral muscles

SYMPTOMS AND SIGNS

Ban 斑	Macule (in tongue diagnosis, red spots)
Ban Shen Bu Sui 半身不遂	Hemiplegia
Ben 本	Root
Bi Yuan 鼻淵	'Nose pool' (sinusitis)
Biao 标	Manifestation
Cao Za 嘈杂	Gnawing hunger
Chuan 喘	Breathlessness
Dao Han 盗汗	Night sweating
Dian 点	Red points (on the tongue)
Duan Qi 短气	Shortness of breath
Duo Qi 夺气	Robbing of Qi (very feeble voice with interrupted speech)
E Xin 恶心	Nausea
Fan Wei 反胃	Regurgitation of food
Fan Zao 烦燥	Mental restlessness
Feng Tuan 风团	Wheal
Feng Yin Zhen 风瘾疹	Wind hidden rash (urticaria)
Feng Zhen 风疹	Wind rash (German measles)
Fu 腐	Mouldy
Gan Ou 干呕	Short retching with low sound
Han Re Wang Lai 寒热往来	Alternation of chills and fever
Han Zhan 汗颤	Shivers

Hu Re 湖热	Tidal fever		*Ru E* 乳蛾	Milky moth (swollen tonsils)
Hua 滑	Slippery (tongue coating)		*Shang Qi* 上气	Rebellious-Qi breathing
Ji 肌	Blood masses		*Shen Chong* 身重	Feeling of heaviness of the body
Jia 瘕	Qi masses		*Shi* 实	Full, Fullness, Excess
Jiao Qi 脚气	Leg Qi		*Shi E* 石蛾	Stone moth (swollen tonsils)
Jie 结	Accumulation (or nodules)		*Shi Zhen* 湿疹	Eczema
Jing Ji 惊悸	Fright palpitations		*Shou Chan* 手颤	Tremor of the hands
Ju 聚	Qi masses		*Shou Zhi Luan* 手指挛	Contraction of the fingers
Jue 厥	Breakdown		*Shui Dou* 水痘	Waterpox (chickenpox)
Jue Han 厥汗	Sweating from collapse		*Shui Pao* 水泡	Vesicle
Kou Chuang 口疮	Mouth ulcers		*Shui Zhong* 水肿	Water oedema
Kou Yan Wai Xie 口眼歪斜	Deviation of eye and mouth		*Si Ni* 四逆	Four Rebellious
Li Ji 里急	Internal urgency (or tension of lining)		*Tai Qi Shang Ni* 胎气上逆	Fetus' Qi rebelling upwards
Li Ji Hou Zhong 里急後重	Difficulty in defecation		*Tan Yin* 痰饮	Phlegm-Fluids (or Phlegm-Fluids in Stomach and Intestines)
Liu Lei 流泪	Streaming eyes		*Tou Chong* 头重	Feeling of heaviness of the head
Ma Mu 麻木	Numbness/tingling		*Tou Fa Bian Bai* 头发变白	Greying of the hair
Ma Zhen 麻疹	Hemp rash (measles)		*Tou Fa Tuo Luo* 头发脱落	Alopecia
Man 满	Feeling of fullness			
Men 闷	Feeling of oppression		*Tou Qing* 头倾	Drooping head
Mu Chan 目颤	Quivering eyeball		*Tou Yun* 头晕	Dizziness
Mu Hua 目花	Floaters		*Tu* 吐	Vomiting (without sound)
Mu Hun 目昏	Blurred vision		*Tuo* 脱	Collapse
Mu Xuan 目眩	Blurred vision		*Wu Chi* 五迟	Five Retardations
Nao Ming 脑鸣	Brain noise		*Wu Feng* 恶风	Aversion to wind
Ni 腻	Sticky (tongue coating)		*Wu Han* 恶寒	Aversion to cold
Ni Jing 逆经	Reverse period		*Wu Han Fa Re* 恶寒发热	(Simultaneous) Aversion to cold and fever
Nong Pao 脓泡	Pustule		*Wu Ruan* 五软	Five Flaccidities
Ou Tu 呕吐	Vomiting (with sound)		*Wu Xin Fa Re* 五心发热	Five-palm heat
Pao 泡	Vesicle			
Pi 痞	Feeling of stuffiness		*Xiao* 哮	Wheezing
Qi Shao 气少	Weak breathing		*Xin Fan* 心烦	Mental restlessness
Qi Zhong 气肿	Qi oedema		*Xin Zhong Ao Nong* 心中懊脑	Heart feeling vexed
Qing 青	Bluish-greenish (colour)			
Qiu Zhen 丘疹	Papule			
Re Du 热毒	Toxic Heat		*Xu* 虚	Empty, Emptiness, Deficiency

Xuan Yin 玄饮	Phlegm-Fluids in the hypochondrium
Xuan Yun 眩晕	Dizziness
Yan Chi 眼眵	Discharge from the eyes
Yan Shi 厌食	Aversion to food
Yi Yin 溢饮	Phlegm-Fluids in the limbs
Yu Zheng 郁症	Depression
Yue 哕	Long retching with loud sound
Zhan Han 颤汗	Shiver sweating
Zhang 涨	Feeling of distension
Zhen 疹	Rash
Zheng 症	Blood masses
Zheng Chong 怔忡	Panic palpitations
Zhi Yin 支饮	Phlegm-Fluids above the diaphragm
Zu Chan 足颤	Tremor of the feet

DISEASE SYMPTOMS

Beng Lou 崩漏	Flooding and trickling
Bi Jing 闭经	No periods
Bi Zheng 痹症	Painful Obstruction Syndrome
Dian Kuang 癫狂	Manic depression
Dian Xian 癫痫	Epilepsy
Fei Xu Lao 肺虚芳	Lung Exhaustion
Feng Zhen 风疹	German measles
Gan 疳	Childhood Nutritional Impairment
Gao Lin 膏淋	Sticky Painful-Urination Syndrome
Jing Jian Qi Chu Xue 经间期出血	Bleeding between periods
Jue Zheng 蕨症	Breakdown Syndrome
Lao Lin 芳淋	Fatigue Painful-Urination Syndrome
Lin Zheng 淋症	Painful Urination Syndrome
Ma Zhen 麻疹	Measles
Mian Tan 面瘫	Facial paralysis

Qi Lin 气淋	Qi Painful-Urination Syndrome
Re Lin 热淋	Heat Painful-Urination Syndrome
Shi Lin 石淋	Stone Painful-Urination Syndrome
Shi Zhen 湿疹	Eczema (dermatitis)
Shui Dou 水痘	Chickenpox
Tan Huan 瘫缓	Paralysis
Wei Zheng 痿症	Atrophy Syndrome
Wen Bing 温病	Warm disease
Wu Chi 五迟	Five Retardations
Wu Ruan 五软	Five Flaccidities
Xu Lao 虚芳	Exhaustion
Xu Sun 虚损	Exhaustion
Xue Lin 血淋	Blood Painful-Urination Syndrome
Ye Ge 噎膈	Diaphragm choking
Yin Zhen 瘾疹	Urticaria
Yu Zheng 郁症	Depression pattern
Yue Jing Guo Duo 月经过多	Heavy periods
Yue Jing Guo Shao 月经过少	Scanty periods
Yue Jing Hou Qi 月经後期	Late periods
Yue Jing Xian Hou Wu Ding Qi 月经先後无定期	Irregular periods
Yue Jing Xian Qi 月经先其	Early periods
Zhong Feng 中风	Wind-stroke
Zi Lin 子淋	Painful-urination pregnancy
Zi Yun 子晕	Dizziness of pregnancy
Zi Zhong 子肿	Oedema of pregnancy

VITAL SUBSTANCES

Hou Tian Zhi Qi 后天之气	Postnatal Qi
Hun 魂	Ethereal Soul

Jing 精	Essence
Jun Huo 君火	Emperor Fire
Ming Men 命门	Gate of Life
Ming Men Huo 命门火	Fire of the Gate of Life
Po 魄	Corporeal Soul
Shen 神	Mind (the Shen of the Heart) or Spirit (the complex of Heart-Shen, Corporeal Soul, Ethereal Soul, intellect and will-power)
Tian Gui 天癸	Heavenly Gui
Wei Qi 卫气	Defensive Qi
Xian Tian Zhi Qi 先天之气	Prenatal Qi
Xiang Huo 相火	Minister Fire
Yi 意	Intellect
Ying Qi 营气	Nutritive Qi
Yuan Qi 原气	Original Qi
Zhen Qi 真气	True Qi
Zheng Qi 正气	Upright Qi
Zhi 志	Will-power
Zhong Qi 中气	Central Qi
Zong Qi 宗气	Gathering Qi (of the chest)

EMOTIONS

Bei 悲	Sadness
Jing 精	Shock
Kong 恐	Fear
Nu 怒	Anger
Si 思	Pensiveness
Xi 喜	Joy
You 忧	Worry

CHANNELS AND POINTS

Bao Luo 胞络	Uterus channel
Bao Mai 胞脉	Uterus vessel
Chong Mai 冲脉	Penetrating Vessel

Cou Li 腠里	Space between skin and muscles
Dai Mai 带脉	Girdle Vessel
Du Mai 督脉	Governing Vessel
Fu Luo 浮络	Superficial Connecting channel
Hui Xue 会穴	Gathering point
Jing Bie 经别	Divergent channel
Jing Jin 经筋	Muscle channel
Jue Yin 厥阴	Terminal Yin
Luo Mai 络脉	Connecting channel
Luo Xue 络穴	Connecting point
Mu Xue 募穴	Front Collecting points
Ren Mai 任脉	Directing Vessel
Shao Yang 少阳	Lesser Yang
Shao Yin 少阴	Lesser Yin
(Bei) Shu Xue 背输穴	Back Transporting points
Sun Luo 孙络	Minute Connecting channel
Tai Yang 太阳	Greater Yang
Tai Yin 太阴	Greater Yin
Wu Shu Xue 五输穴	Five Transporting points
Xi Xue 郄穴	Accumulation point
Yang Ming 阳明	Bright Yang
Yang Qiao Mai 阳跷脉	Yang Heel Vessel
Yang Wei Mai 阳维脉	Yang Linking Vessel
Yin Qiao Mai 阴跷脉	Yin Heel Vessel
Yin Wei Mai 阴维脉	Yin Linking Vessel
Yuan Xue 原穴	Source point

PULSE POSITIONS

Chi 尺	Rear (pulse position)
Cun 寸	Front (pulse position)
Guan 关	Middle (pulse position)

PULSE QUALITIES

Chang 长	Long
Chen 沉	Deep
Chi 尺	Slow
Cu 促	Hasty
Da 大	Big
Dai 代	Irregular or Intermittent
Dong 动	Moving
Duan 短	Short
Fu 浮	Floating
Fu 伏	Hidden
Ge 革	Leather
Hong 洪	Overflowing
Hua 滑	Slippery
Huan 缓	Slowed-Down
Ji 肌	Hurried
Jie 结	Knotted
Jin 筋	Tight
Kou 芤	Hollow
Lao 牢	Firm
Ru 濡	Soggy
Ruan 软	Soggy
Ruo 弱	Weak
San 散	Scattered
Se 涩	Choppy
Shi 实	Full
Shu 数	Rapid
Wei 微	Minute
Xi 细	Fine
Xian 弦	Wiry
Xu 虚	Empty

METHODS OF TREATMENT

An Tai 安胎	Calm the Fetus
Bu 补	Tonify (or reinforce as a needle technique)

Gong Yu 功瘀	Dispel stasis (of Blood)
Gu 固	Consolidate
Gu Tuo 固脱	Consolidate collapse
Hua Shi 化湿	Resolve Dampness
Hua Tan 化痰	Resolve Phlegm
Hua Yu 化瘀	Eliminate stasis (of Blood)
Huan Ji 缓急	Moderate urgency
Huo Xue 活血	Invigorate Blood
Jie (Biao) 解表	Release (the Exterior)
Jie Yu 解郁	Eliminate stagnation (of Qi)
Li Qi 理气	Move Qi
Li Shi 利水	Resolve Dampness
Li Shui 利水	Transform Water
Ping Gan 平肝	Calm the Liver
Po Xue 破血	Break up Blood
Qing (Re) 清热	Clear Heat
Qu (Feng) 去风	Expel (external Wind)
Qu Yu 去瘀	Eliminate stasis (of Blood)
San Han 散寒	Scatter Cold
San Jie 散结	Dissipate accumulation or dissipate nodules
Sheng Xin 生新	Promote healing of tissues
Shu (Gan) 疏肝	Pacify (the Liver)
Tiao He Ying Wei 调和营卫	Harmonize Nutritive and Defensive Qi
Tiao Jing 调经	Regulate the period
Tong Luo 通络	Remove obstructions from the Connecting channels
Tong Qiao 通窍	Open the orifices
Tong Ru 通乳	Remove obstructions from the breast's Connecting channels
Wen Jing 温经	Warm the menses
Xi Feng 熄风	Extinguish Wind (internal)
Xie 泻	Reduce (as a needle technique)
Xie 泄	Clear (Heat)
Xie 泻	Drain (Fire)
Xie Xia 泻下	Move downwards

Xin Kai Ku Jiang 辛开苦降	Use pungent herbs to open and bitter ones to make Qi descend
Xuan Fei 宣肺	Restore the diffusing of Lung-Qi
Yang (Xue) 养血	Nourish (Blood)

PATHOGENIC FACTORS

Feng Han 风寒	Wind-Cold
Feng Re 风热	Wind-Heat
Han 寒	Cold
Huo 火	Fire

Re 热	Heat
Re Du 热毒	Toxic Heat
Shi 实	Dampness
Shu 暑	Summer-Heat
Tan 痰	Phlegm
Tan Yin 痰饮	Phlegm-Fluids in general and also Phlegm-Fluids in the Stomach
Xuan Yin 悬饮	Phlegm-Fluids in the hypochondrium
Yi Yin 溢饮	Phlegm-Fluids in the limbs
Zao 燥	Dryness
Zhi Yin 支饮	Phlegm-Fluids in the diaphragm

Bibliography

1979 The Yellow Emperor's Classic of Internal Medicine – Simple Questions (*Huang Di Nei Jing Su Wen* 黄帝内经素问), People's Health Publishing House, Beijing. First published c. 100BC.

1981 Spiritual Axis (*Ling Shu Jing* 灵枢经), People's Health Publishing House, Beijing, first published c. 100BC.

Beijing College of Traditional Chinese Medicine 1980 Tongue Diagnosis in Chinese Medicine (*Zhong Yi She Zhen* 中医舌诊), People's Health Publishing House, Beijing.

Chen Jia Yuan 1988 Eight Secret Books on Gynaecology (*Fu Ke Mi Shu Ba Zhong* 妇科秘书八种), Ancient Chinese Medicine Texts Publishing House, Beijing. Chen's book, written during the Qing dynasty (1644–1911), was entitled 'Secret Gynaecological Prescriptions' (*Fu Ke Mi Fang* 妇科秘方).

Chen You Bang 1990 Chinese Acupuncture Therapy (*Zhong Guo Zhen Jiu Zhi Liao Xue* 中国针灸治疗学), China Science Publishing House, Beijing.

Cheng Bao Shu 1988 An Annotated Translation of the Study of the Pulse from Pin Hu Lake (*Pin Hu Mai Xue Yi Zhu* 濒湖脉学译注), Ancient Chinese Medical Texts Publishing House, Beijing. 'The Study of the Pulse from Pin Hu Lake' was first published in 1564.

Cheng Shao En 1994 Diagnosis, Patterns and Treatment in Chinese Medicine (*Zhong Yi Zheng Hou Zhen Duan Zhi Liao Xue* 中医证候诊断疗学), Beijing Science Publishing House, Beijing.

Cheng Xin Nong 1987 Chinese Acupuncture and Moxibustion (*Zhong Guo Zhen Jiu Xue* 中国针灸学), Foreign Languages Press, Beijing.

Chinese Medicine Research Institute and Guangzhou College of Chinese Medicine 1980 Concise Dictionary of Chinese Medicine (*Jian Ming Zhong Yi Ci Dian* 简明中医辞典), People's Health Publishing House, Beijing.

Chinese Medicine Research Institute and Guangzhou College of Chinese Medicine 1981 Great Dictionary of Chinese Medicine (*Zhong Yi Da Ci Dian* 中医大辞典), People's Health Publishing Company, Beijing.

Cong Chun Yu 1989 Gynaecology in Chinese Medicine (*Zhong Yi Fu Ke Xue* 中医妇科学) Ancient Chinese Medicine Texts Publishing House, Beijing.

Deng Tie Tao 1988 Practical Chinese Medicine Diagnosis (*Shi Yong Zhong Yi Zhen Duan Xue* 实用中医诊断学), Shanghai Science Publishing House, Shanghai.

Fuzhou City People's Hospital 1988 A Revised Explanation of the Pulse Classic (*Mai Jing Jiao Shi* 脉经校释), People's Health Publishing House, Beijing. The 'Pulse Classic' was written by Wang Shu He and was first published in AD280.

Gu Yi Di 1986 Illustrated Collection of Diagnostic Methods in Chinese Medicine (*Zhong Yi Zhen Fa Tu Pu* 中医诊法图谱), Publishing House of the Shanghai College of Traditional Chinese Medicine, Shanghai.

Guang Dong College of Chinese Medicine 1979 Diagnosis in Chinese Medicine (*Zhong Yi Zhen Duan Xue* 中医诊断学) Shanghai Science Publishing House, Shanghai.

Guo Zhen Qiu 1985 Chinese Medicine Diagnosis (*Zhong Yi Zhen Duan Xue* 中医诊断学), Hunan Science Publishing House, Changsha.

He Ren 1981 A New Explanation of the Synopsis of Prescriptions from the Golden Cabinet (*Jin Gui Yao Lue Xin Jie* 金匮要略新解), Zhejiang Science Publishing House, Zhejiang.

Heilongjiang Province National Medical Research Group 1984 An Explanation of the Great Compendium of Acupuncture (*Zhen Jiu Da Cheng Jiao Shi* 针灸大成校释), People's Health Publishing House, Beijing. The 'Great Compendium of Acupuncture' itself was published in 1601.

Huang Shi Lin 1989 Research in Chinese Medicine Pulse Diagnosis (*Zhong Yi Mai Xiang Yan Jiu* 中医脉象研究), People's Health Publishing House, Beijing.

Li Dong Yuan 1976 Discussion on Stomach and Spleen (*Pi Wei Lun* 脾胃论), People's Health Publishing House, Beijing. First published in 1246.

Li Jing Wen 1994 Illustrated Collection of Tongue Images in Frequently-Seen Diseases of the Digestive System (*Chang Jian Xiao Hua Xi Ji Bing She Xiang Tu Pu* 常见消化系疾病舌图谱), People's Health Publishing House, Beijing.

Lin Zhi Han 1987 The Essential Four Diagnostic Examinations (*Si Zhen Jue Wei* 四诊抉微), Chinese Bookshop Publishing House, Beijing. First published in 1723.

Ling Yao Xing 1994 Practical Dictionary of Words and Phrases from the Nei Jing (*Shi Yong Nei Jing Ci Ju Ci Dian* 实用内经辞句辞典), Shanghai Chinese Pharmacology University Publishing House, Shanghai.

Liu Guan Jun 1981 Pulse Diagnosis (*Mai Zhen* 脉诊), Shanghai Science Publishing House, Shanghai.

Lu De Ming 1993 Illustrated Collection of Diagnosis and Treatment of External Diseases in Chinese Medicine (*Zhong Yi Wai Ke Zhen Liao Tu Pu* 中医外科诊疗图谱), Publishing House of the Shanghai College of Traditional Chinese Medicine, Shanghai.

Ma Zhong Xue 1989 Great Treatise of Chinese Diagnostic Methods (*Zhong Guo Yi Xue Zhen Fa Da Quan* 中国医学诊法大学), Shandong Science Publishing House, Shandong.

Nanjing College of Traditional Chinese Medicine 1978 A Study of Warm Diseases (*Wen Bing Xue* 温病学), Shanghai Science Publishing House, Shanghai.

Nanjing College of Traditional Chinese Medicine 1979 A Revised Explanation of the Classic of Difficulties (*Nan Jing Jiao Shi* 难经校释), People's Health Publishing House, Beijing. First published c. AD100.

Pei Zheng Xue 1980 A Commentary on the Discussion of Blood Syndromes (*Xue Zheng Lun Ping Shi* 血证论评释), People's Health Publishing House, Beijing. The Discussion on Blood Syndromes (*Xue Zheng Lun* 血证论) by Tang Zong Hai was originally published in 1885.

Shang Han Lun Research Group of the Nanjing College of Traditional Chinese Medicine 1980 An Explanation of the Discussion of Cold-induced Diseases (*Shang Han Lun Jiao Shi* 伤寒论校释), Shanghai Science Publishing House, Shanghai. 'The Discussion of Cold-induced Diseases' was written by Zhang Zhong Jing in c. 220BC.

Wang Ke Qin 1988 Theory of the Mind in Chinese Medicine (*Zhong Yi Shen Zhu Xue Shuo* 中医神主学说), Ancient Chinese Medical Texts Publishing House.

Wang Luo Zhen 1985 A Compilation of the Study of the Eight Extraordinary Vessels (*Qi Jing Ba Mai Kao Jiao Zhu* 奇经八脉考校注), Shanghai Science Publishing House, Shanghai. The 'Study of the Eight Extraordinary Vessels' (*Qi Jing Ba Mai Kao*) by Li Shi Zhen was published in 1578.

Wang Xue Tai 1995 Great Treatise of Chinese Acupuncture (*Zhong Guo Zhen Jiu Da Quan* 中国针灸大全), Henan Science and Technology Publishing House, Henan.

Wu Qian 1977 Golden Mirror of Medicine (*Yi Zong Jin Jian* 医宗金鉴), People's Health Publishing House, Beijing, Vol. 2. First published in 1742.

Yang Ji Zhou 1980 Great Compendium of Acupuncture (*Zhen Jiu Da Cheng* 针灸大成), People's Health Publishing House, Beijing. First published in 1601.

Yang Jia San 1988 Great Dictionary of Chinese Acupuncture (*Zhong Guo Zhen Jiu Da Ci Dian* 中国针灸大辞典), Beijing Physical Training College Publishing House, Beijing.

Zhai Ming Yi 1979 Clinical Chinese Medicine (*Zhong Yi Lin Chuang Ji Chu* 中医临床基础) Henan Publishing House, Henan, p. 132.

Zhang Bo Yu 1986 Chinese Internal Medicine (*Zhong Yi Nei Ke Xue* 中医内科学), Shanghai Science Publishing House, Shanghai.

Zhang Jie Bin 1982 Classic of Categories (*Lei Jing* 类经), People's Health Publishing House, Beijing, p. 99. First published in 1624.

Zhang Jie Bin (also called Zhang Jing Yue) 1986 Complete Works of Jing Yue (*Jing Yue Quan Shu* 景岳全书), Shanghai Science Publishing House, Shanghai. First published in 1624.

Zhang Shu Sheng 1995 Great Treatise of Diagnosis by Observation in Chinese Medicine (*Zhong Hua Yi Xue Wang Zhen Da Quan* 中华医学望诊大全), Shanxi Science Publishing House, Taiyuan.

Zhang Yuan Kai (editor) 1985 Medical Collection of Four Families from Meng He (*Meng He Si Jia Yi Ji* 孟河四家医集), Jiangsu Science Publishing House, Nanjing.

Zhao Jin Duo 1985 Identification of Patterns and Diagnosis in Chinese Medicine (*Zhong Yi Zheng Zhuang Jian Bie Zhen Duan Xue* 中医证状鉴别诊断学), People's Health Publishing House, Beijing.

Zhao Jin Duo 1991 Differential Diagnosis and Patterns in Chinese Medicine (*Zhong Yi Zheng Hou Jian Bie Zhen Duan Xue* 中医证候鉴别诊断学), People's Health Publishing House, Beijing.

Zhao Jin Ze 1991 Differential Diagnosis and Patterns in Chinese Medicine (*Zhong Yi Zheng Hou Jian Bie Zhen Duan Xue* 中医证候鉴别诊断学), People's Health Publishing House, Beijing.

Zhu Qi Shi 1988 Discussion on Exhaustion (*Xu Lao Lun* 虚劳论), People Health Publishing House, Beijing, p. 19. First published c. 1520.

Zhu Wen Feng 1999 Diagnosis in Chinese Medicine (*Zhong Yi Zhen Duan Xue* 中医诊断学), People's Health Publishing House, Beijing.

Chinese chronology

Xia: 21st to 16th century BC

Shang: 16th to 11th century BC

Zhou: 11th century to 771BC

Spring and Autumn period: 770–476BC

Warring States period: 475–221BC

Qin: 221–207BC

Han: 206BC–AD220

Three Kingdoms period: AD220–280

Jin: 265–420

Northern and Southern dynasties: 420–581

Sui: 581–618

Tang: 618–907

Five dynasties: 907–960

Song: 960–1279

Liao: 906–1125

Jin: 1115–1234

Yuan: 1271–1368

Ming: 1368–1644

Qing: 1644–1911

Republic of China: 1912–1949

People's Republic of China: 1949–

INDEX

Note:
Page numbers in *italics* denote figures; **bold** denotes main entries; *plate* denotes colour photographs

A

abdomen
abnormal feelings in 741–742
areas influenced by organs 510, *510*
areas of 145, *513*, 513–516
borborygmi 742–743
central-lower 516
channels influencing 145
see also specific channels
cold feeling in 741–742
distension (bloating) *see* distension
(bloating)
energy rising feeling in 742
epigastrium *see* epigastrium
flatulence *273*, 743
fullness *see* fullness
hypochondrium *see* hypochondrium
interrogation **326–335**
kidneys reflection 146
large 146, 745
lateral-lower, areas and palpation
515–516, *516*
lumps/masses 146–147, 511–512,
856–857
contracted ears and 584
gynaecological symptoms 856–857
symptoms and signs 744–745
types *147*, *512*
observation **143–147**
oedema 146, 745
pain *see* abdominal pain
palpation 510–512, 513–516
patterns *334*
sagging lower 146, 745
size 146, 745
skin signs 147
distended veins 147, 743
lines *147*, 743
maculae *147*, 743–744
stomach and spleen reflection 146
symptoms and signs 326–327,
735–745
temperature 510–511
tenderness 511, *511*

texture 511, *511*
thin 146, 745
umbilical area *see* umbilicus
xyphoid process *see* xyphoid process
abdominal pain
after childbirth 844
case histories
central–lower abdominal area
332–333
constipation 273
epigastric pain 330
hypochondrial pain 331, *332*
tongue/pulse diagnosis 244
diagnosis 327
evacuation related 273–274
fullness *see* fullness
location 327–335, *328*, *334*
area under xyphoid process
328–329, *329*, 736–737
see also xyphoid process
central–lower abdominal area
332–333, 739–740
epigastrium *see* epigastrium
hypochondrium *see* hypochondrial
pain
lateral lower abdominal area 740
left-lateral lower abdominal area
334–335
right-lateral lower abdominal area
333, 333–334
umbilical area 332, 738–739
see also umbilicus
menstrual pain 401–404
oppression 735
patterns *334*
pregnancy 838
stagnant Cold in Uterus 1002
stuffiness 327, 736
abortion 408
see also miscarriage
Accumulation Disorder 868–869
breath odour 550, *550*
creases on index finger 195, 196, 197

crying in babies 544
with Spleen deficiency, hot palms and
soles 866
temple palpation in babies 519
ACE inhibitors, effect on pulse 508
aches
back *see* backache
earache 357, *357*, 413, 582
head *see* headache
limbs 671
nose 595
shoulder 656
teeth 306–307, *307*, 615
whole body 317–318, *318*, 709–710,
833
acne 71
inflammatory *plate 21.24*
occurrence 182
papular-pustular *plate 21.21*
pathology and diagnosis
Chinese 183, *183*
Western 182–183
pustular *plate 21.22*
scarring *plate 21.23*
symptoms and signs 569, 783–784
acne rosacea *plate 21.55*
acupuncture
accumulation of Blood 966
Attack of Wind 965
Bladder deficient and Cold 926
Blood rebelling upwards after
childbirth 1003
Cold transformation 968
Dampness and Phlegm in Uterus 1002
Directing and Penetrating Vessels
deficient and Cold 999
Directing and Penetrating Vessels
empty 999
Directing and Penetrating Vessels
unstable 999
fetus Heat 1003
Full-Heat in Directing and Penetrating
Vessels 1000

acupuncture *(contd.)*
  Heart-Qi and Heart-Yin deficiency
      881
  Heart-Yang collapse 880
  Heat transformation 968
  Heat victorious agitates Blood 957
  Heat victorious stirring Wind 957
  Kidney- and Liver Yin deficiency with
      Empty Heat 909
  Kidney and Heart not harmonized
      (Kidney- and Heart-Yin
      deficiency with Heart
      Empty-Heat) 909
  Kidney-Yang (predominant) and
      Kidney-Yin deficiency 907
  Kidney-Yang and Kidney-Yin
      deficiency (predominant) 907
  Kidney-Yang deficiency, Water
      overflowing 906
  Kidney-Yin deficiency 906
  Kidney-Yin deficiency , Empty Heat
      blazing 907
  Kidney-Yin deficiency with Phlegm
      907
  Liver-Blood deficiency generating Wind
      895
  Liver-Blood stasis 893
  Liver-Fire Blazing Upwards 893
  Liver-Fire generating Wind 894
  Liver-Heat stirs Wind 970
  Liver-Wind harbouring Phlegm 895
  Liver-Yang rising 892
  Liver-Yang rising deriving from
      Liver-Yin deficiency 894
  Liver-Yang rising generating Wind
      894
  Lung
      invasion by Wind-Cold 901
      invasion by Wind-Dryness 901
      invasion by Wind-Heat 901
  Lung-Heat 902, 955
  Lung-Qi collapse 903
  Lung-Qi deficiency 899
  Lung-Qi deficiency with Phlegm
      899–900
  Lung-Qi stagnation 903
  Lung-Yang deficiency 900
  Lung-Yin deficiency 900
  Lung-Yin deficiency with Empty-Heat
      900
  Obstruction of Spleen by Dampness
      with stagnation of Liver-Qi
      889
  Phlegm misting Mind 882
  Phlegm obstructing Middle Burner
      888
  Rebellious Liver Qi 892
  Small Intestine deficient and Cold 912
  Small Intestine Qi tied 912
  Spleen- and Liver-Blood deficiency
      889
  Spleen- and Lung-Qi deficiency 889
  Spleen-Blood deficiency 886
  Spleen Damp-Heat 970
  stagnant Cold in Uterus 1002
  Stomach Blood stasis 915
  Stomach-Qi rebelling upwards 916
  Uterus deficient and Cold 1002
  Water Overflowing to Heart 883
  Wind-Cold invasion (Cold prevalent)
      965
  Yang Heel Vessel *(Yang Qiao Mai)*
      1004
  Yin Heel Vessel *(Yin Qiao Mai)* 1004
  Yin Linking Vessel *(Yin Wei Mai)* 1005
  see also individual points
acupuncture points
  back transporting *(Bei Shu)* points
      522
  front collecting *(Mu)* points 521–522
  palpation 520–522
  source *(Yuan)* points 522
  see also individual points
adenoids, swollen 111
adolescence, Five Stages of Life 417
adverse drug reactions 429
agalactia 408, *408*
age/aging
  Five Stages of Life 417–418
  pulse 450, 470
  see also elderly
Ah Shi points 520, 527–528
Ai Fu Nuan Gong Wan 1025
alae nasi, flapping 90, 598
alcoholism, hand tremor 130, 156
allergic rhinitis 304, 305, 546, 1017,
      1019
alopecia 72, *72*, 566
  see also hair loss
amenorrhoea 400, 401, 829, 845
An Shen Ding Zhi Wan 1025
anger 385–386, 420–423, *423*
  propensity to 791
  pulse indication 452
  sighing 545
anorexia 319
antibiotics
  residual pathogenic factors 974
  tongue 204, *204*
antidepressants, effect on pulse
      507–508
anus
  fissure 762
  fistula 762
  haemorrhoids 761–762
  itching 761
  prolapse 762
  symptoms and signs **761–763**

ulcers 763
anxiety 384–385
  patterns *384, 385*
  in pregnancy 840
  symptoms and signs 792–793,
      799–800
  see also fear; mental-emotional
      symptoms; worry
apical pulse 512, *512*
appetite 264–265
  aversion to food 264, 721
  excessive hunger 264, 720
  hunger but no desire to eat 265, 721
  poor 719–720
  see also hunger
armpits *see* axillae
arms
  symptoms/signs **679–692**
  tremor 341
  see also limbs
arthritis, rheumatoid 138
asthma
  hand lines 134, *134*
  mouth open 97
atopic eczema *see* eczema
atrial fibrillation, pulse indication 460
atrophy
  dorsum of hands 130, 685–686
  legs 160, 694–695
  limbs 153–154, *154*, 338, *338*,
      674–675
  muscles along spine 116, 705
  thenar eminence of hands 130, 685
Attack of Cold 945, *945*, 965
Attack of Cold/Wind differentiation
      369–370, *370, 370*, 966
Attack of Wind 945, *945*, 965
Auspitz's sign 184
axillae
  rash 785
  sweating in 779

B

Ba Xian Chang Shou Wan 1025
Ba Zhen Tang 1026
Ba Zheng San 1026
babies
  convulsions 155
  crying 413, 544, 868
  effect of childbirth 412
  feeding 412
  fontanelles
      late closure in babies 70, 872
      raised 871–872
      sunken 871
  index finger observation 1057
  see also index finger creases
      (children)

period in womb 411, 412
prenatal shock 411–412
sleeping problems 413
temple palpation 518–519, *519*
weaning 412
see also children
back
aches *see* backache
boils on 119, 706
buttocks *see* buttocks
channels influencing 115, *115, 116*
lower
dryness and redness 119, 706
feeling of cold and heaviness 704
rigidity 116, 705
skin marks 119, 706
stiffness 705
symptoms and signs **703–715**
vesicles on 119, 706
weakness with knee weakness
704–705
yellow colour 119, 706
observation **115–120**
pustules on *118,* 118–119
sciatica 704
skin signs 118–119, 706–707
spots on *118,* 118–119, 706
stiffness like tight belt 657
upper
carbuncles 788
cold 656
hot 656
see also spine
backache
lower 318, *318,* 703–704
upper 656
bad breath (halitosis) 111, 729
Bai He Gu Jin Tang 1026
Bai Hu Tang 1026
Bai Tou Weng Tang 1026
Ban 176, 177
Ban Xia Hou Po Tang 1026
Ban Xia Tang 1026
Bao He Wan 1026
Bao Jin Jian 1026–1027
Bao Yuan Tang 1027
Bei Mu Gua Lou San 1027
belching
diagnosis by sound 546, *546*
patterns 266
symptoms and signs 717–718
Bell's palsy (facial paralysis) 60–61, 573,
plate 4.1
beta blockers, effect on pulse 508
Big Head Warm Disease 564
Big pulse *see* pulse qualities
birth *see* childbirth
bitter taste 726–727
see also taste

BL-23 Shenshu 119, 706
BL-40 Weizhong 533, *533*
Bladder **925–926**
channels 995
injury during childbirth 845
invasion of external Dampness
949–950
urinary difficulty 845
Bladder channel 995
abdomen 145
back 115, *115, 116*
ears relationship 105, *106*
eyes relationship 78
neck 109, *109*
palpation 533, *533*
blood vessel 533
skin 533
Bladder deficient and Cold 926
bleeding
ears 583
eyes, between iris and pupil 649
gums 101, 307, *307,* 619
menstrual *see* menstrual bleeding
vaginal *see* vaginal bleeding
see also Blood loss
blepharoconjunctivitis 643–644
blindness, sudden 630–631
bloating (distension) *see* distension
(bloating)
blocked nose 304, *304,* 591–592,
1017
see also rhinitis
Blood
accumulation of 966
see also Blood stasis
Empty-Blood 990
Heat victorious agitates Blood 957
levels 957
Latent Heat *960*
oedema 179
pattern identification 930–932
pulse diagnosis 434, 454, 463, 497
rebelling upwards after childbirth
1003
stasis *see* Blood stasis
in urine 839
see also entries beginning Blood (below);
individual organs
Blood and Qi deficient, clinical
manifestations 932–933
Blood and Yin deficiency with
Empty-Wind, convulsions after
childbirth 848
Blood-Cold, clinical manifestations 931
Blood collapse 931–932
clinical manifestations 931–932
Blood deficiency 930
abnormal lip colour in pregnancy 624
amenorrhoea 829

after miscarriage 845
body aches 709
during menstruation 833
breast distension 849
breast milk 847
breech presentation 842
case histories 1015
chronic fever 375, 815
clinical manifestations 930
cold hands and feet 672
coldness 364
complexion colours, sallow white 51
constipation 749
dizziness
during menstruation 835
in pregnancy 840
dry, cracked and peeling palms
684–685
eclampsia 841
with Empty-Heat 302, 376
Five-Palm Heat 817
genital eczema (female) 858
habitual miscarriage 842
headache 290, 561–562
hot palms and soles 866
infertility (female) 855
insomnia 348, 807
itching 713
late (long cycle) periods 827
lines on the face 574
Liver- and Heart-Blood deficiency 898
lochia 844
milky nipple discharge 851
miscarriage 841
numbness of face 572
oedema after childbirth 846
pain in hands 682
pale eye corners 636
pale eyelids 638
pale gums 620
pale helix 585
pale menstrual blood 825
post-chemotherapy fever 817
Qi deficiency and *see* Qi and Blood
deficiency
sallow complexion 578
scanty periods 828
severe, abnormal lip colour in
pregnancy 624
skin eruptions during menstruation
834
slow fetal growth 842
small breasts 852
Spleen Qi and Spleen-Blood deficiency
804
tongue diagnosis 205, 228
watery menstrual blood 826
weight loss 319
white/pale complexion 575

Blood deficiency and Intestines Dryness, anal fissure 762
Blood deficiency generating Empty-Wind, anal itching 761
Blood deficiency in Penetrating Vessel, restless legs 700
Blood deficiency with Cold in Uterus, purple menstrual blood 826
Blood deficiency with Dryness
    eczema 783
    genital eczema (women) 858
    small breasts 852
    warts 787
    with Wind in the skin, psoriasis 783
Blood deficiency with Empty-Heat, red complexion 577
Blood deficiency with Empty-Wind
    quivering eyeball 644
    trembling lips 623
Blood deficiency with internal Wind
    flapping eyelids 639
    itching ears 582
Blood deficiency with Wind
    dry, cracked and peeling palms 685
    skin, itching hands 683
Blood-Dryness 931
    clinical manifestations 931
Blood-Heat
    clinical manifestations 815, 931
    dark philtrum 626
    distended abdominal veins 743
    early (short cycle) periods 827
    fever during menstruation 833
    habitual miscarriage 842
    heavy periods 827–828
    infertility (female) 855
    itching 713
    lochia 844
    maculae on abdomen 743
    macular eruptions 573
    malignant melanoma 788
    menstrual clots 826
    miscarriage 841
    naevi (moles) 787
    pattern identification 931
    post-chemotherapy fever 817
    psoriasis 783
    red philtrum 626
    rosacea 785
    urticaria 785
    vaginal bleeding 838
    warts 787
Blood-Heat from Liver-Fire
    alopecia 566
    fainting 560
    hair falling out 566
Blood-Heat in Heart 931
Blood-Heat in Liver 931

Blood-Heat in Lungs, papules on nose 599
Blood-Heat in Stomach 931
Blood-Heat with Damp-Heat, malignant melanoma 788
Blood-Heat with Wind and Dryness, psoriasis 783
Blood levels, Latent Heat *960*
Blood loss
    clinical manifestations 931
    dry and brittle hair 566
Blood stagnation
    generating Wind *see* Wind
    tongue 231
Blood stasis 930
    abdomen 326
    abdominal masses 856
    acne 569
    in back, lower backache 704
    blood vessels distended on ear 586
    body aches 709
        during menstruation 833
    chronic, numbness of the tongue 614
    chronic and severe, dry skin 782
    chronic fever 375
    clinical manifestations 815, 930
    collapse after childbirth 847–848
    contraction
        of fingers 686
        of limbs 677
    crying out 822
    Damp-Heat with *see* Damp-Heat
    dark helix 585
    dark nails 692
    digestive symptoms 262
    dizziness after childbirth 846
    dry and cracked lips 623
    dry nostrils 594
    epigastric lumps 744
    excessive pubic hair 860
    facial pain 571
    fever in cancer 816
    flattening of lumbar spine 708
    frozen shoulder 656
    habitual miscarriage 842
    in head, hot and painful eyes 632
    headache 290, 561
        during menstruation 832
    helix dry and contracted 584
    herpes zoster 786
    hyperactivity 805
    infertility (female) 856
    in Intestines, blood in stools 751
    jaundice 714
    knotted in the Interior, abdominal masses (gynaecological symptom) 856–857
    list of spine 708
    lochia 844

    maculae on abdomen 744
    malignant melanoma 788
    menopausal syndrome 856
    mid-cycle menstrual bleeding 830
    naevi (moles) 788
    with oedema, protruding umbilicus 147
    oedema after childbirth 846
    pain in ribs 324
    post-chemotherapy fever 817
    psoriasis 783
    purple lips 621
    purple palate 625
    purple tongue 212, 213, *213*
    rigidity of lower back 705
    rosacea 785
    sallow complexion 578
    severe
        contracted ears with abdominal masses 584
        dark complexion 578
    in skin, urticaria 784
    stiff philtrum 625
    Stomach 915
    swollen fingers 686
    tidal fever 816
    tongue diagnosis 210
    Toxic Heat with *see* Toxic Heat with Blood stasis
    warts 787
    yellow complexion 576–577
    yellow sclera 635
    see also entries beginning Blood stasis (below)
Blood stasis from Cold
    abnormal lip colour in pregnancy 624
    bluish-greenish helix 585
    dark helix 585
    lines on abdomen 743
    purple complexion 578
Blood stasis from Heat
    bluish-greenish helix 585
    purple complexion 578
    yellow helix 585
Blood stasis from Qi deficiency, distension feeling in limbs 674
Blood stasis in Bladder
    abdominal pain - central, lower 739
    urination painful 755
Blood stasis in Directing and Penetrating Vessels 1000
Blood stasis in Liver and Spleen, distended abdominal veins 743
Blood stasis in Liver channel
    Peyronie's disease 772
    vulvar sores 858
Blood stasis in Lower Burner
    blood in sperm 768
    inability to ejaculate 768

pain and itching of penis 771
urination difficult 756
Blood stasis in Lungs, sense of smell
loss 598
Blood stasis in Stomach
epigastric pain 737
purple gums 620
reddish-purple nose 591
regurgitation of food 718
swallowing difficulty (diaphragm
choking) 726
venules on the thenar eminence
685
vomiting of blood 725
Blood stasis in Uterus
early (short cycle) periods 827
fever during menstruation 833
heavy periods 828
menstrual bleeding stopping and
starting 830
menstrual clots 826
scanty periods 828
sticky menstrual blood 826
Blood stasis knotted in Interior,
abdominal masses 856–857
Blood stasis with Blood-Heat, lines on
abdomen 743
Blood stasis with Damp-Heat
helix dry and contracted 584
in Liver channel, purple scrotum
770–771
yellow complexion 576
Blood stasis with Damp-Phlegm, in skin,
acne 784
Blood stasis with Heat in Uterus, purple
menstrual blood 825
Blood stasis with Phlegm
excessive pubic hair 773, 860
goitre 604
hoarse voice 606, 820
staggering gait 696
unilateral sweating 777
wide neck 655
Blood stasis with Phlegm-Heat, redness
and erosion of pharynx
603
Blood stasis with Spleen-Qi sinking,
sunken umbilicus 745
Blood stasis with Wind and Dryness,
psoriasis 783
blurred vision 360, *360*, 628
blushing, face 579
body
aches 317–318, *318*, 709–710
menstrual symptoms 833
loss of feeling 710–712
observation
body, mind and complexion **1–66**
body movements **59–66**

body shape, physique and
demeanour **11–29**
parts **67–200**
see also individual parts
body build (physique)
classification 12, 25–27
compact type 25–26, *26*
muscular type 26, *26*
observation **11–29**
overweight type 27, *27*
robust type 25, *25*
thin type 26–27, *27*
see also body shape
Body Fluids
deficiency 935
pattern identification 927–928,
935–938
body hair 176
see also pubic hair
body movements
children 194
face 60–61
head 59–60
limbs/body 61–65
observation **59–66**
body odour 549–550
constitutional 549, 550
diagnosis by 549–550
Five Elements 549–550
body part observation **67–200**
body shape
abundant in Yang *12*, 12–13
abundant in Yin *13*, 13–14
classification *see* body shape
classification
deficient in Yang 14, *14*
deficient in Yin 14, *14–15*
Earth type 17–18, *18*
Fire type 16–17, *17*
high pain/drug tolerance 27–28
low pain/drug tolerance 28
Metal type 19, *19*
observation **11–29**
strong postnatal Qi 23, 23–24
strong prenatal constitution *22*
Water type 19–20, *20*
weak postnatal Qi 24, 24–25
weak prenatal constitution 23, *23*
Wood type 15–16, *16*
Yin/Yang in balance 15, *15*
see also body build (physique)
body shape classification 11–29
body build 12, 25–27
Five Elements 11, 15–21
pain/drug tolerance 12, 27–28
prenatal/postnatal influences 11,
21–25
by Yin and Yang 11, 12–15
boiling cauldron pulse 506

boils
back (BL-23 Shenshu) 119, 706
eyelid 639
scalp 70, 568, 788
borborygmi 742–743
bouncing stone pulse 507
bowel movements, pain 258
brain noise 298, *298*
breast(s) **849–853**
gynaecomastia 145, 669–670
nipples *see* nipple(s)
nodularity and tenderness 122
observation **121–125**
organs influencing 397
pain 398, 850
palpation 513
peau d'orange skin 125, 852
premenstrual distension 398, 399,
832–833, 1016
redness and swelling 122, 850
size 122
small 122, 852–853
steaming, fever after childbirth 847
swollen 122, 850
symptoms 397–398
tongue areas 123
breast cancer 123, 397, 397–398,
462
see also cancer
breast milk
after childbirth 847
agalactia 408, *408*
overfeeding, vomiting 864
breastfeeding
agalactia 408, *408*
lactation 408, *408*
breath
foul 111, 729
shortness of (Duan Qi) 545, 661
smell diagnosis 550, *550*
breathing
diagnosis by hearing 544–545
equalizing, pulse taking 447
pathological sounds 545, *545*
rebellious-Qi (Shang Qi) 545, 661
sighing 545, 670
weak (Qi Shao) 545, 661
yawning 670
breathlessness (Chuan) 545
symptoms and signs 661–662
breech presentation 842
Bright Hall 87
Bright-Yang channels
acute fevers 373
headache 562
patterns 967
acupuncture 967
clinical manifestations 967
prescription 967

Bright-Yang organ patterns
  acupuncture 967
  clinical manifestations 967
  prescription 967
  tidal fever 816
Bu Fei Tang 1027
Bu Gan Tang 1027
Bu Shen Gu Chong Wan 1027
Bu Shen Yang Xue Tang 1027
Bu Zhong Yi Qi Tang 1027
buttocks
  pustules and papules 119, 707
  ulcers on 706–707

C

calves, cramp 344, 700–701
cancer
  breast 123, *397*, 397–398, 462
  chemotherapy 244, 817
  fever 816–817
  hand lines 136, *136*
  hoarse voice 543
  lung 457
  malignant melanoma *see* malignant
    melanoma
  nasal carcinoma 596
  pulse diagnosis 462–463
  tumours, abdominal cavity 128
  Western treatments 462
candida *plate 21.46, plate 21.47*
  occurrence 187
  pathology and diagnosis
    Chinese 187–188
    Western 187, *187*
  symptoms and signs 787
Cang Er Bi Dou Yan Fang 1027–1028
Cang Fu Dao Tan Wan 1028
cannabis 429–430
carcinoma *see* cancer
carotid artery, pulsation 110, 655
case histories **1013–1024**
  abdominal pain
    central–lower abdominal area
      332–333
    constipation 273
    epigastric pain 330
    hypochondrial pain 331, *332*
    tongue/pulse diagnosis 244
  alternating feeling of heat/cold
    370–371
  arm tremor 341
  Blood deficiency 1015
  breast lumps 123–124
  constipation/abdominal distension
    273
  Damp-Heat in Stomach and Spleen
    1014
  defensive Qi 1019–1020

Deficiency–Excess conditions 1023
  depression 1022
  diabetes mellitus 278–279
  diarrhoea 272
  eczema 182
  emotional states 1022, 1023
  Empty-Heat 1022
  feeling of cold 1018
  fertility 406–408
  gnawing hunger 722
  hair loss 1020, 1022
  infertility (female) 407–408,
    1013–1015, 1017–1015
  leg oedema 160
  limbs
    arm tremor 341
    generalized joint pain *340*
  Liver- and Heart-Blood deficiency
    1015
  Liver-Blood deficiency 1024
  Liver-Blood stasis 1024
  Liver patterns 1024
  Liver-Qi stagnation 1024
  Liver-Yang rising 1024
  menstrual bleeding 399–400
  menstrual pain 402–404
  otitis media 1021
  palpitations 1014
  panic attacks 385
  period pain 1016
  Phlegm 1020
  Phlegm-Heat 1022
  premenstrual breast distension 398,
    1016
  pulse and clinical application 457,
    459, 460
  pulse diagnosis 1020
  stress 1020, 1022
  thirst 278–279
  tinnitus 356
  tiredness 1022, 1023
    acute onset 1023
  tongue/pulse diagnosis 243–248,
    1022
    abdominal extension and pain 244
    benign positional vertigo 247–248
    joint pain 243
    premenstrual tension 244–246
  ulcerative colitis 272
  Yin deficiency 1021–1022
cataract 651
catarrh, chronic, children 413
causes of disease
  climate 428, *428*
  diagnosis **415–430**
  diet 427–428
  drugs as *see* drugs as causes of disease
  emotions 420–427
  excessive sexual activity 430

Five Stages of Life 417–418
  heredity 418–419
  immunizations 429
  interactions between *416*
    emotional problems at puberty and
      overwork 416–417
    hereditary weak constitution with
      diet 416
    trauma and climate 416
    weak Heart constitution and
      emotional problems 417
  medicinal drugs 429
  overwork 427
  recreational drugs 429–430
  trauma 428–429
Chai Hu Shu Gan Tang 1028
Chang Tai Bai Zhu San 1028
channel diagnosis, historical aspects
  1056–1058
channel patterns
  Bright-Yang 967
  Greater Yang stage 965–966
  Heat in Bright Yang -, fevers, acute
    373
channels
  abdomen 145
  back 115, *115*, 116
  bladder 995
  breasts *121*, 121–122, *122*
  chest 143, *143*
  Chinese terms 1064
  connecting *see* Connecting channels
  Dampness 950
  ears 105, *106*
  eyes 76, *77*, 78
    corners of 84–85, *85*
  gall-bladder 996
  genitalia *149*, 149–150, *150*
  gums 99
  heart 994
  invasion of external Dampness 950
  kidneys 995
  large intestine 993–994
  liver 996
  lungs 993
  mouth and lips 93–94, *94*
  muscles *see* Muscle channels
  nose 87–88, *88*
  pain, organ *vs.* channel pain 259
  palpation of 525–538
  pericardium 995
  philtrum 101
  Phlegm in the channels 937
  skin 174
  small intestine 994–995
  spleen 994
  stomach 994
  teeth 99, *99*
  throat and neck 109–110, *110*

Triple Burner 995–996
see also Eight Extraordinary Channels;
Twelve Channels; *specific channels*
cheeks/cheek-bones, red 54, *plate 3.21,*
plate 3.22, plate 3.23, plate 3.24
chemotherapy, fever 817
Chen Xiang Jiang Qi Tang (Stomach-Qi
stagnation) 1028
chest
abnormal shape 668–669
apical pulse palpation 512, *512*
areas influenced by organs 510, *510*
breasts *see* breast(s)
breathlessness *see* breathlessness
(Chuan)
channels influencing 143, *143*
cough *see* cough/coughing
distension feeling 664–665
feeling of heat 325, *325*
feeling of oppression/tightness 324,
324
gynaecomastia 145, 669–670
heat feeling 665
interrogation **321–326**
observation **143–147**
oppressive feeling in 664
pain *see* chest pain
palpation of 512–513
palpitations *see* palpitations
patterns 334
protruding 144, *144*, 145, *145*, 668
on one side 669
protruding sternum 144, *144*, 669
rib pain 664
sunken 144, *144, 145*, 668–669
sunken on one side 669
sweating 778
symptoms and signs **659–670**
tenderness 512–513, *513*
wheezing *see* wheezing *(Xiao)*
xyphoid process *see* xyphoid process
chest pain **323–324**, *324*, 663–664
case history 387–388
patterns 334
ribs 664
chickenpox 180, *180*, 870
shingles after *see* herpes zoster
(shingles)
childbirth 406–408, *408*
breech presentation 842
convulsions after 155
effect on baby 412
gynaecological symptoms and signs
843–848
lochia observation after 166–167
postpartum problems 412, **843–848**
abdominal pain 844
agalactia 408, *408*

Blood rebelling upwards after 1003
breast milk 847
collapse 847–848
constipation 845–846
convulsions 848
dizziness 846
fever 846–847
lactation 408, *408*
lochia 843–844
oedema 846
pain 844–845
post-natal depression/psychosis 847
retention of placenta 843
sweating 846
urinary difficulty 845
vaginal bleeding 845
see also pregnancy
problems during pregnancy 841–842
slow fetal growth 842
urticaria after 185
see also pregnancy
childhood, Five Stages of Life 417
Childhood Nutritional Impairment
eyelids loss of control 640
itching nose 593
swollen nose 596
Childhood Nutritional Impairment
Nebula 648
children
Accumulation Disorder *see*
Accumulation Disorder
body movements 194
childhood diseases 412
chronic catarrh 413
chronic cough 198
communicating with 411
complexion colours
bluish-greenish 192
pale 192
red 191
yellow 191–193
congenital kyphosis 708
constipation 867
constitutional weakness 866–867
convulsions 198, 199, 870–871
coughs/wheezing 413
crying 868
diarrhoea 865
digestive symptoms 412
disturbed sleep 868
ear problems 865
earache 413, 865
ears 192, *192*
eyes 192, *192*
feet, palpation 520
fetus toxin 871
fever 863–864
fingers palpation 520
Five Flaccidities 869

Five Retardations 869
flapping of nostrils 870
fontanelles 871–872
gums, lips and throat 193, *194*
hands, palpation 520
hot palms and soles 866
illnesses, residual pathogenic factors
975
immunizations 412
index finger creases *see* index finger
creases (children)
infections 870
inflammations 869–870
jaundice 870
learning difficulties 804
limbs
atrophy 153
flaccidity 154
long penis 872
mouth 193, *194*
nose 192–193, *193*
itching 593
root of 199, *199*
swollen 596
observation **191–200**
orifices 192–194
respiratory problems 412–413, 865
sleeping problems 413
slow development 413, *413*
spinal muscles 194
swollen tonsils 193
symptoms 411–413
urination problems 867
vomiting 864–865
white membrane on pupil 648
white spots on palate/tongue 872
worm infestation 199, 597, 869
see also babies
choking 114, 726
Choppy pulse *see* pulse qualities
chronic fatigue syndrome *see* postviral
fatigue syndrome
Chuan see breathlessness *(Chuan)*
circling fish pulse 506–507
Clear Yang not ascending, clinical
manifestations 932
climate 416, 428, *428*
coccyx, pain 705
coeliac disease, tiredness 284–285
Cold
Attack of 945, *945*, 965
Blood stasis from *see* Blood stasis
in channels, stiff knees 699
climate 428
Empty-Cold *see* Empty-Cold
exterior 946, 946–947, *947*
Heat in Interior 988
external, invading Stomach, vomiting
724

Cold (*contd.*)
  fetus Cold 1003
  flattening of lumbar spine 708
  frozen shoulder 656
  Full *see* Full-Cold
  interior 947
  internal
    bluish-greenish lips 622
    bluish-greenish nose 590
    bluish-greenish philtrum 626
    bluish-greenish sclera 635
    small or absent lunulae on nails 692
    strabismus 629
    with Yang deficiency *see* Yang
      deficiency
  invasion
    elbow pain 679
    joint pain 710
    knee pain 697
  invasion, lower backache 318, 947
  invasion of Lungs by Wind-Cold
    901–902
  list of spine 708
  lochia 844
  pain
    characteristics *259*
    in hands 682
    in limbs 672
  pathogenic factors 946–947
  stagnant Cold in Uterus 1002–1003
  stagnation *see entries beginning Cold
    Stagnation*
  Stomach *see* Stomach-Cold
  Stomach deficient and Cold
    (Stomach-Yang deficiency)
    913–914
  stuffiness feeling under Heart 666
  tongue diagnosis 230–231
  true Cold–false Heat 988, 989
  true Heat–false Cold 814, 989, *989*,
    1022
  Uterus deficient and Cold 1002
  Wind-Cold invasion (Cold prevalent)
    965
  see also specific organs
cold, feeling of 361–367, **813–814**
  alternating with heat 370–371
  aversion to cold 363, 365, 367–368
  aversion to wind 362–363
  case history 1018
  cold conditions 986–987
  cold feet 344
  cold hands 342–343, *343*
  contradictory feelings of Cold/Heat
    817–818
  depression 381
  in exterior conditions 365–366, *366*,
    813–814
    external invasions 365, 813, 946

fear of cold 363
  in interior conditions 363–364, *364*,
    366, *366*, 814
  shivers 363, 365, 813–814
  with simultaneous fever *367*,
    367–370, *817–818*
  Wind-Cold *vs* Wind-Heat 366, *366*
Cold-Dampness
  contraction of fingers 687
  contraction of limbs 677
  invasion
    elbow pain 679
    hip pain 697
    knee pain 697
  jaundice in children 870
  limb oedema 676
  location/sites *see entries beginning
    Cold-Dampness*
  oedema of the feet 694
  paralysis 711
  sticky/metallic taste 728
  thigh pain 697
  unilateral sweating 778
  white vaginal discharge 857
  yellow sclera 634
Cold-Dampness in back
  cold and heaviness 704
  see also Cold-Dampness in lower back
Cold-Dampness in Bladder channel
  anal itching 761
  coccyx pain 705
Cold-Dampness in channels, stiff knees
  699
Cold-Dampness in Gall-Bladder, jaundice
  714
Cold-Dampness in Intestines
  abdominal fullness 741
  blood and mucus in stools 750
  dark urine 754
  diarrhoea or loose stools 747–748
Cold-Dampness in Large Intestine,
  abdominal pain, lateral-lower
  740
Cold-Dampness in lower back
  lower back and knee weakness 705
  lower backache 703
  stiffness of lower back 705
Cold-Dampness in lower back and legs,
  sciatica 704
Cold-Dampness in Lower Burner
  cold genitals in men 769
  itching scrotum 771
  swelling and pain in testicles 773
Cold-Dampness in Spleen 887
  acupuncture 887
  clinical manifestations 887
  prescription 887
Cold-Dampness in Stomach
  epigastric pain 737

nausea 723
  sour regurgitation 718
  thin pointed fingers 687
  vomiting 724–725
Cold-Dampness in Stomach and
    Intestines, diarrhoea with
    vomiting 748
Cold-Dampness in Stomach and Spleen
  nose polyps 598
  poor appetite 720
  sense of smell loss 597
  yellow lips 622
Cold-Dampness in Uterus, watery
    menstrual blood 826
Cold-Dampness on Exterior, absence of
    sweating 780
Cold fetus, Five Retardations 869
cold food, excess 427
Cold-Heat in Lungs, wheeze in children
    865
Cold in Bladder, pale and abundant urine
    754
Cold in Interior, raised fontanelles 872
Cold in Intestines
  constipation 749
  umbilical pain 738–739
Cold in Liver channel
  abdominal pain, lateral-lower 740
  cold of head 563
  Peyronie's disease 772
Cold in Lower Burner
  cold-watery sperm 768
  five-colour vaginal discharge 858
  swelling and pain in testicles 773
Cold in Stomach
  absence of thirst 733
  epigastric pain 737
  gnawing hunger 721
  hiccup 719
  nausea 723
  regurgitation of food 718
  retching 725
  vomiting 724
Cold in Uterus
  after childbirth 844
  constipation after childbirth 846
  infertility (female) 855
  late (long cycle) periods 827
  menstrual bleeding stopping and
    starting 830
  menstrual clots 826
  retention of placenta 843
  scanty periods 828
Cold invading Stomach 916
  acupuncture 916
  clinical manifestations 916
  prescription 916
Cold on Exterior, Heat in Interior, absence
    of sweating 780

Cold-Phlegm
  clinical manifestations 936
  dark eyelids 638
  swollen eyelids 639
Cold-Phlegm in Lungs 902
  acupuncture 902
  breathlessness 662
  chronic cough 660
  clinical manifestations 902
  prescription 902
  spoon-shaped fingers 687
  wheeze in children 865
  wheezing 662
Cold retention, vulvar sores 858
cold sores 97, 97, 309, 610–611,
    plate 21.48
  see also herpes simplex
Cold stagnation, distended abdominal
    veins 743
Cold stagnation in Liver channel 895
  acupuncture 895
  clinical manifestations 895
  cold genitals in men 769
  contraction of scrotum 769
  dark scrotum 771
  feeling of cold in abdomen 742
  prescription 895
Cold stagnation in Uterus, painful
    periods 828
Cold transformation 968
colicky pain 256
collapse, after childbirth 847–848
complexion colours
  bluish/greenish 55–56, 577–578,
    plate 3.32
  bluish-purple 57
  changes during chronic disease 49
  children see children
  conforming/opposing colour 44–46,
    48–49
    clinical significance 46
    Five Elements 45, 45
    patterns 44–45, 45, 46
  dark 56, 578
  depression 381
  distinct/obscure colour 42–43,
    plate 3.3, plate 3.4, plate 3.30,
    plate 3.31
  dominant colours 40–41
  emotions and spirit 49–50
  environmental/lifestyle factors 40,
    50
  floating red 54, plate 3.25
  greenish/bluish 55–56
  guest colours 40–41
  lustre/lustreless colour 44, 47
  normal 50–51, plate 3.9
  observation **39–58**
    body, mind and complexion **1–66**

complexion colour **39–58**
  different aspects of 42–50
  prognosis determination 47–49
    Simple Questions 47
  purple 56–57, 578
  red 54, 577, plate 3.1, plate 3.2,
    plate 3.3, plate 3.4, plate 3.5,
    plate 3.6, plate 3.26, plate 3.27,
    plate 3.28
  reddish-purple 56–57
  sallow 52, 578–579
  scattered/concentrated colour 43,
    plate 3.5, plate 3.6
  Simple Questions 47
  spirit and emotions 36, 37
  superficial/deep colour 42, plate 3.28,
    plate 3.29
  symptoms and signs **575–579**
  thin/thick colour 43–44, 48, plate 3.7,
    plate 3.8, plate 3.26, plate 3.27
  white 51–52, 575–576
    bluish white 52
    bright white 51, plate 3.10
    dull white 51, plate 3.11
    pale white 51, plate 3.12
    sallow white 51, plate 3.13,
      plate 3.14
  yellow 52–54, 576–577, plate 3.7
    ash-like yellow 53, plate 3.19
    bluish-yellow 52
    bright yellow (jaundice) 53–54
    dry-yellow 53, plate 3.18
    dull yellow 52, plate 3.15
    floating reddish-yellow 53
    floating yellow 53, plate 3.17
    greyish-yellow 52, plate 3.16
    rich-yellow 53, plate 3.20
    Yang yellow 53
    Yin yellow 54
    see also jaundice
concentration difficulties 804
concha see ear(s)
Connecting channels 525–527
  body cavities 526
  energetic layers 525–526, 526
  palpation 526–527
    pressing 527
    stroking 527
    techniques 527
    touching 527
constipation 270–271
  after childbirth 845–846
  case history 273
  in children 867
  definition 748
  loose stools alternation 749–750
  in pregnancy 839–840
  premenstrual symptoms 405, 834
  symptoms and signs 748–749

constitutional traits
  and diet, causes of disease 416
  observation 9–10
  prenatal constitution, body shape 22,
    23, 23
  and spirit 34–36
    strong spirit /strong constitution 35
    strong spirit /weak constitution
      36
    weak spirit /strong constitution
      35
    weak spirit /weak constitution 35
  weakness 866–867
    constipation in children 867
    and diet 416
    heart deficiency 866
contraceptive pill 396–397
contraction
  fingers 63, 65, 130–131, 131,
    686–687
  limbs 155, 155
convulsions
  after childbirth 848
  in children
    acute 870–871
    chronic 870–871
  children, index finger creases 198,
    199
  fetus toxin 871
  limbs 155–156, 156
  pregnancy (eclampsia) 841
cornea see eye(s)
coronary heart disease, hand lines 134,
    134
corticosteroids, effects on tongue 204
Cou Li 169, 169–170, 525
cough/coughing **322–323**, 323
  acute 322, 323, 659–660
  blood 660–661
  case history 323
  children 413
  in children 865
  chronic 322, 323, 660
  diagnosis by 545–546, 546
  in pregnancy 840
cramp, calves 344, 700–701
Crane Knee Wind, atrophy 153
craving 426, 426
  for sweets 722
Crohn's disease 272
crying out 543, 822
cutaneous regions 5
cysts, breast 122

D

Da Bu Yin Wan 1028
Da Bu Yuan Jian 1028
Da Ding Feng Zhu 1028

Damp-Cold
  frozen shoulder 656
  retention, rigidity of lower back 705
  shoulder ache 656
  upper backache 656
Damp-Cold in Bladder 925–926
  acupuncture 925
  clinical manifestations 925
  prescription 926
Damp-Cold in Gall Bladder 918
  acupuncture 918
  clinical manifestations 918
  prescription 918
Damp-Dryness, Lungs, chronic cough
    660
Damp-Heat 370
  abdominal masses 744
  acupuncture 955
  brain noise 298
  candida 787
  case history 1014, 1015
  chronic, yellow complexion 576
  climate 428
  clinical manifestations 954–955
  crying out 822
  elbow pain 679
  external invasion, tinea (ringworm) of
    hands 684
  facial pain 302, 303, 571
  fever in cancer 816
  five-colour vaginal discharge 857
  Gall-Bladder and Liver, pain in ribs
    324
  greasy hair 567
  greasy skin 781–782
  head, feeling of heaviness 297
  heaviness feeling
    in legs 699
    in limbs 673
  hot hands and feet 672–673
  invasion of, diarrhoea in children 865
  irritability 802
  itching hands 683
  jaundice in children 870
  knee pain 697
  limb oedema 676
  low-grade fever in children 864
  mid-cycle menstrual bleeding 829
  naevi (moles) 787
  numbness/tingling in limbs 673
  numbness/tingling of hands 683
  oedema after childbirth 846
  oedema of the feet 693
  pain in foot 697
  pain in limbs 672
  paralysis 711
  patterns 893
  prescription 955
  red complexion 577

  red eye corners 637
  red-white vaginal discharge 857
  retention, vesicles on lower back 706
  in specific systems *see entries beginning*
    Damp-Heat (below)
  spots on the back 706
  sticky/metallic taste 728
  stiff knees 699
  thigh pain 696–697
  tinea 786
  tiredness 285, 286
  ulcers on lower leg 701
  vaginal discharge 857
  white vaginal discharge 857
  yellow sclera 634
  yellow sweat 777
  yellow vaginal discharge 857
Damp-Heat and Toxic Heat in Liver
    channel, swelling of vulva
    858–859
Damp-Heat in abdomen, sunken
    umbilicus 745
Damp-Heat in Bladder 925
  abdominal pain - central, lower 739
  acupuncture 925
  anal fissure 762
  blood in urine 758
  clinical manifestations 925
  dark urine 753
  dribbling of urine 757
  frequent urination 756
  painful urination 839
  papules or pustules on buttocks 707
  prescription 925
  red sclera 635
  scanty and difficult urination 755
  sperm in urine 759
  urination difficult 755
  urination painful 754
  urine retention 839
Damp-Heat in Bladder channel
  anal itching 761
  anal prolapse 762
  coccyx pain 705
  haemorrhoids 761–762
Damp-Heat in Directing and Penetrating
    Vessels 1001
  bleeding on intercourse 860
Damp-Heat in Ears 977
Damp-Heat in Gall-Bladder 917–918
  acupuncture 918
  bleeding from ears 583
  blood vessels distended on ear 586
  clinical manifestations 917–918
  concha swelling and redness 586
  ear discharge 583
  earache 582
  itching ears 582
  itching eyes 631

  jaundice 714
  prescription 918
  rash in axillae 785
  sense of smell loss 597
  swollen ears 584
  wax production excess 583
  yellow helix 585
Damp-Heat in Gall-Bladder, Liver,
    Stomach and Spleen, aversion
    to food 721
Damp-Heat in Gall-Bladder and Liver
    374, 893, 917
  abdominal pain (hypochondrial area)
    738
  acupuncture 893, 917
  bad smell sensation 597
  bitter taste 727
  blocked nose 592
  clinical manifestations 893, 917
  distension feeling in eyes 642
  herpes zoster 786
  prescription 893, 917
  protruding eyeball 643
  red helix 586
  rib pain 664
  sweating in axillae 779
  thirst 731–732
  yellow nails 691
Damp-Heat in Governing Vessel, anal
    itching 761
Damp-Heat in Head 977–978
  hot and painful eyes 632
Damp-Heat in Intestines
  abdominal fullness 741
  blood and mucus in stools 750
  blood in stools 751
  borborygmi (bowel sounds) 743
  diarrhoea or loose stools 747
  difficulty in defecation 751
  mucus in stools 751
  red philtrum 626
  straining in defecation 752
  umbilical pain 739
Damp-Heat in joints, joint pain 710
Damp-Heat in Large Intestine 921
  abdominal pain, lateral-lower 740
  cold sores 611
  tooth cavities 616
  toothache 615
Damp-Heat in Liver 893
  acupuncture 893
  blood in urine 758
  clinical manifestations 893
  dark urine 753
  leukoplakia 859
  prescription 893
Damp-Heat in Liver channel
  boils on scalp 568
  dandruff 567

genital eczema (female) 858
genital eczema (women) 858
herpes simplex 786
itching scalp 567
leukoplakia 859
long penis in children 872
premature ejaculation 766
priapism 768
red scrotum 770
redness and swelling of glans penis 772
sticky yellow nipple discharge 851
stiffness of back like tight belt 657
swollen and oozing scrotum 770
ulcers on penis 772
ulcers on the scalp 568
vaginal itching 858
vulval swelling 858–859
warts 787
Damp-Heat in lower back, lower back and knee weakness 705
Damp-Heat in lower back and legs, sciatica 704
Damp-Heat in Lower Burner
blood in sperm 768
dark philtrum 626
impotence 765
itching scrotum 771
nocturnal emissions 767
pain and itching of penis 771
Damp-Heat in Penetrating Vessel, gynaecomastia 670
Damp-Heat in skin
acne 569, 783
herpes simplex 785
herpes zoster 786
itching 713
Damp-Heat in Spleen
acupuncture 887, 956, 970
clinical manifestations 887, 956, 970
heat of the face/hot flushes 570
prescription 887, 956, 970
red grains inside eyelids 641
sweet taste 727
yellow nose 589–590
Damp-Heat in Spleen and Kidneys, yellow colour on lower back 706
Damp-Heat in Spleen channel, itching nose 593
Damp-Heat in Stomach 916
acupuncture 916, 956
clinical manifestations 916, 956
cold sores 610
epigastric pain 737
hot hands 681
hunger with no desire to eat 721
prescription 916, 956
red, itching and swollen fingers 785
regurgitation of food 718

sore throat 601
sour regurgitation 718
thin pointed fingers 687
toothache 615
venules on the thenar eminence 685
Damp-Heat in Stomach and Intestines 374, 815
Damp-Heat in Stomach and Spleen 977
blocked nose 592
boil on head 788
carbuncles on neck 788
case history 1014
contracted pupils 650
dry mouth 733
flat philtrum 625
inverted eyelashes 650
itching around mouth 611
limb flaccidity 675
night sweating 776
nose polyps 598
poor appetite 720
red eyelids 637
runny nose 592
sense of smell loss 597
stye on eyelids 637
sweating of hands and feet 778
swollen lips 623
swollen nose 596
thirst 731
tooth cavities 616
ulcers on nose 598
vomiting in children 864
yellow and dry teeth 618
yellow fluid between iris and pupil 649
yellow lips 622
yellow nails 691
Damp-Heat in Stomach channel, nose pain 595
Damp-Heat in Stomach steaming upwards, sweating on head 778
Damp-Heat in Stomach with Spleen-Qi deficiency, mouth ulcers during menstruation 834
Damp-Heat in Uterus
painful periods 829
sticky menstrual blood 826
Damp-Heat invasion in Gall-Bladder and Liver channels, ear problems in children 865
Damp-Heat invasion in Lesser-Yang channels, ear problems in children 865
Damp-Heat with predominance of Dampness, eczema 783
Damp-Heat with predominance of Heat, eczema 782
Damp-Heat with Toxic-Heat
herpes simplex 786

warts 787
withered and thickened nails 690
Damp-Heat with Toxic-Heat and Liver-Fire, vulvar sores 858
Damp-Phlegm
abdominal distension (bloating) 327
abdominal masses 744, 857
gynaecological symptom 857
acne 569
chronic cough 323
clinical manifestations 936
glue ear 865
greasy skin 781
head heaviness feeling 561
hemiplegia 711
numbness of half the body 712
numbness of head 563
obesity 319
pain in foot 698
Damp-Phlegm in Intestines, borborygmi (bowel sounds) 743
Damp-Phlegm in Lower Burner
sagging lower abdomen 745
scrotum drooping to one side 769
vulval swelling 858
Damp-Phlegm in Lungs 902, 976
acupuncture 902, 976
breathlessness 662
chronic cough 660
clinical manifestations 902, 976
cough in pregnancy 840
prescription 902, 976
snoring 811, 821
swollen nose 596
wheezing 662–663
Damp-Phlegm in Middle Burner, epigastric lumps 744
Damp-Phlegm in skin, acne 784
Damp-Phlegm in Spleen, sleepiness after eating 723
Damp-Phlegm in Spleen and Lungs, streaming eyes 633
Damp-Phlegm in Uterus
amenorrhoea 829
late (long cycle) periods 827
pale menstrual blood 825
sticky menstrual blood 826
Damp-Phlegm obstructing Spleen
abdominal distension (bloating) 741
loss of taste 728
nodules within eyelids 640
Damp-Phlegm with Qi deficiency, obesity 714
Dampness 948, **977–978**
abdomen 326
acute 950
body aches 709
candida 787
chronic 950

Dampness (*contd.*)
  climate 428
  clinical manifestations *948, 949*
  concentration difficulties 804
  digestive symptoms 262
  external *949, 949–950*
  glue ear 865
  greasy hair 566–567
  greasy skin 781
  groaning 822
  groin pain 698
  head, feeling of distension 297
  head heaviness feeling 561
  headache 561
  heaviness feeling in legs 699
  heaviness feeling in limbs 673
  internal 950
  invasion, joint pain 710
  itching hands 343, 683
  joint pain 318
  muzziness (fuzziness) of head 563
  numbness of half the body 712
  numbness/tingling in limbs 673
  numbness/tingling of hands 683
  oedema of body 713
  pain in foot 697
  pain in hands 682
  pain in limbs 672
  pathogenic factors **948–950**
  Spleen-Yang deficiency with
      Dampness, somnolence 810
  stiff knees 699
  tongue diagnosis 230
  Turbid Dampness surrounding the
      heart 883
  yellow complexion 576
  see also Cold-Dampness; *entries
      beginning Dampness (below)*;
      Wind-Dampness
Dampness and Phlegm in Uterus
      1002
Dampness in Bladder, turbid urine 754
Dampness in channels,
      numbness/tingling 712
Dampness in Gall-Bladder, otitis media
      1021
Dampness in Intestines
  constipation 749
  mucus in stools 751
Dampness in Lower Burner
  with Blood stasis in Liver channel,
      Peyronie's disease 772
  dyspareunia 859
  infertility (female) 855
  lack of libido (female) 860
  libido, lack of in women 860
Dampness in muscles
  muscle ache in limbs 671
  retention

  limb paralysis 677
  paralysis of legs 695
Dampness in nasal passage, nasal voice
      821
Dampness in skin, itching 713
Dampness in Spleen, pain in soles of feet
      698
Dampness in Stomach 1019
Dampness in Stomach and Spleen 977
  absence of thirst 733
  yellow palate 625
Dampness obstructing Middle Burner,
      loss of taste 728
Dan Shen Yin 1028–1029
Dan Zhi Xiao Yao San 1029
dandruff 73, *73*
  hair 567
Dang Gui Ji Xue Teng Tang 1029
Dang Gui Long Hui Wan 1029
Dang Gui Shao Yao San 1029
Dang Gui Si Ni Tang 1029
Dang Gui Zhi Tang 1029
dangerous conditions, indication by pulse
      qualities 506–507
Dao Chi Qing Xin Tang 1029
Dao Chi San 1029–1030
Dao Han (night sweating) 776
daytime pain 257
daytime sweating 351, *351*
deafness 355, 356–357, *357*
  see also tinnitus
Deep Connecting channels 526
  see also Connecting channels
Deep pulse *see* pulse qualities
defecation
  difficulty in 751–752
  interrogation 269, 270
  straining in 752
  symptoms and signs **747–752**
  see also stools
Defensive Qi *see* Qi, Defensive
Deficiency, pain characteristics 259
Deficiency–Excess conditions 1023
Deficient Yang floating, red complexion
      577
demeanour, observation **11–29**
depression
  antidepressants, effect on pulse
      507–508
  case history 1022
  in Chinese medicine 381–382
  definition 380–381
  diagnosis 381
  with manic behaviour *see* mania
  patterns 382–384, *383, 384*
  post-natal 847
  signs 381
  symptoms and signs 381, 797–798
  tiredness 283, 284

  see also mental-emotional
      symptoms
dermatitis *see* eczema
dermographism 181, *plate 21.10*
Di Sheng Tang 1030
Di Tan Tang 1030
diabetes mellitus, thirst, case histories
      278–279
diagnosis
  of causes of disease **415–430**
  by hearing and smelling **539–552**
  by interrogation **233–251**
  microsystems 8, *8–9*
  by observation **1–233**
  by palpation **431–538**
Diaphragm
  choking 114, 726
  Phlegm-Fluids 937
  residual Heat in, insomnia 808
Diaphragm-Heat
  anxiety 800
  depression 798
diarrhoea 271
  case history 272
  in children 865
  loose stools 747–748
  menstrual symptoms 833–834
  premenstrual symptoms 405
  vomiting with 748
diet 427–428
  cold food 427
  eating habits 428, *428*
  food choice 427, *428*
  greasy food 427
  hereditary weak constitution with
      diet 416
  hot food 427
  not eating enough 427
digestive symptoms *263*
  children 412
  main patterns 262–263, *263*
Ding Xiang Shi Di Tang 1030
Directing and Penetrating Vessels
  Blood stasis in 1000
  Damp-Heat in 1001
  deficient and cold 999–1000
  empty 999
  Empty-Heat in 1001
  Full-Cold in 1001–1002
  Full-Heat in 1000–1001
  Stagnant Heat in 1001
  unstable 999
Directing Vessel (*Ren Mai*) **998**
  abdomen 145, 146, 515
  chest 143, 513
  Damp-Heat in the Directing and
      Penetrating Vessels 860
  Directing and Penetrating Vessel
      disharmony *see* Penetrating

Vessel and Directing Vessels
disharmony
genitalia 149, 150
mouth 93, *94*
neck and throat 109, *109*
see also Directing and Penetrating
Vessels; Penetrating Vessel
(*Chong Mai*)
disease
causes of disease *see* causes of disease
diagnosis of causes **415–430**
distending pain ('*Zhang Tong*') 255–256
distension (bloating)
abdomen 146, *146*, 255–256, 264,
326–327
fullness *vs* 511, 740–741
symptoms and signs 735, 740–741
case history 244
see also fullness
diuretics, effect on pulse 508
dizziness **295–296,** 559–560
after childbirth 846
interrogation **295–296**
menstrual symptoms 835
in pregnancy 840
underlying patterns 296
dreaming 347
excessive 348, 349, *350*, 808–809
recurrent 348
significance of dreams *809*
see also sleep
drinks/drinking
hot/cold drink preference 279
interrogation **277–279**
pain 258
symptoms and signs **731–733**
see also thirst
drug tolerance, body shape 27–28, *28*
drugs as causes of disease
adverse drug reactions 429
medicinal drugs 429
recreational drugs 429–430
dry and brittle hair 72–73, *73*, 566
dry eyes 360, *360*
Dry-Heat 370, 955
clinical manifestations 955
intestines 955
Dry-Heat in Intestines, fever in children
863–864
Dry-Heat in Lungs 645
itching nose 593
nosebleed 595
dry mouth 279
Dry-Phlegm
chronic cough 322
clinical manifestations 936
Dry-Phlegm in Lungs 811, 821
Dryness 901, 951, *951*
injuring Lungs 593

pathogenic factors **950–951**
Dryness in Intestines and Liver-Blood
deficiency 752
Dryness in Lungs 782
Dryness invading Lungs 605
Duan Qi (shortness of breath) 545, 661
Duo Ming San 1030
Dupuytren's contracture 63
dyspareunia 859

E

E Jiao Ji Zi Huang Tang 1030
ear(s) **355–357**
abnormal colour 107–108
abnormal size 107, 584
bleeding 583
blood vessels distended 108, 586
channels influencing 105, *106*
children 192, *192*, 413, 865–866
concha, swelling and redness 108,
586–587
contracted 107, 584
Damp-Heat 977
discharge 108, *108*, 583
earache 357, *357*, 413, 582
helix
abnormal colour 107, 585–586
dry and contracted 107, 584
interrogation **355–357**
itching 357, *357*, 582
large 106
as microsystem 8
normal 106
observation **105–108,** 1056
problems in children 865–866
red back of 108, 586
red helix *plate 9.2*
signs 106, *106*
size 106–107
small 106
sores 107, 584
swollen 107, 584, *plate 9.1*, *plate 9.2*
symptoms and signs **581–588**
tinnitus *see* tinnitus
warts 107, 585
wax production, excess 108, 583–584
see also deafness
earache 357, *357*, 413, 582
Earth
Water insulting Earth 1009
Wood overacting on Earth 1008
Earth insulting Wood 1009
Earth not generating Metal 1008
Earth overacting on Water 1008
Earth Rampart *79*
Earth type
abdomen size 146
body odour 549, *550*

body shape 17–18, *18*
face *plate1.4*
Fire not generating Earth 1008
voice 542, *542*
eclampsia 841
eczema *plate 21.13, plate 21.14, plate*
21.15, plate 21.17
acute *plate 21.11*
case history 182
chronic *plate 21.12, plate 21.18, plate*
21.20
genital (women) 858
pathology and diagnosis
Chinese 181–182
Western 181
scales on skin 179, 181
symptoms and signs 782–783
Eight Extraordinary Channels
combined Directing/Penetrating Vessel
999–1003
Directing Vessel (*Ren Mai*) **998**
combined Penetrating Vessel
patterns **999–1003**
Girdle Vessel (*Dai Mai*) **1003–1004**
Governing Vessel (*Du Mai*) **997–998**
pattern identification 981,
997–1006
Penetrating Vessel (*Chong Mai*)
998–999
combined Directing Vessel pattern
999–1003
Yang Heel Vessel (*Yang Qiao Mai*)
1004
Yang Linking Vessel (*Yang Wei Mai*)
1005
Yin Heel Vessel (*Yin Qiao Mai*) **1004**
Yin Linking Vessel (*Yin Wei Mai*) **1005**
Eight Principles 497–498, 927
Full–Empty 988–991
Hot–Cold 985–988
interior/exterior 984–985
pattern identification 981, **983–991**
Yin–Yang **991**
Eight Ramparts 79, *79*
ejaculation
excessive sexual activity 430
inability 767–768
nocturnal emissions 393, *393*, 767
premature 393, *393*, 766–767
tiredness/dizziness after 393, 768
elbows, painful 342, *342*, 679
elderly
body odour 550
diaphragm choking 114, 726
dizziness 295
Five Stages of Life 418
headache 288
kyphosis 708
limbs

elderly (*contd.*)
   contraction 155
   rigidity 154
pulse variation in 450, 461
emotional states
   case histories 1022, 1023
   patient interrogation 250
   voice reflection 542
emotional symptoms
   oppression feeling in chest 664
   puberty and overwork 416–417
   pulse clinical application 458–459, 459
   pustules on back 118
   worry/overthinking 386–387
   see also mental-emotional symptoms
emotions 420–427
   anger *see* anger
   anxiety *see* anxiety
   Chinese terms 1064
   craving 426, *426*
   fear *see* fear
   grief 424–425, *425*
      see also grief
   guilt 426–427, *427*
   hatred 426, *426*
   inappropriate laughter 795
   and internal organs *422*
   joy 423, *423*
      excess 388, *389*, 794
      see also mania
   love (obsessional/misdirected) 425–426, *426*
   observation of mind, spirit and emotions **31–38**
   pensiveness 424, *424*
   puberty and overwork 416–417
   sadness *see* sadness
   severe timidity 795
   shock *see* shock
   and spirit 36–37
      complexion 36, 37
      eyes 36, 37, 75, 80
      tongue 36, 37
   startled easily 793–794
   symptoms and signs **791–795**
   weak Heart constitution and 417
   worry *see* worry
emotions line 133, *133*
emphysema
   heartbeat 128
   spoon-shaped fingers 131, *131*
Emptiness of Sea of Marrow
   brain noise 298, 564
   drooping head 563–564
   leaning of head to one side 564
   learning difficulties (children) 804
Empty-Blood 990
Empty-Cold 364

anal fistula 762
   vs Full-Cold 947
   interior 947
   pale philtrum 625–626
Empty-Cold in Liver channel
   glaucoma 641
   streaming eyes 633–634
Empty-Cold in Lower Burner 769
Empty-Cold in Uterus 838
Empty-Cold with Qi stagnation 147
Empty-Fire 951
   vs Full-Fire 952
Empty-Heat **986**, *986*
   anal fistula 762
   case history 1022
   dry skin 782
   face 301
   vs Full-Heat 371
   Heart- and Kidney-Yin deficiency with Heart Empty-Heat, insomnia 808
   Heart-Yin deficiency with Empty-Heat
      excessive dreaming 809
      sleep talking 810
   hot flushes 302
   Kidney- and Liver Yin deficiency with 909
   Kidney- and Lung-Yin deficiency with 909–910
   Kidney and Heart not harmonized (Kidney- and Heart-Yin deficiency with Heart Empty-Heat) 803, 909
   Kidney-Yin deficiency with 906
   Liver-Yin deficiency with 896
      sleep talking 810
   Liver-Yin deficiency with Empty-Heat
      excessive dreaming 809
      sleep walking 811
   Lung-Yin deficiency with 900
      red palms of hands 681
   Stomach-Yin deficiency with 914
   venules on the thenar eminence 685
   Yin deficiency with Empty Heat 932
Empty-Heat from Yin deficiency
   chronic fever *374*
   fever, chronic *374*, 815
Empty-Heat in Directing and Penetrating Vessels 1001
Empty Latent Heat *960*
Empty pulse *see* pulse qualities
Empty-Qi 990
Empty-Wind
   eclampsia 841
   Liver 970–971
Empty-Wind agitating in Interior
   acupuncture 957
   clinical manifestations 957
   prescription 957

Empty-Yang 990
Empty-Yin 990
endometriosis, hand lines 135
energetic layers
   channels 525–526, *526*
   skin 516, *517*
energy levels 281–286
   patient interrogation 250
   see also exhaustion (*Xu Lao*)
epigastrium 145, *145*, 146
   areas and palpation 515, *515*
   lumps 147, 744–745
   pain in 329, *329*, 737–738
      case histories 330
      patterns *331*
   spleen/stomach relationship 515
   see also abdomen
epilepsy
   convulsions 155–156
   tremor/spasticity 62
Er Chen Tang 1030
Er Zhi Wan 1030
erectile dysfunction 392, *392*
   hand lines 135, *135*
   symptoms/signs 765–766
erosion, skin 179, *179*
erysipelas 870
Ethereal Soul (*Hun*)
   depression 382
   Mind and mood 382, *382*
   movement of 382, *382*, 383, *383*
excess joy 388, *389*, 794
excessive dreaming 348, 349, *350*, 808–809
excretions
   lochia *see* lochia
   menstrual blood *see* menstrual bleeding
   nasal discharge 164, *164*
   observation **163–167**
   smell 550–551
   sputum *see* sputum
   stools *see* stools
   sweat *see* sweat/sweating
   urine *see* urine
   vaginal discharge *see* vaginal discharge
exhaustion (*Xu Lao*) 282
   dark nose 591
   historical aspects 282
   see also tiredness
exterior Wind *see* Wind, exterior
external invasion
   contraction of fingers 687
   fever in children 863–864
external pathogens, pulse 468
external toxins, convulsions/fever after childbirth 846, 848
External Wind-Cold, channels of face
   eye and mouth deviation 573

facial paralysis 573
facial tic 573
Extreme Heat generating Wind 893–894
　acupuncture 894
　clinical manifestations 893–894, 945
　prescription 894
eye(s) **357–360**
　area around, greenish/bluish
　　　complexion 55
　areas of 78, *78–79*
　bladder and 78
　blepharoconjunctivitis 643–644
　blurred vision 360, *360*
　breast lumps and 123
　cataract 651
　channels influencing *see* channels
　children 192, *192*
　closed 650
　control of 36, 80–81
　cornea 646–647
　　opacity 646–647
　　scarring after opacity 647
　corners 78, 79, 81
　　abnormal colours 84–85, *85*,
　　　636–637
　　pale 636
　　red 636–637
　deviation of 71, 573
　discharge from 84, *84*, 634
　distension feeling 641–642
　drooping red membrane 645–646
　dry 360, *360*, 631–632
　ecchymosis under conjunctiva
　　　644–645
　Eight Ramparts 79, *79*
　eye/mouth deviation 60, *60*
　feeling of distension 360
　Five Wheels 78–79, *79*
　floaters 358, 628
　gall-bladder and 77–78
　glaucoma 641
　heart 75, 77
　inability to shut or open 650
　internal organ relationship 76–78, *78*
　interrogation **357–360**
　itching 359, *359*, 631
　kidneys and 77
　lashes, inverted 650–651
　liver and 76–77
　lustre 36, 75, 80, *plate 6.1*
　movement of 80–81
　normal 81
　observation **75–86**
　open 650
　painful *358*, 358–359, *359*
　　hot and 632–633
　　menstrual symptoms 835
　pathological signs 81–85
　protruding 82, *83*, 642–643

pupils *see* pupil(s)
quivering 644
red veins/membrane 645–646
scaly 643–644
sclera *see* sclera colour
small intestine 78
sockets 85, *85*
spirit and emotions 36, 80
staring and fixed 83, 123, 650
stomach and spleen 77
strabismus 83, *83*
streaming 84, *84*, 360, *360*,
　　633–634
sunken 82–83, 643
symptoms and signs **627–652**
system 79, 79–80
turning up 644
veins *plate 12.1*
vision *see* vision
see also eyelids
Eye System 79, 79–80
eyelids 78, 79
　abnormal colour 83, *83*–84, 637–638
　area around, greenish/bluish
　　　complexion 55
　boil on 639
　dark 638
　drooping 640
　flapping 639
　green 638
　loss of control 640
　lower redness 641
　nodules within 640–641
　pain 639
　pale 638
　red 637–638
　red grains inside 641
　stye 637
　swollen 84, *84*, 638–639
　see also eye(s)

F

face **301–309**
　acne *see* acne
　blushing 579
　complexion colour *see* complexion
　　　colours
　eye/mouth deviation 60, *60*
　feeling heat of face/hot flushes
　　　569–571
　feeling of heat in 302, *302*
　feeling of numbness/tingling 303,
　　　572
　internal organs relationship 3, *3*
　interrogation 301–309
　lines 71, 574
　as microsystem 7–8
　movements 60–61

observation **69–74**
　constitution of person 69
　diagnostic signs 70–71, *71*
　reading 87
oedema 71, 572
pain in **302–303**, 303, *303*,
　　571–572
paralysis (Bell's palsy) 60–61, 573,
　　plate 4.1
redness and swelling 573
symptoms and signs **569–574**
tics 61, 572–573
ulcers (below zygomatic arch) 71,
　　574
warts *plate 21.52*
see also eye(s); mouth; philtrum
faeces *see* stools
fainting **296–297**, 560–561
　underlying patterns 297
falls, miscarriage 841
false spirit 34
Fan Guan Mai, pulse 451
Fan Zao (mental restlessness) 794
fasciculation (muscle twitching) 63,
　　714–715
fear 384–385, 425, *425*
　of cold 363
　patterns *385*
　symptoms and signs 792–793
　see also anxiety
febrile diseases *see* fever
feet
　cold 344, 519, *520*, 672, 694
　hot 672–673
　little finger correspondence *142*, 142
　oedema 345, 693–694
　pain 697–698
　painful 344–345, *345*
　palpation 519–520
　soles of *see* soles of feet
　sweaty 778–779
　toe ulcers 701
　tremor 64–65
Fen Rou 169, *169*
Feng Tuan 177
Feng Yin Zhen 185
Feng Zhen 180
fertility 406–408
　case histories 406–408
fetus
　breech presentation 842
　problems during pregnancy 841–842
　slow growth 842
fetus Cold 1003
fetus Heat 867, 1003
fetus toxin 871
fever 361–377, 814–816
　acute 814–815
　　closed eyes 650

fever (*contd.*)
  contracted ears 584
  convulsions 155
  after chemotherapy 817
  after childbirth 846–847
  in cancer 816–817
  in children 863–864
    low-grade 864
  chronic **374–375**, 815–816
    Blood deficiency 375, 815
    Blood stasis 375, 815
    Empty-Heat from Yin deficiency
      374, 815
    Qi deficiency 374–375, 815
    Stagnant Liver-Qi turned into Heat
      375, 815
  Damp-Heat *see* Damp-Heat
  degrees of 369, *369*
  in exterior patterns 368
  Four Levels 373, *373*
  head tilted backwards 565
  Heat at Blood level 374
  Heat at Nutritive-Qi level 374
  Heat in Bright Yang -channel pattern
    373
  Heat in Bright Yang -organ pattern
    374
  Heat in the Lungs (Qi level) 373
  interior *372*, 372–375
  menstrual symptoms 833
  origin *372*, 372–373
  pathology 368
  Phlegm-Heat in the Lungs (Qi level)
    373
  purple gums 621
  purple lips 622
  red lips 621
  with simultaneous cold feeling *367*,
    367–370
  tidal 816
  withered and brittle nails 690
  see also Heat
fibroadenoma 122
fibrocystic disease 122
Fine pulse *see* pulse qualities
finger(s) 130–132
  cocoon like 132
  contraction of 63, 65, 130–131, *131*,
    686–687
  cracked 132, 687–688
  index *see* index finger(s); index finger
    creases (children)
  little *142*, 142
  middle 141, *141*
  observation of **130–132**
    babies 1057–1058
  palpation 520
  pulse taking *see* pulse, method of
    taking

ring 141, *142*
shriveled and wrinkled 132, 688
spoon-shaped 131, *131*, 687
swollen 131–132, *132*, 686
  red and itching 785
symptoms/signs **686–688**
thickened 132, 688
thin pointed 131, *131*, 687
thumbs 140, *140*
tuberculosis (TB) 131, *131*
see also hands; index finger(s); index
  finger creases (children); nails
Fire
  characteristics 951
  Empty-Fire 951, 952
  Full-Fire 951, 952
  Metal insulting Fire 1009
  not generating Earth 1008
  pathogenic factors **951–952**
  Qi levels 956
  Water overacting on Fire 1008
  Wood not generating Fire 1007–1008
  see also Dry-Heat
Fire in Intestines, anal fissure 762
Fire injuring Yin 799
Fire insulting Water 1009
Fire overacting on Metal 1008
Fire Rampart 79
Fire types
  body odour 549, 550, *550*
  body shape 16–17, *17*
  face *plate 1.3*
  voice 542, *542*
Firm pulse *see* pulse qualities
fissures
  anal 762
  skin 180
fistula, anal 762
Five Elements
  body shape classification 11,
    15–21
  Earth insulting Wood 1009
  Earth not generating Metal 1008
  Earth overacting on Water 1008
  Fire insulting Water 1009
  Fire not generating Earth 1008
  Fire overacting on Metal 1008
  generating sequence patterns
    1007–1008
  insulting sequence patterns **1009**
  Metal insulting Fire 1009
  Metal not generating Water 1008
  Metal overacting on Wood 1008
  overacting sequence patterns **1008**
  pattern identification **1007–1009**
  Water insulting Earth 1009
  Water not generating Wood 1008
  Water overacting on Fire 1008
  Wood insulting Metal 1009

  Wood not generating Fire 1007–1008
  Wood overacting on Earth 1008
  see also individual elements
Five Flaccidities 869
Five-Palm Heat 376, *376*, 817
Five Retardations 869
  children's development *413*
five senses, internal organs and nine
    orifices relationship 2, *2*
Five Stages of Life 417–418
  adolescence 417
  childhood 417
  middle age 418
  old age 418
  young adulthood 417–418
Five Wheels 78–79, *79*
flaccidity
  limbs 154, *154*, 338, *338*
  pores 172
flatulence 273, 743
floaters 358, 628
Floating pulse *see* pulse qualities
flushed cheeks 189
Fo Shou San 1030
fontanelles
  late closure in babies 70, 872
  raised 871–872
  sunken 871
food
  allergies 264
  aversion to 264, 721
  cold, excess 427
  constantly picking 722
  craving 722
    see also craving
  interrogation **261–267**
  intolerance 264
  pain 258
  regurgitation *see* regurgitation
  sleepiness after eating 722–723
  stagnation, accumulation disorder
    869
  swallowing difficulty (diaphragm
    choking) 114, 726
  see also appetite; digestive symptoms;
    taste
Food-Essences, atrophy 153
Food-Phlegm, clinical manifestations
    936–937
food poisoning
  aversion to food 721
  diarrhoea with vomiting 748
  gnawing hunger 721
  nausea 723
  poor appetite 720
  umbilical pain 739
  vomiting 725
food retention
  abdominal fullness 741

abdominal pain below xyphoid process 736
acupuncture 916
after childbirth 844
aversion to food 721
belching 717
clinical manifestations 916
convulsions in children 871
crying in children 868
diarrhoea 748
  in children 865
  with vomiting 748
digestive symptoms 262–263
disturbed sleep 868
epigastric pain 738
fainting 560
fever after childbirth 847
foul breath 729
grinding teeth 616–617
headache 562
in Intestines, constipation 749
low-grade fever in children 864
pale eyelids 638
prescription 916
regurgitation of food 719
retching 725
sour regurgitation 718
sour taste 728
Spleen-Qi deficiency with, accumulation disorder 869
with Stomach-Heat in children, sweating on head 778
vomiting 725, 748
white membrane on pupil in children 648
foot *see* feet
forearm
  connecting channels 526–527
  diagnosis 517–518
  organ correspondence 518, *518*
  palpation 176, 517–518
  skin 176
  see also limbs
forehead
  skin palpation 517
  temperature 517
foul breath 111, 729
Four Levels 373, *373*, 958
  Blood level 957
  clinical manifestations 958
  Defensive Qi level 954–955
  Latent Heat 958–962
  Nutritive Qi level 956
  pattern identification **939–952, 953–964**
  Qi level 955–956
  relationship to
    Six Stages 962, *963–964*
    Three Burners *941*, 962, *963–964*

summary of 957–958, *958*
tongue appearance *958*
four limbs *see* limbs
frozen shoulder 656
Fu 169, *169*, 526
Fu Tu Dan 1030–1031
Fu Zi Li Zhong Wan 1031
Full-Cold 986–987, *987*
  bluish/greenish complexion 577
  characteristics 363, *363*
  vs Empty-Cold *947*, *988*
  internal, purple lips 622
  pale philtrum 625
  white/pale complexion 575
Full-Cold in Directing and Penetrating Vessels 1001–1002
  acupuncture 1002
  clinical manifestations 1001
  prescription 1002
Full-Fire *vs* Empty-Fire *951*, *952*
Full-Heat **985–986**, *986*
  anal fistula 762
  dry and cracked lips 622
  dry skin 782
  vs Empty Heat *371*, *987*
  red complexion 577
  red dorsum of hands 681
  red lips 621
  red nails 691
  red palate 625
  redness inside lower eyelids 641
  severe, dark sclera 636
  Small Intestine 911
  spontaneous sweating 775
  venules on the thenar eminence 685
  see also Heat
Full-Heat in Directing and Penetrating Vessels 1000–1001
Full-Heat in Small Intestine 615
Full-Heat with Blood stasis 622
Full Latent Heat *960*
Full pulse *see* pulse qualities
Full–Empty **988–991**
fullness
  digestive symptoms 262–263
  vs distension 511, 740–741
  with pain 256, 327, *327*
  pain characteristics *259*
  symptoms and signs 735, 740–741
  see also distension (bloating)
furuncle *see* boils

G

gait 161, 695–696
  festination 161, 695
  shuffling 161, 696
  staggering 161, 696
  stepping 161, 696

unstable 161, 695–696
Gall-Bladder
  channels 996
  Damp-Heat in *see* Damp-Heat
  Damp-Heat patterns 917–918
  Heat in *see* Heat in Gall-Bladder
  invasion of external Dampness 950
  pattern identification **917–919**
  Phlegm 937
  tongue coating distribution 223, *223*, *plate 26.2*
Gall-Bladder channel 996
  abdomen 145
  breasts 121, *121*
  chest 143
  Damp-Heat in *see* Damp-Heat
  ears relationship 105, *106*
  eyes relationship *76*, *77*, *77–78*
  neck 109, *109*
  palpation 536, *536*
    blood vessel 536
    skin 536
Gall-Bladder deficiency 918
  acupuncture 918
  clinical manifestations 918
  excessive dreaming 809
  fear/anxiety 793
  insomnia 808
  prescription 918
  severe timidity 795
  sleep disturbances 348
Gall-Bladder-Heat 918
  acupuncture 918, 956
  clinical manifestations 918, 955–956
  prescription 918, 956
  sleep talking 810
  tiredness 286
Gall-Bladder-Heat pattern (Qi level of four levels) 605
Gall-Bladder stagnation with Phlegm-Heat 918–919
  acupuncture 918–919
  clinical manifestations 918
  prescription 919
Gan Cao Gan Jiang Tang 1031
Gan Lu Xiao Du Dan 1031
Gan Yi 648
gastritis, hand lines 133, *133*
Gate of Life 80
Gathering-Qi 127, *128*, 512
GB-2 Tinghui 536, *536*
GB-24 Riyue 522
GB-25 Jingmen 522
Ge 169, *169*
Ge Gen Qin Lian Tang 1031
Ge Xia Zhu Yu Tang 1031
genitalia
  channels influencing *149*, 149–150, *150*

genitalia (*contd.*)
female, inflammation 858–859
genital eczema (female) 858
herpes simplex 188
male **765–774**
cold 769
ejaculation *see* ejaculation
penis *see* penis
scrotum *see* scrotum
testicles 737
observation **149–151**
pubic hair *see* pubic hair
thrush (candida) 187
vagina *see entries beginning* vaginal
vulva *see* vulva
warts *plate 21.53*
German measles 180, *180*
Girdle Vessel (*Dai Mai*) **1003–1004**
abdominal pain, lateral-lower 740
acupuncture 1004
clinical manifestations 1003–1004
herbs 1004
pathology
skin marks on back 119, 706
stiffness of back like tight belt 657
pathology (Damp-Heat), groin pain 698
prescription 1004
glaucoma 641
glue ear 865
goitre 110, *110*, 315–316, *316*, 604
Governing Vessel (*Du Mai*) **997–998**
acupuncture 997
back 115, *115*, 116
clinical manifestations 997
genitalia 149, *149, 150*
gums 99
heat in *see* Heat
herbs 998
mouth 93–94, *94*
neck 109, *109*
nose flow 87, 88, *88*
philtrum 101
greasy food, excess 427
greasy hair 73, 566–567
greasy skin 179, 781–782
Greater-Yang channels, headache 562
Greater Yang stage
channel patterns 965–966
organ patterns 966–967
pattern identification **965–967**
Greater-Yin channels, headache 562
Greater Yin stage
acupuncture 967
clinical manifestations 967
prescription 967
greying prematurely 73, *73*, 565
grief **387–388**, 424–425, *425*
case history 387–388

patterns *388*
Plum Stone Syndrome 314
pulse indication 452, 459
tiredness 283
groaning 542, 543, 822
groin pain 698
Gu Tai Jian 1031
Gui Pi Tang 1031
Gui Shen Wan 1031
Gui Zhi Fu Ling Wan 1032
Gui Zhi Tang 1032
guilt 426–427, *427*
gums **306–308**
abnormal colour 101, *101*, 620–621
bleeding 101, 307, *307*, 619
channels influencing 99, *99*
children 193, *194*
inflamed 101, 307, 618–619
observation **100–101**
oozing pus 101, 620
pale 620
problems 101, *101*
purple 620–621
receding 101, 307–308, *308*, 619–620
red 620
signs *100*
symptoms and signs **618–621**
see also teeth
Gun Tan Wan 1032
gynaecological history 395, *396*, 396–397
gynaecological problems **823–860**
see also menstruation, problem symptoms
gynaecomastia 145, 669–670

H

H$_2$-receptor antagonists, pulse 508
haemorrhoids 761–762
hair
body 176
see also pubic hair
dandruff 73, *73*, 567
development 71–72
dry and brittle 72–73, *73*, 566
falling out *see* hair loss
greasy 73, 566–567
observation of **69–74**
premature greying 73, *73*, 565
hair loss 72, *72*, 565–566
alopecia 72, *72*, 566
case histories 1020, 1022
halitosis 111, 729
hallucinations, visual 76
hand line(s) 133–136
abnormal signs on 133, *133*
cancer 136, *136*

circulatory diseases 134, *134*
coronory heart disease 134, *134*
description of 133
digestive system diseases 133, *133*
diseases indicated on 133–136
emotions 133, *133*
head 133, *133*
Jade Pillar 133, *133*, 135
life 133, *133*
main 133, *133*
reproductive system diseases 135, *135*
respiratory diseases 134, *134*
urinary system diseases 135, *135*
hands
abnormal colour 129
alcoholics 130
cold 519, *520*, 672, 680
coldness 342–343, *343*
dorsum
muscle atrophy 130, 685–686
palm comparison 520
red 129, 681
fingers *see* finger(s)
hot 672–673, 680–681
hotness 343, *343*
itching 343, *343*, 683
knuckles deformed 132, *132*, 684
numbness/tingling 343, *343*, 683
observation **129–136**
oedema 343, 684
pain in 682–683
painful 342, *342*
pale 129, 681
palms
dorsum comparison 520
dry, cracked and peeling 132, 684–685
red 129, 681
sweaty 133, 681–682, 779
palpation 519–520
respiratory diseases 134, *134*
sweating 778–779
symptoms and signs **680–686**
thenar eminence
atrophy 130, 685
venules 130, 685
tinea (ringworm) *see* tinea (ringworm)
tremor 64, 130, *130*, 156, 684
tuberculosis (TB) *134*
warts *plate 21.51*
Hao Qin Qing Dan Tang 1032
Hasty pulse *see* pulse qualities
hatred 426, *426*
HE-1 Jiquan 531, *531*, 532
HE-7 Shenmen 531, *531*, 532
head
body movements 59–60
brain noise 298, 564
constitution of patient 69

development 71–72
drooping 563–564
face *see* face
fainting 560–561
feeling of
  cold in 298, 563
  distension 297, *297*, 562
  dizziness 559–560
  heat in 299, *299*, 563
  heaviness 297, *297*
  muzziness (fuzziness) 297, *298*, 563
  skin numbness/tingling 299, *299*
fontanelle closure delay, babies 70
hair on *see* hair
headache 561–562
interrogation 287–299
leaning to one side 70, 564
neck rigidity 59–60
numbness 563
observation **69–74**
  signs *70*
scalp *see* scalp
sweaty 778
swelling 70, 564
symptoms and signs **559–569**
thumbnail correspondence 140, *140*
tilted backwards 70, 565
tremor 59, 70, 564
ulcers 70, 564–565
see also scalp
Head, Damp-Heat 977–978
head line 133, *133*
headache **288–294**, 561–562
  ameliorating/aggravating factors 289
  case histories 291–294
  character of pain 288–289
  classification *290*
  elderly 288
  external origin *290*, 291
  hypertension 288
  internal origin 289–291, *290*
  interrogation **237–238, 288–294**
  location 288, *289*
  menstrual symptoms 405, 832
  migraine, case history 291–293
  onset 288
  patterns underlying *294*
  post-orgasm 394
  premenstrual symptoms 405
  time 288
health line 133, *133*
hearing (listening), diagnosis by **541–548**
belching 546, *546*
breathing 544–545
  see also breathing
coughing and sneezing 545–546, *546*
crying in babies 544

hiccup 546, *546*
speech *see* speech/talking
voice *see* voice
vomiting 547, *547*
Heart
  apical pulse palpation 512, *512*
  combined patterns **883**
  feeling vexed (*Xin Zhong Ao Nong*) 665–666
  Heart- and Kidney-Yin deficiency with Heart Empty-Heat, insomnia 808
  left front pulse position *500*, 500–501, *501*
  lunula correspondence 140
  palpitations under 666–667
  pathology, spots on back 118
  pattern identification **879–883**
  Phlegm-Fire harassing the Heart 882
    insomnia 808
  Phlegm-Heat in *see* Phlegm-Heat
  Phlegm-Heat in the Heart 1016–1017
  Phlegm misting Heart 937
  problems, pulse diagnosis 459–460
  Qi deficiency of Spleen and Heart with floating Yang, hyperactivity 804
  sexual symptoms 391
  skin relationship 173
  stuffiness feeling under 666
  Turbid Dampness surrounding the Heart 883
  Turbid Phlegm in the Heart 803
  voice influence 542
  Water overflowing to the Heart 883
  Yang deficiency of Heart and Lungs, feeling of cold 814
Heart- and Gall-Bladder-Qi deficiency 800
Heart- and Kidney-Yang deficiency 578
Heart- and Kidney-Yang deficiency with Water overflowing
  to Heart, pulsation of carotid artery 655
  heartbeat displaced upwards 667–668
Heart- and Kidney-Yin deficiency
  amenorrhoea 829
  cataract 651
  insomnia 808
  itching tongue 613
  menopausal syndrome 856
  tinnitus 581
  upper teeth moist, lower teeth dry 618
Heart- and Kidney-Yin deficiency with Empty-Heat
  anxiety 800
  depression 798
  hot hands and feet 673
  nocturnal emissions 767

Heart- and Kidney-Yin deficiency with Heart Empty-Heat
  inappropriate laughter 795
  insomnia 808
  libido, lack of in women 860
  upper teeth moist, lower teeth dry 618
Heart- and Liver-Blood deficiency 898
  acupuncture 898
  case history 1015
  clinical manifestations 898
  post-natal depression 847
  prescription 898
Heart- and Liver-Fire
  insomnia during menstruation 835
  premature greying 565
  premenstrual tension 831
  sticky menstrual blood 826
Heart- and Liver-Yin deficiency
  Phlegm with goitre 604
  post-natal depression/psychosis 847
Heart- and Lung-Qi deficiency (deficiency of Gathering-Qi) 903–904
  acupuncture 904
  clinical manifestations 903–904
  prescription 904
  sadness 792
  tinnitus 582
Heart- and Lung-Yang deficiency *363*
Heart- and Spleen-Blood deficiency
  amenorrhoea 829
  depression 798
  depression and manic behaviour 799
  insomnia during menstruation 835
  irregular periods 827
  lack of libido in men 766
  schizophrenia 802
  severe timidity 795
  tiredness/dizziness after ejaculation 768
Heart- and Spleen-Qi deficiency
  propensity to worry 791–792
  severe timidity 795
  sighing 670
  sweating on chest 778
  vomiting of blood 725–726
Heart- and Spleen-Yang deficiency
  impotence 765
  premature ejaculation 766–767
Heart and Gall-Bladder deficiency
  excessive dreaming 809
  startled easily 793
Heart-Blood deficiency 365, 880
  acupuncture 880
  anxiety 799
  blurred vision and floaters 628
  case history 1014
  chest symptoms 322
  clinical manifestations 880
  cold hands 680

Heart-Blood deficiency (*contd.*)
  coldness 364
  concentration difficulties 804
  craving for sweets/constant picking
    722
  depression 797–798
  difficulty in finding words 822
  fainting 560
  feeling of cold 814
  hot and painful eyes 633
  insomnia 807
  irritability 801
  lack of libido in men 766
  numbness of the tongue 614
  pale hands 681
  prescription 880
  propensity to worry 792
  sadness 792
  sleep talking 810
  slurred speech 821
  startled easily 793
  stuttering 822
  tinnitus 582
  visual acuity decreased 630
Heart-Blood stasis 882
  acupuncture 882
  anxiety 800
  chest pain 663
  clinical manifestations 882, 930
  depression 798
  heartbeat below xyphoid process 668
  irritability 801
  poor memory 804
  post-natal depression/psychosis 847
  prescription 882
  reddish-purple nose 591
Heart channels 994
  abdomen 145
  breasts 121, *121*
  chest 143, *143*
  eyes relationship 75, 77
  mouth relationship 94, *94*
  palpation *531*, 531–532
    blood vessel 531
    skin 531–532
Heart cracks 36, 37, *217*, 217–218,
    plate 25.6, *plate 25.7*
Heart deficiency
  constitutional weakness 866
  crying in children 868
Heart Empty-Heat, excess joy 794
Heart-Fire
  anxiety 799–800
    in pregnancy 840
  bitter taste 727
  blood in urine 758, 839
  craving for sweets/constant picking
    722
  disturbed sleep 868

dryness and redness of skin on lower
    back 706
excess joy 794
excessive dreaming 808
eye discharge 634
Heart feeling vexed 665
heat feeling in chest 665
heat of the face/hot flushes 569–570
hot and painful eyes 632
hot hands 680
inappropriate laughter 795
insomnia 808
irritability 801
itching eyes 631
itching tongue 613
loud voice 819
mental restlessness 794
morning sickness 837
mouth open 612
mouth ulcers 610
nocturnal emissions 767
pain and itching of penis 771
painful tongue 613
painful urination 839
premenstrual tension 831
protruding eyeball 642
rash in axillae 785
red eye corners 636
red helix 586
red membrane in corner of eye 646
red sclera 635
red veins in eyes 645
redness on throat 607
sleep talking 810
staring, fixed eyes 650
startled easily 793
streaming eyes 633
stuttering 822
sweating in axillae 779
sweaty palms 682
swollen nose 596
thirst 731
tongue ulcers 614
urination painful 754
urticaria 784
Heart-Fire blazing 881–882
  acupuncture 882
  clinical manifestations 881–882
  prescription 882
Heart-Heat
  blood vessels distended on ear 586
  blushing 579
  crying in babies 868
  crying in children 868
Heart-Qi, reflection of, pulse diagnosis
    445, 459
Heart-Qi and Heart-Blood deficiency 880
  acupuncture 880
  clinical manifestations 880

prescription 880
Heart-Qi and Heart-Yin deficiency 881
Heart-Qi deficiency
  acupuncture 879
  clinical manifestations 879
  heartbeat below xyphoid process 668
  lack of libido (female) 860
  libido, lack of in women 860
  morning sickness 837
  mouth open 612
  prescription 879
  sweating of the palms 779
  sweaty palms 682
Heart-Qi deficiency with Blood stasis
    669
Heart-Qi deficiency with Heart-Blood
    stasis
  heartbeat displaced downwards 667
  heartbeat displaced to the right 668
Heart-Qi stagnation 881
  abdominal pain (area below xyphoid
    process) 736
  acupuncture 881
  clinical manifestations 881
  nausea 723–724
  prescription 881
Heart Vessel Obstruction 882–883
  acupuncture 883
  clinical manifestations 882–883
  prescription 883
Heart-Yang deficiency
  acupuncture 879
  chest pain 663
  clinical manifestations 879
  cold hands 680
  depression 798
  lack of libido in men 766
  pain in hands 682
  pale hands 681
  palpitations under the Heart 667
  patterns 879–880
  prescription 879
  sweating of the palms 779
  sweaty palms 682
  swollen scrotum 770
Heart-Yang deficiency with Phlegm 880
  acupuncture 880
  chest pain 663
  clinical manifestations 880
  oppression feeling in chest 664
  prescription 880
Heart-Yang deficiency with Water
    overflowing, muscle twitching
    715
Heart-Yin and Heart-Yang deficiency
    881
  acupuncture 881
  clinical manifestations 881
  prescription 881

Heart-Yin deficiency
  acupuncture 880
  anxiety 799
  clinical manifestations 880
  dry eyes 632
  fainting 560
  insomnia 807
  pain in hands 683
  patterns 880–881
  prescription 880
  propensity to worry 792
  startled easily 793
  sweaty palms 682, 779
  thirst 732
Heart-Yin deficiency with Empty-Heat
  acupuncture 881
  anxiety 799
  blushing 579
  clinical manifestations 881
  excessive dreaming 809
  Heart feeling vexed 665
  heat feeling in chest 665
  heat of the face/hot flushes 570
  hot hands 680
  irritability 802
  itching tongue 613
  painful tongue 613–614
  palpitations under the Heart 667
  prescription 881
  propensity to worry 792
  red eye corners 636
  red membrane in corner of eye 646
  red veins in eyes 645
  redness on throat 607
  scaly eyeballs 643–644
  sleep talking 810
  sweating in axillae 779
  swollen nose 596
  thirst 732
  tongue ulcers 614–615
Heartbeat
  below xyphoid process 128, 668
  displacement
    left and right 128, 668
    upwards and downwards 128,
      667–668
  intercostal space 127, 128
  observation **127–128**
  pulsation of Xu Li 127–128, 512
  see also pulse
Heat
  acute interior, dry and white teeth
    617
  Blood-Heat see Blood-Heat
  Blood level (Four Levels)
    purple nails 692
    sudden blindness 631
  Blood stasis from see Blood stasis
  climate 428

contradictory feelings of Cold/Heat
    817–818
  Damp-Heat see Damp-Heat
  disturbed sleep 868
  with Dryness, lines on the face 574
  Empty-Heat see Empty-Heat
  face 301
  fetus Heat 1003
  Five-Palm Heat 817
  Full see Full-Heat
  Full-Heat see Full-Heat
  generating Wind see Wind
  injuring Body Fluids, indented nails
    689
  Latent see Latent Heat
  in Lung see Lung-Heat
  Nutritive-Qi level, limb flaccidity 675
  pain characteristics 259
  Phlegm-Heat see Phlegm-Heat
  see also fever; Wind-Heat; specific organs
heat, feeling of 361–377
  alternating with cold 370–371,
    376–377
  internal causes 371–372
    see also fever
Heat - chronic, dark helix 585
Heat at Blood level 374
  fever in children 864
Heat at Defensive-Qi level 869–870
Heat at Ying level 863–864
Heat generating Wind see Wind
Heat in Bladder
  incontinence of urine 757
  urine retention in infants 867
Heat in Bright Yang
  abdominal fullness 741
  acupuncture 970
  channel pattern 373
  clinical manifestations 815, 970
  constipation 748–749
  fever in children 863–864
  organ pattern 374
  prescription 970
  umbilical pain 739
Heat in Exterior, Cold in Interior 988
Heat in Gall-Bladder 979
  blocked nose 592
  blurred vision and floaters 628
  depression 798
  swollen ears 584
Heat in Governing Vessel, ulcers on the
    scalp 569
Heat in Heart and Small Intestine, dark
    urine 753
Heat in Intestines
  blood in stools 751
  dark urine 754
  straining in defecation 752
Heat in Kidneys

acupuncture 970
  clinical manifestations 970
  prescription 970
Heat in Large Intestine
  cold sores 611
  toothache 615
Heat in Lesser-Yang channels, red helix
    586
Heat in Liver and Gall-Bladder
  dry throat 605
  sores on ear 584
  vomiting 724
  warts on ear 585
Heat in Liver and Stomach, neck ulcers
    789
Heat in Lung channel, red membrane in
    corner of eye 646
Heat in Lungs 373
Heat in Lungs (Qi level) 969–970
  acupuncture 969
  clinical manifestations 815, 969
  prescription 969–970
Heat in Lungs and Spleen
  drooping red eye membrane 646
  eyelid pain 639
  stye on eyelids 637
Heat in Lungs and Stomach
  acne 569, 784
  eyelid pain 639
  redness and swelling of pharynx 602
  rosacea 785
  stye on eyelids 637
  white purulent spots in throat
    606–607
Heat in Lungs with Dryness 978
Heat in Nutritive-Qi level 374
  acupuncture 956, 970
  clinical manifestations 956, 970
  fever in cancer 816
  prescription 956, 970
Heat in Pericardium
  acupuncture 956, 970
  clinical manifestations 956, 970
  delirious speech 822
  prescription 956
Heat in Spleen and Heart
  tongue/palate white spots 872
  toothache 615
Heat in Stomach 978–979
Heat in Stomach and Intestines, redness
    and erosion of pharynx 603
Heat in Stomach and Kidneys, plaque 617
Heat in Stomach and Spleen
  dribbling from mouth 612
  dry throat 605
  red membrane in corner of eye 646
  red ring around pupil 648
  sweet taste 727
  yellow fluid between iris and pupil 648

Heat stagnating in Interior
  cold hands and feet 672
  feeling of cold 814
  white/pale complexion 576
Heat victorious stirring Wind (Blood
       level), limb convulsions 678
Heaven Rampart 79
heaviness 949
Hei Dan 175
Hei Shen San 1032
helix see ear(s)
hemiplegia 64, 155, 711–712
  see also paralysis
Hemp Rash 180
herbs
  Yang Heel Vessel (Yang Qiao Mai)
       1004
  Yin Heel Vessel (Yin Qiao Mai) 1004
  Yin Linking Vessel (Yin Wei Mai) 1005
heredity 418–419
  causes of disease 416
  Weak-Heart constitution 419
  Weak-Kidney constitution 420
  Weak-Liver constitution 419–420
  Weak-Lung constitution 419
  Weak-Spleen constitution 419
herpes simplex plate 21.49
  pathology and diagnosis 188, 188
  symptoms and signs 785–786
  types 188
  see also cold sores
herpes zoster (shingles) plate 21.50
  occurrence 188
  pathology and diagnosis 188–189,
       189
hiccup 546, 546, 719
hip pain 343–344, 697
historical aspects **1051–1060**
  channel diagnosis 1056–1058
  pulse diagnosis 1051–1055
  tongue diagnosis 1058–1059
hot conditions 985–988
  see also Heat
hot flushes (menopausal) 301, 302,
       401, 569–571
hot food, excess 427
hot hands 343, 343
Hua Chong Wan 1032
Hua Gan Jian 1032
Huang Lian E Jiao Tang 1032
Huang Qi Jian Zhong Tang 1032
Hun (Ethereal Soul) see Ethereal Soul
       (Hun)
hunger
  but no appetite 265, 721
  case history 722
  excessive 264, 720
  gnawing 721–722
  poor appetite 719–720

see also appetite
Huo Po Xia Ling Tang 1033
Huo Xiang Zheng Qi San 1033
Hurried pulse see pulse qualities
hyperactivity 804–805
hyperopia 629–630
hypertension
  hand lines 134, 134
  headache 288
hypnotics, pulse 507
hypochondrial pain 331–332, 332, 738
  after childbirth 844–845
  case history 331, 332
hypochondrium 145, 145
  areas and palpation 514, 514
  lumps 147, 744
  Phlegm-Fluids 668, 738, 937
  see also abdomen

I

ichtyosis 179
identification of patterns see pattern
       identification
images (Xiang) 1
immunizations
  causes of disease 429
  children 412
impotence see erectile dysfunction
incoherent speech 821
incontinence
  stools 750
  urine 757
index finger(s) 140, 141
  analysis (children) 194–199
    see also index finger creases
       (children)
  babies 1057–1058
  creases see index finger creases
       (children)
  gates (children) 194, 194
  see also finger(s)
index finger creases (children) 195–199
  bow facing inside 196, 196
  bow facing outside 196, 197
  branching out 199, 199
  curved 197, 198
  diagonal 197, 197
  fish-bone 198, 198
  flowing pearl 195, 196
  hook 197, 198
  long pearl 195, 196
  long vertical 197, 197
  needle 197, 197
  s-shaped 198, 198
  snake going away 195, 196
  snake returning 195–196, 196
  spear 197, 197
  three 197–198, 198

three squiggly 199, 199
  worm 197, 198
  see also finger(s)
infants see babies; children
infertility (female) 855–856
  case histories 407–408, 1013–1015,
       1017–1015
inflammation
  in children 869–870
  female genitalia 858–859
insomnia 348, 348–349, 349, 807–808
  menstrual symptom 835
  patterns 350
  premenstrual symptoms 405, 835
insulin, effect on pulse 508
interior, Eight Principles 984–985
Intermittent pulse see pulse qualities
internal organs
  Dampness 949–950, 950
  facial areas relationship 3
  five tissues relationship 3–4, 4
  nine orifices and five senses
       relationship 2, 2
  pattern identification **877–926**
  see also individual organs
interrogation 235
  10 traditional questions 249–250
    limitations 249
  16 questions 250–251
  abdomen **326–335**
  asking the right questions 237–238
  avoiding pitfalls 239–240
  body 317–319
  chest **321–326**
  children's symptoms **411–413**
  diagnosis by **233–251**
  ears **355–357**
  emotional state 250
  energy levels 250
  eyes **357–360**
  face 301–309
  feeling of cold, heat and fever
       361–377
  food and taste **261–267**
  head 287–299
  integration with observation 242
  limbs **337–345**
  mental–emotional symptoms
       379–389
  neck **311–316**
  nose **303–306**
  pain **253–260**
  patient expressions 239
  pattern identification 242, 242
  procedure 240–241
  pulse diagnosis integration 243–248
  sexual life 250
  sexual symptoms 391–394
  sleep disturbances **347–350**

stools and urine **261–267**
styles, Western vs Chinese 236–237
sweating **351–354**
symptom timescales 241
terminology, Western vs Chinese 238–239, 255
thirst and drink **277–279**
throat **311–316**
tiredness 281–286
tongue diagnosis integration 243–248
trigger events 241
women's symptoms **395–409**
see also questions
intestinal gas 551
intestinal worms *see* worm infestation
Intestine(s)
  deficient and Cold, abdominal pain 739
  Dry-Heat (Fire) 955
  invasion of external Dampness 950
  large *see* Large Intestine
  Phlegm-Fluids 937
  small *see* Small Intestine
invasion
  absence of sweating 780
  acute cough 659
  cold upper back 656
  contraction of limbs 677
  flapping eyelids 639
  headache 291, 562
  lower backache 704
  nasal voice 820
  numbness/tingling in limbs 673
  runny nose 592
  stiff neck 653
  streaming eyes 634
  upper backache 656
  white/pale complexion 576
irregular pulse *see* pulse qualities
irritability 385–386
  patient expressions *386*
  patterns 385
  symptoms and signs 800–802
  see also anger; mental-emotional symptoms
itching 319, *319*, 713
  anus 761
  ears 357, *357*, 582
  eyes 359, *359*, 631
  fingers 785
  hands 343, *343*, 683
  mouth 611
  nose 304, *304*, 593
  penis 771
  scalp 287, 567
  scrotum 771
  throat 313, 605
  tongue 613

J

vaginal 858
see also urticaria

Jade Pillar 133, *133*, 135
  see also hand line(s)
jaundice 174, 175
  children 870
  complexion colours 53–54
  fetus toxin 871
  signs 714
Ji
  masses 146, 147, 511
  skin 169, *169*
Ji Ju 146, 147, 511
Ji Yin Jian 1034
Jian Ling Tang 1033
Jie Du Huo Xue Tang 1033
Jin Gui Shen Qi Wan 1033
Jin Jia Wan 1048
Jin Ling Zi San 1033
Jin Suo Gu Jing Wan 1033
Jing Fang Si Wu Tang 1033
Jing Jin see Muscle channels
Jing Mai 525
jogging, slow pulse 471–472
joint(s)
  contraction 64
  pain in 254, 318, *318*, 710
    after childbirth 844
  pain in, case histories
    generalized joint pain *340*
    tongue/pulse diagnosis 243
joy 423, *423*
  excess 388, *389*, 794
  see also mania
Ju 146, 147, 511
Ju He Wan 1034
Ju Pi Zhu Ru Tang 1034
Jue 539

K

KI-3 Taixi 533–534, *534*
Kidney(s)
  abdominal reflection of state 146, 515
  Body Fluid deficiency 935
  channels 995
  combined patterns 908–910
  eyes relationship 77
  failing to receive Qi 908
  gums relationship 99
  lunula correspondence 140
  pathology, spots on back 118
  pattern identification **905–910**
    combined patterns 908–910
  Phlegm 937
  pulse position
    left rear *502*, 502–503, *503*

    right rear 506, *506*
  skin relationship *172*, 172–173, *173*
  voice influence 541, *542*
Kidney- and Liver-Yin deficiency 908–909
  acupuncture 909
  amenorrhoea 829
  atrophy of legs 694
  bleeding on intercourse 859–860
  breast lumps 851
  cataract 651
  clinical manifestations 908–909
  constipation 749
  contraction of limbs 677
  dark sclera 636
  distended abdominal veins 743
  dyspareunia 859
  early (short cycle) periods 827
  heartbeat displaced downwards 667
  heavy periods 828
  impotence 765–766
  incontinence of urine 757
  kyphosis 708
  leg weakness 699
  leukoplakia 859
  limb atrophy 674–675
  limb paralysis 677
  limb rigidity 676
  Liver-Yang rising generating Wind 894
  lordosis 707
  myopia 629
  night vision decreased 630
  painful periods 829
  paralysis 710
    of legs 695
  premenstrual tension 832
  prescription 909
  restless legs 700
  small breasts 852
  staggering gait 696
  straining in defecation 752
  ulcers on lower leg 701
  vaginal itching 858
  watery menstrual blood 826
  weak knees 699
  white specks on sclera 647
Kidney- and Liver-Yin deficiency and Liver-Blood deficiency, giving rise to Liver-Wind, limb convulsions 678
Kidney- and Liver-Yin deficiency with Blood deficiency, bleeding between iris and pupil 649
Kidney- and Liver-Yin deficiency with Blood Empty-Heat, heavy periods 828

Kidney- and Liver-Yin deficiency with
    Blood-Heat, swollen fingers
    686
Kidney- and Liver-Yin deficiency with
    Empty-Heat 909
  anxiety in pregnancy 840
  blood in stools 751
  convulsions in children 871
  distension feeling in eyes 642
  fever during menstruation 833
  five-colour vaginal discharge 857
  menstrual bleeding returning after
    menopause 830
  mid-cycle menstrual bleeding 829
  psoriasis 783
  red sclera 635
  red-white vaginal discharge 857
  streaming eyes 633
  ulcers on penis 773
Kidney- and Liver-Yin deficiency with
    internal Wind
  gait festination 695
  limb paralysis 677
  paralysis 710
  stepping gait 696
  unstable gait 695–696
Kidney- and Liver-Yin deficiency with
    Liver-Qi stagnation,
    premenstrual breast distension
    832
Kidney- and Liver-Yin deficiency with
    Liver-Yang rising
  dizziness
    during menstruation 835
    in pregnancy 840
  hyperactivity 804
  menopausal syndrome 856
Kidney- and Liver-Yin deficiency with
    Wind-Phlegm in channels,
    shuffling gait 696
Kidney- and Lung-Yin deficiency 909
Kidney- and Lung-Yin deficiency with
    Empty-Heat 909–910
  acupuncture 910
  clinical manifestations 909–910
  prescription 910
Kidney- and Spleen-Yang deficiency 910
  acupuncture 910
  clinical manifestations 910
  prescription 910
Kidney- Yin deficiency and Kidney-Yang
    deficiency *see* Kidney-Yang and
    Kidney- Yin deficiency
Kidney and Heart not harmonized
    (Kidney- and Heart-Yin
    deficiency with Heart Empty-
    Heat) 909
Kidney channel
  abdomen 145

gums 99
palpation 533–534, 534
  blood vessel 533
  skin 534
pathology in pregnancy, hoarse voice
    820
Kidney deficiency
  chronic diarrhoea 271
  coccyx pain 705
  concentration difficulties 804
  constitutional 869
  constitutional weakness 867
  dark eyelids 638
  dark nails 692
  deafness 356–357
  difficulty in finding words 822
  dizziness 559
    after childbirth 846
  ears 355
  eyeball turning up 644
  Five Flaccidities 869
  flapping of nostrils 870
  flat philtrum 625
  hair falling out 565–566
  headache 291, 562
  hot and painful eyes 633
  impotence 392, 392
  infertility (female) 855
  irregular periods 827
  joint pain 710
  knee pain 697
  late (long cycle) periods 827
  loose teeth 616
  lower backache 318
  miscarriage 841
  pain in foot 697
  poor memory 803
  sexual symptoms 391
  stiff neck 653
  tinnitus 581
  tooth cavities 616
Kidney deficiency with Blood stasis,
    scoliosis 707
Kidney deficiency with Dampness
  pain in soles of feet 698
  ulcers on penis 773
Kidney deficiency with Phlegm, boils on
    BL-23 Shenshu (back) 706
Kidney-Essence, tongue spirit 209
Kidney-Essence deficiency
  atrophy of legs 695
  children, kyphosis 708
  dark complexion 578
  deviated neck 654
  elderly, kyphosis 708
  hyperopia 629
  impotence 766
  late closure of fontanelles 872
  limb atrophy 674–675

lordosis 707
loss of pubic hair 773, 860
nocturnal emissions 767
premature greying 565
quivering eyeball 644
red veins in eyes 645
scoliosis 707
strabismus 628–629
thin and brittle nails 689
Kidney-Essence deficiency with weakness
    of Governing Vessel, spine bent
    forward 707–708
Kidney-Qi deficiency 905
  acupuncture 905
  clinical manifestations 905
  failing to receive Qi 908
  lochia 843
  prescription 905
  retention of placenta 843
  sweating after childbirth 846
  urinary difficulty after childbirth 845
  vaginal bleeding, after childbirth 845
Kidney-Qi deficient and sinking
  prolapse of uterus 859
  urine retention 839
Kidney-Qi not firm 907–908
  acupuncture 908
  clinical manifestations 907–908
  cold-watery sperm 768
  dribbling of urine 756
  ejaculation during sleep 767
  incontinence of urine 757
  premature ejaculation 766
  prescription 908
  prolapse of vagina 859
  sperm in urine 759
Kidney-Yang and Kidney- Yin deficiency
  Kidney- Yin deficiency predominant
    907
  patterns 907
Kidney-Yang deficiency 905–906
  acupuncture 905–906
  anal prolapse 762
  clinical manifestations 905
  cold and heaviness in lower back 704
  cold feet 694
  coldness 364
  constipation 749
    after childbirth 845
    in pregnancy 839
  dark scrotum 771
  depression 797
  diarrhoea 747
    during menstruation 834
  dilated pupils 649
  fear/anxiety 793
  feeling of cold in abdomen 742
  frequent urination 756
  habitual miscarriage 842

impotence 392, 392, 765
lack of libido
    female 860
    male 766
leg weakness 699
leukoplakia 859
libido, lack of in women 860
limb oedema 675
limb weakness 674
loose scrotum 769
lower back and knee weakness 704
lower backache 703
menopausal syndrome 856
nighttime urination 758
nocturnal enuresis 757, 867
obesity 319
oedema
    of abdomen 745
    after childbirth 846
    of body 713
    of feet 693
    in pregnancy 838
pain in soles of feet 698
pale and abundant urine 754
paralysis 710
patterns 905–906
Peyronie's disease 772
premenstrual constipation 834
prescription 906
regurgitation of food 719
runny nose 592
salty taste 727
scanty and difficult urination 755
scanty periods 828
severe, dark complexion 578
severe timidity 795
with simultaneous Kidney-Yin
        deficiency 376
sneezing 591
soft and withered penis 771–772
soft neck 654
somnolence 810
stiff knees 699
stiffness of lower back 705
streaming eyes 633
sunken chest 669
thigh pain 697
tiredness/dizziness after ejaculation
        768
turbid urine 754
urination difficult 756
vaginal bleeding 838
weak knees 698
weak voice 820
white purulent spots in throat 607
white vaginal discharge 857
Kidney-Yang deficiency with
        Dampness
    heaviness feeling in legs 700

heaviness feeling in limbs 674
sciatica 704
Kidney-Yang deficiency with deficiency of
        Original Qi, fainting 560
Kidney-Yang deficiency with Empty-Cold,
        purple lips 621–622
Kidney-Yang deficiency with Heart-Heat
        905–906
Kidney-Yang deficiency with Liver-Blood
        deficiency, premenstrual breast
        distension 833
Kidney-Yang deficiency with Liver-Blood
        stasis, abdominal masses 744
Kidney-Yang deficiency with Phlegm
    breathlessness 662
    wheezing 663
Kidney-Yang deficiency with Water
        overflowing 906
    to Heart, palpitations 666, 667
    increased salivation 733
    to Lungs, breathlessness 662
Kidney-Yang rising, blurred vision and
        floaters 628
Kidney-Yin and Kidney-Yang deficiency
    menopausal syndrome 856
    protruding eyeball 643
Kidney-Yin deficiency 906
    acupuncture 906
    anxiety 800
    atrophy of muscles in dorsum of hands
        685
    atrophy of thenar eminence 685
    bluish-greenish sclera 635
    blurred vision and floaters 628
    clinical manifestations 906
    congenital 872
        long penis in children 872
    constipation
        after childbirth 845
        in pregnancy 839
    contracted ears 584
    corneal opacity 647
    dry and brittle hair 566
    dry and dull teeth 617
    dry eyes 632
    dry scalp 568
    dry skin 782
    dry throat 605
    fear/anxiety 793
    frequent urination 756
    habitual miscarriage 842
    helix dry and contracted 584
    irritability 801
    leg weakness 699
    limb flaccidity 675
    lower back and knee weakness 705
    lower backache 703
    menopausal syndrome 856
    nocturnal enuresis 758

obstruction feeling in throat 607
pain in soles of feet 698
patterns 906–907
plaque 617
prescription 906
salty taste 727
scanty and difficult urination 755
scanty periods 828
scarring after corneal opacity 647
with simultaneous Kidney-Yang
        deficiency 376
soft and withered penis 771
sweating after childbirth 846
thirst 732
tiredness/dizziness after ejaculation 768
turbid urine 754
visual acuity decreased 630
voice loss 840
withered and brittle nails 690
yellow and dry teeth 618
Kidney-Yin deficiency , Empty Heat
        blazing 906–907
    acupuncture 907
    clinical manifestations 906–907
    prescription 907
Kidney-Yin deficiency with Bladder-Heat,
        urinary difficulty after
        childbirth 845
Kidney-Yin deficiency with Blood
        Empty-Heat, infertility (female)
        856
Kidney-Yin deficiency with Empty-Heat
        906
    acupuncture 906
    bleeding from ears 583
    bleeding gums 619
    blood in sperm 768
    blood in urine 758, 839
    burning sensations in soles of feet 701
    clinical manifestations 906
    concha swelling and redness 586–587
    dark urine 753
    dilated pupils 649
    dry and dull teeth 617
    ear discharge 583
    ecchymosis under conjunctiva
        644–645
    excessive pubic hair 774, 860
    feeling of heat in head 299
    glaucoma 641
    grey teeth 618
    heat of head 563
    heat of the face/hot flushes 570
    hyperopia 629
    inability to ejaculate 767–768
    irritability 801–802
    itching ears 582
    itching scrotum 771
    lochia 844

Kidney-Yin deficiency with Empty-Heat
(*contd.*)
  loose teeth 616
  mouth ulcers during menstruation
    834
  nosebleed 594
  pain and itching of penis 771
  painful urination 839
  premature greying 565
  prescription 906
  priapism 768–769
  receding gums 619–620
  red eye corners 637
  red helix 586
  red membrane in corner of eye 646
  redness of pharynx 602
  sperm in urine 759
  swollen nose 596
  vaginal bleeding 838
  wax production excess 584
Kidney-Yin deficiency with internal
    Wind, tremor of legs 700
Kidney-Yin deficiency with Liver-Yang
    rising, menopausal syndrome
    856
Kidney-Yin deficiency with Phlegm 907
Kidneys not receiving Qi
  breathlessness 661
  pulsation feeling under umbilicus 742
knees
  painful 344, *344*, 697
  stiff 699
  weakness in 344, 698–699, 704–705
Knotted pulse *see* pulse qualities
knuckles, deformed 132, *132*, 684
Ku ('bitter'), terminology problems 239
kyphosis *117*, 117–118, 708

L

lactation 408, *408*
Large Intestine
  Body Fluid deficiency 935
  Damp-Heat in 921
  deficient and Cold
    abdominal pain, lateral-lower 740
    blood and mucus in stools 750
  Heat in *see* Heat
  heat patterns 921–922
  pattern identification **921–923**
  pulse diagnosis, discrepancies 444
Large Intestine channel 993–994
  abdomen 145
  ears 105, *106*
  mouth 93, *94*
  nose 88, *88*
  palpation 528–529, *529*
    blood vessel 528–529
    skin 529

philtrum 101
throat 109, *109*
larynx 311
Latent Heat **958–962**, *959*
  Bright-Yang type 961–962
  clinical manifestations 959, *959*, *960*
  Full/Empty 960
  Lesser-Yang type 961
  Lesser-Yin type *960*, 962
  tiredness 285, 1023
  types *960*
Latent Heat in Lesser Yin, Five-Palm Heat
  817
Latent Heat invasion *vs* Wind-Heat 960
laughter, inappropriate 795
leaking roof pulse 507
learning difficulties (children) 804
Leather pulse *see* pulse qualities
legs
  arched 160, *160*, 696
  atrophy 160, 694–695
  calves, cramp 344, 700–701
  circulatory problems, pulse diagnosis
    435
  gait *see* gait
  groin pain 698
  heaviness feeling in 699–700
  inner, plucking of veins 1056–1057
  knees *see* knees
  observation **159–162**
  oedema 159–160, 713
    case history 160
  paralysis 160, 695
  restless 700
  symptoms and signs **693–701**
  thigh pain 696–697
  tremor 700
  ulcers (lower leg) 701
  weakness 699
  see also feet; limbs
Lesser-Yang pattern (Six Stages)
  bitter taste 727
  dry throat 605
  night sweating 776
Lesser-Yang stage
  acupuncture 967, 979
  clinical manifestations 813, 967,
    979
  Latent Heat 961
  prescription 967, 979
  tiredness 284
Lesser-Yang syndrome, abdominal pain
  738
Lesser-Yin channels, headache 562
Lesser-Yin stage 968
  Latent Heat *960*, 962
leukoplakia 151, 859
Li 857
LI-4 Hegu 528, 529, *529*

Li Ji Hou Zhong (difficulty in defecation)
  751
Li Yan Cha 1034
LI-5 Yangxi 528–529, *529*
Li Zhong An Hui Tang 1034
Li Zhong Tang 1034
Lian Mei An Hui Tang 1034
Lian Po Yin 1034
Liang Di Tang 1034–1035
Liang Fu Wan 1035
Liang Ge San 1035
Liang Shou Tang 1035
libido, lack of
  female 393–394, *394*, 860
  male 392–393, *393*, 766
Life Gate 194, *194*
life line 133, *133*
limbs
  abnormal feelings 673–674
  atrophy/flaccidity 153–154, *154*,
    338, *338*, 674–675
  Blood stasis 931
  calves 344
  children *see* children
  cold feet 344
  contraction 63–64, 155, *155*, 677
  convulsions 155–156, *156*, 678
  elbow pain 342, *342*
  feeling of distension *338*, 338–339,
    674
    causes *338*
  feeling of heaviness 339
  flaccidity 154, *154*, 675
  generalized joint pain 339–340,
    340
  hand pain 342, *342*
  heaviness feeling 673–674
  hip pain 343–344, 697
  interrogation **337–345**
  knee pain 344, *344*
  movements 155–156, 676–677
  muscle ache 339, 671
  numbness/tingling 339, *339*, 673
  observation **153–157**
  oedema 156–157, *157*, 675–676,
    713
  pain in 672
  painful feet 344–345, *345*
  Painful Obstruction Syndrome 64
  paralysis 154–155, *155*, 676–677
  Phlegm-Fluids 937
  rigidity 154, *154*, 676
  shoulders 341–342
  swelling 157, *157*, 675–676
  symptoms and signs **671–715**
  thigh pain 344, 696–697
  tremor 340–341
  tremor/spasticity 61–65, 156, *156*,
    678

weakness 338, *338*, 674
see also arms; legs
Lin Xiao 179
lines, face 71, 574
Ling Gan Wu Wei Jiang Xin Tang 1035
Ling Gui Zhu Gan Tang 1035
Ling Jiao Gou Teng Tang 1035
lips 308–309
  abnormal colouring 94–96, *95, 96*
    bluish-greenish 95, *95*, 622
    pale 94–95, *95*, 621
    pregnancy 95–96, *96*, 624
    purple 95, *95*, 621–622
    red 95, *95*, 621
    yellow 95, *95*, 622
  channels 93–94, *94*
  children 193, *194*
  cold sores 309
  drooping 96, 624
  dry or cracked 96, *96*, 622–623
  inverted lips 96, 624
  macules *plate 21.2*
  observation **93–104**
  peeled 96, 623
  swollen 96, 623
  symptoms and signs **621–624**
  trembling 96, 623
  voice influence 541, 542
  see also mouth
list of spine 118, *118*, 708
listening *see* hearing (listening)
Liu Jun Zi Tang 1035
LIV-3 Taichong 536–537, *537*
LIV-9 Yinbao 536–537
LIV-10 Wuli 536–537, *537*
LIV-13 Zhangmen 521
LIV-14 Qimen 522
Liver
  Body Fluid deficiency 935
  channels 996
  combined patterns 897–898
  Damp-Heat in *see* Damp-Heat
  Ethereal Soul, movement *383*
  Heat in *see* Heat
  left middle pulse position *501,*
    501–502, 502
  Liver-Blood deficiency patterns 895
  nails relationship 137
  pattern identification **891–898**
    combined patterns 897–898
  Phlegm-Fire *see* Phlegm-Fire
  Rebellious Liver Qi *see* Rebellious Liver
    Qi
  skin relationship 173
Liver- and Heart-Yin deficiency, post-
    natal depression 847
Liver- and Kidney-Yin deficiency *see*
    Kidney- and Liver-Yin
    deficiency

Liver- and Spleen-Blood deficiency
  dull-pale palate 624
  pale-white nails 691
Liver- and Spleen deficiency, Five
    Retardations 869
Liver and Kidney deficiency
  amenorrhoea 829
  congenital, arched legs 696
  drooping eyelids 640
  hemiplegia 711
  pain in limbs 672
  premature greying 565
Liver-Blood and Kidney-Yang deficiency,
    joint pain after childbirth 844
Liver-Blood and Liver-Yin deficiency with
    internal Wind, trembling
    mouth 612
Liver-Blood deficiency
  abdominal pain
    after childbirth 844
    in pregnancy 838
  acupuncture 895
  anxiety 800
  atrophy of muscles in dorsum of hands
    685
  atrophy of thenar eminence 685
  blurred vision and floaters 628
  case histories 1024
  clinical manifestations 895, 930, 946
  cold feet 694
  constipation
    after childbirth 845
    in pregnancy 839
  contraction
    of fingers 686
    of limbs 677
  convulsion of limbs 678
  cracked fingers 687
  cramps in calves 700
  dandruff 567
  depression 798
  dizziness 559
    after childbirth 846
  dry and brittle hair 566
  dry and cracked lips 623
  dry and dull teeth 617
  dry skin 782
  eye pain during menstruation 835
  eye symptoms 358
  fainting 560
  fear/anxiety 793
  feeling of cold 364, 366, 814
  fever after childbirth 847
  hair falling out 565
  headache 291, 294
    during menstruation 832
  hot and painful eyes 632
  hypochondrial pain, after childbirth
    844

insomnia 807
irritability 801
itching eyes 631
itching scalp 567
joint pain 710
  after childbirth 844
lack of libido (female) 860
leukoplakia 859
Liver-Yang rising 894
muscle ache in limbs 671
myopia 629
night vision decreased 630
numbness of half the body 712
numbness of head 563
numbness/tingling 712
  of hands 683
  in limbs 673
pale hands 681
pale lips 621
pale nose 589
patterns 895
premature greying 565
premenstrual constipation 834
prescription 895
propensity to worry 792
restless legs 700
ridged nails 688
sadness 792
scalp itching 299
severe, dry eyes 632
strabismus 629
streaming eyes 633
tinnitus 582
twisted nails 691
vaginal bleeding 838
visual acuity decreased 630
weight loss 714
withered and brittle nails 689
yellow complexion 576
yellow sclera 635
Liver-Blood deficiency generating
    Liver-Wind 678
Liver-Blood deficiency generating Wind
    894–895
  acupuncture 895
  clinical manifestations 894, 895
  eye pain during menstruation 835
  prescription 895
  tremor of hands 684
  tremor of legs 700
Liver-Blood deficiency with Empty
    internal Wind, swollen scrotum
    770
Liver-Blood deficiency with Empty-Wind
  cramps in calves 700–701
  dry skin 782
  itching around mouth 611
Liver-Blood deficiency with internal Cold,
    bluish-greenish nails 691–692

Liver-Blood deficiency with internal
Wind, urticaria 784
Liver-Blood deficiency with Liver-Heat,
streaming eyes 633
Liver-Blood deficiency with Liver-Wind
dandruff 567
facial tic 572
itching scalp 567
Liver-Blood deficiency with Phlegm 895
acupuncture 895
clinical manifestations 895
prescription 895
Liver-Blood deficiency with secondary
Liver-Qi stagnation,
premenstrual tension 832
Liver-Blood stasis 892–893
abdominal masses 744
abdominal pain 738
after childbirth 844, 845
central, lower 739
lateral-lower 740
acupuncture 893
alopecia 566
amenorrhoea after miscarriage 845
bluish-greenish nails 692
bluish-greenish nose 590
breast pain 850
case histories 1024
clinical manifestations 892–893
Connecting channels of Brain (Eye
system), contracted pupils 649
cracked fingers 687
cracked nails 688
cramps in calves 701
dyspareunia 859
eye pain during menstruation 835
fever after childbirth 847
gynaecomastia 670
hypochondrial lumps 147, 744
irritability 801
joint pain, after childbirth 844
limb paralysis 677
Liver-Qi stagnation with see Liver-Qi
stagnation
lochia 844
nose pain 595–596
nosebleed 595
painful periods 828
paralysis 710–711
of legs 695
premenstrual breast distension 832
prescription 893
protruding chest 668
purple nails 692
purple scrotum 770
reddish-purple nose 591
retention of placenta 843
rib pain 664
sleep walking 811

sudden blindness 630
thickening of nails 688
thin and brittle nails 689
vaginal bleeding after childbirth 845
withered and brittle nails 690
yellow nose 590
Liver-Blood stasis with Phlegm
breasts, peau d'orange 852
inverted nipples 852
Liver-Blood stasis with Water
overflowing, heartbeat
displaced to the left 668
Liver channels
abdomen 145
breasts 121, 121, 122
chest 143
Damp-Heat in see Damp-Heat
Empty-Cold in see Empty-Cold
eyes relationship 76–77, 77
genitalia 149, 149, 150
mouth relationship 93, 94
palpation 536–537, 537
blood vessel 536–537
skin 537
stagnation of Cold in 895
Wind-Heat in see Wind-Heat
Liver deficiency, constitutional weakness
867
Liver Empty-Wind 970–971
acupuncture 970
clinical manifestations 970
prescription 971
Liver-Fire
abdominal pain - central, lower 739
anxiety 800
in pregnancy 840
bitter taste 727
blazing with Phlegm-Heat, goitre
604
bleeding between iris and pupil 649
bleeding from ears 583
blurred vision and floaters 628
blushing 579
boils on scalp 568
brain noise 298
breast milk 847
burning sensations in soles of feet 701
constipation 748
contracted pupils 649
dandruff 567
dark nose 591
distension feeling in eyes 641
distension of head feeling 562
disturbed sleep 868
dizziness 560
drooping red eye membrane 646
dry eyes 632
dryness and redness of skin on lower
back 706

dyspareunia 859
earache 582
ecchymosis under conjunctiva 644
excessive dreaming 808
eye discharge 634
facial pain 303, 571
feeling of heat in head 299
Five-Palm Heat 817
glaucoma 641
haemorrhoids 762
head, feeling of distension 297
headache 288, 290, 561
during menstruation 832
heat of head 563
heat of the face/hot flushes 569
heavy periods 828
hot and painful eyes 632
hyperactivity 805
insomnia 808
insulting Lungs
breathlessness 662
chronic cough 660
nosebleed 594
invading Stomach
epigastric pain 738
vomiting of blood 725
irritability 801
itching eyes 631
itching scalp 567
loud voice 819
mouth ulcers 610
nocturnal enuresis 757, 867
pain in soles of feet 698
painful tongue 614
propensity to anger 791
protruding eyeball 642
red eye corners 636
red membrane in corner of eye 646
red nose 590
red ring around pupil 648
red sclera 635
red veins in eyes 645
redness and pain of scalp 568
redness on throat 607–608
sour taste 727–728
streaming eyes 633
sudden blindness 630
sweating on head 778
swollen nose 596
thickening of nails 688
thirst 731
tinnitus 581
ulcers
in mastoid region 565
on nose 598
on penis 773
on scalp 568
urination painful 754–755
weight loss 714

wide neck 655
withered and brittle nails 690
Liver-Fire Blazing Upwards 893
Liver-Fire generating Wind 894
Liver-Fire insulting Lungs 897–898
   acupuncture 897–898
   clinical manifestations 897
   prescription 898
Liver-Fire insulting the Lungs 897–898
Liver-Heat stirs Wind 970
Liver patterns, case histories 1024
Liver Phlegm-Fire 896
   acupuncture 896
   clinical manifestations 896
   prescription 896
Liver-Qi
   constipation in pregnancy 840
   Rebellious see Rebellious Liver-Qi
Liver-Qi deficiency 896
   acupuncture 896
   clinical manifestations 896
   empirical prescription by Dr Chen Jia
      Xu 1030
   fear/anxiety 793
   lack of libido (female) 860
   prescription 896
   severe timidity 795
   soft and withered penis 771
Liver-Qi invading Spleen
   borborygmi (bowel sounds) 742
   craving for sweets/constant picking
      722
   diarrhoea or loose stools 747
   eyelids loss of control 640
   flatulence 743
   grinding teeth 616
   quivering eyeball 644
   sour taste 728
   straining in defecation 752
Liver-Qi invading Stomach
   belching 717
   epigastric pain 737
   gnawing hunger 721
   hiccup 719
   nausea 723
   poor appetite 720
   retching 725
   sour regurgitation 718
   sour taste 728
   vomiting 724
Liver-Qi stagnation
   abdominal distension (bloating) 741
   abdominal masses 744, 856
   abdominal pain
      central, lower 739
      lateral-lower 740
      in pregnancy 838
   abdominal pain (hypochondrial area)
      738

after childbirth 844
acupuncture 891
amenorrhoea after miscarriage 845
anxiety 800, 840
bluish-greenish complexion 578
bluish-greenish philtrum 626
brain noise 564
breast milk 847
breasts
   distension 849
   lumps 850
   skin, peau d'orange 852
breech presentation 842
case histories 1024
chest pain 663
chest symptoms 321
clinical manifestations 891
cold hands 680
constipation 749
contraction of fingers 687
depression 382, 797
deviated neck 654
deviation of the mouth 613
distension feeling
   in chest 664
   in eyes 642
eye and mouth deviation 573
facial tic 573
fainting 560
flatulence 743
headache 561
hoarse voice 820
inverted nipples 852
irregular periods 827
irritability 801
lack of libido
   female 860
   male 766
loud voice 819
lower backache 318
menstrual bleeding stopping and
      starting 830
milky nipple discharge 851
miscarriage 841
muscle ache in limbs 671
neck pain 654
obstruction feeling in throat 607
oedema of hands 684
oppression feeling in chest 664
pain
   in hands 682
   in ribs 324
patterns 891–892
period pain 828
premenstrual breast distension 832
premenstrual tension 831
prescription 891
propensity to anger 791

protruding eyeball 643
rib pain 664
rigidity of neck 654
scanty and difficult urination 755
severe
   breast pain 850
   chest protruding on one side 669
   protruding chest 668
sighing 670
stiff neck 653
tiredness 285
   case histories 284
upper backache 656
urinary difficulty 756
   after childbirth 845
urination painful 755
urine retention 839
yawning 670
see also entries beginning Stagnant
      Liver-Qi
Liver-Qi stagnation - turned into Heat
   spots on the back 706
   yellow sweat 777
Liver-Qi stagnation - turned into Heat
      rebelling upwards
   depression 797
   energy rising feeling in abdomen 742
   glaucoma 641
Liver-Qi stagnation - turned into
      Liver-Fire
   menstrual bleeding returning after
      menopause 830
   nosebleed during menstruation 834
   painful periods 829
   premenstrual breast distension 832
Liver-Qi stagnation invading Intestines,
      premenstrual constipation 834
Liver-Qi stagnation invading Spleen
   constipation and loose stools
      alternation 749–750
   diarrhoea during menstruation 833
Liver-Qi stagnation invading Spleen with
      Dampness, constipation and
      loose stools alternation 750
Liver-Qi stagnation invading Stomach,
      vomiting during menstruation
      835
Liver-Qi stagnation with Blood deficiency,
      startled easily 793–794
Liver-Qi stagnation with Blood-Heat, rash
      in axillae 785
Liver-Qi stagnation with Blood stasis,
      breast lumps 850
Liver-Qi stagnation with Damp-Heat in
      Liver channel
   five-colour vaginal discharge 858
   red-white vaginal discharge 857
Liver-Qi stagnation with Liver-Blood
      deficiency, paralysis 711

Liver-Qi stagnation with Liver-Blood
    stasis
  protruding eyeball 643
  ulcers on neck 789
Liver-Qi stagnation with Phlegm 892
  acupuncture 892
  breast pain 850
  clinical manifestations 892
  prescription 892
  protruding eyeball 642
  swollen breasts 850
Liver-Qi stagnation with Phlegm-Heat,
    swollen breasts 850
Liver-Qi stagnation with Qi-Phlegm,
    depression 797
Liver-Qi with Liver-Blood stagnation,
    neck ulcers 789
Liver-Wind
  alopecia 566
  arm tremor *341*
  bluish/greenish complexion 578
  bluish-greenish sclera 635
  contracted pupils 649
  contraction of fingers 687
  deviation of the mouth 613
  distension feeling in eyes 642
  dizziness 295, 560
  Extreme Heat generating Wind
      893–894
  eye and mouth deviation 573
  eye pain during menstruation 835
  facial tic 572
  headache 290, 561
  hemiplegia 711
  hot and painful eyes 632
  itching eyes 631
  limb convulsions 678
  limb rigidity 676
  Liver-Blood deficiency giving rise to
      Wind 894–895
  Liver-Fire generating Wind 894
  Liver-Yang rising deriving from
      Liver-Blood deficiency 894
  Liver-Yang rising generating Wind
      894
  neck pain 654
  numbness
    of face 572
    of half the body 712
    of head 563
    of tongue 614
  numbness/tingling
    of hands 683
    in limbs 673
  opisthotonos 715
  patterns 893–895
  protruding eyeball 642
  rigidity of neck 654
  stiff neck 653

strabismus 629
sudden blindness 631
trembling mouth 612
tremor of hands 684
tremor of head 564
tremor/spasticity of limbs 678
Liver-Wind agitating within, eclampsia
    841
Liver-Wind and Phlegm
  deviation of the mouth 613
  dilated pupils 649
  eye and mouth deviation 573
  facial tic 572
  headache 290
  tremor of hands 684
Liver-Wind harbouring Phlegm 895
Liver-Wind with Phlegm-Heat,
        protruding eyeball 642
Liver-Yang deficiency 896–897
  acupuncture 897
  clinical manifestations 896–897, 897
  prescription 897
Liver-Yang rising 892
  acupuncture 892
  anxiety 800
  blurred vision and floaters 628
  blushing 579
  case histories 1024
  clinical manifestations 892
  distension feeling
    in eyes 642
    of head 562
  dizziness 295, 559
  headache 288, 289–290, 291, 292,
      293, 294, 561
    during menstruation 832
  heat of the face/hot flushes 569
  hot and painful eyes 632
  insomnia before menstruation 835
  irritability 801
  limb rigidity 676
  neck pain 654
  prescription 892
  propensity to anger 791
  red complexion 577
  redness on throat 607–608
  rigidity of neck 654
  stiff neck 653
  strabismus 629
  tinnitus 581
  upper backache 656
Liver-Yang rising deriving from Liver-
    Blood deficiency 894
Liver-Yang rising deriving from Liver-Yin
    deficiency 894
Liver-Yang rising generating Liver-Wind,
    limb convulsions 678
Liver-Yang rising generating Wind 894,
    945

Liver- and Kidney-Yin deficiency
    894
Liver-Yin deficiency 894
Liver Yin and Kidney- deficiency *see*
    Kidney- and Liver-Yin
    deficiency
Liver-Yin deficiency
  abdominal distension (bloating)
      741
  abdominal pain (hypochondrial area)
      738
  acupuncture 896
  anxiety 800
  blurred vision and floaters 628
  clinical manifestations 895–896
  contraction of fingers 686
  dry eyes 631–632
  dry scalp 568
  dry skin 782
  dry throat 605
  fainting 560
  insomnia 808
  itching eyes 631
  itching scalp 567
  Liver-Yang rising deriving from 894
  patterns 895–896
  prescription 896
  ridged nails 688
  sleep talking 810
  sleep walking 810–811
  thin and brittle nails 689
  thirst 732
  visual acuity decreased 630
  withered and brittle nails 689
  withered and thickened nails 690
Liver-Yin deficiency generating Wind
  tremor of hands 684
  tremor of legs 700
Liver-Yin deficiency with Empty-Heat
    896
  acupuncture 896
  blood in urine 839
  clinical manifestations 896
  excessive dreaming 809
  prescription 896
  red eye corners 636
  red veins in eyes 645
  sleep talking 810
  sleep walking 811
  sweating in axillae 779
lochia 843–844
  observation 166–167
  smell 551
  see also vaginal discharge
Long Chi Qing Hun Tang 1035–1036
Long Dan Bi Yuan Fang 1036
Long Dan Xie Gan Tang 1036
Long pulse *see* pulse qualities
lordosis 117, *117*, 707

Loss of Body Fluids
  dull-white nails 691
  shriveled and wrinkled fingers 688
love (obsessional/misdirected) 425–426,
    426
lower back *see* back
Lower Burner
  finger disease reflection 141
  pattern identification 970–971
  pulse diagnosis
    Foot section 437, *438*
    position assignment 443
    state of *434, 435*
Lown–Ganong–Levine (LGL) Syndrome,
    pulse indication 460
LU-1 Zhongfu 521, 528, *528*
LU-4 Xiabai 528, *528*
Lu Jiao Tu Si Zi Wan 1036
Lui Wei Di Huang Wan 1035
lumbar flattening, spine *117, 118,*
    708
Lung(s)
  Body Fluid deficiency 935
  channels 993
  Cold-Phlegm in 902
  combined patterns 903–904
  Damp-Phlegm in *see* Damp-Phlegm
  Dry-Heat in *see* Dry-Heat
  Dryness *see* Dryness
  emphysema
    heartbeat 128
    spoon-shaped fingers 131, *131*
  Heart- and Lung-Qi deficiency
      (deficiency of Gathering-Qi)
      903–904
  Heat in *see* Heat
  Heat in Lungs (Qi level) 969–970
  pattern identification **899–904**
    combined patterns 903–904
  Phlegm *see* Phlegm
  Phlegm-Dryness in 902–903
  Phlegm-Fluids in the Lungs 903
  Phlegm-Heat in *see* Phlegm-Heat in
      Lungs
  Phlegm patterns 902–903
  right front pulse position *503,*
    503–504, 504
  skin relationship 170–172
  thumb lunula correspondence 140
  Toxic Heat in *see* Toxic Heat
  voice influence 541, *542*
  Wind-Heat in Lung Defensive-Qi
      portion 969
  Yang deficiency of Heart and, feeling of
      cold 814
Lung- and Heart- Yang deficiency *363*
Lung- and Heart-Qi deficiency *see*
      Heart- and Lung-Qi deficiency
      (deficiency of Gathering-Qi)

Lung- and Kidney - constitutional
      deficiency, protruding sternum
      669
Lung- and Kidney-Yang deficiency
  blocked nose 592
  bluish/greenish complexion 578
  Empty-Heat with, sore throat 601
Lung- and Kidney-Yin deficiency
  dry eyes 632
  hoarse voice 606, 820
  spoon-shaped fingers 687
  sunken chest 669
Lung- and Kidney-Yin deficiency with
      Empty-Heat
  nosebleed during menstruation 834
  redness and swelling of pharynx 602
  white purulent spots in throat 606
Lung- and Spleen-Qi deficiency
  aching nose 595
  blocked nose 591
  constipation 749
  cough in children 865
  coughing blood 661
  dry nostrils 594
  frequent urination 756
  incontinence
    faecal 750
    urinary 757
  inverted eyelashes 650
  loss of sense of smell 597
  nasal voice 821
  Phlegm in the Lungs with, snoring
      811
  severe and chronic, sunken eyeball
      643
  snoring 811, 821
  straining in defecation 752
  urinary difficulty after childbirth 845
  yellow sweat 777
Lung- and Spleen-Yang deficiency,
      swollen fingers 686
Lung- and Stomach-Heat, nose pain 595
Lung- and Stomach-Qi stagnation,
      obstruction feeling in throat
      607
Lung-Blood stasis 930–931
lung cancer 457
  see also cancer
Lung channel
  back 115
  chest 143, *143*
  nose 87–88, *88*
  palpation 528, *528*
    blood vessel 528
    skin 528
Lung cracks 205, *205*
Lung deficiency
  constitutional weakness 867
  flapping of nostrils 870

Lung deficiency with Phlegm-Heat, blood
      vessels distended on ear 586
Lung-Dryness 901
  chronic cough 660
  itching throat 605
Lung-Heat 902
  acupuncture 902, 955
  acute
    flapping alae nasi (nostrils) 598
    nosebleed 594
  acute cough 659–660
  blocked nose 591–592
  Blood Level (Four Levels), coughing
      blood 661
  breathlessness 662
  clinical manifestations 902, 955
  coughing blood 660–661
  dry nostrils 593
  heat feeling in chest 665
  heat of the face/hot flushes 570
  hoarse voice/loss of voice 606
  hot hands 680
  hot upper back 656
  irritability 801
  loud voice 819
  mental restlessness 794
  papular eruptions 573
  papules on nose 599
  prescription 902, 955
  red eye corners 636
  red helix 586
  red nose 590
  red sclera 635
  redness on throat 607
  scaly eyeballs 643
  sweaty palms 682
  swollen nose 596
  thirst 732
  tongue diagnosis 205, *205*
  ulcers on nose 598
Lung-Qi, rebellious 643
Lung-Qi and Kidney-Yang deficiency
      (Governing Vessel deficient)
  breathlessness 662
  itching nose 593
  kyphosis 708
Lung-Qi and Lung-Yin deficiency
      900–901
  acupuncture 901
  clinical manifestations 900–901
  Heart- and Lung-Qi deficiency
      (deficiency of Gathering-Qi)
      903–904
  prescription 901
Lung-Qi collapse 903
Lung-Qi deficiency 899
  acupuncture 899
  breathlessness 661
  chronic cough 322, 660

Lung-Qi deficiency (*contd.*)
  clinical manifestations 899
  itching nose 593
  limb oedema 675
  nocturnal enuresis 758
  not descending, scanty and difficult
      urination 755
  oedema of the face 572
  patterns 899–900
  prescription 899
  propensity to worry 792
  sneezing 304, 591
  spontaneous sweating 775
  sunken chest 668–669
  sweaty palms 681, 779
  urination difficult 755
  weak voice 820
Lung-Qi deficiency with Damp-Heat, bad
      smell sensation 597
Lung-Qi deficiency with Empty-Cold
  dribbling from mouth 612
  runny nose 592
Lung-Qi deficiency with Phlegm
      899–900
  acupuncture 899–900
  breathlessness 662
  clinical manifestations 899
  mouth open 612
  prescription 900
  wheezing 663
Lung-Qi stagnation 903
  acupuncture 903
  breast distension 849
  breathlessness 661
  chest, feeling of oppression/tightness
      324
  chest pain 663
  clinical manifestations 903
  distension feeling in chest 665
  hoarse voice 820
  irritability 801
  loud voice 819
  oppression feeling in chest 664
  premenstrual breast distension 833
  prescription 903
  propensity to worry 792
  sadness 792
  sighing 670
  yawning 670
Lung-Qi stagnation with Phlegm
  phlegm in throat 603
  premenstrual breast distension 833
Lung-Yang deficiency 900
  clinical manifestations 900
  cold hands 680
  oedema of hands 684
  pain in hands 682
  pale hands 681
  Phlegm with *see* Phlegm

prescription 900
  spontaneous sweating 775
  sweaty palms 681
Lung-Yang deficiency with Phlegm,
      wheezing 663
Lung-Yang deficiency with Water
      overflowing, muscle twitching
      715
Lung-Yin and Blood deficiency,
      amenorrhoea 829
Lung-Yin deficiency
  acupuncture 900
  breathlessness 661
  chest sunken on one side 669
  chronic cough 322, 660
  clinical manifestations 900
  cough in pregnancy 840
  dry skin 782
  dry throat 605
  hoarse voice/loss of voice 606
  hot upper back 656
  itching throat 605
  Kidney- and Lung-Yin deficiency 909
  Kidney- and Lung-Yin deficiency with
      Empty-Heat 909–910
  obstruction feeling in throat 607
  pain in hands 683
  patterns 900
  prescription 900
  sunken chest 669
  sweaty palms 681, 779
  thirst 732
  voice loss 840–841
Lung-Yin deficiency with Empty-Heat
  acupuncture 900
  blushing 579
  chronic cough 660
  clinical manifestations 900
  coughing blood 661
  dry nostrils 593
  flapping alae nasi (nostrils) 598
  heat feeling in chest 665
  heat of the face/hot flushes 570
  hot hands 680
  nose pain 595
  prescription 900
  red eye corners 636
  redness of pharynx 602
  redness on throat 607–608
  thirst 732
Lung-Yin deficiency with Phlegm 900
  acupuncture 900
  clinical manifestations 900
  prescription 900
  wheezing 663
Lungs
  invasion by Wind 901–902
  invasion by Wind-Cold 901
  invasion by Wind-Dryness 901

invasion by Wind-Heat 901
  invasion by Wind-Water 901–902
    acupuncture 902
    clinical manifestations 901–902
    prescription 902
lunulae *see* nails
Luo channels
  connecting 525
  see also Connecting channels
  skin 174
Luo Mai 525
lurking pain *(Yin Tong)*, pain
      classification 257
lustre
  body skin 175
  complexion 40
    lustre/lustreless colour 44, 47
  eyes 37, 75, 80
    spirit and emotion 36, 37, 40, 80,
      plate 6.1

M

Ma Huang Tang 1036
Ma Mu 299
Ma Xing Shi Gan Tang 1036
Ma Zhen 180
Ma Zi Ren Wan 1036
macules 176–177, *177, 178, plate 21.1,
      plate 21.2*
  black 177
  connecting channels 174
  eruptions 573
  purple 177, *plate 21.1*
  red 177
  shape and density 177
  vs vesicles/papules 958
  white 177
  Yang 176
  Yin 177
Mai Men Dong Tang 1036
malignant melanoma 186, *186,
      plate 21.37*
  nodular *plate 21.36, plate 21.38*
  pathology and diagnosis, Western *vs*
      Chinese 186
  superficial spreading *plate 21.35,
      plate 21.38, plate 21.39*
  symptoms and signs 788
  see also cancer
mania 388, 799
  depression patterns 382, 383,
      798–799
  depressive phase 798–799
  see also joy, excess
mastoid ulcers 70
ME (myalgic encephalomyelitis) *see*
      postviral fatigue syndrome
measles 180, *180,* 586

melanoma *see* malignant melanoma
memory, poor 803–804
Men ('feeling of oppression') 664
  terminology problems 238–239
menarche 396
menopause
  hot flushes 301, 302, 401, 569–571
  menstrual bleeding returning after
    830
  night sweating 401
  symptoms/signs 856
menstrual bleeding **825–826**
  case history 399–400
  colour 166, *166*, 400, *400*, 825–826
  consistency 166, *166*, 400, *400*
  intermittent 830
  menstrual clots 826
  mid-cycle bleeding 829–830
  pale 825
  post-menopause 830
  purple 825–826
  quantity 399–400, *400*, 403
  sticky 826
  watery 826
menstrual pain 401–404, *404*,
    828–829
  case histories 402–404, 1016
  nature of pain 402–404
  time of pain 401–402
  see also menstruation, problem
    symptoms
menstruation 398–406
  age of menarche 396, 399, 401
  amenorrhoea 400, 401, 829
  bleeding *see* menstrual bleeding
  early (short cycle) 827
  gynaecological symptoms and signs
    827–830, 831–835
  heavy 827–828
  irregular 827
  late (long cycle) 827
  menstrual cycle 396, 396–397, 399,
    401
    irregularities 400–401
  mid-cycle bleeding 829–830
  pain *see* menstrual pain
  premenstrual breast distension 398,
    399
  premenstrual symptoms *see*
    premenstrual symptoms
  problem symptoms 831–835
    body aches 833
    diarrhoea 833–834
    dizziness 835
    eye pain 835
    fever 833
    headache 832
    insomnia 835
    mouth ulcers 834

  nosebleed 834
  oedema 833
  skin eruptions 834
  vomiting 835
  pulse and 451
  scanty 828
  symptoms and signs **827–835**
  tension before *see* premenstrual
    symptoms
  see also menstruation, problem
    symptoms
mental difficulties
  concentration difficulties 804
  hyperactivity 804–805
  learning difficulties (children) 804
  poor memory 803–804
  symptoms/sign **803–805**
  see also mental-emotional symptoms
mental-emotional symptoms **379–389**
  depression *see* depression
  emotional problems at puberty and
    overwork 416–417
  excess joy 388, 389, 794
    see also mania
  fear/anxiety *see* anxiety; fear
  irritability/anger 385
    see also irritability
  menopause 401
  mental restlessness 388–389
  miscarriage 408
  sadness/grief 387–388
    see also grief
  schizophrenia 802
  symptoms and signs **797–802**
  weak Heart constitution and
    emotional problems 417
  worry/overthinking 386–387
  see also emotional symptoms;
    emotions; mental difficulties
mental restlessness 251, **388–389**
  patterns 389
  symptoms and signs 794
Metal
  Fire overacting on Metal 1008
  Wood insulting Metal 1009
Metal insulting Fire 1009
Metal not generating Water 1008
Metal overacting on Wood 1008
Metal type
  abdomen size 146
  body odour 549, *550*
  body shape 19, *19*
  Earth not generating Metal 1008
  face *plate 1.5*
  voice 542, *542*
metallic taste 728
microsystems 8, 8–9
  ears 8
  face 7–8

micturition *see* urination (micturition)
middle age, Five Stages of Life 418
Middle Burner
  finger disease reflection 140, *141*
  pattern identification 970
  pulse diagnosis
    Gate section 437, *438*
    position assignment 443
    state of *434*, *435*
  see also Three Burners (Triple Burner)
migraine
  case histories 291–293
  see also headache
Mind
  depression 798
  mood and Ethereal Soul 382, *382*
  observation
    body, mind and complexion **1–66**
    eyes **75**, *76*
    mind, spirit and emotions **31–38**,
      1016
  Phlegm misting the Mind 882
  relationship with Ethereal Soul 383,
    383
  spirit/body relationship 32, 347, 542
Ming Men (Fire of the Gate of Life) 80,
    766
Ming Tang 87
Ming Tang (nose) 303
Minister Fire, tongue red points 211
Minister Fire blazing upwards, nocturnal
    emissions 767
Minister Fire deficiency
  cold genitals in men 769
  see also Kidney-Yang deficiency
Minute Connecting channels 526
  see also Connecting channels
Minute pulse *see* pulse qualities
miscarriage 408
  amenorrhoea following 845
  habitual 842
  threatened 84
moles 185–186
monoamine oxydase inhibitors (MAOI)
    508
mood swings 1016
morning sickness 406, 837–838
motivation, lack of 1022
motor-neurone disease 61, 153
Mountain Rampart 79
mouth 308–309
  channels 93–94, *94*
  children 193, *194*
  cold sores 97, *97*, 309, 610–611
  cracked corners 97, *97*, 611
  deviation of 71, 97–98, *98*, 573
    signs 613
  dribbling from corners 98, *98*, 612
  dry 279, 732–733

mouth (*contd.*)
  eye/mouth deviation 60, *60*
  increased salivation 733
  itching 611
  observation **93–104**
  open 97, *97*, 612
  oral thrush (candida) 187
  palate
    abnormal colour 98–99, *99*,
      624–625
    symptoms and signs **624–625**
    white spots 872
    Yin organs 98, *98*
  philtrum *see* philtrum
  saliva 94
  symptoms and signs **609–613**
  trembling 612
  ulcers 97, *97*, 308, 308–309,
    609–610, 834
  see also gums; lips; teeth; tongue
Moving pulse *see* pulse qualities
Mu Xiang Liu Qi Yin 1036–1037
Mu Xuan ('blurred vision') 360
mucus, in stools 271
multiple sclerosis 62
mumps 870
muscle ache, limbs 339
Muscle channels 527
  characteristics 527
  functions 527
  palpation 527
muscle twitching (fasciculation) 63,
    714–715
muscles
  limbs *see* limbs
  space between skin and 176
  spinal
    atrophy 116, 705
    children 194
myalgic encephalomyelitis (ME) *see*
      postviral fatigue syndrome
myomas 135
myopia 629

N

naevi (moles) *plate 21.34*
  differentiation of 186
  pathology and diagnosis, Western *vs*
      Chinese 185–186
  symptoms and signs 787–788
nails
  abnormal colour 139, *140*, 691–692
  bluish-greenish 139, 691–692
  coarse and thick 138, 688
  cracked 138, 688
  curling 139, 690
  dark 139, 692
  dry skin and 178

dull-white 139, 691
falling off 139, 689
flaking 138, 690
indented 137, *138*, 689
lunulae 140
  large 692
  men and women 140
  small or absent 692
normal 137
observation **137–142**
onset of disease indication 137
organ system correspondence
    140–142
pale-white 139, 691
palpation 520
purple 139, 692
red 139, 691
ridged 137, 688
surface abnormalities 137–138,
    139
symptoms and signs **688–692**
thickening 138, 688
thin and brittle 138, 689
twisted 139, 691
white spots 139, 691
withered and brittle 138, 689–690
withered and thickened 138, 690
yellow 139, 691
  see also finger(s); hands
nasal discharge 164, *164*
  see also rhinitis
nasal voice 543, 820–821
nausea
  morning sickness 406
  patterns 266
  premenstrual symptoms 405
  retching 725
  symptoms and signs 723–724
  see also vomiting
neck
  carbuncles 788
  channels influencing *109*, 109–110,
      110, 312
  deviated 113, *113*, 654
  goitre 315–316, *316*
  interrogation **311–316**
  length 112
  long 112, *112*
  observation **109–114**
  pain 316, *316*, 654
  rigidity 112–113, 654
  rigidity/stiffness 59–60, 316, *316*
  short 112, *112*
  soft 113, 654
  stiff 653
  swollen glands 114, *114*, 655
  symptoms and signs **653–656**
  thin 114, *114*
  ulcers 789

wide 113, *113*, 655
  see also throat
Nei Bu Wan 1037
nephritis, hand lines 135
night sweating 251, 351–352, *352*,
      385, 776
  menopause 401
nighttime pain 257
nine orifices, internal organs and five
      senses relationship 2, *2*
nipple(s) 851–852
  abnormalities 124–125
  bloody discharge 851–852
  cracked 125, 852
  discharge 124, *124*
  inverted 125, 852
  milky discharge 851
  sticky yellow discharge 851
nocturnal emissions 393, *393*, 767
nocturnal enuresis 274, 275, 757–758,
      867
Nong Pao 178
nose **303–306**
  abnormal colour 89, 89–90, *90*,
      589–591
    bluish-greenish 89, *89*, 590
    dark 90, *90*, 591
    pale 89, *89*, 589
    red 89, *89*, 590
    reddish-purple 89–90, *90*, 591
    yellow 89, *89*, 589–590
  aching 305, *305*, 595
  bad smell sensation 597
  bleeding 90, 594–595
  blocked 304, *304*
  carcinoma 596
  channels influencing 87–88, *88*
  children *see* children
  discharge from 164, *164*
  dry nostrils 306, *306*
  face reading 87
  internal organ relationship 88, 88–89
  itching 304, *304*, 593
  nostrils *see* nostrils
  observation **87–92**
  organs influencing 304
  pain 595–596
  pain in 305, *306*
  papules on 90, 598–599
  polyps in 90, 598
  rhinitis 87
  runny 305, *305*, 592–593
  sinusitis 87
  sneezing *see* sneezing
  swollen 90, 596–597
  symptoms and signs **589–600**
  ulcers on 90, 598
  Yang convergence 87
  see also smell/smelling (olfaction)

nosebleed 90, 594–595
  menstrual symptoms 834
nostrils 90
  dry 90, 306, *306*, 593–594
  flapping 90, 598, 870
Nu Lao Dan 175
Nuan Gan Jian 1037
numbness/tingling 319, *319*
  half of body 712
  hands 343, *343*
  limbs 339, *339*, 673, 712
Nutritional Impairment Patterns,
      inflamed gums 619
Nutritive and Defensive Qi not
      harmonized
  fever during menstruation 833
  unilateral sweating 778
Nutritive and Defensive Qi obstructed,
      yellow sweat 777

O

obesity 319, 713–714
observation
  babies 1057–1058
  body, mind and complexion **1–66**
  body movements **59–66**
  body shape, physique and demeanour
      11–29
  complexion colour **39–58**
  constitutional traits 9–10
  diagnosis by **1–233**
  integration with interrogation 242
  mind, spirit and emotions **31–38**
  parts of the body **67–200**
    back **115–120**
    breasts **121–125**
    chest and abdomen **143–147**
    children **191–200**
    ears **105–108**
    excretions **163–167**
    eyes **75–86**
    face **69–74**
    genitalia **149–151**
    hair **69–74**
    hands **129–136**
    head **69–74**
    heartbeat **127–128**
    legs **159–162**
    limbs **153–157**
    mouth and lips **93–104**
    nails **137–142**
    nose **87–92**
    skin **169–190**
    throat and neck **109–114**
    see also individual entries
  tongue diagnosis **201–232**
Obstruction of Spleen by Dampness with
      stagnation of Liver-Qi 889

odour, diagnosis by *see* smell/smelling
oedema
  abdomen 146, 745
  after childbirth 846
  blood 179
  clinical manifestations 935
  face 71, 572
  feet 345
  hands 343
  legs 159–160, 713
    case history 160
  limbs 156–157, *157*, 675–676, 713
  menstrual symptoms 833
  in pregnancy 406, 838
  premenstrual 405
  skin 179, *179*
old age
  Five Stages of Life 418
  see also elderly
olfaction *see* smell/smelling (olfaction)
opisthotonos 63, 715
oppression, abdominal pain 735
  see also Men ('feeling of oppression')
optic nerve 80
oral thrush 187
organ patterns
  Bright-Yang 967
  Greater Yang stage 966–967
  Heat in Bright Yang 374
orgasm
  female
    anorgasmia 393–394
    excessive sexual activity 430
    headache after 394
  male *see* ejaculation
Original Qi deficiency
  and kidney-Yang deficiency 560
  urine retention in infants 867
otitis media, case history 1021
ovarian cysts, hand lines 135
Overflowing pulse *see* pulse qualities
overthinking 386–387
  patterns 387
overwork 282, 416–417, 974

P

paediatric symptoms/signs **861–872**
  see also children
pain
  abdominal *see* abdominal pain
  bluish/greenish complexion 578
  bowel movements 258, 270, 273
  breast(s) 398
  character of, headache 288–289
  classification 255–260
  coccyx 705
  continuous 257
  daytime 257

effect of eating/drinking 258, 264
  elbows 342, *342*, 679
  epigastric 329, *329*
  eyelids 639
  eyes 358, *358–359*, *359*, 632–633,
      835
  face 571–572
  factors affecting 254–255, 258–259
  feet 344–345, *345*
  groin 698
  hands 342, *342*, 682–683
  hips 343–344, 697
  hypochondrial pain *see* hypochondrial
      pain
  intermittent 257
  interrogation **253–260**
  joints 710
  knees 344, *344*, 697
  localized 255
  movement/rest 258–259
  moving 255
  nature of 254, 255–257
    boring pain 257
    colicky pain 256
    cutting pain 257
    distending pain ('*Zhang Tong*')
      255–256
    lurking pain (*Yin Tong*) 257
    pulling pain 257
    pushing pain 257
    soreness 255
    spastic pain 256
    throbbing pain 257
  neck 654
  nighttime 257
  nose 595–596
  organ *vs.* channel pain 259, *259*
  pressure 258
  in ribs 324, *324*, 664
  scalp 69, 568
  shoulders 341–342, *342*
  soles of feet 345, 698
  temperature 258
  testicles 773
  thighs 344, 696–697
  timing 254, 257
  tolerance 27–28
  tongue 613–614
    in tongue 309
  umbilical 332, 738–739
  during urination 839
  xyphoid process 328–329, *329*,
      736–737
pain tolerance, body shape 27–28, *28*
Painful Obstruction Syndrome 64, 113,
      214, 985
  case histories 1020
  channel palpation in 527–528
  Chronic, deformed knuckles 684

Painful Obstruction Syndrome (*contd.*)
  Cold, rigidity of neck 654
  Cold-Dampness, swelling of fingers
    686
  Damp, swelling of joints in limbs
    676
  Damp-Heat, swelling of fingers 686
  deformed knuckles 132
  generalized joint pain *340*
  neck pain/stiffness 316
  organ *vs.* channel pain 259
  shoulder 341
  swelling of joints 157
  Wind-Damp
    neck pain 654
    stiff neck 653
    swelling of fingers 686
  withered and brittle nails 138
palate *see* mouth
paleness, tongue-body colour 210
palms *see* hands
palpation 509–524
  abdomen 510–512, 513–516
    see also abdomen
  acupuncture points 520–522
  babies temples 518–519, *519*
  breasts 513
  channels 525–538
  chest 512–513
    see also chest
  diagnosis by **431–538**
  feet and hands 519–520
    see also feet; hands
  forearm 517–518
  forehead 517
  pressing 509, 510, 527
  skin 516–519
    see also skin
  stroking 509, 510, 527
  techniques 509–510, 527
  touching 509, 510, 527
palpitations 322, 325–326, 385,
    666–667
  case history 325–326, 1014
  Heart-Blood deficiency, case history
    1014
panic attacks, case history 385
papules
  eruptions 71, 174, 573
  nose 90, 598–599
  skin on body 177–178, *178*
  vs vesicles/macules *958*
paralysis 61–62, 710–711
  facial (Bell's palsy) 60–61, 573
  hemiplegia 64
  legs 160, 695
  limbs 154–155, *155*, 676–677
  motor-neurone disease 61
  multiple sclerosis 62

pathogenic factors
  Chinese terms 1066
  Cold **946–947**
  Dampness **948–950**
  Deficiency–Excess conditions 1023
  Dryness **950–951**
  Fire **951–952**
  pattern identification **939–952**
  residual *see* residual pathogenic factors
  Summer-Heat **948**
  Wind **943–946**
patient expressions 239
patient questioning *see* interrogation;
    questions
pattern identification **873–1009**
  Blood **930–932**
  Body Fluids **927–933**
  combined Qi, Blood, Yin and Yang
    874–875, **932–933**
  Eight Principles 875, 981, **983–991**
    interior/exterior 984–985
  Five Elements 875, 982, **1007–1009**
    see also Five Elements
  internal organs 874, **877–926**
    bladder 925–926
    Gall-Bladder 917–919
    Heart 879–883
    heart 879–883
    Large Intestine 921–923
    Liver 891–898
    Lung(s) 899–904
    Small Intestine 911–912
    Spleen 885–889
    Stomach 913–916
  interrogation 242, *242*
  pathogenic factors 875, 939–940,
    943–952
    Cold 946–947
    Dampness 948–950
    Dryness 950–951
    Fire 951–952
    pattern identification 939–952
    Summer-Heat 948
    Wind 943–946
  Qi **929–930**
  Three Burners 875, 940, *941*,
    969–971
  Yang **932**
  Yin **932**
pattern identification, Eight
    Extraordinary Channels 981,
    997–1006
  combined Directing/Penetrating Vessel
    999–1003
  Directing Vessel (*Ren Mai*) 998
  Girdle Vessel (*Dai Mai*) 1003–1004
  Governing Vessel (*Du Mai*) 997–998
  Penetrating Vessel (*Chong Mai*)
    998–999

  Yang Heel Vessel (*Yang Qiao Mai*)
    1004
  Yang Linking Vessel (*Yang Wei Mai*)
    1005
  Yin Heel Vessel (*Yin Qiao Mai*) 1004
  Yin Linking Vessel (*Yin Wei Mai*) 1005
pattern identification, Four Levels 875,
    940, *941*, **953–964**
  Blood level 957
  Defensive Qi level 954–955
  Latent Heat 958–962
  Nutritive Qi level 956
  Qi level 955–956
pattern identification, Six Stages 875,
    940, *941*, **965–968**
  Bright-Yang stage 961–962
  Greater Yang stage 965–967
  Greater Yin stage 967
  Lesser-Yang stage 967
  Lesser Yin stage 968
  Terminal-Yin stage 968
pattern identification, Twelve Channels
    981, **993–996**
  bladder 995
  gall-bladder 996
  heart 994
  kidneys 995
  large intestine 993–994
  liver 996
  lungs 993
  pericardium 995
  small intestine 994–995
  spleen 994
  stomach 994
  Triple Burner 995–996
P-6 Neiguan 664
PE-8 Laogong 534–535, *535*
peau d'orange skin (breasts) 852
pecking bird pulse 507
Penetrating Vessel (*Chong Mai*)
    998–999
  abdomen 145, 146
    lateral-lower region 515–516
    umbilical region 515
  area under xyphoid process 328–329,
    329, 513
  Blood stasis in Directing and
    Penetrating Vessels 1000
  breasts 121, *121, 122*, 513
  chest 143
  Damp-Heat in Directing and
    Penetrating Vessels 860,
    1001
  Directing and Penetrating Vessel
    disharmony 376, 851
  Directing and Penetrating Vessels
    deficient and cold 999–1000
  Directing and Penetrating Vessels
    Empty 999

Directing and Penetrating Vessels
    unstable 999
disharmony of 376
Empty-Heat in Directing and
    Penetrating Vessels 1001
Full-Cold in Directing and Penetrating
    Vessels 1001–1002
Full-Heat in Directing and Penetrating
    Vessels 1000–1001
genitalia 149
mouth 93, 94
Rebellious Qi *see* Rebellious Qi in
    Penetrating Vessel
Stagnant Heat in Directing and
    Penetrating Vessels 1001
see also Directing and Penetrating
    Vessels
Penetrating Vessel and Directing Vessels
    deficient and cold 742
Penetrating Vessel and Directing Vessels
    disharmony 376, 851
acne 569, 784
feeling of heat in face 302
itching around mouth 611
urticaria 784
penis
    glans, redness and swelling 150
    long, in children 150, 872
    pain and itching 771
    Peyronie's disease 150, 772
    priapism 150, 768–769
    redness and swelling 150, 772
    soft and withered 150, 771–772
    ulcers on 150, 772–773
    see also genitalia
pensiveness 424, *424*
Pericardium
    channels 995
    Heat 956, 970
Pericardium channel
    breasts 121, *121*
    palpation 534–535, *535*
        blood vessel 534
        skin 534–535
period pain *see* menstrual pain
periods *see* menstruation
Peyronie's disease 150, 772
pharynx 311
    dryness 111
    erosion 111, 602–603
    observation 110–111
    red 110–111, 602–603
    signs *111*
    swelling 111, 602
    ulcers 111
    see also throat
philtrum
    abnormal colour 102, 625–626
    channels 101

fertility *101*, 102
flat 102, *102*, 625
observation **101–102**
shape 102
stiff 102, *102*, 625
symptoms and signs **625–626**
Phlegm
    Blood stasis and *see* Blood stasis with
        Phlegm
    breast distension 849
    breast lumps 851
    chest symptoms 321–322
    Cold *see* Cold-Phlegm
    cold hands and feet 672
    Cold-Phlegm, clinical manifestations
        936
    Cold-Phlegm in the Lungs 902
    concentration difficulties 804
    confusing/complicated conditions
        1020
    contraction of limbs 677
    cough 322, 323
    Damp-Phlegm *see* Damp-Phlegm
    Damp-Phlegm in the Lungs 902, 976
    Dampness and Phlegm in Uterus 1002
    dark sclera 636
    difficulty in finding words 822
    digestive symptoms 262
    dizziness 295, 559
    Dry-Phlegm, clinical manifestations
        936
    excess wax production 583
    excessive pubic hair 860
    fainting 560
    fever in cancer 816
    Food-Phlegm, clinical manifestations
        936
    Gallbladder 937
    goitre 315
    greasy hair 567
    head, feeling of heaviness 297
    headache 238, 290, 291, 293
    in joints 937
        thin and brittle nails 689
    Kidney deficiency with 706
    Liver-Blood deficiency with Phlegm
        895
    Liver-Qi stagnation with *see* Liver-Qi
        stagnation with Phlegm
    Liver-Wind harbouring Phlegm 895
    Liver-Wind with *see* Liver-Wind and
        Phlegm
    menopausal syndrome 856
    muzziness (fuzziness) of head 563
    nasal voice 821
    numbness/tingling of hands 683
    pattern identification 936–938
    Phlegm-Fluids 937
    Phlegm in the channels 937

    Phlegm misting Heart 937
    Qi-Phlegm 936
    Qi stagnation and *see* Qi stagnation
        with Phlegm
    residual pathogenic factors 976–977
    Shock-Phlegm 937
    slurred speech 821
    Spleen-Qi deficiency with, somnolence
        810
    sticky/metallic taste 728
    stuffiness feeling under Heart 666
    thickening of nails 688
    in throat 603–604
    tongue diagnosis 230
    Turbid *see* Turbid Phlegm
    ulcers on neck 789
    Wine-Phlegm 938
    withered and brittle nails 690
    yellow nails 691
Phlegm accumulation 837
Phlegm and Blood stasis in Lower Burner
    872
Phlegm and Blood stasis in Middle
    Burner 744–745
Phlegm and retention of food 744
Phlegm-Dryness in Lungs 902–903
    acupuncture 903
    clinical manifestations 902–903
    prescription 903
Phlegm-Fire
    hemiplegia 711
    hyperactivity 805
Phlegm-Fire affecting Heart 799
Phlegm-Fire harassing Heart 882
    acupuncture 882
    anxiety 800
    bipolar disorder 388
    clinical manifestations 882
    depression 798
    excess joy 794
    excessive dreaming 808–809
    inappropriate laughter 795
    incoherent speech 821
    insomnia 808
    painful tongue 614
    palpitations under the Heart 667
    prescription 882
    schizophrenia 802
    startled easily 793
Phlegm-Fire harassing Mind 840
Phlegm-Fire harassing upwards 841
Phlegm-Fire in Stomach 808–809
Phlegm-Fluids
    bluish-greenish nose 590
    clinical manifestations 937
    pale nose 589
    stuffiness feeling under Heart 666
    yellow nose 590
Phlegm-Fluids in abdomen 742

Phlegm-Fluids in chest and
    hypochondrium 668, 738
Phlegm-Fluids in Lungs 903
    acupuncture 903
    chest protruding on one side 669
    chest sunken on one side 669
    chronic cough 660
    clinical manifestations 903
    prescription 903
Phlegm-Fluids in Lungs with Blood stasis
    669
Phlegm-Fluids in Stomach 738
Phlegm-Fluids obstructing Heart 667
Phlegm-Heat
    case histories 1022
    chest pain with sputum 324
    clinical manifestations 936
    convulsions in children 871
    dark eyelids 638
    facial pain 571
    greasy skin 781–782
    hot and painful eyes 632
    nodules under skin 788
    red sclera 635
    spontaneous sweating 775
    stagnation of the Gall Bladder with
        918–919
    voice loss 840–841
    Wind and, phlegm in throat 604
Phlegm-Heat in Heart 1016–1017
    Heart feeling vexed 665
    staring, fixed eyes 650
    sudden blindness 631
Phlegm-Heat in Liver, sudden blindness
    631
Phlegm-Heat in Lungs 373, 902,
        976–977
    aching nose 595
    acupuncture 902
    acute cough 659
    bad smell sensation 597
    breathlessness 661–662
    chest pain 663
    clinical manifestations 902, 976–977,
        977
    cough in children 865
    cough in pregnancy 840
    coughing blood 661
    flapping of nostrils 870
    foul breath 729
    prescription 902
    snoring 811, 821
    spoon-shaped fingers 687
    sticky/metallic taste 728
    thirst 732
    wheezing 662
Phlegm-Heat in muscles, muscle ache in
    limbs 671
Phlegm-Heat in Stomach

dry mouth 733
    epigastric pain 737
Phlegm-Heat in Stomach and Heart 794
Phlegm-Heat in the Lungs 902
Phlegm-Heat obstructing Spleen
        640–641
Phlegm-Heat rising 564
Phlegm in channels 937
    cold hands 680
    numbness/tingling 712
Phlegm in Gallbladder 937
Phlegm in Interior 814
Phlegm in joints 676, 937
Phlegm in Kidneys 937
Phlegm in Limbs
    heaviness feeling in limbs 674
    numbness/tingling in limbs 673
Phlegm in Lower Burner, cold feet 694
Phlegm in Lungs
    chest, feeling of oppression/tightness
        324
    chronic, protruding chest 668
    nose polyps 598
    oppression feeling in chest 664
    protruding sternum 669
    pulsation of carotid artery 655
    snoring 821
    white specks on sclera or pupil 647
Phlegm in Lungs and Spleen
    distension feeling in eyes 642
    strabismus 629
Phlegm in Lungs with Lung- and
        Spleen-Qi deficiency, snoring
        811
Phlegm in Stomach, abdominal pain 736
Phlegm misting Heart 937
Phlegm misting Mind 882
Phlegm obstructing clear orifices
        603–604
Phlegm obstructing Heart 614
Phlegm obstructing Middle Burner 888
Phlegm obstructing Mind orifices 821
Phlegm obstructing Spleen, large
        abdomen 745
Phlegm obstructing Stomach
    nausea 723
    poor appetite 720
    vomiting 724
Phlegm obstructing Uterus, scanty
        periods 828
Phlegm patterns 882
Phlegm under skin 937
Phlegm with Blood stasis 937
Phlegm with Lung-Qi stagnation
    breast distension 850
    breast lumps 851
physique see body build (physique)
Pi ('feeling of stuffiness') 736
Ping Wei San 1037

pinworms 869
    see also worm infestation
placenta, retention of 843
plaque
    skin 177–178, plate 21.4
    teeth 100, 617
pleuritis, heartbeat displacement 128
plucking of veins of inner leg
        1056–1057
Plum Stone Syndrome 314
points/channels, Chinese terms 1064
polycystic ovary syndrome 407, 1022
polyps, nose 90, 598
Pool Rampart 79
poor memory 803–804
post-natal depression/psychosis 847
Postnatal Qi 261
    abdomen 146
postviral fatigue syndrome
    aches 317–318
    pulse and clinical application
        457–458
    residual pathogenic factors 974
    tiredness 286
pregnancy 406–408, **837–842**
    abdominal pain 838
    anxiety 840
    aversion to food 721
    breech presentation 842
    childbirth 408, 408
    constipation 839–840
    convulsions 841
    cough 840
    dizziness 840
    eclampsia 841
    epileptic attacks during 155–156
    feeling of suffocation 841
    fertility 406–408
    gynaecological symptoms and signs
        837–842
    hoarse voice 543, 820
    lips abnormal colour 95–96, 96,
        624
    loss of voice 840–841
    miscarriage
        habitual 842
        threatened 84
    morning sickness 406, 837–838
    oedema during 406, 838
    problems during 837–842
    problems with fetus 841–842
        slow fetal growth 842
    pulse 451
    urination problems 839
    vaginal bleeding 838
    see also childbirth; childbirth,
        postpartum problems
premature ejaculation 393, 393,
        766–767

premenstrual symptoms 404–406, *405, 406*
  breast distension 398, *399,* 832–833, 1016
  constipation 405, 834
  diarrhoea 405
  headaches 405
  insomnia 405, 835
  nausea 405
  premenstrual tension 404–405
    case histories, tongue/pulse diagnosis 244–246
    pulse clinical application 458
    symptoms and signs 831–832
  water retention 405
  see also menstruation; menstruation, problem symptoms
prenatal constitution, body shape *22, 23, 23*
Prenatal Qi, abdomen 146
priapism 150, 768–769
prognosis determination, complexion colours 47–49
prolapse
  anal 762
  uterus 859
  vagina 151, 859
prostatic hypertrophy, hand lines 135
prostatitis, hand lines 135
protruding eyeball *82, 83,* 642–643
psoriasis
  with bright-red plaques *plate 21.29*
  differential diagnosis 184, *184*
  occurrence 183
  with pale and dry-scaly plaques *plate 21.31*
  with pale plaques *plate 21.28*
  pathology and diagnosis
    Chinese *184,* 184–185
    Western *183,* 183–184, *184*
  with purple lesions *plate 21.30*
  pustular *plate 21.26*
  scalp *plate 21.27*
  with scaly plaques *plate 21.25*
  symptoms and signs 783
  types 183, *183–184*
psychosis, post-natal depression 847
pterygium 646
puberty, emotional problems and overwork 416–417
pubic hair
  excessive 150, 773–774, 860
  loss of 150, 773, 860
pulse, method of taking 446–449
  equalizing breathing 447
  fingers
    arranging 447–448
    five movements 448–449
    moving 448–449

pushing *449,* 456, 457
  rolling 448, *448, 449,* 456–457
leveling the arm 446–447, *447*
time 446
pulse diagnosis 237, **433–464**
  accuracy in 461
  acupuncturist's and herbalist's perspective 444
  acute *vs* chronic conditions 445
  anger 452, 458
  assignment of position to organs 438–445
    Classic of Difficulties 438–439, *439, 440*
    different authors on 438, *439*
    Golden Mirror of Medicine *439,* 441–442, *442*
    modern China 442–443
    Pulse Classic *439,* 439–441
    Study of the Pulse from Pin Hu Lake *439,* 441
  blood, state of 434, 455, 463
  cancer 462–463
  case histories 457, 459, 460
  case history 1020
  Classic of Difficulties 435–436
  clinching a diagnosis 457
  clinical application 457–463
    acute *vs* chronic conditions 445
  clinical presentation of symptoms absence of 461–462
    disharmonies indicated beyond 461
  deep level 445, 445–446, *446*
  Deficiency and Excess differentiation 457–458
    in cancer 462
  emotional problems 458–459, *459*
  epigastric pain 330
  external and internal, interpretation 443, *443*
  Foot position, submerging Yin 452–453
  Foot section 436–437, *437, 438*
  front, middle and rear sections 437
  Gate section 436–437, *437, 438*
    Yang and Yin boundary 452–453
  heart problems 459–460
  Heart-Qi reflection 445
  historical aspects 1051–1055
  Inch section 436–437, *437, 438*
    emerging Yang 452–453
  integration with interrogation 243–248
  interpretation 445
  limitations 464
  Lower Burner *see* Lower Burner
  method of taking 435
  Middle Burner *see* Middle Burner
  middle level 445, 445–446, *446*

  nine regions *434,* 434–435
  organ and pattern disharmony 434
  organ problems 457, 459
  postviral fatigue syndrome 457–458
  premenstrual tension 458
  pressure application 445, 446
  Qi state 434, 455
  radial artery 436, *436*
  reconciling different arrangements 443–445
  sadness and grief 452, 459
  significance 434, 444–445
  skills required 434
  small and large intestine, discrepancies 444
  subjections to 464
  superficial level 445, 445–446, *446*
  three levels *445,* 445–446, *446*
    feeling *455, 455*
  three sections 436–437, *438*
  Tongue diagnosis, integration 463–464
  Toxic Heat 462, 463
  treatment principle determination 458
  Upper Burner *see* Upper Burner
  Yellow Emperor's Internal Classic *434,* 434–435
  Yin and Yang organs reflection 443–444
  see also Yang; Yin
pulse interpretation guidelines 454–457
  feeling overall quality 456
  feeling quality, strength and level 456–457
  feeling with three fingers 454
  pulse rate counting 457
  spirit, Stomach-Qi and root feeling 454
  three levels feeling *455, 455*
  three positions, feeling together and individually 454
pulse positions, Chinese terms 1064
pulse qualities **465–508**
  ACE inhibitors on 508
  antidepressants 507–508
  apical 512
  arrangement of 466, *467*
  basic eight 467–479
  beta blockers 508
  boiling cauldron 506
  bouncing stone 507
  Chinese terms 1064
  circling fish 506–507
  classification 496–498
    basic eight 496
    different aspects for 497
    Eight Principles 497–498
    Four Levels patterns 498, *498,* 605

pulse qualities (*contd.*)
    Qi, blood and body fluids patterns 497
    Six Stages patterns 498, *498*, 605
    Triple Burner patterns *499*
  complete set of *466*, 467
  dangerous conditions indication 506–507
  diuretics 508
  drugs effect on 507–508, *508*
  empty type 479–485
  external pathogens 468
  factors affecting 449–451, *451*
    age 450, 461
    body build 450–451
    Fan Guan Mai 451
    gender 550, *550*
    menstruation 451
    pregnancy 451
    season *449*, 449–450
    short term 446
    Xie Fei Mai 451
  feeling and identifying 466–467
  full type 485–491
    in cancer 462
    elderly 461
  H$_2$-receptor antagonists 508
  Insulin 508
  leaking roof 507
  non-traditional 494–496
  normal attributes 451–453, *452*, *454*
    root 452–535
      see also root
    spirit 451
      see also spirit
    Stomach-Qi 451–452
      see also Stomach-Qi
    wave qualities 452–453, *453*
  pecking bird 507
  positions 499–506
    left front (Heart) *500*, 500–501, *501*
    left middle (Liver) *501*, 501–502, *502*
    left rear (Kidneys) *502*, 502–503, *503*
    right front (Lungs) *503*, 503–504, *504*
    right middle (Stomach and Spleen) *504*, 504–505, *505*
    right rear (Small Intestine and Kidneys) 506, *506*
  rate counting 457
  sesame seed hasty 507
  spinning bean 507
  swimming shrimp 507
  terminology of 498, *499*
  tranquillizers and hypnotics 507
  umbilical 515, *515*

untying rope 507
upturned knife 507
warfarin on 508
without wave 452, 459
see also pulse qualities, *individual attribute*; symptoms and signs
pulse qualities, Big 488–489
  clinical manifestations *489*
  clinical significance 488
  combinations 489
  description 488
  differentiation of similar pulses 489
  with strength 488–489
  without strength 489
pulse qualities, Choppy
  clinical significance 478, *478*
  combinations 478
  description 477–478, *478*
  differentiation of similar pulses 478–479
  heart problems 460
  left front (Heart) position 501
  position significance 479
pulse qualities, Deep 462, 469–470
  clinical significance 470
  combinations 470
  description 469–470
  differentiation of similar pulses 470
  full and weak differentiation 470
  left middle (Liver) position 501
  left rear (Kidneys) position 502
  position significance 470
pulse qualities, Empty 474–475
  clinical significance 474–475, *475*
  combinations 475
  description 474
  differentiation of similar pulses 475
  position significance 446, 475
pulse qualities, Fine 480
  clinical significance 480, *480*
  combinations 480
  description 480
  differentiation of similar pulses 480
  left rear (Kidneys) position 503
  position significance 480
  right middle (Stomach and Spleen) position 505
pulse qualities, Firm 489–490
  clinical significance 489, *489*
  combinations 489
  definition 445–446, 497
  description 489
  differentiation of similar pulses 489–490
pulse qualities, Floating 445, 467–469
  clinical significance 467–468
  combinations 468–469
  description 467
  differentiation of similar pulses 469

  Empty 445, 455, 468, 469
  exterior conditions 468
  interior conditions 468–469
  left front (Heart) position 500–501
  left middle (Liver) position 501
  left rear (Kidneys) position 502
  position significance 469
  right front (Lungs) position 504
  right middle (Stomach and Spleen) position 505
  right rear (Small Intestine and Kidneys) position 506
  Western disease conditions 469, *469*
pulse qualities, Full 475–476
  combinations 476
  common conditions manifesting 476, *476*
  description 475
  differentiation of similar pulses 476
  position significance 476
pulse qualities, Hasty 492
  clinical significance 492, *492*
  combinations 492
  description 492
  differentiation of similar pulses 492
pulse qualities, Hidden 483–484
  clinical significance 483–484, *484*
  combinations 484
  description 483
  differentiation of similar pulses 484
  position significance 484
pulse qualities, Hollow 482
  clinical significance 482, *482*
  combinations 482
  description 482
  differentiation of similar pulses 482
  left front (Heart) position 501
  left rear (Kidneys) position 503
  right front (Lungs) position 504
  right middle (Stomach and Spleen) position 505
pulse qualities, Hurried 492–493
  clinical significance 492–493, *493*
  combinations 493
  description 492
  differentiation of similar pulses 493
pulse qualities, Intermittent 493–494
  clinical significance 493, *493*
  combinations 493
  description 493
  differentiation of similar pulses 494
pulse qualities, Irregular 494–495
  clinical significance 494, *495*
  combinations 495
  description 494
  differentiation of similar pulses 495
  heart disharmony 445, 459–460
  rate or rhythm 491–494, 497

pulse qualities, Knotted
  clinical significance 491, *491*
  combinations 491–492
  description 460, 491
  differentiation of similar pulses 492
  with strength 491
  without strength 491
pulse qualities, Leather
  clinical significance 483, *483*
  combinations 483
  description 482–483, 497
  differentiation of similar pulses 483
pulse qualities, Long 490
  clinical significance 490, *490*
  combinations 490
  description 490
  differentiation of similar pulses 490
  wave flow 453
pulse qualities, Minute
  clinical significance 480, *480*
  combinations 481
  differentiation of similar pulses 481
  heart problems 460
  position significance 481
  pulse description 480
pulse qualities, Moving 490–491
  clinical significance 490–491, *491*
  combinations 491
  description 490
  differentiation of similar pulses 491
pulse qualities, Overflowing 487–488
  clinical significance 487, *488*
  combinations 488
  description 487
  differentiation of similar pulses 488
  emotional problems 458
  left front (Heart) position 500
  left middle (Liver) position 502
  left rear (Kidneys) position 503
  position significance 488
  right front (Lungs) position 504
  with strength 487
  Toxic Heat 463
  without strength 488
pulse qualities, Rapid 472–474
  clinical significance 472–474
  combinations 474
  common conditions manifesting 473, *473*
  description 472
  differentiation of similar pulses 474
  emotional problems 458–459
  heat and non-heat reasons for 473–474, *473–474*
  position significance 474
  tongue not red with 463
  Toxic Heat 462, 463
pulse qualities, Sad 495–496
  clinical significance 496, *496*

combinations 496
  description 495–496
  differentiation of similar pulses 496
  position significance 496
pulse qualities, Scattered 484–485
  clinical significance 484, *484*
  combinations 484
  description 484, 497
  differentiation of similar pulses 484–485
  heart problems 460
  position significance 485
pulse qualities, Short 481–482
  clinical significance 481–482, *482*
  combinations 482
  description 481
  differentiation of similar pulses 482
  left front (Heart) position 500
  wave flow 453
pulse qualities, Slippery 457, 460, 462, 476–477
  clinical significance 476–477, *477*
  combinations 477
  common conditions manifesting 476
  description 476
  differentiation of similar pulses 477
  left front (Heart) position 501
  left middle (Liver) position 501–502
  left rear (Kidneys) position 502
  position significance 477
  right front (Lungs) position 504
  right middle (Stomach and Spleen) position 505
  right rear (Small Intestine and Kidneys) position 506
pulse qualities, Slow 470–472
  clinical significance 470–471
  cold conditions and heat symptoms 471, *471*
  combinations 472
  common conditions manifesting 471, *471*
  contradictory manifestations 471, *471*
  description 470
  differentiation of similar pulses 472
  jogging 471–472
  life situations causing 472, *472*
  position significance 472
  tongue red with 463
pulse qualities, Slowed-down 494
  clinical significance 494, *494*
  combinations 494
  description 494
pulse qualities, Soggy (Weak-Floating)
  clinical significance 481, *481*
  combinations 481
  description 481, 497
  differentiation of similar pulses 481
  position significance 481

right middle (Stomach and Spleen) position 505
pulse qualities, Stagnant 495
  clinical significance 495, *495*
  combinations 495
  description 495
  differentiation of similar pulses 495
  position significance 495
pulse qualities, Tight 486–487
  clinical significance 486, *486*
  combinations 486–487
  description 486
  differentiation of similar pulses 487
  position significance 487
pulse qualities, Weak 479
  clinical significance 479, *479*
  combinations 479
  description 479
  differentiation of similar pulses 479
  left front (Heart) position 500
  left rear (Kidneys) position 502–503
  levels 445
  position significance 479
  right middle (Stomach and Spleen) position 505
  right rear (Small Intestine and Kidneys) position 506
pulse qualities, Wiry 485–486
  clinical significance 485, *485*
  combinations 485–486
  description 485
  differentiation of similar pulses 486
  elderly 461
  left front (Heart) position 501
  left middle (Liver) position 502
  position significance 486
  right middle (Stomach and Spleen) position 505
  right rear (Small Intestine and Kidneys) position 506
pupil(s)
  bleeding between iris and 649
  contracted 649–650
  dilated 649
  red ring around 647–648
  white membrane in children 648
  white specks 647
  yellow fluid between iris and 648–649
  see also eye(s)
Purple Leg and Teeth Nutritional Impairment Pattern, inflamed gums 619
pustules 174, 178, *178*, *plate 21.6*

Q

Qi
  body shape *23*, *23–24*, *24*, *24–25*
  clinical manifestations 958

Qi (*contd.*)
  defensive
    case history 1019–1020
    clinical manifestations 958
    cold 367
    deficiency, Lungs and Kidneys,
        wheeze in children 865
    invasion of external Dampness 950
    levels 954–955
    Wind-Heat in Lung Defensive-Qi
        portion 969
  Empty-Qi 990
  nutritive 815, 956, 958, 970
  pattern identification 929–930
  pulse diagnosis
    feeling levels 455
    state of 434, 454
    see also pulse diagnosis
  pulse qualities classification 497
  rebellious *see entries beginning*
        Rebellious Qi
  Rebellious Qi *see entries beginning*
        Rebellious Qi
  role of spleen 262
  strong postnatal, body shape *23,
      23–24*
  upright, residual pathogenic factors
      974, 975
  weak postnatal, body shape *24, 24–25*
  see also individual organs
Qi, Original, deficiency
  and kidney-Yang deficiency 560
  urine retention in infants 867
Qi and Blood deficiency
  atrophy of legs 694
  carbuncles on neck 788
  chronic, small or absent lunulae on
      nails 692
  clinical manifestations 932–933
  contraction of scrotum 769
  corneal opacity 647
  deviation of the mouth 613
  drooping eyelids 640
  dry and brittle hair 566
  dull-pale palate 624
  eye and mouth deviation 573
  eye discharge 634
  facial pain 303, 571
  fear/anxiety 792–793
  fever during menstruation 833
  grinding teeth 617
  hyperopia 629–630
  indented nails 689
  limb atrophy 674–675
  limb paralysis 677
  limb weakness 674
  muffled voice 820
  night vision decreased 630
  oedema of body 713

pain in foot 697
pain in limbs 672
painful periods 829
paralysis 710
paralysis of legs 695
poor memory 803
premature greying 565
protruding eyeball 643
receding gums 307, *308*, 619
sense of smell loss 597
severe
  soft neck 654
  thin neck 655
  with Toxic Heat, gums oozing pus
      620
severe and chronic, strabismus 629
thickened fingers 688
thin abdomen 745
thin and brittle nails 689
unilateral sweating 777–778
Qi and Blood deficiency of Heart, night
    sweating 776
Qi and Blood deficiency of Spleen, pale
    lips 621
Qi and Blood deficiency of Spleen and
    Heart
  brain noise 564
  dizziness 560
Qi and Blood deficiency with Blood stasis,
    curling nails 690
Qi and Blood deficiency with dryness of
    Blood
  coarse and thick nails 688
  cracked nails 688
Qi and Blood deficiency with internal
    Wind
  gait festination 695
  stepping gait 696
  unstable gait 696
Qi and Phlegm stagnation
  depression and manic behaviour 798
  schizophrenia 802
Qi and Yang deficiency of Stomach,
    swallowing difficulty
    (diaphragm choking) 726
Qi and Yin collapse, sweating from
    collapse 776
Qi and Yin deficiency
  boil on eyelid 639
  clinical manifestations 933
  dilated pupils 649
  hot and painful eyes 633
  sore throat 601
Qi and Yin deficiency of Heart, Heart
    feeling vexed 665
Qi and Yin deficiency of Stomach,
    regurgitation of food 719
Qi and Yin deficiency of Stomach and
    Spleen, sweet taste 727

Qi and Yin deficiency with Toxic Heat,
    swollen neck glands 655
Qi collapse
  clinical manifestations 929
  Lung-Qi collapse 903
Qi collapse with deficiency of Blood,
    collapse after childbirth 847
Qi deficiency
  amenorrhoea after miscarriage 845
  breast distension 849
  breast milk 847
  breech presentation 842
  chronic fever 374–375, 815
  clinical manifestations 929
  digestive symptoms 262
  dizziness in pregnancy 840
  early (short cycle) periods 827
  exhaustion (*Xu Lao*) 282
  headache 561
  Heart- and Lung-Qi deficiency
      (deficiency of Gathering-Qi)
      903–904
  heavy periods 827
  insomnia 807
  lochia 844
  low-grade fever in children 864
  Lung- and Spleen-, Phlegm in the
      Lungs with 811
  menstrual clots 826
  milky nipple discharge 851
  miscarriage 841
  nails with white spots 691
  oedema after childbirth 846
  pale menstrual blood 825
  pale philtrum 625
  paralysis 62
  post-chemotherapy fever 817
  severe, weak voice 820
  slow fetal growth 842
  small breasts 852
  Spleen-and Heart-Qi deficiency,
      somnolence 810
  Spleen Qi and Spleen-Blood deficiency
      804
  tidal fever 816
  tongue 227, 230
  tremor/spasticity 63
  watery menstrual blood 826
  white/pale complexion 575
Qi deficiency of Central 712
Qi deficiency of Spleen and Heart with
    floating Yang, hyperactivity
    804
Qi deficiency with Blood stasis
  hemiplegia 711
  limb flaccidity 675
  limb oedema 676
  oedema of the feet 694
  thigh pain 697

Qi deficiency with internal Wind 648
Qi Gate 194, *194*
Qi Ju Di Huang Wan 1037
Qi levels 955–956, *956*
   Heat in Lungs 969–970
   Heat *vs.* Fire 956
   Latent Heat *960*
Qi obstructed 930
   clinical manifestations 930
Qi oedema 179
Qi-Phlegm, clinical manifestations 936
Qi Shao (weak breathing) 545, 661
Qi sinking, clinical manifestations 929
Qi stagnation
   abdomen 326
   abdominal distension (bloating) *327*
   abdominal masses 856
   body aches 709
   breast distension 849
   breast lumps 851
   clinical manifestations 929–930
   cold hands/feet 363–364, 365,
      672
   digestive symptoms 262
   feeling of cold 814
   flattening of lumbar spine 708
   groaning 822
   infertility (female) 855
   limbs
      feeling of distension *338*, *338*
      oedema 676
   list of spine 708
   lochia 844
   menopausal syndrome 856
   oedema
      after childbirth 846
      body 713
      limbs 676
      during menstruation 833
      in pregnancy 838
   post-chemotherapy fever 817
   sore throat 602
   swollen fingers 686
   tongue 231
Qi stagnation and Blood stasis
   abdominal masses (gynaecological
      symptom) 856
   amenorrhoea 829
   blocked nose 592
   bluish-greenish lips 622
   drooping eyelids 640
   earache 582
   herpes zoster 786
   hip pain 697
   invasion, elbow pain 679
   joint pain 710
   knee pain 697
   limb rigidity 676
   numbness/tingling 712

   of hands 683
   in limbs 673
   oedema of body 713
   oedema of the feet 693
   pain in hands 682
   scarring after corneal opacity 647
   sciatica 704
   shoulder ache 656
   stiff knees 699
   stiffness of lower back 705
   ulcers on lower leg 701
   upper backache 656
   yawning 670
Qi stagnation and Blood stasis in Bladder
      channel, haemorrhoids 762
Qi stagnation and Blood stasis in
      descending branch of
      Penetrating Vessel, thigh pain
      697
Qi stagnation and Blood stasis in
      Liver channel, groin pain 698
Qi stagnation and Blood stasis in
      Penetrating Vessel 697, 740
Qi stagnation and Blood stasis in Uterus,
      purple menstrual blood 825
Qi stagnation in Bladder, abdominal pain
      - central, lower 739
Qi stagnation in Intestines, difficulty in
      defecation 751
Qi stagnation in Lower Burner, swelling
      and pain in testicles 773
Qi stagnation in Stomach and Intestines,
      umbilical pain 738
Qi stagnation with Dampness
   distended abdominal veins 743
   distension feeling in limbs 674
Qi stagnation with deficiency of Blood
      and Kidneys, feeling of
      suffocation 841
Qi stagnation with disharmony of Liver
      and Spleen, feeling of
      suffocation 841
Qi stagnation with Phlegm
   abdominal pain (area below xyphoid
      process) 737
   goitre 604
   menopausal syndrome 856
   obstruction feeling in throat 607
   premenstrual breast distension 832
   in Stomach, regurgitation of food 718
   trembling mouth 612
   wide neck 655
Qi transportation sites, Yin organs
      relationship 4
Qi Zhong 179
Qing 175
Qing E Wan 1037
Qing Gan Tou Ding Tang 1037
Qing Gu San 1037

Qing Hai Wan 1038
Qing Hao Bie Jia Tang 1038
Qing Jing San 1038
Qing Luo Yin 1038
Qing Qi Hua Tan Tang 1038
Qing Re An Tai Yin 1038
Qing Re Gu Jing Tang 1038
Qing Re Tiao Xue Tang 1038–1039
Qing Wei San 1039
Qing Ying Tang 1039
Qing Zao Jiu Fei Tang 1039
Qing Zao Run Chang Tang 1039
Qiu Zhen 177
Qu Tiao Tang 1039
questions
   Simple Questions, complexion colours
      47
   16 questions 250–251
   10 traditional questions 249–250
      limitations 249
   see also interrogation
Quivering tongue 219

R

Rapid pulse *see* pulse qualities
rash(es), skin 180, *180*, 319, 869–870,
      953–954
Rebellious Liver Qi 892
   clinical manifestations 892, 930
   prescription 892
Rebellious Liver-Qi invading Spleen 897
   acupuncture 897
   clinical manifestations 897, 930
   prescription 897
Rebellious Liver-Qi invading Stomach
   acupuncture 897
   clinical manifestations 897, 930
   prescription 897
Rebellious Lung-Qi (Lung-Qi not
      descending), protruding eyeball
      643
Rebellious Qi
   clinical manifestations 930
   digestive symptoms 262
Rebellious-Qi breathing (Shang Qi) 545,
      661
Rebellious Qi in Penetrating Vessel 238
   abdomen 328
   abdominal pain (area below xyphoid
      process) 736
   affecting Heart, palpitations 666
   breathlessness 662
   chest, feeling of oppression/tightness
      324, *324*, 664
   chest pain 663
   energy rising feeling in abdomen 742
   headache after orgasm 394
   pain with a distressing feeling 256

Rebellious Qi in Penetrating Vessel
    (*contd.*)
  palpitations under the Heart 667
  panic attacks 385
  in pregnancy, aversion to food 721
  pulsation feeling under umbilicus 742
  stuffiness feeling under Heart 666
recreational drugs 429–430
redness on 110, 607–608
regurgitation
  sour 267, 718
  symptoms and signs 718–719
Ren-3 Zhongji 522
Ren-4 Guanyuan 521–522
Ren-5 Shimen 522
Ren-12 Zhongwan 521
Ren-14 Juque 521
Ren-17 Shanzhong
  chest tenderness 512
  palpation 522
Ren Shen Bu Fei Tang 1039
residual, in Diaphragm, insomnia 808
Residual Damp-Heat invasion in
    Lesser-Yang channels, ear
    problems in children 865
Residual Damp-Heat with Qi deficiency,
    swollen neck glands 655
Residual dryness and Phlegm in Lungs
    660
Residual dryness in Lungs 660
Residual Heat in Diaphragm
  Heart feeling vexed 665–666
  heat feeling in chest 665
  insomnia 808
Residual Heat in Lungs, low-grade fever
    in children 864
residual pathogenic factors **973–979**
  diagnosis 975
  disturbed sleep 868
  effects 975, 976
  formation 973–975, 974
  phlegm 976–977
  tongue signs 976
  treatment 975–976
  types 975, 979
  upright Qi 974, 975
Residual Phlegm in Lungs with Lung-Qi
    deficiency, wheeze in children
    865
Residual Phlegm in Lungs with Spleen-Qi
    deficiency, wheeze in children
    865
respiratory problems
  asthma
  in children 865
retching 725
rheumatoid arthritis, withered and brittle
    nails 138
rhinitis 87, 592–593

see also allergic rhinitis
ribs, pain in 324, *324*, 664
ringworm *see* tinea (ringworm)
Root of Post-Heaven Qi 261
root pulse
  interpretation 454
  normal attribute 452–453
rosacea *plate 21.54*, *plate 21.55*
  occurrence 189
  pathology and diagnosis 189, *189*
  symptoms and signs 785
Rou Fu Bao Yuan Tang 1039
roundworms 869
  see also worm infestation

S

Sad pulse *see* pulse qualities
sadness **387–388**, 424–425, *425*
  patterns *388*
  pulse indication 452, 459
  symptoms and signs 792
salpingitis, hand lines 135
salty taste 727
San Jia Fu Mai Tang 1039
San Miao Hong Teng Tang 1040
San Ren Tang 1040
San Zi Yang Qin Tang 1040
Sang Ju Yin 1040
Sang Piao Xiao San 1040
Sang Xing Tang 1040
scalp
  boils 70, 568
  dry 69, 568
  erosions 70
  itching 287, 299, *299*, 567
  psoriasis *plate 21.27*
  redness and pain of 69, 568
  ulcers 70, 568–569
  see also head
Scattered pulse *see* pulse qualities
schizophrenia 802
sciatica 704
sclera colour
  abnormal 81, 81–82, *82*, 634–636
  bluish-greenish 82, *82*, 635
  dark 82, *82*, 636
  red 81, 81–82, 635
  white specks 82, *82*, 647
  yellow 81, *81*, 634–635
  see also eye(s)
scoliosis 117, *117*, 707
scrotum
  abnormal colour 151
  contracted 150, 769
  dark 151, 771
  drooping on one side 151, 769
  itching 771
  loose 151, 769

oozing 151, 770
pale 151, 770
purple 151, 770–771
red 151, 770
swollen 151, 770
see also genitalia
Sea of Marrow, Emptiness of *see*
    Emptiness of Sea of Marrow
selective serotonin reuptake inhibitors
    (SSRI), effect on pulse 507
semen (sperm)
  blood in 768
  cold and watery 768
sesame seed hasty pulse 507
sexual intercourse
  bleeding (female) 859–860
  pain (female) 859
sexual life
  patient interrogation 250
  sexual activity
    excessive 118–119, 430
    frequency 392
sexual problems 391–394
  anorgasmia 393–394
    see also orgasm
  female 393–394
  impotence *see* erectile dysfunction
  lack of libido *see* libido, lack of
  male 392–393, **765–774**
  nocturnal emissions 393, *393*, 767
  premature ejaculation 393, *393*,
    766–767
  tiredness/dizziness after ejaculation
    393, 768
Sha Shen Mai Dong Tang 1040
Shang 539
Shang Qi (Rebellious-Qi breathing) 545,
    661
Shao Fu 145, 515
Shao Fu Zhu Yu Tang 1040
Shao Yao Tang 1040–1041
She Gan Ma Huang Tang 1041
Shen 31, 207, 209, 451
Shen Fu Tang 1041
Shen Ge San 1041
Shen Ling Bai Zhu San 1041
Shen Qi Si Wu Tang 1041
Sheng Hua Tang 1041
Sheng Mai San 1041
Sheng Yang Tang 1041
Sheng Yu Tang 1041
Shi Pi Yin 1042
Shi Xiao San 1042
shingles *see* herpes zoster (shingles)
shivers 363, 365, 813–814
  with sweating 353
shock 425, *425*, 1022
  affecting Heart, palpitations 666
  convulsions in children 871

crying in children/babies 868
  disturbed sleep 868
Shock-Phlegm 937
Short pulse *see* pulse qualities
shortness of breath *(Duan Qi)* 545, 661
Shou Tai Wan 1042
shoulder(s)
  ache 656
  frozen 656
  inability to raise 341–342, *342*
  pain 341–342, *342*
  problems and channel palpation 528
  symptoms and signs **653–656**
  see also limbs
Shui Dou 180
Shui Pao 178
Shui Zhong 179
SI-16 Tianchuang 532, *532*
Si Hai Shu Yu Wan 1042
Si Jun Zi Tang 1042
Si Mo Tang 1042
Si Ni Tang 1042
Si Wu Ma Zi Ren Wan 1042
Si Wu Tang 1042
Sick Sinus Syndrome 460
sighing 545, 670
signs and symptoms *see* symptoms and
    signs
Simple Questions, complexion colours,
    prognosis 47
sinusitis 87, 1017, 1019
  Damp-Heat in Head *978*
  Sick Sinus Syndrome 460
Six Stages
  Bright-Yang stage 961–962
  Greater Yang stage 965–967
  Greater Yin stage 967
  Lesser-Yang stage 967
  Lesser Yin stage 968
  pattern identification **939–952**
  relationship to
    Four Levels 962, 963–964
    Three Burners 962, *962*, 963–964
  Terminal-Yin stage 968
skin
  acne *see* acne
  body hair 176
  breasts, peau d'orange 852
  candida *see* candida
  carbuncles 788
  complexion *see* complexion colours
  connecting channels 174
  Cou Li 176
  cutaneous regions 5
  Dampness 949, 950
  dermographism 181
  diseases 181–190
    pathology and diagnosis 181–190
    see also individual diseases

dry 178–179, *179*, 517, 782
eczema *see* eczema
energetic layers 516, *517*
erosion 179, *179*
eruptions 782–785
  menstrual symptoms 834
feet *see* feet
fissures 180
forearm *see* forearm
forehead *see* forehead
furuncle *see* boils
greasy 179, 517
growths and masses 787–789
hands *see* hands
herpes simplex *see* herpes simplex
herpes zoster *see* herpes zoster
    (shingles)
infections 785–787
internal organs influence 170–173,
    173
  heart 173
  kidneys *172*, 172–173, *173*
  liver 173
  lungs 170–172
  stomach and spleen 172
layers *169*, 169–170
lesion types 170, *170–171*
lesions/signs *plates 21.1–21.22*
lustre 175
  see also lustre
macules *see* macules
malignant melanoma *see* malignant
    melanoma
moisture 176, 517
moles *see* naevi (moles)
nodules under 640–641, 788–789
observation **169–190**
oedema 179, *179*
palpation 516–519
  see also palpation
papules *see* papules
Phlegm under skin 937
plaque 177–178
psoriasis *see* psoriasis
pustules 174, 178, *178*
rashes 180, *180*, 319, 785, 869–870,
    953–954
rosacea *see* rosacea
scales 179, *179*, 181, 184, *plates 21.7*
signs 174–181
space between muscles and 176
swelling 179, *179*
symptoms and signs **781–789**
temperature 516, *516*
texture 175–176, 517
tinea *see* tinea (ringworm)
ulcers *see* ulcers
urticaria *see* urticaria
vesicles 174, 178, *178*

warts *see* warts
wheals 177, 185
skin colour (body) 174–175, *175*
  bluish-greenish 175
  dark 175
  pale 174
  race variation consideration 174
  red 174
  yellow 174–175, *175*
sleep
  duration 347
  interrogation **347–350**
  see also dreaming; insomnia; sleep
      problems
sleep problems **807–811**
  in children 413, 868
  excessive dreaming *see* dreaming
  insomnia *see* insomnia
  sleep talking 544, 810
  sleep walking 810–811
  snoring 543, 811, 821
  somnolence 349, 810, 1022
    after eating 722–723
Slippery pulse *see* pulse qualities
Slow pulse *see* pulse qualities
slurred speech 544, 821
Small Intestine
  channels 994–995
  Full-Heat 911
  pattern identification 911–912
  pulse diagnosis, discrepancies 444
  right rear pulse position 506, *506*
  worm infestation 912
Small Intestine channel
  abdomen 145
  ears relationship 105, *106*
  eyes relationship 78
  palpation 532, *532*
    blood vessel 532
    skin 532
Small Intestine deficient and Cold 912
Small Intestine Qi pain 911–912
  acupuncture 912
  clinical manifestations 911
  prescription 912
Small Intestine Qi tied 912
smell/smelling (olfaction)
  diagnosis by **549–552**
    body odour *see* body odour
    breath 550, *550*
    intestinal gas 551
    odour of bodily secretions 550–551
    sputum 550
    sweat 550
    urine and stools 550–551
    vaginal discharge and lochia 551
  loss of sense 306, *306*, 597–598
  yin organs 540
  see also nose

sneezing 304, *304*
  diagnosis by 546, *546*
  symptoms and signs 591
snoring 543, 811, 821
  see also sleep problems
Soggy pulse *see* pulse qualities
soles of feet 345, *345*
  burning sensations 345, 701
  pain in 345, 698
somnolence 349, 810
  patterns *350*
  see also sleep
sore throat 110, *313*, 601–602
  external origin 312
  internal origin 312–313
sound, voice *see* voice
sour regurgitation 718
  patterns 267
sour taste 727–728
SP-11 Jimen 530–531, *531*
SP-12 Chongmen, Spleen channel
  530–531, *531*
spasticity, limbs 62–63, 156, *156*
speech/talking 544, *544*
  delirious 822
  difficulty in finding words 822
  dislike of 544
  incoherent, incessant 821
  sleep 544
  slurred 544, 821
  stuttering 543, 822
  see also voice
sperm *see* semen (sperm)
spine
  bent forward 116, 707–708
  childrens muscles along 194
  coccyx pain 705
  curve abnormalities 116–118, *118*,
    707–708
  kyphosis *117*, 117–118, 708
  list of 118, *118*, 708
  lordosis 117, *117*, 707
  lumbar flattening *117*, 118, 708
  muscle atrophy along 116, 705
  scoliosis 117, *117*, 707
  see also back
spinning bean pulse 507
spirit
  aspects of 32–33
  body/mind relationship *32*
  conditions 33–34
    false 34
    strong 33–34
    weak 34
  and constitution 34–36
    strong spirit /strong constitution 35
    strong spirit /weak constitution 36
    weak spirit /strong constitution 35
    weak spirit /weak constitution 35

embodiment of 32
and emotions 36–37
  complexion 36
  eyes 36, 37, 75, 80
  tongue 36, 37
lustre of 33
observation, mind, spirit and emotions
  31–38
pulse
  interpretation 454
  normal attribute 451
tongue spirit 207
vitality of 32–33
Spleen
  abdominal reflection of state 146
  channels 994
  Damp-Heat in *see* Damp-Heat
  Dampness 977
  epigastrium relationship 515
  Heat in *see* Heat
  invasion of Cold, diarrhoea in children
    865
  lunula correspondence 140
  pattern identification **885–889**
  Postnatal Qi 261
  Qi deficiency of Spleen and Heart with
    floating Yang, hyperactivity
    804
  Qi transformation/transportation 262
  right middle pulse position *504*,
    504–505, *505*
  skin relationship 172
  voice influence 541, 542
  Yang deficiency of Stomach and
    Spleen, feeling of cold 814
Spleen- and Heart-Blood deficiency
  888–889
  acupuncture 889
  clinical manifestations 888–889
  learning difficulties (children) 804
  prescription 889
Spleen- and Heart-Qi deficiency,
  somnolence 810
Spleen- and Kidney-Yang deficiency
  amenorrhoea 829
  atrophy of legs 694
  blood in urine 758
  borborygmi (bowel sounds) 743
  breast distension 849
  cold feet 694
  convulsions in children 871
  craving for sweets/constant picking
    722
  distended abdominal veins 743
  drooping lips 624
  dull-white nails 691
  heavy periods 828
  hiccup 719
  incontinence of faeces 750

loss of pubic hair 773, 860
mid-cycle menstrual bleeding 830
milky nipple discharge 851
muscle twitching 714–715
night vision decreased 630
nighttime urination 758
oedema during menstruation 833
pale menstrual blood 825
pale scrotum 770
phlegm in throat 604
poor appetite 720
premenstrual tension 832
protruding umbilicus 147
severe, sagging lower abdomen 745
slow fetal growth 842
straining in defecation 752
sunken fontanelles 871
swallowing difficulty (diaphragm
  choking) 726
swollen scrotum 770
umbilical pain 739
vomiting in children 864
vomiting of blood 726
watery menstrual blood 826
wax production excess 583
white membrane on pupil in children
  648
yawning 670
Spleen- and Kidney-Yang deficiency with
    Liver-Qi stagnation,
    premenstrual breast distension
    833
Spleen- and Kidney-Yang deficiency with
    Phlegm
  breast lumps 851
  swollen breasts 850
Spleen- and Kidney-Yin deficiency,
    tongue/palate white spots
    872
Spleen- and Liver-Blood deficiency 889
Spleen- and Lung-Qi deficiency 889
  clinical manifestations 889
  nocturnal enuresis 867
  prescription 889
Spleen- and Stomach-Qi deficiency 888
Spleen and Kidney deficiency with
    Dampness, flaking nails 690
Spleen-Blood deficiency 886
Spleen channel
  abdomen 145
  eyes relationship 77
  mouth 93
  palpation 530–531, *531*
    blood vessel 530
    skin 530–531
  skin 174
Spleen Combined Patterns 888–889
  Spleen- and Heart-Blood deficiency
    888–889

Spleen- and Stomach-Qi deficiency 888
Spleen Damp-Heat
  clinical manifestations 970
  prescription 956, 970
Spleen deficiency
  constitutional, Five Flaccidities 869
  constitutional weakness 867
  late closure of fontanelles 872
Spleen deficiency with accumulation
      disorder, hot palms and soles
      866
Spleen deficiency with Liver-Yang rising
      and Phlegm, dizziness in
      pregnancy 840
Spleen deficient and Cold 868
Spleen deficient and Cold, crying in
      babies 868
Spleen Empty-Heat, red gums 620
Spleen-Heat 888
  acupuncture 888
  clinical manifestations 888
  craving for sweets/constant picking
      722
  heat of the face/hot flushes 570
  peeled lips 623
  prescription 888
  red eyelids 637
  red gums 620
  red nose 590
  swollen eyelids 638
  tiredness 285
  yellow complexion 576
  yellow nose 590
Spleen not controlling Blood 886–887
  acupuncture 886–887
  clinical manifestations 886
  prescription 887
Spleen-Qi 262
Spleen-Qi and Heart-Blood deficiency,
      ejaculation during sleep 767
Spleen Qi and Spleen-Blood deficiency
      804
Spleen-Qi deficiency 885
  abdominal distension (bloating) *327,*
      741
  acupuncture 885
  bleeding between iris and pupil 649
  bleeding from ears 583
  bleeding from gums 619
  bleeding on intercourse 860
  blurred vision and floaters 628
  boil on eyelid 639
  breast milk 847
  chronic
    candida 787
    sallow complexion 578
    tinea 787
    yellow complexion 576

chronic with retention of Dampness,
      yellow nose 590
  clinical manifestations 885
  craving for sweets/constant picking
      722
  diarrhoea during menstruation 833
  diarrhoea in children 865
  diarrhoea or loose stools 747
  difficulty in defecation 752
  dribbling from mouth 612
  fever after childbirth 846
  flatulence 743
  following food poisoning, sunken
      eyeball 643
  habitual miscarriage 842
  with Lung-Qi deficiency *see* Lung- and
      Spleen-Qi deficiency
  menstrual bleeding returning after
      menopause 830
  muscle atrophy along spine 705
  night vision decreased 630
  nosebleed 594
  nosebleed during menstruation 834
  numbness of the tongue 614
  obesity 319
  oedema after childbirth 846
  painful urination 839
  pale gums 620
  patterns 885–886
  prescription 885
  severe, constipation and loose stools
      alternation 750
  severe with internal Wind (children),
      bluish-greenish nails 692
  sleepiness after eating 722
  tiredness 285
  trembling lips 623
  turbid urine 754
  urinary difficulty after childbirth 845
  vaginal bleeding 838
  weak voice 820
  white membrane on pupil in children
      648
  white vaginal discharge 857
  yellow vaginal discharge 857
Spleen-Qi deficiency with Blood
      deficiency, jaundice 714
Spleen-Qi deficiency with Damp-Heat
  bad smell sensation 597
  boil on eyelid 639
  candida 787
  herpes simplex 785
Spleen-Qi deficiency with Damp-Heat in
      Stomach, mouth ulcers during
      menstruation 834
Spleen-Qi deficiency with Dampness
      885–886
  acne 569, 784
  acupuncture 885–886, 886

breech presentation 842
  clinical manifestations 885
  ear discharge 583
  eczema 783
  heaviness feeling in legs 700
  heaviness feeling in limbs 673–674
  leukoplakia 859
  prescription 886
  sallow complexion 578
  sleepiness after eating 723
  stye on eyelids 637
  tinea 786
  ulcers on lower leg 701
  vaginal itching 858
  white membrane on pupil in children
      648
Spleen-Qi deficiency with Dampness and
      secondary Liver-Qi stagnation,
      premenstrual tension 832
Spleen-Qi deficiency with Liver-Qi
      stagnation
  goitre 604
  yellow complexion 576
Spleen-Qi deficiency with Phlegm 886
  acupuncture 886
  clinical manifestations 886
  dizziness during menstruation 835
  nodules under skin 788
  prescription 886
  somnolence 810
  vomiting during menstruation 835
  wheezing 663
Spleen-Qi deficient and sinking
  anal prolapse 762
  diarrhoea or loose stools 748
  drooping eyelids 640
  drooping lips 624
  haemorrhoids 762
  nocturnal enuresis 757–758
  urine retention 839
Spleen-Qi sinking 886
  acupuncture 886
  clinical manifestations 886
  leaning of head to one side 564
  long penis in children 872
  loose scrotum 769
  prescription 886
  prolapse of uterus 859
  prolapse of vagina 859
  sunken umbilicus 745
Spleen-Yang and Liver-Blood deficiency,
      painful periods 829
Spleen-Yang deficiency 886
  acupuncture 886
  clinical manifestations 886
  cold hands 680
  coldness *364*
  Kidney- and Spleen-Yang deficiency
      910

Spleen-Yang deficiency (contd.)
    limb oedema 675
    oedema in pregnancy 838
    oedema of abdomen 745
    oedema of body 713
    oedema of hands 684
    oedema of the face 572
    oedema of the feet 693
    prescription 886
Spleen-Yang deficiency with Dampness
    scanty and difficult urination 755
    somnolence 810
Spleen-Yang deficiency with Empty-Cold
    pale gums 620
    pale lips 621
    purple lips 621
Spleen-Yin deficiency 887
    acupuncture 887
    clinical manifestations 887
    gnawing hunger 722
    patterns 887
    prescription 887
    retching 725
Spleen-Yin deficiency with Empty-Heat
    heat of the face/hot flushes 570
    loose teeth 616
    peeled lips 623
    swollen eyelids 638
sprain, back, lower backache 703
sputum
    chest pain 324
    diagnosis by smell 550
    observation 163–164, 164
ST-9 Renying 529, 530
ST-25 Tianshu 521
ST-40 Fenglong 664
ST-42 Chongyang, Stomach channel
    529, 530, 530
Stagnant Cold in Uterus 1002–1003
Stagnant Heat in Directing and
        Penetrating Vessels 1001
Stagnant Liver-Qi see Liver-Qi stagnation
Stagnant Liver-Qi invading Stomach,
    morning sickness 837
Stagnant Liver-Qi turned Heat 891–892
    acupuncture 892
    bloody nipple discharge 852
    chronic fever 375
    clinical manifestations 815, 891–892
    prescription 892
Stagnant Liver-Qi turned into Fire
    breast lumps 851
    cracked nipples 852
Stagnant Liver-Qi turned into Heat
    breasts, redness and swelling 850
    fever in cancer 816
Stagnant Liver-Qi turning into Heat with
        Blood Stasis, breasts, redness
        and swelling 850

Stagnant pulse see pulse qualities
stagnation, depression 381–382
stagnation of Qi see Qi stagnation
staring, fixed eyes 83, 123, 650
steaming breast, fever after childbirth
        847
sternum, protruding 144, 144, 669
Stomach
    abdominal reflection of state 146
    Body Fluid deficiency 935
    channels 994
    Cold invading 916
    Damp-Heat in see Damp-Heat
    Dampness 977
    Dampness in Stomach 1019
    epigastrium relationship 515
    food retention 916
    invasion of Cold, vomiting in children
        864
    invasion of external Dampness 950
    pattern identification **913–916**
    Phlegm-Fluids 937
    Postnatal Qi 261
    pulse influence 452
    Rebellious Liver-Qi invading the
        Stomach 897
    right middle pulse position 504,
        504–505, 505
    skin relationship 172
    Toxic Heat in see Toxic Heat
    Yang deficiency of Stomach and
        Spleen, feeling of cold 814
Stomach- and Heart-Fire, grinding teeth
        616
Stomach- and Intestines-Yin deficiency,
        constipation 749
Stomach- and Intestines-Yin deficiency
        with Empty-Heat, blood and
        mucus in stools 750
Stomach- and Liver-Fire, vomiting 724
Stomach- and Spleen-Heat, sweet taste
        727
Stomach- and Spleen-Qi deficiency
    abdominal masses 744
    atrophy of legs 694
    atrophy of muscles in dorsum of hands
        686
    atrophy of thenar eminence 685
    belching 717
    blood in stools 751
    cataract 651
    chronic, yellow palate 625
    dizziness 560
    dribbling of urine 756
    drooping head 563
    dry and brittle hair 566
    epigastric pain 737
    flapping eyelids 639
    headache 291

leg weakness 699
limb atrophy 674
limb flaccidity 675
limb paralysis 676–677
loss of taste 728
open eyes 650
pale palate 624
paralysis 710
paralysis of legs 695
poor appetite 720
severe, withered and thickened nails
        690
sweating of hands and feet 778–779
thin pointed fingers 687
tooth cavities 616
toothache 615
urination difficult 756
urticaria 784
vomiting during menstruation 835
weak knees 699
weight loss 319, 714
Yin Fire with, mouth ulcers 610
Stomach- and Spleen-Qi deficiency and
        sinking, drooping eyelids 640
Stomach- and Spleen-Qi deficiency with
        Cold in Stomach, loss of taste
        728
Stomach- and Spleen-Qi deficiency with
        Dampness, heaviness feeling in
        limbs 674
Stomach- and Spleen-Qi deficiency with
        Heart-Heat, abdominal pain
        (area below xyphoid process)
        736
Stomach- and Spleen-Yang deficiency
    absence of thirst 733
    convulsions in children 871
    with Empty-Cold, pale nose 589
    feeling of cold in abdomen 742
    pale palate 624
Stomach- and Spleen-Yin deficiency
    dry and cracked lips 622
    sweating of hands and feet 779
Stomach and Intestines deficient and
        cold, diarrhoea with vomiting
        748
Stomach and Pericardium Fire,
        depression and manic
        behaviour 799
Stomach and Spleen deficiency
    congenital, arched legs 696
    lordosis 707
Stomach and Spleen deficient and cold
    abdominal fullness 741
    borborygmi (bowel sounds) 743
    increased salivation 733
    poor appetite 720
    yellow fluid between iris and pupil
        648–649

Stomach and Spleen Fluids injured, paralysis 711
Stomach-Blood stasis 915, 931
Stomach channel
  abdomen 145
  area under xyphoid process 513
  breasts 121, *121*, 122
  Damp-Heat in *see* Damp-Heat
  eyes relationship 77, *77*
  heart 127–128
  mouth 93, *94*
  neck and throat 109, *109*
  palpation 529–530, *530*
    blood vessel 529
    skin 529–530
  teeth and gums 99
Stomach-Cold
  green eyelids 638
  venules on the thenar eminence 685
Stomach cracks, tongue diagnosis 229, *229*, 330, *plate 25.5*
Stomach Damp-Heat 916
  acupuncture 916, 956
  clinical manifestations 916, 956
  prescription 916, 956
Stomach deficient and cold
  belching 718
  venules on the thenar eminence 685
  vomiting 724
Stomach deficient and Cold
      (Stomach-Yang deficiency)
      913–914
  acupuncture 913–914
  clinical manifestations 913–914
  prescription 914
  Stomach-Yang and Stomach-Yin
      deficiency 914
Stomach Empty-Heat, yellow complexion
      576
Stomach-Fire 915
  acupuncture 915
  bleeding gums 619
  clinical manifestations 915
  epigastric pain 737
  excessive hunger 720
  gums oozing pus 620
  mouth ulcers during menstruation 834
  nosebleed 594
  nosebleed during menstruation 834
  numbness of face 572
  painful tongue 614
  prescription 915
  receding gums 619
  toothache 307, 615
  trembling lips 623
  vomiting of blood 725
  warts on ear 585
  see also Stomach Phlegm-Fire
Stomach-Heat 915

abdominal pain (area below xyphoid
      process) 736
  acupuncture 915, 955
  belching 717
  body aches 710
  burning sensations in soles of feet 701
  clinical manifestations 915, 955
  cold sores 610
  cracked mouth corners 611
  disturbed sleep 868
  drooping eyelids 640
  dry and white teeth 617
  dry nostrils 593
  epigastric pain 737
  excessive hunger 720
  foul breath 729
  gnawing hunger 721
  headache 561
  heat of the face/hot flushes 570
  hiccup 719
  hot hands 680
  hot hands and feet 673
  inflamed gums 618
  irritability 801
  itching around mouth 611
  loose teeth 616
  morning sickness 837
  mouth ulcers 609
  nausea 723
  pain in soles of feet 698
  papules on nose 598–599
  plaque 617
  prescription 915, 955
  red eyelids 637
  red gums 620
  redness of pharynx 602
  retching 725
  sleep talking 810
  sour taste 728
  thirst 731
  trembling mouth 612
  urticaria 785
  vomiting 724
  weight loss 714
  yellow complexion 576
  see also Heat
Stomach Phlegm-Fire 915
  acupuncture 915
  clinical manifestations 915
  prescription 915
Stomach-Qi 262
  pulse
    interpretation 454
    normal attribute 451–452
  tongue coating 207, 221, 222, 228
Stomach-Qi deficiency 913
  acupuncture 913
  breast milk 847
  clinical manifestations 837, 913

hiccup 719
limb weakness 674
nausea 723
pain in soles of feet 698
prescription 913
small breasts 852
vomiting 724
  in children 864
Stomach-Qi deficiency with Dampness,
      pain in soles of feet 698
Stomach-Qi rebelling upwards 916
Stomach-Qi stagnation 914–915
    abdominal pain (area below xyphoid
        process) 736
  acupuncture 914
  clinical manifestations 914
  prescription 914–915
Stomach strong - Spleen weak, hunger
      with no desire to eat 721
Stomach-Yang and Stomach-Yin
      deficiency 914
  prescription 914
Stomach-Yang deficiency 913–914
  acupuncture 913–914
  clinical manifestations 913–914
  pain in hands 682–683
  prescription 914
  Stomach-Yang and Stomach-Yin
      deficiency 914
Stomach-Yin deficiency 914
  acupuncture 914
  belching 718
  clinical manifestations 914
  cracked mouth corners 611
  dry throat 605
  epigastric pain 737
  hiccup 719
  morning sickness 837
  nausea 723
  patterns 914
  poor appetite 720
  prescription 914
  restless legs 700
  scarring after corneal opacity 647
  swallowing difficulty (diaphragm
      choking) 726
  thirst 732
  vomiting 724
  vomiting in children 864
Stomach-Yin deficiency with Blood
      dryness, regurgitation of food
      719
Stomach-Yin deficiency with Empty-
      Cold, morning sickness 837
Stomach-Yin deficiency with Empty-Heat
      914
  acupuncture 914
  bleeding gums 619
  clinical manifestations 914

Stomach-Yin deficiency with Empty-Heat (*contd.*)
  cold sores 610–611
  cracked mouth corners 611
  dry nostrils 594
  excessive hunger 720
  heat of the face/hot flushes 570
  hot hands 680–681
  hot hands and feet 673
  inflamed gums 618
  painful tongue 614
  prescription 914
  red gums 620
  thirst 732
  toothache 615
  vomiting of blood 725
stools
  blood and mucus in 750–751
  blood in 751
  colour 164–165, *165*, 272–273
  consistency 165, *165*, 271
  defecation of *see* defecation
  foul smelling 271, 273, 550
  frequency 270–271
  incontinence 750
  interrogation **261–267**
  loose 747–748
    constipation alternation 749–750
  mucus in 271, 751
  normal 164, *272*
  observation 164–165
  odour 273
  shape 165, *165*, 272, *272*
  smell diagnosis 550–551
  see also constipation; diarrhoea
strabismus 83, *83*
  symptoms/signs 628–629
streaming eyes 84, *84*, 360, *360*, 633–634
stress, case histories 1020, 1022
stroke, hemiplegia 155
stroking, palpation technique 509, *510*
stuffiness, abdominal pain 327, 736
stuffiness feeling under Heart 666
stuttering 543, 822
Su He Xiang Wan 1042–1043
Su Zi Jiang Qi Tang 1043
sublingual veins 213–214, 1057, *plate 24.10*
suffocation, feeling of, pregnancy 841
Summer-Heat 370
  acupuncture 954
  carbuncles on upper back 788
  clinical manifestations 815, 948, 954
  with Dampness 950
  pathogenic factors 948, *948*
  prescription 954
  tidal fever 816
  Summer-Heat invasion

diarrhoea with vomiting 748
  spontaneous sweating 776
Summer-Heat with Toxic Heat, boil on head 788
Sun 526
sunken eyeball 82–83, 643
sunken fontanelles 871
Suo Gong Zhu Yu Tang 1043
Suo Quan Wan 1043
Superficial Connecting channels 526
  see also Connecting channels
swallowing difficulty (diaphragm choking) 726
sweat/sweating **351–354**
  absence of 353–354, 780
  after childbirth 846
  body area 353
  chest 778
  classification 353
  clinical significance 352
  from collapse 776–777
  daytime 351, *351*, 353
  exterior patterns 352
  hands and feet 778–779
  head 778
  interior patterns 352, *352*
  localized 777–779
  nighttime 351–352, *352*, 776
  observation **164**, *164*
  pathology 352–353
  shivering 353
  smell diagnosis 550
  spontaneous 775–776
  symptoms and signs **775–789**
  unilateral 777–778
  yellow 777
sweet craving 722
sweet taste 727
swimming shrimp pulse 507
symptoms and signs **601–608**
  Chinese terms 1061–1063
  gynaecological problems **823–860**
    breast signs **849–853**
    childbirth **843–848**
    menstrual bleeding **825–826**
    menstrual cycle **827–830**
    menstruation, problem symptoms **831–835**
    miscellaneous **855–860**
    pregnancy **837–842**
    see also individual entries
  parts of the body **557–822**
    abdomen **735–745**
    anus **761–763**
    arms **679–692**
    chest **659–670**
    cold feeling, shivering **813–814**
    defecation **747–752**
    digestive system and taste **717–729**

ears **581–588**
    emotions **791–795**
    eyes **627–652**
    face colour (complexion) **575–580**
    fever **814–817**
    gynaecological **823–860**
    head and face **559–574**
    heat feeling **817–818**
    legs **693–701**
    limbs **671–678**
    lips **621–624**
    lower back **703–715**
    mental difficulties **803–805**
    mental-emotional symptoms **797–802**
    mouth, tongue, teeth, gums and lips **609–624**
    nails **688–692**
    neck and shoulders **653–656**
    nose **589–600**
    palate and philtrum **624–626**
    sexual and genital symptoms in men **765–774**
    skin **781–789**
    sleeping problems **807–811**
    sweating **775–789**
    thirst and drink **731–733**
    throat **601–608**
    voice **819–821**
    see also individual entries
  timescales 241

T

tachycardia, pulse indication 459
Tao He Cheng Qi Tang 1043
Tao Hong Si Wu Tang 1043
taste
  bitter 726–727
  classification 265
  food and **261–267**
  interrogation **261–267**
  loss of 728
  salty 727
  sour 727–728
  sticky/metallic 728
  sweet 727
TB-22 Heliao 535, 535–536
techniques 509–510
teeth 99–100, 306–308
  abnormal colour 100, *100*
  bad *100*
  channels influencing 99, *99*
  dry and dull 100, 617
  dry and white 100, 617
  grey 100, 618
  grinding 616–617
  loose 100, 616–617
  observation **99–100**

plaque 100, 617
symptoms and signs 99, **615–618**
teethmarks *plate 25.8*
tooth cavities 99, 616
toothache 615
upper moist and lower dry 100, 618
yellow and dry 100, 618
see also gums
temperature
pain 258
see also Cold; Heat
temples palpation, babies 518–519, *519*
see also fontanelles
Terminal-Yin channels, headache 562
Terminal-Yin stage
acupuncture 968
clinical manifestations 968
prescription 968
testicles, swelling and pain in 773
thenar eminence 1056
thighs
pain in 344, 696–697
see also limbs
thirst
absence of 279, 733
case histories, diabetes mellitus
278–279
dry mouth 279, 732–733
hot/cold drink preference 279
interrogation **277–279**
symptoms and signs **731–733**
see also drinks/drinking
thorax *see* chest
Three Burners (Triple Burner)
blood strength indication in 454
channels 995–996
ears relationship 105, *106*
Lower Burner 970–971
Middle Burner 970
neck 109, *109*
palpation (channel) 535, 535–536
blood vessel 535
skin 535
pattern identification 939–940,
969–971
pulse qualities classification 499
Qi strength
reflection 444–445
three levels 455, *455, 456*
relationship to
Four Levels *941, 962, 963–964*
Six Stages *962, 962, 963–964*
skin 172, 172–173, *173*
Upper Burner 969–970
see also individual elements
throat
carotid artery pulsation 110, 655
channels influencing *109,* 109–110,
110, 312

children 193, *193*
dry 313, *313,* 605–606
feeling of obstruction 314, *314*
foul breath 111
goitre 110, *110,* 604
hoarse voice 313–314, *314*
interrogation **311–316**
itching 313, 605
observation **109–114**
obstruction feeling 607
Phlegm 603–604
see also neck; pharynx; tonsils
thrush *see* candida
thumbs 140, *140*
Thunder Rampart *79*
Tian Di Jian 1043
Tian Gui (sperm/menstrual blood) 430
Tian Ma Gou Teng Yin 1043
Tian Tai Wu Yao San 1043
Tian Wang Bu Xin Dan 1044
Tiao Wei Cheng Qi Tang 1044
Tiao Zheng San 1044
tics, facial 61, 572–573
tidal fever 816
Tight pulse *see* pulse qualities
timidity, severe 795
tinea (ringworm)
hands 130, 684
pathology and diagnosis
Chinese 187, *187*
Western 186, *187*
symptoms and signs 786–787
tinea capitis *plate 21.43*
tinea corporis (ringworm) *plate 21.40,*
plate 21.41
tinea cruris *plate 21.45*
tinea manuum *plate 21.42*
tinea pedis *plate 21.44*
tingling
see numbness/tingling
tinnitus 355, *357,* 581–582
case history 356
headache 288
see also deafness
tiredness 281–286
acute onset 1023
case histories 282–286, 1022, 1023
depression 381
patterns causing 282–286
see also exhaustion *(Xu Lao)*
toe(s)
ulcers 701
see also feet
tolerance *see* drug tolerance; pain
tolerance
Tong You Tang 1044
tongue 309
appearance comparison
Four Levels 958

residual pathogenic factors 976
breast areas 123
clinical significance 206–207
colour
external factors affecting 204, *204*
purple (sides) 205, 206, *206*
see also tongue-body colour
Heart cracks 36, 37, 217, *217–218*
internal/external Wind 231
itching 309, 613
numbness 309, 614
pain in 309, 613–614
Qi/blood stagnation 231
Qi deficiency 227
spirit and emotions 36, 37
Stomach cracks 229, *229*
sublingual veins 213–214, 1057,
plate 24.10
symptoms and signs **613–615**
teethmarks *plate 25.8*
ulcers 614–615
white spots 872
tongue-body colour 206, **209–214**
bluish-purple *plate 24.7*
external factors affecting 204, *204*
pale 210, *plate 24.1*
purple 212–213, *213, plate 24.8,*
plate 24.9
red 210, *210, 211, plate 24.2*
with slow pulse 463
red points 211–212, *212, plate 24.5*
red tips *plate 24.3*
reddish-purple *plate 24.6*
tongue-body shape 206, **215–220**
cracked *217, 217–218, 218,* 463,
plate 25.4
deviated 218, *218,* 231
flaccid 217
long/short 217
moving 218
quivering 219
stiff 216, *plate 25.3*
swollen/partially swollen 216, *216,*
plate 25.1, plate 25.2, plate 27.1
thin 215–216
toothmarked 219, *219*
tongue coating 206–207, **221–225,**
plate 26.2
appearance 958
clinical significance 221–222
distribution 223, *223*
epigastrium 330
external diseases 224–225
formation 207
moisture 223
mouldy 224
physiology 221
presence/absence 222
slippery 224

tongue coating (*contd.*)
 sticky 123, 224, *plate 26.3*
 texture 224
 thickness 223
 with/without root 222–223, *223,*
  plate 26.1
 yellow 111
tongue diagnosis **201–232**, 230, 237
 case histories 1015, 1016, 1022
 examination conditions 203–204
 historical aspects 1058–1059
 integration with interrogation
  243–248
 lighting 203
 observation techniques 203–204
 pulse diagnosis integration 463–464
 tongue areas 204, 204–206, *205,*
  206
tongue images/patterns **227–231**
 Blood-deficiency 228
 Qi deficiency 227
 Yang deficiency 227–228
 Yin deficiency 228–230, *229*
tongue spirit 207, 209
tonsillitis 314–315
 acute 314
 case history 315, *315*
 chronic 314–315
tonsils 314–315, 979
 abnormal colour 111–112
 exudate 112
 greyish 112
 red and swollen 111–112
 signs *112*
 swollen 111, 603
 see also throat
tooth *see* teeth
toothache 306–307, *307*, 615
touching, palpation technique 509, 510
Toxic *see* Toxic Heat
Toxic Heat
 anal ulcers 763
 Blood level (Four Levels)
  contracted pupils 650
  swollen nose 596
 bloody nipple discharge 851
 breast lumps 851
 breast pain 850
 breasts, redness and swelling 850
 buttock ulcers 706–707
 cancer 462, 463
 channels of face
  deviation of the mouth 613
  eye and mouth deviation 573
 Chickenpox 870
 concha swelling and redness 587
 corneal opacity 647
 crying out 822
 dandruff 567

epidemic on Exterior, white purulent
  spots in throat 606
epidemic on Interior, white purulent
  spots in throat 606
external
 buttock ulcers 707
 red, itching and swollen fingers 785
 toe ulcers 701
face, redness and swelling of face
  573–574
fever in cancer 816
five-colour vaginal discharge 858
head
 boils on scalp 568
 head swelling 564
Heart invasion, heartbeat displaced
  downwards 667
herpes zoster 786
Intestines
 blood and mucus in stools 750
 blood in stools 751
invasion
 herpes simplex 786
 redness and swelling of face 573
 with Wind-Heat *see* Wind-Heat
itching 713
Liver
 nails falling off 689
 ulcers on nose 598
Liver and Gall-Bladder, ear discharge
  583
Lower Burner, blood in sperm 768
Lungs
 dry nostrils 594
 itching nose 593
 swollen nose 596
Lungs and Stomach, runny nose
  592–593
measles, eye discharge 634
mouth ulcers 610
Nutritive-Qi level, swollen nose 596
protruding eyeball 643
raised fontanelles 871–872
rash in axillae 785
redness, erosion and swelling of
  pharynx 602
rosacea 785
skin
 acne 569, 783–784
 tinea (ringworm) of hands 684
 urticaria 784
Stomach
 boil on eyelid 639
 ulcers below zygomatic arch 574
Stomach and Intestines, swollen tonsils
  603
Stomach and Spleen, swollen lips 623
strabismus 629
throat at Qi level, swollen tonsils 603

tinea 786
toe ulcers 701
ulcers on penis 773
Wind-Heat invasion with *see*
  Wind-Heat, invasion with Toxic
  Heat
yellow sclera 635
toxic heat, tonsils 979
Toxic Heat at Qi level 870
Toxic Heat in Interior, erysipelas 870
Toxic Heat in Liver channel
 red scrotum 770
 redness and swelling of glans penis
  772
 swollen and oozing scrotum 770
 vulval swelling 858–859
Toxic Heat in Lower Burner, swelling and
  pain in testicles 773
Toxic Heat in Stomach, red, itching and
  swollen fingers 785
Toxic Heat in Stomach and Lungs
 carbuncles on upper back 788
 neck ulcers 789
Toxic Heat in tonsils 979
Toxic Heat in Uterus, menstrual bleeding
  returning after menopause
  830
Toxic Heat on Exterior, erysipelas 870
Toxic Heat with Blood stasis
 acne 784
 breasts, peau d'orange 852
 inverted nipples 852
 swollen neck glands 655
Toxic Heat with Empty-Heat in Stomach,
  carbuncles on neck 788
Toxic Heat with Liver-Fire and
  Damp-Heat, vulvar sores 858
Toxic Heat with stagnation of Qi and
  stasis of Blood 584
toxins, external, convulsions/fever after
  childbirth 846, 848
trachoma 645–646
tranquillizers, effect on pulse 507
trauma 428–429
 climate 416
 coccyx pain 705
 miscarriage 841
 vaginal bleeding 838
tremor
 arms 341
 feet 64–65
 hands 64, 130, *130*, 156, 684
 head 59, 70, 564
 legs 700
 limbs 62–63, 156, *156*, 340–341,
  678
tricyclic antidepressants, effect on pulse
  507
trigeminal neuralgia 303

Triple Burner *see* Three Burners (Triple Burner); *individual elements*
true Cold–false Heat 988, *988*
true Heat–false Cold 814, 988, *989*, 1022
Tu Si Zi Wan 1044
tuberculosis (TB)
    health line 134, *134*
    spoon-shaped fingers 131, *131*
tumours, abdominal cavity 128
    see also cancer
Turbid Dampness surrounding Heart 883
    acupuncture 883
    clinical manifestations 883
    prescription 883
Turbid Phlegm
    head
        blurred vision and floaters 628
        headache 561
        visual acuity decreased 630
    lungs, purple lips 622
    throat, white purulent spots 606
Turbid Phlegm in Heart 803
Turbid Yin not descending, clinical manifestations 932
Twelve Channels
    bladder 995
    gall-bladder 996
    heart 994
    kidneys 995
    large intestine 993–994
    liver 996
    lungs 993
    pattern identification **993–996**
    pericardium 995
    small intestine 994–995
    spleen 994
    stomach 994
    Triple Burner 995–996

U

ulcerative colitis
    case history 272
    hands lines 133
ulcers
    anal 763
    buttocks 706–707
    face (below zygomatic arch) 71, 574
    foot *plate 21.8, plate 21.9*
    head 70, 564–565
    lower leg 701
    mouth 97, *97, 308,* 308–309, 609–610, 834
    neck 789
    nose 90, 598
    pathology and diagnosis, Western *vs* Chinese 180
    penis 150, 772–773

pharynx 111
scalp 70, 568–569
skin 180–181, *181*
toes 701
tongue 614–615
umbilicus
    pain 332, 738–739
    pulsation feeling under 742
    pulse 515, *515*
    regions 515, *515*
    signs 147
        protruding 147, 745
        sunken 147, 745
untying rope pulse 507
Upper Burner
    pattern identification 969–970
    pulse diagnosis
        Inch section 437, *438*
        position assignment 443
        state of *434,* 435
    see also Three Burners (Triple Burner)
upper respiratory infections, children 112
Upright Qi, deficiency 462
upturned knife pulse 507
urinary infections, hand lines 135
urination (micturition)
    difficulty with 275, 755–756, 845
    frequent 756
    nighttime 758
    nocturnal enuresis 274, 275, 757–758, 867
    painful 275, 754–755
    problems in children 867
    problems in pregnancy 839
urine 274–275
    blood in 758, 839
    cloudiness 275
    colour 165, *165,* 274
    dark 753–754
    dribbling 756–757
    frequency 274
    incontinence 275, 757
    interrogation **261–267**
    observation 165, *166*
    odour 275
    pale and abundant 754
    quantity 275
    smell diagnosis 550–551
    sperm in 759
    turbid 754
urine retention 274, 275, 839
    in infants 867
urticaria *plate 21.32*
    chronic *plate 21.33*
    dermographism 181, *plate 21.10*
    pathology and diagnosis, Western *vs* Chinese 185, *185*
    symptoms and signs 784–785

wheals 185
    see also itching
Uterus
    Dampness and Phlegm 1002
    invasion of external Dampness 950
    prolapse 859
    stagnant cold 1002
Uterus-Blood stasis 931
Uterus deficient and cold 1002

V

vagina
    leukoplakia 859
    prolapse 151, 859
vaginal bleeding
    after childbirth 845
    on intercourse 859–860
    in pregnancy 838
    trauma 838
    see also menstrual bleeding
vaginal discharge 409, *409,* 857–858
    case history 396
    five-colour 857–858
    observation 166–167, *167*
        colour 166, *167,* 857
        consistency 166, *167*
        lochia *see* lochia
    red-white 857
    smell 551
    white 857
    yellow 857
    see also lochia
vaginal itching 858
vaginal prolapse 151, 859
veins
    eyes *plate 12.1*
    inner leg, plucking of 1056–1057
veins (children) 194–195
    colour 195, *195*
    differentiation criteria 194, *194*
    length and thickness 195, *195*
    movement 195, *195*
    visibility 195
vertigo, benign positional
    case histories 247–248, 295–296
    see also dizziness
vesicles 174, 178, *178, plate 21.5*
    vs macules/papules 958
vision disorders 628–631
    blurred 360, *360*
        with floaters 628
    decreased night vision 630
    decreased visual acuity 630
    hyperopia 629–630
    myopia 629
    strabismus 83, *83,* 628–629
    sudden blindness 630–631
    see also eye(s)

visual hallucinations 76
vital substances, Chinese terms
    1063–1064
voice 541–544
    baby's cry 544
    crying out 543, 822
    Five-Elements 542
    groaning 542, 543, 822
    hoarseness 313–314, *314*, 543, 606,
        820
    internal organs influencing 541,
        542
    laughing 542
    loss of 606
        in pregnancy 840–841
    loud 819
    mind and spirit, reflection of state 542
    muffled 820
    nasal 543, 820–821
    normal 542
    pitch 542
    shouting 542
    singing 542
    snoring 543, 821
    strength and quality 542, 543–544,
        544
    symptoms and signs **819–821**
    weak 820
    weeping 542
    see also hearing (listening), diagnosis
        by; speech/talking
vomiting
    blood 725–726
    in children 864–865
    diagnosis by sound 547, *547*
    diarrhoea with 748
    menstrual symptoms 835
    patterns 266
    symptoms and signs 724–725
    see also nausea
vulva
    leukoplakia 151, 859
    sores 151, 858
    swelling 151, 858–859

W

Walking Crow Teeth Nutritional
        Impairment Pattern 619
walking difficulties 338, *338*
warfarin, effect on pulse 508
warts 189, *plate 21.51, plate 21.52*
    ears 107, 585
    genital *plate 21.53*
    genitalia 189
    infection route 189
    pathology and diagnosis 189, *189*
    presentation 189
    symptoms and signs 787

Water
    accumulation of 179, 966
        see also oedema
    Earth overacting on Water 1008
    Fire insulting Water 1009
    invasion of Lungs by Wind-Water
        901–902
    Metal not generating Water 1008
Water insulting Earth 1009
Water not generating Wood 1008
Water overacting on Fire 1008
Water Overflowing, swollen eyelids 638
Water Overflowing to Heart 883
Water Pox 180
Water Rampart 79
water retention, premenstrual symptoms
        405
    see also oedema
Water type
    body odour 549, 550
    body shape 19–20, *20, plate1.7*
    faces *plate1.6*
    voice 542, *542*
weak breathing (*Qi Shao*) 545, 661
Weak-Heart constitution
    disease heredity 419
    emotional problems 417
Weak-Kidney constitution, disease
        heredity 420
weak knees 344
Weak-Liver constitution, disease heredity
        419–420
Weak-Lung constitution, disease heredity
        419
Weak pulse *see* pulse qualities
Weak-Spleen constitution, disease
        heredity 419
weakness, constitutional 866–867
    constipation in children 867
    heart deficiency 866
    hereditary weak constitution and
        diet 416
weakness of limbs 338, *338*
Wei Ling San 1044
Wei Ling Tang 1044
Wei syndrome 61
weight change 713–714
    see also obesity
weight loss 319, 714
Wen 539
Wen Dan Tang 1044–1045
Wen Pi Tang 1045
Wen Yang Bu Gan Jian 1045
wheals 177, *plate 21.3*
wheezing (*Xiao*) 545
    in children 413, 865
    symptoms and signs 662–663
white purulent spots in 606–607
whooping cough 545

Wind
    Attack of 945, *945*
        acupuncture 965
        clinical manifestations 965
        prescription 965
    aversion to 362–363
    Blood stagnation generated 644
    body aches 709
    in channels, hemiplegia 711
    climate 428
    clinical manifestations 944, *944*
    coarse and thick nails 688
    convulsions 155
    dizziness 295
    Empty
        tremor of the head 564
        tremor/spasticity of limbs 678
    Empty-Wind agitating in the Interior
        957
    exterior 362, *944*, **944–945**
        Wind-Cold 944–945
    external invasion
        dribbling from mouth 612
        grinding teeth 617
        numbness/tingling of hands 683
        tongue 231
        toothache 615
    Heat generated
        eyeballs turning up 644
        tremor of hands 684
        tremor/spasticity of limbs 678
    Heat victorious stirring Wind 957
    interior 945–946
        see also Extreme Heat generating
            Wind; Liver-Blood deficiency;
            Liver-Yang rising generating
            Wind
    internal
        bluish-greenish helix in children
            585
        contraction of limbs 677
        eyeball turning up 644
        generation 155
        head tilted backwards 565
        numbness/tingling 712
        with Qi deficiency 648
        quivering eyeball 644
        tongue 231
    internal Empty, grinding teeth 617
    invasion of Lungs by 901–902
    invasion of Lungs by Wind-Cold
        901
    invasion of Lungs by Wind-Dryness
        901
    invasion of Lungs by Wind-Water
        901–902
    in joints
        joint pain 710
        limb rigidity 676

Liver-Blood deficiency giving rise to
Wind 894–895
Liver-Fire generating Wind 894
Liver-Heat stirs Wind 970
Liver-Wind *see* Liver-Wind
pain in hands 682
pain in limbs 672
pathogenic factors **943–946**
in skin
dry skin 782
itching 713
Wind-Cold invasion (Wind prevalent)
965
Wind and Heat in skin, psoriasis 783
Wind and Phlegm in channels
limb paralysis 677
paralysis of legs 695
Wind-Cold *369*, **369–370**, 944–945,
945
Wind-Cold in channels, facial pain 571
Wind-Cold in skin, urticaria 784
Wind-Cold invasion 965
cough in children 865
facial pain 302, 303
fever after childbirth 846
Wind-Dampness, clinical manifestations
945
Wind-Dampness in Girdle Vessel,
unilateral sweating 778
Wind-Dampness invasion
head, feeling of heaviness 297
headache 291, 562
nasal voice 820
yellow complexion 577
Wind-Dampness on Exterior,
spontaneous sweating 776
Wind-Dampness retention, channels of
back
lordosis 707
scoliosis 707
Wind-Dryness
acute cough 659
dry nostrils 594
dry throat 606
Wind-Dryness invading the Lungs, dry
skin 782
Wind Gate 194, *194*
Wind-Heat *369*, **369–370**
acupuncture 954
clinical manifestations 369, 954,
959
Dry-Heat 370
external invasion
fever in children 863–864
tinea (ringworm) of hands 684
headache 291
invasion in Blood, skin eruptions
during menstruation 834
invasion in Lesser-Yang channels

sores on ear 584
tinnitus 582
invasion with Dryness
dandruff 567
hoarse voice/loss of voice 606
invasion with Phlegm, mouth ulcers
610
invasion with Toxic Heat
gums oozing pus 620
swollen neck glands 655
swollen tonsils 603
Liver and Lung channels, drooping red
eye membrane 646
Liver channel
corneal opacity 647
eyelids loss of control 640
prescription 954
skin, swollen lips 623
Spleen channel, red grains inside
eyelids 641
Summer-Heat 370
tinea 786
vs Wind-Cold *945*, 954
feeling of cold *366*, *366*
Wind-Heat at Defensive-Qi level
Chickenpox 870
skin rash 869–870
Wind-Heat in channels, facial pain 571
Wind-Heat in Lung Defensive-Qi portion
acupuncture 969
clinical manifestations 969
flapping of nostrils 870
prescription 969
Wind-Heat in skin
herpes zoster 786
urticaria 784
Wind-Heat invasion
aching nose 595
acupuncture 966
acute cough 659
boil on eyelid 639
clinical manifestations 966
cold sores 610
contracted pupils 650
cough in children 865
coughing blood 661
distension of head feeling 562
dry and white teeth 617
dry nostrils 594
dry throat 605
ear discharge 583
earache 582
ecchymosis under conjunctiva 645
eye discharge 634
facial pain 302–303
fever after childbirth 846
flapping alae nasi (nostrils) 598
headache 562
herpes simplex 786

hoarse voice 820
hot and painful eyes 633
inflamed gums 618
inverted eyelashes 651
itching ears 582
itching eyes 631
itching tongue 613
vs Latent Heat *960*
nosebleed 595
prescription 966
red back of ear (children) 586
red eye corners 637
red eyelids 637–638
red lips 621
red nose 590
red philtrum 626
red sclera 635
redness and pain of scalp 568
redness/swelling of pharynx 602
runny nose 592
scaly eyeballs 644
sense of smell loss 597
sore throat 601
streaming eyes 634
swollen eyelids 638
yellow complexion 577
Wind-Heat invasion in Lesser-Yang
channels, ear problems in
children 865
Wind-Heat with Toxic Heat, spots on
back 706
Wind invasion
blocked nose 591
drooping eyelids 640
hot hands 681
itching hands 683
itching throat 605
joint pain 318, *318*
joint pain after childbirth 844
muffled voice 820
neck pain 654
nose itching 593
nose pain 595
numbness of face 572
red complexion 577
sneezing 304, 591
see also residual pathogenic factors
Wind invasion with penetration of Heat
at Qi level, convulsions in
children 871
Wind on Exterior, acute invasion
984–985
Wind-Phlegm
clinical manifestations 936
contraction of fingers 687
cramps in calves 701
dark eyelids 638
distension feeling in limbs 674
dribbling from mouth 612

Wind-Phlegm (contd.)
  headache 290, 561
  hemiplegia 711
  limb rigidity 676
  nodules under skin 789
  numbness/tingling 712
    of face 572
    of hands 683
    in limbs 673
  slurred speech 821
  tremor/spasticity of limbs 678
  unilateral sweating 777
  see also Phlegm
Wind Rampart 79
Wind Rash 180
Wind-stroke 650
Wind-Water invasion
  clinical manifestations 945
  cold and heaviness feeling in lower
    back 704
Wind-Water invasion in Lungs
  oedema of body 713
  oedema of limbs 676
  oedema of the face 572
  swollen ears 584
  swollen fingers 686
Wine-Phlegm 938
Wiry pulse see pulse qualities
Wolff–Parkinson–White (WPW)
    Syndrome 460
women-fatigue jaundice 175
women's symptoms **395–409**
Wood
  Earth insulting Wood 1009
  Metal overacting on Wood 1008
  Water not generating Wood 1008
Wood insulting Metal 1009
Wood not generating Fire 1007–1008
Wood overacting on Earth 1008
Wood types
  body odour 549, 550, 550
  body shape 15–16, 16, plate1.2
  face plate1.1
  voice 542, 542
worm infestation 199, 597
  children 869
  index finger creases 197, 198
  pinworms 869
  prescriptions 912
  roundworms 869
worry 386–387, 423–424, 424
  depression 798
  patterns 387
  propensity to 791–792
  see also anxiety
Wu Hu Tang 1045
Wu Ling San 1045
Wu Mei Wan 1045
Wu Ren Wan 1045

Wu Yao San 1045
Wu Zhu Yu Tang 1045
Wu Zi Yan Zong Wan 1046

X

Xi Jiao Di Huang Tang 1046
Xiang (images) 1
Xiang Leng Wan 1046
Xiao see wheezing (Xiao)
Xiao Chai Hu Tang 1046
Xiao Fu 145, 516
Xiao Jian Zhong Tang 1046
Xiao Qing Long Tang 1046
Xiao Yao San 1046
Xie Bai San 1046
Xie Fei Mai 451
Xie Huang San 1046
Xie Xin Tang 1047
Xin Fan ('mental restlessness') 239
Xin Yi Qing Fei Yin 1047
Xin Zhong Ao Nong (Heart feeling vexed)
    665–666
Xing Su San 1047
Xiong Men 324
Xu Lao (exhaustion) 282
Xu Li 127–128, 512
Xuan Fu 169, 170
Xuan Fu Dai Zhe Tang 1047
Xue Fu Zhu Yu Tang 1047
xyphoid process
  abdominal pain 328–329, 329,
    736–737
  area under 513, 513
  heartbeat below 128, 668

Y

Yan Hu Sou Tang 1047
Yang
  body shape classification 11, 12–15
  Empty-Yang 990
  Greater Yang stage **965–967**
  nose convergence 87
  pulse
    feeling levels 455
    organs 443–444, 445, 445
    positions of 452–453
  see also individual organs
Yang, Bright- see Bright-Yang
Yang, Clear, not ascending 932
Yang, Lesser-
  Latent Heat 961
  pattern 284
Yang and Yin see Yin and Yang
Yang channels, ears 105
Yang collapse
  clinical manifestations 932
  contraction of scrotum 769

dilated pupils 649
hemiplegia 711
hoarse voice 820
sweating from collapse 776–777
white/pale complexion 575–576
Yang deficiency
  body shape 14, 14
  clinical manifestations 932
  cold hands and feet 672
  cold upper back 656
  with Empty-Cold 688
  fever in cancer 816
  floating upwards, sweating on head
    778
  Heart and Lungs 814
  Kidney 814
  muscle twitching 63
  pale eye corners 636
  pale eyelids 638
  pale helix 585
  paralysis 62
  severe, inverted lips 624
  small or absent lunulae on nails 692
  of Stomach and Spleen 814
  tiredness, acute onset 1023
  tongue-body colour 206, 210
  tongue patterns 227–228
  white/pale complexion 575
Yang Heel Vessel (Yang Qiao Mai) **1004**
Yang Linking Vessel (Yang Wei Mai)
    1005, **1005**
Yang yellow 53
Yang Yin Qing Fei Tang 1047
yawning 670
Ye Ge (diaphragm choking) 114, 726
Yellow Emperor's Internal Classic 434,
    434–435
Yi Gan San 1047–1048
Yi Guan Jian 1048
Yi Jia Zheng Qi San 1048
Yi Wei Tang 1048
Yi Yin Jian 1048
Yin
  body shape classification 11, 12–15
  collapse
    contraction of scrotum 769
    hemiplegia 711
    hoarse voice 820
  Empty-Yin 990
  organs
    musical correlation 539, 539–540,
      540
    smell correlation 540
  pulse
    feeling levels 455
    organs 443–444, 445, 445
    positions of 452–453
  see also individual organs
Yin, Lesser see Lesser-Yin

Yin, Turbid, not descending, clinical
      manifestations 932
Yin and Qi deficient, clinical
      manifestations 933
Yin and Yang
    collapse
        nosebleed 595
        sunken eyeball 643
    deficient, clinical manifestations 932
Yin Chen Hao Tang 1048
Yin-Cold in abdomen, energy rising
      feeling in abdomen 742
Yin collapse
    acupuncture 957
    clinical manifestations 932, 957
    prescription 957
Yin deficiency
    body shape *14*, 14–15
    case history 1021–1022
    chronic, thin neck 655
    clinical manifestations 932
    cracked nails 688
    dry mouth 732–733
    hot palms and soles 866
    insomnia 348
    low-grade fever in children 864
    night sweating 776
    paralysis 62
    Qi deficiency with *see* Qi and Yin
        deficiency
    severe
        inverted lips 624
        redness and erosion of pharynx 603
    thin abdomen 745
    tidal fever 816
    tongue-body colour 206
    tongue patterns 228–230, *229*
    weight loss 319, 714
Yin deficiency generating Empty-Wind
      (Blood level), limb convulsions
      678

Yin deficiency with Blood-Heat, cracked
      nipples 852
Yin deficiency with Empty-Heat
    clinical manifestations 932, 1022
    dry and cracked lips 622
    eye discharge 634
    facial pain 571
    fever in cancer 816
    Five-Palm Heat 817
    and internal Wind, facial pain 571
    large lunulae on nails 692
    mental restlessness 794
    mouth ulcers 610
    night sweating 776
    red complexion 577
    red lips 621
    redness and erosion of pharynx
        603
    redness inside lower eyelids 641
Yin deficiency with Empty-Heat and
      Damp-Heat, herpes simplex
      786
Yin deficiency with Empty-Heat and
      Dampness, yellow sweat
      777
Yin deficiency with Phlegm-Fire and
      Empty-Heat, schizophrenia
      802
Yin deficiency with Phlegm-Heat, facial
      pain 571–572
Yin excess, closed eyes 650
Yin-Fire
    heat of the face/hot flushes 570
    pathology *375*, *375*, 376
    red complexion 577
Yin-Fire from deficiency of Stomach and
      Spleen and Original Qi 888
    acupuncture 888
    clinical manifestations 888
    prescription 888
Yin Heel Vessel *(Yin Qiao Mai)* **1004**

Yin Linking Vessel *(Yin Wei Mai)* *1005*,
      1005
Yin organs
    manifestations 4–5, *5*
    Qi transportation sites relationship 4
Yin Qiao San 1048
Yin Tong (lurking pain), pain
      classification 257
Yin/Yang balance, body shape *15*,
      15
Yin yellow 54
Yin Yu ('gloominess/depression') 381
Yin–Yang 991
You Gui Wan 1048–1049
Yu 539
Yu Nu Jian 1049
Yu Zheng ('depression pattern') 381
Yue Ju Wan 1049

Z

Zeng Ye Tang 1049
Zhang ('distension') 740
    see also distension (bloating)
'Zhang Tong' (distending pain) 255–256
Zhen 180
Zhen Gan Xi Feng Tang 1049
Zhen Ren Yang Zang Tang 1049
Zhen Wu Tang 1049
Zheng Jia 147, 511
Zheng Qi Tian Xiang San 1049
Zhi 539
Zhi Bo Di Huang Wan 1049
Zhi Gan Cao Tang 1050
ZhI Shi Dao Zhi Wan 1050
Zhi Shi Gua Lou Gui Zhi Tang 1050
Zho Jin Wan 1050
Zhu Ye Shi Gao Tang 1050
Zong Qi see Gathering-Qi
Zuo Gui Wan 1050
Zuo Gui Yin 1050

Notes

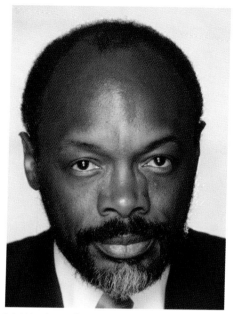

Plate 1.1 Wood-type face (© Roger Ressmeyer/CORBIS)

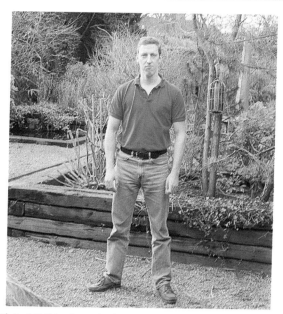

Plate 1.2 Wood-type body

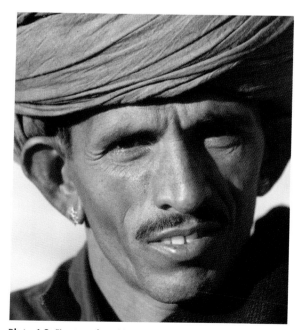

Plate 1.3 Fire-type face (© Dave Bartruff/CORBIS)

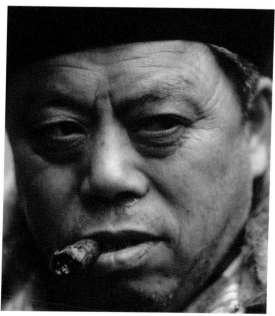

Plate 1.4 Earth-type face (© Arnie Hodalic/CORBIS)

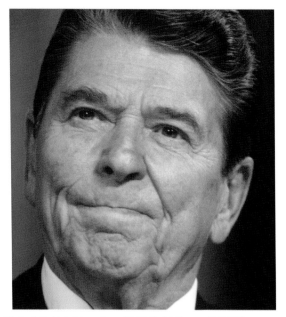

Plate 1.5 Metal-type face (© Wally McNamee/CORBIS)

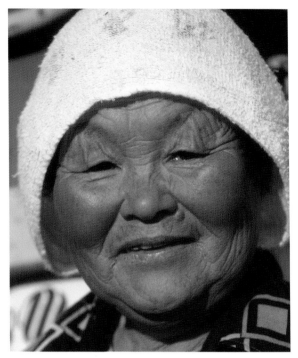

Plate 1.6 Water-type face (© Ric Ergenbright/CORBIS)

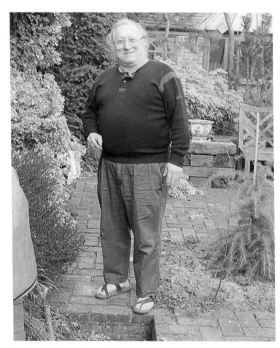

Plate 1.7 Water-type body

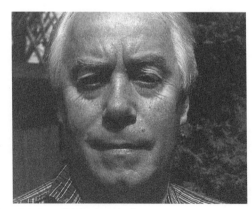

Plate 3.1 Superficial colour (red)

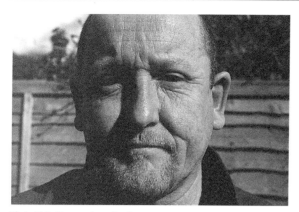

Plate 3.2 Deep colour (red)

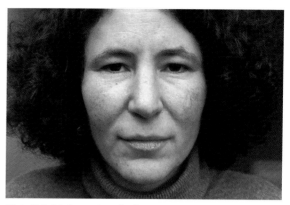

Plate 3.3 Distinct colour (red)

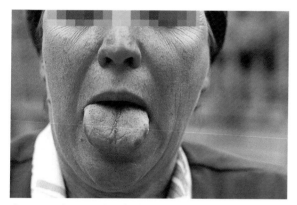

Plate 3.4 Obscure colour (red)

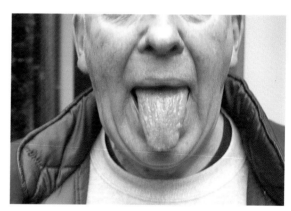

Plate 3.5 Scattered colour (red)

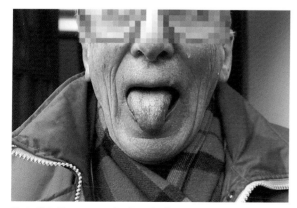

Plate 3.6 Concentrated colour (red)

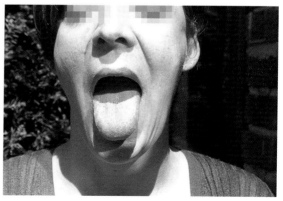

Plate 3.7 Thin colour (yellow)

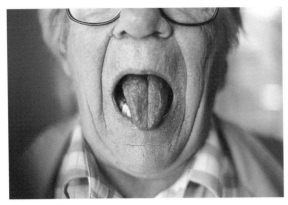

Plate 3.8 Thick colour (yellow)

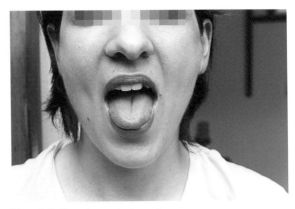

Plate 3.9 Normal complexion colour

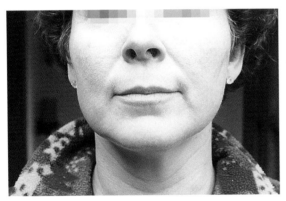

Plate 3.10 Bright-white complexion colour

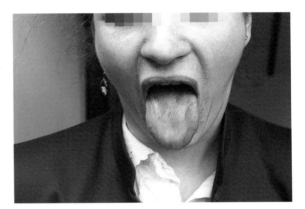

Plate 3.11 Dull-white complexion colour

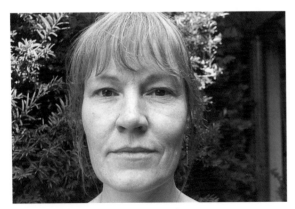

Plate 3.12 Pale-white complexion colour

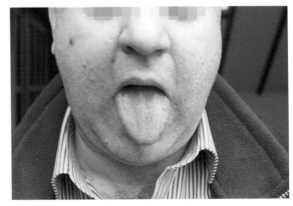

Plate 3.13 Sallow-white complexion colour

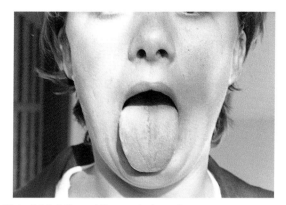

Plate 3.14 Sallow-white complexion colour

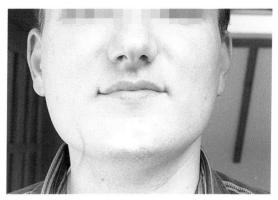

Plate 3.15 Dull-yellow complexion colour

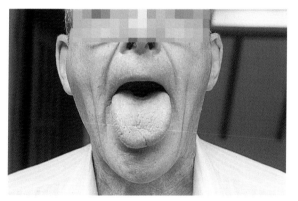

Plate 3.16 'Greyish-yellow complexion

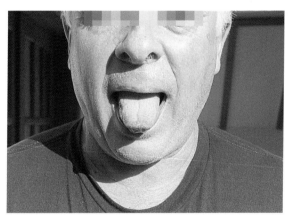

Plate 3.17 Floating-yellow complexion colour

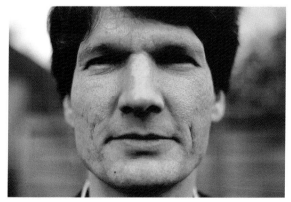

Plate 3.18 Dry-yellow complexion colour

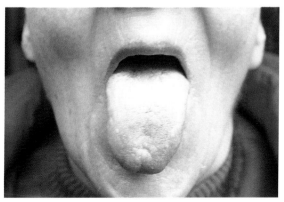

Plate 3.19 Ash-like yellow complexion colour

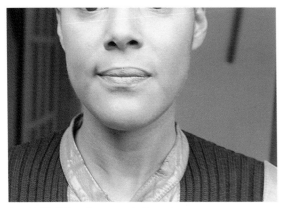

Plate 3.20 Rich-yellow complexion colour

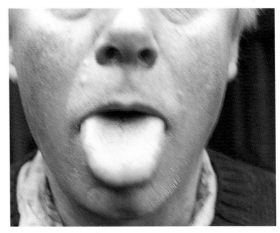

Plate 3.21 Red cheeks

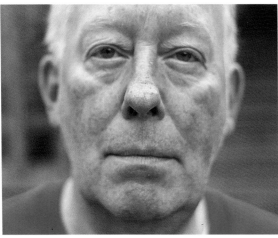

Plate 3.22 Red cheeks

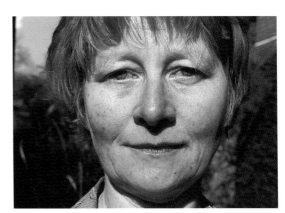

Plate 3.23 Red cheekbones

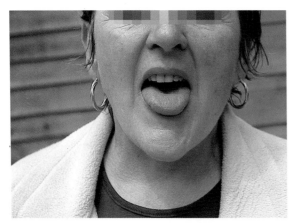

Plate 3.24 Red cheekbones

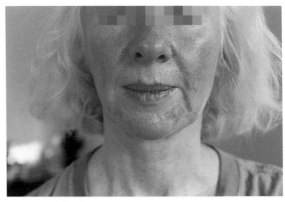

Plate 3.25 Floating-red complexion colour

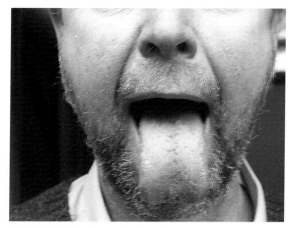

Plate 3.26 Thin-red complexion colour

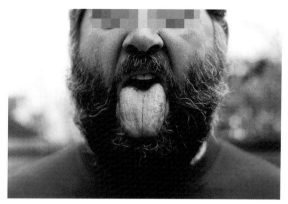

Plate 3.27 Thick-red complexion colour

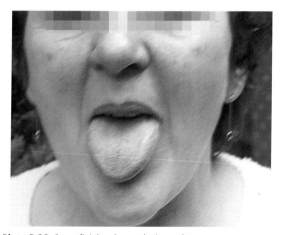

Plate 3.28 Superficial-red complexion colour

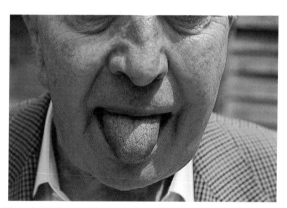

Plate 3.29 Deep-red complexion colour

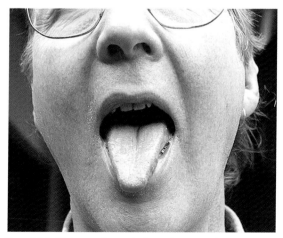

Plate 3.30 Distinct-red complexion colour

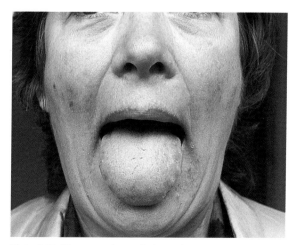

Plate 3.31 Obscure-red complexion colour

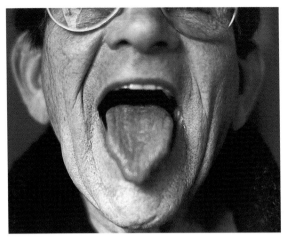

Plate 3.32 Bluish-Greenish complexion colour

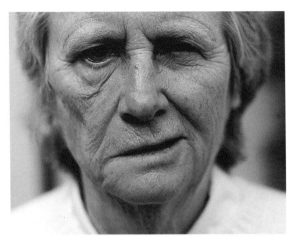

Plate 4.1 Bell's palsy (facial paralysis)

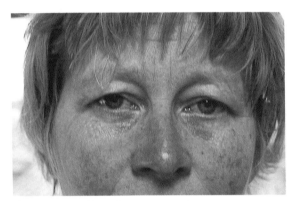

Plate 6.1 Eyes without lustre

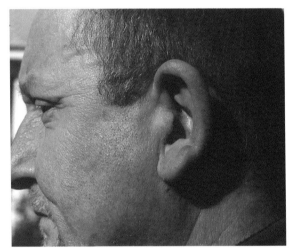

Plate 9.1 Swollen ear (also red helix)

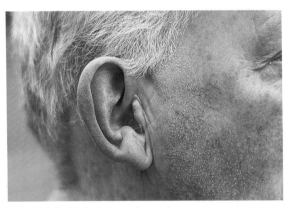

Plate 9.2 Red helix (also swollen ear)

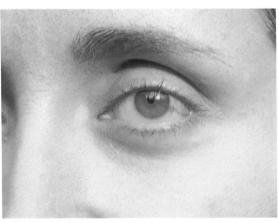

Plate 12.1 Horizontal vein in the left eye

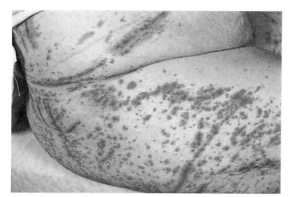

Plate 21.1 Purple macules (Reproduced with permission from Gawkrodger D 1992 An Illustrated Colour Text of Dermatology, Churchill Livingstone, Edinburgh)

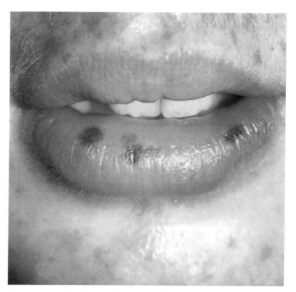

Plate 21.2 Macules on lips (Reproduced with permission from Wilkinson J D and Shaw S 1998 Dermatology, Churchill Livingstone, Edinburgh)

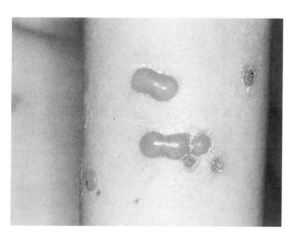

Plate 21.3 Wheals (Reproduced with permission from Gawkrodger D 1992 An Illustrated Colour Text of Dermatology, Churchill Livingstone, Edinburgh)

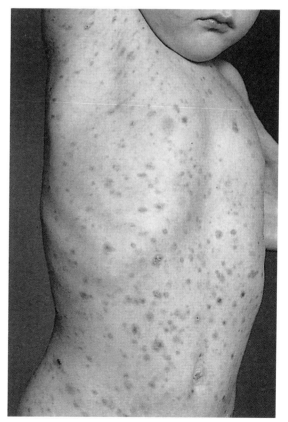

Plate 21.4 Papules (Reproduced with permission from Gawkrodger D 1992 An Illustrated Colour Text of Dermatology, Churchill Livingstone, Edinburgh)

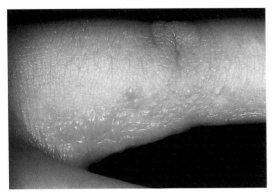

Plate 21.5 Vesicles (Reproduced with permission from Wilkinson J D and Shaw S 1998 Dermatology, Churchill Livingstone, Edinburgh)

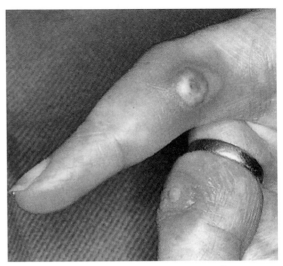

Plate 21.6 Pustule (Reproduced with permission from Gawkrodger D 1992 An Illustrated Colour Text of Dermatology, Churchill Livingstone, Edinburgh)

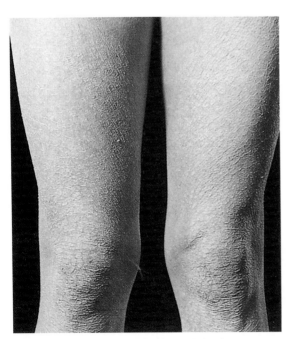

Plate 21.7 Scales (Reproduced with permission from Gawkrodger D 1992 An Illustrated Colour Text of Dermatology, Churchill Livingstone, Edinburgh)

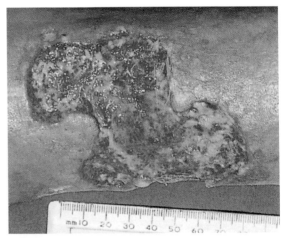

Plate 21.8 Venous ulcer on the ankle (Reproduced with permission from Gawkrodger D 1992 An Illustrated Colour Text of Dermatology, Churchill Livingstone, Edinburgh)

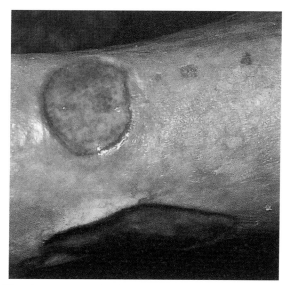

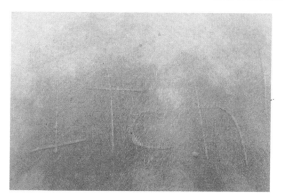

Plate 21.10 Dermographism (Reproduced with permission from Wilkinson J D and Shaw S 1998 Dermatology, Churchill Livingstone, Edinburgh)

Plate 21.9 Necrotic ulcer (Reproduced with permission from Gawkrodger D 1992 An Illustrated Colour Text of Dermatology, Churchill Livingstone, Edinburgh)

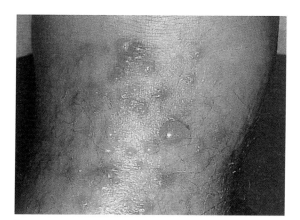

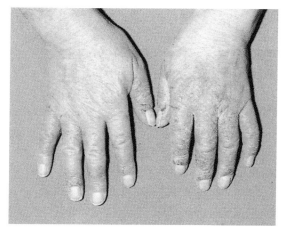

Plate 21.11 Acute eczema (dermatitis) (Reproduced with permission from Gawkrodger D 1992 An Illustrated Colour Text of Dermatology, Churchill Livingstone, Edinburgh)

Plate 21.12 Chronic eczema (dermatitis) (Reproduced with permission from Gawkrodger D 1992 An Illustrated Colour Text of Dermatology, Churchill Livingstone, Edinburgh)

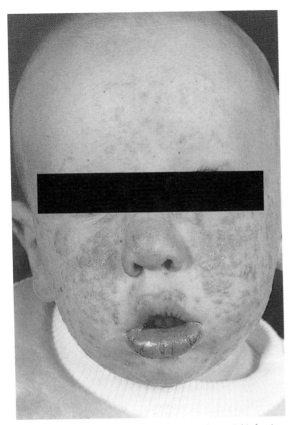

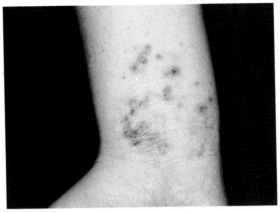

Plate 21.14 Atopic eczema with excoriations and lichenification (Reproduced with permission from Gawkrodger D 1992 An Illustrated Colour Text of Dermatology, Churchill Livingstone, Edinburgh)

Plate 21.13 Atopic eczema with secondary bacterial infection (Reproduced with permission from Gawkrodger D 1992 An Illustrated Colour Text of Dermatology, Churchill Livingstone, Edinburgh)

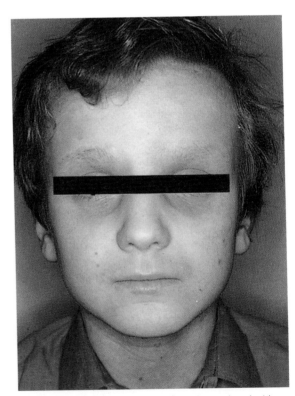

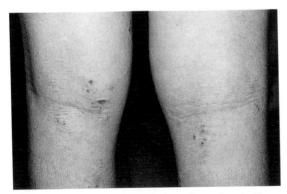

Plate 21.15 Atopic eczema on the knee (Reproduced with permission from Gawkrodger D 1992 An Illustrated Colour Text of Dermatology, Churchill Livingstone, Edinburgh)

Plate 21.16 'Dry' pruritic atopic eczema (Reproduced with permission from Gawkrodger D 1992 An Illustrated Colour Text of Dermatology, Churchill Livingstone, Edinburgh)

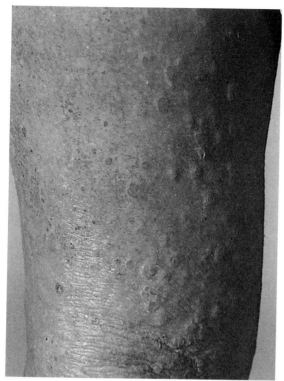

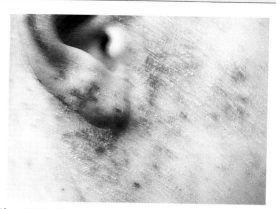

Plate 21.18 Chronic atopic eczema

Plate 21.17 Atopic eczema with extensive lichenification (Reproduced with permission from Gawkrodger D 1992 An Illustrated Colour Text of Dermatology, Churchill Livingstone, Edinburgh)

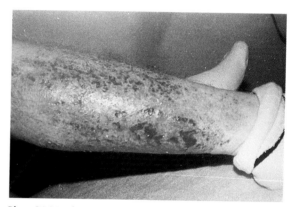

Plate 21.20 Chronic eczema (infected)

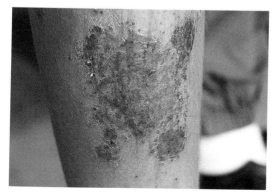

Plate 21.19 Chronic eczema (infected)

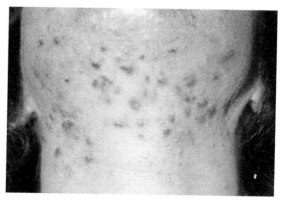

Plate 21.21 Papular-pustular acne (Reproduced with permission from Gawkrodger D 1992 An Illustrated Colour Text of Dermatology, Churchill Livingstone, Edinburgh)

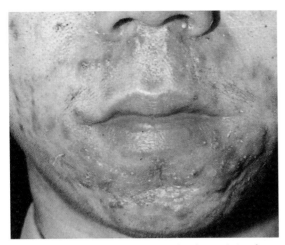

Plate 21.22 Pustular acne (Reproduced with permission from Gawkrodger D 1992 An Illustrated Colour Text of Dermatology, Churchill Livingstone, Edinburgh)

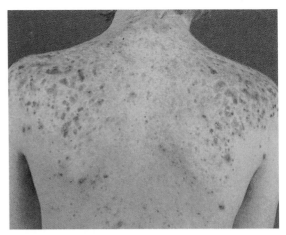

Plate 21.23 Scarring acne (Reproduced with permission from Gawkrodger D 1992 An Illustrated Colour Text of Dermatology, Churchill Livingstone, Edinburgh)

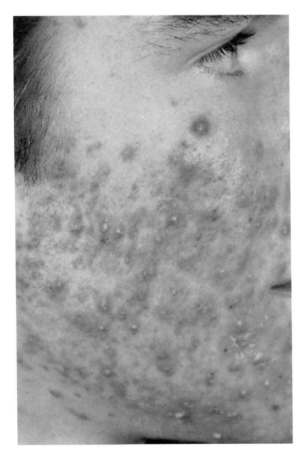

Plate 21.24 Inflammatory acne (Reproduced with permission from Wilkinson J D and Shaw S 1998 Dermatology, Churchill Livingstone, Edinburgh)

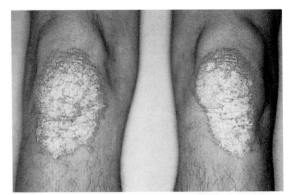

Plate 21.25 Psoriasis with scaly plaques (Reproduced with permission from Gawkrodger D 1992 An Illustrated Colour Text of Dermatology, Churchill Livingstone, Edinburgh)

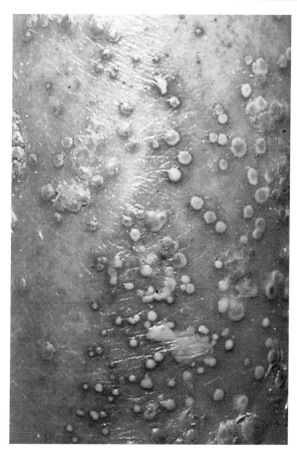

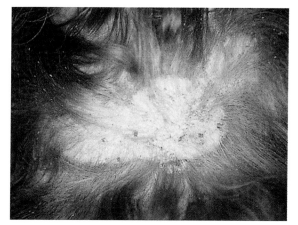

Plate 21.27 Psoriasis of scalp (Reproduced with permission from Gawkrodger D 1992 An Illustrated Colour Text of Dermatology, Churchill Livingstone, Edinburgh)

Plate 21.26 Pustular psoriasis (Reproduced with permission from Wilkinson J D and Shaw S 1998 Dermatology, Churchill Livingstone, Edinburgh)

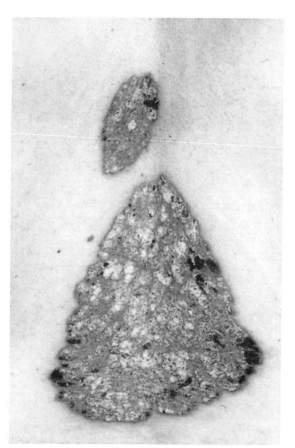

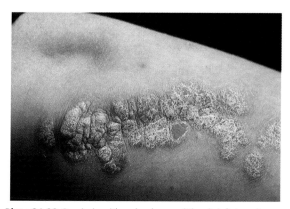

Plate 21.28 Psoriasis with pale plaques (Blood deficiency)

Plate 21.29 Psoriasis with bright-red plaques (Blood-Heat and Dryness) (Reproduced with permission from Wilkinson JD and Shaw S 1998 Dermatology, Churchill Livingstone, Edinburgh)

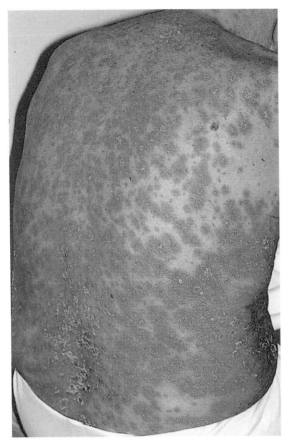

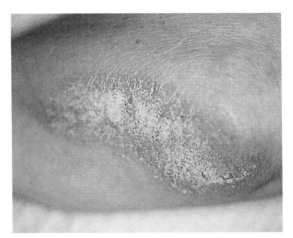

Plate 21.31 Psoriasis with pale and dry-scaly plaques (Blood deficient and dry with Wind) (Reproduced with permission from Gawkrodger D 1992 An Illustrated Colour Text of Dermatology, Churchill Livingstone, Edinburgh)

Plate 21.30 Psoriasis with purple lesions (Blood-Heat and Blood stasis) (Reproduced with permission from Gawkrodger D 1992 An Illustrated Colour Text of Dermatology, Churchill Livingstone, Edinburgh)

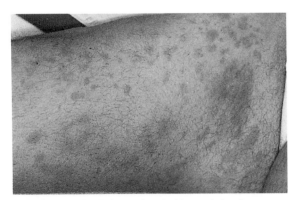

Plate 21.32 Urticaria (Reproduced with permission from Gawkrodger D 1992 An Illustrated Colour Text of Dermatology, Churchill Livingstone, Edinburgh)

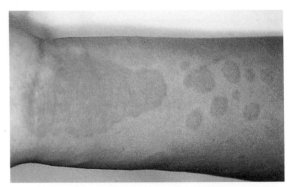

Plate 21.33 Chronic urticaria (Reproduced with permission from Gawkrodger D 1992 An Illustrated Colour Text of Dermatology, Churchill Livingstone, Edinburgh)

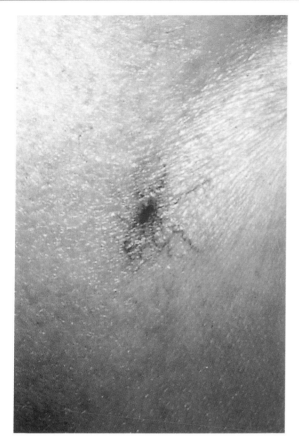

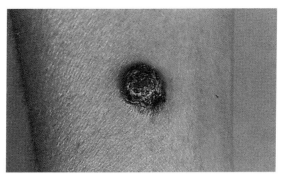

Plate 21.36 Nodular malignant melanoma (Reproduced with permission from Gawkrodger D 1992 An Illustrated Colour Text of Dermatology, Churchill Livingstone, Edinburgh)

Plate 21.34 Naevus (spider angioma) (Reproduced with permission from Wilkinson J D and Shaw S 1998 Dermatology, Churchill Livingstone, Edinburgh)

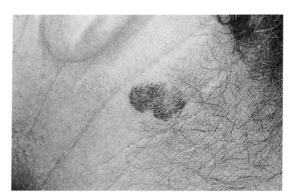

Plate 21.35 Superficial spreading malignant melanoma (Reproduced with permission from Gawkrodger D 1992 An Illustrated Colour Text of Dermatology, Churchill Livingstone, Edinburgh)

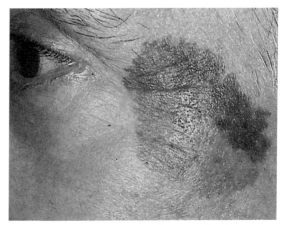

Plate 21.37 Malignant melanoma (lentigo maligna) (Reproduced with permission from Gawkrodger D 1992 An Illustrated Colour Text of Dermatology, Churchill Livingstone, Edinburgh)

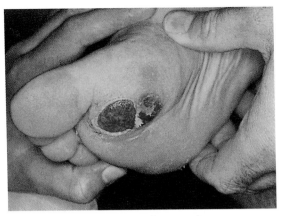

Plate 21.38 Acral lentiginous malignant melanoma (Reproduced with permission from Gawkrodger D 1992 An Illustrated Colour Text of Dermatology, Churchill Livingstone, Edinburgh)

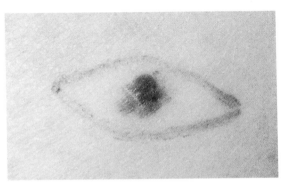

Plate 21.39 Superficial spreading malignant melanoma (Reproduced with permission from Gawkrodger D 1992 An Illustrated Colour Text of Dermatology, Churchill Livingstone, Edinburgh)

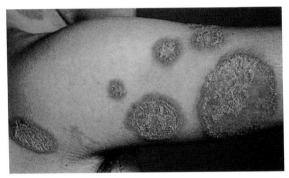

Plate 21.40 Tinea corporis due to ringworm (Reproduced with permission from Gawkrodger D 1992 An Illustrated Colour Text of Dermatology, Churchill Livingstone, Edinburgh)

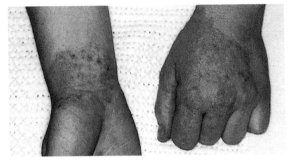

Plate 21.41 Tinea corporis with central clearing (Reproduced with permission from Gawkrodger D 1992 An Illustrated Colour Text of Dermatology, Churchill Livingstone, Edinburgh)

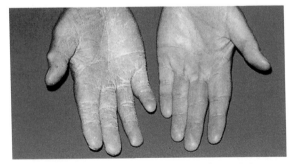

Plate 21.42 Tinea manuum (Reproduced with permission from Gawkrodger D 1992 An Illustrated Colour Text of Dermatology, Churchill Livingstone, Edinburgh)

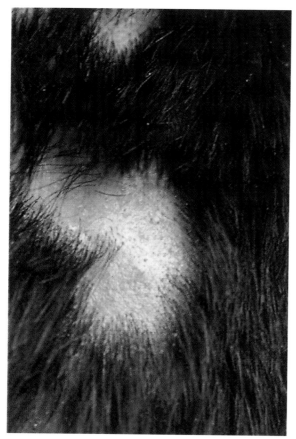

Plate 21.43 Tinea capitis (Reproduced with permission from Wilkinson J D and Shaw S 1998 Dermatology, Churchill Livingstone, Edinburgh)

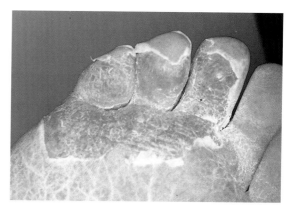

Plate 21.44 Tinea pedis (Reproduced with permission from Wilkinson J D and Shaw S 1998 Dermatology, Churchill Livingstone, Edinburgh)

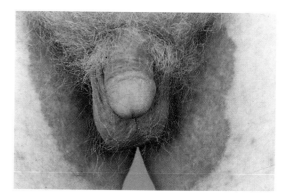

Plate 21.45 Tinea cruris (Reproduced with permission from Wilkinson J D and Shaw S 1998 Dermatology, Churchill Livingstone, Edinburgh)

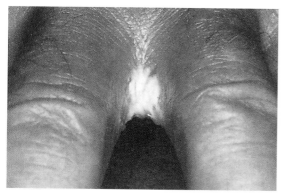

Plate 21.46 *Candida albicans* in the interdigital cleft (Reproduced with permission from Gawkrodger D 1992 An Illustrated Colour Text of Dermatology, Churchill Livingstone, Edinburgh)

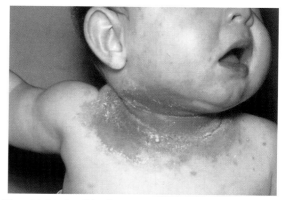

Plate 21.47 *Candida albicans* on the neck (Reproduced with permission from Wilkinson J D and Shaw S 1998 Dermatology, Churchill Livingstone, Edinburgh)

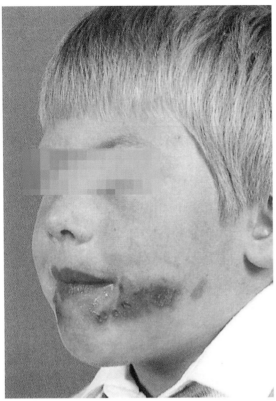

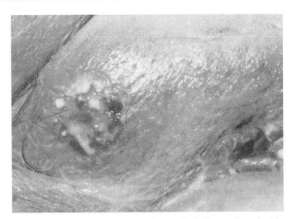

Plate 21.49 Herpes simplex on the genitals (Reproduced with permission from Gawkrodger D 1992 An Illustrated Colour Text of Dermatology, Churchill Livingstone, Edinburgh)

Plate 21.48 Herpes simplex on the cheek (Reproduced with permission from Gawkrodger D 1992 An Illustrated Colour Text of Dermatology, Churchill Livingstone, Edinburgh)

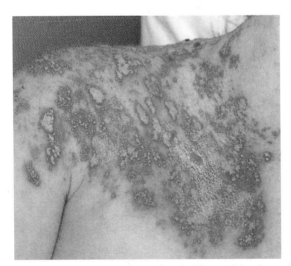

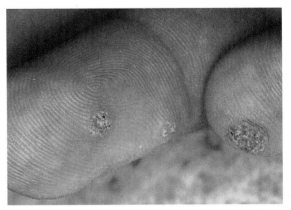

Plate 21.50 Herpes zoster (Reproduced with permission from Gawkrodger D 1992 An Illustrated Colour Text of Dermatology, Churchill Livingstone, Edinburgh)

Plate 21.51 Wart on hand (Reproduced with permission from Gawkrodger D 1992 An Illustrated Colour Text of Dermatology, Churchill Livingstone, Edinburgh)

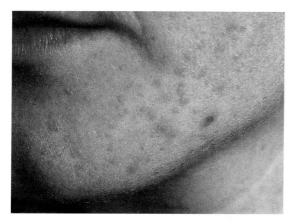

Plate 21.52 Plane viral warts (Reproduced with permission from Gawkrodger D 1992 An Illustrated Colour Text of Dermatology, Churchill Livingstone, Edinburgh)

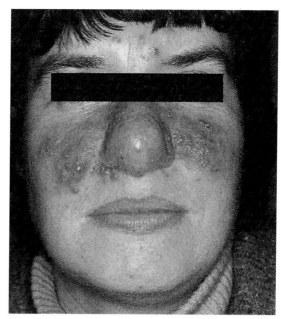

Plate 21.54 Rosacea (Reproduced with permission from Gawkrodger D 1992 An Illustrated Colour Text of Dermatology, Churchill Livingstone, Edinburgh)

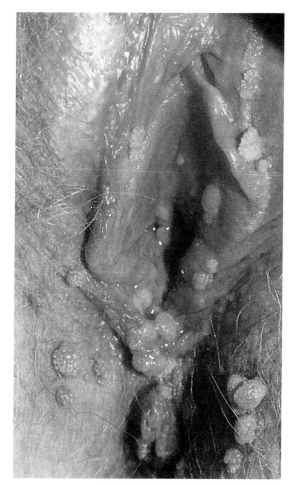

Plate 21.53 Genital warts (Reproduced with permission from Gawkrodger D 1992 An Illustrated Colour Text of Dermatology, Churchill Livingstone, Edinburgh)

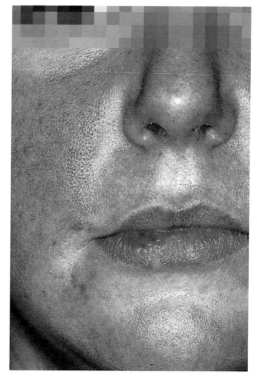

Plate 21.55 Acne rosacea (Reproduced with permission from Wilkinson J D and Shaw S 1998 Dermatology, Churchill Livingstone, Edinburgh)

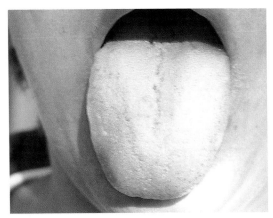

Plate 24.1 Pale tongue

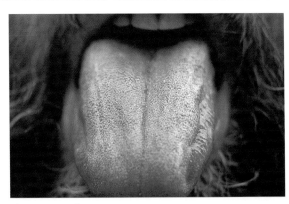

Plate 24.2 Red tongue

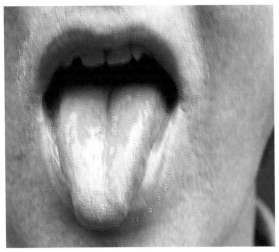

Plate 24.3 Red tip

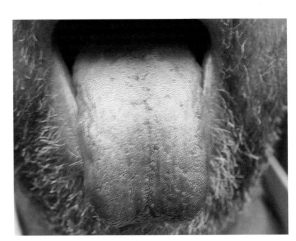

Plate 24.4 Red sides (Liver areas)

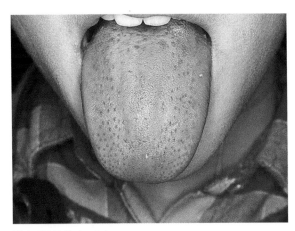

Plate 24.5 Red points

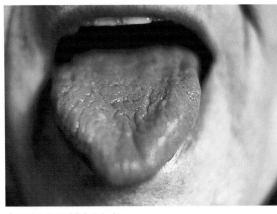

Plate 24.6 Reddish-Purple tongue

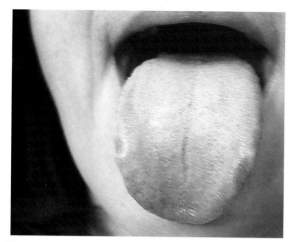

Plate 24.7 Bluish-Purple (right side) tongue

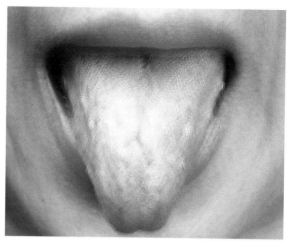

Plate 24.8 Purple colour in Liver areas

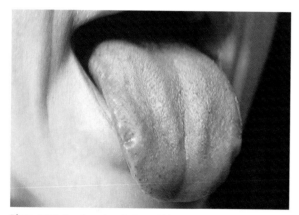

Plate 24.9 Purple colour in breast/chest area

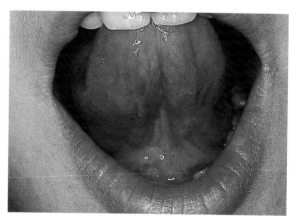

Plate 24.10 Sublingual veins

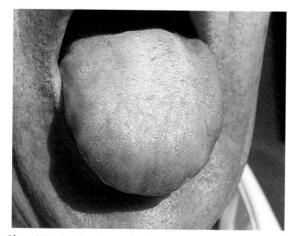

Plate 25.1 Swollen tongue body

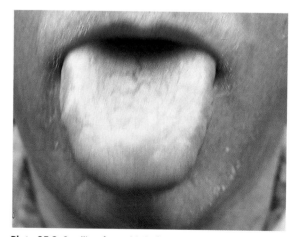

Plate 25.2 Swelling front third of tongue (Lung area)

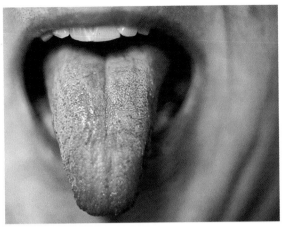

Plate 25.3 Stiff tongue body (this tongue is also very Purple)

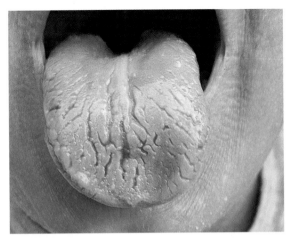

Plate 25.4 Irregular cracks

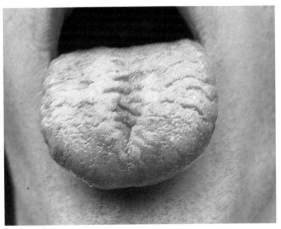

Plate 25.5 Stomach crack

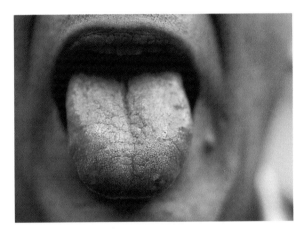

Plate 25.6 Heart crack

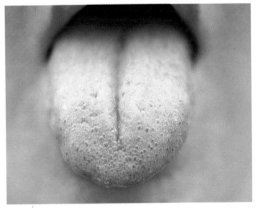

Plate 25.7 Heart crack

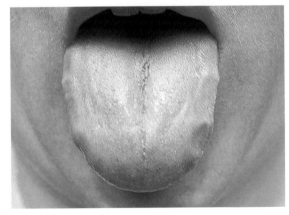

Plate 25.8 Teethmarks

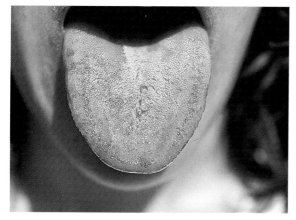

a

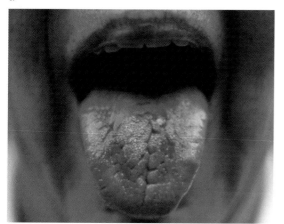

b

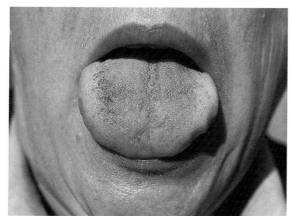

c

Plate 26.1a,b Coating without root; **c** Coating without root (in Gall-Bladder area)

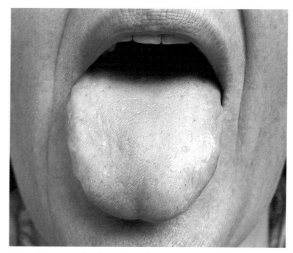

Plate 26.2 Coating in Gall-Bladder area

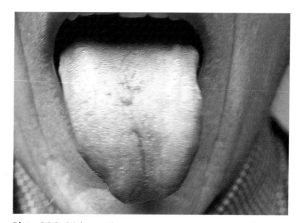

Plate 26.3 Sticky coating

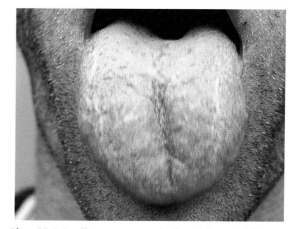

Plate 27.1 Swelling on tongue sides from Spleen-Qi deficiency